Workbook to Accompany
Mosby's

PARAMEDIC TEXTBOOK

Third Edition

Kim D. McKenna, RN, BSN, CEN, EMT-P

Chief Medical Officer
Florissant Valley Fire Protection District
Florissant, Missouri
Adjunct Instructor
St. Louis Community College
St. Louis, Missouri

Mick J. Sanders, MSA, EMT-P

EMS Training Specialist
St. Charles, Missouri

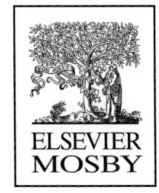
ELSEVIER
MOSBY

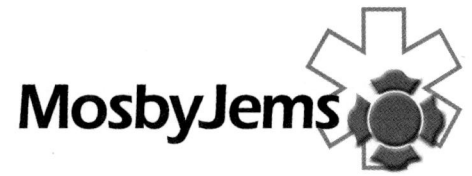
MosbyJems

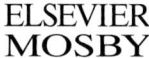

ELSEVIER
MOSBY

11830 Westline Industrial Drive
St. Louis, Missouri 63146

WORKBOOK TO ACCOMPANY MOSBY'S PARAMEDIC TEXTBOOK, EDITION 3   0-323-02788-1
Copyright © 2005, Mosby Inc.

Previous editions copyrighted 1994, 2001

International Standard Book Number 0-323-02788-1

Acquisitions Editor: Linda Honeycutt
Development Editor: Laura Bayless
Publishing Services Manager: Melissa Lastarria
Project Manager: Rich Barber

Printed in the United States

Working together to grow
libraries in developing countries

www.elsevier.com | www.bookaid.org | www.sabre.org

ELSEVIER   BOOK AID International   Sabre Foundation

Last digit is the print number: 9 8 7 6 5 4 3 2 1

To my children—Ginny, Becky, Maggie, Grant—and to my husband, Don.

Thanks for helping me remember to enjoy life.

KDM

Preface

The *Workbook to Accompany Mosby's Paramedic Textbook,* third edition, has been written to enhance the paramedic student's understanding and retention of the material presented in the textbook. This has been accomplished using a variety of questions designed to encourage the various levels of learning necessary in this field, from recall and memorization to application of concepts. Some of the features of this workbook include the following:

- A special section on studying and test-taking skills (see p. viii) so that good habits can begin early in the program
- A format that follows *Mosby's Paramedic Textbook,* third edition, chapter by chapter, with answers referenced to the appropriate objective
- Summaries from the textbook chapters to refresh key information
- An entirely new *Wrap It Up* section in each chapter that offers an additional opportunity to use learning in context
- Matching questions that reinforce key terms or content within the chapters
- Extensive use of case study–based questions to help visualize the real-life application of information
- Self-assessment sections that offer the opportunity to review material using multiple-choice questions, a testing format often used by instructors for examinations
- Complete rationale for all answers that ensures understanding of material
- A programmed review of basic math skills that precedes the drug dose calculation section
- Illustrations for student identification of anatomy, patient management techniques, and special equipment
- Paramedic career opportunities section (see p. xi) that introduces some of the choices in the paramedic profession

Electrocardiogram and drug flashcards at the end of the book can be removed for easy reference and study purposes. Flashcards are completed by the students and are keyed to questions in the workbook. The electrocardiogram flashcards show actual patient rhythms, and the drug flashcards are based on patient care scenarios. Three blank drug flashcards will allow students to create cards for regional drugs.

Before completing each chapter of the workbook, you should read the accompanying chapter in *Mosby's Paramedic Textbook,* third edition, and review the learning objectives. When you encounter areas of difficulty while completing the questions, reread the text and attempt the questions again. We hope that this workbook, when used effectively, will facilitate mastery of the complex knowledge necessary to become a paramedic. Enjoy!

Workbook to Accompany
Mosby's

PARAMEDIC TEXTBOOK

Third Edition

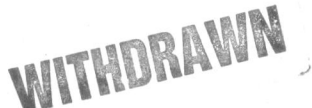

About the Authors

Kim D. McKenna, RN, BSN, CEN, EMT-P is the Chief Medical Officer for the Florissant Valley Fire Protection District in Florissant, Missouri, and an Adjunct Instructor for St. Louis Community College in St. Louis, Missouri. Her past experiences include intensive care and emergency nursing. She has been involved in prehospital education since 1985, including 4 years as the primary instructor of a paramedic training program.

Mick J. Sanders, MSA, EMT-P received his paramedic training in 1978 from St. Louis University Hospitals. He earned a Bachelor of Science degree in 1982 and a Master of Science degree in 1983 from Lindenwood College in St. Charles, Missouri. He has worked in various health care systems as a field paramedic, emergency department paramedic, and EMS instructor. For 12 years, Mr. Sanders served as Training Specialist with the Bureau of Emergency Medical Services, Missouri Department of Health, where he oversaw EMT and paramedic training and licensure in St. Louis City and the surrounding metropolitan area.

Acknowledgments

This workbook, of course, would never have been possible without the terrific manuscript of *Mosby's Paramedic Textbook,* third edition, written by Mick J. Sanders. His commitment to excellence is reflected throughout the text, and his encouragement and suggestions made the completion of the workbook possible.

Many thanks to Catherine Parvensky, who wrote the studying and test-taking tips and the paramedic career opportunities sections of the workbook.

For the original patient electrocardiogram strips, I am indebted to the staff of the intensive care unit and especially to my former colleagues in the emergency department at St. John's Mercy Medical Center. A debt of gratitude goes to Gary Denton of Acute Coronary Syndrome Consultants, Inc., and to Wolff Medical Publishing, Inc. for the 12-lead electrocardiogram tracings included in this edition of the text.

To all of my paramedic students, past and present, I sincerely appreciate all that you have taught me and your suggestions for the content of this workbook.

And to the fellow paramedics and EMTs with whom I work in the field, thanks for showing me where the textbook ends and reality begins.

I am also grateful to the reviewers of this and past editons: Bob Nixon, BA, EMT-P; Monroe Yancie, NREMT-P; Jeff DeGraffenreid, Johnson County Medical Action Emergency Medical Services, Olathe, Kansas; and Janet Fitts, RN, EMT-P for their suggestions and fresh ideas.

Thanks to the staff at Elsevier, especially Laura Bayless, who worked so diligently to make this project happen; to Rich Barber whose attention to detail is evident throughout the text; and to Joy Knobel in Marketing who cheered us all on. We are forever grateful.

Kim D. McKenna
Mick J. Sanders

Study Tips

For all the emphasis placed on furthering education, little guidance is given for how to be a good student. Learning the following studying and test-taking tips can help you get the most out of your paramedic course and other classes in the future.

STUDY SESSIONS

The way that an individual studies may determine the likelihood of successful completion of a training program. You need to develop a routine pattern for studying and stick to it. The following are methods to increase the effectiveness of study sessions:

- Set a regular time for studying each day.
- Pace yourself by scheduling a specific amount of time for each subject or chapter.
- Take periodic breaks to prevent burnout.
- Read lesson information before each session and review notes immediately after the class.
- Do not wait until the last minute and expect to cram information and do well. Instead, pace yourself throughout the course.
  - Be aware of distractions, internal and external.
  - Internal distractions include hunger, tension, fatigue, illness, glucose levels, and daydreaming and getting sidetracked.
  - External distractions include room temperature (hot or cold), noise levels, and lighting.
- Make a game of it; drill the information by using the following:
  - Flash cards for memorizing facts
  - Jeopardy cards
  - Trivial Pursuit cards
- When frustration sets in, do the following:
  - Take a break.
  - Have a snack. (Sugar helps.)
  - Take a walk. (Increased cardiovascular activity increases blood flow to the brain.)
  - Take a few deep breaths and relax.

WHERE AND WHEN DO YOU STUDY BEST?

Everyone has a particular time and place in which they are most productive. For some it is late at night, and for others it is early in the morning. Determine when you are at your peak and study daily at that time.

- Where do you do the best work?
  - At a desk or table?
  - In front of the television? (Some people need background noise to focus.)
- Decide whether you work better studying alone or in work groups. Sometimes, work sessions are a great motivation for studying.

- Decide what form of studying works best for you:
  - Writing notes from the book
  - Highlighting information in the book
  - Taking copious notes
  - Listening to the instructor and asking questions

INCREASING RETENTION

There are many ways to increase retention of material, including association, mnemonics, imagery, and recitation. Try them all and see what works best for you:

Association—Relate information to something you understand. Build new information on what is already known.

Mnemonics—Use letters or words to remember facts. For example, use "AVPU" to determine a patient's level of consciousness: *A*lert, *V*erbal, *P*ainful stimuli, or *U*nconscious.

Imagery—Visualize a picture of the information. Memorize a chart or picture of the body and associated organs, and then remember that picture for questions on anatomy.

Recitation—Read notes out loud or discuss the information with peers. Hearing information repeatedly helps retention.

TEST-TAKING TIPS

Test taking is a skill that can be learned. Most state examinations are multiple-choice questions and are graded solely on the number of correct answers. There is no penalty for guessing, so do not leave any questions unanswered because they will be marked incorrect.

Multiple-choice questions are made up of two parts: the stem (question) and possible answers. These types of questions can be factual or situational:

Factual: During one-person cardiopulmonary resuscitation, the ratio of compressions to ventilations is
a. 15 to 2
b. 5 to 1
c. 10 per minute
d. 20 per minute

Situational: A 55-year-old man was shoveling his driveway when he developed shortness of breath and pain in the middle of his chest. He is most likely suffering from which of the following?
a. Myocardial infarction
b. Congestive heart failure
c. Emphysema
d. Angina pectoris

When answering a question, thoroughly analyze it. To accomplish this, do the following:
- Read the stem without looking at the answers. Evaluate the question, looking for key words such as *not, except, first,* or *final.*
- Identify key content words such as *one rescuer, adult victim, radiating pain, slurred speech,* or *conscious victim.*
- Think of a correct answer and then look at all the choices to see whether your answer is there. If not, find the next *best answer.*
- Do not read into the question.
- Eliminate obviously wrong answers and select from those remaining.
- Do not change answers. Your first hunch is usually correct.

PREPARING FOR TESTS

You can take some simple steps to prepare yourself for a test:
- Get a good night's sleep before the examination.
- Avoid milk products because they tend to induce sleep.
- Eat a good meal but not too much before the examination. (Blood flow is forced to the digestive tract the first hour after eating a large meal, which tends to induce sleep.)

- Exercise moderately to increase blood supply to the brain.
- Layer clothes so that you can add or remove layers as necessary to be comfortable during the examination.
- Use a wristwatch to pace yourself.
- Sit away from friends or other distractions.
- Be prepared and be positive. If you have studied properly, you know the material and will do well on the examination.

STRATEGIES FOR INCREASING TESTING PERFORMANCE

If you use the following strategies, you are sure to improve your performance during tests:
- Pace yourself to make certain that you have enough time to answer all questions.
- Use scrap paper to work through questions.
- At the end, make certain you have answered *all* questions. Do not change answers unless you initially misread the question.
- Make sure that you complete the answer sheet correctly. Fill in circles completely, and do not leave stray marks. Make certain that you check the number on the answer sheet against the number on the test every 10 questions to avoid the unnecessary stress of finding yourself on the wrong line.

Paramedic Career Opportunities

Since its inception in 1967, emergency medical services (EMS) has developed into a sophisticated profession with various levels of care that result in improved care of the sick and injured. With the evolution of EMS have come career opportunities for emergency medical technicians, paramedics, nurses, and physicians. Although specific job opportunities depend on geographical locations, in general, opportunities for prehospital emergency responders have emerged from volunteer to paid career positions. For a certified EMT-Paramedic, many options are available.

OTHER AREAS OF INTEREST

Aside from traditional prehospital roles, some paramedics have taken on expanded duties. Although much controversy has surrounded the use of paramedics within the emergency department, some hospitals in the United States employ paramedics to use their full skills and knowledge. Others may hire them as orderlies, pathology assistants, intravenous team members, phlebotomists, suture technicians, and respiratory therapists.

Some hospitals also have extended emergency departments in which paramedics have an expanded function. These facilities offer treatment for minor illnesses or injuries, physical examinations, and health screenings. They often are located within industrial settings, universities, or stand-alone buildings not part of hospitals.

Finally, paramedics who pursue advanced education can find additional opportunities. Many universities offer credit hours toward a bachelor's degree for any individual with a paramedic certification. For a field paramedic with experience, other advanced opportunities may include training as a nurse or physician's assistant.

POSITION

A *field paramedic* requires current certification as an EMT-Paramedic. Some states and organizations also require National Registry certification.

A *paramedic supervisor* usually requires substantial experience as a field provider and supervisory experience.

A *flight paramedic* usually requires substantial experience as a field provider and the ability to work under pressure. Additional certifications or training may be required by the individual service.

An *interhospital transport medic* usually requires certification/licensure as a paramedic. Additional specialized training may be required or provided by the employer.

An *EMS administrator,* in addition to paramedic certification/licensure, often requires advanced degrees in EMS, business, or health care administration.

An *EMS educator* usually requires paramedic certification and experience as an instructor.

Specialized training in education to meet the minimum requirements set forth by each state usually is needed. Advanced-degree certification often is desired for high-level training programs.

DESCRIPTION

Many paramedics enjoy the day-to-day operations of a field provider, administering emergency care to the sick and injured. Roles and responsibilities of paramedics undoubtedly will grow as the emergency department extends into the community through advanced life support personnel.

An advanced life support supervisor is usually an experienced paramedic with administrative or management skills. Responsibilities for this position generally include recruitment, scheduling, discipline, and supervision of emergency care personnel.

Flight paramedics use their knowledge and skills to care for victims who require air medical evacuation and rapid transport to hospitals. A flight crew usually is composed of a pilot, a flight medic, and a flight nurse. Some organizations hire paramedics to assist with the interhospital, intercontinental, or international transfer of patients requiring monitored transportation. Responsibilities for this position generally include monitoring of patients during transport and initiation of emergency care when necessary. Additional training for specialty skills often is necessary in this role to meet the needs of high-risk infants, children, or other patients who are critically ill or injured.

Experienced paramedics with backgrounds in management can act in administrative capacities within various organizations. Although advanced training often is necessary, administrative positions in hospitals, government emergency services organizations, and independent companies are possibilities.

Many colleges and universities offer programs in EMS, including paramedic certification programs, associate's degrees, bachelor's degrees, and even master's degrees. Paramedics with experience in education can obtain positions as instructors for such programs.

Contents

PART ONE

IN THIS PART

EMS Systems: Roles and Responsibilities

READING ASSIGNMENT

Chapter 1, pages 1-21, in *Mosby's Paramedic Textbook,* ed. 3

OBJECTIVES

Upon completion of this chapter, the paramedic student will be able to do the following:
1. Outline key historical events that influenced the development of emergency medical services (EMS) systems.
2. Identify the key elements necessary for effective EMS systems operations.
3. Differentiate among training and roles and responsibilities of the four nationally recognized levels of EMS licensure/certification: first responder, EMT-Basic, EMT-Intermediate, and EMT-Paramedic.
4. List the benefits of membership in professional EMS organizations.
5. Describe the benefits of continuing education.
6. Differentiate among professionalism and professional licensure, certification, and registration.
7. Describe the paramedic's role in patient care situations as defined by the U.S. Department of Transportation.
8. Describe the benefits of each component of off-line (indirect) and online (direct) medical direction.
9. Outline the role and components of an effective, continuous quality improvement program.
10. Identify the key components of prehospital research and its benefits to the EMS system.

SUMMARY

- The roots of prehospital emergency care may date back to the military.
- In the early twentieth century through the mid-1960s, prehospital care in the United States was provided in a few ways. Care was provided mostly by urban hospital-based systems. These systems later developed into municipal services. Care also was provided by funeral directors and volunteers who were not trained in these services.
- The operations of an effective EMS system include citizen activation, dispatch, prehospital care, hospital care, and rehabilitation.
- The various levels of providers have their own distinct roles and duties. These roles include telecommunicators (dispatchers), first responders, EMT-Basics, EMT-Intermediates, and EMT-Paramedics. These levels combine to make an effective prehospital EMS system.
- Many professional groups and organizations help to set the standards of EMS. These groups exist at the national, state, regional, and local levels. The groups take part in development, education, and implementation. Being active in such a group helps to promote the status of the paramedic.
- Continuing education is crucial. It provides a way for all health care providers to maintain basic technical and professional skills.

- Professionalism refers to the way in which a person conducts himself or herself. Professionalism also refers to how one follows the standards of conduct and performance established by the profession.
- The roles and duties of the paramedic can be divided into two categories. These groups are *primary* and *additional* duties.
- The two types of medical direction are online (direct) and off-line (indirect) medical direction. Both are equally important. They help to ensure that the components of quality medical care are in place in an EMS system.
- A CQI program identifies and attempts to resolve problems in areas such as medical direction, financing, training, communication, prehospital management and transportation, interfacility transfer, receiving facilities, specialty care units, dispatch, public information and education, audit and quality assurance, disaster planning, and mutual aid.
- Quality EMS research helps shed light on the efficacy, effects, and cost-effectiveness of EMS interventions. The research is based on experimental data. Such research can lead to changes in professional standards and training. The research also can lead to changes in equipment and procedures.
- When planning research, the researcher should consider involving an institutional review board.

REVIEW QUESTIONS

1. While working late, a 56-year-old man develops chest pain. The man is alone in his office when the chest pain increases, and he falls to the floor, suffering a cardiac arrest.

   Identify the missing components of the EMS system in Fig. 1-1 that are necessary to effectively resuscitate this victim and return him to a productive role in society.

   a. _____

   b. _____

   c. _____

   d. _____

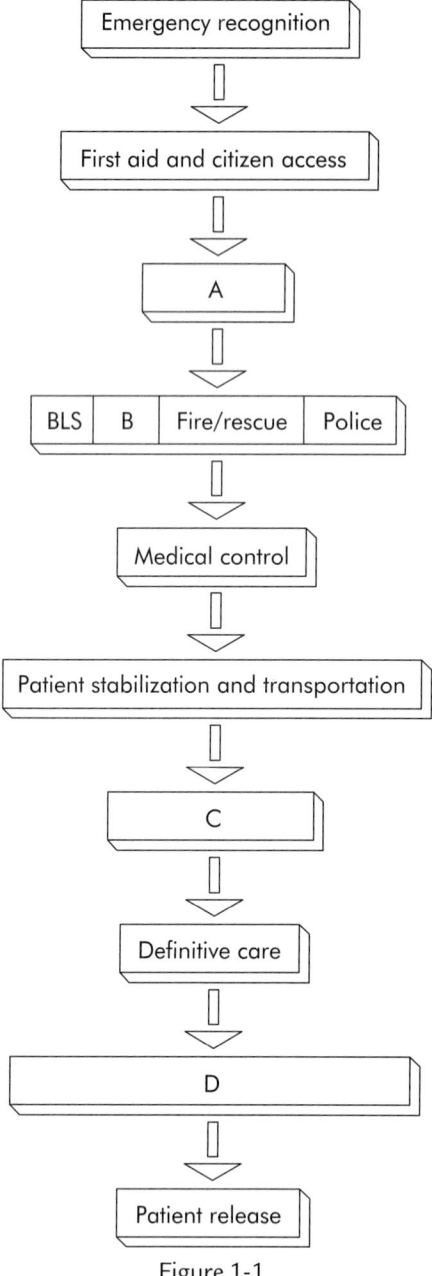

Figure 1-1

Questions 2 and 3 pertain to the following case study:

After attending a continuing education lecture on advances in trauma care, you report to work for your 12-hour shift. You carefully check out your vehicle for equipment and mechanical readiness for a call and then head to the company fitness room to exercise. Just as you finish your workout, the tones sound. You are dispatched to a nursing home for a person with "difficulty breathing." The street alarm is activated, and as you pull out, you carefully glance to ensure that traffic has come to a stop before proceeding onto the busy roadway in front of your station. Upon arrival at the nursing home, you obtain a rapid history from the nursing home staff and begin your assessment of the 87-year-old patient. She is in obvious respiratory distress, and you recognize the need for rapid interventions to prevent further deterioration of her condition. Your partner administers oxygen and prepares to insert an intra-venous (IV) line as you contact on-line medical direction. You briefly describe your patient's condition and request orders for nitroglycerin and furosemide. The physician advisor agrees with your treatment plan. As soon as your partner secures the IV line, you administer the drugs, carefully checking for allergies and appropriate dosing before giving them. A repeat assessment of the patient in 5 minutes shows some improvement. You continue plans to transfer her into the ambulance. The nursing home staff tells you she should be transported to the city hospital. This is consistent with your medical protocols, so you agree. As you depart, another evaluation demonstrates even more improvement. On arrival at the hospital, you give a report and transfer care of the patient to the nursing staff and then complete your patient report. You ask the physician about another drug that you had considered requesting, but she agrees that in this patient's circumstance, the treatment plan you had chosen was appropriate. Back at base, you restock the vehicle with the drugs and equipment used on the call. Then you head down to the classroom to help teach the 8 pm community cardiopulmonary resuscitation (CPR) class.

2. List 10 primary responsibilities of the paramedic that were demonstrated in this simulated call.

a.

b.

c.

d.

e.

f.

g.

h.

i.

j.

3. List two additional responsibilities of the paramedic that were demonstrated in this scenario.

a.

b.

Match the historical role in EMS in column I with the appropriate person or event in column II. Use each answer only once.

Column I	Column II
4. _____ First use of helicopter for medical evacuation during an armed conflict.	**a.** American Red Cross
5. _____ Demonstrated the value of mouth-to-mouth ventilation.	**b.** Belfast, 1966
6. _____ Twentieth century battlefield ambulance corps developed.	**c.** Korean conflict
7. _____ Dr. Eugene Nagel trains firefighters as paramedics.	**d.** Miami, 1967
8. Earliest documented mobile coronary unit performs prehospital defibrillation.	**e.** Napoleonic Wars
9. _____ Clara Barton performs battlefield emergency medical care and brings this organization to the United States.	**f.** Peter Safar, MD, 1958
10. _____ Jean Larry transports wounded in covered cart.	**g.** World War I
11. _____ Fixed-wing medical transports were developed in this conflict.	**h.** World War II
	i. Vietnam conflict

Match the description in column I with the appropriate licensure and certification level in column II. Use each answer only once.

Column I	Column II
12. _____ Trained in basic life support, including defibrillation	**a.** EMT-B
13. _____ Trained in all aspects of basic and advanced life support	**b.** EMT-I
14. _____ Trained in all aspects of basic life support and IV therapy	**c.** EMT-P
	d. First responder

Match the activity in column I with the appropriate term in column II. You may use each term *more* than once.

Column I	Column II
15. _____ Education and training of EMS personnel	**a.** Continuing education
16. _____ Personnel selection for employment	**b.** Continuous quality improvement
17. _____ Appropriate equipment choice selection	**c.** Medical direction
18. _____ Clinical protocol guidance and direction	**d.** Professional associations
19. _____ Clinical problem resolution	
20. _____ Interface among EMS systems	
21. _____ Advocacy within medical community	
22. _____ On-line communication with physicians and EMS	
23. _____ Patient care report reviews	
24. _____ Establish standards of care	
25. _____ Serve as resource experts	
26. _____ Introduction of new information	

Questions 27 to 35 pertain to the following research abstract, which was published in *Prehospital Emergency Care*, 2(3), 1998. Read the abstract carefully and then answer each question.

Efficacy of Midazolam for Facilitated Intubation by Paramedics
Authors: Edward T. Dickinson, MD, NREMT-P
Jason E. Cohen, BA, EMT-P
C. Crawford Mechem, MD

Affiliation: Department of Emergency Medicine, University of Pennsylvania School of Medicine, Philadelphia, Pennsylvania

Objective: The use of pharmacological agents by paramedics to facilitate endotracheal intubation (ETI) is becoming increasingly common. This study was done to determine the efficacy of intravenous midazolam, a short-acting benzodiazepine, as a drug to facilitate ETI in patients resistant to conventional ETI.

Methods: The study was conducted in a suburban municipal EMS system over a 22-month period. All paramedics were trained in the use of midazolam for facilitated intubation prior to allowing the use of midazolam in the system. All calls in which midazolam was used were reviewed on a monthly basis by investigators via retrospective review of the prehospital care reports.

Results: During the study period, 13,212 emergency responses occurred, resulting in 154 ETIs by paramedics. Midazolam was used to facilitate 20 (13%) of these ETIs. "Clenched teeth" and failed intubation attempt were the most commonly cited indications for facilitated intubation. Eleven patients had medical complaints, and nine were trauma patients. Successful ETI with midazolam was achieved in 17 of 20 (85%) cases. In 88% (15 of 17) of these cases, a single dose of midazolam was sufficient for ETI; mean dose 3.6 mg (standard deviation [SD] 1.1 mg). The three patients with failed ETI received multiple doses of midazolam; mean dose 5 mg (SD 2 mg).

Conclusion: The prehospital use of single-dose IV midazolam is generally effective in accomplishing facilitated ETI in patients resistant to conventional (nonpharmacological) endotracheal intubation.

27. What was the purpose of this study (i.e., what problem or question are the authors trying to solve)?

_____

_____

28. Is the hypothesis stated in this abstract? _____ If you answered yes, what is it? If you answered no, what do you think it is?

_____

29. What is the study population?

_____

30. What are the sample and sample size for this research?

_____

31. Was a random sampling procedure used? Yes/No Explain your answer.

_____

32. Did this study use a qualitative or quantitative approach?

_____

33. The study indicates a standard deviation for the mean dose of 1.1 mg. What does that mean?

_____

34. What are some weaknesses or unanswered questions related to this research?

_____

35. Are the findings of this study important to the EMS community?

_____

STUDENT SELF-ASSESSMENT

36. Which federal law enabled creation of the U.S. Department of Transportation and the National Highway Traffic Safety Administration and provided funding for EMS?
  a. Accidental Death and Disability Act
  b. Consolidated Omnibus Reconciliation Act
  c. Emergency Medical Services Systems Act
  d. Highway Safety Act

37. Which of the following is _not_ a component of the EMS system?
  a. Disaster planning   **c.** Intensive care units
  b. Insurance providers   **d.** Paramedic training

38. How has health care reform affected emergency medical services?
  a. It results in larger reimbursement amounts for each call.
  b. It may increase the distance for transport based on insurance restrictions for hospitals.
  c. It has caused a decrease in emergency ambulance transports.
  d. It will restrict the scope of practice for the EMS provider.

39. Which of the following describes the manner in which a paramedic follows the practice, guidelines, and ethical considerations of prehospital emergency care?
  a. Certification   **c.** Professionalism
  b. Licensure   **d.** Registration

40. Which of the following is _not_ a role of the paramedic as defined by the U.S. Department of Transportation?
  a. Assessing and providing emergency patient care
  b. Coordinating collection of outstanding patient bills
  c. Documenting and communicating patient care
  d. Making sure the ambulance is adequately stocked

41. The EMS physician medical director is responsible for which of the following:
  a. Ensuring maintenance of ambulances and equipment
  b. Monitoring the quality of EMS care
  c. Negotiating staff salary and benefit disputes
  d. Providing patient care in the field on advanced life-support units

42. A man who claims to be an emergency department physician is attempting to direct care in an inappropriate manner on a cardiac arrest call. You should do which of the following:
  a. Contact on-line medical direction for instructions
  b. Follow his orders because he has appropriate credentials

    c. Ignore him and carry on as you see appropriate

    d. Immediately ask the police to arrest him

43. Which of the following demonstrates a prospective method of a continuous quality improvement model?

    a. Continuing education programs

    b. Listening to audio tapes of EMS reports

    c. Observation of prehospital care by the medical director

    d. Reviewing prehospital patient care records

44. You are conducting research for a drug to treat cardiac arrest. Only you and your partner have been trained to gather the data, so the drug will be used only on days that you work. This type of subject selection is called which of the following:

    a. Alternative time sampling   **c.** Statistical table sampling

    b. Convenience sampling   **d.** Systemic sampling

45. You are doing a study on the variability of scene response times according to time of day. Here are the data you collected (in minutes) for one group: 1, 2, 3, 4, 4, 4, 4, 4, 5, 5, 5, 5, 6, 6, 6, 7, 7, 8, 9. What is the mode for this set of data?

    a. 4

    b. 5

    c. 6

    d. 7

46. Before your research is approved by an institutional review board, what must you prove?

    a. Consent will be obtained.

    b. The hypothesis is true.

    c. No risks will be incurred.

    d. Your sample is large enough.

WRAP IT UP

Your rural EMS service responds to a call for a vehicle accident with possible rescue. Your ambulance arrives on the scene first, and you provide the scene size-up on the radio for the incoming units: "4017 on the scene, two vehicles involved, major damage, investigating." A bystander shouts to you that he called 9-1-1 on his cell phone and that there is a guy "hurt real bad" in one of the cars. You and your EMT partner split up, going to separate cars to triage the injured. Major damage to the car prevents access through the doors, so you break a window to gain access. The driver, an unrestrained teenage boy, has trauma to the head. He is taking agonal gasps and has a rapid radial pulse. You shout to your partner that you have a critical patient and immediately call dispatch to send a helicopter and a second ambulance. As you begin to manage the patient's airway and to ventilate him, the rescue pumper arrives. Your partner tells you that there are two patients in the second car: a woman with minor lacerations and her 9-year-old daughter, who has significant cervical spine tenderness and is hysterical. The second ambulance crew arrives, and you tell them that extrication is needed. You direct the paramedic on the rescue pumper to manage the two patients in the second car while you and your partner care for your critically injured patient as extrication efforts proceed. Your patient has apparent head, chest, and abdominal injuries. Dispatch notifies you that the helicopter has a 2-minute estimated time of arrival (ETA). Police have blocked the highway for safety and are assisting with the landing zone. Moments before the helicopter lands, rescue crews remove the car door, and you perform rapid extrication. You carefully move the patient to the spine board, secure him, and move him to your ambulance. With your partner's assistance, you intubate the patient using in-line spinal immobilization. Then, as your partner ventilates the patient, you initiate an IV line while firefighters assist with monitoring and assessment of vital signs. The air medical crew arrives. You give them a rapid, thorough report and direct them to take the patient to the closest level I trauma center. The rescue pumper paramedic reports that the two patients from the second vehicle are being transported by ground past the local hospital to the trauma center. You quickly clean your rig and return in service to the station to write your patient care report.

  1. What role did citizens play in this call?

_____

  2. What steps did dispatch take to coordinate the activities in this call?

_____

3. What role, if any, did medical direction play in this call?

_____

4. Why was the use of the helicopter indicated in this situation when the other two patients were taken by ground to the same facility?
- **a.** The male patient needed intubation.
- **b.** The ETA of the second ambulance was delayed.
- **c.** Prolonged extrication was needed.
- **d.** Multiple trauma patients were involved.

5. Why were the patients taken to the trauma center rather than a closer hospital?
- **a.** Definitive care is rapidly available for the trauma patient at a trauma center.
- **b.** Mileage charges are greater to a more distant hospital.
- **c.** Helicopters transport only to trauma centers.
- **d.** Local hospitals have poorer quality of care.

6. Why were you performing the advanced skills on this call rather than your partner?
- **a.** The attending paramedic always performs the skills.
- **b.** The first person reaching the patient performs invasive skills.
- **c.** Your partner is an EMT, and these skills exceed his license in many states.
- **d.** The most experienced crew member is designated to perform skills.

7. Rank the attributes of the professional paramedic that you think would be most important on this call from 1 to 11, with 1 the most important and 11 the least important.

_____ Integrity	_____ Empathy
_____ Self-motivation	_____ Appearance and personal hygiene
_____ Self-confidence	_____ Communication
_____ Time management	_____ Teamwork and diplomacy
_____ Respect	_____ Patient advocacy
_____ Careful delivery of service	

8. Would your rankings from the question above change for the following situations? If you answer yes, indicate how they would change.
- **a.** A 75-year-old patient who is despondent over the loss of his wife is threatening to kill himself. Yes/No

_____

_____

- **b.** A 27-year-old woman has just miscarried a 20-week pregnancy; this is her sixth miscarriage in 2 years. Yes/No

_____

_____

- **c.** A 54-year-old patient in the mayor's chambers has chest pain, and electrocardiogram (ECG) readings suggest a heart attack. He does not want to be transported to the hospital. Yes/No

_____

_____

9. Place a ✔ beside the roles/responsibilities of the paramedic used on this call.

_____ Preparation	_____ Response
_____ Scene assessment	_____ Patient assessment
_____ Recognition of injury or illness	_____ Patient management
_____ Appropriate patient disposition	_____ Patient transfer
_____ Documentation	_____ Returning to service

CHAPTER 1 ANSWERS

REVIEW QUESTIONS

1. a. Dispatcher; b. Advanced life support; c. Hospital delivery; d. Patient rehabilitation and education
    (Objective 2)

2. a. Physical preparation for the job (exercise program)
    b. Having appropriate equipment and supplies
    c. Responding to the scene in a safe manner
    d. Performing a quick patient assessment to determine priorities for care
    e. Contacting medical direction for assistance with the care plan
    f. Managing the emergency in the appropriate manner
    g. Stabilizing the patient in the field
    h. Providing transport by the appropriate means to the correct facility
    i. Reporting to the staff regarding the patient's condition on arrival
    j. Replacing equipment and debriefing the call
    (Objective 7)

3. a. Advocating citizens' role in the EMS system by teaching community programs such as CPR.
    b. Continuing personal professional development by attending continuing education programs
    (Objective 7)

4. c
5. f
6. g
7. d
8. b
9. a
10. e
11. h
    (Questions 4-11: Objective 1)

12. a or d
13. c
14. b
    (Questions 12-14: Objective 3)

15. a, b, c, d
16. c
17. a, b, c
18. b, c, d
19. a, b, c, d
20. c, d
21. c, d
22. b, c
23. b, c
24. b, c, d
25. c, d
26. a, c, d
    (Questions 15-26: Objectives 4, 5, 8, 9)

27. To determine the efficacy of IV midazolam to aid in prehospital intubations that failed conventional methods
28. No. No hypothesis is stated. The hypothesis could have been that the use of midazolam will facilitate intubation in patients who could not be intubated by conventional means.

29. The study population is the 154 ETIs that occurred within the study period.
30. The sample is the patients who could not be intubated by conventional means (sample size is 20 patients).
31. No. Random sampling was not done. All patients who met the criterion (failed intubation) were included.
32. Descriptive statistics were used to report the findings in this quantitative paper.
33. This means that about 65% of the patients received 3.6 mg ± 1.1 mg of midazolam in the successful ETI group.
34. Many other things could be considered. For example, did the age of the patients affect the success? Were the missed patients trauma or medical patients, and did that influence success rates? Is 20 a large enough sample size to make a broad generalization to all EMS patients? What was the experience level of the paramedics in the "success" group versus the "fail" group?
35. The use of any drug is associated with potential risks and complications. Objective data on the effectiveness of drugs, especially in the unique prehospital environment, support the standards and practice of paramedic care. (Questions 27-35: Objective 10)

STUDENT SELF-ASSESSMENT

36. d. This act, passed in 1966, required states to develop effective EMS programs or lose federal construction funds. It enabled large amounts of money to be spent for development of EMS and advanced life support (ALS) pilot programs. Accidental Death and Disability: the Neglected Disease of Modern Society (the "white" paper) was not an act but a report published by the National Academy of Sciences–National Research Council through its Committee on Trauma and Shock. The committee's recommendations paved the way for the Highway Safety Act of 1966. The EMSS act of 1973 developed regional EMS organizations. It identified 15 required components of the EMS system. The Consolidated Omnibus Reconciliation Act (COBRA) eliminated federal funds for EMS and redistributed them under state block grants.
(Objective 1)

37. b. Although insurance reimbursement is necessary for many EMS systems to operate, the insurance providers are not considered a part of the system.
(Objective 2)

38. b. Patients' health plans now often restrict their choice of hospitals. Except in life-threatening emergencies, patients must seek care from their preferred provider or lose reimbursement. In some places this has resulted in expanded transport areas if EMS agencies are to meet the needs of the health care consumers they serve. Generally, the health care changes have resulted in decreases rather than increases in reimbursement.
(Objective 2)

39. c. Certification authorizes a person who has met specific qualifications to participate in an activity. Licensure grants a license to practice a profession. Registration is the act of enrolling a person's name in a book of record.
(Objective 6)

40. b. Although this role may fall to the paramedic in some systems, it is not defined by the government as an integral role.
(Objective 3)

41. b. Other personnel should assume patient care and administrative and maintenance duties. The primary role of the EMS physician medical director is to ensure quality patient care.
(Objective 8)

42. a. On-line medical direction should be contacted to attempt to arbitrate the situation. If this is impossible, police intervention may be recommended. Written policies addressing this issue should be prepared by the medical director so that actions to be taken in this situation are clearly defined.
(Objective 8)

43. a. The continuing education program can be offered to introduce new material, concepts, or skills so that appropriate patient care is delivered when that knowledge or skill is needed. This is done to ensure quality before a problem occurs. Direct observation of care is a concurrent method of CQI, and review of records and tapes is done after the actual care is delivered (retrospectively).
(Objective 9)

44. b. Alternative time sampling selects participants based on a predetermined time interval (e.g., day of the week, month). Sampling using a statistical table involves selection of patients based on a table that predetermines which patient will be following a selected protocol. Systemic sampling enrolls patients in the order in which they are encountered. For example, it may be established that every other patient encountered gets the test intervention.
(Objective 10)

45. a. The number 4 occurs most frequently. The *mean,* or average of the sum of the times, is 5, as is the *median,* or middle of the group.
(Objective 10)

46. a. Although traditional informed consent is not always possible, an acceptable alternative must be demonstrated to the IRB before your project is approved. The purpose of the research is to prove or disprove the hypothesis; this can be determined only after the study is completed. If risks are associated with the research, you must demonstrate that the potential benefit of the study warrants the risk. The primary responsibility of the IRB is to consider ethical, not procedural, issues with the research.
(Objective 11)

WRAP IT UP

1. Citizens recognized the emergency, called 9-1-1, and provided information to responding EMS units.
(Objective 2)

2. Dispatch identified the nature of the emergency, dispatched the proper apparatus to the correct location, dispatched the helicopter and an additional ambulance when directed, and updated the scene crew on the status of the helicopter.
(Objective 2)

3. Although no on-line medical direction was identified on this call, undoubtedly the crews notified on-line medical direction of their status. In addition, on-line medical direction should have had a role in determining the treatment protocols used, the protocol for using air medical services, and the protocol determining use of the trauma center. Medical direction also should be involved in a review of the call at a later time to monitor quality of care.
(Objective 8)

4. c. Most systems provide for dispatch of air medical crews when prolonged extrication is likely and the patient's condition warrants it. In other situations, even when the patient's condition is critical, the time to the appropriate hospital and other factors would be considered and should be established by protocol in collaboration with medical direction.
(Objective 2)

5. a. Protocols should define when patients are taken to a trauma center. Typically these are based on the mechanism of injury, the anatomical injuries involved, and the patient's physiological status. Definitive care (surgery) for the trauma can be most effectively delivered at a trauma center, where appropriate resources (personnel and equipment) are readily available.
(Objective 2)

6. c. In many states, advanced invasive skills such as intubation and vascular access are not within the scope of practice of an EMT.
(Objective 3)

7. Responses will vary by individual opinion; however, careful delivery of service, time management, self-confidence, and communication likely would rank very high on this type of call.
(Objective 6)

8. All attributes are critical for the paramedic; however, responses will vary by individual opinion. The following attributes are more likely to be ranked higher.
   a. Yes. Communication, respect, empathy, and patient advocacy
   b. Yes. Empathy, respect, and careful delivery of service
   c. Yes. Careful delivery of service, communication, teamwork and diplomacy, and appearance and personal hygiene.
(Objective 6)

9. All of these roles and responsibilities are used on this call.
(Objective 7)

The Well-Being of the Paramedic

READING ASSIGNMENT
Chapter 2, pages 22-41, in *Mosby's Paramedic Textbook*, ed. 3

OBJECTIVES
Upon completion of this chapter, the paramedic student will be able to do the following:
1. Describe the components of wellness and associated benefits.
2. Discuss the paramedic's role in promoting wellness.
3. Outline the benefits of specific lifestyle choices that promote wellness, including proper nutrition, weight control, exercise, sleep, and smoking cessation.
4. Identify risk factors and warning signs of cancer and cardiovascular disease.
5. Identify preventive measures to minimize the risk of work-related illness or injury associated with exposure, lifting and moving patients, hostile environments, vehicle operations, and rescue situations.
6. List signs and symptoms of addiction and addictive behavior.
7. Distinguish between normal and abnormal anxiety and stress reactions.
8. Give examples of stress-reduction techniques.
9. Outline the 10 components of critical incident stress management.
10. Given a scenario involving death or dying, identify therapeutic actions you may take based on your knowledge of the dynamics of this process.
11. List measures to take to reduce the risk of infectious disease exposure.
12. Outline actions to be taken following a significant exposure to a patient's blood or other body fluids.

SUMMARY
- Wellness has two main aspects: physical well-being and mental and emotional health.
- As health care professionals, paramedics have a responsibility to serve as role models in disease prevention.
- Physical fitness can be described as a condition that helps individuals look, feel, and do their best.
- Sleep helps to rejuvenate a tired body.
- Steps to reduce cardiovascular disease include the following: improving cardiovascular endurance, eliminating cigarette smoking, controlling high blood pressure, maintaining a normal body-fat composition, maintaining good total cholesterol/high-density lipoprotein ratio, monitoring triglyceride levels, controlling diabetes, avoiding excessive alcohol, eating healthy foods, reducing stress, and making a periodic risk assessment.
- Most common cancers are linked to one of three environmental risk factors: smoking, sunlight, and diet.

- Injuries on the job can be minimized. Knowledge of body mechanics during lifting and moving is helpful. Also, being alert for hostile settings is key. Prioritization of personal safety during rescue situations is wise. In addition, paramedics must practice safe vehicle operations. They must use safety equipment and supplies as well.
- The misuse and abuse of drugs and other substances may lead to chemical dependency (addiction). This may have a wide range of effects on physical and mental health.
- "Good" stress is eustress. Eustress is a positive response to stimuli and is considered protective. "Bad" stress is distress. Distress is a negative response to environmental stimuli and is the source of anxiety and stress-related disorders.
- Adaptation is a process where persons learn effective ways to deal with stressful situations. This dynamic process usually begins with using defense mechanisms. Next, one develops coping skills, followed by problem solving, and culminating in mastery.
- Critical incident stress management is designed to help emergency personnel understand their reactions. The process reassures them that what they are experiencing is normal and may be common to others involved in the incident.
- Often news of a sudden death must be given to a family. The paramedic's initial contact can influence the grief process greatly.
- The paramedic's duty is to be familiar with laws, regulations, and national standards that address issues of infectious disease. The paramedic also must take personal protective measures to guard against exposure.
- Actions to take after a significant exposure include disinfection, documentation, incident investigation, screening, immunization, and medical follow-up.

REVIEW QUESTIONS

Complete the following table to describe your wellness behaviors, analyze risks or benefits associated with those behaviors, and identify opportunities to improve them.

Behavior	Current practice	Risk/benefit of this behavior	Improvement plan
Diet (fats, vitamins, carbohydrates)			
Weight			
Cardiovascular endurance			
Strength/flexibility			
Sleep (hours/day)			

Continued

Behavior	Current practice	Risk/benefit of this behavior	Improvement plan
Cardiovascular disease risk factors			
Cancer risk factors			
Injury prevention			
Substance abuse			
Smoking			

Match the defense mechanism in column II with the appropriate example in column I. Use each defense mechanism only once.

Column I

1. _____ A rape victim who cannot recall anything from the time she was abducted until the police find her
2. _____ A paramedic who, when passed over for a promotion, states that the boss always plays favorites
3. _____ A paramedic who is upset by a violent death and washes all the vehicles in the garage
4. _____ A victim of an automobile accident who refuses to acknowledge that he cannot move his legs
5. _____ An EMT who gave poor care, yet complains about the patient's hospital treatment
6. _____ A 10-year-old who begins to suck his thumb en route to the hospital after sustaining a fracture from a fall

Column II

a. Compensation
b. Denial
c. Isolation
d. Projection
e. Rationalization
f. Reaction formation
g. Regression
h. Repression
i. Substitution

Questions 7 to 11 pertain to the following case study:

You respond to a call for an assault. Police on the scene tell you that an 18-year-old man has been stabbed. You find the patient, who turns out to be your nephew, at a party on the fourth floor of an apartment complex that has no working elevators. The patient is alert and crying and has a briskly bleeding puncture wound in the midaxillary line. He complains of having severe difficulty breathing and abdominal pain, and he has a rapid radial pulse. Oxygen is administered, and as you prepare for rapid transport and treatment, some party goers begin to get belligerent.

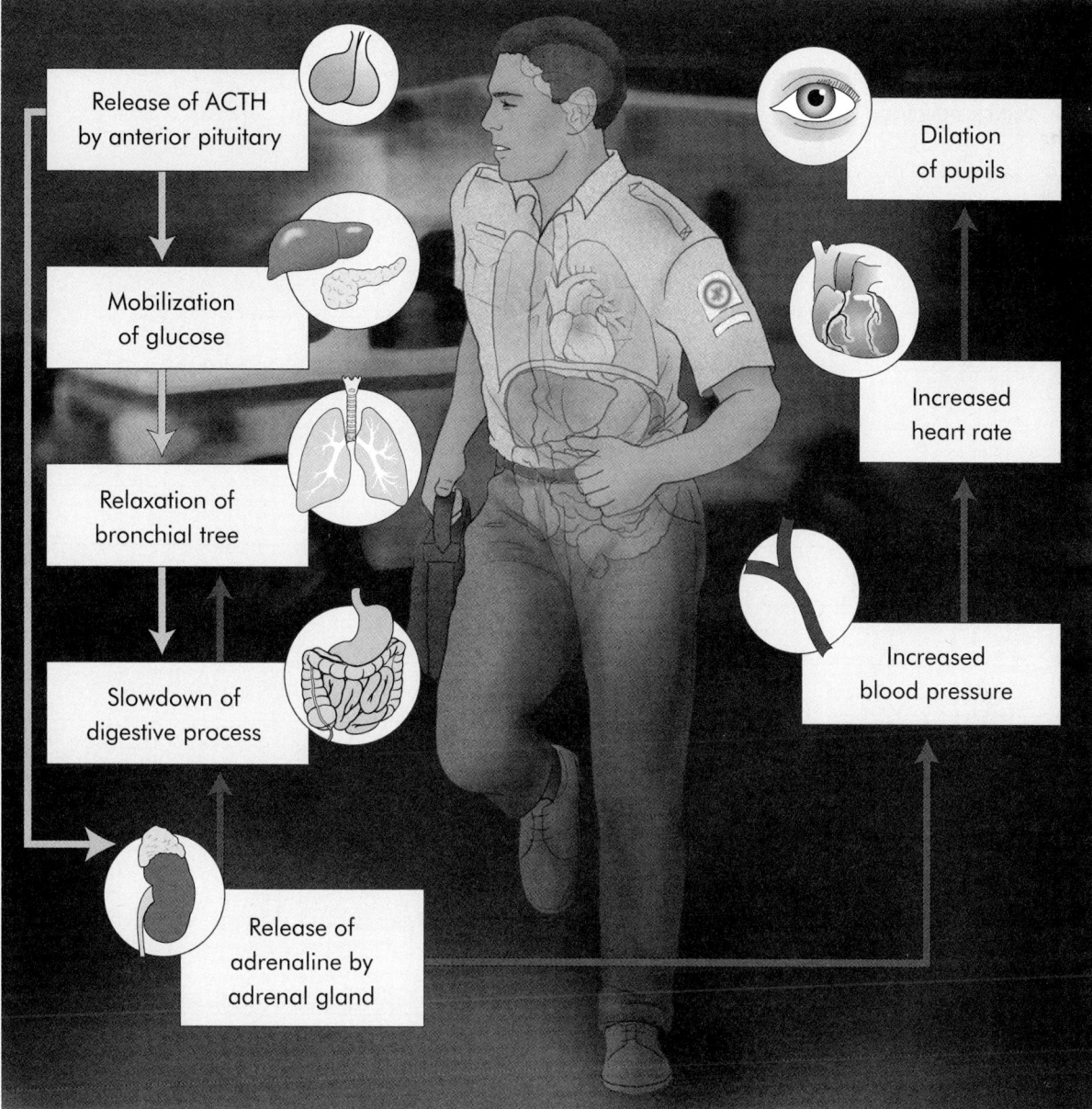

Figure 2-1

7. Describe three measures that you should take to reduce the risk of work-related illness and injury on this type of call in each of the following areas:

   a. Infectious disease

   _____

   b. Lifting and moving

   _____

    c. Hostile environments

_____

    d. Vehicle operation

_____

8. Briefly explain how each area of the body labeled in Fig. 2-1 responds to stress during the alarm reaction in this type of situation.

    a. _____

    b. _____

    c. _____

    d. _____

    e. _____

    f. _____

    g. _____

    h. _____

9. Describe two daily wellness practices that may benefit you as a paramedic when you respond to this type of situation.

    a.

    b.

10. List two reasons you, your crew, or both might use the services of the critical incident stress debriefing team after this call.

_____

_____

11. Which of the services that can be provided by a critical incident stress debriefing team may be of benefit after this call?

_____

12. List five causes of stress that are job related and five that are not job related.

    a. Job-related stressors:

_____

    b. Non–job-related stressors:

_____

13. List three potential symptoms of decompensation from the effects of long-term stress.

   a.

   b.

   c.

14. Name five effective stress-management techniques that can minimize the effects of EMS job-related stress. (After you complete this, survey paramedics you know to see what strategies they use.)

   a.

   b.

   c.

   d.

   e.

Questions 15 to 17 pertain to the following case study:

> You arrive at a family gathering where you find a 46-year-old man in full cardiopulmonary arrest. His mother is crying and begging, "Please, Lord, don't take him, take me." His wife is distraught, pacing and saying, "It's going to be OK; it's not as bad as it seems." The brother yells at you as you enter, "What took you so long? Hurry up! What are you waiting for?"

15. Identify which of the stages of grief described by Dr. Kubler-Ross each family member is exhibiting in this situation.

   a. Mother:

   b. Wife:

   c. Brother:

16. How should you care for these family members to promote normal grieving?

_____

_____

_____

17. How can you deal with the pent-up emotions you must suppress while caring for dying patients and their families on calls like this?

_____

_____

18. Identify which of the following situations represents an exposure to blood or body fluids. If exposure is involved, describe a measure that could have prevented it.

   a. After using a lancet to obtain a blood sample from your patient for dextrose measurement, you puncture your hand with the lancet. Exposure? Yes/No
Preventive measure:

_____

b. Blood sprays from a patient's endotracheal tube, hitting you in the face. You aren't sure if any got in your eyes or mouth. Exposure? Yes/No

Preventive measure:

_____

c. Your bare forearm brushes against a bloody sheet. You have no open wounds on your arm. Exposure? Yes/No

Preventive measure:

_____

d. You put the IV bag in your mouth to hold it up as you move the patient, and your partner points out that blood is splattered over the bag. Exposure? Yes/No

Preventive measure:

_____

19. At the scene of a motor vehicle collision, glass punctures your glove and cuts your finger. The patient's blood penetrates the glove and comes in contact with your cut. List at least four actions you should take after this exposure.

   a.

   b.

   c.

   d.

STUDENT SELF-ASSESSMENT

20. Which of the following is true regarding a healthy diet?
    a. Amino acids are produced by the body in the liver.
    b. Fats should be completely eliminated from the diet.
    c. Vitamin supplements are necessary for normal health.
    d. Water is one of the most important nutrients.

21. Which of the following is true regarding a routine physical fitness program?
    a. A decrease in muscle mass and metabolism will occur.
    b. A decrease in resting blood pressure may occur.
    c. A decrease in resistance to injury will occur.
    d. It should not be done if you have any preexisting illness.

22. Which of the following is a lifestyle modification associated with a decreased risk of heart disease?
    a. Reducing cigarette smoking
    b. Maintaining blood pressure at 120/80 mm Hg
    c. Reducing the very-low-density lipoprotein (VLDL) triglyceride level to 400 mg/dL
    d. Maintaining the low-density lipoprotein (LDL) cholesterol level at 190 mg/dL

23. Which of the following signs or symptoms is commonly listed as a warning sign of cancer?
    a. Indigestion or change in bowel habits
    b. Irregular heart beats or palpitations
    c. Lifelong presence of warts or moles
    d. Persistent nasal congestion

24. Actions that may prevent you from becoming infected with a communicable disease while practicing as a paramedic include which of the following?
    a. Annual skin testing for tuberculosis
    b. Frequent hand washing during all patient care activities
    c. Recapping of needles after patient use
    d. Use of body substance isolation for high-risk patients

25. How can you minimize your risk of injury while lifting or moving patients?
    a. Bend at the hips and knees
    b. Hold the load 18 inches from your body
    c. Lift with your back, not your legs
    d. Move backward rather than forward
26. Which of the following may indicate the potential for addiction or addictive behavior?
    a. Your partner asks you to drive him home from a bar because he feels he has had too much to drink.
    b. Your partner tells her husband she only had six beers instead of the 12 she actually drank.
    c. Your partner mentions that he is going out to have a few beers with some friends after work.
    d. Your partner says she can't handle booze the way she used to and now prefers beer to hard liquor.
27. You are called to a scene to assume care from a rescue unit. You immediately recognize the paramedic caring for the patient as an individual with whom you consistently disagree over patient care issues. What type of stress is this call likely to produce?
    a. Environmental   c. Personality
    b. Managerial   d. Psychosocial
28. Generalized feelings of apprehension are known as:
    a. Anxiety   c. Reaction formation
    b. Phobias   d. Stress
29. A paramedic student has just failed his practical examination station because of improper airway management technique. He states, "Well, I would have done it, but we never practiced it in class this way." This is an example of which defense mechanism?
    a. Projection   c. Regression
    b. Rationalization   d. Sublimation
30. Critical incident stress debriefing is most helpful for which of the following?
    a. New employees after every critical patient situation
    b. Selected high-risk employees with psychological problems
    c. Mass casualty incidents involving more than 10 patients
    d. Situations in which a high degree of stress is perceived
31. When dealing with the family of a patient who is dying, you can best interact with them by doing which of the following?
    a. Reassuring them that no one you ever care for dies
    b. Changing the subject every time someone brings up death
    c. Allowing the family to remain with the patient if possible
    d. Avoiding direct communication with the immediate family
32. Which response to the death of a close family member would not be expected in a preschool child?
    a. The child acts as though nothing has happened.
    b. The child asks when the family member will come back.
    c. The child fears that other family members will also die.
    d. The child thinks that he or she was responsible for the death.
33. School-age children (7 to 12 years old) feel that death:
    a. Is temporary and reversible
    b. Happens to others, not themselves
    c. Is a punishment for their bad thoughts
    d. Is the same as severe illness
34. Which of the following is an appropriate action to take after a needle-stick injury of the finger?
    a. Complete the exposure report and turn it in at the end of your shift.
    b. Determine whether the patient is high risk to decide whether you need to report the incident.
    c. Report the exposure to your supervisor and the receiving facility immediately.
    d. Squeeze out as much blood as possible and suck on your finger.

WRAP IT UP

Today is your worst nightmare. At about 1430 you are dispatched to a government building for a report of an explosion. It's your third day of a 72-hour shift, and you were just joking about taking the world record for most hours without sleep. En route, you see a plume of thick black smoke in the direction you are headed, and dispatch updates that there have been multiple calls and it appears there is major damage. You begin to review triage principles in your head, and you notice that your mouth is dry and you can feel your own heart pounding—sensations you haven't felt since your first rides as a paramedic student. Arriving on the scene, you see a multistory commercial structure with half of the side blown off. Command directs you and your partner to begin triage. There is mass confusion; people are moving all over the place. You attempt to set up a triage area, but bystanders are everywhere, rushing out with patients. Seven long hours later, 125 patients, some critically injured, have been triaged, treated, and transported. Among the casualties were your overweight captain, who was taken to the hospital with chest pains, and an out of shape co-worker, who strained his shoulder trying to free a trapped patient.

After the incident, things just got worse. One of your best friends just seems to be falling apart; she's drinking too much and in jeopardy of losing her job because of tardiness, frequent "sick" call-ins, and poor work performance. She keeps blaming everything on others and won't admit that she has a problem. The first few days after the incident, everyone pulled together, but now the stress level at work is high. Some people just keep to themselves; others are blaming co-workers for things that go wrong; and many of your colleagues don't even want to talk about the call.

1. What caused the dry mouth and palpitations that the paramedic experienced en route to this call?
   a. Cardiac irregularity
   b. Panic attack
   c. Parasympathetic release
   d. Stress reaction
2. After the incident, which defense mechanisms were observed in the paramedic's co-workers? (Check all that apply.)

   _____ Compensation   _____ Denial
   _____ Isolation   _____ Projection
   _____ Rationalization   _____ Reaction formation
   _____ Regression   _____ Repression
   _____ Substitution

3. What wellness activities may have reduced the chance of workplace illness or injury on this call?
   a. Balanced diet
   b. Cardiovascular endurance exercises
   c. Stretching and weight training
   d. All of the above
4. What stress reduction techniques might be helpful

   a. Before a call such as this:

   _____

   b. After a call such as this:

   _____

5. What strategies can paramedics use to increase their chance of sleep between calls on long shifts?

   _____

   _____

CHAPTER 2 ANSWERS

REVIEW QUESTIONS

1. h
2. e
3. i
4. b
5. d
6. g
(Questions 1-6: Objective 8)

7. a. To reduce the risk of acquiring an infectious disease, the paramedic should obtain appropriate immunizations, maintain good personal health and hygiene, use universal precautions during patient care (in this case gloves, goggles/mask, and gown if there is a risk of splash or spray), avoid recapping needles, dispose of contaminated sharps in an appropriate container, wash hands thoroughly after completing patient care, and appropriately dispose of soiled linens, equipment, and trash.

    b. To reduce the risk of injury from moving and lifting this patient, the paramedic should maintain good physical conditioning, obtain assistance in moving the patient if the person's size is too great for the paramedic and a partner, pay attention when walking, move forward when possible, take short steps, bend at the knees and hips, lift with the legs, keep the load close to the body, keep the patient's body in line when moving, and use the appropriate device for the situation (e.g., stair chair versus long back board).

    c. To reduce the risk of injury when providing care in a hostile environment, the paramedic should coordinate activities with law enforcement, scan the area for the fastest escape route, stay alert and move the patient out of the hostile area as quickly as possible, and leave the area if the situation becomes too dangerous. The best policy is to avoid entering the scene until the police have it under control.

    d. To ensure maximum safety when leaving this scene and transporting the patient to the hospital, the paramedic should use lights and sirens as dictated by local policy, proceed carefully through intersections, and maintain due regard for the safety of others.
    (Objectives 5, 11)

8. (a.) The pituitary gland releases adrenocorticotropic hormone, stimulating the sympathetic nervous system. (b.) Adrenal glands release epinephrine and norepinephrine, which (c) cause a rise in blood pressure by increasing systemic vascular resistance; (d) slow the digestive tract; (e) dilate the bronchioles, allowing deeper breathing; (f) stimulate glucose production in the liver; (g) dilate the pupils; and (h) increase the rate and strength of the heart's contractions.
(Objective 7)

9. Good physical conditioning permits rapid movement of the patient out of this hostile situation with reduced risk of injury to the paramedic. Good emotional health practices facilitate the use of healthy coping mechanisms in dealing with the personal stressors involved in this call.
(Objective 2)

10. Situations that pose a threat to rescuers' lives may be perceived as stressful, depending on the situation and the individuals involved. Having a critically injured patient who is a close relative or acquaintance often creates a very stressful situation.
(Objective 10)

11. Individual consultation may be necessary if only one person was overwhelmed by the call. If the event was perceived as very stressful by the whole group, defusing immediately after the incident, critical incident stress debriefing within 24 to 72 hours, and follow-up services after debriefing may be needed.
(Objective 9)

12. a. Working in hazardous situations; dealing with injured or dying children; working in an uncontrolled, unpredictable environment; dealing with emotionally upset, unpredictable patients; needing to make life and death decisions quickly. b. Physical illness of oneself or a close family member; loss of a job or starting a new job; personal financial troubles; the death of a loved one; and marital troubles, among others.
(Objective 7)

13. Irritability, apathy, chronic fatigue, feelings of not being appreciated, difficulty sleeping, drinking or drug abuse, decline in social activities, appetite changes, desire to quit work, and physical complaints.
(Objective 7)

14. Early recognition of signs and symptoms of stress, awareness of personal limitations, peer counseling, group discussions, proper diet, sleep, exercise, and pursuit of positive activities outside EMS.
(Objective 8)

15. a. Bargaining: The mother is bargaining her life for her son's life. b. Denial: The wife is denying the severity of the problem. c. Anger: The brother's anger is directed at the EMS personnel.
(Objective 10).

16. You should tell the family that the patient is critically ill and that you are going to do everything possible to help him. Remain calm and try to let the family remain close if patient care is not compromised. Assign tasks to the angry brother (e.g., stay with his mother and care for her).
(Objective 10)

17. Paramedics should be encouraged to talk about particularly distressing situations with other crew members and to avail themselves of resources available through medical direction and employee assistance programs.
(Objective 8)

18. a. Yes. Use accessible sharps containers and safety lancets.
    b. Yes. Wear a mask, eye protection, and gown when there is a risk of splash or spray.
    c. No exposure involved. You should wash your arm thoroughly.
    d. Yes. Do not place objects in your mouth when biohazards are present.
    (Objective 11)

19. a. Wash the area thoroughly.
    b. Document the exposure.
    c. Immediately report to the appropriate personnel.
    d. Complete the medical follow-up.
    (Objective 12)

STUDENT SELF-ASSESSMENT

20. d. Cellular function depends on a fluid environment. Amino acids are essential for body growth and cellular life and are not produced by the body. Polyunsaturated fats can help reduce high blood cholesterol levels if included as part of a low-fat diet.
(Objective 1)

21. b. An increase in muscle mass, metabolism, and resistance to injury should be anticipated with a carefully planned fitness program. Fitness programs can be tailored to accommodate the needs of individuals with preexisting medical conditions (e.g., arthritis, heart disease) and are encouraged.
(Objective 1)

22. b. Cigarette smoking should be eliminated to reduce the risk of heart disease. The triglyceride level should not exceed 200 to 300 mg/dL, and the LDL cholesterol level should be below 160 mg/dL.
(Objective 4)

23. a. The other signs listed by the American Cancer Society are a sore throat, unusual bleeding or discharge, thickening or a lump in the breast or elsewhere, obvious change in a wart or mole, and a nagging cough or hoarseness.
(Objective 4)

24. b. Annual skin testing is an excellent measure for detecting exposure to tuberculosis so that it can be appropriately treated; however, it does not prevent infection. Needle recapping is never advised because this greatly increases the risk of injury and exposure. Body substance isolation measures should be used for all patients, not just those that might be high risk.
(Objective 5)

25. a. To minimize the risk of injury, you should also hold the load close to your body, lift with your legs (not your back), and move forward rather than backward when possible.
(Objective 5)

26. b. Lying about using a substance indicates guilt about using the substance; this is a warning sign.
(Objective 6)

27. d. Environmental stress results from factors such as siren noise and weather. Personality stress relates to the way individuals feel about themselves. Managerial stress is not a distinct entity.
(Objective 7)

28. a. *Phobias* are unrealistic fears. *Reaction formation* is a defense mechanism in which unacceptable desires are suppressed by accentuating opposite behaviors. *Stress* is a generalized response to certain situations.
(Objective 7)

29. b. *Projection* occurs when one's own undesirable feelings are attributed to someone else. *Regression* is a return to an earlier stage of emotional adjustment. *Sublimation* occurs when unacceptable urges are modified to become socially acceptable.
(Objective 7)

30. d. New paramedics may be at greater risk for high stress after a critical call; however, veterans will continue to be vulnerable to unusually stressful calls. Multiple patient situations may not always trigger stress responses in rescuers; it depends on the individual situation. A high-risk employee with psychological problems probably will require care in addition to the critical incident stress debriefing program.
(Objective 9)

31. c. If the family raises the issue of death, a realistic description of the seriousness of the patient's condition should be briefly given. Direct eye contact and touch, if appropriate, may be used to convey concern and caring.
(Objective 10)

32. a. The family should watch for behavioral changes at home and at school, as well as difficulty eating or sleeping, and should encourage the child to express his or her feelings.
(Objective 10)

33. b. School-age children have begun to understand the concept of the finality of death; however, they still feel that it happens only to others.
(Objective 10)

34. c. All needle-stick injuries should be reported immediately so that appropriate source testing and follow-up can be completed in a timely manner.
(Objective 12)

WRAP IT UP

1. d. These are normal sympathetic responses to stress.
   (Objective 7)

2. Denial, rationalization, and substitution (the paramedic who shows poor performance); isolation (co-workers who keep to themselves); and repression (responders who don't want to talk about the call).
   (Objective 7)

3. d. Diet and exercise can reduce weight and improve cardiovascular fitness. Musculoskeletal injuries can be reduced by improving strength and flexibility.
   (Objective 3)

4. a. Exercise, meditation, and positive social connections can help in the management of stress on a daily basis.
   b. Critical incident stress debriefing, one-on-one counseling, exercise, reframing, controlled breathing, progressive relaxation, guided imagery, proper diet, and sleep are all techniques that may assist in the management of stress.
   (Objective 8)

5. Take some quiet time to relax before trying to sleep (reading, meditation, exercise); avoid stimulants; eat simple carbohydrates to release serotonin; select a dark sleeping area; try to pick a "normal" nap time (often difficult at work).
   (Objective 2)

CHAPTER

3

Injury Prevention

READING ASSIGNMENT
Chapter 3, pages 42-53, in *Mosby's Paramedic Textbook*, ed. 3

OBJECTIVES
Upon completion of this chapter, the paramedic student will be able to do the following:
1. Identify roles of the emergency medical services community in injury prevention.
2. Describe the epidemiology of trauma in the United States.
3. Outline the aspects of the emergency medical services system that make it a desirable resource for involvement in community health activities.
4. Describe community leadership activities that are essential to enable the active participation of emergency medical services in community wellness activities.
5. List areas with which paramedics should be familiar to participate in injury prevention.
6. Evaluate a situation to determine opportunities for injury prevention.
7. Identify resources necessary to conduct a community health assessment.
8. Relate how alterations in the epidemiological triangle can influence injury and disease patterns.
9. Differentiate among primary, secondary, and tertiary health prevention activities.
10. Describe strategies to implement a successful injury prevention program.

SUMMARY
- EMS providers are members of the community's health care system. They can be an important resource for injury prevention.
- Unintentional injuries are the fifth leading cause of death, exceeded only by heart disease, cancer, stroke, and chronic obstructive pulmonary disease.
- The United States has more than 600,000 EMS providers. This valuable human resource plays a major role in public education, a component of health promotion that seems only fitting.
- EMS workers play an active role in protecting and promoting the health of a community. The community, in turn, must protect EMS workers from injury. It also must provide them with a strong education in their field. Furthermore, the community should support and promote the collection and use of injury data. In addition, it must obtain resources for primary injury prevention activities. The community must empower EMS workers to provide primary injury prevention.
- All EMS workers must have a basic knowledge of personal injury prevention. They also should know about maladies and injuries common to various age groups, recreational activities, workplaces, and other facilities in the community.
- Paramedics must be able to identify the signs and symptoms of abuse and abusive situations. They also must be able to recognize potentially dangerous situations.
- Paramedics should identify and use outside community resources. They also should properly document primary injury data. They should be able to recognize and use the teachable moment.

- EMS providers must maximize their time and resources. Therefore they should identify targets for community health education. They can do this by performing a community health assessment.
- To identify community education goals, the paramedic must understand that illness and injury are influenced by several factors: (1) the degree of exposure to an agent; (2) the strength of the agent; (3) the susceptibility of the individual (host); and (4) the biologic, social, and physical environment.
- *Primary* injury prevention is characterized by efforts to prevent the occurrence of an injury. *Secondary* prevention and *tertiary* prevention involve efforts to help prevent the development of further problems from an event that has already occurred.
- A good injury prevention program must serve the whole target population in a community. An effective program also takes into account reading level and age. These are the marks of a successful program. The EMS provider can present community health education in diverse ways. These can include verbal, written/static material, and dynamic visual presentations.

REVIEW QUESTIONS

Questions 1 to 9 pertain to the following case study:

At 1400 the tones sound, and you are dispatched to the home of an elderly resident who has slipped and fallen. On arrival at the emergency department, the physician confirms your suspicion—the patient's hip is broken. As you ride back to the base, you remark to your partner how this is the fourth patient you've transported this month with a broken hip. These calls really bother you, because your own grandmother was institutionalized and then died of pneumonia shortly after a similar injury just 6 months ago. By the time you arrive back at your station, you have resolved to do something about the problem. You approach the chief, who listens to your idea. He tells you to return when you have some solid information about the target population, the magnitude of the problem, your goals, and the cost involved.

1. Injury accounts for about what percentage of emergency department (ED) visits in the United States?

_____

2. The initial visit to the emergency department for this type of injury has a high price. List two other "costs" associated with this type of injury.

_____

_____

3. Give at least three reasons why EMS is ideally suited to perform community prevention activities with the elderly.

   a.

   b.

   c.

4. What additional information would you need to be able to provide prevention for this type of injury in this group?

_____

5. What will you need from your boss before moving ahead with this project?

_____

6. List three community resources you may need to contact to identify the number of elderly individuals living in your district, the incidence of hip fractures, the morbidity and mortality rates associated with this injury, and costs associated with such fractures.

   a.

   b.

   c.

7. You decide that the causes of fall injury in the elderly are most likely the result of the host and environmental factors of the epidemiological triangle. List two host and two environmental factors that may contribute to falls in the elderly.

Host:

a. _____

b. _____

Environmental:

a. _____

b. _____

After careful evaluation of the problem, you decide that the best plan would be to have EMS crews visit elderly residents' homes with a checklist that would identify risk factors for falls in the home. A brief educational pamphlet with specific recommendations would then be given to the resident.

8. Is your plan an example of a primary, secondary, or tertiary intervention?

_____

9. List at least four factors you should consider in preparing the written educational materials to be distributed to the community.

_____

_____

Each of the examples in questions 10 to 18 represents a factor that could cause or increase susceptibility to illness and injury. Indicate whether the example is an *agent* factor (causative), a *host* factor (influences exposure, susceptibility, or response to agents), or an *environmental* factor (influences existence of the agent, exposure, or susceptibility).

Example	Agent, Host, or Environmental Factor
10. Fatigue	
11. Firefighter	
12. Carbon monoxide	
13. Gender	
14. Hepatitis	
15. Malnutrition	
16. Poor personal hygiene	
17. Flood	
18. Cholesterol	

19. List at least four injury prevention strategies a paramedic might use to help reduce neurological injury.

a.

b.

c.

d.

STUDENT SELF-ASSESSMENT

20. A total of 10 people in your EMS district have been killed in motor vehicle collisions thus far this year. Where do deaths from unintentional causes such as this rank in the United States?
  a. First
  b. Third
  c. Fifth
  d. Seventh

21. The number of drownings in your community rose last year. The health department asks your EMS agency to assist with an educational plan to help reduce the incidence of drowning. Why are EMS providers ideal for this type of program?
  a. They have more time than other health care providers to teach these programs.
  b. Paramedics and EMTs will be welcomed into homes and public places to present educational programs.
  c. EMS agencies have abundant financial resources to fund these programs.
  d. EMS providers are the best authorities on preventing such tragedies.

22. How can EMS safety be enhanced during emergency care and transportation?
  a. Educate the public to pull to the right when they see emergency traffic
  b. Ticket people who fail to yield to emergency traffic
  c. Establish a policy of parking upwind from all HAZMAT spills
  d. Ensure that police assume all responsibility for scene safety

23. How can EMS agencies promote the involvement of staff members in community wellness programs?
  a. Penalize those who decline to participate
  b. Ask everyone on duty to participate
  c. Offer it as an alternative to a less desirable chore
  d. Provide a salary for off-duty injury prevention work

24. You respond to a call for domestic violence. You find a woman with bruising around her face, and she and her husband are yelling at each other. She screams at you to leave her alone when you try to examine her, and he is staggering and cursing at you. What is your primary goal in this situation?
  a. To restrain the patient and ask medical direction for permission for involuntary transport
  b. To ask the police to arrest both of them so that they can be contained in a controlled space
  c. To maintain the safety of your crew and to diffuse the situation calmly without violence
  d. To forcibly remove the man from the situation so that the woman will not be afraid of treatment

25. Which of the following patient situations would likely present a teachable moment?
  a. A hysterical mother being transported with her child, who just fell down a flight of stairs
  b. An elderly patient who refuses care after falling in a dimly lit stairway and injuring her wrist
  c. A child with minor injuries who was struck by a car that crossed the median onto the sidewalk
  d. A cyclist without a helmet who fell off his bike during a race and is confused during transport

26. You believe that you are running many more calls related to heart problems in the elderly. What community resources can you use as sources of information to determine whether the makeup of your community is changing?
  a. Census data
  b. Chamber of commerce
  c. Fire service
  d. Local newspaper

27. It is a cold, wintry day, and the trees are glistening after the ice storm last night. Your crew alone has run four calls to the local sledding hill to care for patients with injuries ranging from broken extremities to lumbar fractures. Which element in the epidemiological triangle is most likely having the greatest influence on the injuries you are seeing in this situation?
  a. Physical environment
  b. Social setting
  c. Strength of the agent
  d. Susceptibility of the host

28. Which of the following is an example of a primary health prevention activity with which a paramedic may be involved?
    a. You check the blood pressure of residents diagnosed with hypertension each week.
    b. You coordinate a stop smoking program for a group of your fellow employees.
    c. You coordinate a drunk-u-drama at the high school before prom week.
    d. You arrange a support group for EMS personnel recovering from alcohol abuse.
29. You are preparing a presentation on drug use for the young people in your area. How can you make sure your audience will understand your message?
    a. You test it on a teen patient during an EMS call.
    b. You ask your crew if it appeals to them.
    c. You include slides to increase the likelihood of retention.
    d. You make sure the language and reading level suit the audience.
30. Which of the following injury prevention strategies is associated with the greatest reduction in injury and death after a vehicle crash?
    a. Automatic airbag deployment on crash impact
    b. Driver education programs for senior citizens
    c. Fines for driving without wearing seatbelts
    d. Television advertising promoting safe driving techniques

WRAP IT UP

As you arrive on the scene of a "pedestrian struck" call, you observe a child whose life has changed forever. The 8-year-old boy, who had been riding his bike without a helmet, had careened down a hill into an intersection and was struck by a small truck. The distraught driver tells you that the boy flew up and hit the windshield with his head. You note that the windshield is starred and that the front quarter panel of the truck is dented. It's immediately evident that the child is seriously injured. He has a forehead laceration and is combative. You quickly immobilize him and load him into the ambulance while maintaining the airway. En route to the local trauma center, you continue your assessments, intubate the trachea, insert an intravenous (IV) line, and notify the trauma team of your assessment and your estimated time of arrival (ETA). The boy's condition worsens as you roll him into the trauma room. Later, during the postincident review, you are told that although he survived, he will have severe cognitive impairment. He is in rehabilitation, and it is unclear whether he will ever function normally again. You are angry and frustrated. You have many long discussions about the call with your captain. After much thought, and with the captain's approval, you decide to start a helmet program in your community. You plan to hold clinics at which you will properly fit helmets for those who have one and sell helmets for $5 (your cost to buy them) to those who don't. You also plan to develop brochures and deliver presentations in the local elementary schools.

1. a. What is the goal of a program such as this?

_____

_____

   b. Is this goal consistent with the mission of an EMS organization? _____

_____

_____

2. Why would EMS providers be suitable professionals to initiate such a program?

_____

_____

3. Where can you find information to justify the cost of this program to your chief?

_____

_____

4. Could you tie in on-scene education to a program like this?

_____

_____

5. Place a ✔ beside the components of a community health assessment that could be helpful in your research for this program.

_____ Population demographics   _____ Morbidity statistics

_____ Mortality statistics   _____ Crime and fire information

_____ Community resource allocation   _____ Hospital data

_____ Senior citizen needs   _____ Education standards

_____ Recreational facilities   _____ Environmental conditions

_____ Other factors

6. Would this program be a primary, secondary, or tertiary community health intervention?

_____

_____

7. Where can you seek funding to support your program?

_____

_____

8. What must you consider in developing your brochure and your presentation?

_____

_____

CHAPTER 3 ANSWERS

REVIEW QUESTIONS

1. About 42% of ED visits are related to injury.
(Objective 2)

2. In addition to the initial ED visit, other costs related to injury include lost quality of life, loss of income, and long-term hospitalizations/care.
(Objective 2)

3. EMS providers are ideally suited for educating elderly people in their community because they are welcomed into the home. Also, they are viewed as experts who are medically educated; they are considered to have people's best interests at heart; and they may be the first to identify situations that pose a risk.
(Objectives 1, 3)

4. Injury prevention material specific to falls in the elderly would need to be obtained.
(Objective 4)

5. You will need financial support, endorsement of your agency, and possibly assistance from your boss to identify other community resources.
(Objective 4)

6. Census data should reflect the number of elderly; the area health department should have statistics on mortality and injury frequency and type; your own EMS system could provide information about the number of elderly patients transported as a result of fall-related injuries; and national agencies such as the Centers for Disease Control and Prevention (CDC) and the National Safety Council can provide cost data and are accessible either through the Internet or the library.
(Objective 7)

7. Host: Poor eyesight, impaired balance secondary to medication use, decreased sensation. Environmental: poor lighting, loose area rugs, absence of or poorly maintained railings, icy walkways.
(Objective 8)

8. This is a primary intervention if it involves people who have not had injuries from a fall.
(Objective 8)

9. You will need to consider the following factors: the cost of the materials (who will pay for them); whether someone in the community already has materials you could use (e.g., hospital, health department); the reading levels of the audience; whether you need to prepare bilingual materials if you have a large group that does not read English; and the type size of the material (to accommodate clients with poor vision).
(Objective 10)

10. Host. Fatigue may result in a shortened attention span, which may lead to an injury.
11. Environment. Firefighters are placed in hostile environments by their work, which increases their susceptibility to injury or illness.
12. Agent. Carbon monoxide is a poisonous gas that can cause illness or death.
13. Host. Certain diseases are more prevalent in one gender than the other (e.g., rheumatoid arthritis is more prevalent in women).
14. Agent. Hepatitis is a virus that causes disease.
15. Host. Malnutrition deprives the body of essential nutrients necessary to maintain health.
16. Host. Poor personal hygiene predisposes an individual to infection.
17. Environmental. Floods may cause water contamination and increase the risk of the epidemic spread of disease.
18. Agent. Excess cholesterol is associated with an increased risk of heart disease.
(Questions 10-18: Objective 8)

19. Helmet, seatbelt, senior fall prevention, safe bicycle riding programs
20. c. Unintentional injuries are the top cause of death for persons between 1 and 38 years of age and the fifth leading cause of death overall. (Objective 2)

STUDENT SELF-ASSESSMENT

21. b. Residents of a community usually have a high level of trust in EMS providers and will let them in to speak about these issues. The amount of time paramedics have in any given EMS system depends on the call volume and other commitments, such as training or other departmental duties. EMS agencies do not always have financial resources but may have a community partner to fund the support materials for the program. EMS providers often have baseline knowledge about injury prevention but can be educated on specific injury prevention materials.
(Objective 3)

22. a. Ticketing people who fail to yield may be helpful, but it affects only those who may have caused injury to EMS providers or their patients. Education is more desirable.
(Objective 4)

23. d. Penalizing personnel or forcing them to participate in an activity may be necessary, but it does not promote maximum participation in activities. Rewards and incentives are helpful.
(Objective 4)

24. c. Situations involving domestic violence are volatile and complicated. Measures to diffuse, rather than escalate, the situation should be used unless the circumstances pose an immediate danger to your crew, your patient, or the police.
(Objective 5)

25. b. This patient is calm and cooperative, but she probably realizes that her injury could have been more serious. A few words about appropriate lighting and specific recommendations for accomplishing it would likely be taken quite seriously at that moment. For the child hit by a car, calming may be a greater priority, and there is no evidence of a need to teach him anything specific to relate to this incident. In *a* and *d,* the parent or patient is not in an appropriate mental state to be taught.
(Objective 6)

26. a. Census data, which may be obtained through the Internet or the library, provide information about population demographics, including age and income levels. The area health department can give you specific information about deaths in your community and their causes. The local paper may refer you to information sources but won't likely have specifics. Fire departments have very specific call data related to fires and whether they also provide EMS and illness or injury information. The chamber of commerce has economic data and information about industry, religious organizations, and cultural opportunities in a community.
(Objective 7)

27. a. The icy conditions undoubtedly are having the greatest influence on the situation. The ice prevented the host from controlling the speed or direction of the sled, and it caused the crash.
(Objective 8)

28. c. The drunk-u-drama will attempt to teach students how to prevent injuries from occurring. You are performing secondary interventions on the hypertensive group and the smokers; both these groups already have a condition you are attempting to control or stop. Tertiary activities, designed to rehabilitate, would include the support group activities.
(Objective 9)

29. d. Although brief opportunities for teaching occur during an EMS call, a formal educational plan wouldn't be appropriate. Your crew members may think the program is great, but the target audience may not relate to it at all. Slides are appropriate, but depending on your audience and your message, they may not be desirable or possible. For example, if your program is to be delivered to youth groups on a street corner, you would have to choose a different method.
(Objective 10)

30. a. Engineering safety controls, which do not offer the user a choice whether to use them, are more effective.

WRAP IT UP

1. a. The goal would be to reduce injury and death for those riding bicycles and other wheeled recreational toys.
b. For most EMS agencies, this goal should be consistent with their mission, which is to reduce death and disability.
(Objective 1)

2. EMS providers are medically educated, are high-profile role models, are welcome in schools and homes, and are considered "experts" on injury and prevention. Therefore they are ideal providers of injury prevention programs.
(Objective 3)

3. Information on the costs of unintentional injuries can be obtained from National Safety Council statistics, some state data, trauma centers, and trauma organizations.
(Objective 7)

4. On-scene education could be included in such a program by (1) giving helmets to children who have been in collisions while on bikes, scooters, or roller blades; (2) by offering to properly fit them for a helmet; or (3) by encouraging them to wear their helmet (or wear it properly).
(Objective 9)

5. Population demographics, mortality statistics, morbidity statistics, hospital data, recreational facilities (e.g., a skateboard park in your district), and other factors (e.g., funding sources, a local police bicycle rodeo at which you could implement your program) could be helpful in creating your presentation.
(Objective 7)

6. This is mainly a primary injury prevention program; it prevents the injury from happening.
(Objective 9)

7. Funding could be sought through federal grants, local service clubs (Kiwanis, Lions, Optimists, Rotary), SafeKids coalitions, and hospitals. If you can establish the program with seed money and then sell your helmets for cost, the program may perpetuate itself, with little additional funding needed.
(Objectives 7, 10)

8. In developing the materials for your program, you must consider (1) the money available; (2) the reading level of the target audience; (3) the likes and dislikes of the target audience; (4) the attention span of the target audience; and (5) ethnic, cultural, and religious considerations for the target audience. After the program has been put together, someone from your target audience should "preview" the material and give you their opinion.
(Objective 10)

CHAPTER

4

Medical/Legal Issues

READING ASSIGNMENT
Chapter 4, pages 54-71, in *Mosby's Paramedic Textbook,* ed. 3

OBJECTIVES
Upon completion of this chapter, the paramedic student will be able to do the following:
1. Describe the basic structure of the legal system in the United States.
2. Relate how laws affect the paramedic's practice.
3. List situations that the paramedic is legally required to report in most states.
4. Describe the four elements involved in a claim of negligence.
5. Describe measures paramedics may take to protect themselves from claims of negligence.
6. Describe the paramedic's responsibilities regarding patient confidentiality.
7. Outline the process for obtaining expressed, informed, and implied consent.
8. Describe legal complications relating to consent.
9. Describe actions to be taken in a refusal-of-care situation.
10. Describe legal considerations related to patient transportation.
11. Outline legal issues related to specific resuscitation situations.
12. List measures the paramedic should take to preserve evidence when at a crime or accident scene.
13. Detail the components of the narrative report necessary for effective legal documentation.
14. Define common medical/legal terms that apply to prehospital situations involving patient care.

SUMMARY
- The structure of the legal system in the United States is composed of five types of law: legislative law, administrative law, common law, criminal law, and civil law.
- To safeguard against litigation, the paramedic must be knowledgeable of legal issues. The paramedic also must know about the effects of these issues.
- Paramedics and health care workers may be required by law to report some cases. These include cases of abuse or neglect of children and older adults and spouse abuse. They also include cases that involve rape, sexual assault, gunshot wounds, stab wounds, animal bites, and some communicable diseases.
- Lawsuits that have to do with patient care usually result from civil claims of negligence. This refers to the failure to act as a reasonable, prudent paramedic would act in such circumstances.
- Most legal authorities stress that protection against claims of negligence has three elements. The first is training. The second is competent patient care skills. The third is full documentation of all patient care activities.
- Some state and federal regulations provide protection for the paramedic with respect to notification of infectious disease exposure, immunity statutes, and special crimes against EMS personnel.

- Confidential information is threefold. For the most part, confidential information includes any details about a patient that are related to the patient's history. Any assessment findings also are included. Any treatment given is included as well. As a rule, the release of these details requires written permission from the patient or legal guardian. (There are some exceptions.)
- A mentally competent adult has the right to refuse medical care. This is the case even if the decision could result in death or permanent disability.
- Four other legal complications related to consent are abandonment, false imprisonment, assault, and battery.
- A competent patient has certain rights. The patient has the right to decide what medical care (and transportation) to receive. This is a basic concept of law and medical practice.
- Legal responsibilities for the patient continue until patient care is transferred to another member of the health care system (or it is clear that the patient no longer requires care). Legal issues related to patient transport include level of care during transportation, use of the emergency vehicle operating privileges, choice of patient destination, and payer protocols.
- Resuscitation issues that relate directly to EMS include withholding or stopping resuscitation, advance directives, potential organ donation, and death in the field.
- Emergency medical services play two important roles when responding to crime scenes: (1) focusing on patient care and (2) preserving evidence at the scene when possible.
- In the legal field the general belief is that "if it was not written down, it was not done." Thus thoroughness and attention to detail are vital in documentation.

REVIEW QUESTIONS

Match the legal term in column II with its definition in column I. Use each answer only once.

Column I

1. _____ Forcefully restraining the arm of an alert, competent patient while an intravenous line is placed
2. _____ As a joke, advising the emergency department staff that the patient is a prostitute
3. _____ Telling a friend that you treated a nurse you both know for a drug overdose
4. _____ Restraining an alert, conscious adult with an obvious fracture and transporting him by ambulance against his will
5. _____ Documenting that the patient is homosexual and remarking, "Now let's see them get insurance"
6. _____ Leaving a patient in the emergency department to go on another call before you have an opportunity to give a report to the nurse or physician on duty

Column II

a. Abandonment
b. Assault
c. Battery
d. False imprisonment
e. Libel
f. Invasion of privacy (libel)
g. Malpractice
h. Slander

7. Violations of state motor vehicle codes by a paramedic can result only in civil lawsuits. True/False. If you answered false, explain why.

_____

_____

8. Good Samaritan legislation may protect off-duty EMS providers from litigation if no negligence or reckless disregard is involved. True/False. If you answered false, explain why.

_____

_____

9. Group insurance policies protect EMS providers from lawsuits arising from negligent acts. True/False. If you answered false, explain why.

_____

_____

10. List four situations that most states require a paramedic to report to the authorities.

   a.

   b.

   c.

   d.

11. List the four elements necessary to prove negligence.

   a.

   b.

   c.

   d.

12. A 40-year-old patient involved in a motor vehicle collision complains of mild neck pain and tingling in her fingers. She is quickly assessed and signs a refusal of care form at the urging of the paramedic crew. Later that day she loses sensation and movement in all extremities, stops breathing, and dies. Which, if any, of the four elements in question no. 11 could be used to prove negligence in this situation and why?

_____

_____

_____

13. Name three effective means by which the paramedic can avoid claims of liability when providing patient care.

   a.

   b.

   c.

14. You are called to treat an alert, 72-year-old patient who is experiencing chest pain. The patient exhibits classic signs and symptoms of myocardial infarction. You explain to him that he needs to go to the hospital because you feel that his symptoms could be those of a heart attack, and proper medicine could be given to help his condition. He states that he wants his wife to drive him instead of going by ambulance. You advise him that if his condition worsens in the car, his wife would be unable to help him and he might die. You again urge him to come with you. Fill in the blanks below with the type of consent that best applies to the situation.
The patient can now make a(n)

   a. _____ consent. He tells you that he has decided to go in the ambulance. This constitutes a(n)

   b. _____ consent. If he had lost consciousness before agreeing to ambulance transport, his consent is said to be a(n)

   c. _____ consent, and treatment could be rendered.

15. You respond to the scene of an automobile collision, where you find an awake, alert, 24-year-old man complaining of neck pain and tingling in his right arm. His vital signs are stable. The patient's vehicle was struck from behind and sustained considerable damage. The patient refuses transport to the hospital. What five things should be done or explained to this patient and documented on the patient care report regarding his refusal of care?

a.

b.

c.

d.

e.

Questions 16 to 21 refer to the following case study:

You are dispatched to an expensive rural home for an "accidental injury." When you arrive, you find two patients, a man and a woman. The man, who appears to be approximately 30 years old, apparently had been shot in the head at close range. He had been found pulseless and breathless by a family member, who found both patients 20 minutes before your arrival. The male patient has a large exit wound with brain matter extruding. After your initial assessment, you decide not to resuscitate him. The female patient is a woman whom you recognize as a local celebrity. She has a gunshot wound to the abdomen, is unconscious, and has no radial pulse. You note a plastic bag of white powder and a hypodermic needle next to her. A handgun is lying on the floor next to the man. The family wants you to take the woman to the closest local hospital so that they can "keep things quiet." The nearest trauma center is an equal distance away.

16. What type of consent applies in this situation?

_____

17. List four facts you must document about the male patient to ensure legal compliance.

a.

b.

c.

d.

18. Describe actions you should take to preserve evidence at this scene with regard to the following:

a. Clothing

_____

b. Weapon

_____

c. Blood on the floor

_____

d. Documentation of the scene

_____

e. Positioning of the ambulance

_____

19. Should you transport the patient to the hospital the family wants or to the trauma center? Explain your answer.

_____

_____

20. Why shouldn't you document, "Drugs found lying next to patient"?

_____

_____

21. To which of the following personnel is it appropriate to tell the facts of this case?
  a. Police officers assigned to the case   Yes/No
  b. A paramedic from another service   Yes/No
  c. The press   Yes/No
  d. Medical personnel caring for the patient   Yes/No
  e. Hospital staff in the smokers' area   Yes/No

STUDENT SELF-ASSESSMENT

22. Which branch of law is also referred to as _tort law?_
  a. Administrative law   **c.** Criminal law
  b. Civil law   **d.** Legislative law

23. In which of the following situations may abandonment be alleged when a paramedic relinquishes care to an EMT?
  a. A patient being transferred with an infusion of blood
  b. A patient going from a nursing home to a hospital for a wrist injury
  c. A hysterical, uninjured patient from a mass casualty situation
  d. A dialysis patient being transported for routine care

24. Which of the following is necessary for successful prosecution of a criminal law case?
  a. Criminal intent must be proved.
  b. Injury must be demonstrated.
  c. A patient must sue for financial gain.
  d. A statute must be violated.

25. You are called to a private residence, where you find an elderly man suffering from heat-related illness. The family evidently left this chronically confused individual at home with no air conditioning and all the windows closed. What legal issue must you remember on this call?
  a. You should not remove the patient's clothes so that you can preserve the chain of evidence.
  b. This patient can't give consent, therefore you must contact the next of kin before transport.
  c. Writing the neighbors' statements in the patient care report may constitute libel.
  d. You are required to report this situation to the appropriate legal or social agency.

26. The Ryan White Act provides protection for the paramedic with regard to which of the following?
  a. Good Samaritan acts   **c.** Infectious disease
  b. Governmental immunity   **d.** Violent acts

27. A paramedic finds an unconscious patient who has a strong odor resembling alcohol on the breath. No care is initiated, and during transport the patient aspirates. On arrival at the hospital, the patient is found to have a dangerously low blood sugar level, and a lengthy hospitalization ensues. Why could this patient claim negligence?
  a. The paramedic violated a law while providing care.
  b. The paramedic committed malfeasance while providing care.
  c. The patient suffered damage from the negligent act.
  d. Evidence existed of conflicting views of causation.

28. Patient confidentiality would be breached in most states if a paramedic discussed the patient's comments and care with which of the following?
    a. Lawyers in court
    b. Emergency department personnel
    c. Personal friends
    d. A quality assurance committee
29. When a patient agrees to treatment verbally or in writing, it is known as which of the following?
    a. Expressed consent
    b. Implied consent
    c. Informed consent
    d. Referred consent
30. You are caring for an elderly patient who experienced a syncopal episode. He now refuses care. What actions must you take to ensure legal compliance during this refusal process?
    a. Force the patient to sign the refusal form before release.
    b. Tell the patient that if he changes his mind, he can call you again for transport.
    c. Do not give the patient any additional advice or you may be liable.
    d. Transport the patient against his will because his condition involved a loss of consciousness.
31. What do EMS traffic right-of-way privileges usually include?
    a. The right to travel as fast as necessary to get to the hospital quickly
    b. The ability to proceed without slowing through intersections
    c. The right to override the directions of a traffic officer
    d. Definitions of appropriate use of lights and sirens
32. According to the American Heart Association, what criteria must be met to stop resuscitation in the prehospital setting after you have initiated advanced life support procedures?
    a. Persistent asystole or agonal rhythm is present and no reversible causes are identified.
    b. The family assures you that there is a "do not resuscitate" order, but it can't be found.
    c. Endotracheal intubation and IV access can't be established, therefore you are unable to give drugs.
    d. Trauma is a factor, and your transport time will be 20 minutes or longer.
33. You respond to a stabbing at a local bar. What actions should you take during your care of the patient to preserve evidence?
    a. Cut the clothing through the knife hole to minimize other damage
    b. Give the clothes to a bystander so that evidence will remain at the scene
    c. Move the knife, if present, so that EMS personnel will not step on it
    d. Follow the same path to and from the ambulance and patient
34. Which of the following should be included in the narrative portion of the patient care report?
    a. Care rendered
    b. History
    c. Physical findings
    d. All of the above

WRAP IT UP

Your ambulance is dispatched at 0500 to a party at a local bar. The patient is a 35-year-old woman who was involved in a fight. She has a large laceration, made by a broken bottle, that extends into her eye. You control the bleeding with 5 × 9 dressings and a Kerlix wrap. The patient is awake, alert, and oriented to person, place, and time. She refuses transport. You recognize the seriousness of her wound due to its depth and involvement with her eye, and you attempt at length to persuade her to be transported. She is rude and belligerent and persistently refuses care. You decide to take her forcibly because of the seriousness of her wound. You and your partner pick her up and carry her to the ambulance, secure her with straps and soft wrist restraints, and take her to the hospital. Patients are lined up three deep in the halls in the emergency department (ED). You wait 30 minutes to give a report to a nurse, but they are all busy. Finally, because it is a busy night and you must get back into service, you give the patient care report and your verbal report to the registration clerk, along with your phone number so that the nurse can contact you with any questions. You call an acquaintance whom you know is a co-worker of this patient, because you know that the woman will need a ride home from the hospital because of her impaired vision. After you leave the ED, the patient, whom you left restrained supine, vomits and aspirates. This results in pneumonia, which requires a 2-week hospitalization.

1. Were the actions of the paramedic within his or her scope of practice?

_____

_____

_____

2. Is the paramedic protected under the Good Samaritan rules in this case? If not, why not?

_____

_____

_____

3. Is the paramedic protected by immunity statutes in this case? If not, why not?

_____

_____

_____

4. Is this a mandatory reportable situation under most state laws?

_____

_____

_____

5. Place a ✔ beside any term that may describe a legal rule the paramedic may have violated in this situation. Explain each violation.

_____ Abandonment	_____ Negligence
_____ Assault	_____ Battery
_____ False imprisonment	_____ Libel
_____ Slander	_____ Civil rights violation

CHAPTER 4 ANSWERS

REVIEW QUESTIONS

1. c. Physical force against individuals against their will and without legal justification is battery.
2. h. Making statements about a person with malicious intent is slander.
3. f. You released information about the nurse that could cause ridicule, embarrassment, or notoriety.
4. d. Forcible restraint and confinement against one's will is false imprisonment.
5. f. Making false written statements about a person with malicious intent is libel.
6. a. Failure to appropriately turn over care of the patient to a qualified individual may be considered abandonment.
   (Questions 1-6: Objectives 7, 8, 14)

7. False. If a criminal law is violated, a paramedic could be charged under that statute as well. For example, in the past, EMS personnel have been charged with manslaughter when someone died as a result of a vehicular collision involving the ambulance.
   (Objective 2)

8. True.
   (Objective 4)

9. False. The lawsuit may be filed regardless of the presence of insurance. However, the insurance may protect the paramedic's personal assets. This is controversial; some sources advise against carrying insurance.
   (Objective 6)

10. Child abuse or neglect; elder abuse or neglect; rape; animal bites; gunshot or stab wounds.
    (Objective 3)

11. Duty to act; breach of duty; damage to the patient; and proximate cause are the four elements that must be proven to win a negligence suit.
    (Objective 5)

12. Duty to act: The unit was on duty and was called to care for this patient.
    Breach of duty: The standard of care would have indicated immobilizing and transporting this patient; the crew failed to act as the standard of care dictated.
    Damage to the patient: The patient lost movement, stopped breathing, and died after being abandoned by the paramedic crew.
    Proximate cause: The patient apparently died from spinal cord damage; the paramedic crew did not immobilize and protect the cervical spine, which might have prevented death.
    (Objective 5)

13. The paramedic may reduce the risk of liability claims by obtaining appropriate training, delivering competent patient care, and ensuring thorough documentation.
    (Objective 6)

14. a. Informed
    b. Expressed
    c. Implied
    (Question 14: Objective 8)

15. You must document the following: the patient's level of consciousness (awake and alert); that you explained to the patient the risks of refusing care, including paralysis or death; that you had the patient sign a refusal form, noting any witnesses; any follow-up instructions you gave the patient; and that you told the patient to call EMS again if his condition worsened or he changed his mind.
    (Objective 9)

16. Implied consent is assumed because the patient is unconscious.
(Objective 8)

17. The absence of a heart rate (ECG) strip in several leads; the absence of respirations, pulse, and spontaneous movement; fixed and dilated pupils; and the condition of the body (specifically the wounds) should be documented. In addition, the known time that the patient was breathless and pulseless with no care before your arrival should be documented.
(Objective 11)

18. a. You should take care not to cut the clothing through the bullet hole. If the clothes are removed, you should not shake them. If removed on the scene, the clothes should be given only to the police. If removed in the ambulance, the clothes should be placed in a paper bag and given to a police officer at the hospital, if possible. b. You should not touch the weapon unless it poses a danger to your crew. c. Try not to step in the blood on the floor, if possible. d. Carefully and objectively document your findings on the scene. Note the specific location and position of both patients and the location of the weapon. Any other unusual scene findings should also be listed. e. Your ambulance should be parked away from any obvious evidence if it does not interfere with scene safety.
(Objective 12)

19. Typically you may override a family's wishes for specific cases when state protocols indicate that patients may be taken to specialty centers such as trauma centers, which are known to improve survival for specific injuries.
(Objective 10)

20. Unless you have proof that the bag contains drugs, you should note only what you specifically observed; that is, that a bag containing a white powdery substance and a syringe with a needle were found to the right of the patient.
(Objective 13)

21. a. Yes
b. No, not unless the paramedic has a legitimate medical or legal reason to know the information.
c. No. Specific department regulations about information to be released to the press should be followed.
d. Yes. Medical direction needs to know the facts of the case for quality improvement reasons.
e. No. Only hospital staff directly involved in the patient's care should be informed of the details of the case.
(Objective 7)

STUDENT SELF-ASSESSMENT

22. b. *Administrative law* refers to regulations that are developed by a government agency to provide details about the process of the law. *Criminal laws* are enacted by federal, state, or local government to protect society. *Legislative laws* are made by legislative branches of government and are determined by statutes and constitutions.
(Objective 1)

23. a. A patient who needs continuing advanced care should not be released by a paramedic to someone with lesser training.
(Objective 2)

24. d. Criminal law violations need not involve injury or criminal intent. The patient sues for damages in civil suits. A criminal law violation is based on proof that a statute has been violated.
(Objective 1)

25. d. If you have any suspicion of elder abuse or neglect, you are obligated to report it. You should remove clothing if necessary for care. Implied consent is indicated on this call.
(Objective 3)

26. c. The Ryan White Comprehensive AIDS Resources Emergency Act of 1990 (PL 101-381) describes reporting requirements for hospitals to EMS providers who have been exposed to certain communicable diseases and lists other organizational responsibilities for infectious disease reporting.
(Objective 4)

27. c. The patient suffered damage, as evidenced by the long hospitalization. This could result in loss of income if the person was employed. This was more likely a breach of duty or nonfeasance (failure to perform a required act or duty) rather than malfeasance (performing a wrongful or unlawful act). Although the potential exists that the paramedic's actions violated EMS law, the failure to provide standard of care is usually not legislated.
(Objective 5)

28. c. Privileged patient information should never be given to personnel with no legal right to know it.
(Objective 7)

29. a. *Implied consent* permits a paramedic to render lifesaving care if the patient is unable to agree because of a lack of mental competence. *Informed consent* means that the patient has been told the implications of the injury and illness, the treatment needed, and potential complications. There is no such thing as referred consent.
(Objective 8)

30. b. You should ask the patient to sign a refusal of care form; however, if he refuses to do so, document his refusal and witness it. Be sure to advise the patient about further care for his condition. If he is awake and alert now, he may legally refuse transport.
(Objective 9)

31. d. EMS agencies are typically permitted to travel moderately faster (often 10 mph) than regular traffic; however, excessive speed is hazardous. Crews should slow down or stop until they are certain that traffic has stopped and then proceed cautiously though intersections. Traffic officers' instructions should be followed. If a dispute occurs, supervising officers should be contacted immediately.
(Objective 10)

32. a. In most cases a written rather than verbal "do not resuscitate" order is required to stop resuscitation. If airway or IV access can't be established, resuscitation efforts should not be terminated in the field. In some cases specific time limits may be placed on the provision of resuscitation; these should be determined in cooperation with medical direction, and they usually are used only with very long transports.
(Objective 11)

33. d. Do not cut through the stab hole. Do not give clothing to bystanders other than authorized law enforcement personnel. Do not move the knife unless it is essential for crew safety.
(Objective 12)

34. d. The patient care report should be as detailed as possible to paint a picture of the clinical findings and the care given.
(Objective 13)

WRAP IT UP

1. The care of the patient's wound was within the scope of practice; however, the actions related to the patient's consent were not.
(Objective 2)

2. No. Good Samaritan protections do not typically extend to those on duty.
(Objective 5)

3. No. Immunity statutes typically apply only to government agencies and do not always protect individual employees of those agencies.
(Objective 5)

4. No. Most states would not consider this type of assault "reportable"; however, for the safety of the EMS crew, it is prudent to have law enforcement present on all scenes that involve a violent crime.
(Objective 3)

5. Abandonment: The paramedic crew left the patient in the care of a clerical employee, not a person of equal or higher license.
Negligence: The paramedics had a duty to act (monitor a restrained patient until relieved by a qualified person); they breached that duty (turned the patient over to the registration clerk); there was injury (pneumonia secondary to aspiration); and there was proximate cause (the plaintiff likely could prove that the injury was caused by the paramedics' restraint and abandonment of the patient).
Assault: The paramedics told the patient they would transport her against her will.
Battery: The paramedics forcibly restrained the patient against her will.
False imprisonment: The paramedics restrained the patient to the stretcher against her will.
Slander: The paramedic called the patient's co-worker to tell her of the situation.
(Objectives 4, 6, 14)

Ethics

READING ASSIGNMENT
Chapter 5, pages 72-79, in *Mosby's Paramedic Textbook,* ed. 3

OBJECTIVES
Upon completion of this chapter, the paramedic student will be able to do the following:
1. Define ethics and bioethics.
2. Distinguish between professional, legal, and moral accountability.
3. Outline strategies to use to resolve ethical conflicts.
4. Describe the role of ethical tests in resolving ethical dilemmas in health care.
5. Discuss specific prehospital ethical issues including allocation of resources, decisions surrounding resuscitation, confidentiality, and consent.
6. Identify ethical dilemmas that may occur related to care in futile situations, obligation to provide care, patient advocacy, and the paramedic's role as physician extender.

SUMMARY
- Ethics is the discipline relating to right and wrong, moral duty and obligation, moral principles and values, and moral character. Bioethics is the science of medical ethics. Morals refers to social standard or customs.
- Paramedics must meet a standard established by their level of training and regional practice. Paramedics must abide by the law when ethical conflicts occur.
- A paramedic must act in a way that is seen as morally acceptable.
- The rapid approach to ethical issues is a process. The process involves reviewing past experiences; deliberation (if possible); and performing the impartiality test, universalization test, and interpersonal justifiability test to reach an acceptable decision.
- Two concepts of ethical health care are to provide patient benefit and to do no harm.
- All resources must be allocated fairly. This is an accepted bioethical value.
- Advance directives, living wills, and other self-determination documents can help the paramedic to make decisions about the appropriateness of resuscitation in the prehospital setting.
- A health care professional is not allowed to reveal details supplied by the patient to others without the patient's consent. This is the principle of confidentiality.
- In some cases, patients refuse lifesaving care. These cases can produce legal and ethical conflicts.
- Other areas that are likely to raise ethical questions in the prehospital setting include providing care in futile situations, the paramedic's obligation to provide care, patient advocacy, and the paramedic's role as physician extender.

REVIEW QUESTIONS

Match the term in column II with its description in column I. Use each term only once.

Column I

1. _____ Working to benefit others
2. _____ The study of right, wrong, and morality
3. _____ To do no harm
4. _____ A person's ability to make rational decisions independently
5. _____ Moral duty or obligation related to medicine
6. _____ Maintaining the privacy of personal patient information

Column II

a. Autonomy
b. Beneficence
c. Bioethics
d. Confidentiality
e. Ethics
f. Nonmaleficence
g. Rationality

Questions 7 to 9 pertain to the following case study.

A fellow paramedic who is a close friend calls you and is very upset. Her daughter was involved in a vehicle collision. She is fine, but a person in the other car was injured and has been taken to the hospital. You transported the injured patient, and your friend wants to know the extent of injuries, what the patient said, and details related to the crash.

7. **a.** What should you tell your friend about the patient's injuries?

_____

b. Is your decision ethically correct with regard to the patient and your friend?

_____

Your friend's daughter has been charged with reckless driving. You believe that the patient you transported was intoxicated; in fact, he admitted to using alcohol and cocaine before the incident. Despite his serious injuries, he was laughing and making inappropriate comments.

8. Will this affect your decision about disclosing patient information? Why or why not?

_____

_____

9. Did you make your decision about this problem based on professional, legal, or moral accountability?

_____

_____

10. Think about how you would respond to each of the following situations and state whether *professional, legal,* or *moral* accountability issues would prompt your actions.

a. You are leaving the hospital after transporting a patient. You notice that your partner has picked up some towels, although you didn't use any on the patient. He says, "Oh, these are for me. I want to wash my car this afternoon."

_____

_____

b. As you depart from a scene, you hear your partner make an inappropriate racial comment about the patient.

_____

_____

c. You notice that an on-duty co-worker has an alcoholic drink while attending your annual department awards banquet.

_____

_____

d. Your partner administers a slightly different dose of pain medicine than that ordered by medical direction because he feels that the doctor was being "too conservative."

_____

_____

e. Your teenage niece is experiencing severe vomiting in her first trimester of pregnancy. It is clear that she needs IV fluids to relieve her dehydration, but she has no insurance, and you know it will cost your brother hundreds of dollars if she is seen in the emergency department. He asks whether you can get some supplies from work and come to the house to give her the fluids.

_____

_____

Question 11 pertains to the following case study:

You and your partner are caring for a 55-year-old patient who is in respiratory arrest. You have called for assistance and are told it will be 10 minutes. After intubation, the patient is stable as long as you ventilate regularly. You are preparing for transport when suddenly your partner collapses and is pulseless.

11. a. The circumstances allow you to care for only one patient or the other. Who will you choose to resuscitate? Why?

_____

_____

b. How did you reach the above decision? Try using the ethical tests in the rapid approach to emergency medical problems to see whether they would assist you in this situation.

(1) Have you experienced a similar problem in the past?

(2) Can you buy time for deliberation or to consult with others?

(3) Would you accept the action if you were in the patient's place?

(4) Would you feel comfortable having the action performed in all similar circumstances?

(5) Can you provide good reasons to justify and defend your actions to others?

12. State which of the following factors is the cause of the ethical dilemma in each of the following situations. Then give an action you could take.

Allocation of resources	Care in futile situations
Decisions regarding resuscitation	Obligation to provide care
Confidentiality	Physician extender role
Consent	

a. You request pain medicine to care for your patient's very painful single extremity injury. On-line medical direction refuses.

Cause of ethical dilemma: _____

Possible action: _____

_____

b. Your patient has a severe headache, is vomiting, and has a numb right hand. Blood pressure is 220/140 mm Hg. Despite your detailed explanations, the patient is refusing treatment or transport.

Cause of ethical dilemma: _____

Possible action: _____

_____

c. You are triaging at a mass casualty situation. You evaluate a child, the same age as yours, whose skin is warm. Bystanders say she just stopped breathing a few moments ago.

Cause of ethical dilemma: _____

Possible action: _____

_____

d. You respond to a private residence. The patient has a legally executed living will. Hysterical family members are begging you to resuscitate the patient.

Cause of ethical dilemma: _____

Possible action: _____

_____

STUDENT SELF-ASSESSMENT

13. What are the standards of honorable behavior to which paramedics are expected to conform in the EMS profession?
    a. Certifications   **c.** Laws
    b. Ethics   **d.** Morals

14. Which of the following determines moral accountability in the practice of EMS?
    a. Laws and regulations
    b. Personal beliefs and values
    c. Professional licensure
    d. Standards related to education and skills

15. During a call, you find yourself in a situation that involves an ethical dilemma. What strategy can you use to resolve the problem?
    a. Let the patient's family tell you what to do.
    b. Ask yourself which action you would prefer if you were in the patient's place.
    c. Abide by your partner's opinion in the situation.
    d. Rely on your policies and procedures for guidance.

16. Which of the ethical tests can help correct for your personal bias about a situation?
    a. Would you accept the action if you were in the patient's place?
    b. Would you feel comfortable having this action performed under similar circumstances?
    c. Can you justify and defend your actions to others?
    d. Have you experienced a similar problem in the past?

17. On a call, you are faced with an unusual situation that falls just on the fringe of your legal and professional boundaries. You decide to take action because you are able to provide clear reasons explaining and defending your actions to others. What type of ethical test have you used?
    a. Autonomy
    b. Impartiality
    c. Interpersonal justifiability
    d. Universalizability
18. Which of the following situations involves an ethical decision? The patient has a living will and is pulseless.
    a. The family asks you to abide by the living will.
    b. The patient is cold and has rigor mortis.
    c. A signature is in the wrong place on the living will document.
    d. The nursing home staff think that a living will exists but cannot locate it.
19. You are transporting a patient and her doctor from an outpatient surgery center to the hospital because a complication has occurred. The patient's respirations are very slow, and her chest is barely moving. You note the need to ventilate, but the physician strongly disagrees. If you elect to proceed, you are acting on which ethical principle?
    a. Allocation of resources
    b. Autonomy
    c. Care in futile situations
    d. Patient advocacy

WRAP IT UP

You are dispatched at 1500 to a home in a quiet residential neighborhood to "check the welfare with possible forcible entry." Out of town adult family members report that they have been unable to contact their father for a day and a half, and they are concerned for his health. On arrival you note that the man's car is in the garage. Two newspapers are in the driveway, and neighbors tell you that they haven't seen him in 2 days. You circle the home, knocking loudly and looking in windows. Through the kitchen window, you are able to see feet protruding from behind the counter. The captain elects to force a door to gain entry. Once in, you find a 79-year-old man who tells you he slipped and fell 2 days ago and is unable to get up. You examine him and are unable to find any injuries, although he appears somewhat dehydrated, his heart rate is elevated, and his clothing is soaked with urine. He is very thin, and when you check the refrigerator and cabinets, you find little food.

The patient is alert and oriented; however, he seems slow to respond, his speech is slightly slurred, and he has weakness on the left side. He tends to repeat information. He adamantly refuses to be transported. According to your protocol, you can't forcibly transport him based on the information you have provided. Repeated attempts to reach medical control are not successful. You decide to transport the patient anyway.

1. Why does this call present an ethical conflict?

_____

_____

2. Answer all the tests of ethical decision making to see how they would apply to this situation. Explain your answers.

    a. Impartiality test: Would you accept this action if you were in the patient's place?

_____

_____

    b. Universalizability test: Would you feel comfortable having this action performed in all relevantly similar circumstances?

_____

_____

c. Interpersonal justifiability test: Are you able to provide good reasons to justify and defend your actions to others?

   _____

   _____

3. Answer the following ethical questions regarding this call.
   a. What is the patient's best interest?
   b. What are the patient's rights?
   c. Does the patient understand the issues at hand?
   d. What is the paramedic's professional, legal, and moral accountability?

   a. _____

   b. _____

   c. _____

   d. _____

4. **a.** Put a ✔ beside the bioethical values you would be following if you leave the patient unattended at the scene.
   b. Put an ✗ beside the bioethical values you would be following if you arrange either for someone to come and provide temporary care for the patient or for the Division of Aging to come and evaluate him within 12 hours.

   _____ Autonomy   _____ Beneficence
   _____ Confidentiality   _____ Allocation of resources
   _____ Nonmaleficence   _____ Personal integrity

CHAPTER 5 ANSWERS

REVIEW QUESTIONS

1. b
(Objective 4)

2. e
(Objective 1)

3. f
(Objective 4)

4. a
(Objective 4)

5. c
(Objective 4)

6. d
(Objective 1)

7. a. You can disclose nothing about the patient's injuries except what is permitted by departmental policy.
b. Your feelings about whether this is ethical will be personal.

8. Your legal obligation would not change regardless of your decision.

9. Your legal obligation prevents you from disclosing information. (Questions 7 to 9: Objective 2)

10. a. Legal (theft), professional, and moral conflicts may come into play here.
b. Professional and moral conflicts may be involved as you make a decision about how to respond to this situation.
c. Legal (working/driving while under the influence), professional, and moral standards are involved in the paramedic's actions and in your response to them.
d. Professional and moral issues are involved in this situation.
e. Legal (theft of equipment), professional (actions without medical direction), and moral (allocation of resources) issues are involved in this situation.
(Objective 2)

11. The answers to each of these questions are personal. Discuss your answers with a fellow student. How do your views compare?
(Objective 3)

12. a. Physician extender role. Possible actions: Clarify and repeat request for orders. Ask for a call review/critique to discuss the issue.
b. Consent. Possible actions: Have on-line medical direction speak to the patient. Talk to the family to see if they can convince the patient. If not, provide detailed follow-up instructions and try to leave the patient in the supervised care of family or friends.
c. Allocation of resources. Possible actions: Reevaluate your resources to determine whether resuscitation should proceed. Ask for a change of assignment if possible.
d. Decisions regarding resuscitation. Possible actions: Contact medical direction. Remove the family from the area and calmly explain the wishes of their loved one.
(Objectives 3-5)

STUDENT SELF-ASSESSMENT

13. b. Certification is a professional standard. Laws are legal standards. Morals are social standards.
(Objective 1)

14. b. Laws and regulations relate to legal accountability. Professional licensure and standards relate to education. Skills relate to professional accountability.
(Objective 2)

15. b. This is known as the impartiality test.
(Objective 3)

16. b. This is known as the universalizability test.
(Objective 3)

17. a. The impartiality test can correct partiality or personal bias. The universalizability test helps eliminate moral decision difficulty. The interpersonal justifiability test requires reasons for your actions and approval from others of those reasons.
(Objective 4)

18. c. If the family concurs and the living will is legal, no ethical question exists. If the patient has obvious signs of death, no ethical dilemma exists. If the living will document cannot be produced, legally it cannot be recognized.
(Objective 5)

19. d. Allocation of resources is an issue when the patient's health care needs can't be met because of inadequate resources. Autonomy is a person's ability to make decisions. Care in futile situations arises when the care you are about to give serves no purpose.
(Objective 6)

WRAP IT UP

1. An ethical conflict exists because a disparity clearly exists between what you can legally do and what you know needs to be done for this man.
(Objective 2)

2. a. Assuming the patient is lucid, he may not accept it.
   b. This is a question each student should answer individually.
   c. Could you justify your actions? What rationale would you use? Are other options available?
   (Objective 4)

3. a. Do you have enough information to determine whether this is in the patient's best interest?
   b. An alert, oriented patient has the right to refuse care. Are other social service agencies available that you could involve that might help make the determination whether the patient is presently competent to make this decision? Can local police assist you?
   c. Did you explain and have the patient verbalize his understanding of the risks of leaving him alone?
   d. Professionally you have a responsibility to care for patients and to ensure their safety; however, you also have a responsibility to follow protocols. Legally your state law and your local protocols may state that the patient has the right to refuse. Moral questions will be answered individually. Involve medical direction to help resolve the situation on-line.
   (Objective 2)

4. a. Autonomy, possibly personal integrity
   (Objective 5)
   b. Beneficence, nonmaleficence
   (Objective 5)

PART TWO

CHAPTER 6

Review of Human Systems

READING ASSIGNMENT
Chapter 6, pages 80-149, in *Mosby's Paramedic Textbook,* ed. 3

OBJECTIVES
Upon completion of this chapter, the paramedic student will be able to do the following:
1. Discuss the importance of human anatomy as it relates to the paramedic profession.
2. Describe the anatomical position.
3. Properly interpret anatomical directional terms and body planes.
4. List the structures that compose the axial and appendicular regions of the body.
5. Define the divisions of the abdominal region.
6. List the three major body cavities.
7. Describe the contents of the three major body cavities.
8. Discuss the functions of the following cellular structures: the cytoplasmic membrane, the cytoplasm (and organelles), and the nucleus.
9. Describe the process by which human cells reproduce.
10. Differentiate and describe the following tissue types: epithelial tissue, connective tissue, muscle tissue, and nervous tissue.
11. For each of the 11 major organ systems in the human body, label a diagram of anatomical structures, list the functions of the major anatomical structures, and explain how the organs of the system interrelate to perform the specified functions of the system.
12. For the special senses, label a diagram of the anatomical structures of the special senses, list the functions of the anatomical structures of each sense, and explain how the structures of the senses interrelate to perform their specialized functions.

SUMMARY
- The paramedic must understand human anatomy fully. This understanding will help the paramedic to organize a patient assessment by body region. Knowledge of anatomy also will help the paramedic to communicate well with medical direction and other members of the health care team.
- The anatomical position refers to a patient standing erect with the palms facing the examiner.
- Directional terms are expressed in anatomical terminology. Examples of these are *up* or *down, front* or *back,* and *right* or *left*. These terms always refer to the patient, not the examiner. Internal body structure is classified into anatomical planes of the human body. These planes can be thought of as imaginary straight-line divisions.

56

- The appendicular region of the body includes the limbs, or extremities. The axial region consists of the head, neck, thorax, and abdomen.
- The abdomen usually is divided into four quadrants: upper right, lower right, upper left, and lower left.
- The three major cavities of the human body are the thoracic cavity, the abdominal cavity, and the pelvic cavity.
- The thoracic cavity contains the trachea, esophagus, thymus, heart, great vessels, lungs, and the cavities and membranes that surround them. The abdominopelvic cavity is surrounded by membranes and contains organs and blood vessels.
- The cytoplasmic membrane encloses the cytoplasm. The membrane forms the outer boundary of the cell.
- Cytoplasm lies between the cytoplasmic membrane and the nucleus. Specialized structures in the cell (organelles) are located in the cytoplasm. These organelles perform functions key to the survival of the cell. The nucleus is a large, membrane-bound organelle. It ultimately controls all other organelles in the cytoplasm.
- All human cells, with the exception of the reproductive (sex) cells, reproduce by a process known as mitosis. In this process, cells divide to multiply.
- Four main types of tissue make up the many organs of the body. These are epithelial, connective, muscle, and nervous. Epithelial tissue covers surfaces and forms structures. Connective tissue is made of cells separated from each other by intercellular material. This material is known as the extracellular matrix. Muscle tissue is contractile tissue and is responsible for movement. The nervous tissue has the ability to conduct electrical signals. These signals are known as action potentials.
- A system is a group of organs arranged to perform a more complex function than any one organ can perform alone. The eleven major organ systems in the body are the integumentary, skeletal, muscular, nervous, endocrine, circulatory, lymphatic, respiratory, digestive, urinary, and reproductive.
- The integumentary system consists of the skin and accessory structures such as hair, nails, and a variety of glands. The functions of the integumentary system include protecting the body against injury and dehydration, defense against infection, and temperature regulation.
- The skeletal system consists of bone and associated connective tissues, including cartilage, tendons, and ligaments. The skeletal system provides a rigid framework for support and protection. It also provides a system of levers on which muscles act to produce body movements.
- The three primary functions of the muscular system are movement, postural maintenance, and heat production.
- The nervous and the endocrine systems are the major regulatory and coordinating systems of the body. The nervous system rapidly sends information. It does this by means of nerve impulses conducted from one area of the body to another. The endocrine system sends information more slowly. It does this by means of chemicals secreted by ductless glands into the bloodstream.
- The heart and cardiovascular system are responsible for circulating blood throughout the body. Blood transports nutrients and oxygen to tissues. Blood carries carbon dioxide and waste products away from tissues. In addition, blood carries hormones produced in endocrine glands to their target tissues. Blood also plays a key role in temperature regulation and fluid balance. Blood also protects the body from bacteria and foreign substances.
- The lymphatic system includes lymph, lymphocytes, lymph nodes, tonsils, spleen, and thymus gland. The lymphatic system has three basic functions. The first is to help maintain fluid balance in tissues. The second is to absorb fats and other substances from the digestive tract. The third is to play a role in the immune defense system of the body.
- The organs of the respiratory system and the cardiovascular system move oxygen to cells. They move carbon dioxide from cells to where it is released into the air. The entrance to the respiratory tract begins at the nasal cavity and includes the nasopharynx, oropharynx, laryngopharynx, and larynx. Below the glottis are the structures of the lower airway and lungs. These structures include the trachea, the bronchial tree, the alveoli, and the lungs.
- The digestive system provides the body with water, electrolytes, and other nutrients used by cells. The gastrointestinal tract is an irregularly shaped tube. Associated accessory organs (mainly glands) secrete fluid into the digestive tract.
- The urinary system works with other body systems to maintain homeostasis. It does this by removing waste products from the blood. It also does this by helping to maintain a constant body fluid volume and composition. The contents of the urinary system include two kidneys, two ureters, the urinary bladder, and the urethra.
- The purpose of the male reproductive system is to make and transfer spermatozoa to the female. The purpose of the female reproductive system is to make oocytes and to receive the spermatozoa for fertilization, conception, gestation, and birth. The male reproductive system consists of the testes, epididymis, ductus deferens, urethra, seminal vesicles, prostate gland, bulbourethral glands, scrotum, and penis. The female reproductive

organs consist of the ovaries, uterine (or fallopian) tubes, uterus, vagina, external genital organs, and mammary glands.

- Senses provide the brain with information about the outside world. Four senses are recognized as special senses: smell, taste, sight, and hearing and balance.

REVIEW QUESTIONS

Match the cellular structure from column II with its definition in column I. Use each answer only once.

Column I

1. _____ Cytoplasmic "canals" that transport proteins and other substances

2. _____ Phospholipid layer that forms the outer boundary of the cell
3. _____ Organelles that contain enzymes capable of digesting proteins and lipids
4. _____ Mass of a cell that lies between the cytoplasmic membrane and nucleus

5. _____ Sacs that package materials for secretion from the cell

6. _____ Control center of the cell; contains genetic material
7. _____ Structures composed of ribonucleic acid and protein that manufacture enzymes
8. _____ Powerhouse of the cell, responsible for production of adenosine triphosphate

Column II

a. Centrioles
b. Cytoplasm
c. Cytoplasmic membrane
d. Endoplasmic reticulum
e. Golgi apparatus
f. Lysosomes
g. Mitochondria
h. Nucleus
i. Ribosomes

9. Label Fig. 6-1 with the appropriate cellular structures listed in column II of question 8.

a.

b.

c.

d.

e.

f.

g.

10. All human cells divide by the process of mitosis throughout the life of a human organism. True/False. If this is false, explain why.

_____

_____

11. Describe the anatomical position.

_____

12. Circle the appropriate directional terms in boldface in the following sentences.

    a. The wrist lies **distal/proximal** to the elbow.

    b. The right nipple is located **medial/lateral** to the sternum.

    c. The cervical spine is **superior/inferior** to the lumbar spine.

    d. The umbilicus is located on the **dorsal/ventral** surface of the body.

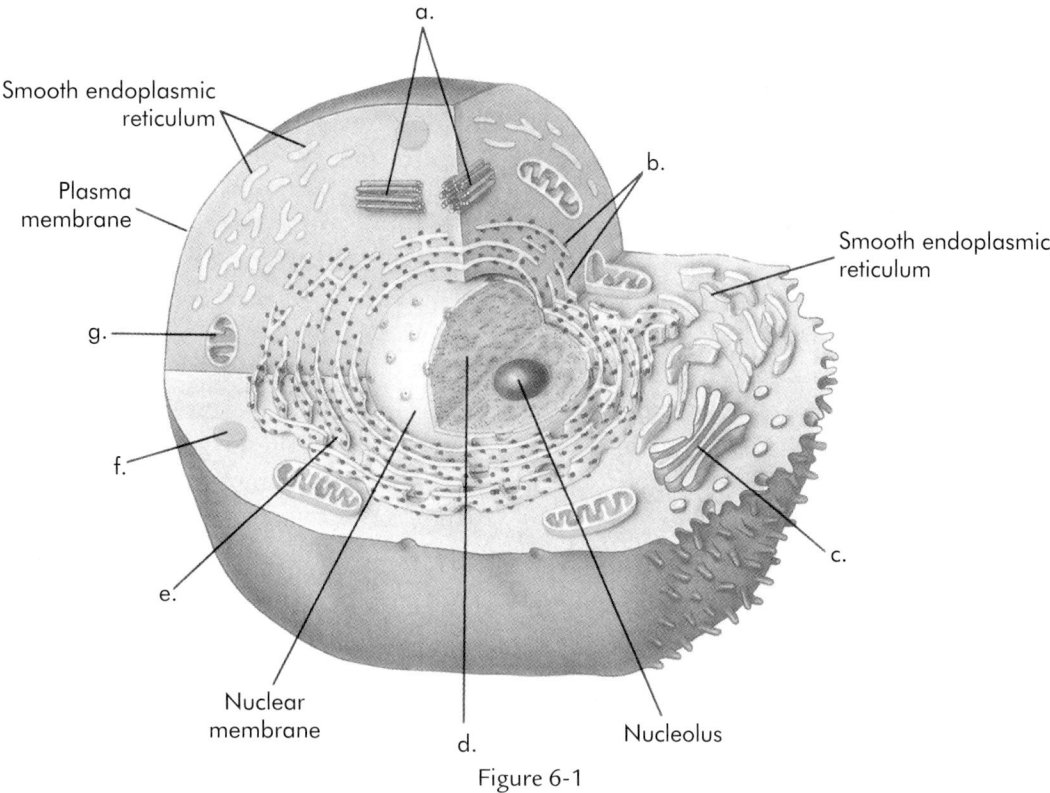

a.

Smooth endoplasmic
reticulum

Plasma
membrane

b.

Smooth endoplasmic
reticulum

g.

f.

c.

e.

Nuclear
membrane

d.

Nucleolus

Figure 6-1

13. List the structures that make up the following regions of the body.

    a. Appendicular region:

_____

    b. Axial region:

_____

14. Name the anatomical landmarks that divide the abdomen into four quadrants.

_____

Questions 15 to 19 pertain to the following case study:

    You respond to a call for a burn. You determine that the scene is safe and then approach the patient. She is lying on her right side, moaning, and has burned sites over several areas. You begin your assessment and care and roll her supine. As you carefully remove her clothing, you can better observe the burns, as shown in Fig. 6-2.

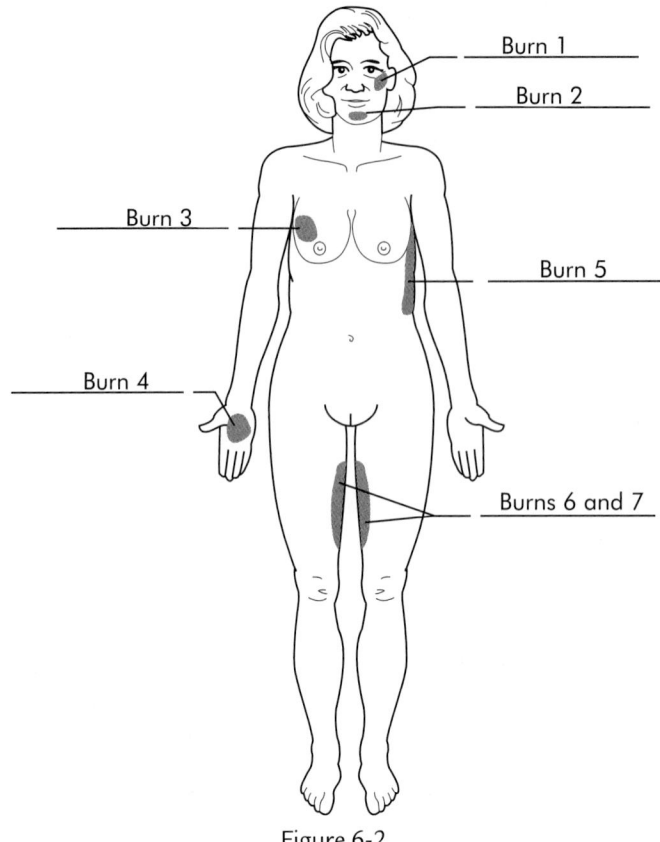

Burn 1

Burn 2

Burn 3

Burn 5

Burn 4

Burns 6 and 7

Figure 6-2

15. What directional term describes the patient's position when you arrived?

_____

16. Using appropriate directional terms, describe where

    a. Burn (1) is located relative to the left eye

_____

    b. Burn (2) is located relative to the mouth

_____

    c. Burn (3) is located relative to the nipple

_____

    d. Burn (4) lies relative to the right hand

_____

    e. Burn (5) lies relative to the axilla

_____

    f. Burns (6 and 7) are located

_____

17. Burn (5) encroaches on what abdominal quadrant?

_____

18. List the major body cavities under each wound.

    a. Burn (3)

_____

    b. Burn (5)

_____

19. Have these wounds affected the axial or appendicular regions of the body?

_____

20. For each of the following subgroups of tissues, list the tissue type (epithelial, connective, muscle, or nervous), one area of the body where it is found, and at least one specialized function it performs.

Subgroup	Type	Body Area	Function
Striated voluntary tissue			
Bone			
Epithelium			
Adipose tissue			
Hemopoietic tissue			
Striated involuntary tissue			
Neurons			
Cartilage			
Areolar tissue			
Nonstriated involuntary tissue			
Neuroglia			

21. List the 11 major body systems.

    a.

    b.

    c.

    d.

    e.

    f.

g.

h.

i.

j.

k.

22. Label the structures of the skin shown in Fig. 6-3 and list two functions of each.

	Structure	Functions
a.		
b.		
c.		

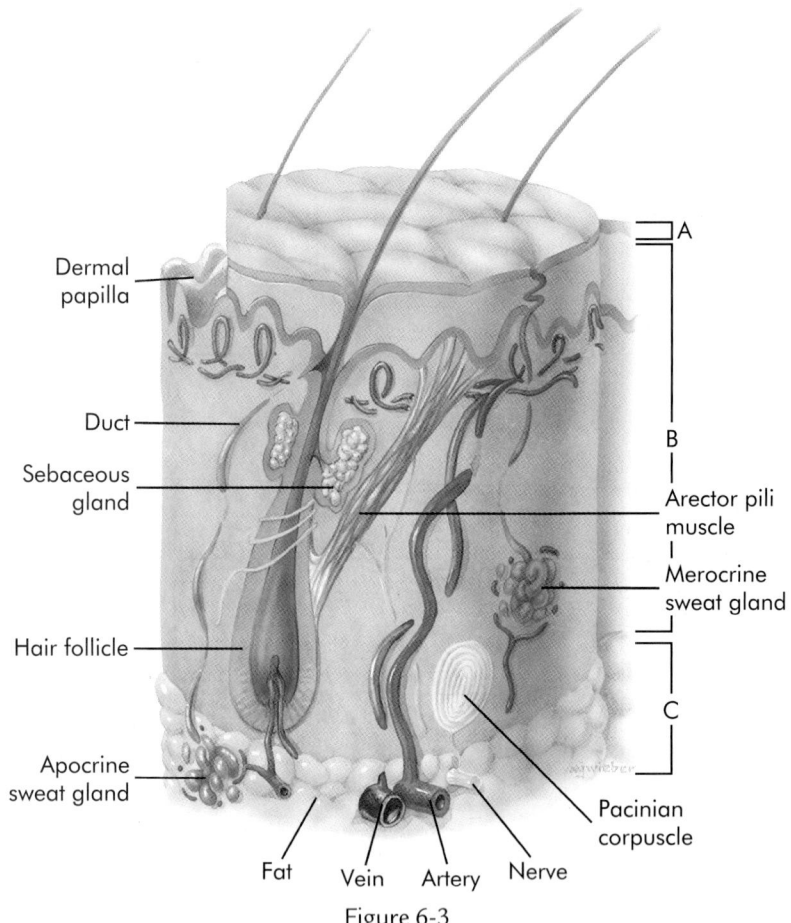

Dermal papilla

Duct

Sebaceous gland

Hair follicle

Apocrine sweat gland

Fat   Vein   Artery   Nerve

A

B

Arector pili muscle

Merocrine sweat gland

C

Pacinian corpuscle

Figure 6-3

23. List three functions of the glands located in the skin.

a.

b.

c.

24. Describe the effect on the skin's function of a large, third-degree (full-thickness) burn that destroys all the layers of the dermis.

_____

_____

25. Label the bones of the human skull shown in Fig. 6-4.

    a.

    b.

    c.

    d.

    e.

    f.

    g.

    h.

    i.

    j.

    k.

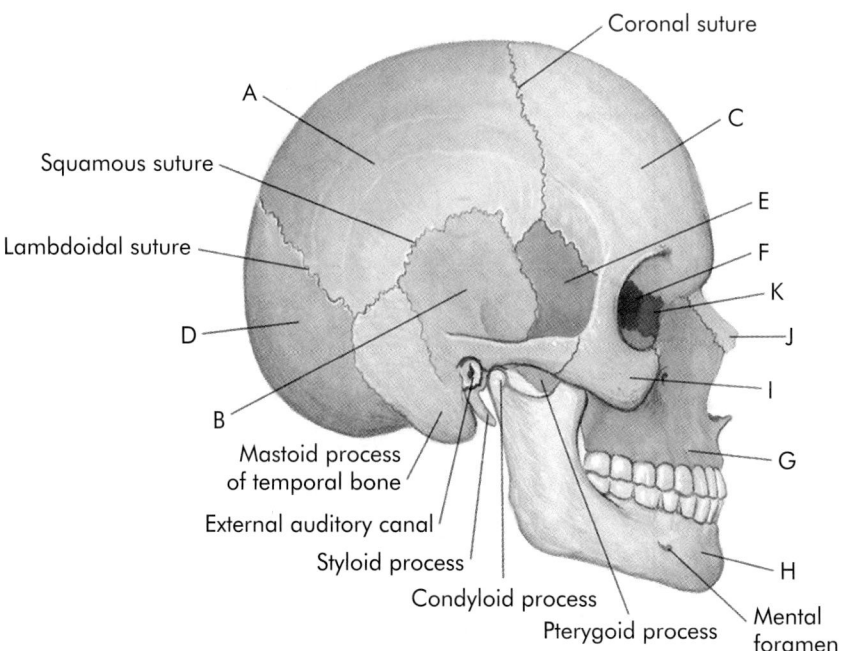

Figure 6-4

26. Label the bony regions of the vertebral column shown in Fig. 6-5 and indicate the number of vertebrae in each region.

Region	**Number of Vertebrae**
a.	
b.	
c.	
d.	
e.	

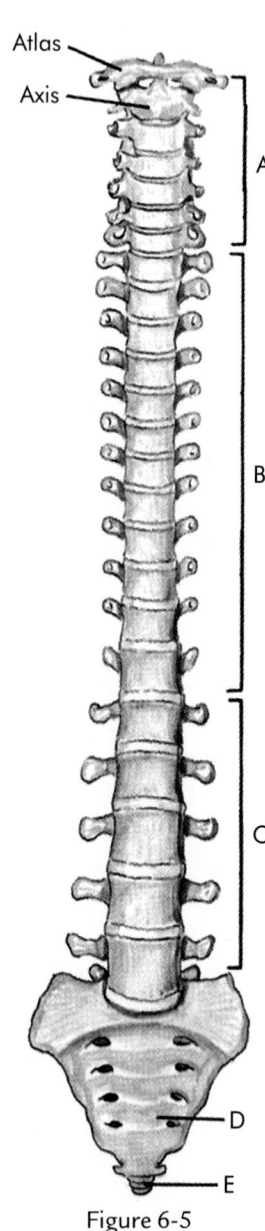

Figure 6-5

27. List two functions of the thoracic cage.

a.

b.

28. Label the structures of the thoracic cage shown in Fig. 6-6.

a.

b.

c.

d.

e.

f.

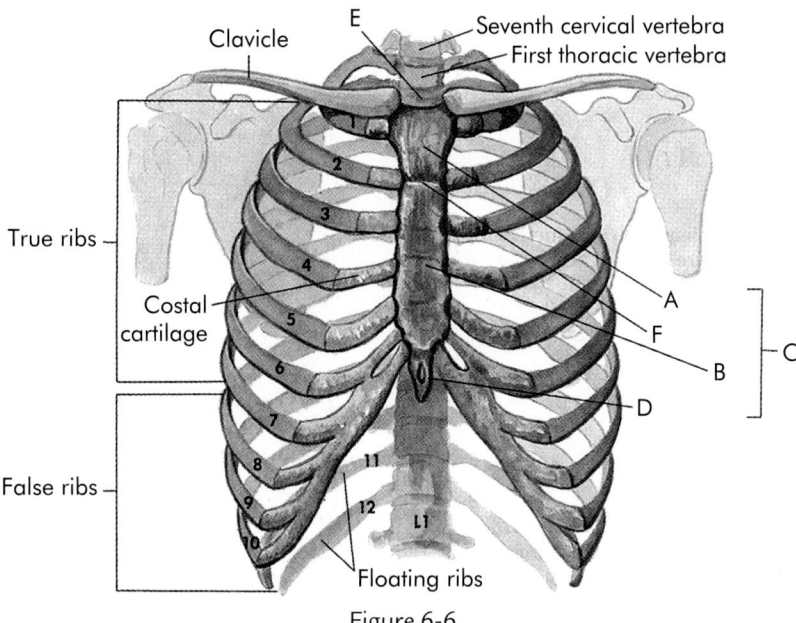

Figure 6-6

29. What problems can occur when a patient sustains a traumatic injury that results in a fractured sternum and multiple fractured ribs?

_____

30. Complete the following sentences, which relate to the skeletal system.

The pectoral girdle is composed of the **(a)** _____ and **(b)** _____. Its function

is to **(c)** _____.

The point of attachment of the appendicular and axial skeleton occurs at the **(d)** _____

_____ joint.

31. Label the diagram of the upper extremity shown in Fig. 6-7.

a.

b.

c.

d.

e.

f.

g.

h.

i.

j.

k.

l.

m.

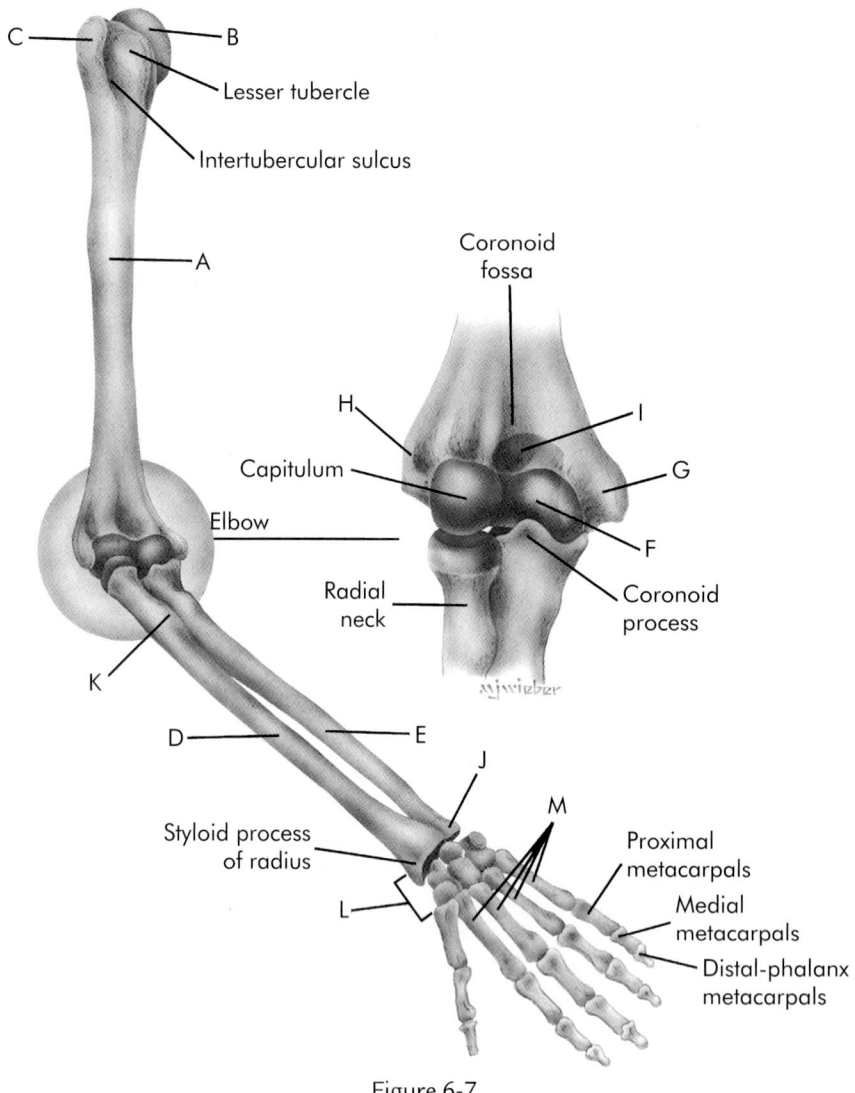

Figure 6-7

32. Label the parts of the pelvic girdle shown in Fig. 6-8.

    a.

    b.

    c.

    d.

    e.

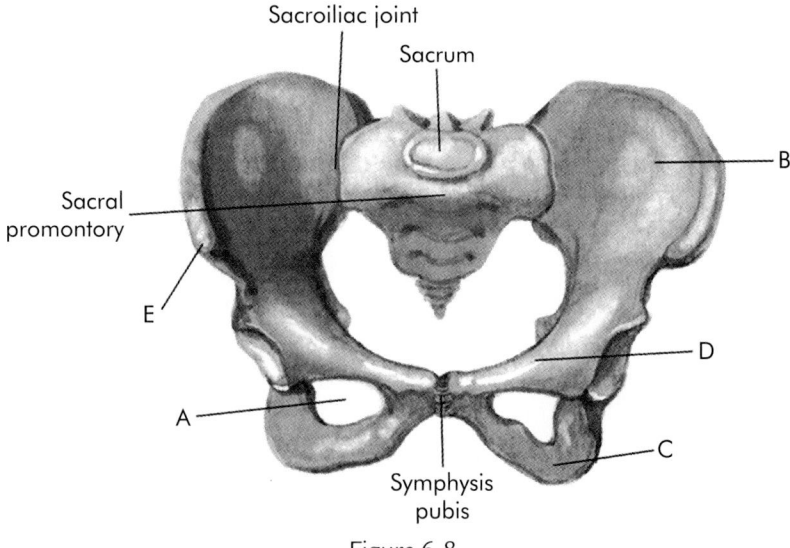

Figure 6-8

33. What are the functions of the pelvic girdle?

_____

_____

34. Label the bones of the lower extremity shown in Fig. 6-9.

    a.

    b.

    c.

    d.

    e.

    f.

    g.

    h.

    i.

    j.

    k.

    l.

m.

n.

o.

p.

q.

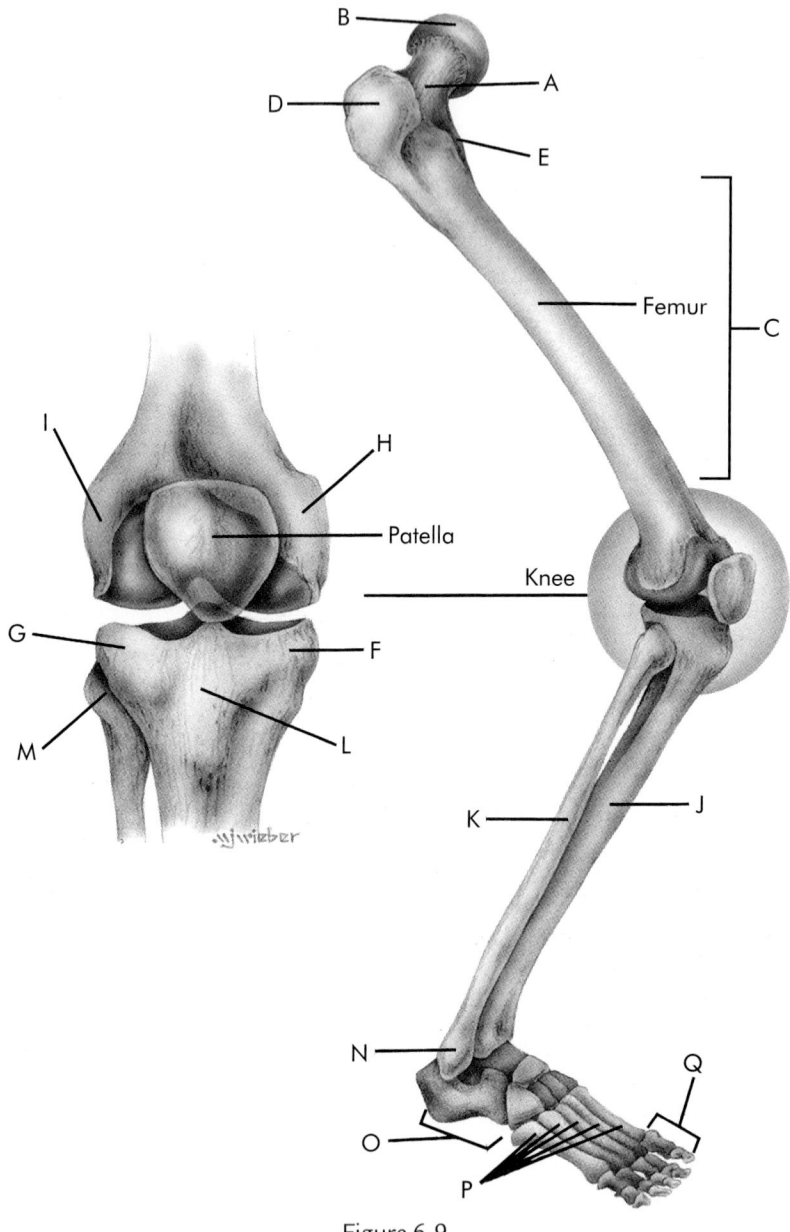

Figure 6-9

35. Complete the blanks in the following statements about joints.

The three major classifications of joints are **(a)** _____, _____, and

_____. Fibrous joints have **(b)** _____ movement. Fibrous joints can

be further divided into sutures, found in the **(c)** _____, syndesmoses found between the

(d) _____ and _____, and a gomphosis joint, which consists of a peg in

a socket, such as the joints between (e) _____ and _____. A synchondrosis is
a cartilaginous joint that allows only slight movement. One can be found in the chest between the ribs and the

(f) _____. Symphysis joints, another example of cartilaginous joints, can be found in the

chest at the (g) _____, in the pelvis at the (h) _____, and in the spine at the

(i) _____. Synovial joints are classified into six divisions, all of which contain (j) _____

_____. Joints consisting of two opposed, flat surfaces, such as the articular processes between vertebrae,

are (k) _____ joints. Joints that consist of two saddle-shaped, articulating surfaces that allow

movement in two planes (e.g., the carpometacarpal joint in the thumb) are (l) _____. Joints
that consist of a convex cylinder of bone that fits into a corresponding concavity in another bone and permit

movement in one plane, such as the elbow and knee, are known as (m) _____ joints. A cylindrical bony process that rotates within a ring composed of bone and ligament, such as the head of the radius where
it articulates with the ulna, is a(n) (n) _____ joint. A wide range of motion is permitted by
shoulder and hip joints, where the head of one bone fits into the socket of an adjacent bone. These are known as

(o) _____ joints. The atlantooccipital joint is an example of a modified

ball and socket joint known as a(n) (p) _____ joint.

36. Replace the boldface words in the following sentences with the correct terms from the following list. Use each
term only once.

Abduction	Excursion	Opposition
Adduction	Extension	Pronation
Depression	Flexion	Rotation
Eversion	Inversion	Supination

a. The patient has sustained an injury to his elbow and is unable to rotate his forearm so that the anterior surface is up or rotate his forearm so that the anterior surface is down.

_____ or

_____

b. To determine whether the patient had intact neurological function, the paramedic had **her move her
thumb and little finger toward each other.**

_____

c. After he injured his knee, the soccer player had pain when he **bent** and **stretched out** his lower leg.

_____ and

_____

d. An older woman with a hip fracture has a leg that looks shortened and shows **external movement about its
axis.**

_____

e. A person with a shoulder separation has limited ability to **move the arm from the midline.**

_____

f. A patient with a posterior hip dislocation has the following physical findings: the leg is shortened, internally rotated, and slightly **moved toward the midline.**

_____

g. Ankle sprains are frequently produced by turning the ankle **inward** or turning it **outward.**

_____   or

_____

h. Newer splints for the foot can sometimes make casting unnecessary when the desired effect is to prevent **movement from side to side.**

_____

i. The blow to the head with a baseball bat **produced movement of the temporal bone in an inferior direction.**

_____

37. List the three primary functions of the muscular system.

a.

b.

c.

38. Complete the following sentences pertaining to the muscular system.

The specialized contractile cells of the muscles are called **(a)** _____. Each muscle fiber is filled

with thick and thin threadlike structures known as **(b)** _____. These are composed of the

proteins **(c)** _____ and _____. The contractile unit of skeletal muscle fibers

is the **(d)** _____. During muscle contraction, the two myofilaments slide toward each other and

shorten the sarcomere fueled with energy from **(e)** _____.

39. Define the following terms.

a. Isometric muscle contraction:

_____

b. Isotonic muscle contraction:

_____

c. Muscle tone:

_____

40. Describe the role the muscular system plays in maintaining body temperature.

_____

_____

41. Briefly describe the function of the nervous system.

_____

_____

42. List the primary components of the following:

   a. Central nervous system:

_____

   b. Peripheral nervous system:

_____

43. List the two subdivisions of the efferent division of the nervous system and briefly describe the function of each.

   a. _____

   b. _____

44. Label the parts of the brain shown in Fig. 6-10.

   a.

   b.

   c.

   d.

   e.

   f.

   g.

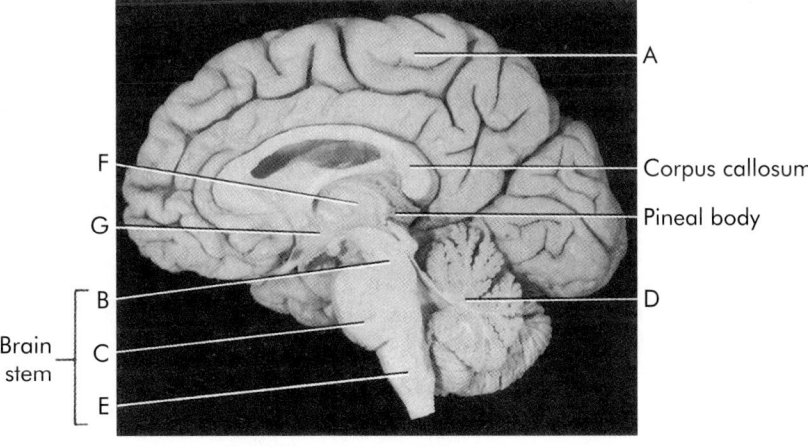

Figure 6-10

45. Briefly describe the functions of each of the following areas of the brain stem.

   a. Medulla:

_____

b. Pons:

_____

c. Midbrain:

_____

d. Reticular formation:

_____

e. Hypothalamus:

_____

f. Thalamus:

_____

46. Label the parts of the cerebrum shown in Fig. 6-11 and list one important function of each area.

Area	Function
a.	
b.	
c.	
d.	

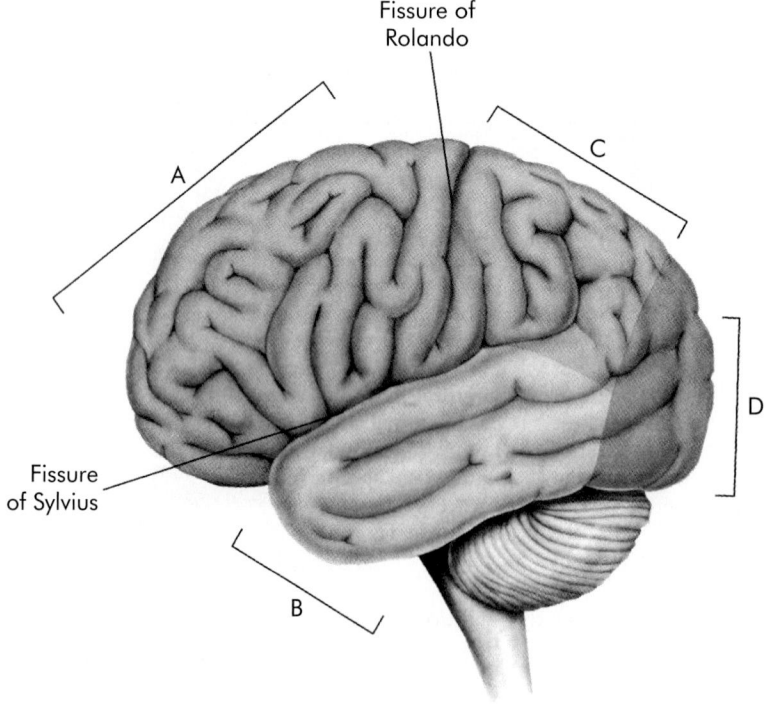

Figure 6-11

47. Briefly describe the major functions of the cerebellum.

_____

_____

48. List two functions of the spinal cord.

    a.

    b.

49. Complete the following sentences about the meninges.

Cerebrospinal fluid bathes and cushions the **(a)** _____ and _____. It is

formed in a network of brain capillaries known as the **(b)** _____.

50. List the three functional categories of the 12 cranial nerves.

    a.

    b.

    c.

51. For each of the following organs or body systems, describe the effects of stimulation by each division of the autonomic nervous system.

Affected Organ	Sympathetic	Parasympathetic
Heart		
Lungs		
Pupils		
Intestine		
Blood vessels		

52. Describe the function of the endocrine system.

_____

_____

53. For each of the following hormones, list the primary target tissue and one action the hormone may have on that tissue.

Hormone	Target	Action
Epinephrine		
Aldosterone		
Antidiuretic hormone		
Parathyroid hormone		
Calcitonin		
Insulin		
Glucagon		
Testosterone		
Thymosin		
Oxytocin		
Thyroid hormone		

54. Describe how hormones reach their target tissues.

_____

_____

55. List five functions of the circulatory system.

   a.

   b.

   c.

   d.

   e.

56. Complete the following sentences regarding the components of blood.

   About 95% of the formed elements in blood are red blood cells, also known as **(a)** _____.

   The primary component of red blood cells is **(b)** _____. This gives blood its red color and allows it

   to transport **(c)** _____ from the lungs to the tissues and to transport

(d) _____ from the tissues to the lungs. The remaining 5% of the formed elements in

blood consists of white blood cells, called **(e)** _____ and platelets, known as

(f) _____. The primary function of white blood cells is

(g) _____. Platelets help prevent blood loss by activating the formation of

(h) _____ to seal off wounds in the blood vessels. The pale yellow fluid that surrounds these

formed elements is **(i)** _____.

57. Label the structures of the heart indicated on Fig. 6-12 and draw arrows to show the path taken by the blood from the point where it enters the heart from the body until it returns to the body from the heart.

a.

b.

c.

d.

e.

f.

g.

h.

i.

j.

k.

l.

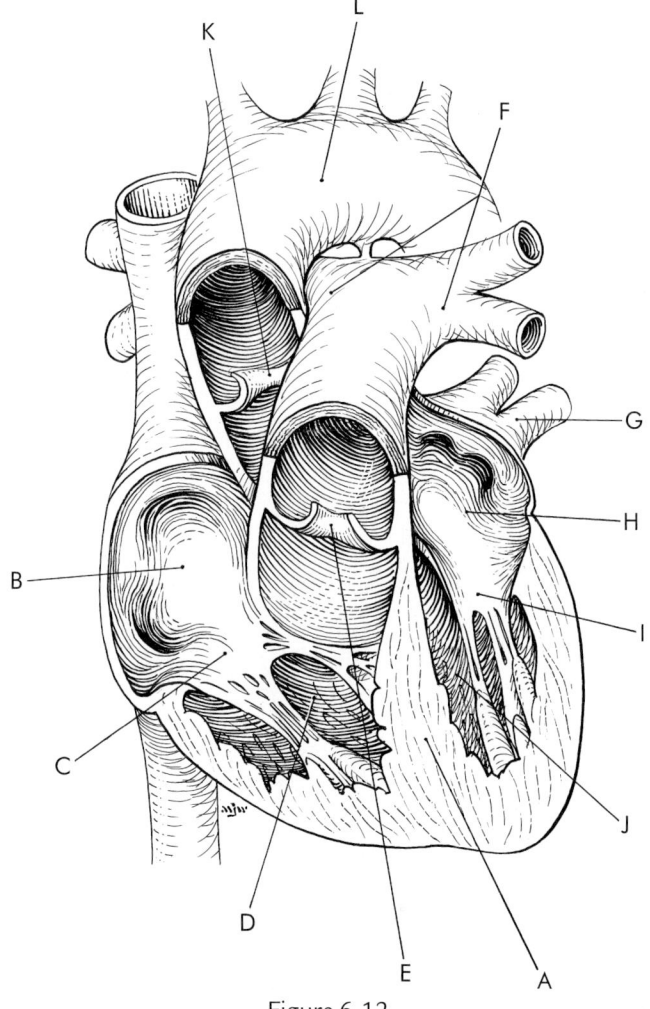

Figure 6-12

58. Name the branches of the circulatory system from the aorta to the cellular level and back to the vena cava.

_____

_____

59. Briefly describe the characteristics of blood vessels that permit vasodilation and vasoconstriction.

_____

_____

60. What structural feature of some veins inhibits the back flow of blood?

_____

61. What is the purpose of an arteriovenous anastomosis (arteriovenous shunt)?

_____

_____

62. List the three basic functions of the lymphatic system.

   a.

   b.

   c.

63. Describe the flow of lymph from its beginning in the tissues until it empties into the circulatory system.

_____

_____

_____

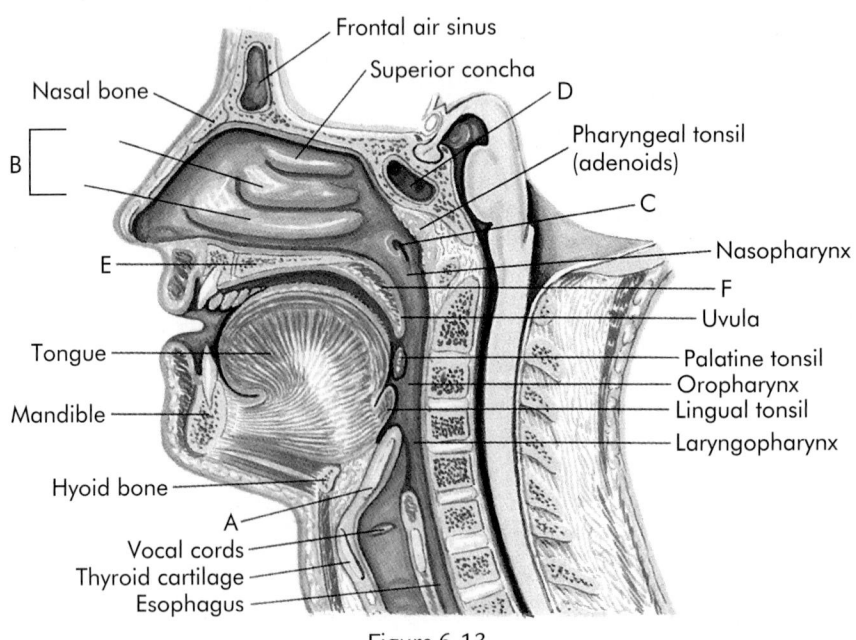

Figure 6-13

76

64. Label the parts of the upper airway shown in Fig. 6-13 and list one function of each structure.

Structure	Function
a.	
b.	
c.	
d.	
e.	
f.	

65. Label the parts of the larynx shown in Fig. 6-14.

　a.

　b.

　c.

　d.

　e.

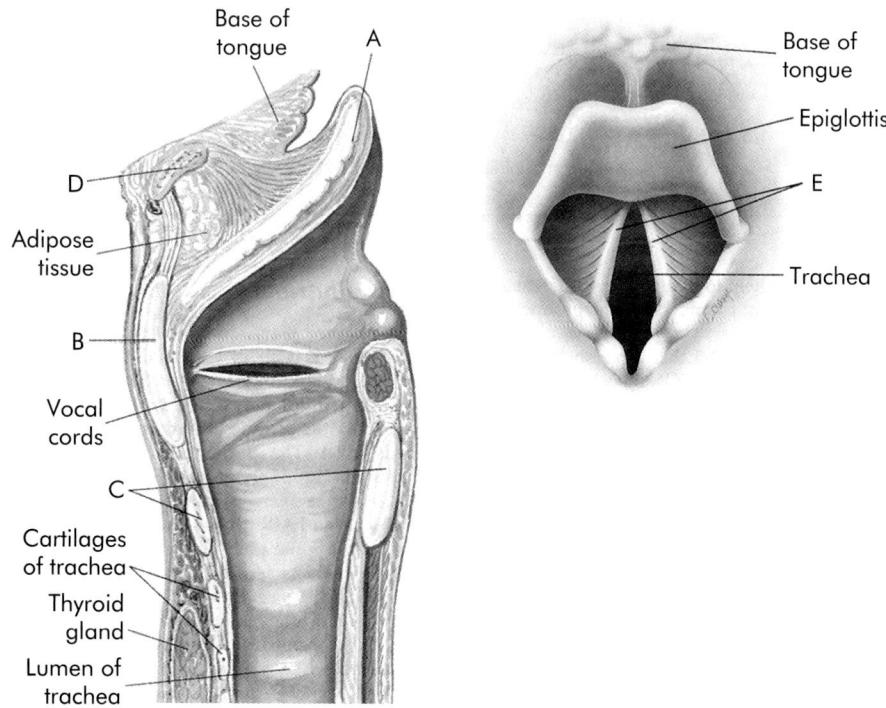

Figure 6-14

66. Label the parts of the lower airway shown in Fig. 6-15.

    a.

    b.

    c.

    d.

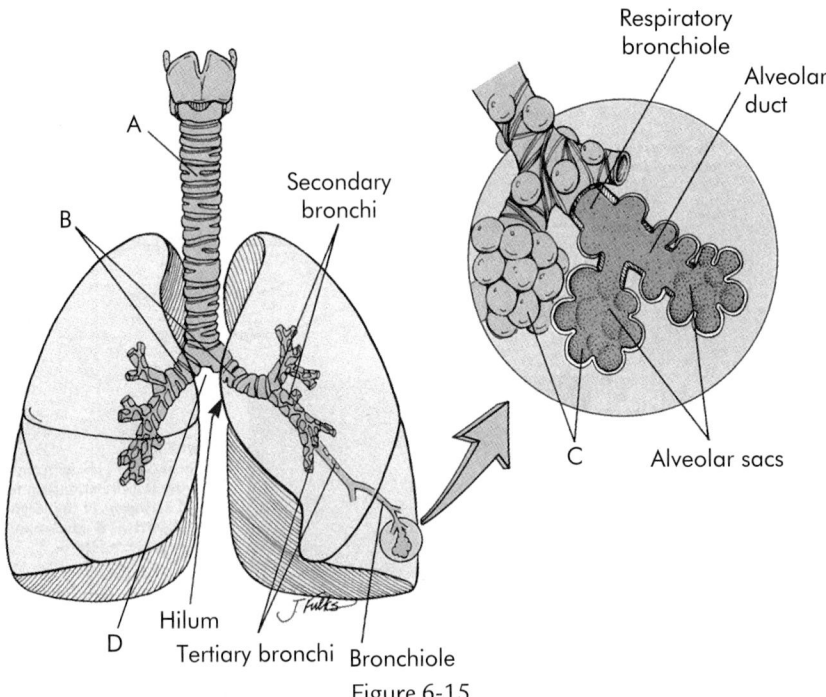

Figure 6-15

67. Describe how the structure of the trachea protects the airway.

_____

_____

68. Describe what happens to the bronchioles that causes wheezing during an asthma attack.

_____

_____

69. Describe the anatomical feature of the alveoli that performs the following functions.

    a. Permits the movement of oxygen to the blood and carbon dioxide (CO_2) from the blood:

_____

    b. Prevents collapse of the alveoli:

_____

70. Describe the location of the lungs in the chest cavity.

_____

_____

71. List the divisions of the following:

   a. Right lung:

_____

   b. Left lung:

_____

72. Describe the functions of the following:

   a. Pleural space:

_____

   b. Pleural fluid:

_____

73. List the functions of the digestive system.

_____

74. As a cheeseburger passes through the digestive tract, many digestive juices act on it to convert the food into a usable form for the body. For each area of the digestive tract listed, name a digestive juice excreted and briefly describe its function.

Area	Digestive Juice	Function
Mouth		
Stomach		
Pancreas		
Liver		
Large intestine		

75. List the functions of the urinary system.

_____

_____

76. List two specific functions of the kidneys in addition to urine production.

   a.

   b.

77. The basic functional unit of the kidney is the **(a)** _____. It produces urine by a three-step

process: **(b)** _____, **(c)** _____, and **(d)** _____.

78. State whether each of the following increases or decreases urine production.

a. Aldosterone:

b. Atrial natriuretic factor:

c. Large increase in blood pressure:

d. Shock:

79. Label the parts of the male reproductive system shown in Fig. 6-16.

a.

b.

c.

d.

e.

f.

g.

h.

i.

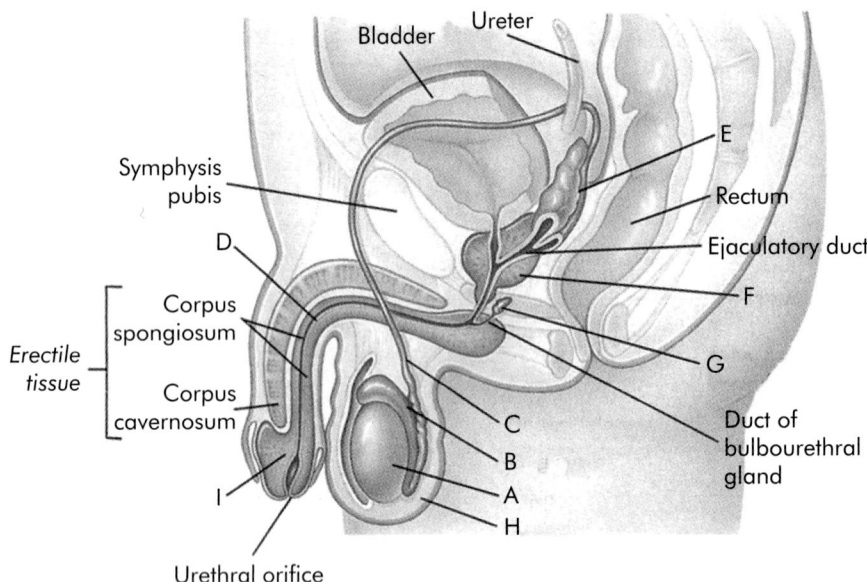

Figure 6-16

80. Label the parts of the female reproductive system shown in Fig. 6-17.

    a.

    b.

    c.

    d.

    e.

    f.

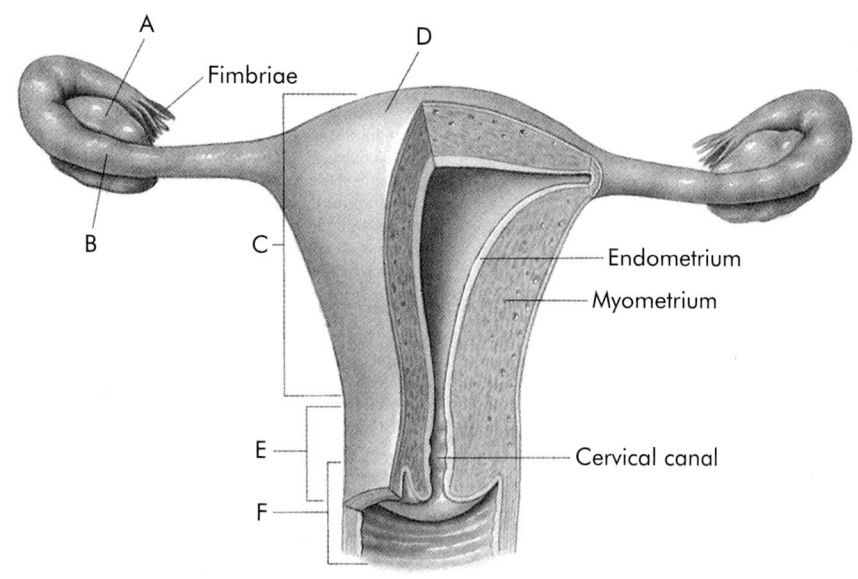

Figure 6-17

81. Label the parts of the female perineum shown in Fig. 6-18.

    a.

    b.

    c.

    d.

    e.

    f.

    g.

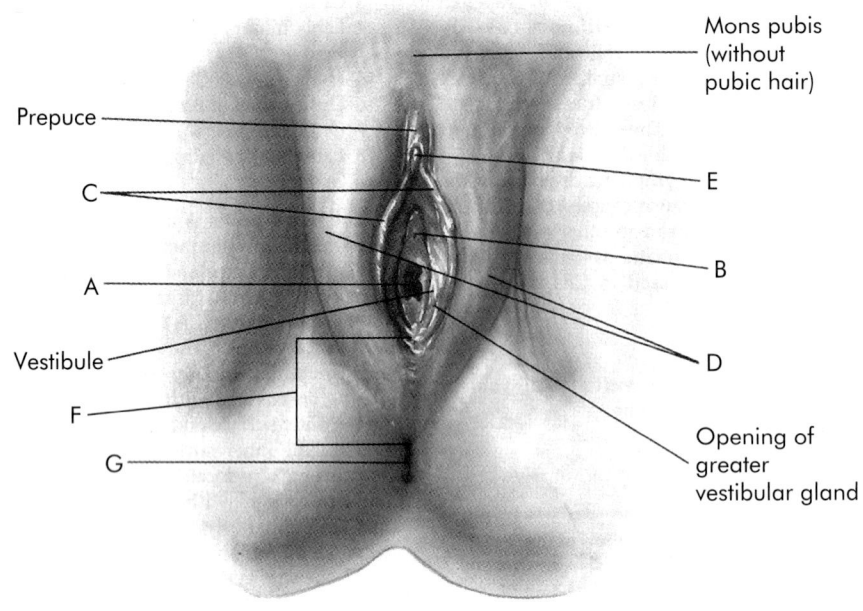

Prepuce

Mons pubis (without pubic hair)

C

E

A

B

Vestibule

D

F

Opening of greater vestibular gland

G

Figure 6-18

82. Complete the following sentences pertaining to the olfactory sense.

Receptors for the olfactory nerves lie in the upper part of the **(a)** _____ cavity. When olfactory cells

are stimulated by airborne molecules, the nerve impulses travel in the olfactory bulb and **(b)** _____.

The brain interprets the impulses as specific odors in the **(c)** _____ and **(d)** _____ centers.

83. Complete the following sentences pertaining to the sense of taste.

Sensory structures that detect taste stimuli in the mouth are **(a)** _____ _____.

Taste buds are most commonly found in the mouth on the **(b)** _____. However, they are also

found on the **(c)** _____, _____, and _____. The four basic tastes

that are detected are **(d)** _____, _____, _____, and

_____.

84. Complete the following sentences pertaining to the sense of vision.

The sensation of vision is transmitted from the eye to the brain by way of the **(a)** _____ nerve.

Impulses that travel from the brain to control the movements of the eye are relayed by the **(b)** _____

nerve. The avascular, transparent structure that bends and refracts light as it enters the eye is the **(c)** _____ .

The size of the pupil and therefore the amount of light that enters the eye through it is controlled by the

(d) _____. The inner sensory layer of the retina contains two types of photoreceptor cells. The receptors responsible for night vision are the **(e)** _____, and the receptors that permit daytime and color vision are the **(f)** _____. The eye has two compartments. The anterior chamber is filled with **(g)** _____ humor, and the posterior chamber contains **(h)** _____ humor. The humor in both chambers helps maintain **(i)** _____ _____.

85. List the function of each of the following accessory structures of the eye.

   a. Eyebrows:

_____

   b. Eyelids:

_____

   c. Lacrimal glands:

_____

86. Complete the following sentences pertaining to the tissues associated with hearing and balance.

The external and middle ear are involved in **(a)** _____, and the inner ear plays a role in **(b)** _____ and _____. The senses of hearing and balance are transmitted by the **(c)** _____ nerve. Sound is picked up by the external ear prominence, known as the **(d)** _____, and transmitted through the external auditory meatus into the **(e)** _____ canal. At the end of the canal, vibration of the **(f)** _____ _____ is produced. These vibrations are picked up and transmitted to the oval window by the auditory ossicles of the middle ear. These three bones are the **(g)** _____, _____, and _____. Finally, in the inner ear inside the cochlea lies the hearing sense organ, called the **(h)** _____. The two other structures in the inner ear involved in balance are the **(i)** _____ and **(j)** _____ _____.

STUDENT SELF-ASSESSMENT

87. You find your patient lying face up on his back. This is which position?
   a. Anatomical
   b. Lateral recumbent
   c. Prone
   d. Supine

88. A teenage football player has collapsed after a sharp blow to the left upper quadrant of the abdomen. You suspect injury to which of the following?
   a. Appendix
   b. Gallbladder
   c. Liver
   d. Spleen

89. Which of the following structures is located in the mediastinum?
    a. Diaphragm
    b. Lungs
    c. Thyroid
    d. Trachea
90. Cardiac muscle cells are which of the following?
    a. Striated voluntary
    b. Striated involuntary
    c. Nonstriated voluntary
    d. Nonstriated involuntary
91. The actual conducting cells of the nervous system are which of the following?
    a. Dendrites
    b. Neuroglia
    c. Neurons
    d. Synapses
92. Which of the following is a function of the integumentary system?
    a. Collection of lymph
    b. Movement
    c. Production of vitamin C
    d. Temperature regulation
93. The scapula and clavicle make up which of the following?
    a. Pectoral girdle
    b. Pelvic girdle
    c. Thorax
    d. Vertebral disks
94. An indoor soccer player has sustained an injury resulting in marked swelling and pain at the inner aspect of the ankle. You would describe this to an on-line physician as pain and swelling in which area?
    a. Lateral malleolus
    b. Medial malleolus
    c. Olecranon
    d. Patella
95. Muscle fiber contractions are initiated when stimulated by which of the following?
    a. Actin and myosin
    b. Motor neurons
    c. Myofilaments
    d. Sarcomeres
96. Which of the following is the primary action of the frontal lobe of the cerebral cortex?
    a. To receive and integrate visual input
    b. To evaluate olfactory and auditory input
    c. To receive and interpret sensory information
    d. To initiate voluntary motor function
97. The spinal cord ends at which vertebra?
    a. Twelfth thoracic
    b. Second lumbar
    c. Sacral
    d. Coccygeal
98. What is the innermost meningeal layer (mater), which adheres to the brain and spinal cord?
    a. Arachnoid
    b. Choroid
    c. Dura
    d. Pia
99. Which component of the endocrine system transmits information from the gland to its target body part?
    a. Enzyme
    b. Hormone
    c. Neurotransmitter
    d. Synapse
100. Which of the following is the formed element in blood that contains hemoglobin and carries oxygen?
    a. Erythrocyte
    b. Immunoglobulin
    c. Leukocyte
    d. Platelet
101. Which blood vessel (or vessels) carry blood from the heart to the systemic circulation?
    a. Aorta
    b. Pulmonary arteries
    c. Pulmonary veins
    d. Vena cava
102. Cardiac electrical impulse conduction is normally initiated in which of the following structures?
    a. Atrioventricular node
    b. Bundle of His
    c. Purkinje fibers
    d. Sinoatrial node
103. Lymph nodes filter foreign substances and are located in all the body regions listed below except which?
    a. Axillary
    b. Cervical
    c. Inguinal
    d. Temporal
104. Which of the following is the airway division that is involved in the production of speech and that serves as a protective sphincter to prevent liquids and solids from entering the lungs?
    a. Larynx
    b. Retropharynx
    c. Pharynx
    d. Trachea

105. The functional unit of the respiratory system where gas exchange occurs between the lungs and the blood is which of the following?
    a. Alveolus
    b. Bronchus
    c. Capillary
    d. Trachea
106. The major site of nutrient absorption in the intestines is which of the following?
    a. Colon
    b. Duodenum
    c. Ileum
    d. Jejunum
107. Liver function includes all the following actions except:
    a. Bile production
    b. Drug detoxification
    c. Hormone secretion
    d. Plasma protein synthesis
108. Which of the following statements is true with regard to renal function?
    a. All fluid filtered from the glomerulus becomes urine.
    b. Healthy people produce 180 L of urine per day.
    c. Water and other nutrients are reabsorbed in the tubules.
    d. Potassium and ammonia are secreted into the blood.
109. Which of the following hormones influences urine production?
    a. Aldosterone
    b. Glucagon
    c. Oxytocin
    d. Testosterone
110. Where does sperm production occur?
    a. Epididymis
    b. Prostate
    c. Seminal vesicle
    d. Testes
111. When the nasal receptors of the olfactory neurons are stimulated, messages are sent for interpretation to the olfactory and_____centers of the brain.
    a. Frontal
    b. Medullary
    c. Pontine
    d. Thalamic
112. The hearing sense organ is which of the following?
    a. Cochlea
    b. Organ of Corti
    c. Semicircular canal
    d. Vestibule

WRAP IT UP

You are dispatched to a rural emergency department to transfer a patient to the regional trauma center. The nurse gives you the following patient report: The 27-year-old female was thrown off her all-terrain vehicle (ATV) and struck a tree. She is lying on her back in full spinal immobilization. She has a laceration on her forehead above her right eyebrow; a fracture of her right forearm; a fracture in her right upper thigh; a pelvic fracture; several rib fractures on the left anterior side of her chest; and possible internal abdominal injuries. The nurse also tells you that the patent's erythrocyte count is low; her urine output is 10 mL/hour, which is draining through the urinary catheter; she has a nasogastric tube because she vomited earlier; and she is receiving high-concentration oxygen because her oxygen saturation level dropped and she was dyspneic. The woman is conscious but slightly confused and can't feel anything below her umbilicus. She is unable to move below her waist but can bend and straighten her arms.

1. Fill in the appropriate anatomical terms to describe this patient.

She is lying **(a)** _____ on the long spine board. Her laceration is **(b)** _____to her

eyebrow. Her forearm fracture is **(c)** _____ to her elbow and could be in one of two long bones,

the **(d)** _____ or _____. The fracture in her upper thigh is in the

(e)_____, and the bones of the pelvis that could be fractured are the **(f)** _____,

_____, _____, or _____.

2. What structures underlie the fractured ribs that could also be injured?

_____

3. List the abdominal organs that could be involved if the patient's injuries are in the following places.

    a. Upper right quadrant: _____

    b. Upper left quadrant:_____

    c. Lower right quadrant:_____

    d. Lower left quadrant: _____

4. What region of the brain lies under her facial injury? _____

5. a. What are erythrocytes?

_____

    b. What is the significance of a low erythrocyte count?

_____

6. The loss of sensation below her umbilicus signals likely injury to what level of the spinal cord?

_____

7. a. Is she producing too much, too little, or a normal amount of urine?

_____

    b. What could cause a change in urine output?

_____

_____

8. The urinary catheter passes through what anatomical structures?

_____

9. What medical terms could you substitute for "can bend and straighten her arms"?

_____

10. Put a ✔ beside the body systems that are affected in some way by this patient's condition (either directly or by the body's compensatory mechanisms).

    _____Integumentary system   _____Skeletal system
    _____Muscular system   _____Nervous system
    _____Endocrine system   _____Circulatory system
    _____Lymphatic system   _____Digestive system
    _____Urinary system   _____Reproductive system
    _____Respiratory system

REVIEW QUESTIONS

1. d
2. c
3. f
4. b
5. e
6. h
7. i
8. g
   (Questions 1-8: Objective 8)

9. a. centrioles; b. ribosomes; c. Golgi apparatus; d. nucleus; e. endoplasmic reticulum; f. lysosome; g. mito-chondrion
   (Objective 8)

10. False. Some cells, such as those of the nervous system, divide only until birth.
    (Objective 9)

11. The person is standing erect with palms and feet facing the examiner.
    (Objective 2)

12. a. Distal; b. lateral; c. superior; d. ventral
    (Objective 3)

13. a. Extremities and their girdles; b. head, neck, thorax, and abdomen
    (Objective 4)

14. Horizontally through the umbilicus and vertically from the xiphoid process through the symphysis pubis
    (Objective 5)

15. You initially found the patient in the right lateral recumbent position.
    (Objective 3)

16. a. Burn (1) is inferior and lateral to the left eye.
    b. Burn (2) is inferior to the mouth.
    c. Burn (3) is superior and lateral to the right nipple.
    d. Burn (4) is on the ventral aspect (or palmar surface) of the hand.
    e. Burn (5) is inferior to the axilla.
    f. Burns (6) and (7) are on the medial aspect of both thighs.

17. Burn (5) encroaches on the left upper quadrant of the abdomen.
    (Objective 5)

18. a. Burn (3) overlies the thoracic cavity.
    b. Burn (5) overlies the thoracic and abdominal cavities.

19. The wounds affect both the axial and appendicular regions of the body.
    (Objective 4)

20. Conduction of action potentials

Subgroup	Type	Body Area	Function
Striated voluntary tissue	Muscle	Skeletal muscle	Movement of bones
Bone	Connective	Bones of body	Support and protection
Epithelium	Epithelial	Skin, glands	Protection, lining of body cavities
Adipose tissue	Connective	Subcutaneous tissue	Insulation, protection, storage of energy
Hemopoietic tissue	Connective	Marrow cavities, spleen, tonsils	Formation of blood and lymph cells
Striated involuntary tissue	Muscle	Cardiac muscle	Contraction of the heart
Neurons	Nervous	Nervous system	Conduction of action potentials
Cartilage	Connective	Articulating surface	Smooth movement of bones; ear, nose
Areolar tissue	Connective	Around organs, under skin	Cushioning and affixing
Nonstriated involuntary tissue	Muscle	Smooth muscle of viscera	Vegetative muscle functions
Neuroglia	Nervous	Nervous system	Support cells, nourishment, protection, insulation

(Objective 10)

21. Integumentary, skeletal, muscular, nervous, endocrine, circulatory, lymphatic, respiratory, digestive, urinary, and reproductive
(Objective 11)

22. a. Epidermis: barrier against infection, protection, prevention of fluid loss
b. Dermis: sense organ, contains sweat glands
c. Subcutaneous layer: insulation, storage of energy, shock layer, absorption
(Objective 11)

23. Lubrication to prevent drying, excretion of water and wastes, and temperature regulation
(Objective 11)

24. Decreased ability to perceive pain, decreased ability to regulate temperature, and decreased ability to preserve body fluids
(Objective 11)

25. a. Parietal; b. temporal; c. frontal; d. occipital; e. sphenoid; f. ethmoid; g. maxilla; h. mandible; i. zygomatic; j. nasal; k. lacrimal
(Objective 11)

26. a. Cervical spine (7); b. thoracic spine (12); c. lumbar spine (5); d. sacrum (1 fused); e. coccyx (1 fused)
(Objective 11)

27. Protection for the organs of the thorax (and some abdominal organs) and maintenance of lung inflation
(Objective 11)

28. a. Manubrium; b. body; c. sternum; d. xiphoid process; e. jugular notch; f. sternal angle
(Objective 11)

29. Injury to underlying organs, impaired ventilation, and blood loss
(Objective 11)

30. a. Scapula; b. clavicle; c. attach the upper extremity to the axial skeleton; d. sternoclavicular joint
(Objective 11)

31. a. Humerus; b. head; c. greater tubercle; d. radius; e. ulna; f. trochlea; g. medial epicondyle; h. lateral epicondyle; i. olecranon; j. styloid process; k. radial tuberosity; l. carpals; m. metacarpals
(Objective 11)

32. a. Obturator foramen; b. ilium; c. ischium; d. pubis; e. anterior superior iliac spine
(Objective 11)

33. Protection of the pelvic organs and point of attachment for the lower extremity to the axial skeleton
(Objective 11)

34. a. Neck; b. head; c. shaft; d. greater trochanter; e. lesser trochanter; f. medial condyle; g. lateral condyle; h. medial epicondyle; i. lateral epicondyle; j. tibia; k. fibula; l. tibial tuberosity; m. head of fibula; n. lateral malleolus; o. tarsal bones; p. metatarsals; q. phalanges
(Objective 11)

35. a. Fibrous, cartilaginous, synovial; b. little or no; c. skull; d. radius, ulna; e. teeth, mandible (or maxilla); f. sternum; g. sternal angle; h. symphysis pubis; i. intervertebral disks; j. synovial fluid; k. plane (or gliding); l. saddle joints; m. hinge; n. pivot; o. ball and socket; p. ellipsoid
(Objective 11)

36. a. Supinate (supination) or pronate (pronation); b. opposition; c. flexion and extension; d. rotation; e. abduction; f. adduction; g. inversion or eversion; h. excursion; i. depression
(Objective 11)

37. Movement, muscle tone, and heat production
(Objective 11)

38. a. Muscle fibers; b. myofilaments; c. actin, myosin; d. sarcomere; e. adenosine triphosphate (ATP)
(Objective 11)

39. a. Isometric muscle contraction maintains constant length of the muscles in the body. b. During an isotonic contraction, the amount of muscle tension is constant, but the length of the muscle changes, causing movement of a body part. c. Muscle tone is the constant tension of muscles responsible for posture and balance.
(Objective 11)

40. Excess energy from adenosine triphosphate in a muscle contraction is released as heat. If the body temperature falls below a certain level, muscles begin shivering, which can increase heat production up to 18 times the normal resting level.
(Objective 11)

41. Regulation and coordination of the body to maintain homeostasis
(Objective 11)

42. a. Brain and spinal cord; b. nerves and ganglia
(Objective 11)

43. The somatic division transmits impulses from the central nervous system to skeletal muscle. The autonomic division transmits impulses from the central nervous system to smooth muscle, cardiac muscle, and certain glands.
(Objective 11)

44. a. Cerebral cortex; b. midbrain; c. pons; d. cerebellum; e. medulla; f. thalamus; g. hypothalamus
(Objective 11)

45. a. Serves as conduction pathway for ascending and descending nerve tracts and regulates heart rate, blood vessel diameter, breathing, swallowing, vomiting, coughing, and sneezing. b. Ascending and descending nerve tracts pass through and relay information from cerebrum to cerebellum and sleep and respiratory center. c. Involved in hearing and visual reflexes, regulates some automatic functions, such as muscle tone. d. Important for arousal and consciousness, sleep/wake cycle. e. Temperature regulation, water balance, sleep cycle control, appetite, sexual arousal. f. Relays information from sense organs to cerebral cortex, influences mood.
(Objective 11)

46. a. Frontal lobe: voluntary motor function, motivation, aggression, and mood. b. Temporal lobe: olfactory and auditory input, memory. c. Parietal lobe: reception and evaluation of sensory information (except smell, hearing, and vision). d. Occipital lobe: reception and integration of visual input.
(Objective 11)

47. Coordination, balance, and smooth, flowing movement
(Objective 11)

48. Reflex center; also transmits impulses to and from the brain and the rest of the body
(Objective 11)

49. a. Brain, spinal cord; b. choroid plexus
(Objective 11)

50. Sensory, somatomotor and proprioception, and parasympathetic
(Objective 11)

51. Affected

Affected Organ	Sympathetic	Parasympathetic
Heart	Increased rate, contractility	Decreased rate and electrical activity contractility conduction speed
Lungs	Bronchodilation	Bronchoconstriction
Pupils	Dilation	Constriction
Intestine	Decreased peristalsis	Increased peristalsis
Blood vessels	Constriction	No effect

(Objective 11)

52. Coordinates with the nervous system to regulate and control multiple body functions, including metabolic activities and body chemistry
(Objective 11)

53.

Hormone	Target Tissue	Action
Epinephrine	Heart, blood vessels, liver, lungs	Increases heart rate, contractility, blood flow to heart, and release of glucose and fatty acids into blood Bronchodilation
Aldosterone	Kidneys	Regulates water and electrolyte balance
Antidiuretic hormone	Kidneys	Stimulates water retention by kidneys
Parathyroid hormone	Bone, kidney	Increases bone breakdown, helps maintain blood calcium levels
Calcitonin	Bone	Decreases breakdown of bone; maintains blood calcium levels
Insulin	Liver	Promotes glucose entry into cells
Glucagon	Liver	Increases blood glucose by glycogenolysis
Testosterone	Most cells	Produces male sex characteristics, behavior, spermatogenesis
Thymosin	Immune tissues	Promotes development of immune system
Oxytocin	Uterus, mammary gland	Causes uterine contractions, milk expulsion from breasts
Thyroid hormone	Most cells	Increases metabolic rate

(Objective 11)

54. Hormones are secreted into blood and travel to all tissues of the body but act only on the target tissues.
(Objective 11)

55. Transports nutrients, carries hormones, transports wastes, regulates temperature and fluid balance, and provides protection from bacteria
(Objective 11)

56. a. erythrocytes; b. hemoglobin; c. oxygen; d. carbon dioxide; e. leukocytes; f. thrombocytes; g. defense; h. clots; i. plasma
(Objective 11)

57. a. septum; b. right atrium; c. tricuspid valve; d. right ventricle; e. pulmonic valve; f. pulmonary arteries; g. pulmonary veins; h. left atrium; i. mitral or bicuspid valve; j. left ventricle; k. aortic valve; l. aorta
(Objective 11)

58. Aorta, smaller arteries, arterioles, capillaries, venules, veins, venae cavae, and right atrium
(Objective 11)

59. Blood vessels have smooth muscle walls; this allows them to dilate (increasing their diameter) or constrict (decreasing their diameter). This allows blood flow to be directed away from less vital organs to the heart and brain during emergencies.
(Objective 11)

60. Many veins, especially in the lower extremities, have valves that prevent the back flow of blood in this low-pressure system.
(Objective 11)

61. The arteriovenous shunt can selectively allow blood to bypass the capillaries. This is useful to help maintain body temperature.
(Objective 11)

62. Maintains tissue fluid balance, absorbs fats and other substances from the digestive tract, and enhances the body's defense system.
(Objective 11)

63. Lymph is gathered from the tissues by lymph capillaries that have one-way valves to prevent the back flow of lymph into tissues. It flows to larger lymph capillaries that resemble veins. Then it passes through the lymph nodes (in the groin, axilla, and neck), where microorganisms and foreign substances are removed. The lymph vessels meet to enter the right or left subclavian vein, where the lymph reenters the blood.
(Objective 11)

64. a. Epiglottis: protection of lower airway; b. conchae and turbinates: warming and filtering of air; c. eustachian and auditory tube: joining of nasopharynx to ear; d. sinuses: production of sound and mucus; e. hard palate: separation of oropharynx from sinuses; f. soft palate: prevents food from entering nasal cavities.
(Objective 11)

65. a. Epiglottis; b. thyroid cartilage (or Adam's apple); c. cricoid cartilage; d. hyoid bone; e. vocal folds
(Objective 11)

66. a. Trachea; b. bronchi; c. alveoli; d. carina
(Objective 11)

67. Cartilage rings maintain patency of the airway. Goblet cells in the ciliated epithelium of the trachea sweep mucus, bacteria, and other small particles toward the larynx.
(Objective 11)

68. The small bronchioles are surrounded by smooth muscle. Irritants cause constriction of that muscle, the airway size decreases, and a wheeze is produced as air is forced through a very tight airway.
(Objective 11)

69. a. Alveoli are only one cell thick, allowing gases to diffuse easily from within them into the pulmonary capillaries. b. Pulmonary surfactant reduces surface tension in the alveoli, which inhibits collapse of the alveoli.
(Objective 11)

70. The bases of the lungs rest on the diaphragm; the apex extends to a point 2.5 cm superior to the clavicles.
(Objective 11)

71. a. Three lobes, which are further divided into 10 lobules; b. Two lobes, which are further divided into nine lobules
(Objective 11)

72. a. A potential space that forms a vacuum and causes the lung to adhere to the chest wall and remain expanded; b. a lubricant that allows the pleural membranes to slide across one another and that helps the visceral and parietal pleurae to adhere to one another.
(Objective 11)

73. Provides the body with water, nutrients, and electrolytes
(Objective 11)

74.

Area	Digestive Juice	Function
Mouth	Salivary amylase	Begins digestion of carbohydrates
Stomach	Hydrochloric acid, mucus	Produces chyme (intrinsic factor, gastrin, semisolid mixture), pepsinogen
Pancreas	Amylase, sodium bicarbonate	Neutralizes stomach acid, continues digestion
Liver	Bile	Dilutes stomach acid, emulsifies fat
Large intestine	Mucus	Aids movement of feces

(Objective 11)

75. Removes wastes from the body and helps maintain normal body fluid volume and composition
(Objective 11)

76. Control of red blood cell production and vitamin D metabolism
(Objective 11)

77. a. Nephron; b. filtration; c. reabsorption; d. secretion
(Objective 11)

78. a. Decreases; b. increases; c. increases; d. decreases
(Objective 11)

79. a. Testis; b. epididymis; c. ductus deferens and vas deferens; d. urethra; e. seminal vesicles; f. prostate gland; g. bulbourethral glands; h. scrotum; i. penis
(Objective 11)

80. a. Ovary; b. fallopian tube; c. uterine body; d. fundus; e. cervix; f. vagina
(Objective 11)

81. a. Vagina; b. urethra; c. labia minora; d. labia majora; e. clitoris; f. clinical perineum; g. anus
(Objective 11)

82. a. Nasal; b. olfactory tract; c. thalamic; d. olfactory
(Objective 12)

83. a. Taste buds; b. tongue; c. palate, lips, throat; d. sweet, sour, bitter, salt
(Objective 12)

84. a. Optic; b. oculomotor; c. cornea; d. iris; e. rods; f. cones; g. aqueous; h. vitreous; i. intraocular pressure
(Objective 12)

85. a. Shade eyes from direct sun and prevent perspiration from entering eyes; b. protect against foreign objects; c. moisten the eye, lubricate the eyelids, and wash away foreign objects
(Objective 12)

86. a. Hearing; b. hearing, balance; c. vestibulocochlear; d. pinna; e. auditory; f. tympanic membrane; g. incus, stapes, malleus; h. organ of Corti; i. vestibule; j. semicircular canals
(Objective 12)

STUDENT SELF-ASSESSMENT

87. d. The anatomical position is standing erect with palms forward. A person lying in the lateral recumbent position is reclining on the right or left side. The prone position refers to a patient who is lying on the stomach.
(Objective 2)

88. d. The liver and gallbladder are located in the right upper quadrant, and the appendix is in the right lower quadrant.
(Objective 5)

89. d. The lungs are found in the thoracic cavity, and the diaphragm separates the thoracic cavity from the abdominal cavity. The thyroid gland is found in the neck.
(Objective 7)

90. b. Striated voluntary muscle is skeletal muscle, and nonstriated involuntary muscles are found in the viscera. Nonstriated muscles are always involuntary.
(Objective 10)

91. c. A *dendrite* is a component of the neuron. *Neuroglia* are types of nerve cells that support the cells in the nervous system. *Synapses* are the gaps or spaces between nerve cells or effector tissues.
(Objective 10)

92. d. Lymph is collected by the lymphatic system and drains into the circulatory system. Movement is a function of the musculoskeletal system. Vitamin C is ingested by food sources. A form of vitamin D is produced in the skin when exposed to light.
(Objective 11)

93. a.
(Objective 4)

94. b. The lateral malleolus is on the outside of the ankle, the olecranon is at the elbow, and the patella is over the knee.
(Objective 3)

95. b. *Actin* and *myosin* are the actual myofilaments (thin, threadlike structures) that pull together to cause movement. A *sarcomere* is the contractile unit that contains actin and myosin.
(Objective 10)

96. d. The other actions described are attributed to the occipital lobe (a), temporal lobe (b), and parietal lobe (c).
(Objective 11)

97. b
(Objective 11)

98. d. The layers, from innermost to outermost, are the pia, arachnoid, and dura. The choroid plexus is where the cerebrospinal fluid is manufactured.
(Objective 11)

99. b
(Objective 11)

100. a. Immunoglobulins are antibodies, leukocytes are white blood cells, and platelets are cell fragments that aid in hemostasis.
(Objective 11)

101. a. Pulmonary arteries carry deoxygenated blood from the heart to the lungs. Pulmonary veins carry oxygenated blood from the lungs to the heart, and the vena cava carries blood from the systemic circulation to the heart.
(Objective 11)

102. d. Sinoatrial node impulses travel to the atrioventricular node, the bundle of His, and then to the Purkinje fibers.
(Objective 11)

103. d.
(Objective 11)

104. a.
(Objective 11)

105. a. The trachea and bronchus convey air to the alveoli. The capillary is not part of the respiratory system.
(Objective 11)

106. d. Absorption occurs in the other areas of the small intestine (duodenum and ileum) and to a much lesser extent in the colon; however, the primary site of absorption is the jejunum.
(Objective 11)

107. c
(Objective 11)

108. c. Roughly 180 L per day is filtered from the glomerulus; however, all but approximately 2 L of this is reabsorbed into the blood. Potassium and ammonia are secreted from the blood into the urine.
(Objective 11)

109. a. Glucagon promotes conversion of glycogen stored in the liver back to glucose. Oxytocin is a female sex hormone that stimulates uterine contractions and plays a role in lactation. Testosterone is the male sex hormone responsible for male sexual characteristics.
(Objective 11)

110. d. Final maturation (but not production) of the sperm occurs in the epididymis. The prostate and seminal vesicle produce seminal fluid.
(Objective 11)

111. d. Thalamic
(Objective 12)

112. b. The organ of Corti lies within the cochlea. The semicircular canals and vestibule are involved in balance.
(Objective 12)

WRAP IT UP

1. a. supine; b. superior; c. distal; d. radius, ulna; e. femur; f. sacrum, pubis, ilium, ischium
(Objectives 2, 3, 11)

2. aorta, lungs, heart, spleen
(Objective 7)

3. a. liver, intestines; b. spleen, stomach, liver, pancreas, intestines; c. intestines; d. intestines
(Objectives 5 through 7)

4. Frontal
(Objective 11)

5. a. red blood cells; b. A drop in the number of red blood cells reduces the blood's ability to carry oxygen to the cells. It is an indication of blood loss.
(Objective 11)

6. Injuries to the lower thoracic or upper lumbar vertebrae can cause these symptoms.
(Objective 11)

7. a. There is too little urine output. Normal urine output should be approximately 40 to 80 mL/hour (1 to 2 L/day).
b. Urine production could be reduced by increased secretion of aldosterone or antidiuretic hormone (ADH); by a drop in arterial blood pressure; or by sympathetic nervous stimulation.
(Objective 11)

8. The urinary catheter passes through the urethra and into the urinary bladder.
(Objective 11)

9. Flex and extend
(Objective 3)

10. Integumentary system (wound above her eye); skeletal system (fractures); muscular system (damage surrounding fractures); nervous system (motor/sensory deficit in lower extremities); endocrine system (hormone secretion to limit urine output); lymphatic system (if splenic injury is present); respiratory system (increased respiratory rate to compensate for decrease in red blood cells and circulatory shock); digestive system (decreased peristalsis); urinary system (decreased urinary output)
(Objective 11)

CHAPTER 7

General Principles of Pathophysiology

READING ASSIGNMENT
Chapter 7, pages 150-195, in *Mosby's Paramedic Textbook*, ed. 3

OBJECTIVES
Upon completion of this chapter, the paramedic student will be able to do the following:
1. Describe the normal characteristics of the cellular environment and the key homeostatic mechanisms that strive to maintain an optimal fluid and electrolyte balance.
2. Outline pathophysiological alterations in water and electrolyte balance and list their effects on body functions.
3. Describe the treatment of patients with particular fluid or electrolyte imbalances.
4. Describe the mechanisms in the body that maintain normal acid-base balance.
5. Outline pathophysiological alterations in acid-base balance.
6. Describe the management of a patient with an acid-base imbalance.
7. Describe the changes in cells and tissues that occur with cellular adaptation, injury, neoplasia, aging, or death.
8. Outline the effects of cellular injury on local and systemic body functions.
9. Describe changes in body functions that can occur as a result of genetic and familial disease factors.
10. Outline the causes, adverse systemic effects, and compensatory mechanisms associated with hypoperfusion.
11. Describe the ways in which the inflammatory and immune mechanisms respond to cellular injury or antigenic stimulation.
12. Explain how changes in immune status and the presence of inflammation can adversely affect body functions.
13. Describe the impact of stress on the body's response to illness or injury.

SUMMARY
- Two facts illustrate the importance of body water. First, body water is the medium in which all metabolic reactions occur. Second, the precise regulation of the volume and composition of body fluids is essential to health. Water follows osmotic gradients established by changes in sodium concentrations. Thus, sodium and water balance are closely related.
- Two abnormal states of body-fluid balance can occur. If the water gained exceeds the water lost, a state of water excess, or overhydration, exists. If the water lost exceeds the water gained, a state of water deficit, or dehydration, exists.
- In addition to fluid imbalances, disturbances in the balance of electrolytes (other than sodium) may occur. These electrolytes include potassium, calcium, and magnesium. Imbalances of these electrolytes can interfere with neuromuscular function. They may even cause cardiac rhythm disturbances.

- The treatment of isotonic dehydration may include volume replacement with isotonic or occasionally hypotonic solutions. The treatment of hypotonic dehydration may involve intravenous replacement with normal saline or lactated Ringer solution. Occasionally hypertonic saline (e.g., in seizures caused by hyponatremia) is used. Interventions for overhydration depend on the cause. These interventions may include water restriction, administration of a diuretic, or, if hyponatremia is present, administration of saline.
- In-hospital treatment of hypokalemia involves intravenous or oral potassium replacement. Management of hyperkalemia may involve potassium restriction, enteral administration of a cation exchange resin, or intravenous administration of glucose and insulin, sodium bicarbonate, or calcium.
- Treatment of hypocalcemia involves intravenous administration of calcium ions. The management of hypercalcemia may include controlling the underlying disease, hydration, and, occasionally, drug therapy such as with furosemide and other calcium-lowering drugs.
- Hypomagnesemia typically is corrected by the administration of intravenous magnesium sulfate. The most effective treatment for hypermagnesemia is hemodialysis. Calcium salts that antagonize magnesium may also be given.
- The healthy body is sensitive to changes in the concentration of hydrogen ions (pH). It tries to maintain the pH of extracellular fluid at 7.4. This is accomplished through three interrelated compensatory mechanisms: carbonic acid–bicarbonate buffering, protein buffering, and renal buffering.
- Metabolic acidosis occurs when the amount of acid generated exceeds the body's buffering capacity. The four most common forms of metabolic acidosis encountered in the prehospital setting are lactic acidosis, diabetic ketoacidosis, acidosis resulting from renal failure, and acidosis caused by ingestion of toxins. Treatment for metabolic acidosis is aimed at correcting the underlying cause.
- Loss of hydrogen is the initial cause of metabolic alkalosis. This may be caused by vomiting (hydrochloric acid loss), gastric suction, or increased renal excretion of hydrogen ion in the urine. Treatment is directed at correcting the underlying condition. Volume depletion, if present, should be corrected with isotonic solutions.
- Respiratory acidosis is caused by the retention of carbon dioxide. This leads to an increase in the Pco_2. This condition usually is caused by an imbalance in the production of carbon dioxide and its elimination through alveolar ventilation. Treatment for respiratory acidosis involves improving ventilation quickly to eliminate carbon dioxide.
- Hyperventilation may produce respiratory alkalosis by decreasing the Pco_2. Treatment of respiratory alkalosis is directed at correcting the underlying cause of the hyperventilation. An initial approach is to place the patient on low-concentration oxygen. Another is to provide calming measures to assist the patient with slow, controlled breathing.
- An understanding of the processes of disease is crucial. This requires a knowledge of the structural and functional reactions of cells and tissues to injurious agents. Changes in cells and tissues can be caused by adaptation, injury, neoplasia, aging, or death.
- An injured cell may have an abnormal physical shape or size. Cell injury has both cellular and systemic indications.
- Certain factors cause disease. For the most part, these factors may be classified as genetic or environmental. However, a strong interaction occurs between the two.
- The term *hypoperfusion* is used to describe inadequate tissue circulation. Hypoperfusion may result from decreased cardiac output. Decreased cardiac output can lead to shock, multiple organ dysfunction syndrome, and other disease states associated with impaired cellular metabolism. Negative feedback mechanisms important in maintaining cardiac output and tissue perfusion are baroreceptor reflexes, chemoreceptor reflexes, the central nervous system ischemia response, hormonal mechanisms, reabsorption of tissue fluids, and splenic discharge of stored blood.
- The external barriers are the body's first line of defense against illness and injury. These barriers include the skin and the mucous membranes of the digestive, respiratory, and gastrointestinal tracts. When these barriers are breached, chemicals, foreign bodies, or microorganisms are allowed to penetrate cells and tissues. Then the second and third lines of defense are activated. These are the inflammatory response and the immune response. Both the external barriers and the inflammatory response respond to all organisms using the identical nonspecific mechanism. The immune response is specific to individual pathogens.
- Immune responses usually are protective. They help to protect the body from harmful microorganisms and other injurious agents. At times these responses may be inappropriate. They may even have undesirable effects. Examples of inappropriate responses include hypersensitivity and immunity or inflammation deficiencies.
- Many immune-related conditions and diseases are associated with stress. However, the exact cause of these illnesses has not yet been clearly defined. It is believed that the immune, nervous, and endocrine systems communicate through complex pathways. They may be affected by factors involved in the stress reaction.

REVIEW QUESTIONS

Match the mechanism of cellular injury in column I with the appropriate cause in column II.

Column I

1. _____ Inadequate perfusion of oxygenated blood to an organ
2. _____ Group of proteins that kill or help kill bacteria
3. _____ Presence of air or oxygen
4. _____ Amount of blood returning to the ventricle
5. _____ Total resistance against which blood is pumped
6. _____ Substance that causes an antibody to form
7. _____ Osmotic concentration of a solution
8. _____ Ion with a negative charge
9. _____ Volume of blood ejected from a ventricle with each heart beat

Column II

a. Aerobic
b. Afterload
c. Anerobic
d. Anion
e. Antigen
f. Complement system
g. Ischemia
h. Osmolality
i. Preload
j. Stroke volume

Match the mechanism of cellular injury in column I with the appropriate cause in column II.

Column I

10. _____ Skin burns resulting from prolonged contact with gasoline
11. _____ Bruising caused by a blow from a tire iron
12. _____ Unconsciousness resulting from a drop in blood sugar
13. _____ Death secondary to septic shock
14. _____ Tissue death in a leg after occlusion of a blood vessel
15. _____ Severe wheezing that develops after a bee sting

Column II

a. Chemical injury
b. Genetic factors
c. Hypoxic injury
d. Immunological injury
e. Infectious injury
f. Nutritional imbalances
g. Physical agents

16. Complete the following sentences, which refer to the fluid compartments of the body.
The water found outside the cells that includes the water in plasma, bone, tendon, and fascia is the

(a) _____ fluid. The water outside the vascular bed that lies between the tissue cells is known as

(b) _____ fluid. The fluid found inside the cells of the skeletal muscle, intestine, viscera, bone

marrow, glands, and red blood cells is the **(c)** _____ fluid.

17. For each of the following ions, state its name, indicate whether it is a cation or an anion, and state where it is most plentiful in the body (extracellular fluid [ECF] or intracellular fluid [ICF]).

Ion	Name	Cation or Anion	ECF or ICF
PO_4^-			
K^+			
Na^+			
HCO_3^-			
Mg^{++}			
Cl^-			

18. Briefly define the following terms:

  a. Cell membrane permeability:

  _____

  _____

  b. Diffusion:

  _____

  _____

  c. Concentration gradient:

  _____

  _____

  d. Osmosis:

  _____

  _____

  e. Active transport:

  _____

  _____

  f. Facilitated diffusion:

  _____

  _____

19. For each of the following patient situations, choose the suspected fluid or electrolyte imbalance from the list provided and describe appropriate assessments and/or interventions.

  a. You are transporting an older patient for chest pain. After an intravenous (IV) line has been inserted, 500 mL is accidentally infused rapidly. The patient becomes very short of breath, and evaluation reveals moist crackles in the lungs.
  Imbalance: Hyponatremia, hypermagnesemia, or overhydration?

  _____

  Management:

  _____

  _____

  b. Your patient is a 65-year-old adult who complains of vomiting and diarrhea. Home medications include a diuretic. The physical examination reveals a blood pressure of 100/70 mm Hg, a weak pulse, decreased reflexes, and shallow respirations.
  Imbalance: Hyperkalemia, hypocalcemia, or hypokalemia?

  _____

Management:

_____

_____

c. You are called to the airport to evaluate an obviously malnourished child flown to the United States from India for adoption. The chaperone reports that the child has shown abnormal behavior and complains of muscle cramps, abdominal cramps, and tingling of the extremities. As you begin to assess the vital signs, the patient has a grand mal seizure.
Imbalance: Hypernatremia, hypocalcemia, or hypomagnesemia?

_____

Management:

_____

_____

d. A father calls you to evaluate an infant who has been vomiting for 36 hours. The father states that the child has not had a wet diaper in 8 hours. The anterior fontanelle is depressed, and the skin and mucous membranes are dry.
Imbalance: Hypercalcemia, hypermagnesemia, or isotonic dehydration?

_____

Management:

_____

_____

e. Your patient is a 13-year-old bulimic girl who admits to frequent use of water enemas for weight control. You were called for a chief complaint of abdominal pain; however, on arrival you find the patient diaphoretic with a rapid, thready pulse and cyanosis. There is no indication of bleeding.
Imbalance: Hyperkalemia, hyponatremic dehydration, or overhydration?

_____

Management:

_____

_____

f. The family of an older patient with chronic renal failure says that she is confused and very weak. The physical examination reveals shallow, slow respirations that become progressively worse.
Imbalance: Hypermagnesemia, hypocalcemia, or hypokalemia?

_____

Management:

_____

_____

20. Describe the mode of action of the three acid-base buffer systems in the body. Begin with the fastest mechanism and end with the slowest one.

a. _____

b. _____

c. _____

_____

_____

21. For each case presented, indicate which one of the four acid-base disturbances listed below is the cause. State at least one prehospital intervention for management of the imbalance.

Respiratory acidosis   Respiratory alkalosis
Metabolic acidosis   Metabolic alkalosis

a. A 17-year-old student complains of dizziness and tingling in the hands and around the mouth during a college entrance examination. The medical history and physical examination are unremarkable. The respiratory rate is 28 breaths/min and deep.

Imbalance: _____
Intervention:

_____

b. A 72-year-old resident of an extended care facility has been treated with gastric suction.

Imbalance: _____
Intervention:

_____

c. A 30-year-old diabetic woman has had influenza. She has taken no insulin in 2 days and appears dehydrated. Respirations are deep and rapid.

Imbalance: _____
Intervention:

_____

d. A 46-year-old patient who took an overdose of a barbiturate has shallow respirations at a rate of 8 breaths/min.

Imbalance: _____
Intervention:

_____

22. The following arterial blood gas values were obtained in a patient who had had a stroke. State whether each is normal or abnormal. Discuss any action that may be taken in the field to correct any abnormalities identified.

a. pH: 7.25   Normal/Abnormal
   Actions: _____

b. Po_2: 60 mmHg   Normal/Abnormal
   Actions: _____

c. Pco_2: 53 mmHg   Normal/Abnormal
   Actions: _____

23. For each of the following cellular adaptations, give the cause, the effect on the cell, and an example.

Adaptation	Cause	Effect on Cell	Example
Atrophy			
Dysplasia			
Hyperplasia			
Hypertrophy			
Metaplasia			

24. For each of the following situations, explain why cardiac output will increase or decrease in an otherwise healthy individual.

   a. The patient has had a myocardial infarction with necrosis of 50% of the heart muscle.

_____

_____

   b. A dehydrated patient is given 500 mL of normal saline intravenously.

_____

_____

   c. The patient's normal heart rate is 80 and suddenly drops to 40.

_____

_____

   d. A paramedic student enters a testing station.

_____

_____

25. Describe the physiological effects of the baroreceptor response to compensate in each of the following situations.

   a. A 47-year-old adult has a sudden increase in blood pressure to 170/110 mm Hg.

_____

_____

   b. A 22-year-old adult is thrown from a horse and suffers a pelvic fracture. The paramedic's findings are significant internal bleeding and a sudden drop in blood pressure to 60 mm Hg systolic by palpation.

_____

_____

26. Describe the physiological effects of chemoreceptor stimulation in the following situations.

    a. A 36-year-old adult has a massive hemothorax from a gunshot wound. Blood pressure is 76/60 mm Hg.

_____

_____

    b. A 17-year-old patient who took a drug overdose has a shallow respiratory rate of 8 breaths/min. Arterial blood gas tests reveal a Pco_2 of 60 mm Hg

_____

_____

27. A 47-year-old man who suffered a large inferior myocardial infarction has progressively deteriorated. He is now unconscious and has a weak carotid pulse and no obtainable blood pressure. Describe the physiological effects that ensue when the central nervous system ischemia response is initiated.

_____

_____

28. A 65-year-old alcoholic man states that he had a sudden onset of vomiting. The emesis contains bright red blood, and he continues to vomit. Vital signs are: blood pressure, 94/78 mm Hg; pulse, 132 beats per minute (bpm); and respirations, 28 breaths/min. Describe the effects of the following three hormonal mechanisms, which will be activated.

    a. Adrenal medullary mechanism

_____

_____

    b. Renin-angiotensin-aldosterone mechanism

_____

_____

    c. Vasopressin mechanism

_____

_____

29. Multiple organ dysfunction syndrome (MODS) begins with **(a)** _____ _____ damage

caused by **(b)** _____ and _____, which are released into the circulation. This causes the

vascular **(c)** _____ to become **(d)** _____, which allows fluid and cells to leak into the

(e) _____ spaces, increasing **(f)** _____ and _____. Three plasma enzyme cascades

are then activated. They are **(g)** _____, _____, and _____/_____.

Phagocytes cause further damage to the endothelium, causing uncontrolled **(h)** _____ and the

formation of microvascular **(i)** _____ and tissue ischemia. Bradykinin contributes to low

(j) _____ _____ _____. The overall effect of the three complement systems is

(k) _____ formation, **(l)** _____, and **(m)** _____ _____. Initially the

body compensates for these changes, but ultimately tissue hypoxia causes **(n)** _____ _____,

_____ _____. Finally, multiple **(o)** _____ failure occurs.

30. Your partner is off sick with a diagnosis of strep throat. Describe whether the following signs and symptoms experienced during this illness are local or systemic and give at least one inflammatory mechanism that causes the sign or symptom.

Sign or Symptom	Local or Systemic Response	Cause
Edematous throat		
Purulent drainage		
Fever		
Red throat		
Difficulty swallowing		

31. For the following patient blood types, list all safe donor types.

Blood Type	Donors
a. A positive	
b. O negative	
c. AB positive	
d. B negative	

32. For each statement below, note which one of three types of altered immunological reaction has occurred: allergy, autoimmunity, or isoimmunity.

   a. Your patient is agitated and complains of severe low back pain a few moments after you begin to transfuse a unit of blood. _____

   b. You are dispatched to a private residence to care for a 46-year-old woman who began to experience dyspnea, a swollen face, and hives after taking a penicillin tablet prescribed by her dentist. _____

   c. You are transferring a patient to a dialysis center for care after his body rejected his kidney transplant. _____

   d. You notice that your eyes water and get puffy and your hands become very red and itchy when you wear Latex gloves at work. _____

e. Your patient, a 30-year-old woman, is having chest pain. The family tells you she has systemic lupus erythematosus with cardiac and pulmonary involvement. _____

Match the probable cause of immune suppression in column II with the statement in column I.

Column I	Column II
33. _____ An elderly woman develops pneumonia several months after the death of her husband.	**a.** Acquired immune deficiency
34. _____ A cancer patient becomes septic after a course of chemotherapy.	**b.** Deficiencies caused by stress
35. _____ A young girl suffering from anorexia nervosa repeatedly becomes ill with viral illness.	**c.** Deficiencies caused by trauma
	d. Iatrogenic deficiencies
36. _____ A patient infected with the human immunodeficiency virus (HIV) develops Kaposi sarcoma.	**e.** Nutritional deficiencies

37. Fill in the missing information relating to the stress response.

Hormone or Receptor	Location	Action
a.	Found in plasma	Stimulates gluconeogenesis; suppresses immune cell activity
Alpha-1 receptors	Postsynaptic located on effector organs	**b.**
Beta-1 receptors	**c.**	Increased pulse rate
d.	Lungs and arteries	Bronchodilation

38. For each of the following diseases, list a factor that may contribute to its development. Identify whether the factor is environmental or genetic.

Disease	Factor	Environmental or Genetic
Stroke		
Cervical cancer		
Oral cancer		
Melanoma (skin cancer)		
Depression		

STUDENT SELF-ASSESSMENT

39. Which mechanism of cellular transport moves substances against a concentration gradient and requires the use of energy?
    a. Active transport
    b. Diffusion
    c. Facilitated diffusion
    d. Osmosis

40. Which of the following electrolytes is found predominantly in the intracellular fluid?

   a. Bicarbonate   **c.** Potassium

   b. Chloride   **d.** Sodium

41. A solution that has a concentration of solute particles equal to that inside the cells is a(n) _____ solution.

   a. Atonic   **c.** Hypotonic

   b. Hypertonic   **d.** Isotonic

42. Which of the following causes the normal flow of fluid through the interstitial space?

   a. Capillary hydrostatic pressure filters fluid from the interstitial space through the capillary wall.

   b. Oncotic pressure exerted by blood proteins attracts fluid from the vascular space back into the interstitial space.

   c. Capillary permeability determines the ease with which fluid can pass through the capillary wall.

   d. The lymphatic channels close to prevent entry of capillary fluid pushed out by hydrostatic pressure.

43. Your patient is being transferred from a nursing home to a hospital for admission for an intestinal obstruction. His skin is dry, and his tongue has furrows. What fluid and electrolyte imbalance do you suspect?

   a. Hypernatremic dehydration   **c.** Isotonic dehydration

   b. Hyponatremic dehydration   **d.** Osmotic dehydration

44. You are called to transport a 56-year-old patient with a history of renal failure who missed his last dialysis session. He complains of nausea, abdominal distention, weakness, and irritability. Which of the following do you suspect?

   a. Hypercalcemia   **c.** Hypernatremia

   b. Hyperkalemia   **d.** Hyperuria

45. Which of the following is true regarding hypomagnesemia?

   a. It is often accompanied by hypercalcemia.

   b. It results from antacid abuse.

   c. It causes hypoactive reflexes.

   d. It causes cardiac dysrhythmias.

46. Your patient has metabolic acidosis. Which of the following compensatory mechanisms uses proteins in an attempt to rapidly restore normal acid-base balance?

   a. Carbonic acid–bicarbonate buffering

   b. Excretion of hydrogen ions to acidify the urine

   c. Exhalation of excess carbon dioxide

   d. Recovery of bicarbonate in the renal tubules

47. Which acid-base disturbance would you anticipate in a patient with severe flail chest?

   a. Metabolic acidosis   **c.** Respiratory acidosis

   b. Metabolic alkalosis   **d.** Respiratory alkalosis

48. Lactic acidosis is harmful to the body because it

   a. Increases the basal metabolic rate

   b. Decreases the force of cardiac contraction

   c. Increases the response to catecholamines

   d. Can cause severe hypertension

49. Increasing the rate of ventilations for a patient with metabolic acidosis and inadequate stroke volume typically causes which of the following?

   a. Decreased pH and decreased Pco_2

   b. Decreased pH and increased Pco_2

   c. Increased pH and decreased Pco_2

   d. Increased pH and increased Pco_2

50. Which cellular change, which may occur with aging, results in shrinkage of the brain and may cause a delay in the signs and symptoms associated with subdural hematoma (blood clot on the brain).

   a. Atrophy   **c.** Metaplasia

   b. Dysplasia   **d.** Hypertrophy

51. The process of cellular self-destruction is known as _____.

   Autolysis   Necrosis

   MODS   Osmosis

52. Which of the following changes would be expected early after cellular injury?
    a. Accelerated cellular reproduction
    b. Decreased intracellular hydrostatic pressure
    c. Increased intracellular oxygen accumulation
    d. Swelling of cells from increased osmosis
53. Sympathetic vasoconstriction during shock results in which of the following?
    a. Tachycardia
    b. Pupil dilation
    c. Increased container size
    d. Pale, cool skin
54. The central nervous system ischemic response is initiated when
    a. Blood pressure falls below 90 mm Hg systolic.
    b. Aortic and carotid chemoreceptors are stimulated.
    c. Bradycardia and vasodilation are present.
    d. Blood flow decreases in the vasomotor center.
55. Which of the following hormonal mechanisms increases urine production?
    a. Adrenal medullary mechanism
    b. Atrial natriuretic mechanism
    c. Renin-angiotension-aldosterone mechanism
    d. Vasopressin mechanism
56. An elderly patient calls 9-1-1 complaining of chest discomfort and difficulty breathing. Electrocardiographic changes on arrival at the hospital are consistent with acute myocardial infarction. The patient is showing signs of hypoperfusion. What type of shock does this likely represent?
    a. Anaphylactic
    b. Cardiogenic
    c. Hypovolemic
    d. Septic
57. Which of the following situations represents natural immunity in a fellow paramedic?
    a. Immunity to feline leukemia virus
    b. Immunity to measles after immunization
    c. Immunity to chicken pox after having them
    d. Immunity to hepatitis after immunoglobulin administration
58. Which of the following is true regarding hypersensitivity?
    a. It occurs only when the body encounters foreign antigens.
    b. The response always occurs immediately after exposure to the antigen.
    c. It may produce either minor or life-threatening consequences.
    d. It is a normal immune response resulting from exposure to an antigen.
59. Which hormone increases the level of blood glucose and acts as an immunosuppressant by reducing the number of selected leukocytes?
    a. Cortisol
    b. Dopamine
    c. Epinephrine
    d. Norepinephrine

WRAP IT UP

You are dispatched to an industrial accident where people reportedly are trapped. When you arrive, the incident commander tells you that a floor collapsed during erection of a high-rise building. A worker is trapped under the rubble, and the rescue squad is attempting to free him. The commander allows one person to approach the scene. You ask your partner to set up the ambulance and then meet you with a stretcher as close as he can approach the scene. You take the long spine board, immobilization supplies, an airway kit, and your primary resuscitation bag and move carefully toward the patient. He is conscious but very pale, and complains of a burning pain in his lower extremities. The extrication is dangerous; with every piece of debris removed, the entire pile becomes unstable. It is 4 hours before the patient is released. You immobilize him and quickly move him to the ambulance. His skin is pale and cool, he is breathing rapidly, and he has a puncture wound of unknown depth over his right upper abdomen. His lower extremities are gray and pale, but no crepitus or deformity is noted. His vital signs are: BP, 80/56 mm Hg; P, 136/min; R, 32/min; and an oxygen saturation (Sao_2) that won't register a reading. The monitor shows a sinus tachycardia with tall-tented T waves. You administer oxygen by nonrebreather mask at 15 L/min; initiate two large-bore IVs and infuse them at a rapid rate; and quickly begin transport to the trauma center.

1. What fluid should be started on this patient? Explain your answer.
   a. D_5W
   b. D_5NS
   c. LR
   d. NS
   Explanation:

   _____

   _____

2. a. If the electrocardiographic (ECG) change indicates excessive amounts of potassium in the blood, what additional signs or symptoms might this patient experience?

   _____

   b. What could explain this patient's hyperkalemia?
      (1) Abdominal puncture releases potassium into the blood.
      (2) Crushed cells release potassium into the blood.
      (3) Lack of oxygen related to shock causes the release of potassium.
      (4) Potassium production is stimulated during hypoperfusion.

3. What acid-base imbalance will this patient most likely experience? Explain your answer.
   a. Metabolic acidosis
   b. Metabolic alkalosis
   c. Respiratory acidosis
   d. Respiratory alkalosis
   Explanation:

   _____

   _____

4. How will the body attempt to compensate for this acid-base imbalance?

   _____

   _____

5. For each of the following compensatory mechanisms used by the body during shock, put a ✔ on the line if the mechanism directly increases heart rate or contractility; put an ✗ if it acts directly on the blood vessels to cause constriction; and put a ★ if it conserves body water.
   _____ Parasympathetic stimulation   _____ Sympathetic stimulation
   _____ Adrenal medullary mechanism   _____ Renin-angiotensin-aldosterone mechanism
   _____ Vasopressin mechanism   _____ Tissue fluid reabsorption
   _____ Splenic discharge of blood

6. What stage of shock does this patient's signs and symptoms appear to indicate?
   a. Compensated
   b. Multiple organ dysfunction syndrome
   c. Terminal
   d. Uncompensated

CHAPTER 7 ANSWERS

REVIEW QUESTIONS

1. g
(Objective 10)

2. f
(Objective 11)

3. a
(Objective 5)

4. i
(Objective 10)

5. b
(Objective 10)

6. c
(Objective 11)

7. h
(Objective 1)

8. d
(Objective 5)

9. j
(Objective 10)

10. a
11. g
12. f
13. e
14. c
15. d
(Questions 10-15: Objective 7)

16. (a) Extracellular; (b) interstitial; (c) intracellular (Objective 1)

17. PO_4^-: phosphate, anion, intracellular; K+: potassium, cation, intracellular; Na+: sodium, cation, extracellular; HCO_3^-: bicarbonate, anion, extracellular; Mg^{++}: magnesium, cation, intracellular; Cl⁻: chloride, anion, extracellular
(Objective 1)

18. a. The property of a cell membrane that freely permits the passage of water but selectively allows the passage of solute particles. This permits the cell to maintain a relatively constant internal environment. b. A passive process that allows molecules or ions to move from an area of higher concentration to an area of lower concentration in an attempt to achieve a state of equilibrium. c. A situation in which the solute concentration is greater at one point than another in a solvent. Solutes diffuse from the area of higher concentration to the area of lower concentration until equilibrium is achieved. d. The diffusion of water across a selectively permeable membrane from an area of higher water concentration to an area of lower water concentration. e. A rapid, carrier-mediated process that can move a substance across a selectively permeable membrane from an area of low concentration to an area of high concentration. This process requires energy. f. A carrier-mediated process (faster than diffusion) that can move a substance from an area of higher concentration to an area of lower concentration. This process does not require energy.
(Objective 1)

19. a. Overhydration; fluid restriction, normal saline given intravenously to keep the vein open.

b. Hypokalemia; lactated Ringer solution given intravenously to keep the vein open, preparation to assist ventilations, and high-flow oxygen. In-hospital treatment may include oral or IV potassium.

c. Hypocalcemia; possibly calcium ions (calcium chloride) given intravenously, airway management, seizure precautions, IV anticonvulsant therapy.

d. Isotonic dehydration; evaluation of airway, breathing, and circulation; assessment for shock, IV therapy with an isotonic solution.

e. Hyponatremic dehydration; evaluation of the effectiveness of ventilations, high-flow oxygen, IV therapy with lactated Ringer solution or normal saline, and evaluation of vital signs. Occasionally hypertonic saline may be administered.

f. Hypermagnesemia; open airway, assistance with ventilations as necessary, high-flow oxygen, evaluation of vital signs, IV line with normal saline to keep the vein open, possibly IV calcium salts. The most effective treatment is hemodialysis. (Objective 2)

20. a. Buffers produce an immediate response to changes in the hydrogen ion concentration (pH). They represent the body's ability to adjust the concentration of bicarbonate and carbon dioxide in the blood to maintain a relationship of 1 mEq of carbonic acid to 20 mEq of base bicarbonate. If this relationship is maintained, the pH stays within normal limits.

b. The respiratory system can increase alveolar ventilation within minutes in response to an increase in the hydrogen ion concentration. Hydrogen ions combine with bicarbonate to form carbonic acid, which in turn breaks down into carbon dioxide and water. Therefore, by increasing the amount of carbon dioxide the body eliminates, the process can be accelerated and the hydrogen ion concentration reduced.

c. The renal system takes hours to days to act. It restores normal pH by reabsorbing or excreting bicarbonate or hydrogen ions. (Objective 4)

21. a. Respiratory alkalosis; treat cause of underlying hyperventilation.

b. Metabolic alkalosis; initiate IV administration of lactated Ringer solution or normal saline.

c. Metabolic acidosis; initiate IV administration of normal saline.

d. Respiratory acidosis; assist ventilations. (Objectives 5, 6)

22. a. Abnormal; for acidosis caused by an increase in the Pco_2, increase ventilations. b. Abnormal; increase oxygen delivery to the patient. c. Abnormal; increase rate of ventilations.
(Objective 6)

23.

Adaptation	Cause	Effect on Cell	Example
Atrophy	Diminished function, inadequate hormonal or nervous stimulation, reduced blood supply	Decrease or shrinkage in cellular size	Shrinkage of muscle size in a casted limb or from neuro-muscular disease; brain atrophy in old age
Dysplasia	Chronic irritation or inflammation	Abnormal changes in mature cells	Precancerous changes of the cervix or lungs
Hyperplasia	Response to an increase in demand	Increase in the number of cells in a tissue or organ	Cellular or endometrial hyperplasia
Hypertrophy	Increased demand for work by a cell	Increase in the size (but not number) of cells	Large muscles of a body builder or enlarged heart or kidneys
Metaplasia	Cellular adaptation to adverse conditions	Conversion or replacement of normal cells by other cells	Bronchial metaplasia secondary to cigarette smoke

(Objective 7)

24. a. Muscle is lost, therefore contractility and stroke volume decrease, lowering cardiac output.

b. The additional fluid volume improves preload, thereby increasing stroke volume and cardiac output.

c. A sudden drop in the heart rate results in a decrease in cardiac output.

d. Fear and anxiety cause a rise in heart rate and stroke volume, which in turn increases cardiac output.

(Objective 10)

25. a. The vasoconstrictor center of the medulla is inhibited, and the vagal center is excited, resulting in peripheral vasodilation and a decrease in heart rate and the strength of contraction. This results in a decrease in blood pressure.

b. Vagal stimulation is reduced, resulting in a sympathetic response that causes an increase in peripheral vasoconstriction and in the heart rate and strength of contraction. This results in an increase in blood pressure.

(Objective 10)

26. a. The low pressure results in a decrease in oxygen to the chemoreceptor cells; this in turn stimulates the vasomotor center of the medulla, resulting in peripheral vasoconstriction.

b. Chemoreceptors are also stimulated by an increase in the Pco_2, which causes vasoconstriction and an increase in blood flow to the lungs, enhancing their ability to eliminate carbon dioxide. (Objective 10)

27. The central nervous system ischemic response is initiated when blood pressure drops below 50 mm Hg; it triggers intense vasoconstriction in an attempt to improve perfusion to the brain. If the ischemia lasts longer than 10 minutes, the vagal center may be activated, resulting in peripheral vasodilation and bradycardia.

(Objective 10)

28. a. Increased sympathetic stimulation causes the adrenal medulla to release epinephrine and norepinephrine, which results in an increase in heart rate, stroke volume, and vasoconstriction.

b. Low flow to the kidneys results in a release of renin, which by a series of chemical reactions causes plasma proteins to synthesize angiotensin II. Angiotensin II causes vasoconstriction and initiates the release of aldosterone. Aldosterone causes increased retention of sodium and water by the kidneys.

c. The hypothalamic neurons are stimulated by a drop in blood pressure or an increase in plasma solutes, and the secretion of antidiuretic hormone (vasopressin) is increased. This results in vasoconstriction and a decreased rate of urine production.

(Objective 10)

29. (a) vascular endothelial

(b) endotoxins, inflammatory mediators

(c) endothelium

(d) permeable

(e) interstitial

(f) hypotension, hypoperfusion

(g) complement, coagulation, kallikrein/kinin

(h) coagulation

(i) thrombus

(j) systemic vascular resistance

(k) edema

(l) cardiovascular instability

(m) clotting abnormalities

(n) cellular acidosis, impaired cellular function

(o) organ

(Objective 10)

30.

Sign or Symptom	Local or Systemic Response	Cause
Edematous throat	Local	Cellular accumulation of sodium causes edema. Also, hyperemia increases filtration pressure and capillary permeability, causing fluid to leak into interstitital spaces.
Purulent drainage	Local	Bacteria are destroyed by phagocytosis. Then macrophages clear and destroy tissues of dead cells. Destruction of leukocytes is initiated by phagocytosis. Dead tissues plus dead leukocytes plus fluid that leaks into the area form pus.
Fever	Systemic	Mast cell degranulation and an increase in the metabolic rate caused by the inflammatory process
Red throat	Local	Dilation of arterioles, venules, and capillaries in the area of cellular injury
Difficulty swallowing	Local	A consequence of the edema described above

(Objective 11)

31. a. O positive, O negative, A positive, A negative; b. O negative; c. O positive, O negative, A positive, A negative, B positive, B negative, AB positive; AB negative; d. O negative, B negative
(Objective 11)

32. a. Isoimmunity. The body is reacting to beneficial foreign cells.
   b. Allergy. The body is responding to the introduction of a foreign protein (antigen) that it recognizes as harmful.
   c. Isoimmunity. The body rejects helpful foreign tissue that it sees as harmful.
   d. Allergy. The body may be reacting to the protein (antigen) in the Latex.
   e. Autoimmunity. It is thought that systemic lupus erythematosus and other diseases such as dermatomyositis, periarteritis nodosa, scleroderma, and rheumatoid arthritis may be caused by an autoimmune response.[1]
(Objective 12)

33. b. Prolonged emotional or psychological stress can result in physical illness.
34. d. Patients undergoing chemotherapy or radiation therapy for cancer may experience significant suppression of the immune system.
35. e. Severe deficits in calorie or protein intake can seriously impair the immune system.
36. a. The human immunodeficiency virus (HIV) attacks the immune system, making the body easy prey for opportunistic infections and malignancies. (Questions 25-28: Objective 10)
37. a. Cortisol
   b. Vasoconstriction
   c. Heart
   d. Beta-2 receptors

Anderson KN, Anderson LE, Glanze WD: *Mosby's medical nursing and allied health dictionary,* ed 6, St Louis, 2002, Mosby.

38.

Disease	Factor	Environmental or Genetic
Stroke	Hypertension, high cholesterol, smoking	Environmental
Cervical cancer	Infection with gonorrhea	Environmental
Oral cancer	Chewing smokeless tobacco	Environmental
Melanoma (skin cancer)	Excessive exposure to sun	Environmental
Depression	Familial tendency	Genetic
	Metabolic disturbance, drug reaction, nutritional disorder, situational crisis	Environmental

(Objective 9)

STUDENT SELF-ASSESSMENT

39. a. Diffusion is a passive process involving the movement of molecules from an area of high concentration to an area of lower concentration. Facilitated diffusion uses a carrier molecule to move molecules rapidly down a concentration gradient. Osmosis is a process that causes the movement of fluid from an area of low solute concentration to an area of high solute concentration.
(Objective 1)

40. c. All others are found chiefly in the extracellular fluid.
(Objective 1)

41. d. *Atonic* means without tone. A *hypertonic* solution has a greater solute concentration than that inside the cells; a *hypotonic* solution is less concentrated than that inside the cells.
(Objective 1)

42. c. Capillary hydrostatic pressure filters fluid from the blood through the capillary wall. Oncotic pressure exerted by blood plasma proteins attracts fluid from the interstitial space into the blood. The lymph channels open and collect some of the fluid forced out of the capillaries by hydrostatic pressure and return it to the circulation.
(Objective 2)

43. c. Hypernatremic dehydration is associated with an intake of sodium that exceeds sodium losses. Hyponatremic dehydration typically manifests with cramps, seizures, a rapid, thready pulse, diaphoresis, and/or cyanosis. There is no such classification as osmotic dehydration.
(Objective 3)

44. b. A patient in renal failure is frequently hypocalcemic, not hypercalcemic.
(Objective 2)

45. d
(Objective 2)

46. c. Both hydrogen and carbon dioxide bind to hemoglobin, which carries them to the lungs for exhalation.
(Objective 4)

47. c. Ventilation (due to a reduced tidal volume) is frequently severely decreased in these patients. This inhibits the excretion of carbon dioxide from the lungs, causing an increase in carbonic acid and a decrease in the pH.
(Objective 5)

48. b. Lactic acid reduces the peripheral response to catecholamines and can cause severe hypotension.
(Objective 5)

49. c. A decreased pH and increased Pco_2 are signs of respiratory acidosis. An increased pH and decreased Pco_2 are signs of respiratory alkalosis. An increased pH and increased Pco_2 are signs of metabolic alkalosis.
(Objective 6)

50. a. The decrease in cell size that occurs secondary to atrophy of brain cells causes the brain to shrink in size. *Dysplasia* is an abnormal change in a mature cell. *Metaplasia* is the substitution of one cell type for another. *Hypertrophy* is an increase in cell size that results in an increase in organ size.
(Objective 7)

51. Autolysis. *MODS* is the progressive failure of two or more organ systems secondary to severe illness or injury. *Necrosis* refers to the cellular changes that occur after local cell death. *Osmosis* is the movement of water across a semipermeable membrane.
(Objective 7)

52. d. Sodium rushes into the injured cells, increasing the osmotic pressure, which draws more water into the cell.
(Objective 8)

53. d. Tachycardia and pupil dilation are sympathetic responses but do not occur secondary to vasoconstriction. The container size should decrease because of vasoconstriction.
(Objective 10)

54. d. When blood flow to the vasomotor center of the medulla is reduced to the point of ischemia, this response initiates profound vasoconstriction.
(Objective 10)

55. b. All other mechanisms decrease urinary output to conserve blood volume.
(Objective 10)

56. b. If sufficient cardiac muscle is destroyed in myocardial infarction, the stroke volume and therefore cardiac output can be markedly decreased. Anaphylactic shock occurs secondary to exposure of a sensitized individual to an allergen, resulting in dyspnea, wheezing, shock, urticaria, erythema, angioedema, and other dramatic signs and symptoms. Septic shock occurs secondary to a bacterial infection that releases harmful endotoxins.
(Objective 10)

57. a. Feline leukemia virus is a disease to which humans have a natural immunity. Acquired immunity occurs after immunization for measles and after having chicken pox (for most patients). Temporary acquired immunity is conferred if hepatitis B immunoglobulin is administered, but vaccination is needed to ensure acquired long-term immunity.
(Objective 11)

58. c. Hypersensitivity can occur secondary to foreign antigens (allergy, isoimmune reactions) or, in the case of autoimmunity, when the body attacks its own tissues. The response may be immediate or delayed up to several days. Hypersensitivity represents an abnormal immune response.
(Objective 12)

59. a. Dopamine exerts effects on the blood vessels. It causes renal and mesenteric dilation at low levels, beta effects at midrange levels, and strong alpha stimulation at high levels. Epinephrine stimulates alpha and beta cells, causing an increase in the heart rate and contractility and in bronchiolar dilation; it also increases blood glucose by glycogenolysis. It does not suppress white blood cells, as cortisol does. Norepinephrine exerts effects similar to those of epinephrine; however, its alpha effects predominate.
(Objective 13)

WRAP IT UP

1. d. Normal saline (NS) is an isotonic fluid that remains in the intravascular space, available for the heart to pump longer than either of the fluids containing dextrose (D_5W, D_5NS). Lactated Ringer solution (LR) contains potassium, which would not be indicated in this patient.
(Objective 3)

2. a. Cardiac conduction disturbances, irritability, abdominal distention, nausea, diarrhea, oliguria, weakness or paralysis.
(Objective 3)

   b. (2). Intracellular potassium levels are very high. When cells break open, such as during an extensive crush injury or electrical injury, large amounts of potassium are released into the blood.
(Objective 3)

3. a. The prolonged crush forces create an accumulation of lactic acid in the tissues that is released into the general circulation when the patient is freed. In addition, the presence of systemic hypoperfusion creates anaerobic metabolism in some tissues, resulting in the production of lactic acid.
(Objective 5)

4. The respiratory rate will increase, the kidneys will excrete hydrogen ions, and the carbonic acid–bicarbonate buffering system will try to compensate for the metabolic acidosis.
(Objective 4)

5. Parasympathetic stimulation: None
   Sympathetic stimulation: Increases heart rate and contractility, constricts blood vessels
   Adrenal medullary mechanism: Increases heart rate and contractility, constricts blood vessels
   Renin-angiotensin-aldosterone mechanism: Constricts blood vessels, conserves body water
   Vasopressin mechanism: Constricts blood vessels, conserves body water
   Tissue fluid reabsorption: Moves fluid from interstitial to intravascular space (doesn't conserve it)
   Splenic discharge of blood: Releases blood from spleen (doesn't conserve it) (Objective 10)

6. d. The blood pressure is low, therefore the compensatory mechanisms are no longer sufficient to resolve the patient's hypoperfusion.
(Objective 10)

CHAPTER

8

Life Span Development

READING ASSIGNMENT

Chapter 8, pages 196-211, in *Mosby's Paramedic Textbook*, ed. 3

OBJECTIVES

Upon completion of this chapter, the paramedic student will be able to:

1. Describe the normal vital signs and body system characteristics of the newborn, neonate, infant, toddler, preschooler, school-aged child, adolescent, young adult, middle-aged adult, and older adult.
2. Identify the psychosocial features of the infant, toddler, preschooler, school-aged child, adolescent, young adult, middle-aged adult, and older adult.
3. Explain the effect of parenting styles, sibling rivalry, peer relationships, and other factors on a child's psychosocial development.
4. Discuss the physical and emotional challenges faced by the older adult.

SUMMARY

- The newborn is a baby in the first hours of life. A neonate is a baby younger than 28 days. An infant is a child 28 days to 1 year of age.
- The newborn normally weighs 3 to 3.5 kg (7 to 8 pounds). This weight typically triples in 9 to 12 months. The infant's head accounts for about 25% of the total body weight.
- At birth, structures unique to fetal circulation constrict and normally close within the first year of life. Fluid is expelled from the lungs during the first few breaths. Respiratory muscles and alveoli are not fully developed.
- Infants are born with protective reflexes related to breathing, eating, and stress or discomfort.
- At birth the anterior and posterior fontanelles are open. Bone growth occurs at the epiphysis of the bones.
- Some passive immunity is conferred at birth and through the mother's breast milk.
- The caregiver is the major factor in the infant's psychosocial development.
- Temperament is a person's behavioral style. It is the way the person interacts with the environment.
- Toddlers are children 1 to 3 years of age. Preschoolers are 3 to 5 years of age.
- The hemoglobin level in toddlers and preschoolers approaches that of adults. The brain in this age group is about 90% of the adult brain weight. Muscle mass and bone density increase. Walking occurs by age 2, and fine motor skills develop. Control of bowel and bladder is achieved.
- Parenting styles can be described as authoritarian, authoritative, or permissive.
- Sibling rivalry, peer relationships, divorce, and exposure to aggression and violence affect a child's development.

- School-aged children range from 6 to 12 years of age. Physical growth slows, but brain function and the ability to learn quickly develop in this age group. Many children reach puberty during this time. Self-esteem and moral development are critical at this age.
- Adolescents are 13 to 19 years of age. The growth of bone and muscle mass is nearly complete in this age group. Reproductive maturity has been reached. Adolescence often involves some emotional turmoil, and antisocial behavior may be seen.
- Early adulthood spans the period from 20 to 40 years of age. Lifelong habits and routines develop. Body systems are at their optimal performance.
- Middle adulthood extends from 41 to 60 years of age. The physiological aspects of aging become more apparent in this age group. Menopause in women occurs during this stage.
- People reach late adulthood at 61 years of age. Body system changes vary widely from person to person, but the systemic changes of aging become apparent. Some adults in this age group face financial, physical, and emotional challenges.

Match the age range in Column I with the appropriate age in Column II.

Column I	Column II
1. _____ Infant	a. First few hours of life
2. _____ Neonate	b. Younger than 28 days
3. _____ Newborn	c. 28 days to 1 year
4. _____ Preschool	d. 1 to 3 years
5. _____ School age	e. 3 to 5 years
6. _____ Toddler	f. 6 to 12 years

Match the reflex in Column II with the appropriate description in Column I.

Column I	Column II
7. _____ Head turns toward facial stimulation.	a. Babinski's
8. _____ Lips pucker when mouth contacts nipple.	b. Babkin
9. _____ Toes spread up and out when sole stroked.	c. Moro
10. _____ Mouth opens if palm is pressed when supine.	d. Palmar grasp
11. _____ Infant stretches and then hugs self after loud noise.	e. Rooting
	f. Stepping
	g. Sucking

Circle toddler (1 to 3 years) or preschooler (3 to 5 years) to indicate the most common age that children achieve the following social milestones.

12. Can state name of friend	Toddler or Preschooler
13. Speech is understandable to strangers	Toddler or Preschooler
14. Follows directions	Toddler or Preschooler
15. Shows sympathy when appropriate	Toddler or Preschooler
16. Points to a named part of the body	Toddler or Preschooler

17. Fill in the blanks related to the physiological changes associated with late adulthood.

Blood pressure rises as blood vessels (a) _____, (b) _____ resistance increases, and

(c) _____ sensitivity decreases. Blood flow to organs (d) _____. Increased workload

on the heart causes (e) _____, changes in the mitral and aortic (f) _____,

and decreased (g) _____ elasticity. The number of pacemaker cells in the heart (h) _____,

resulting in (i) _____. Blood volume, red blood cells, and platelet count (j) _____.

Lung function and lung capacity (k) _____. Pain (l) _____ and reaction

(m) _____ decrease. Secretion of (n) _____ and gastric juices decreases. Intestinal

sphincters lose (o) _____. About 50% of the nephrons in the (p) _____ are lost.

18. List two causes of each of the following stressors that affect the older adult's lifestyle.
   a. Financial burdens:

_____

_____

   b. Physical and emotional challenges:

_____

_____

19. A heart rate of 140 beats per minute at rest would be considered normal for what age range?
   a. Newborn
   b. Preschool
   c. School age
   d. Toddler

20. Which of the following physiological changes occurs at birth?
   a. Ductus venosus dilates.
   b. Pulmonary vascular resistance decreases.
   c. Right ventricular pressure increases.
   d. Systemic vascular resistance decreases.

21. Which is true regarding the infant's respiratory system?
   a. Bones are the primary chest support.
   b. Body heat and fluids can be lost through respirations.
   c. The number of alveoli is close to the adult.
   d. Tracheal bifurcation occurs lower than the adult.

22. Which is a protective survival reflex in the infant?
   a. Babinski's
   b. Moro
   c. Palmar grasp
   d. Rooting

23. For which type of temperament might low intensity of reactions and a negative mood be observed?
   a. Difficult
   b. Easy
   c. Slow to warm up
   d. Temperamental

24. Which statement is true regarding the toddler?
   a. Hemoglobin approaches adult levels.
   b. Ear, nose, throat structures are similar to the adolescent.
   c. Passive immunity protects children of this age.
   d. Visual acuity averages 20/20.

25. Which parenting style tends to produce children who are responsible, assertive, and self-reliant?
   a. Authoritarian
   b. Authoritative
   c. Permissive
   d. Traditional

26. Which is true regarding the development of peer relationships in the toddler/preschool age group? They are formed with others _____.
   a. At the same age level
   b. Of same school age
   c. Who are adult caregivers
   d. Younger than they are

27. Which is true regarding the school-age child?
   a. Growth rates are faster than toddlers.
   b. Lymphatic tissue is small relative to adults.
   c. Primary tooth growth is beginning.
   d. Skull growth is 95% complete.
28. Conventional reasoning is a stage in which phase of the psychosocial development of a child?
   a. Moral
   b. Peer relationships
   c. Self-concept
   d. Self-esteem
29. What stimulates the release of hormones that initiate the physical changes of puberty in girls?
   a. Gonadotropin
   b. Follicle-stimulating hormone
   c. Luteinizing hormone
   d. Progesterone
30. Which is true regarding psychosocial issues in teenagers?
   a. Anorexia nervosa is a depressive disorder seen in this age group.
   b. Appearance is not a major concern for teens.
   c. Suicide is the leading cause of death in gay and lesbian teens.
   d. Depression rarely is seen in this age group.
31. On which developmental issue do early adults often focus?
   a. Losing weight
   b. Health concerns
   c. Retirement planning
   d. Selecting a mate
32. Which health-related concern is common in the middle-aged adult?
   a. Dementia
   b. Diverticulitis
   c. Hypercholesterolemia
   d. Stroke

WRAP IT UP

You find yourself in a difficult situation. You are the only paramedic on the rescue squad at the scene of a fire at a home day care and have been assigned to care for a group of children until the next ambulances arrive; ETA is 20 to 30 minutes. The caregiver, a 60-year-old woman, and one child sustained significant smoke inhalation and are being rushed to the hospital. You are left with four children: a 5-week-old infant, a 13-month-old boy, a 3-year-old girl, and a 5-year-old girl. The baby is sleeping quietly, and the other children are upset and crying. You manage quickly to obtain the following vital signs with the help of another firefighter:

5-week-old: BP 78/60 mm Hg, P 124/min, R 28/min, SaO$_2$ 99%
13 month-old: BP 80/64 mm Hg, P 120/min, R 28/min, SaO$_2$ 100%
3-year-old: BP 94/66 mm Hg, P 112/min, R 24/min, SaO$_2$ 98%
5-year-old: BP 96/68 mm Hg, P 104/min, R 20/min, SaO$_2$ 98%

When you examine the baby, you note that he is pink with a 1-second capillary refill and is using abdominal muscles to breath, and you can feel a soft diamond-shaped depression at the top of his skull that appears to pulsate with each heartbeat. When he awakens, he turns his face toward you and tries to suck when you stroke his cheek, but he does not cry or seem upset.

The 13-month-old wants nothing to do with you. He screams when you approach him and tries to run, but falls, striking his head on the corner of the bench on which you are seated. His abdomen is protruding, and you note that he has a wet diaper.

The 3-year-old is calmed by the time you try to examine her. She asks what happened to her caregiver, "mo-mo," and you explain that there was a fire and the smoke made her sick.

The 5-year-old girl is trying to be helpful, watching the younger children. She denies feeling sick or hurt and wants her parents to come. You explain that you will call them to come and get her as quickly as they can, but it may take a few minutes.

As you complete your exam, a bystander comes over and explains that she saw the smoke coming from the basement and ran in and got these kids from the family room upstairs where there was no smoke or fire. By then, the children's caregiver ran up the stairs from the basement with the other child and collapsed on the lawn. You continue to monitor the children until the ambulance arrives. In consultation with medical direction and the children's parents, it is decided to leave the children in the care of their parents with detailed follow-up instructions.

1. Place a check mark beside the age groups for which you were responsible on this call.
   a. _____ Newborn   d. _____ Toddler
   b. _____ Neonate   e. _____ Preschooler
   c. _____ Infant   f. _____ School age

2. Identify the abnormal findings that you encountered in each of the following children:
   a. 5-week-old

   _____

   _____

   b. 13-month-old

   _____

   _____

   c. 3-year-old

   _____

   _____

   d. 5-year-old

   _____

   _____

   _____

3. Which of the following is true regarding the 5-week-old child's behavior?
   a. He should have cried when he awoke and did not recognize you.

   _____

   _____

   b. He should be able to track your finger with his eyes.

   _____

   _____

   c. He should grasp your finger if you place it in his hand.

   _____

   _____

   d. He should be saying some single-syllable words.

   _____

   _____

CHAPTER 8 ANSWERS

REVIEW QUESTIONS

1. c

2. b

3. a

4. e

5. f

6. d
(Objective 1)

7. e
(Objective 1)

8. g
(Objective 1)

9. a
(Objective 1)

10. b
(Objective 1)

11. c
(Objective 1)

12. Preschooler
(Objective 2)

13. Preschooler
(Objective 2)

14. Toddler
(Objective 2)

15. Preschooler
(Objective 2)

16. Toddler
(Objective 2)

17. a. Thicken
(Objective 1)

   b. Peripheral
(Objective 1)

   c. Baroreceptor
(Objective 1)

   d. Decreases
(Objective 1)

e. Cardiomyopathy
(Objective 1)

f. Valves
(Objective 1)

g. Myocardial
(Objective 1)

h. Decreases
(Objective 1)

i. Dysrhythmias
(Objective 1)

j. Decrease
(Objective 1)

k. Decreases
(Objective 1)

l. Perception
(Objective 1)

m. Time
(Objective 1)

n. Saliva
(Objective 1)

o. Tone
(Objective 1)

p. Kidney
(Objective 1)

18. a. Reduced income at retirement; increased health care costs (insurance, drugs); costs of assisted living needs
(Objective 4)

b. Decreased mobility; disease processes; cognitive loss; death of a companion (Objective 4)

19. a. The heart rate for each of the other ages can increase to 140 beats/min during serious illness or injury.
(Objective 1)

20. b. The ductus venosus constricts, right ventricular pressure decreases, and systemic vascular resistance increases at birth.
(Objective 1)

21. c. The bones are not fully formed, and so muscles provide much support to the chest. The infant has significantly fewer alveoli than the adult. The tracheal bifurcation is higher in the infant.
(Objective 1)

22. d. Rooting reflex allows the baby to move toward food.
(Objective 1)

23. c. Easy children are characterized by regularity of body functions and acceptance of new situations. Difficult children display intense reaction and withdrawal from new stimuli.
(Objective 2)

24. a. The ear, nose, and throat structures are shorter and more susceptible to infection than the adolescent's. Passive immunity wanes early in infancy. Visual acuity is typically 20/30 in this age group.
(Objective 1)

25. b. Authoritarian parenting style tends to produce children who have low motivation and self-esteem. Children reared by permissive parents may be discontented, distrustful, and self-centered.
(Objective 3)

26. a. Peer relationships are formed with children near the same age and level of maturity.
(Objective 2)

27. d. Growth rates are slower than infants and toddlers. Lymphatic tissue is larger relative to adults until about age 10. Primary teeth are lost, and replacement with permanent teeth begins.
(Objective 1)

28. a. One theory of moral development lists three stages: preconventional reasoning, conventional reasoning, and postconventional reasoning. Self-concept, self-esteem, and peer relationships are also critical in the development of children.
(Objective 2)

29. b. Gonadotropin is released from the hypothalamus and subsequently stimulates the release of luteinizing and follicle-stimulating hormones from the pituitary. These in turn stimulate the release of progesterone (breast development and menstrual cycle) and estrogen (female secondary sex characteristics).
(Objective 1)

30. c. Suicide is the third leading cause of death for teens 15 to 19, but gay and lesbian teens are 2 to 3 times more likely to attempt suicide. Anorexia nervosa is an eating disorder. Depression is common. Appearance is important to teens.
(Objective 1)

31. d. Other key issues in this age group include rearing children, managing a home, finding a social group, leisure activities, and selecting a stable occupation.
(Objective 2)

32. c. Dementia, diverticulitis, and stroke can occur in this age group but are much more common in older adults.
(Objective 2)

WRAP IT UP

1. c, d, e, f
(Objective 1)

2. No abnormal findings were identified in any of the children.
(Objectives 1 and 2)

3. c. This is known as the palmar grasp reflex.
(Objective 1)

PART THREE

Therapeutic Communications

READING ASSIGNMENT
Chapter 9, pages 214-225 in *Mosby's Paramedic Textbook,* ed. 3

OBJECTIVES
1. Define therapeutic communication.
2. List the elements of effective therapeutic communication.
3. Identify internal factors that influence effective communication.
4. Identify external factors that influence effective communication.
5. Explain the elements of an effective patient interview.
6. Summarize strategies for gathering appropriate patient information.
7. Discuss methods of assessing the individual's mental status during the patient interview.
8. Describe ways the paramedic can improve communication with a variety of patients. Such patients include (1) those who are unmotivated to talk; (2) hostile patients; (3) children; (4) older adults; (5) hearing-impaired patients; (6) blind patients; (7) patients under the influence of drugs or alcohol; (8) sexually aggressive patients; and (9) patients whose cultural traditions are different from those of the paramedic.

SUMMARY
- Therapeutic communication is a planned act. It is also a professional act. The paramedic, working with the patient, obtains information that is used to meet patient care goals.
- Communication is a dynamic process. It has six elements: the source, encoding, the message, decoding, the receiver, and feedback.
- To effectively communicate with patients, paramedics must genuinely like people. They must be able to empathize with others. They also must have the ability to listen.
- Good communication calls for a favorable physical environment. Factors such as privacy, interruption, eye contact, and personal dress are external influences. These factors can be controlled. This allows the paramedic to better communicate with the patient.
- The patient interview often decides the direction of the physical examination. Good care means that the paramedic sees each patient as an individual. It also means that the patient's needs are met in a caring, concerned, and receptive way.
- Open-ended and closed (direct) questions can be used to get information from the patient. Techniques include resistance, shifting focus, recognizing defense mechanisms, and distraction.

- The first step with any patient is to assess mental status. This can be done by observing the patient's appearance and level of consciousness. The paramedic also can look for normal or abnormal body movements. During normal conversation, the patient should be able to show clear thinking, a normal attention span, and the ability to concentrate on and understand the discussion. The patient's responses to the environment (i.e., affect) should be appropriate to the situation.
- Difficult interviews generally arise from four situations: (1) the patient's condition may affect the ability to speak; (2) the patient may fear talking because of psychological disorders, cultural differences, or age; (3) a cognitive impairment may be present; or (4) the patient may want to deceive the paramedic.

REVIEW QUESTIONS

Match the communication response in column II with the description in column I. Use each response only once.

Column I	Column II
1. _____ Making associations or implying a cause	a. Clarification
2. _____ Paraphrasing a patient's words	b. Confrontation
3. _____ Pausing for several moments	c. Empathy
4. _____ Reviewing with open-ended questions	d. Explanation
5. _____ Having the patient rephrase a word	e. Interpretation
6. _____ Providing information	f. Reflection
7. _____ Refocusing on one aspect of the interview	g. Silence
	h. Summary

8. Identify selected elements of the communication process in the following example:

You tell your patient that you plan to take his temperature. He says, "Where are you going to take it to?" You clarify that you are going to put a thermometer under his tongue to see whether he has a fever.
   a. Who is the source?
   b. Who did the encoding in the initial message?
   c. Was the decoding effective?
   d. Who was the receiver?
   e. Why was feedback needed?

9. You are caring for a patient who is very emotionally upset. List six actions you can use to convey that you are actively listening to the patient.

   a.

   b.

   c.

   d.

   e.

   f.

10. A patient was assaulted and is found in the midst of a large crowd. How can you control external factors to enable effective communication with this patient?

_____

_____

11. Rewrite the following questions into an open-ended format:

a. Do you feel bad?

_____

b. Does your chest hurt here?

_____

c. Did this problem start today?

_____

d. Are you taking any medicine on a daily basis?

_____

12. Can you identify the problem in each of the following statements if they were made by a paramedic?

a. I know you can't move your legs right now, but don't worry; everything will be just fine.

_____

b. You know you won't have this trouble breathing if you quit smoking.

_____

c. We believe your substernal chest pain may be causing an ischemic area in your myocardium that is going to result in myocardial infarction.

_____

d. Why didn't you take your blood pressure medicine?

_____

13. You are called to a residence for a woman who fell down the stairs. You begin your assessment and patient management, and by the time you get in the back of the ambulance, you realize that her injuries are not consistent with the mechanism of injury she describes. The patient is reluctant to give you much information, and you strongly suspect domestic violence was the cause of her injuries.

a. What reasons may this patient have for resistance regarding information?

_____

b. What statements might you make to begin to talk about this issue?

_____

c. If she tells you she was beaten up by her husband but doesn't want to leave him or have him arrested, how should you respond?

_____

14. You are called to a college dorm for an "overdose." As you arrive on the scene, the patient is walking toward you.

a. What is the first step in your mental status examination of this patient?

_____

b. As you begin your conversation with the patient, what observations will you make regarding mental status?

_____

15. For each of the following difficult situations, identify three strategies that you may use to attempt to communicate with the patient.
    a. A 72-year-old man has paralysis on the right side. He appears to be awake and alert, but he is not responding to your questions appropriately.

    _____

    b. You have been called to a jail to care for a patient who has expressed a wish to kill a number of people. He is sitting with his arms folded, and his voice is getting progressively louder.

    _____

16. Describe your approach when interviewing a 3-year-old and his father.

    _____

17. You are caring for a patient in the ambulance who makes inappropriate and sexually suggestive remarks. What should you do?

    _____

STUDENT SELF-ASSESSMENT

18. Which of the following best describes therapeutic communication?
    a. Verbal and nonverbal behavior that conveys a message
    b. Planned act to communicate and obtain information
    c. Spoken or written words to express ideas or feelings
    d. Decoding and encoding from a messenger to a receiver
19. When a message is put into an understandable format, it is considered which of the following?
    a. Decoded   c. Received
    b. Encoded   d. Sourced
20. When you try to see the situation from another person's point of view, you are demonstrating which of the following?
    a. Cultural imposition c. Ethnocentrism
    b. Empathy   d. Sympathy
21. Which of the following would convey a confident, open attitude during the patient interview in the prehospital setting?
    a. Speaking loudly and quickly
    b. Standing with your arms folded on your chest
    c. Looking into the patient's eyes as the patient speaks
    d. Not invading the patient's personal space
22. Which of the following would demonstrate an effective patient communication strategy?
    a. Beginning questions with "How"
    b. Demonstrating personal bias
    c. Interrupting to get to the point
    d. Using medical terminology
23. Which of the following is a normal finding during the mental status examination?
    a. The patient demonstrates long pauses and rapid shifts in conversation.
    b. The patient has an upright posture and is well groomed.
    c. You repeat questions several times before the patient understands you.
    d. The patient is trembling and clenching and unclenching the fists.
24. Which of the following is the most effective method for communicating with a hearing-impaired patient in the prehospital setting?
    a. Lipreading
    b. Sign language
    c. Whatever method the patient prefers
    d. Note writing

WRAP IT UP

You are working on LSV 4097 and are dispatched to a quiet residential neighborhood for an "unknown nature." The local police community officer meets you on the scene and says that he is worried about the resident. The officer has been working with the resident to improve his living conditions. A month ago, he found the 70-year-old patient living without electricity or running water. He was using the nearby creek for toileting, and he used candles to light his home. Currently the patient is living in a nearby community while trying to clean up his home. This morning a sore on his leg began to bleed, and he is unable to control the bleeding. You note a dirty, ulcerated wound that is red and swollen on the patient's lower leg. He tells you that he is diabetic and not to worry, he will take care of it. He then walks over to a dirty basin of water in the yard and begins to clean the wound with a dirty rag.

You take a short history and do a brief physical examination. You determine that the patient needs to be transported for care of his wound. His compliance with his diabetic medicines is questionable, and you are unsure how well his basic nutritional and hygiene needs are being met. The patient adamantly refuses transport; he is afraid he won't ever be able to come home. Your partner begins to argue with him, and the patient becomes progressively more angry and agitated.

1. What message were you trying to encode to the patient?

_____

2. What information did he decode from your message?

_____

3. What strategy do you think will be most successful for communicating with this patient?
   a. Empathy
   b. Pity
   c. Sympathy
   d. Threats
4. How can you show that you are listening effectively?
   a. Look for weak spots in his arguments that you can debate
   b. Prepare your answer while you listen so you can respond fast
   c. Try to ignore the body language, voice tone, and just listen to his words
   d. Summarize the patient's statements to clarify meaning if you are unsure
5. What are six techniques that you can use from the beginning of the patient interview to improve the chance for an effective patient encounter?
   a.
   b.
   c.
   d.
   e.
   f.
6. Which of the following statements would likely be most effective in this situation?
   a. "Living like this isn't healthy for a human being. You should find somewhere else to live. We need to take you to the hospital to get you to a cleaner place."
   b. "Why are you living in these conditions? Don't you know this isn't healthy?"
   c. "The impaired circulation secondary to your diabetes will prohibit normal mechanisms of healing, leading to possible sepsis. You need immediate medical interventions."
   d. "It looks as though you need some help to heal this wound. Let's take you to the doctor so you can get better quickly and get back to your work here at home."
7. Which of the statements in question 6 appear judgmental?

8. Which of the following would not be helpful in responding to this patient's anger?
   a. "I know you're angry because it seems as if we're telling you what to do. We would just like you to get some care for your wound so you can get home quickly."
   b. You ignore the patient's anger and continue more forcefully with your attempts to make him go to the hospital
   c. "It seems as though you're angry because you're worried you won't be able to come home if you go to the hospital. Our goal is just the opposite; we know how important your home is to you, and we want you to be healthy so you can stay here."
   d. "You seem really angry; can you tell us why? We'd like to be here to help you solve your problem."

The patient responds to your partner with a raised voice and tells him he has no business coming on his property and telling him what to do.

   After you calmly sit with the patient for a few minutes and clearly explain your concerns, as well as the actions the hospital may take to get the patient home quickly, he agrees to be transported for care.

CHAPTER 9 ANSWERS

REVIEW QUESTIONS

1. e
2. f
3. g
4. h
5. a
6. d
7. b

8. a. You (the paramedic) are the source.
   b. You did the encoding.
   c. No, the patient did not interpret the message in an appropriate manner.
   d. The patient was the receiver of the first message.
   e. Feedback was needed to clarify the message.
   (Objective 2)

9. a. Face the patient when he or she speaks.
   b. Maintain eye contact.
   c. Avoid crossing your legs or arms.
   d. Avoid distracting body movements.
   e. Nod in acknowledgment at appropriate times.
   f. Lean toward the patient.
   (Objective 3)

10. Move the patient into the ambulance as quickly as possible for more privacy. Try to avoid interruptions until the interview is finished.
    (Objective 4)

11. a. "How do you feel?"
    b. "Describe (or show me) where your chest hurts."
    c. "Tell me when this problem began."
    d. "What medicines do you take on a daily basis?"
    (Objective 5)

12. a. You shouldn't offer false reassurance.
    b. Showing disapproval and offering unsolicited advice impair effective communication.
    c. Using professional jargon impairs the patient's ability to understand you.
    d. "Why" questions may be viewed as accusations.
    (Objective 5)

13. a. Her resistance may be related to personal pride, fear of loss of self-esteem, or fear of retribution.
    b. Shifting the focus temporarily to her injuries and making statements such as, "I've seen this pattern of injuries before in women who have been hurt by their husbands or boyfriends," may allow her to respond to your comments.
    c. Explain that you recognize she is in a dangerous situation and that you are worried about her. Then give her some information about social service agencies that can provide support or help if she changes her mind later. Report your observations to the hospital staff.
    (Objective 6)

14. a. Observe the patient's appearance, level of consciousness, and gait. Note how he or she is dressed and groomed. Look for any defensive or aggressive postures.
b. Talk to the patient to see if he or she is oriented to person, place, and time. Note the quality of speech and the ability to think clearly, maintain a normal attention span, and concentrate on the discussion.
(Objective 7)

15. a. Consider whether the patient's present illness or a preexisting condition may prevent him from speaking. Tell him that you are there to help. Question family members. See whether the patient can nod to answer questions if he is unable to respond verbally.
b. Make sure you are positioned close to an exit and that law enforcement officers are close by. Try to use normal interviewing techniques. Set limits. Follow protocols for restraint if the patient's behavior becomes violent.
(Objective 8)

16. Ask the father questions first. Offer a distraction to the child and gradually approach and start talking to him. Speak at eye level in a calm, quiet voice. Use short sentences with concrete explanations.
(Objective 8)

17. Inform the patient of your professional role and the inappropriate nature of the comments. Document the situation; if possible, have another caregiver ride in the patient compartment with you.
(Objective 8)

18. b. Each of the other answers describes communication. Therapeutic communication is a planned, deliberate act that uses specific techniques to build a positive relationship and share information to achieve goals for the patient.
(Objective 1)

19. b. Decoding involves interpretation of a message.
(Objective 2)

20. b. *Cultural imposition* means to impose your beliefs or values on people from other cultures. *Ethnocentrism* is viewing your own life as the most acceptable, the best, or superior to others. *Sympathy* is the expression of your feelings about another person's predicament.
(Objective 3)

21. c. Folding your arms may indicate a closed, defensive feeling. Although you need to be aware of a patient's personal space, in the prehospital setting you need to make close contact on most calls to perform an effective examination.
(Objective 5)

22. a. Demonstrating personal bias that leads the patient in an unwanted direction can hamper communications. Interruptions occasionally may be necessary if a life-threatening condition exists, but a more appropriate action is to allow the patient to proceed uninterrupted. Excessive use of medical terminology with patients may impair their ability to understand you.
(Objective 5)

23. b. This observation is just one clue in the examination. All other choices reflect possible abnormal mental status exams.
(Objective 7)

24. c. The paramedic's abilities (regarding sign language) and the circumstances of the call determine which method can be used. Whenever possible, the method that the patient chooses should be used.
(Objective 8)

WRAP IT UP

1. You are trying to encode a message that the patient has a specific medical problem that needs to be cared for in the hospital.
(Objective 2)

2. The message he has decoded tells him that your efforts to get him to go to the hospital will mean that he may never come home again.
(Objective 2)

3. a. Telling the patient that you understand his fear and then clarifying the issues may be effective.
(Objective 2)

4. d. You want him to know that you are listening carefully. You also want to make sure that you understand the meaning of his words.
(Objective 6)

5. Six strategies you can use include the following: face the patient; maintain eye contact; look attentive (don't cross your arms and legs); avoid distracting movements; nod to acknowledge important points; lean toward the speaker.

6. d. You want to use nonthreatening language and acknowledge the patient's chief concern about getting home.
(Objective 6)

7. Responses (a) and (b) sound very judgmental and may make the patient even more angry.
(Objective 6)

8. b. The other answers acknowledge the patient's emotions.
(Objective 6)

CHAPTER

10

History Taking

READING ASSIGNMENT

Chapter 10, pages 226-233, in *Mosby's Paramedic Textbook,* ed. 3.

OBJECTIVES

Upon completion of this chapter, the paramedic student will be able to:
1. Describe the purpose of effective history taking in prehospital patient care.
2. List components of the patient history as defined by the Department of Transportation.
3. Outline effective patient interviewing techniques to facilitate history taking.
4. Identify strategies to manage special challenges in obtaining a patient history.

SUMMARY

- Obtaining a patient history offers structure to the patient assessment. The history often sets priorities in patient care as well.
- Content of the patient history includes date and time, identifying data, source of referral, history, reliability, chief complaint, present illness, past medical history, and review of body systems.
- The paramedic should ensure patient comfort. Several methods are available to accomplish this. The paramedic should avoid entering the patient's personal space. Sensitivity to the patient's feelings and watching for signs of uneasiness also are important. The paramedic should use appropriate language and ask open-ended and direct questions. The paramedic should use therapeutic communications techniques as well.
- Many challenges can affect history taking. One of these challenges is silent or talkative patients. Another is patients with multiple symptoms. Then there are anxious, angry, or hostile patients. The paramedic also may see intoxication, crying, depression, and sexually attractive or seductive patients. False reassurance is a major issue to consider. Patient may present confusing behaviors and histories. Two other issues are developmental disabilities and communication barriers. With these last two, the issue of talking with family and friends can be complex as well.

REVIEW QUESTIONS

Questions 1 and 2 pertain to the following case study:

> You are dispatched to a home to care for a 75-year-old woman who is having chest pain.

1. What additional questions will you need to ask related to her history?

   a. Present illness:

b. Significant medical history:

_____

c. Personal habits and environmental conditions:

_____

d. Family history:

_____

2. What is her chief complaint?

3. Your elderly patient fell and has a painful wrist. Discuss any finding in each of the following elements of the SAMPLE history that may explain a reason for her fall.

   S—

   A—

   M—

   P—

   L—

   E—

4. For each of the following patient complaints, list any personal habits and environmental conditions that are important to know during the patient history:

   a. A 4-year-old child awakens suddenly with a sore throat, fever, muffled voice, dysphagia, and pain on swallowing:

   _____

   b. A 25-year-old soldier complains of fever, night sweats, weight loss, and hemoptysis:

   _____

   c. A 40-year-old is injured in a motor vehicle collision:

   _____

   d. An 18-year-old woman is complaining of abdominal pain:

   _____

   e. A 72-year-old has slurred speech:

   _____

   f. A 45-year-old is complaining of depression:

   _____

   g. A 27-year-old has a heart rate of 50 beats/min:

   _____

   h. A 77-year-old is dirty and has bruises in various stages of healing on the back and arms:

   _____

i. A 16-year-old is extremely thin and frail looking:

_____

5. Describe one technique to use when dealing with each of the following situations during the patient interview:

   a. Your elderly patient clearly is distraught and has a lengthy pause in his conversation as he relates a painful story to you:

_____

   b. The patient begins a long and complex history in much more detail than necessary:

_____

   c. Within the first 60 seconds of your interview, your patient has related at least five different problems of varying severity:

_____

   d. The patient is trembling and tearful despite a relatively minor injury:

_____

   e. The patient asks you to tell her everything will be all right, when you know her condition is critical, and perhaps even lethal:

_____

   f. A patient is verbally venting his anger and frustration about his illness:

_____

   g. The patient strokes your leg in a sexually suggestive manner:

_____

   h. The patient does not speak or understand your language:

_____

STUDENT SELF-ASSESSMENT

6. What is the purpose of obtaining a patient history?
   a. To obtain billing information
   b. To detect signs of injury
   c. To establish priorities of patient care
   d. To make the patient comfortable
7. Which of the following is a routine component of the patient history?
   a. Age   **c.** Religion
   b. Insurance information   **d.** Vital signs
8. Which of the following is true regarding the chief complaint in the patient history?
   a. It is always stated by the patient.
   b. It is usually the reason that emergency medical services was called.
   c. It includes significant medical history.
   d. It will remain the same throughout the call.

9. What might be a good question to ask while taking the history of present illness for a patient who is experiencing difficulty breathing?
   a. Did it start today?
   b. Is your difficulty breathing pretty bad?
   c. Where is your difficulty breathing?
   d. What makes your breathing better or worse?
10. Your patient is complaining of headache and chest tightness after an exposure to an unknown gas at work. What personal habits should you ask about for this patient?
   a. Exercise
   b. Immunizations
   c. Sleep patterns
   d. Smoking history
11. You plan to administer ketorolac tromethamine (Toradol) to a patient. You will not give it if your patient reports anaphylactic reaction to which drug?
   a. Acetaminophen (Tylenol)
   b. Aspirin
   c. Meperidine (Demerol)
   d. Penicillin
12. In which of the following situations is determination of last oral intake important?
   a. An adult with a corneal abrasion
   b. An adult with a small laceration on the forearm
   c. An adult with dizziness
   d. An adult with shoulder pain
13. Which of the following illnesses is not hereditary?
   a. Diabetes
   b. Kidney disease
   c. Sickle cell anemia
   d. Tuberculosis
14. You are called to care for a patient who is very depressed. Which statement may be most helpful?
   a. "Don't worry, we'll take good care of you."
   b. "Everything will be okay when we get you to the hospital."
   c. "My friend was depressed, and he's just fine now."
   d. "It seems as though you are really sad. I'm here to listen."
15. What is a good approach when you are managing the angry or intoxicated patient who does not pose an immediate danger to self or the emergency medical services crew?
   a. Physical restraint
   b. Set limits
   c. Threaten
   d. Yell
16. When interviewing the patient who has developmental delays, you should do which of the following?
   a. Clarify answers.
   b. Not ask the patient.
   c. Omit most questions.
   d. Speak loudly.

WRAP IT UP

At 0900 on a warm spring morning, you are dispatched to a call for "chest pain." On arrival you find a 45-year-old black woman who is complaining of diffuse chest and abdominal pain. She is pale, cool, and diaphoretic. Her husband called you because he was concerned when she said she was too ill to go to work at her law firm, which she had never done before. She is conscious, alert, and oriented and tells you that this began about an hour ago. She is unable specifically to describe the pain but says it is a gnawing sensation sometimes in her chest and left shoulder, and other times in the left lower quadrant of her abdomen. She is nauseated as well. Nothing seems to make the pain change in severity (rated as a 5 to 7), character, or location. She says she is normally healthy, takes Humulin 70/30 insulin for her diabetes, which she was diagnosed with at the age of 6 years. She indicates that she has taken her insulin, has eaten her regular breakfast, and had a normal dinner last evening. Just before your arrival, she says her blood sugar was 80 mg/dL, a normal value for her at this time of day. Her allergies include aspirin and shellfish. She reports no trauma, major surgeries, or hospitalizations since her initial diagnosis of diabetes. She has not traveled recently nor had any occupational exposures to anything unusual. She has two teenage children and is premenopausal with irregular periods (last period 5 weeks ago) and uses rhythm method for birth control. A normal bowel movement was reported this morning. Her parents are both deceased: her father died of an abdominal aneurysm at 48 and her mother of a heart attack at 45 years of age. Vital signs are BP 98/58, P 110, and R 24/min; oxygen saturation is 93%; blood glucose 82 mg/dL; and her electrocardiogram shows a sinus tachycardia. Her physical exam reveals some mild tenderness in the abdomen not specifically localized. Peripheral pulses are weak in all extremities. You apply oxygen at 4 L/min by nasal cannula, initiate an IV of normal saline TKO, and begin transport to the hospital while continuing to monitor the patient's vital signs and level of pain.

1. Which of the following illnesses is a possibility based on the history that she has given to you? List the reasons for your response.

Illness	Yes	No	Reasons (Family History, Signs and Symptoms, Medications)
a. Myocardial infarction			
b. Stroke			
c. Appendicitis			
d. Ectopic pregnancy			
e. Abdominal aortic aneurysm			
f. Urinary tract infection			
g. Gastroenteritis			
h. Hypoglycemia			

2. What could be the significance of neglecting to ask about the following?
   a. Allergies
   b. Menstrual history
   c. Family history

3. Why might the patient be reluctant to call 911 with her history and symptoms?

4. What can you say to the patient if she wants to know what is wrong with her?

CHAPTER 10 ANSWERS

HISTORY TAKING

1. a. Does anything make the pain better or worse? What does the pain feel like? Show me where the pain is. Does it go anywhere else? On a scale of 1 to 10, with 1 being the least and 10 being the worst, where do you rate your pain? When did you first notice your pain?

   b. How is your health in general? Have you been hospitalized for any major illness or injury? Are you having any other signs or symptoms today (difficulty breathing, nausea, vomiting, dizziness, or palpitations)? Do you have any allergies? What medicines do you take? Have you taken anything today? What significant medical history do you have (heart disease, lung disease, high blood pressure, diabetes)? When did you last eat? Was it anything unusual? What were you doing when you first noticed this pain?

   c. Do you smoke? Do you use alcohol or any other drugs?

   d. Are your parents living? Do (Did) they have any heart disease or other major medical problems?
   (Objective 3)

2. Chest pain
   (Objective 2)

3. S—Does the patient have any associated signs or symptoms that may suggest a cardiac or other medical reason for the fall?

   A—Allergies or allergic reactions are unlikely to explain a fall unless the patient becomes hypotensive because of anaphylaxis, loses consciousness, and then falls.

   M—Some daily medicines can cause hypotension (especially orthostatic hypotension) that could lead to a fall. Other sedative, hypnotic, and psychotropic drugs may impair judgment or level of consciousness and predispose a person to a fall. Medications also can suggest preexisting medical conditions such as diabetes, heart disease, or neurological illness that may cause a fall.

   P—Pertinent past medical history may include factors such as heart disease (dysrhythmias), neurological disease (stroke with neurological deficit), diabetes (hypoglycemia), recent surgery, and other conditions that could alter balance, judgment, or consciousness and cause a fall.

   L—If the last meal was not timed correctly and the patient is diabetic or hypoglycemic, a fall could result.

   E—Did the patient have chest pain, visual disturbances, dizziness, palpitations, or any medical reason that could have caused the fall?
   (Objective 3)

4. You should ask about the following:

   a. Immunizations

   b. Tobacco use, alcohol use, screening tests (for tuberculosis), immunizations, home situation, exposure to contagious diseases, travel to other countries

   c. Alcohol or other drugs, use of safety measures (restraint devices)

   d. Diet, exercise, sexual history (possibly physical abuse)

   e. Alcohol and other drugs

   f. Alcohol and other drug use, sleep patterns, home situation, significant other (abuse or violence), sexual history, daily life, patient outlook, and economic condition

   g. Alcohol, drugs, and related substances, exercise and leisure activities

   h. Tobacco use, alcohol, other drugs and related substances, diet, home situation and significant other, physical abuse or violence, daily life, housing, and economic condition

   i. Tobacco use, alcohol, other drugs and related substances, sleep patterns, diet and exercise, and leisure activities
   (Objective 3)

5. a. Remain attentive and listen. Reflect on some of the emotions you sense the patient may be experiencing.

   b. Let the patient talk for a few minutes. Summarize his comments.

   c. Summarize the comments, and ask the patient to select the most pressing ones on which to focus in your examination.

d. Remain calm and caring, and reassure the patient.

e. Reassure the patient that you are listening to her fears, that you are there to care for her, and that you understand her condition.

f. Remain calm and set limits about ways he can express his feelings in an appropriate manner. Be alert for signs of escalation so you can maintain the safety of the patient, yourself, and your crew.

g. Be clear that you are in a caring role and you feel the behavior is unacceptable. If it persists, consider trading roles with your partner if appropriate.

h. Determine whether a family member can translate, or use a translating resource if available.
(Objective 4)

6. c. The history can provide structure and guidance during the physical examination, where you hope to find signs of the illness or injury.
(Objective 1)

7. a. Vital signs are part of the physical assessment.
(Objective 2)

8. b. The patient often states the chief complaint but may not be able to do so if he or she is unconscious. Obtain the medical history after the chief complaint. It may change during the call if the patient's condition changes.
(Objective 3)

9. d. "Did the difficulty start today?" is not an open-ended question. A better way to ask about time of onset is, "Tell me when you noticed that you were having trouble breathing." Answer b. also is not an open-ended question. Asking about location is inappropriate with this chief complaint.
(Objective 3)

10. d. Lung function and laboratory values can be affected by smoking and are important information for this patient.
(Objective 3)

11. b. Allergy to other nonsteroidal antiinflammatory drugs also is a contraindication.
(Objective 3)

12. c. Lack of food intake could lead to hypoglycemia and dizziness.
(Objective 3)

13. d. Tuberculosis may be found in family members because of transmission by close contact.
(Objective 3)

14. d. Offering false reassurances does not benefit the patient.
(Objective 3)

15. b. Establish limits for acceptable behavior.
(Objective 4)

16. a. Use phrases and words that can be understood easily.
(Objective 4)

WRAP IT UP

1. a. Signs and symptoms of present illness, family history of myocardial infarction at early age, diabetes

b. Signs and symptoms do not suggest stroke; however, diabetic and family history are strong for vascular disease.

c. Signs and symptoms vaguely suggest an abdominal condition that may require emergency surgery but may be masked by patient's diabetic history.

d. Ectopic pregnancy is a possible: irregular periods, high-risk birth control method, abdominal pain with radiation to shoulder.

e. Abdominal aneurysm is a possibility based on family history, race (but male sex would be higher risk), weak pulses, diabetes.

f. Urinary tract infection is a high risk in diabetic patients, but you have no report of urinary frequency. Dysuria could be masked by diabetes.

g. Gastroenteritis: mild abdominal symptoms, nausea but no vomiting, no diarrhea reported
(Objective 1)

h. Hypoglycemia: the patient's blood glucose is within the normal range. She does not appear to have other signs or symptoms of hypoglycemia (except tachycardia)

2. a. If myocardial infarction was suspected and aspirin was given without knowledge of the patient's allergy to it, a severe allergic reaction could occur.

b. If a menstrual history was not obtained, the possibility of pregnancy and ectopic pregnancy might not be considered. Patient could have received radiographs and medications harmful to early fetal development, or the possibility of life-threatening ectopic pregnancy might not be considered.

c. The family history is strongly suggestive of two lethal vascular diseases: myocardial infarction and aortic aneurysm. Without the knowledge of this, certain diagnostic tests could be overlooked and the diagnosis missed.
(Objective 1)

3. The patient may be reluctant to call because of fear or denial of illness.
(Objective 4)

4. Tell her your concerns based on her symptoms, history, and physical findings, and explain that further diagnostic tests only available at the hospital will be needed to pinpoint the specific nature of her problem.
(Objective 3)

Techniques of Physical Examination

READING ASSIGNMENT
Chapter 11, pages 234-279, in *Mosby's Paramedic Textbook,* ed. 3

OBJECTIVES
Upon completion of this chapter, the paramedic student will be able to:
1. Describe physical examination techniques commonly used in the prehospital setting.
2. Describe the examination equipment commonly used in the prehospital setting.
3. Describe the general approach to physical examination.
4. Outline the steps of a comprehensive physical examination.
5. Detail the components of the mental status examination.
6. Distinguish between normal and abnormal findings in the mental status examination.
7. Outline the steps in the general patient survey.
8. Distinguish between normal and abnormal findings in the general patient survey.
9. Describe physical examination techniques used for assessment of specific body regions.
10. Distinguish between normal and abnormal findings when assessing specific body regions.
11. State modifications to the physical examination that are necessary when assessing children.
12. State modifications to the physical examination that are necessary when assessing the older adult.

SUMMARY
- The examination techniques commonly used in the physical examination are inspection, palpation, percussion, and auscultation.
- Equipment used during the comprehensive physical examination includes the stethoscope, ophthalmoscope, otoscope, and blood pressure cuff.
- The physical examination is performed in a systematic manner. The exam is a step-by-step process. Emphasis is placed on the patient's present illness and chief complaint.
- The physical examination is a systematic assessment of the body that includes mental status, general survey, vital signs, skin, head, eyes, ears, nose, throat, chest, abdomen, posterior body, extremities, and neurological examination.
- The first step in any patient care encounter is to note the patient's appearance and behavior. This includes assessing for level of consciousness. This may include assessment of posture, gait, and motor activity; dress, grooming, hygiene, and breath or body odors; facial expression; mood, affect, and relation to person and things; speech and language; thought and perceptions; and memory and attention.

- During the general survey, the paramedic should evaluate the patient for signs of distress, apparent state of health, skin color and obvious lesions, height and build, sexual development, and weight. The paramedic also should assess vital signs.
- The comprehensive physical examination should include an evaluation of the texture and turgor of the skin, hair, and fingernails and toenails.
- Examination of the structures of the head and neck involves inspection, palpation, and auscultation.
- A full knowledge of the structure of the thoracic cage is needed. This knowledge aids in performing a good respiratory and cardiac assessment. Air movement creates turbulence as it passes through the respiratory tree. Aire movement produces breath sounds during inhalation and exhalation. In the prehospital setting the paramedic must examine the heart indirectly. However, the paramedic can obtain details about the size and effectiveness of pumping action through a skilled assessment that includes palpation and auscultation.
- The four quadrants of the abdomen and their contents provide the basis for inspection, auscultation, percussion, and palpation of this body region.
- An examination of the genitalia of either sex can be awkward for the patient and the paramedic. The paramedic should inspect the genitalia for bleeding and signs of trauma (if indicated).
- Examination of the anus is indicated in the presence of rectal bleeding or trauma to the area.
- When examining the upper and lower extremities, the paramedic should direct his or her attention to function. The paramedic also should pay attention to structure.
- Assessment of the spine begins with a visual assessment of the cervical, thoracic, and lumbar curves. The assessment continues with a region-by-region examination for pain, swelling, and range of motion.
- A neurological examination may be organized into five categories: mental status and speech, cranial nerves, motor system, sensory system, and reflexes.
- When approaching the pediatric patient, the paramedic should remain calm and confident. The paramedic should observe the child before beginning the physical examination. The paramedic also should make sure to avoid separation of the child and parent. Moreover, the paramedic must establish a rapport with parents and child and must be honest. One caregiver should be assigned to the child.
- The paramedic should not assume that all older adults are victims of disorders related to aging. Individual differences in knowledge, mental reasoning, experience, and personality influence how these patients respond to examination.

REVIEW QUESTIONS

Match the sign in column II with its definition in column I. Use each answer only once.

Column I	Column II
1. _____ Persistent respiratory rate less than 12 breaths/min	**a.** Biot
	b. Bradypnea
2. _____ Normal breath sounds heard over most lung fields	**c.** Cheyne-Stokes
	d. Crackles
3. _____ Low-pitched, rumbling expiratory sounds	**e.** Rhonchi
4. _____ Crowing sound associated with upper airway narrowing	**f.** Stridor
	g. Vesicular
5. _____ Crescendo-decrescendo sequence of respirations followed by apnea	**h.** Wheezes
6. _____ Irregular respirations interrupted by apneic periods	
7. _____ End-inspiratory sounds associated with fluid in the small airways	
8. _____ High-pitched airway noise resulting from lower airway narrowing	

Match the term in column II with the appropriate statement in column I. Use each answer only once.

Column I

9. _____ The child with Down syndrome had a slanted opening between the upper and lower eyelids.
10. _____ The patient said the aliens were controlling him.
11. _____ Third-degree burns affect the skin's resiliency.
12. _____ Malnutrition had caused the man to be very thin.
13. _____ The older patient staggered when he tried to walk.
14. _____ The paralyzed patient had a persistent erection.
15. _____ A semicircle of blood is seen over the iris.
16. _____ The patient's cirrhosis made him look pregnant.
17. _____ After her stroke the woman had trouble making the muscles of her mouth form words.
18. _____ The alcoholic's wife told you that the history he gave you was untrue.

Column II

a. Affect
b. Ascites
c. Ataxia
d. Confabulation
e. Delusions
f. Dysarthria
g. Emaciated
h. Hyphema
i. Hypopyon
j. Macula
k. Palpebral fissures
l. Priapism
m. Turgor

19. Describe the correct method of performing each of the following patient assessment techniques:

   a. Inspection:

   _____

   b. Palpation:

   _____

   c. Auscultation:

   _____

20. For each of the following deviations from normal pupil response, list a cause:

Abnormality	Cause
a. Dilated/unresponsive	
b. Constricted/unresponsive	
c. Unequal/one dilated and unresponsive	
d. Dull/lackluster	

21. Your patient is a teenage assault victim who was struck repeatedly on the head with a baseball bat.

   a. List the 10 steps in the comprehensive physical examination.
      (1)
      (2)
      (3)
      (4)
      (5)
      (6)
      (7)
      (8)
      (9)
      (10)

b. List the components of the mental status examination for this patient.

_____

_____

_____

c. Describe your physical examination of this patient's head and neck, detailing specific examination techniques and the types of normal or abnormal findings you would look for (include ophthalmoscopic and otoscopic examination techniques).

_____

_____

_____

22. You are called to evaluate a patient whose chief complaint is difficulty breathing. Explain your assessment of the thorax.

_____

_____

23. Your 56-year-old patient has a history of right upper quadrant abdominal pain, malaise, nausea, and vomiting. He is jaundiced and complains of itching. Past history reveals heavy alcohol use. You suspect hepatitis. Describe your physical examination of this patient's abdomen.

_____

_____

24. You are examining a patient involved in a motor vehicle collision whose automobile was struck on the side. The patient complains of considerable pain in the pelvic area. The primary survey has been completed. The patient's pulse is elevated, but blood pressure is within normal limits. Describe your examination of this patient's pelvic area.

_____

_____

25. Your crew arrives at the home of an older patient whose family states that she complained of weakness on one side, stumbled, and fell down five steps. No life-threatening conditions are found in the primary survey, and vital sign assessment reveals a moderately elevated blood pressure and pulse. The patient is slightly confused but cooperative. You suspect a stroke. Describe your assessment of this patient's extremities.

_____

_____

26. A painter has fallen approximately 20 feet, striking a scaffold rail with his lower back. Primary survey and vital signs are normal. Outline your physical examination of this patient's back.

_____

_____

27. Provide the information that is missing in the following table, which outlines examination techniques for cranial nerves.

Cranial Nerve Number	Cranial Nerve Name	Assessment Technique
I		Test smell with ammonia inhalants
II		
	Optic	
III	Oculomotor	Test extraocular movements (EOMs) by asking the patient to look up and to the left and right, and diagonally up and down to down, the left and right
IV VI	Trochlear	
V		
	Facial	Note facial symmetry, tics, or abnormal movement; have patient raise eyebrows, frown, show upper and lower teeth, smile, and puff out cheeks; have patient close eyes tightly and resist while you try to open lids
VIII		
IX X		
	Spinal accessory	
XII		

28. List four general guidelines that are helpful when approaching a pediatric patient.

  a.

  b.

  c.

  d.

29. Describe two specific developmental differences that influence patient assessment for the children in each of the following age groups:

  a. Birth to 6 months:

  _____

  b. 7 months to 3 years:

  _____

  c. 4 to 10 years:

  _____

d. Adolescence:

---

30. Describe two special considerations and techniques that may be useful when caring for an older patient.

STUDENT SELF-ASSESSMENT

31. Auscultation is the examination technique that involves which of the following?
   a. Listening with a stethoscope
   b. Feeling for masses and assessing for crepitus
   c. Looking for signs of illness
   d. Tapping the body with your finger

32. Which instrument is used to evaluate the retina, macula, and optic nerve disc?
   a. Ophthalmoscope   **c.** Penlight
   b. Otoscope   **d.** Sphygmomanometer

33. Using an adult blood pressure cuff to evaluate a child's blood pressure can result in which of the following?
   a. False low reading   **c.** Normal reading
   b. False high reading   **d.** Inability to inflate cuff

34. What is the most important information to guide your physical examination of the patient?
   a. Medications and specific doses
   b. Past medical history
   c. Present illness and chief complaint
   d. Vital signs, including blood pressure

35. Which of the following is a component of the comprehensive physical examination?
   a. Chief complaint   **c.** Vascular access
   b. History of present illness   **d.** Vital signs

36. Which of the following is a component of the mental status examination?
   a. Distal pulses   **c.** Speech and language
   b. Pupil reaction   **d.** Visual acuity

37. Which of the following is the clearest way to report an altered level of consciousness?
   a. The patient is obtunded.
   b. The patient is semiconscious.
   c. The patient is stuporous.
   d. The patient is unresponsive to pain.

38. Patient memory and attention can be assessed with which of the following?
   a. AVPU method   **c.** General survey
   b. Digit span   **d.** Glasgow coma scale

39. Your patient walks with a limp. What is this known as?
   a. An abnormal gait   **c.** Bizarre posture
   b. Ataxia   **d.** Cranial nerve palsy

40. An odor of acetone on the breath is associated with which condition?
   a. Alcohol use   **c.** Diabetic conditions
   b. Bowel obstruction   **d.** Poor dental hygiene

41. A patient who tells you that he is very depressed and suicidal but has an expressionless face may be said to have which condition?
   a. Altered affect   **c.** Altered attention
   b. Altered appearance   **d.** Altered emotion

42. Which sign of distress may be found in a patient who has cardiorespiratory insufficiency, pain, or anxiety?
  a. Bradycardia
  b. Cough
  c. Sweating
  d. Wincing

43. Skin color is best assessed by observing the skin on what part of the body?
  a. Arms
  b. Face
  c. Legs
  d. Nail beds

44. When you are taking an axillary temperature using a standard mercury thermometer, what is the minimum time the thermometer should be in place to obtain an accurate temperature?
  a. 4 minutes
  b. 5 minutes
  c. 8 minutes
  d. 10 minutes

45. What is the proper sequence for examination of the abdomen?
  a. Auscultation, inspection, palpation
  b. Inspection, palpation, auscultation
  c. Inspection, auscultation, palpation
  d. Auscultation, palpation, inspection

46. Which of the following findings during examination of the nails is consistent with chronic respiratory or cardiac disease?
  a. Beau lines
  b. Clubbing
  c. Paronychia
  d. Terry nails

47. What should you do to verify that vision is present?
  a. Assess bilateral pupil response to light.
  b. Ask the patient to count fingers at a distance.
  c. Lightly touch the cornea with a cotton swab.
  d. Palpate the globe for firmness.

48. To perform an effective otoscopic examination of the ear, you should pull the ear in what direction?
  a. Down and back in adults
  b. Down and forward in adults
  c. Down and back in infants
  d. Down and forward in infants

49. What physical finding may be encountered in patients who are pregnant, have leukemia, or are taking phenytoin?
  a. Enlarged gums
  b. Nasal bleeding
  c. Swollen eyelids
  d. Tonsillar exudate

50. Chest wall diameter may be increased in patients with what condition?
  a. Heart disease
  b. Implanted cardiac pacemaker
  c. Obstructive pulmonary disease
  d. Rib fractures

51. Which sound may be heard during percussion if hyperinflation due to pulmonary disease, pneumothorax, or asthma is present?
  a. Dullness
  b. Flatness
  c. Resonance
  d. Hyperresonance

52. Which of the following is true regarding assessment of breath sounds?
  a. Normal breath sounds are louder on exhalation.
  b. The stethoscope bell is used to auscultate the lungs.
  c. The patient's mouth should be open.
  d. The patient should be in the supine position.

53. For maximal effectiveness, where should heart sounds be auscultated?
  a. Over the left anterior axillary line
  b. Over the left fifth intercostal space
  c. Over the sternal angle
  d. Over the xiphoid process

54. Simultaneous palpation of the apical and carotid pulses in which each apical beat is not transmitted is known as which of the following?
- **a.** Mean arterial pressure
- **b.** Pulse deficit
- **c.** Pulsus paradoxus
- **d.** Pulse pressure

55. All of the following may cause muffled heart sounds except which one?
- **a.** Cardiac tamponade
- **b.** Obesity
- **c.** Obstructive lung disease
- **d.** Myocardial infarction

56. What is a palpable tremor over a blood vessel called?
- **a.** Bruit
- **b.** Murmur
- **c.** Thrill
- **d.** Vibration

57. During the vascular examination, the anterior surface of the foot should be palpated to detect which pulse?
- **a.** Brachial pulse
- **b.** Dorsalis pedis pulse
- **c.** Popliteal pulse
- **d.** Posterior tibial pulse

58. If a deformity and point tenderness are noted on examination of the pelvis, what condition should you consider?
- **a.** Appendicitis
- **b.** Internal hemorrhage
- **c.** Ruptured ectopic pregnancy
- **d.** Spinal cord injury

59. To evaluate motor function in the lower extremities, you should instruct the patient to do what?
- **a.** Flex and extend the feet and lower and upper legs
- **b.** Lift and hold both legs in the air while lying supine
- **c.** Move the legs laterally as far as possible bilaterally
- **d.** Push the soles of the feet against the paramedic's palms

60. Which of the following is an example of a test to evaluate gait?
- **a.** Have the patient hop in place.
- **b.** Have the patient do the Romberg test.
- **c.** Have the patient touch each heel to the opposite shin.
- **d.** Have the patient touch the finger to the nose, alternating hands.

61. Your patient is a 2-year-old in respiratory distress. Level of consciousness, spontaneous movement, respiratory effort, and skin color can be most effectively evaluated when the child is in which position?
- **a.** Held by the paramedic
- **b.** Held by the parent
- **c.** On the stretcher
- **d.** Sitting in a chair

62. A young child has an obviously fractured lower leg. Which of the following statements is *false* regarding the care of this patient?
- **a.** Remain calm and confident.
- **b.** Separate the parents from the child.
- **c.** Establish rapport with the parents.
- **d.** Be honest with the child and parents.

63. Which of the following statements is *true* regarding the physical examination of a 2-year-old child?
- **a.** Abdominal breathing is normal in this age group.
- **b.** Patient modesty should be a primary concern.
- **c.** Explanations should be given for each activity.
- **d.** Separation anxiety will not be a problem.

64. When examining an older patient, what should you do?
- **a.** Always speak loudly, because most of these patients are deaf.
- **b.** Assume that memory impairment is present.
- **c.** Anticipate numerous health problems and medications.
- **d.** Not expect any variation in the examination.

WRAP IT UP

You are called to a small home for a "person fallen." You arrive on the scene and find an elderly man who has fallen and is lying naked, trapped between the toilet and the bathtub. He is awake but confused. He has cool skin and some injuries to his head and shoulders from trying to wriggle out of his confined space. His family tells you they couldn't get him on the phone for 24 hours so they came by this morning to see what was wrong. You find that he is wedged tightly and you are unable to free him, and a rescue unit is dispatched. They bring hand tools and carefully remove the commode without breaking it to avoid making sharp shards of porcelain that may injure your patient. You extricate him onto the back board after applying a cervical collar and move him to the ambulance. During the rescue your partner checks around the house, looking for medications, signs of drug or alcohol use, or anything unusual, but finds nothing.

The patient's vital signs are: BP 100/60, P 112 irregular, R 20. Oxygen saturation is not detected because of the coolness of the man's extremities, so you administer oxygen by nonrebreather mask at 12 L/min. Your thermometer reads a temp of 97.6° F (36.4° C). The patient's pupils are 4 mm, equal, round, and react to light. Inspection of his head reveals abraded areas where you suspect he was moving his head to free himself. You palpate no deformities or crepitus of the head or face. He follows commands and can move his eyes in the cardinal fields of gaze. There is no tenderness, swelling, or deformity around the nose or frontal or maxillary sinuses. His lips are pale and cracked, as is his tongue. The trachea is midline, neck veins are flat, and the patient denies pain to the posterior aspect of his neck. However, you do not ask him to move it because of your concern about spinal trauma. Inspection of the chest reveals some redness to the left posterior and lateral aspect in a linear fashion. There is considerable tenderness when those areas are palpated. Respiration excursion seems slightly shallow; breath sounds are clear but diminished in all fields. Heart sounds are auscultated with the patient supine, and a normal S1 and S2 are audible. Percussion of the abdomen reveals tympany and dullness in the appropriate locations. The patient winces when his abdomen is palpated but does not seem to be able to localize the pain. His liver and spleen are not palpable. His penis is flaccid, and there is no blood at the urinary meatus. His left shoulder has an abraded area that is tender, but no deformity or crepitus is noted. His hands, wrists, and arms appear to have normal range of motion, but the joints seem somewhat enlarged. Examination of the lower extremities is normal. Palpation of the spine is negative. The patient remains confused and unable to tell you what happened but is cooperative. You ask him to smile, and it exaggerates the facial droop that you noticed earlier in your exam. You also detect some slurring of his speech. Evaluation of muscle strength demonstrates some weakness in his right arm and leg. You initiate an IV TKO, determine that his blood glucose is 110 mg/dL, and monitor his vital signs en route to the hospital. He is later diagnosed with a stroke; however because of his fall and the unknown time of onset, he is not a candidate for fibrinolytic therapy. At the time of follow-up, he is in rehabilitation.

1. Why was it difficult to focus your physical exam on any one area on this patient?

---

2. Why was a temperature assessment indicated in this patient, even though he was found in the house?

---

3. How can you tell whether this patient's confusion is new or normal for him?

---

4. Put a ✔ by each area of the cranial nerve examination where an abnormality was detected and fill in the name of the nerve(s) listed.

Cranial Nerve Number	Cranial Nerve Name(s)
_____Cranial nerve I	
_____Cranial nerve II	
_____Cranial nerves II and III	
_____Cranial nerves III, IV, and VI	
_____Cranial nerve V	
_____Cranial nerve VII	
_____Cranial nerve VIII	
_____Cranial nerves IX and X	
_____Cranial nerve XI	
_____Cranial nerve XII	

5. Why were the liver and spleen not palpable?

_____

CHAPTER 11 ANSWERS

REVIEW QUESTIONS

1. b
2. g
3. e
4. f
5. c
6. a
7. d
8. h
9. k
10. e
11. m
12. g
13. c
14. l
15. h
16. b
17. f
18. d
    (Questions 1-18: Objective 10)

19. a. Observe the environment (scene), general patient appearance, and specific body regions to gather data. b. Use the palmar surface of the hands and fingers to feel for texture, mass, fluid, temperature, and crepitus in various body regions. c. Use a stethoscope or the unaided ear to assess sounds generated by the movement of air or gases within the body.
    (Objective 1)

20.

Abnormality	Cause
a. Dilated/unresponsive	Cardiac arrest, hypoxia, drug use or misuse
b. Constricted/ unresponsive	Injury or disease of the central nervous system, narcotic drug use, use of eye medications
c. Unequal/one dilated	Cerebrovascular accident, direct trauma to the eye, use of eye medications, use of an ocular prosthesis
d. Dull/lackluster	Shock or comatose states

(Objective 6)

21. a. (1) Mental status; (2) general survey; (3) vital signs; (4) skin; (5) head, eyes, ears, nose, and throat (HEENT); (6) chest; (7) abdomen; (8) posterior body; (9) extremities; (10) neurological examination.
    (Objective 7)

    b. Assess whether the patient is alert and responsive to touch and verbal and painful stimuli. Assess the patient's general appearance and behavior. Note verbal and motor responses. If the patient is ambulatory when you arrive, note posture, gait, and motor activity. Observe dress and hygiene and note any body odors, such as alcohol. Note facial expression and determine whether it is appropriate for the situation. Is the patient's affect appropriate for the situation? Is the speech understandable and moderately paced? Assess the quality, rate, loudness, and fluency of the patient's speech. Determine whether the patient has organized thoughts. Determine whether the patient is oriented to person, place, and time. Assess remote and recent memory.
    (Objective 5)

c. Inspect for shape and symmetry of the skull and facial bones. Note bleeding, trauma, deformity, or drainage around the face or from the ears or nose. Inspect the mouth for bleeding and loose or missing teeth. Observe for pupil response to light and assess to see whether the patient's vision is intact. Examine the conjunctiva and sclera by asking the patient to look up while both lower lids are depressed with the thumbs. Palpate the lower orbital rims to determine structural integrity. Use the ophthalmoscope to check the cornea for lacerations, abrasions, or foreign bodies; to check for hyphema in the anterior chamber; to assess the fundus; to see retinal vessels, the optic nerve, and retina; and to assess the vitreous. Palpate the scalp and face for deformities, swelling, indentations, or bleeding, noting pain or tenderness. Inspect the external ear for signs of bruising, deformity, or discoloration. Look for bleeding in the ear canal. Palpate the bones around the ear to see whether the patient feels discomfort. Look for discoloration on the mastoid process. Assess gross auditory acuity by covering one ear at a time and asking the patient to repeat short test words spoken in soft and loud tones. Pull the auricle up and back to perform the otoscopic examination and look at the eardrum. Before applying the cervical collar but while still maintaining cervical immobilization, inspect to ensure that the trachea is midline and note tracheal tugging or obvious symptoms of trauma. Palpate the anterior and posterior neck, noting pain, deformity, malalignment, or subcutaneous emphysema.
(Objective 9)

22. Inspect for chest shape, symmetry, expansion, and the use of accessory muscles. Note the rate, depth, and pattern of respirations. Palpate for tenderness, bulges, depressions, unusual movement, crepitus, and chest expansion. Place both thumbs on the xiphoid process with palms lying flat on the chest wall and palpate for symmetry. Assess the posterior chest wall by placing the thumbs along the spinous processes at the level of the tenth rib. Percuss the chest to detect resonance (normal), hyperresonance (hyperinflation), or dullness or flatness (fluid or pulmonary congestion). Auscultate bilaterally (anterior and posterior) with the patient upright if possible and ask the patient to breathe in and out slowly through the open mouth, noting diminished or adventitious sounds. Palpate the apical impulse. Auscultate the heart at the fifth intercostal space to note frequency, intensity, duration, and timing as well as abnormal sounds such as murmurs.
(Objective 9)

23. Inspect for symmetry, jaundice, or distention and look for surgical scars. Look for smooth movement of the abdomen during respiration. Auscultate all four quadrants for rumblings. Palpate for tenderness, masses, skin temperature, and rigidity and observe for guarding. Percuss all four quadrants of the abdomen to assess for tympany (normal over stomach and intestines) and dullness (over organs and solid masses). Percuss the liver by beginning just above the umbilicus in the right midclavicular line in an area of tympany. Continue in an upward direction until the change from tympany to dullness occurs (usually slightly below the costal margin, which indicates the upper border of the liver). During palpation of the liver the patient should be supine and relaxed. Stand on the patient's right side and place the left hand under the patient in the area of the eleventh and twelfth ribs. Place your right hand on the abdomen, with the fingers pointing toward the patient's head, resting just below the edge of the costal margin. As the patient exhales, press the hand under the patient upward while pushing your right hand gently in and up. If you can feel the liver, it should be firm and nontender. (A healthy adult liver usually cannot be palpated.)
(Objective 9)

24. Inspect for obvious trauma, deformity, symmetry, or bleeding, especially from the urethra. Place the hands on each anterior iliac crest and press down and out, noting movement or crepitus. Place the heel of the hand on the symphysis pubis and press down to determine stability. Palpate the femoral pulses.
(Objective 9)

25. For each extremity, inspect for position, deformity, and obvious signs of trauma, and compare the right extremity with the left. Palpate for structural integrity. Assess grips; have the patient push and pull the paramedic's hands against force, and have the patient push the feet against the opposing force of the paramedic's hands bilaterally to note muscle strength and tone. Assess distal pulse and sensation in all extremities.
(Objective 9)

26. Log roll patient with cervical immobilization. Inspect the neck for midline position. Inspect the back for signs of injury, swelling, discoloration, and open wounds. Palpate the spine, beginning at the neck and proceeding to the sacrum, noting point tenderness or deformity. Place the palm of your hand over the costovertebral angle and strike the hand with your fist, noting any painful reaction.
(Objective 9)

27.

Cranial Nerve Number(s)	Cranial Nerve Name(s)	Assessment Technique
I	Olfactory	Test smell with ammonia inhalants
II	Optic	Test for visual acuity
II	Optic	Inspect the size and shape of the pupils; assess the pupil's response to light
III	Oculomotor	Test EOMs by asking patient to look up and down, to the left and right, and diagonally up and down to the left and right
IV	Trochlear	
VI	Abducens	
V	Trigeminal	Ask patient to clench the teeth while you palpate the temporal and masseter muscles; touch the forehead, cheeks, and jaw to determine sensation
VII	Facial	Note facial symmetry, tics, or abnormal movement; have patient raise eyebrows, frown, show upper and lower teeth, smile, and puff out cheeks; have patient close eyes tightly and resist while you try to open lids
VIII	Acoustic	Assess hearing acuity
IX	Glossopharyngeal	See whether patient can swallow easily and produce saliva and normal voice sounds; ask patient to hold breath and then assess for slowing of the heart rate; test for gag reflex
X	Vagus	
XI	Spinal accessory	Ask patient to raise and lower shoulders and turn the head
XII	Hypoglossal	Ask patient to stick out the tongue and move it in several directions

28. Remain calm and confident; do not separate the parents and child unless absolutely necessary; establish rapport with the parents and child; be honest with the child and parents; if possible, assign one caregiver to stay with the child; observe the patient before the physical examination.
(Objective 11)

29. a. The child is not frightened, the child needs care to maintain body temperature, the child is in constant motion, the child is an abdominal breather, and the paramedic can use the fontanelles to assess overhydration and underhydration. b. Separation anxiety occurs, the child has a fear of strangers, and the paramedic should explain procedures in short sentences. c. The child has a capacity for rational thought, the child can provide a limited history, the paramedic should allow participation in care, the child has a limited understanding of the body, the child fears intrusion into private areas, and the paramedic must explain everything completely. d. The

teenager is concerned about body image and privacy is a major concern, the paramedic should treat the teenager like an adult, and the paramedic must consider sexually transmitted diseases, pregnancy, and drug and alcohol use.
(Objective 11)

30. The patient may have sensory loss that impairs communication, may experience memory loss and confusion, often has numerous health problems that require him or her to take a number of home medications, may have decreased sensory function that can conceal symptoms, and may have fears regarding hospitalization.
(Objective 12)

STUDENT SELF-ASSESSMENT

31. a. Inspection involves looking, palpating involves feeling the body, and selected body areas are tapped during percussion.
(Objective 1)

32. a. The otoscope is used for examining the ears, the penlight can be used to evaluate pupil response, and the sphygmomanometer is used to measure blood pressure.
(Objective 2)

33. a. Blood pressure cuffs that are too wide give a false low reading, and those that are too narrow give a false high reading.
(Objective 2)

34. c. Although all the other information is important, the chief complaint and history of the present illness guide the physical examination and allow the paramedic to focus on key areas.
(Objective 3)

35. d. Chief complaint and history of present illness are historical findings. Vascular access is an intervention.
(Objective 4)

36. c
(Objective 5)

37. d. The other terms are vague and may be interpreted in a variety of ways.
(Objective 3)

38. b. Ask the patient to count from 1 to 10 using only odd numbers. Asking the patient to count by serial sevens or spell a word backward also can be used.
(Objective 5)

39. a. *Ataxia* is a staggering gait, and postural imbalance is associated with central nervous system lesions. Cranial nerve palsy does not cause a limp.
(Objective 6)

40. c. Diabetic ketoacidosis is associated with an odor of acetone on the breath.
(Objective 6)

41. a
(Objective 6)

42. c. Tachycardia, not bradycardia, is a common trait for all three. Cough is not present with pain or anxiety. Wincing is not associated with cardiorespiratory insufficiency.
(Objective 8)

43. d. This area has less pigmentation, and pallor or cyanosis is easier to see.
(Objective 7)

44. d. Oral thermometers should be left in place for 4 to 6 minutes and rectal thermometers for 5 to 8 minutes.
(Objective 7)

45. c. Palpation of the abdomen may create sounds that falsely indicate normal bowel function when none exists.
(Objective 10)

46. b. *Beau lines* are transverse depressions in the nail that inhibit growth and are associated with systemic illness, severe infection, and nail injury. *Paronychia* is an inflammation of the skin at the base of the nail that may result from local infection or trauma. *Terry nails* are transverse white bands that cover the nail except for a narrow zone at the distal tip and are associated with cirrhosis.
(Objective 10)

47. b. Pupil response and corneal touch test the cranial nerves. Palpation of the globe is used to assess for dehydration.
(Objective 9)

48. c. For the adult examination, the auricle should be pulled gently up and back.
(Objective 9)

49. a. This also may be noted if the patient is going through puberty.
(Objective 9)

50. c. This barrel-shaped appearance develops because of air trapping.
(Objective 10)

51. d. Dullness or flatness is heard when fluid is present or pulmonary congestion has occurred. Resonance is usually heard over normal lungs.
(Objective 10)

52. c. Normal breath sounds are louder on inspiration. The diaphragm is used to auscultate the lungs. Ideally, the patient should be sitting if the condition permits.
(Objective 9)

53. b. Ideally, the patient should be sitting up and leaning slightly forward or should be in the left lateral recumbent position.
(Objective 9)

54. b. *Mean arterial pressure* is the diastolic pressure plus one third of the pulse pressure. *Pulsus paradoxus* is a fluctuation in the systolic blood pressure with respiration. *Pulse pressure* is the systolic blood pressure minus the diastolic blood pressure.
(Objective 10)

55. d
(Objective 10)

56. c. *Murmurs* are prolonged extra sounds auscultated with a stethoscope. A *bruit* is an abnormal sound audible over the carotid artery or an organ or gland. A thrill may feel like a tremor or vibration.
(Objective 9)

57. b. The brachial pulse is on the arm, the popliteal pulse is behind the knee, and the posterior tibial pulse is on the medial aspect of the ankle, behind the tibia.
(Objective 9)

58. b. Pelvic fractures are often accompanied by substantial hemorrhage.
(Objective 10)

59. d
(Objective 9)

60. a. Point-to-point movements are evaluated using the heel to shin and finger to nose tests. Stance and balance are tested with the Romberg test.
(Objective 9)

61. b. Anxiety is usually minimized while the child is in the parent's arms. This can minimize respiratory effort and distress and allow for a more effective assessment.
(Objective 11)

62. b. Anxiety can usually be decreased and cooperation increased if the parent and child remain together.
(Objective 11)

63. c
(Objective 11)

64. c. These numerous illnesses can confuse the clinical picture and complicate the paramedic's examination of the patient.
(Objective 12)

WRAP IT UP

1. No history was available, therefore it was unclear whether this was a medical, trauma, or combination call and where the exam should be focused.
(Objective 3)

2. Patients can become hypothermic or hyperthermic in their residence, especially with injury or severe illness.
(Objective 3)

3. Ask relatives and neighbors or call the office of the man's physician if you can find a name on a prescription bottle.
(Objective 3)

4. CN I—not tested—olfactory
CN II, III—normal—optic and oculomotor
CN III, IV, VI—normal—oculomotor, trochlear, abducens
CN V—not tested—trigeminal
CN VII—abnormal (facial droop)—facial
CN VIII—not tested—acoustic
CN IX, X—not tested—glossopharyngeal and vagus
CN XI—not tested—spinal accessory
CN XII—not tested—hypoglossal
(Objective 10)

5. The liver and spleen should not be palpable in a normal adult.
(Objective 10)

Patient Assessment

READING ASSIGNMENT
Chapter 12, pages 280-289, in *Mosby's Paramedic Textbook,* ed. 3

OBJECTIVES
Upon completion of this chapter, the paramedic student will be able to:
1. Identify the components of the scene size-up.
2. Identify the priorities in each component of patient assessment.
3. Outline the critical steps in initial patient assessment.
4. Describe findings in the initial assessment that may indicate a life-threatening condition.
5. Discuss interventions for life-threatening conditions that are identified in the initial assessment.
6. Identify the components of the focused history and physical examination for medical patients.
7. Identify the components of the focused history and physical examination for trauma patients.
8. List the components of the detailed physical examination.
9. Describe the ongoing assessment.
10. Distinguish priorities in the care of the medical versus trauma patient.

SUMMARY
- Sizing up the scene consists of the initial steps performed on every emergency medical services response. These steps help to ensure scene safety. They also provide valuable information to the paramedic.
- Patient assessment comprises five priorities: initial assessment, resuscitation, focused history and physical examination, detailed physical examination, and ongoing assessment.
- The initial assessment includes the paramedic's general impression of the patient, the assessment for life-threatening conditions, and the identification of priority patients requiring immediate care and transport.
- Assessment of life-threatening conditions entails a systematic evaluation of the patient's level of consciousness, airway, breathing, and circulation.
- The paramedic begins resuscitative measures such as airway maintenance, ventilatory assistance, and cardiopulmonary resuscitation immediately after recognizing the life-threatening condition that necessitates each respective maneuver.
- The focused history and physical examination for medical patients are dictated by the patient's overall condition and level of consciousness.
- The paramedic performs a focused history for a trauma patient to reconstruct the mechanism of injury. The paramedic should perform a rapid trauma examination on all patients with a significant mechanism of injury to identify life-threatening conditions.
- The detailed physical examination should be specific to the patient. The exam also should be specific to the injury. The exam should include an assessment of mental status, a general survey, a head-to-toe examination, and baseline vital signs.
- The ongoing assessment is a repeat of the initial assessment.

REVIEW QUESTIONS

Questions 1 to 15 pertain to the following case study:

You are dispatched from your base on a cold, snowy winter night to a motor vehicle crash with injuries on the highway.

1. After ensuring safety, list five priorities during your scene size-up/assessment on this call.

   a.

   b.

   c.

   d.

   e.

   You find one patient, the driver of a car involved in a single-car collision. He was not restrained and has been ejected about 15 feet from the car. You find him lying motionless in a safe location.

2. What are three goals of your initial assessment of this patient?

   a.

   b.

   c.

3. What information have you already gathered to form your general impression of this patient?

   _____

4. What mnemonic can you use to quickly assess his level of consciousness?

   _____

   As you approach the patient, you see some slight movement and note a gurgling sound in his mouth. He responds to pain only.

5. What could be causing gurgling in his airway?

   _____

   _____

6. What personal protective equipment should you be wearing?

   _____

   _____

7. What measures will you use to secure this patient's airway?

   _____

   _____

8. How should you evaluate his breathing?

   _____

   _____

The patient has a dusky color and slow, agonal respirations.

9. What care should you initiate based on this finding?

_____

_____

_____

10. What assessment techniques will you use in the initial assessment to evaluate circulatory status?

_____

_____

You palpate a rapid carotid pulse but _cannot_ detect a radial pulse. His skin is pale and cool, and capillary refill is slow.

11. What criteria for priority patients does this patient meet?

_____

_____

12. List the components of the focused history and physical examination that you will perform on this patient.

_____

_____

You note numerous facial lacerations and crepitus of the facial bones. He has an abrasion on the lateral chest and abdominal area. His left lower arm is deformed, and his left ankle is swollen.

13. What care should you provide before transport for this patient?

_____

14. What should be your goal for scene time on this type of call?

_____

15. Outline the components of the reassessment and the time interval at which they should be performed.

_____

Questions 16 to 20 pertain to the following case study:

You are dispatched to a home for a call of a patient with "difficulty breathing." Your initial scene assessment reveals no hazards, and you enter the patient's bedroom to begin your assessment and care.

16. What information will you gather as you enter the room that will help form your general impression of the patient?

_____

_____

The patient, an elderly black woman, is awake and appears to be in respiratory distress.

17. How will you further assess the following to determine her condition?

   a. Airway

_____

   b. Breathing

_____

   c. Circulation

_____

   You note that the patient is speaking in broken sentences because she must stop often to catch her breath. She has wheezes throughout her lungs and intercostal muscle retractions, and her mucous membranes and nail beds are blue. Her pulse is 124 (regular and strong in the radial artery), and her skin is damp.

18. List two criteria that she meets indicating that she is a priority patient who needs stabilization and rapid transport.

   a.

   b.

19. List four types of information you should gather in the focused history portion of this patient's examination.

   a.

   b.

   c.

   d.

20. How might the care of this patient differ from that given to a critically ill trauma patient?

_____

STUDENT SELF-ASSESSMENT

21. You arrive on the scene of a rollover motor vehicle crash involving a small sports car. Which of the following is a component in scene size-up/assessment on this call?
   a. Begin definitive patient care activities.
   b. Contact medical direction with an initial report.
   c. Initiate a mass casualty plan if indicated.
   d. Notify dispatch to send more resources if needed.

22. During which phase of the patient assessment will the first vital signs be assessed?
   a. Detailed physical examination   **c.** Initial assessment
   b. Focused physical examination   **d.** Ongoing assessment

23. During the initial assessment of a trauma patient, what is the most appropriate method to assess the neurological status?
   a. AVPU
   b. Determination of extraocular muscle function (EOM)
   c. Pupil assessment
   d. Reflex examination

24. Which of the following patient situations represents a life threat identified in the initial assessment of an adult?
   a. Blood pressure in the right arm is much greater than in the left arm.
   b. Heart rate increases by 30 beats/min when the patient stands up.
   c. Stridor is audible.
   d. Temperature is 105.8° F (41° C).

25. You detect that the patient has agonal respirations and a radial pulse during your initial assessment. How should your care and assessment proceed?

   a. Auscultate the chest to determine the proper intervention.

   b. Continue assessment and then manage respiratory failure.

   c. Initiate airway management and ventilation and then proceed.

   d. Treat the respiratory difficulty, and transport with no further examination.

26. What should be the primary determinant of the extent of the focused history and physical examination of the patient?

   a. Patient's overall condition and level of consciousness

   b. Age and preexisting illness

   c. Response time to the closest appropriate hospital

   d. Results of the initial vital sign assessment

27. You respond to a call to aid a person who has fallen 25 feet and is complaining of severe pain in the finger. Which of the following is a component of the focused history and physical examination for this patient?

   a. Continued spinal immobilization

   b. Detailed examination of the finger

   c. Initiation of intravenous fluid therapy

   d. Otoscopic examination of the eyes

28. In which of the following cases is the paramedic most likely to perform a detailed physical examination?

   a. A 2-year-old is acutely dyspneic and cyanotic.

   b. A pale 40-year-old was shot in the chest.

   c. A 59-year-old is weak and diaphoretic.

   d. A 67-year-old patient is in cardiac arrest.

29. What should be included in the ongoing assessment of a patient?

   a. Detailed physical examination

   b. Head-to-toe examination

   c. Repetition of the initial assessment

   d. Vital sign assessment only

30. _____ should *not* be included in the scene management of the critical trauma patient.

   a. Airway control   **c.** Major fracture stabilization

   b. Intravenous fluid therapy   **d.** Spinal immobilization

WRAP IT UP

You are dispatched to respond to a snowmobile collision. On arrival you find a 17-year-old boy who struck a boating dock submerged under the powdery snow while traveling at a high rate of speed. You don the appropriate protective gear and cautiously evaluate the ice conditions and then with great difficulty approach the patient through the waist deep snow. He was not wearing a helmet, and you recognize immediately that he has significant head and facial injuries. His eyes are closed, he is not arousable to voice, and his arms and legs extend when you apply painful stimulus. You radio dispatch and request a rescue unit to assist in extricating him across the snowy lake, and for a helicopter because it is clear that he will need transport to the regional trauma center, located 70 miles away. As you await the rescue, you apply a cervical collar and secure the patient to the long spine board. The patient has a gag reflex and adequate respirations, so you begin high-concentration oxygen administration. You can feel a slow, strong radial pulse, and his pupils are 4 mm, are equal, and react to light. You are unable to remove any of his clothing to perform further assessments because of the frigid conditions. You radio the rescue unit on the truck frequency and instruct them to prepare their stokes unit with sled skids and ask them to set up a landing zone on the road for the incoming helicopter. Dispatch updates you that the air unit has a 7-minute ETA, and you ask them to relay your patient's condition, which you continually reevaluate, to the flight crew. The patient is packaged onto the sled and pulled using a rope and winch to the shore where the flight crew is waiting. You give them a report and help them move the patient into their aircraft. They immediately perform rapid sequence intubation, and noting that one of his pupils is now dilated and nonreactive, begin to hyperventilate the patient. Eight minutes after you give them a report, they are in flight to the trauma center. Later you are told that the patient survived for 2 days in the ICU, was declared brain dead, and donated eyes, bone, skin, liver, heart, and lungs for transplantation.

1. What type of protective gear would be indicated for this situation?

_____

2. Why was it necessary to pause and check ice conditions before proceeding to the patient?

_____

3. What is your highest priority in the scene size-up and assessment?
   a. Forming a general impression
   b. Evaluating resources
   c. Initial patient assessment
   d. Scene safety determination

4. Why were resources called for before patient interventions began?

_____

5. What do you know about the patient's blood pressure?

_____

6. Why was an IV not established or rapid sequence intubation attempted before the patient was moved?

_____

7. Why was a detailed physical examination not performed initially on this patient?

_____

CHAPTER 12 ANSWERS

REVIEW QUESTIONS

1. a. Determine the mechanism of injury.
   b. Find out the number of persons injured.
   c. Determine the need for rescue or hazardous materials resources and request these from dispatch if needed.
   d. Determine the best access for responders you request.
   e. Secure the area, clearing unnecessary persons from the scene.
   (Objective 1)

2. a. Form a general impression of the patient.
   b. Assess for life-threatening conditions.
   c. Identify him as a patient who needs immediate care and transport.
   (Objective 2)

3. The patient is male; has been ejected from a vehicle (a mechanism that is associated with severe injuries); and is not moving, which may indicate severe injury with altered mental status (or death).
   (Objective 3)

4. AVPU (alert, responds to verbal, responds to pain, or unresponsive)
   (Objective 3)

5. Facial or oral bleeding, vomiting, partial obstruction with the tongue and mucus, facial fractures, soft tissue trauma to the face
   (Objective 4)

6. Goggles, mask, gloves, and possibly a gown
   (Objective 1)

7. Open the airway with a modified jaw thrust, suction the secretions, and insert an oral airway if the patient has no gag reflex.
   (Objective 5)

8. Assess the rate, depth, and symmetry of chest movement. Expose the chest wall, inspect for accessory muscle use, and palpate for structural integrity, tenderness, and crepitus. Auscultate for bilateral breath sounds.
   (Objective 4)

9. Begin to assist ventilation with bag-valve device and supplemental oxygen. Hyperventilate and intubate while maintaining in-line cervical immobilization.
   (Objective 5)

10. Assess radial and carotid pulse. Determine skin color, temperature, moisture, and capillary refill (although this determination is not likely to be reliable because of cold environmental conditions).
    (Objective 3)

11. He has a poor general impression and decreased level of consciousness, is unresponsive, has difficulty breathing, and is in shock (likely because of numerous injuries and mechanism of injury [ejection]).
    (Objectives 4 and 7)

12. Continue spinal immobilization and perform a mental status assessment. Inspect and palpate for injuries or signs of injuries of the head, neck, chest, abdomen, pelvis, and extremities. Logroll the patient, and inspect and palpate the posterior surfaces of the body. Obtain baseline vital signs. Determine a brief patient history if anyone is on the scene to provide it.
    (Objective 7)

13. Airway control, ventilation, and spinal immobilization (for spine and fracture immobilization) are first; intravenous therapy can be initiated during transport.
(Objective 10)

14. 10 minutes
(Objective 10)

15. Because the patient is unstable (a priority patient), mental status, airway, breathing, and circulation should be reevaluated at least every 5 minutes during care and transport of this patient.
(Objective 9)

16. You will assess the patient's approximate age, sex, and race; look for obvious injury or indications of medical conditions; note the patient's general level of distress; and ask for the chief complaint.
(Objectives 2 and 3)

17. a. Ask the patient to speak and listen for stridor or gurgling.
b. Evaluate the rate, depth, and symmetry of chest movement. Expose the chest and palpate, observing for respiratory use of the accessory muscles of the neck, chest, and abdomen. Auscultate for breath sounds. Observe for cyanosis, respiratory distress, and distended neck veins. Determine the need to assist ventilations.
c. Assess the patient's skin color, moisture, and temperature, and evaluate the pulse for quality, rate, and regularity.
(Objective 3)

18. a. Poor general impression
b. Difficulty breathing
(Objective 4)

19. a. Chief complaint
b. History of present illness
c. Medical history
d. Current health status
(Objective 6)

20. The priority with the trauma patient is to secure the airway while maintaining spinal immobilization, ventilate with high-flow oxygen, and initiate rapid transport for definitive care. This patient has a patent airway but needs oxygenation and possibly assisted ventilation if the condition deteriorates. Emergency vascular access and drug administration may improve her condition rapidly and may be initiated before transport.
(Objective 10)

21. d. Patient care activities typically begin after the initial scene size-up. Medical direction should be contacted later. A mass casualty incident is unlikely in this setting.
(Objective 1)

22. c. The vital signs should be reassessed during the ongoing assessment.
(Objective 2)

23. a. The other components of the neurological examination are performed later in the assessment.
(Objective 3)

24. c. All other findings are identified later in the examination.
(Objective 4)

25. c. The life threat must be addressed before the examination can proceed.
(Objective 4)

26. a. The speed and focus of the examination are determined rapidly by the condition of the patient as noted in the initial assessment.
(Objective 6)

27. a. Detailed examination can be performed later if no life threats are identified. Otoscopic examination of the eyes is not indicated in this phase of the examination.
(Objective 6)

28. c. In each of the other patients, care in the prehospital setting generally is directed to correction of the life threats.
(Objective 8)

29. c. This should be done every 15 minutes for stable (nonpriority) patients and at least every 5 minutes for unstable (priority) patients.
(Objective 9)

30. b. Intravenous fluid therapy should be initiated only on the scene if it will not delay transport. More often intravenous therapy can be started during transport.
(Objective 10)

WRAP IT UP

1. If this lake were considered a busy traffic way, a helmet and safety goggles would be indicated. A warm turnout coat with reflective strips, slip-resistant waterproof gloves, and boots with steel insoles and steel toe protection should be worn.
(Objective 2)

2. If the ice were unsafe in any part of the scene, it would be critical to know to prevent injury or death to the rescuers and patient.
(Objective 2)

3. d. Evaluation of scene safety throughout all calls is critical.
(Objective 2)

4. Additional resources often take significant time to deploy. Activating them as early as possible is critical to expedite care and rescue.
(Objective 2)

5. A strong radial pulse is palpable, so you can surmise that his systolic blood pressure is close to 80 mm Hg.
(Objective 4)

6. In unsafe situations and in cases of environmental extremes, it is often safer for the crew and the patient to initiate most care in the ambulance. That way proper assessments, visualization, and access can be obtained safely.
(Objective 5)

7. Patient clothing would prevent a detailed physical examination. Priorities were packaging and rescue of the patient; management of the airway, breathing, and circulation; and preventing hypothermia.
(Objective 8)

CHAPTER
13

Clinical Decision Making

READING ASSIGNMENT

Chapter 13, pages 290-297, in *Mosby's Paramedic Textbook*, ed. 3

OBJECTIVES

Upon completion of this chapter, the paramedic student will be able to:
1. List the key elements of paramedic practice.
2. Discuss the limitations of protocols, standing orders, and patient care algorithms.
3. Outline the key components of the critical thinking process for paramedics.
4. Identify elements necessary for an effective critical thinking process.
5. Describe situations that may necessitate the use of the critical thinking process while delivering prehospital patient care.
6. Describe the six elements required for effective clinical decision making in the prehospital setting.

SUMMARY

- The paramedic must be able to do several things at the same time. The paramedic must be able to gather, evaluate, and synthesize information. The paramedic also must be able to develop and implement appropriate patient management plans. The paramedic must apply judgment and exercise independent decision making as well. Lastly, the paramedic must be able to think and work effectively under pressure.
- Protocols, standing orders, and patient care algorithms have several limitations. They may not apply to nonspecific patient complaints that do not fit the model. They also do not address multiple disease etiologies or multiple treatment plans. Moreover, they may promote linear thinking.
- The critical thinking process includes concept formation, data interpretation, application of principle, evaluation, and reflection on action.
- For effective critical thinking, a paramedic must have a solid knowledge base. The paramedic must be able to deal with a large amount of data all at once as well. The paramedic must be able to organize those data, deal with ambiguity, and relate the situation to similar past experience. The paramedic also must be able to reason and construct arguments to support or discount the decision.
- When using assessment-based patient management, the paramedic must analyze a patient's problems, determine how to solve them, carry out a plan of action, and evaluate its effectiveness.
- Effective clinical decision making requires the paramedic to read the patient and the scene. The paramedic also must be able to react, reevaluate, and revise the management plan. Then the paramedic must be able to review performance at a run critique.

REVIEW QUESTIONS

1. List the four key elements of paramedic practice described in this chapter.

   a.

   b.

   c.

   d.

2. Why is it difficult to follow standard protocols, standing orders, and patient care algorithms in the following situations?

   a. A patient does not speak your language. He appears very ill, is pale and diaphoretic, and has a very slow, irregular heartbeat. He gets very anxious and pulls away when you attempt to establish an intravenous line to give medications.

   _____

   b. A patient with chronic obstructive pulmonary disease has signs and symptoms of heart failure and is wheezing.

   _____

   c. An elderly patient with severe kyphosis (hunchback posture) has fallen off a ladder but screams in pain when you attempt to immobilize him on the spine board.

   _____

   d. A child choked on a toy and is stridorous. Each time you approach to assess her, she begins to cry and has increased distress.

   _____

Question 3 pertains to the following case study:

An elderly patient is complaining of chest pain that began 30 minutes ago. She tells you that it began suddenly when she was reading the paper. It is crushing and substernal, rating an "8" on a 1 to 10 scale. It does not radiate, but she feels nauseated and is diaphoretic. Your assessment reveals normal vital signs, clear breath sounds, and no other obvious clinical findings. A 12-lead ECG demonstrates ST segment elevation in leads V_1 and V_2. You and your partner recognize that her presentation is consistent with septal myocardial infarction. You immediately begin oxygen, initiate an intravenous line, and administer nitroglycerin and aspirin. You notify medical direction and transmit the ECG, anticipating the need for cardiac catheterization. You reevaluate her vital signs, breath sounds, and level of pain every 5 minutes during the 15-minute transport to the hospital. During the following shift, your supervisor gives you feedback on the patient's outcome. During the run critique, everyone agrees that the care was good but the scene time was somewhat long. During the ensuing discussion, you identify ways to reduce scene times on future calls.

3. Identify which parts of this scenario demonstrate each of the following phases of the critical thinking process:

   a. Concept formation:

   _____

   b. Data interpretation:

   _____

c. Application of principle:

_____

d. Evaluation:

_____

e. Reflection on action:

_____

4. List five steps that can help paramedics to think clearly in highly stressful situations.

a.

b.

c.

d.

e.

5. List the six "Rs" of effective clinical decision making.

a.

b.

c.

d.

e.

f.

STUDENT SELF-ASSESSMENT

6. To practice effectively as a paramedic, you should be able to do which of the following?
   a. Gather, evaluate, and synthesize information
   b. Know all current medical techniques
   c. Make diagnoses and provide definitive care
   d. Teach your personal values to patients

7. Which of the following is an advantage of protocols, standing orders, and patient care protocols?
   a. They don't work well when numerous disease etiologies coexist.
   b. They may not apply to nonspecific patient complaints that do not fit the model.
   c. They promote a standardized approach to patient care for classic presentations.
   d. They promote linear thinking and cookbook medicine in all situations.

8. You recognize that a patient is hypoglycemic based on the history, physical examination, and blood analysis. What phase of the critical thinking process have you entered when you initiate an intravenous line and administer glucose?
   a. Application of principle
   b. Concept formation
   c. Data interpretation
   d. Reflection on action

9. In which of the following situations is a paramedic most likely to use critical thinking skills?
   a. The monitor shows ventricular fibrillation.
   b. The blood glucose strip reads 40 mg/dL.
   c. The patient stops breathing and becomes cyanotic.
   d. The trauma patient has severe neck pain but is dyspneic when supine.

10. Which of the following is *not* one of the six elements described in the text as being needed for effective clinical decision making?
    a. React
    b. Read the scene
    c. Request consultation with medical direction
    d. Review performance at a run critique

WRAP IT UP

You are dispatched to a residence for a seizure at 2300. When you arrive, you find a 2-year-old child who is drowsy but easily arousable. Her mother says she found her shaking in bed. She has a "cold" that began today but is otherwise quite healthy. The child is becoming progressively more awake, as you assess her vital signs: P 128; R 28; Sao_2 98%. You are questioning the mother when, moments later, the child seizes again. You move her to the ambulance, and you become concerned when her level of consciousness remains significantly depressed 5 minutes after the seizure, with snoring respirations noted. You insert a nasal airway and administer oxygen as your partner initiates an IV into her left antecubital fossa. You place her on an ECG monitor so that you can continuously monitor her heart rate. Her BP is 60/40 mm Hg; you know that's too low for her. Something seems out of place here. After a fluid bolus, her pressure comes up, but she is still very drowsy. You call your report while en route to the pediatric emergency department.

1. What additional measures might you have used to help with your concept formation?

2. Why would it be difficult to follow a standard protocol or algorithm for this child?

3. After interpreting the data you currently have, what are the chief life threats that concern you?

4. How did you react to the data found on this call?

CHAPTER 13 ANSWERS

REVIEW QUESTIONS

1. a. Gather, evaluate, and synthesize information. b. Develop and implement appropriate patient management plans. c. Apply judgment and exercise independent decision making. d. Think and work effectively under pressure.
   (Objective 1)

2. a. The language barrier makes it impossible to explain properly to the patient what needs to be done, yet you cannot forcibly treat the patient. b. Wheezing caused by chronic obstructive pulmonary disease is treated with a beta agonist such as albuterol; however, treatment for congestive heart failure involves furosemide, nitroglycerin, and morphine. Critical thinking is required to identify subtle findings and point you to the correct treatment path for this patient. c. The correct treatment for this patient is to place him on a spine board (because of the mechanism of injury and age); however, this increases his pain and perhaps his injury because of his altered anatomy, therefore critical thinking is required to determine an acceptable compromise to meet this patient's needs. d. Standard of care requires you to perform a patient assessment on this child; however, when you attempt to do this, her condition worsens. You must determine a compromise that will not harm her.
   (Objectives 2, 5)

3. a. Concept formation occurred when the patient assessment was done; b. data interpretation included interpretation of the vital signs, physical findings, history, and ECG to determine the likelihood of myocardial infarction; c. application of principle involved making the interpretation (MI), selecting the appropriate course of care (O_2, intravenous therapy, nitroglycerin, aspirin), and then delivering that care; d. reassessment of pain, vital signs, and breath sounds constitutes the evaluation phase of the process; e. the run critique provided the opportunity for reflection on action.
   (Objective 3)

4. a. Stop and think; b. scan the situation; c. decide and act; d. maintain clear and concise control; e. regularly and clearly reevaluate the patient.
   (Objective 4)

5. a. Read the patient; b. read the scene; c. react; d. reevaluate; e. revise patient management plan; f. review performance at run critique.
   (Objective 6)

STUDENT SELF-ASSESSMENT

6. a. Paramedics must know techniques appropriate within their scope of practice that have been approved by medical direction. Paramedics are not expected to make diagnoses. Although in some cases (such as hypoglycemia) paramedics provide definitive care, in most cases definitive care is delivered at the hospital. Paramedics must recognize that their personal values may be different from those of the patient.
   (Objective 1)

7. c. Each of the other choices represents a possible disadvantage of protocols, standing orders, and patient care protocols.
   (Objective 2)

8. a. Concept formation involves the process of gathering elements to determine the "what" of the patient story. Data interpretation occurs when data are gathered and interpreted to form a field impression.
   (Objective 3)

9. d. The patient has two concurrent serious problems, and the treatments of these conditions conflict. The paramedic must use critical thinking to resolve the problem.
(Objective 5)

10. c. In some situations medical direction is unavailable or is not available in a timely manner to provide assistance in situations that require rapid clinical decision making.
(Objective 6)

WRAP IT UP

1. Check the environment for any medicines; check her blood glucose level; check her skin temperature; complete her exam (e.g., pupils, rashes, and so on).
(Objective 3)

2. With no history of this, it is unclear what is causing the seizures. In this case general measures to ensure airway, breathing, and blood pressure and to manage recurring seizures would be followed.
(Objective 2)

3. Altered level of consciousness; partial airway obstruction; seizures; low blood pressure
(Objective 4)

4. Airway was managed (nasal airway); IV initiated; fluid bolus given; patient monitored; medical direction consulted.
(Objective 6)

CHAPTER

14

Assessment-Based Management

READING ASSIGNMENT
Chapter 14, pages 298-305, in *Mosby's Paramedic Textbook,* ed. 3

OBJECTIVES
Upon completion of this chapter, the paramedic student will be able to:
1. Discuss how assessment-based management contributes to effective patient and scene assessment.
2. Describe factors that affect assessment and decision making in the prehospital setting.
3. Outline effective techniques for scene and patient assessment and choreography.
4. Identify essential take-in equipment for general and selected patient situations.
5. Outline strategies for patient approach that promote an effective patient encounter.
6. Describe techniques to permit efficient and accurate presentation of the patient.

SUMMARY
- Assessment-based management "puts it all together." This means that the paramedic gathers, evaluates, and synthesizes information. The paramedic makes proper decisions based on the information. Then the paramedic takes the appropriate actions required for the patient's care.
- Factors that can affect the quality of assessment and decision making include the paramedic's attitude, the patient's willingness to cooperate, distracting injuries, labeling and tunnel vision, the environment, patient compliance, and considerations of personnel availability.
- Promoting a coherent assessment is the goal. Thus members of the response team should have a preplan for determining roles and responsibilities.
- The paramedic crew should always be prepared for the worst event. They should carry essential equipment to manage every aspect of patient care.
- A calm and orderly manner is essential for the paramedic. This is especially the case when approaching a patient. During the initial assessment the paramedic must look actively for problems that pose a threat to life.
- Presenting the patient in the course of prehospital and hospital care is twofold. Presentation refers to the skills of effective communication. Presentation also refers to the effective transfer of patient information.

REVIEW QUESTIONS
For questions 1 to 5, what is your field impression based on the patterns described in each of the following scenarios (knowing that further assessment is necessary to confirm each)? Describe the key differences in each pair that distinguish the patterns.

1. **a.** A 24-year-old patient with a history of diabetes is found confused and diaphoretic with weakness on the right side.

_____

   b. An 80-year-old patient with a history of hypertension is found confused and diaphoretic with weakness on the right side.

_____

   c. Key differences in patterns:

_____

2. **a.** A 20-year-old woman whose last menstrual period was 8 weeks ago has severe right lower quadrant abdominal pain and signs of shock.

_____

   b. A 12-year-old boy has severe right lower quadrant abdominal pain, fever, and vomiting.

_____

   c. Key differences in patterns:

_____

3. **a.** A 38-year-old man has severe left lower back pain that radiates down into his testicle, and he has hematuria.

_____

   b. A 70-year-old man had a sudden onset of lower back pain described as "ripping." He is pale, wants to have a bowel movement, and has a cool left foot.

_____

   c. Key differences in patterns:

_____

4. **a.** A healthy 4-month-old infant is found pulseless, with rigor mortis, and in bed with no obvious signs of trauma.

_____

   b. A healthy 16-year-old patient is found pulseless, with rigor mortis, and in bed with no obvious signs of trauma.

_____

   c. Key differences in patterns:

_____

5. **a.** A 70-year-old man complains of crushing substernal chest pain. He is diaphoretic and having multifocal premature ventricular contractions. His history includes hypertension, smoking, and diabetes.

_____

b. A 25-year-old woman complains of crushing substernal chest pain. She is diaphoretic and having multifocal premature ventricular contractions. Her chest struck the steering wheel in a motor vehicle crash 10 minutes ago.

_____

c. Key differences in patterns:

_____

Questions 6 and 7 refer to the following case study:

> You are dispatched to an address where the resident is an alcoholic who calls often for minor problems. She curses at you for taking so long to respond, and then says she fell out of bed yesterday, hit her head, and now has a headache. You note a large bruise on the temporal area of her head but no other injuries. Her speech is slurred, and she has a staggering gait. Her vital signs are BP 160/100 mm Hg, P, 64/min, and R 16/min. You advise her that she will be okay, and she declines transport. The next day she is found unconscious and is diagnosed with a large subdural hematoma that resulted in her death.

6. List factors that may have contributed to your decision in this case.

_____

_____

7. Why is this patient at increased risk for intracerebral bleeding?

_____

Questions 8 to 12 refer to the following case study:

> You are dispatched to a call for a stabbing. Your patient is a 17-year-old boy who was stabbed at a street party. It is dark, and the police are trying to control a large, loud, belligerent crowd that has gathered at the scene. Your patient says he cannot breathe, and when you pull his shirt off, you note a stab wound above the right nipple. Breath sounds are equal. You apply an occlusive dressing, and you elect to move the patient to the ambulance for further assessment and care.

8. During the initial contact with this patient, what are the responsibilities for each of the following team members?

a. Team leader

_____

b. Patient care person (as described in this textbook)

_____

_____

9. Should you carry your drug box with you on a call like this? Why?

_____

10. Explain why the contemplative or the resuscitative approach would be appropriate for this call.

_____

_____

When you get in the ambulance, you talk to the patient, assess his airway and breathing, and apply oxygen. Your partner begins transport. As you begin to initiate an IV, you note blood dripping off the side of the ambulance cot. You cut the patient's clothing off and find a wound in the groin spurting blood.

11. List two factors that you think delayed detection of the patient's bleeding.

   a.

   b.

12. What pertinent positives should be included in your patient care report?

STUDENT SELF-ASSESSMENT

13. Which of the following terms describes the process of gathering, evaluating, and synthesizing information; making appropriate decisions based on available information; and taking the appropriate actions required for patient care?
   a. Assessment-based management
   b. Initial assessment
   c. Ongoing assessment
   d. Patient-focused care

14. Field impression of any given situation is based on which of the following factors?
   a. Information gathered before any physical examination
   b. Advice of medical direction and perception of the call
   c. The paramedic's "gut instinct" and pattern recognition
   d. The patient's chief complaint and assessment of the problem

15. What should you rule out if you encounter an uncooperative patient?
   a. Chest pain or dyspnea   **c.** Neuromuscular disorder
   b. Hypoxia or hypoglycemia   **d.** Personality disorder

16. Why is it important to predesignate roles for emergency medical services calls?
   a. To identify who is at fault if a problem occurs on a call
   b. To allow all paramedics to perform the skills at which they excel
   c. To ensure appropriate skills acquisition
   d. To promote coherent, efficient patient care delivery

17. What is the advantage of taking notes while obtaining the patient history?
   a. To obtain adequate billing information
   b. To provide evidence that may be used in court
   c. To prevent the need for repetitive questioning of the patient
   d. To reassure the patient that you are listening

18. In which of the following patient situations would the contemplative approach to patient care be appropriate?
   a. A large bleeding laceration
   b. Cramping abdominal pain
   c. Decreased level of consciousness
   d. Dyspnea and diaphoresis

19. You respond to a call in which you find a 24-year-old woman who is hyperventilating. What is the *last* condition for which you should assess while performing your history and physical exam?
   a. Anxiety attack   **c.** Diabetic ketoacidosis
   b. Asthma   **d.** Pulmonary embolus

20. You are caring for a patient who is seriously injured after a fall. What is a serious consequence of inadequately presenting your patient during your report to the hospital?
   a. Appropriate resources may not be ready.
   b. The nursing staff will be angry with you.
   c. The patient may misunderstand you.
   d. You may have an increased time out of service.

21. Which of the following is a characteristic of an effective patient presentation?
   a. Every assessment finding is described.
   b. It should last no longer than 5 minutes.
   c. It should include the name of the patient and the doctor.
   d. It should follow a standard format and be concise.

WRAP IT UP

Your partner groans as you pull up to the three-story apartment building where you are responding for a "person passed out." You know the address, you know the patient, and you know that this is probably no emergency, because you have been here many times for minor complaints of headache, constipation, and blood pressure checks. "What should we bring?" he asks wearily. "Let's bring it all," you say, grabbing the monitor, airway bag, and jump kit, even though you realize it is probably just an exercise in weight lifting. You enter the apartment, and your patient, a 70-year-old man, is semireclined on the sofa. When you ask what is going on, he tells you he must have pulled something in his back, it has been bothering him all day, and then he "fell out" and when he woke up, he called 911. "Tell me about your pain," you inquire, as vital signs are taken and his medicines (labetolol, hydrochlorothiazide (HydroDIURIL), potassium, aspirin) are recorded. "Well, it's in my back, and it's real bad, kind of like I tore something in there, and it goes down in my leg," he says, grimacing suddenly as he relates his story. You notice his skin is cool, his lips and nails are pale, and when you grab his wrist, his heart rate, while not rapid, is weak. His vital signs are BP 104/64 mm Hg, P 68/min, R 20/min, and SaO_2 93%. "That pressure's a bit low for you," your partner tells the patient as he opens a nasal cannula and places it on his face. On the physical exam, you note a tender pulsatile mass above his umbilicus to the right of the midline. Femoral pulses are weak, and you cannot feel any pulses in his cool, pale feet. You establish a line and send your partner and the police officer to retrieve the stretcher from the ambulance. Your patient is monitored, packaged, and transported to the hospital after you call report. Based on your notification, the ED resuscitation room is setup, and the patient is quickly diagnosed with abdominal aortic aneurysm. He is in surgery by the time you complete your report and is hospitalized for several weeks because of renal complications.

1. What findings fit the "pattern" of abdominal aortic aneurysm in this case study?

_____

2. How would your impression of the situation have changed if the following were true:
   a. The patient were 17 years old, had no medical history (no daily medications), and was unknown to the paramedics.
   b. The patient did not have a pulsating mass.
   c. You found a heart rhythm disturbance before you palpated his abdomen.
3. a. Which vital sign assessment did not fit the "pattern."
   b. What could explain this altered vital sign?
4. Which factor had the potential to have a negative impact on your assessment of this patient?
   a. Distracting environment
   b. Labeling and tunnel vision
   c. Personnel considerations
   d. Uncooperative patient
5. Place a check mark beside the team leader responsibilities that you observed on this call.
   a. _____ Accompanies patient to hospital
   b. _____ Establishes dialogue with patient
   c. _____ Obtains history
   d. _____ Performs physical exam
   e. _____ Presents the patient
   f. _____ Completes documentation
   g. _____ Team leadership

CHAPTER 14 ANSWERS

REVIEW QUESTIONS

1. a. Hypoglycemia (further assessment to rule out stroke would also be needed.)
   b. Stroke
   c. Age (Stroke is more common in the elderly.), history (Patient in *a.* had a history of diabetes); (patient in *b.* had a history of hypertension.)
   (Objective 1)

2. a. Ectopic pregnancy
   b. Appendicitis
   c. Sex (Boy in *b.* would not have gynecological complaints.), age (Appendicitis is common in this age group.), clinical signs (shock in ectopic pregnancy versus fever in appendicitis)
   (Objective 1)

3. a. Nephrolithiasis (kidney stone)
   b. Abdominal aortic aneurysm
   c. Age (Aneurysm is more common in men 60 to 70 years of age.), clinical signs/symptoms (Hematuria is common in kidney stones; urge to defecate, cool extremity, and signs of shock are consistent with aneurysm.)
   (Objective 1)

4. a. Sudden infant death syndrome or child abuse
   b. Drug or alcohol toxicity or suicide
   c. Age (Sudden infant death syndrome and abuse are more common in infants; suicide and drug abuse or overdose are more common in teens).
   (Objective 1)

5. a. Myocardial infarction
   b. Myocardial contusion
   c. Age (Myocardial infarction is more common in older patients; history of *a.* is consistent with risk factors of myocardial infarction; mechanism of injury in *b.* is consistent with myocardial injury.)
   (Objective 1)

6. Your attitude, the patient's willingness to cooperate, and labeling or tunnel vision (the expectation that her signs and symptoms were related to alcohol intoxication) may have contributed to your decision.
   (Objective 2)

7. Chronic alcoholism can impair the clotting mechanisms, putting the patient at risk for bleeding. Poor coordination caused by intoxication increases the risk of injury (falls) in alcoholic patients.
   (Objective 2)

8. a. The team leader establishes contact and begins dialogue with the patient, obtains the history, and performs the physical examination.
   b. The patient care person provides scene cover (watches the crowd), gathers scene information (size/type of weapon), obtains vital signs, and performs skills.
   (Objective 3)

9. When moving into a volatile situation such as this one, you should take the mininum amount of equipment; the drug box would not be indicated based on the dispatch information. (This may vary by agency based on size and contents of drug box.)
   (Objective 4)

10. The resuscitative approach is necessary because a life threat exists.
    (Objective 5)

11. a. The presence of distracting injuries (the chest wound)
    b. The environment (dangerous and dark)
    (Objective 2)

12. The patient is conscious, and breath sounds are present and equal bilaterally.
    (Objective 6)

13. a. Initial assessment and ongoing assessment are components of assessment-based management.
    (Objective 1)

14. c. The field impression is based on a careful history, physical examination, and then analysis and evaluation based on the paramedic's knowledge and past experiences.
    (Objective 2)

15. b. Alcohol or drug intoxication, hypovolemia, and head injury or concussion are other physiological problems that may cause a patient to be uncooperative.
    (Objective 3)

16. d. This becomes especially important when multiple units respond to a scene.
    (Objective 4)

17. c. Taking notes keeps you from forgetting critical information that will be necessary when you complete your patient care report later.
    (Objective 5)

18. b. The contemplative approach is appropriate only when immediate intervention to manage a life threat is not needed.
    (Objective 5)

19. a. All the other conditions represent life-threatening problems associated with hyperventilation; your examination therefore should be tailored to rule out those problems first.
    (Objective 5)

20. a. An inadequate or inaccurate report can result in delayed patient care related to room or resource (medical staff, equipment) unavailability.
    (Objective 6)

21. d. Ideally, the report should be concise, follow a standard format, and include pertinent positives and negatives. The patient's name should not be included if radio communication is used.
    (Objective 6)

WRAP IT UP

1. Patient age, history of hypertension (from medications), description and location of pain, pulsatile mass, location of mass, diminished pulses in extremities, hypotension, syncopal episode
   (Objective 1)

2. a. Aneurysm would be unlikely (but not impossible) in someone that age and with no previous history. The patient would still need similar interventions and urgent transport due to the physical findings (cool skin, weak pulse, low SaO_2 for age).
   b. The treatment and impression should not change. A pulsatile mass is not always palpable.
   c. The history and description of the pain should still lead you to suspect aneurysm.

3. a. Tachycardia would have been expected.
b. Patient was taking a beta-blocker, which will not permit the heart to speed up effectively to compensate for shock.
(Objective 2)

4. b. Having been to many "false alarms," it would be possible to discount the patient's complaints and, if a comprehensive exam was not done, to miss this critical condition.
(Objective 2)

5. a, b, c, d, e, f, g
(Objective 3)

CHAPTER

15

Communications

READING ASSIGNMENT
Chapter 15, pages 298-317, in *Mosby's Paramedic Textbook*, ed. 3

OBJECTIVES
Upon completion of this chapter, the paramedic student will be able to:
1. Outline the phases of communications that occur during a typical emergency medical services (EMS) event.
2. Describe the role of communications in EMS.
3. Define common EMS communications terms.
4. Describe the primary modes of EMS communications.
5. Describe how EMS communications are regulated.
6. Describe the role of dispatching as it applies to prehospital emergency medical care.
7. Outline techniques for relaying EMS communications clearly and effectively.

SUMMARY
- Communications regarding EMS refers to the delivery of information. The patient and scene information is delivered to other key members of the emergency response team.
- Verbal, written, and electronic communications allow the delivery of information between the party requesting help and the dispatcher; between the dispatcher and paramedic; and between the paramedic, hospital, and direct/online medical direction.
- Emergency communications technology has industry-specific terminology.
- The primary modes of EMS communications include simplex mode, duplex mode, multiplex mode, trunking system, digital, and computer.
- In the United States, the FCC regulates communications over the radio. The paramedic must be familiar with the regulatory agencies. The paramedic must follow their guidelines as well.
- The functions of an effective dispatch communications system include receiving and processing calls for EMS assistance, dispatching and coordinating EMS resources, relaying medical information, and coordinating with public safety agencies.
- A standard format of transmission of patient information is a wise idea. The standard allows for the best use of communications systems. The standard also allows physicians to receive details quickly about the patient. In addition, the standard decreases the chance of omitting any critical details.

REVIEW QUESTIONS

Match the communication term in Column II with the appropriate definition in Column I. Use each answer only once.

Column I

1. _____ A unit of frequency equal to one cycle per second
2. _____ The ability to transmit or receive in one direction at a time
3. _____ A grouping of radio equipment that includes a transmitter and receiver
4. _____ Radio frequencies between 300 and 3000 MHz
5. _____ The ability to transmit and receive simultaneously through two different frequencies
6. _____ A unit of frequency equal to 1 million cycles per second
7. _____ Radio frequencies between 30 and 300 MHz
8. _____ A unit that receives transmissions from a mobile radio and retransmits them at higher power on another frequency

Column II

a. Base station
b. Duplex
c. Hertz
d. Kilohertz
e. Megahertz
f. Mobile station
g. Remote console
h. Repeater
i. Simplex
j. UHF
k. VHF

9. A person is stabbed with a knife. List the five phases of communications that occur on most emergency medical services calls such as this.

a.

b.

c.

d.

e.

10. A man is injured seriously at a rural site. Describe the communication process from the time of his injury until the EMS crew returns to service.

_____

_____

_____

_____

11. List three common causes of interference with radio transmissions.

a.

b.

c.

12. Briefly describe four responsibilities of an EMS dispatcher.

a.

b.

c.

d.

13. List three essential pieces of information that the dispatcher must obtain from a bystander who calls in to report a motor vehicle crash.

 a.

 b.

 c.

14. Identify three ways in which the Federal Communications Commission directly influences EMS.

 a.

 b.

 c.

15. Describe six actions the paramedic may take to ensure clear and understandable radio transmissions.

 a.

 b.

 c.

 d.

 e.

 f.

    Johnny Smith, a paramedic who works on City Unit 7, is called to an industrial site. He finds a 30-year-old patient lying on his back on the grass, where he landed after falling 20 feet from a painting platform. On the paramedic's arrival at 1 PM, the patient's vital signs are as follows: blood pressure, 120/80 mm Hg; pulse, 116 per minute; and respirations, 20 per minute. He states he became dizzy and fell. When Smith palpates, the patient complains of pain in the lumbar region of the back and on both heels, which are swollen. Distal pulses, sensation, and movement are present in all extremities. Lung sounds are clear and equal bilaterally. The patient gives Smith his name and knows the date and time and where he is. His skin is warm and dry. The patient weighs about 100 kg and takes ibuprofen prescribed by Dr. Jones for back pain. Smith places him on 100% oxygen via non-rebreather mask, positions him on a backboard with cervical collar, and notifies Dr. Kane, the online medical physician, of the patient's condition and the 15-minute estimated arrival time to City Hospital. Vital signs at 1:25 PM are unchanged. The patient's condition remains the same en route.

16. Write a concise, complete radio report to communicate the appropriate information regarding this patient to the base hospital.

_____

_____

_____

_____

_____

_____

_____

_____

_____

_____

_____

_____

_____

_____

STUDENT SELF-ASSESSMENT

17. What is manipulation of the intended idea for communication known as?
  a. Decoding
  b. Encoding
  c. Feedback
  d. Receiving

18. After being called to an airplane crash with two seriously injured patients, the first arriving EMS crew tells online medical direction, "There are people (meaning bystanders) everywhere." The physician interprets this to indicate a mass casualty situation and activates the mass casualty incident plan. What type of communication error occurred here?
  a. Attributes of the receiver
  b. Selective perception
  c. Semantic problems
  d. Time pressures

19. Which of the following is a component of a simple communication system?
  a. Remote console
  b. Microwave links
  c. Mobile unit
  d. Satellite receivers

20. What is a radio receiver circuit used for suppressing the audio portion of unwanted radio noises or signals called?
  a. Decibel
  b. Frequency modulation
  c. Squelch
  d. Tone

21. What is the term for the number of repetitive cycles per second completed by a radio wave?
  a. Amplitude modulation
  b. Frequency
  c. Range
  d. Wattage

22. What is transmission and reception of electrocardiograms over the radio or telephone called?
  a. Coverage
  b. Hotline
  c. Patch
  d. Telemetry

23. What are the HEAR and EACOM radios used to tie hospitals together and receive and transmit tone pulses known as?
  a. Cellular telephones
  b. Decoders and encoders
  c. Microwave transmitters
  d. Satellite dishes

24. Which component of a communication system receives transmissions from a low-power portable radio on one frequency and simultaneously retransmits it at a higher power on another frequency?
  a. Mobile transceivers
  b. Portable radios
  c. Remote console
  d. Repeaters

25. How is the strongest signal selected when numerous satellite receivers are used?
  a. Base stations
  b. Cellular lines
  c. Decoders
  d. Voting systems

26. What are dispatch services located away from base stations that facilitate communications with field personnel known as?
  a. Complex systems
  b. Mobile transceivers
  c. Portable transceivers
  d. Remote consoles

27. What is an advantage of communication with cellular telephones?
   a. They allow unlimited channel access.
   b. They permit uninterrupted communication.
   c. They provide a secure link between EMS and the hospital.
   d. They transmit simultaneous calls in disaster situations.
28. Which of the following is not a responsibility of the dispatcher?
   a. Dispatching EMS resources
   b. Coordinating with public safety services
   c. Receiving calls for assistance
   d. Providing off-line medical control
29. What is a function of prearrival instructions?
   a. To allow EMS personnel to be disregarded
   b. To determine whether the call is unfounded
   c. To provide life-saving instructions
   d. To allow the EMS crew more time to respond
30. What is the role of the Federal Communications Commission?
   a. To consult with EMS agencies regarding radio equipment
   b. To develop new radio technologies
   c. To monitor frequencies for appropriate usage
   d. To train dispatchers in prearrival instructions
31. Which of the following is a technique for effective radio communication?
   a. Speak at a range of 6 to 8 inches from the microphone.
   b. Speak slowly and clearly and enunciate words distinctly.
   c. Show emotion to demonstrate the urgency of critical situations.
   d. Take your time and include all patient information available.
32. Which is *not* a component of the SOAP format for patient reports?
   a. Assessment data   c. Patient information
   b. Objective data   d. Subjective information

WRAP IT UP

At 0130 the prealert tone sounds in your engine-house, and the lights go on as you hear the dispatcher say, "4017 respond to number 12 Avid Court, chest pain." As you roll out of your bunk, the call is repeated, and then you hear the dispatcher recite the call numbers. Your partner pulls the run direction card as a backup because the computer was down earlier. You are attending this call, so you read the directions and tap the responding key of your on-board computer screen as you pull out of the engine room. The instructions on the screen note the patient's previous heart history. You pull up the global positioning system map to ensure you are proceeding in the correct direction. The dispatcher sends you a note indicating that there is a large dog that the caller has been instructed to secure in a bedroom. You tap the arrival button on your computer screen and proceed in to care for the patient. Based on your patient assessment, you suspect the patient is having an acute myocardial infarction and perform a 12-lead ECG. Your partner connects your monitor to the telephone line, and you transmit a copy of the ECG to medical direction. Then, when you contact medical direction using the cellular telephone for orders, they agree with your interpretation of inferior myocardial infarction. You notify dispatch that you are departing the scene to transport to Central Medical Center. They notify you that the local hospital diversion program indicates that they are on diversion and cannot accept the patient, so you elect to go the other direction to a medical center an equal distance and contact them on your VHF radio with a patient report. You indicate your arrival at the hospital on your dispatch screen. After giving a verbal report to the receiving RN, you proceed to the EMS report room where the fax from dispatch with your call times is waiting. Your partner has brought in your computer, and so you complete your report following the prompts on the screen and then type in the narrative. The patient is now in the cardiac catheterization lab and unable to sign the consent and notice of receipt of the HIPAA forms, so you document that and give the privacy notice to the family member. You obtain the nurse's signature, print your report, and then touch your computer screen to notify dispatch that you are returning in service. As you pull into you station, you pop out the wireless antenna in your laptop computer, and then, when a good signal is detected, press upload, and the report now is securely in the department mainframe and accessible to only the privacy officer and a few designated officers.

1. List all the persons and/or agencies with which the EMS crew communicated on this call.

_____

_____

2. What key information did the dispatcher provide on this call?

_____

_____

3. What modes of communication were used on this EMS call?

_____

_____

4. Identify problems that could have been encountered on this call if any of the following communication errors had occurred.

Communication Error	**Potential Problems**

   a. Dispatcher fails to identify or transmit correct address.

_____

_____

   b. Dispatcher fails to give instructions regarding dog.

_____

_____

   c. Computer fails and no backup system is available.

_____

_____

   d. Incorrect or incomplete information is reported to medical direction.

_____

_____

   e. Fail to report all medications given to receiving RN.

_____

_____

   f. Forget to notify dispatch when returning in service.

_____

CHAPTER 15 ANSWERS

REVIEW QUESTIONS

1. c
(Objective 3)

2. i
(Objective 3)

3. a
(Objective 3)

4. j
(Objective 3)

5. b
(Objective 3)

6. e
(Objective 3)

7. k
(Objective 3)

8. h
(Objective 3)

9. a. Occurrence of the event
   b. Detection of the need for emergency services
   c. Notification and emergency response
   d. EMS arrival, treatment (including consultation with medical direction), and preparation for transport
   e. Preparation of EMS for the next emergency response
   (Objective 1)

10. Emergency medical services response is initiated by bystanders by telephone to a communications center or public safety answering point. The communications specialist obtains the necessary information (often accompanied by digital information) about the origin of the call. The call taker then passes the information by digital technology (if available) to the telecommunicator, who dispatches appropriate emergency personnel and equipment. The EMS crew notifies the communications center while en route and obtains additional information. The EMS crew notifies the communications center on arrival to scene. The EMS crew contacts medical direction for orders and reports. Care is rendered, and the patient is prepared for transport; the EMS crew notifies the communication center when they depart from the scene and arrive at the receiving facility. The ambulance is made ready for the next emergency call and communications is notified when it is available for another call.
(Objective 2)

11. Mountains, dense foliage, and tall buildings
(Objective 4)

12. a. To receive calls for EMS assistance
   b. Dispatch and coordinate EMS resources
   c. Relay medical information
   d. Coordinate with public safety agencies
   (Objective 5)

13. a. Name and callback number of individual who placed the call
   b. Address of emergency and directions including specific landmarks because of the possible rural location
   c. The nature of the emergency (Is the victim trapped, how seriously is he or she injured, and is he or she accessible to the EMS crew?)
   (Objective 5)

14. Licensing and frequency allocation, establishing technical standards for radio equipment, and establishing and enforcing rules and regulations
   (Objective 6)

15. Speak 2 to 3 inches away from and across the microphone, speak slowly and clearly, speak without emotion, be brief, avoid codes (unless approved by system), and advise the receiving party when the transmission has been completed.
   (Objective 7)

16. City Unit 7, paramedic Smith calling City Hospital. We are on the scene at an industrial site with a patient who fell approximately 20 feet onto a grassy area. The patient is a 30-year-old male weighing approximately 100 kg. Patient's chief complaint is back pain. Also complaining of bilateral heel pain. Patient states he became dizzy and fell. Medical history of back pain for which he takes ibuprofen. Patient is awake, alert, and oriented times 3. Lungs are clear bilaterally; skin is warm and dry. Tenderness to palpation in lumbar region of back and bilaterally on heels. Soft tissue swelling present bilaterally at calcaneus. Distal pulse, sensation, and movement present in all extremities. V/S are BP 120/80, P 116, R 20. Patient placed on 100% oxygen by complete non-rebreather mask and immobilized on a backboard with cervical collar. Private physician is Dr. Jones. ETA will be 15 minutes. Standing by for any additional orders, over.
   (Objective 7)

17. b. Decoding is interpretation of a message. Feedback is the response to the initial idea. Receiving indicates the receiver got the message.
   (Objective 2)

18. c. The word *people* was mistakenly interpreted as *patients*.
   (Objective 2)

19. c. All other equipment listed is part of a complex system.
   (Objective 4)

20. c. A decibel is a unit of measurement for signal power levels. Frequency modulation is a deviation in carrier frequency resulting in less noise. A tone is a unique carrier wave used to signal a receiver selectively.
   (Objective 3)

21. b. Amplitude modulation is a radio frequency that fluctuates according to the applied audio. Range refers to the general perimeter of signal coverage. A watt measures power output.
   (Objective 3)

22. d. Coverage refers to the area where radio communication exists. A hotline is a dedicated line activated by merely lifting the receiver. Patching permits communication between different communication modes.
   (Objective 3)

23. b. These tones can be set to all-call for efficient disaster communication. Cellular telephones are used for ambulance-to-hospital contact in some areas. Satellite dishes and microwave transmitters extend transmission distance.
   (Objective 4)

24. d. Mobile transceivers usually are mounted on the vehicle and operate at lower outputs than base stations. Portable radios are handheld devices used when working away from the emergency vehicle. Remote center consoles are located away from base stations and are connected by dedicated telephone line, microwave, or other radio means.
(Objective 4)

25. d. Voting systems automatically select the strongest or best audio signal among numerous satellite receivers.
(Objective 4)

26. d. Remote consoles control all base station functions and are connected by dedicated telephone lines.
(Objective 4)

27. c. No dedicated cell channels exist for EMS, so lines may be busy when an emergency call is being made. In some areas the cell coverage is not good and communication may be terminated abruptly. This does not allow simultaneous communication.
(Objective 4).

28. d. This is the physician medical director's job.
(Objective 5)

29. c. Prearrival instructions complement EMS care but do not include call screening.
(Objective 5)

30. c. They also are responsible for licensure and allocation of frequencies. They establish technical standards for radio equipment and establish and enforce rules and regulations for equipment operation.
(Objective 6)

31. b. You should speak 2 to 3 inches from the microphone, converse without emotion, and be brief.
(Objective 7)

32. c. Plan of patient management is the fourth component.
(Objective 7)

WRAP IT UP

1. Partner, dispatch, patient and their family, medical direction, receiving facility, receiving RN.
(Objective 1)

2. Location of call, nature of call, previous information known about patient, presence of dog, diversion status of hospital, times
(Objective 6)

3. Radio voice, tones, light, computer (dispatch of call); fax (ECG); cellular telephone (medical direction); radio (dispatch, receiving facility); face-to-face (patient, partner, family, receiving RN)
(Objective 7)

4. a. Determining the correct location of a call is a critical element in your response time. Failure to do so could delay your response significantly.
b. Scene safety could have been compromised.
c. Response delays if no backup directions are available.
d. Inappropriate and even dangerous orders may be given if the report to medical direction is not accurate.
e. Duplicate administration of medications is possible if an incomplete report is given. This could cause serious side effects.
f. A call might be given to a more distant unit, delaying response time and leaving their zone without coverage.
(Objective 7)

Documentation

READING ASSIGNMENT

Chapter 16, pages 318-330, in *Mosby's Paramedic Textbook,* ed. 3

OBJECTIVES

Upon completion of this chapter, the paramedic student will be able to:
1. Identify the purpose of the patient care report (PCR).
2. Describe the uses of the patient care report.
3. Outline the components of an accurate, thorough patient care report.
4. Describe the elements of a properly written emergency medical services document.
5. Describe an effective system for documentation of prehospital patient care.
6. Identify differences necessary when documenting special situations.
7. Describe the appropriate method to make revisions or corrections to the patient care report.
8. Recognize consequences that may result from inappropriate documentation.

SUMMARY

- The patient care report is used to document the key elements of patient assessment, care, and transport.
- The three primary reasons for written documentation are that the medical community involved in the patient's care uses it, it is a legal record, and it is essential to data collection.
- The PCR should include dates and response times, difficulties encountered, observations at the scene, previous medical care provided, a chronological description of the call, and significant times.
- A properly written EMS document is accurate, legible, timely, unaltered, and free of nonprofessional or extraneous information.
- Many approaches for writing the narrative can be used. The paramedic should adopt only one approach. The paramedic should use this approach consistently to avoid omissions in report writing.
- Special documentation is necessary when a patient refuses care or transport. Such documentation also is needed in those cases when care or transportation is not needed. Special documentation also is needed for mass casualty incidents.
- Most EMS agencies have separate forms for revisions or corrections to the patient care report.
- Documentation that is inappropriate may have medical and legal implications.

REVIEW QUESTIONS

Questions 1 and 2 pertain to the following case study:

> You are a paramedic working on Unit 4017 and are dispatched to a private residence on a call for a "person down." On arrival at the scene at 1400, you find a 20-year-old woman lying on the lawn in front of the house. She is awake

but is saying inappropriate words. The patient's husband tells you that his wife is diabetic and takes insulin, but she missed lunch. He says he found her confused in the yard. Her skin is pale, cool, and diaphoretic; respiratory rate is 20 breaths per minute and unlabored with clear breath sounds in all fields; radial pulse is 120 per minute; and her blood pressure is 110/70 mm Hg. While your partner initates an IV in the right antecubital space at 1406, you measure the patient's blood glucose level, which is 50 mg/dL. Following your standing orders, you begin an IV of normal saline and then at 1408 administer 25 g (50 mL) of D50W through the IV. Within 2 minutes the patient looks at you and asks, "Why are you here?" She is now alert and answering appropriately, and by the time her husband reminds her what has happened, she is oriented completely to person, place, and time. She agrees to be transported to General Hospital, and the ambulance departs the scene at 1413. While en route, you call a report to Dr. Smith, and at 1416 another set of vital signs reveals the following: BP 118/74, P 96/min, R 20/min with warm, dry, pink skin. She denies allergies to medicine and states she took 10 units of regular and 20 units of Lente insulin at 0700. On arrival to the hospital at 1420, there is no change in the patient's condition, and you note that 100 mL of the IV fluid has been infused. Your partner restocks your bag with the supplies used, which include a 250-mL bag of normal saline, macrodrip IV tubing, an 18G IV catheter, and D50W.

1. Write a narrative documenting your findings on this patient as you would on your state patient care report (assuming there is no check-box format on your report).

_____

_____

_____

_____

_____

_____

_____

_____

_____

2. List at least four activities for which your patient care report from this call may be used.

_____

_____

_____

_____

3. Describe the appropriate method to complete documentation for each of the following situations:
   a. Your patient lacerated his hand. The wound is deep and gaping, and he cannot move two of his fingers. He is refusing care and says he will go to his doctor tomorrow.

   _____

   _____

   _____

   b. You are responding to a call for a "full arrest." Before you arrive on scene, the dispatcher notifies you to disregard the call. You go back in service and return to your station.

   _____

   _____

   _____

   c. More than 100 patients are complaining of burning eyes and throats and difficulty breathing after an industrial gas release. You are providing care in the treatment sector.

   _____

   _____

   _____

   d. You have just returned to your engine house from the hospital when you realize that you did not document some essential information about the patient's history on the patient care report.

   _____

   _____

   _____

4. What is a possible consequence of failure to document the following information in a patient care report?
   a. The trauma patient reports an allergy to tetanus vaccine. He is unconscious when you arrive in the emergency department.

   _____

   _____

   _____

   b. You administered the maximum dosage of lidocaine to a patient who was in ventricular tachycardia but neglected to document it on your patient care report.

   _____

   _____

   _____

c. The patient fell earlier in the day and is unconscious on arrival to the emergency department. You do not document that the patient takes warfarin (Coumadin) daily.

_____

_____

_____

d. You fail to note that a patient had numbness in his arm before spinal immobilization.

_____

_____

_____

STUDENT SELF-ASSESSMENT

5. What is the purpose of the patient care report?
   a. To document patient assessment
   b. To document patient care
   c. To document patient transport
   d. To document all of the above
6. Which of the following is not an appropriate use of the patient care report?
   a. Administrative and billing information
   b. Legal record of sequence of care provided
   c. Research document for the local press
   d. Supply inventory tracking
7. Which of the following should *not* be documented on the patient care report?
   a. Chronological description of events that occurred during the call
   b. Circumstances documenting that the paramedic fell during care of this patient
   c. Difficulties encountered during patient care, treatment, and transport
   d. Time of call, dispatch, arrival at scene, arrival at hospital, and back in service
8. If the respiratory rate section is not completed on the ambulance reporting form, what should the physician assume about patient respirations?
   a. They were not an important vital sign assessment.
   b. They were not pertinent in this patient section.
   c. They were not assessed specifically by the paramedic.
   d. They were within normal limits for the patient age group.
9. When a patient refuses care, what must the paramedic document?
   a. Advice given to the patient regarding the condition
   b. Nothing is needed as long as the patient was alert and oriented.
   c. The detailed physical examination
   d. The patient's insurance information
10. What should you document when your response is canceled en route to the scene?
   a. Canceling authority and time of cancellation
   b. No documentation is needed in this situation.
   c. Scene size-up information
   d. You must still respond and obtain a refusal.
11. You are leaving work and suddenly realize you forgot to document a crucial piece of information about patient care on a patient record. What should you do?
   a. Ask your supervisor to fill in the essential information.
   b. Note the date and time the correction was made on the appropriate form.
   c. Wait until you return to work after your 4-day break to finish it.
   d. You may not add anything after the report is complete.

WRAP IT UP

It seems odd that you would be nervous today. Normally, you are the one who is calm, cool, and collected even on the most serious trauma calls. As you sit waiting to testify at the deposition, you go over the details of the call in your mind. At the time you thought you'd never forget them, but after 5 years the details tend to fade. Thankfully, your attorney says that you will have the benefit of your patient care report to refer to during your testimony. The plaintiff who was thrown off of a motorcycle while apparently intoxicated is alleging that your care led to the long-term disability he is experiencing from nerve damage to his badly fractured leg. You sit around the table with your attorney, the prosecuting attorney, and a court reporter who swears you in. The attorney begins by asking you why your response to the scene of the collision was so slow based on the location from which you responded. You explain, as you documented, that traffic was diverted that evening because of highway construction, resulting in an unavoidable delay in response. He queries you about your statements that the patient was "drunk." You respond that you did not document that the patient was drunk. Rather, you noted that there was a strong odor resembling alcohol on the patient's breath, that he had slurred speech, that he repeatedly was moving his clearly fractured extremity, despite repeated requests for him to hold still so that he would not injure it further until appropriate immobilization could be completed. The attorney asks if that behavior was consistent with a head injury also, and you state that yes it would be; however, as you detailed in your report, the mechanism of injury was not consistent with head injury as evidenced by bystander reports that his leg had been pinned between the bike and a car, and his head never struck the ground. You also note that his helmet was undamaged. The attorney then makes the allegation that you did not follow proper care to his client's injured leg and wonders why you scratched out the word "traction" before splint. You state that, as you noted in your report, there was gross deformity to his lower leg and ankle; however, before, during, and after splinting, there was a good dorsalis pedis and posterior tibial pulse with the last check you noted after you moved the patient to the cot in the resuscitation room at the trauma center. Further, you review with him the policy of your department when an error is made on the report as was done here. Evidently, the word *traction* was written mistakenly, so you crossed through it with a single line and placed your initials beside the strikeout. You also had documented the numbness that the patient reported in his toes and his ability to move them during those pulse checks. In response to his questions regarding your apparently long scene time, you point to your note regarding the patient's repeated attempts to get off the cot and run away. With each series of questions, you were able to answer accurately and thoroughly based on your documentation. After the deposition, your attorney notifies you that, while his client's suit is still proceeding against the hospital, the prosecuting attorney will be dropping your name and your service from the client's claims.

1. List five uses of this patient care report aside from the one already mentioned.

_____

_____

_____

_____

2. Place a check mark beside the components of an accurate, complete patient care report that were mentioned in this case.
    a. _____ Dates
    b. _____ Response times
    c. _____ Difficulties en route
    d. _____ Communication difficulties
    e. _____ Scene observations
    f. _____ Reasons for extended on scene time
    g. _____ Previous care provided
    h. _____ Time of extrication
    i. _____ Time of patient transport
    j. _____ Reason for hospital selection
3. Which is true regarding the correction of a patient care report that was done in this case?
    a. It would have been better to black out the error completely.
    b. It should have been explained thoroughly in the narrative.
    c. It was completed properly.
    d. Individual strikeouts should not be done, the entire sentence should be rewritten.

CHAPTER 16 ANSWERS

REVIEW QUESTIONS

1. At 1400, 4017 arrived to the scene of a residence. Found a 20-year-old woman supine on the lawn, saying inappropriate words. Her husband states she is a diabetic. He found her in the yard confused. Patient's skin is pale, cool, and diaphoretic. Vital signs are BP 110/70, P 120/min, R 20/min with clear breath sounds. Blood glucose determined to be 50 mg/dL. 1406 IV 250 mL NS initiated in the right antecubital space by paramedic Ward. 1408 25 g (50 mL) D50W given IVP by paramedic McKenna. 1410 Patient states, "Why are you here?" 1412 Patient is alert and oriented to person, place, and time. Patient states she took 10 units of regular and 20 units of Lente insulin at 0700 today. 1413 Ambulance en route to General Hospital. Report called to Dr. Smith. No further orders requested. 1416 BP 118/74, P 96/min, R 20/min. Skin is pink, warm, and dry. 1420 Arrival to General Hospital. 100 mL NS infused.
On some patient report forms, check boxes or tables will permit documentation of many of the items included in this narrative report. In that instance, it is often unnecessary to repeat the information on the narrative.
(Objectives 3, 4, 5)

2. Medical continuity of care, quality improvement, legal record, supply tracking, performance evaluation, state reporting, education, and skill tracking
(Objective 2)

3. a. Document the patient's level of consciousness, your advice to the patient (including possible consequences of refusal) medical direction advice to the patient, signatures of the patient and/or witnesses as required in your system, a narrative description of your exam that you told patient to call 9-1-1 again if he changes his mind, and the events that occurred.
b. Note the name of the person/agency that canceled your response, and the time the response was terminated. Ensure that this falls within the scope of your departmental policies.
c. Document care on the appropriate mass casualty incident (MCI) forms (often on triage tags). Record patient condition and disposition on appropriate tracking form (may be done by sector leader).
d. Note the purpose of the revision or correction and why the information did not appear on the original document as soon as possible using the appropriate departmental form. Ensure the correction is made by the original author. Send a copy of the revision to the appropriate parties.
(Objective 6)

4. a. If tetanus vaccine is administered to the patient in the hospital, he will likely have an allergic reaction and be harmed. You could face legal repercussions.
b. If additional lidocaine is administered at the hospital, the patient may have a toxic reaction. When the chart is audited for quality purposes, it will appear that you did not perform a procedure that was indicated. If drug inventory is tracked from the patient report, it will not be replaced, and you may run short. If the patient's bill is itemized, he or she will not be charged for this intervention, and your department may lose revenue needed for operations.
c. The patient's condition could deteriorate quickly, and the medical staff would not recognize the increased risk of bleeding. You could face legal repercussions.
d. If the patient alleges that the numbness developed as a result of your care, you would have no documentation to substantiate your claim that the patient was symptomatic before your care; you could be successfully sued.
(Objective 8)

5. d. All these elements should be recorded in an accurate, legible, understandable manner.
(Objective 1)

6. c. The records should be maintained confidentially and only released to parties other than the hospital after patient consent is given.
(Objective 2)

7. b. This is documented on the appropriate department incident report.
   (Objective 3)

8. c. In a court of law the assumption is that if it is not documented, it was not done.
   (Objective 4)

9. a. Advice to the patient, including risks of refusal and benefits of treatment, should be noted. Additionally, you should document that the patient was instructed to call back if the condition worsened or if he or she reconsidered. A detailed examination generally is not performed on a patient who refuses (document it if it is done).
   (Objective 6)

10. a. A special form may be required to document these situations. You should always keep a record in case subsequent liability results.
    (Objective 6)

11. b. Some agencies and states require separate reports. Patient care information should be completed only by the paramedic on the call. Corrections and revisions should be made as soon as possible.
    (Objective 7)

WRAP IT UP

1. Medical audit, quality improvement, billing and administration, data collection, written record for other health care professionals to reference
   (Objective 2)

2. Dates, response times, difficulties en route, scene observations, reasons for extended on scene time, time of patient transport
   (Objective 3)

3. c. Local and state policy for report correction should be followed.
   (Objective 7)

PART FOUR

IN THIS PART

17

Pharmacology

READING ASSIGNMENT
Chapter 17, pages 332-387 , in *Mosby's Paramedic Textbook,* ed. 3

OBJECTIVES
Upon completion of this chapter, the paramedic student will be able to:
1. Explain what a drug is.
2. Identify the four types of drug names.
3. Outline drug standards and legislation and the enforcement agencies pertinent to the paramedic profession.
4. Describe the paramedic's responsibilities in drug administration.
5. Distinguish among drug forms.
6. Outline autonomic nervous system functions that may be changed with drug therapy.
7. Discuss factors that influence drug absorption, distribution, and elimination.
8. Describe how drugs react with receptors to produce their desired effects.
9. List variables that can influence drug interactions.
10. Identify special considerations for administering pharmacological agents to pregnant patients, pediatric patients, and older patients.
11. Outline drug actions and care considerations for a patient who is given drugs that affect the nervous, cardiovascular, respiratory, endocrine, and gastrointestinal systems.
12. Explain the meaning of drug terms that are necessary to interpret information in drug references safely.

SUMMARY
- A drug may be defined as any substance taken by mouth; injected into a muscle, blood vessel, or cavity of the body; or applied topically to treat or prevent a disease or condition.
- Drugs can be identified by four types of names. These include the chemical name; generic or nonproprietary name; trade, brand, or proprietary name; and official name.
- The Drug Enforcement Agency is the sole legal drug enforcement body in the United States. Other regulatory bodies or services include the FDA; the Public Health Service; the Federal Trade Commission; in Canada, the Health Protection Branch of the Department of National Health and Welfare; and for international drug control, the International Narcotics Control Board.
- Paramedics are held responsible for the safe and effective administration of drugs. In fact, they are responsible for each drug they provide to a patient. They are legally, morally, and ethically responsible.
- Drug allergies can be divided into four classifications based on the mechanism of the immune reaction. They are type I (anaphylactic), type II (cytotoxic), type III (serum sickness), and type IV (contact dermatitis) reactions.
- The parasympathetic and sympathetic nervous systems function continuously. They innervate many of the same organs at the same time. The opposing actions of the two systems balance each other. In general, the sympathetic

system dominates during stressful events. The parasympathetic system is most active during times of emotional and physical calm.

- The degree to which drugs attain pharmacological activity depends partly on the rate and extent to which they are absorbed. Absorption in turn depends on the ability of the drug to cross the cell membrane. The rate and extent of absorption depend on the nature of the cell membrane the drug must cross, blood flow to the site of administration, solubility of the drug, pH of the drug environment, drug concentration, and drug dosage form.

- The route of drug administration influences drug absorption. These routes can be classified as enteral, parenteral, pulmonary, and topical.

- Distribution is the transport of a drug through the bloodstream to various tissues of the body and ultimately to its site of action. After absorption and distribution, the body eliminates most drugs. The body first biotransforms the drug and then excretes the drug. The kidney is the primary organ for excretion; however, the intestine, lungs, and mammary, sweat, and salivary glands also may be involved.

- Many factors can alter the response to drug therapy, including age, body mass, gender, pathological state, genetic factors, and psychological factors.

- Most drug actions are thought to result from a chemical interaction. This interaction is between the drug and various receptors throughout the body. The most common form of drug action is the drug-receptor interaction.

- Many variables can influence drug interactions, including intestinal absorption, competition for plasma-protein binding, biotransformation, action at the receptor site, renal excretion, and alteration of electrolyte balance.

- Narcotic analgesics relieve pain. Narcotic antagonists reverse the narcotic effects of some analgesics. Nonnarcotic analgesics interfere with local mediators released when tissue is damaged in the periphery of the body. These mediators stimulate nerve endings and cause pain.

- Anesthetic drugs are CNS depressants that have a reversible effect on nervous tissue. Antianxiety agents are used to reduce feelings of apprehension, nervousness, worry, or fearfulness. Sedatives and hypnotics are drugs that depress the CNS. They produce a calming effect. They also help induce sleep. Alcohol is a general CNS depressant that can produce sedation, sleep, and anesthesia.

- Anticonvulsant drugs are used to treat seizure disorders. Most notably they treat epilepsy.

- All CNS stimulants work to increase excitability. They do this by blocking activity of inhibitory neurons or their respective neurotransmitters or by enhancing the production of the excitatory neurotransmitters.

- Psychotherapeutic drugs include antipsychotic agents, antidepressants, and lithium. These drugs are used to treat psychoses and affective disorders, especially schizophrenia, depression, and mania.

- Several movement disorders can result from an imbalance of dopamine and acetylcholine. Drugs that inhibit or block acetylcholine are referred to as anticholinergic. Three classes of drugs affect brain dopamine: those that release dopamine, those that increase brain levels of dopamine, and dopaminergic agonists.

- The autonomic drugs mimic or block the effects of the sympathetic and parasympathetic divisions of the autonomic nervous system. These drugs are classified into four groups: cholinergic (parasympathomimetic) drugs, cholinergic blocking (parasympatholytic) drugs, adrenergic (sympathomimetic) drugs, and adrenergic blocking (sympatholytic) drugs.

- Skeletal muscle relaxants can be classified as central acting, direct acting, and neuromuscular blockers.

- Cardiac drugs are classified by their effects on specialized cardiac tissues. Cardiac glycosides are used to treat congestive heart failure and certain tachycardias. Antidysrhythmic drugs are used to treat and prevent disorders of cardiac rhythm. The pharmacological agents that suppress dysrhythmias may do so by direct action on the cardiac cell membrane (lidocaine), by indirect action that affects the cell (propranolol), or both.

- Antihypertensive drugs used to reduce blood pressure are classified into four major categories: diuretics, sympathetic blocking agents (sympatholytic drugs), vasodilators, and ACE inhibitors. Calcium channel blockers also are used to treat persons with hypertension who do not respond to other drug therapies.

- Antihemorrheologic agents are used to treat peripheral vascular disorders. These disorders are caused by pathological or physiological obstruction (e.g., arteriosclerosis). These agents improve blood flow to ischemic tissues.

- Drugs that affect blood coagulation may be classified as antiplatelet, anticoagulant, or fibrinolytic agents. Drugs that interfere with platelet aggregation are known as antiplatelet or antithrombic drugs. Anticoagulant drug therapy is designed to prevent intravascular thrombosis. The therapy decreases blood coagulability. Fibrinolytic drugs dissolve clots after their formation. These drugs work by promoting the digestion of fibrin.

- Hemophilia is a group of hereditary bleeding disorders. These disorders involve a deficiency of one of the factors needed for the coagulation of blood. Replacing the missing clotting factor can help manage hemophilia.

- Hemostatic agents speed up clot formation, thus reducing bleeding. Systemic hemostatic agents are used to control blood loss after surgery. They work by inhibiting the breakdown of fibrin. Topical hemostatic agents are used to control capillary bleeding. They are used during surgical and dental procedures.
- The treatment of choice in managing a loss of blood or blood components is to replace the sole blood component that is deficient. Replacement therapy may include transfusing whole blood (rare), packed red blood cells, fresh-frozen plasma, plasma expanders, platelets, coagulation factors, fibrinogen, albumin, or gamma globulins.
- Hyperlipidemia refers to an excess of lipids in the plasma. Antihyperlipidemic drugs sometimes are used along with diet and exercise to control serum lipid levels.
- Bronchodilator drugs are the primary form of treatment for obstructive pulmonary disease such as asthma, chronic bronchitis, and emphysema. These drugs may be classified as sympathomimetic drugs and xanthine derivatives.
- Mucokinetic drugs are used to move respiratory secretions, excessive mucus, and sputum along the tracheobronchial tree.
- Oxygen is used chiefly to treat hypoxia and hypoxemia.
- Direct respiratory stimulant drugs act directly on the medullary center of the brain. These drugs are analeptics. They increase the rate and depth of respiration.
- Spirits of ammonia is a reflex respiratory stimulant. The drug is administered by inhalation.
- A cough may be prolonged or may result from an underlying disorder. In such a case, treatment with antitussive drugs may be indicated.
- The main clinical use of antihistamines is for allergic reactions. They also are used to control motion sickness or as a sedative or antiemetic.
- Drug therapy for the gastrointestinal system can be divided into drugs that affect the stomach and drugs that affect the lower gastrointestinal tract. Antacids buffer or neutralize hydrochloric acid in the stomach. Antiflatulents prevent the formation of gas in the gastrointestinal tract. Digestant drugs promote digestion in the gastrointestinal tract. They do this by releasing small amounts of hydrochloric acid in the stomach. Drugs used to induce vomiting may be administered as part of the treatment of certain drug overdoses and poisonings. Drugs used to treat nausea and vomiting include antagonists of histamine, acetylcholine, and dopamine and other drugs the actions of which are not understood clearly.
- Cytoprotective agents and other drugs are used to treat peptic ulcer disease by protecting the gastric mucosa. H_2 receptor antagonists block the H_2 receptors. They also reduce the volume of gastric acid secretion and its acid content.
- Two common conditions of the lower gastrointestinal tract may require drug therapy: constipation and diarrhea. Drugs used to manage these conditions include laxatives and antidiarrheals.
- Drugs used to treat eye disorders include antiglaucoma agents, mydriatics, cycloplegics, antiinfective/antiinflammatory agents, and topical anesthetics.
- Drugs used to treat disorders of the ear include antibiotics, steroid/antibiotic combinations, and miscellaneous preparations.
- The endocrine system works to control and integrate body functions. A number of drugs are used to treat disorders of the anterior and posterior pituitary, the thyroid and parathyroid glands, and the adrenal cortex.
- The pancreatic hormones play a key role in regulating the amount of certain nutrients in the circulatory system. The two main hormones secreted by the pancreas are insulin and glucagon. Imbalances in either of these may call for drug therapy. This therapy is meant to correct metabolic derangements.
- Drugs that affect the female reproductive system include synthetic and natural substances such as hormones, oral contraceptives, ovulation stimulants, and drugs used to treat infertility.
- The male sex hormone is testosterone. Adequate amounts of this hormone are needed for normal development. Adequate amounts also are needed for the maintenance of male sex characteristics.
- Antineoplastic agents are used in cancer chemotherapy to prevent the increase of malignant cells.
- Antibiotics are used to treat local or systemic infection. This group includes penicillin, cephalosporins, and related products; macrolide antibiotics; tetracyclines; and miscellaneous antibiotic agents.
- Persons can be infected by bacterial organisms, fungi, and viruses. Examples of antifungal drugs include tolnaftate (Tinactin), fluconazole (Diflucan), and nystatin (Mycostatin).
- Few drugs exist for use in any viral infections. One antiviral drug is acyclovir (Zovirax). This drug is effective against herpes infection. Another one is zidovudine (Retrovir, AZT), which currently is used to treat human immunodeficiency virus infection.

- Drugs used to treat inflammation or its symptoms may be classified as analgesic-antipyretic drugs and non-steroidal antiinflammatory drugs. A number of medications have both properties.
- Immunosuppressant drugs reduce the activity of the immune system. They do this by suppressing the production and activity of lymphocytes. These drugs are prescribed after transplant surgery. They can help to prevent the rejection of foreign tissues. They also are sometimes given to halt the progress of autoimmune disorders.
- Immunomodulating agents are drugs that help the immune system to be more efficient. They do this by activating the immune defenses and by modifying a biological response to an unwanted stimulus.
- Serum contains agents of immunity. These are antibodies. The antibodies can protect against an organism if the serum is injected into someone else. This forms the basis for passive immunization. Vaccines are composed of killed or altered microorganisms. These are administered to a person to produce specific immunity to a disease-causing bacterial toxin, virus, or bacterium (active immunization).

REVIEW QUESTIONS

Match the appropriate drug form in Column II with its description in Column I. Use each drug form only once.

Column I	Column II
1. _____ Semisolid medicine in a greasy base externally applied to the skin	a. Capsule
2. _____ A sweetened alcohol and water solution	b. Elixir
3. _____ Drug ground into loose granules	c. Emulsion
4. _____ Drug compressed into small disks	d. Extract
5. _____ Drug dissolved in sugar and water suspension (magma)	e. Liniment
6. _____ Flat or round medicine held in mouth until dissolved	f. Lotion
7. _____ Gelatin-covered, dry drug preparation	g. Aqueous
8. _____ Suspension of fat or oil in water with an agent that decreases surface tension	h. Ointment
9. _____ Suspension of insoluble particles in water	i. Tablets
	j. Powder
	k. Aqueous solution
	l. Troche

10. Complete the following sentences by listing the appropriate drug name:
    The precise composition and molecular structure of a drug are described in its (a) _____ name. The name that is not protected by law and denotes pharmacologically similar drugs is known as the

    (b) _____ name. The trademarked name of the drug designated by the company

    that manufactures it is the (c) _____ name. The initials *USP* or *NF* follow the

    (d) _____ name.

11. In one sentence, describe how the following drug standards or legislation influence medication administration and distribution in the United States:
    a. Pure Food and Drug Act (1906):

    _____

    b. Federal Drug and Cosmetic Act (1938):

    _____

    c. Harrison Narcotic Act (1914):

    _____

12. List the agency responsible for each of the following aspects of drug control:

  a. It has the power to suppress false or misleading advertising regarding drugs to the general public.

_____

  b. It is responsible for enforcing the federal Food, Drug, and Cosmetic Act.

_____

  c. It monitors the distribution of controlled substances.

_____

  d. It regulates biological products like antitoxins.

_____

13. Refer to the _Physician's Desk Reference_ (PDR) or _Mosby's DRUGConsult,_ common drug reference sources, to find the answers to the following questions.

  a. What is the indication for the drug beclomethasone?

_____

  b. List the contraindications and side effects of this drug.

_____

Questions 14 to 17 pertain to the following case study:

> Dispatch alerts you to respond to a call for an "accidental injury." When you arrive on the scene, you find a 35-year-old man who stumbled and fell, injuring his wrist. There is deformity, swelling, crepitus, and tenderness proximal to his right hand. After application of the appropriate splint and ice, you decide that medication for pain is indicated.

14. What eight points are critical to ensure that you meet your legal, moral, and ethical obligations for safe, effective medication administration to this patient?

  a.

  b.

  c.

  d.

  e.

  f.

  g.

  h.

> After eliciting a careful history and consultation with medical direction, you initiate an intravenous line in the uninjured extremity and administer ketorolac tromethamine (Toradol) intravenous push. Several moments after administration, the patient becomes anxious and states that he feels like "his throat is going to close in." His skin appears flushed, and a large, flat, raised rash is erupting. The patient states he has never taken this drug before.

15. What type of reaction is this patient having?

_____

16. List two emergency drugs that may be used to treat this patient's signs and symptoms.

_____

After you arrive at the emergency department, the patient admits to the physician that he has had a reaction to aspirin in the past (although during your history, he denied allergic reaction). The physician tells you that there is a reported cross-reactivity between aspirin and ketorolac tromethamine.

17. How would you have known that this type of reaction was possible?

_____

18. Select the appropriate drug term from the following list to complete the sentences:

Antagonism
Contraindications
Cumulative action
Depressant
Drug allergy
Drug dependence
Drug interaction
Idiosyncrasy

Potentiation
Side effect
Stimulant
Summation
Synergism
Therapeutic action
Tolerance
Untoward effect

a. An abnormal or peculiar response to a drug that possibly is caused by a genetic deficiency is

_____.

b. Caffeine and methylphenidate (Ritalin) are examples of drugs that exhibit a(n)

_____ effect.

c. A drug action caused by an immunological response to a previous exposure is a(n)

_____ reaction.

d. The desired effect of naloxone on narcotics is attributed to _____.

e. The enhancement of the effects of one drug caused by the concurrent administration of a second drug is

_____.

f. An undesirable effect of a drug that is harmful to the patient is a(n) _____.

g. The combined action of two drugs that is greater than the sum of each individual agent acting

independently is _____.

h. The intense physical or emotional disturbance possibly resulting when a narcotic is withheld from a person

who frequently uses it is a result of _____.

i. A drug that diminishes a person's central nervous system function is a _____.

j. The ability of atropine to increase the heart rate is known as the desired effect, or _____.

k. The list of factors used to describe situations when medication administration would be harmful is the

_____.

l. Concurrent administration of drugs such that one agent modifies the actions of the other is

_____.

m. A decreased response to a drug after repetitive doses, which necessitates higher doses to achieve the desired

effect, is _____.

n. When repeat administration of drugs results in absorption that exceeds metabolism and excretion, the increased effect that results is known as _____.

19. List six factors that influence the rate and extent to which a drug is absorbed in the body.

    a.

    b.

    c.

    d.

    e.

    f.

20. List four groups of drugs that are associated with a high incidence of drug-drug interactions.

    a.

    b.

    c.

    d.

21. You need to administer acetaminophen to a child who has been vomiting repeatedly. What enteral route will you choose?

    _____

22. When giving epinephrine to an asthmatic patient, a slow and sustained effect is desirable to minimize side effects and prolong the effects of the drug. You will administer the drug by the _____ route.

23. Your 76-year-old patient has a heart rate of 34 and a blood pressure of 70 mm Hg by palpation. You wish to give atropine to increase the heart rate. What route will you choose? _____

24. A 3-month-old infant is in hemorrhagic shock after sustaining a gunshot wound to the abdomen. After intravenous attempts are unsuccessful, what route will you consider for fluid volume resuscitation?

    _____

25. Is the rate of drug absorption by the pulmonary route faster or slower than the subcutaneous route?

    _____

26. List the two physiological barriers to drug distribution within the body.

    a.

    b.

27. Circle the appropriate response regarding drug effects in children.
   a. The blood-brain barrier in infants is less/more effective than in adults; therefore the central nervous system effects of drugs will be less/more.

   b. The newborn has a(n) decreased/increased ability to metabolize drugs; therefore drug toxicity is less/more likely to occur.

28. List three physiological factors that may result in altered drug absorption, distribution, biotransformation, or elimination in the older adult.

   a.

   b.

   c.

29. You are called to a sparsely furnished, one-room apartment to care for a 79-year-old woman complaining of difficulty breathing. She states that she has a history of heart disease and "swelling," and she hands you a sack of empty medication bottles that contained furosemide, digoxin, and potassium. She thinks she last took them 5 or 6 days ago. Discuss three possible reasons for the patient's medication noncompliance.

   a.

   b.

   c.

DRUG CLASSIFICATIONS

30. When given the following description and drug name, identify the drug group to which it belongs and give one additional example of another drug from the same group.
   a. Your patient says he takes lorazepam (Ativan) to help him relax.

   Drug group: _____ Example: _____

   b. You arrive in the emergency department with a 65-year-old woman experiencing an acute myocardial infarction. Immediately, the emergency department staff administers tissue plasminogen activator in an attempt to dissolve the clot.

   Drug group: _____ Example: _____

   c. Before your Mediterranean cruise, you take dimenhydrinate (Dramamine) to prevent seasickness.

   Drug group: _____ Example: _____

   d. During a cardiopulmonary arrest or in selected cases of shock, drugs such as epinephrine (Adrenalin) may be used to stimulate the heart.

   Drug group: _____ Example: _____

   e. Your 45-year-old patient is complaining of chest pain. His only home medication is hydrochlorothiazide (HCTZ) for hypertension.

   Drug group: _____ Example: _____

   f. An older patient is taking captopril (Capoten) for her congestive heart failure.

   Drug group: _____ Example: _____

g. A 30-year-old patient with a seizure disorder is taking phenobarbital (Luminal).

Drug group: _____ Example: _____

h. A 52-year-old hospice patient is taking hydromorphone (Dilaudid) to control his pain.

Drug group: _____ Example: _____

i. Diltiazem (Cardizem) is used by a patient who states that she takes it to control a fast heart rhythm.

Drug group: _____ Example: _____

j. A person at risk for developing clots that may cause heart attack or stroke may be prescribed dipyridamole (Persantine).

Drug group: _____ Example: _____

k. Asthmatics may have a large number of home medicines that may include isoetharine hydrochloride (Bronkosol).

Drug group: _____ Example: _____

l. You observe a patient in the emergency department who is drowsy and having difficulty speaking moments after she has been given etomidate (Amidate).

Drug group: _____ Example: _____

m. You will have increased vigilance for evidence of bleeding if a patient tells you he is taking warfarin sodium (Coumadin).

Drug group: _____ Example: _____

n. A 35-year-old patient is experiencing complications following an outpatient surgical procedure. Her only home medication is pentazocine (Talwin).

Drug group: _____ Example: _____

o. Asthmatic patients may be taking a variety of drugs besides bronchodilators in an attempt to control their disease. Examples of these include cromolyn sodium (Intal), beclomethasone dipropionate (Vanceril Inhaler), and ipratropium (Atrovent).

Drug group: _____ Example: _____

p. You are dispatched to a call for an unconscious person. The patient is awake but confused and combative when you arrive and has a medication list that includes ethosuximide (Zarontin).

Drug group: _____ Example: _____

q. You are treating a young woman with a history of depression. She has taken all 20 of her fluoxetine (Prozac) in a suicide attempt.

Drug group: _____ Example: _____

r. When you arrive at the emergency department with a combative, psychotic patient in restraints, the nurse gives the patient an intramuscular injection of haloperidol (Haldol).

Drug group: _____ Example: _____

s. A patient with a chronic pain disorder is taking amitriptyline (Elavil).

Drug group: _____ Example: _____

t. Medications for management of gastroesophageal reflux disease may include esomeprazole (Nexium).

Drug group: _____ Example: _____

u. During your annual physical, a blood test reveals that you have high cholesterol. The doctor prescribes atorvastatin (Lipitor).

Drug group: _____ Example: _____

v. A patient with Parkinson's disease is taking levodopa (Larodopa).

Drug group: _____ Example: _____

w. Your patient is vomiting blood. His home medicines include ranitidine (Zantac).

Drug group: _____ Example: _____

31. List the generic name of one drug and its general mechanism of actions for each of the following groups of antidysrhythmic drugs.

Group	Generic Name	Actions
IA		
IB		
IC		
II		
III		
IV		

32. Fill in the missing information about hypertensive medications in the following table:

Classification	Generic Name	Actions
	Furosemide, hydrochlorothiazide, spironolactone with hydrochlorothiazide (Aldactazide)	
Beta-blocking agents		
		Block sympathetic stimulation, have multiple sites of action
	Diazoxide, hydralazine, minoxidil (arteriolar dilator), sodium nitroprusside, amyl nitrite, isosorbide dinitrate, nitroglycerin (arteriolar and venous dilator drugs)	
Angiotensin II receptor antagonists	Irbesartan (Avapro), losartan (Cozaar, Hyzaar), valsartan (Diovan)	
Calcium channel blockers		Decrease peripheral resistance by inhibiting blockers, decreasing the contractility of vascular smooth muscle

33. Match the drug listed in Column II with the endocrine gland that it affects in Column I. Use each drug only once.

Column I	Column II
_____ Adrenal cortex	**a.** Clomiphene citrate (Clomid)
_____ Ovary	**b.** Dexamethasone (Decadron)
_____ Pancreas	**c.** Iodine products
_____ Parathyroid	**d.** Methyltestosterone (Metandren)
_____ Pituitary	**e.** Glimepiride (Amaryl)
_____ Testes	**f.** Vasopressin
_____ Thyroid	**g.** Vitamin D

STUDENT SELF-ASSESSMENT

34. Any substance taken by mouth; injected into a muscle, blood vessel, or cavity of the body; or applied topically to treat or prevent a disease or condition is a(n)
   a. Antidote
   b. Drug
   c. Parenteral
   d. Vaccine

35. Morphine is regulated under the Controlled Substance Act of 1970 and is a Schedule _____ drug.
   a. I
   b. II
   c. III
   d. IV

36. The blood-brain barrier and placental barrier will allow passage of only
   a. Antibiotics
   b. Lipid-soluble drugs
   c. Undissociated drugs
   d. Water-soluble drugs

37. Agonists are drugs that do which of the following?
   a. Bind to a receptor and cause a specific response.
   b. Bind to a receptor and cause no response.
   c. Cause duplication of specific receptors.
   d. Prevent chemicals from reaching the receptor sites.

38. The measurement of the relative safety of a drug is which of the following?
   a. Biological half-life
   b. Median effective dose
   c. Median lethal dose
   d. Therapeutic index

39. Which of the following drugs is recommended for administration by endotracheal tube?
   a. Bretylium
   b. Hydroxyzine
   c. Diazepam
   d. Naloxone

40. Which of the following drug administration routes will deliver the most rapid effects?
   a. Oral
   b. Intramuscular
   c. Subcutaneous
   d. Transtracheal

41. Your patient is in profound shock following myocardial infarction. The route of choice for drug administration will be which of the following?
   a. Intramuscular
   b. Intravenous
   c. By mouth
   d. Subcutaneous

42. Which of the following is an opioid antagonist?
   a. Butorphanol tartrate
   b. Naloxone hydrochloride
   c. Oxycodone hydrochloride
   d. Pentazocine hydrochloride

43. All of the following drugs have anticonvulsant properties except which one?
   a. Diazepam
   b. Magnesium sulfate
   c. Nalbuphine
   d. Phenytoin

44. You are transporting a patient with a history of narcolepsy. What drugs might you find that he is taking to reduce his symptoms of this disorder?
   a. Methamphetamine (Desoxyn)
   b. Methylphenidate (Ritalin)
   c. Pemoline (Cylert)
   d. Phenmetrazine (Preludin)

45. Drugs such as levodopa (Larodopa) and carbidopa-levodopa (Sinemet) enhance brain dopamine levels and are used to treat which of the following?

    a. Depression   **c.** Myasthenia gravis

    b. Hypotension   **d.** Parkinson's disease

46. You are experiencing severe muscle spasms after injuring your back at work. Which of the following is an anti-spasmodic medication that may be prescribed for you?

    a. Carbamazepine (Tegretol)   **c.** Chlorpromazine (Thorazine)

    b. Chlordiazepoxide (Librium)   **d.** Cyclobenzaprine (Flexeril)

47. The drugs vecuronium (Norcuron) and succinylcholine (Anectine) may be used for rapid sequence induction of intubation in a person who has sustained severe head trauma. The primary action of these drugs in this situation is which of the following?

    a. To decrease intracranial pressure

    b. To dry oral secretions

    c. To paralyze the muscles

    d. To provide pain relief

48. An indirect-acting cholinergic drug that may be used in the management of poisoning from atropine is which of the following?

    a. Glucagon   **c.** Physostigmine

    b. Lorazepam   **d.** Verapamil

49. What is the chief neurotransmitter for the parasympathetic nervous system?

    a. Acetylcholine   **c.** Metaraminol (Aramine)

    b. Epinephrine (Adrenalin)   **d.** Norepinephrine

50. Stimulation of the beta$_2$-adrenergic receptors will cause which of the following?

    a. Negative inotropic effect on the heart

    b. Positive inotropic effect on the heart

    c. Bronchiolar dilation

    d. Peripheral vasoconstriction

51. Epinephrine has which of the following?

    a. Alpha effects only   **c.** Alpha and beta effects

    b. Beta effects only   **d.** Neither alpha nor beta effects

52. Drugs that increase the contractility of the heart have a positive _____ effect.

    a. Chronotropic   **c.** Dromotropic

    b. Cholinergic   **d.** Inotropic

53. You are called to the home of an older man who is complaining of dizziness, nausea, vomiting, weakness, and yellow vision. When questioned about his home medications, he states that he takes a small tablet to help his "weak heart." His pulse is 45 per minute. You suspect he is suffering from which of the following?

    a. Digoxin overdose   **c.** Tricyclic antidepressant overdose

    b. Isoproterenol overdose   **d.** Verapamil overdose

54. Which of the following is a group IV antidysrhythmic drug?

    a. Bretylium tosylate   **c.** Procainamide

    b. Lidocaine   **d.** Verapamil

55. The primary mechanism by which antihypertensives reduce blood pressure is by decreasing which of the following?

    a. Cardiac output   **c.** Myocardial contractility

    b. Intravascular blood volume   **d.** Peripheral vascular resistance

56. Which of the following drugs acts by dissolving a clot that has formed already?

    a. Aspirin   **c.** Heparin

    b. Coumadin   **d.** Streptokinase

57. Which of the following is a beta$_2$-specific bronchodilator?

    a. Albuterol   **c.** Ephedrine

    b. Aminophylline   **d.** Isoproterenol

58. All of the following are indications for antihistamines except which one?

    a. Allergic reactions   **c.** Motion sickness

    b. Asthma   **d.** Nausea and vomiting

59. An elderly patient has a disorder necessitating the use of pilocarpine drops. What is he suffering from?
   a. Conjunctivitis
   b. Glaucoma
   c. Keratitis
   d. Pain

60. Which of the following is true about insulin?
   a. It is secreted by the adrenal glands.
   b. It is secreted only during stress.
   c. It will increase the use of fat for fuel.
   d. It will move glucose into the cells.

61. Your patient states that she is allergic to penicillin. Which of the following drugs can she take safely?
   a. Amoxicillin (Amoxil)
   b. Cefazolin (Ancef)
   c. Dicloxacillin (Dynapen)
   d. Tetracycline (Achromycin)

62. Which of the following is an antiviral drug used in treatment of patients infected with human immunodeficiency virus?
   a. Acyclovir (Zovirax)
   b. Pyrimethamine (Daraprim)
   c. Quinine (Quinamm)
   d. Zidovudine (Retrovir)

63. Isoniazid (INH) and rifampin (Rifadin) are drugs used to treat which of the following?
   a. HIV infection
   b. Leprosy
   c. Malaria
   d. Tuberculosis

WRAP IT UP

You are dispatched to the home of an elderly male who has been "passing out." When you arrive, you find him to be conscious but confused and unable to give you any history. He is pale and sweaty, has vomited, and has the following vital signs: BP 90/54 mm Hg, P 56/min, and R 16/min. When you listen to his lungs, you hear crackles in the bases on both sides. You find a medication list that indicates he is allergic to penicillin and the following list of current medicines: digoxin (Lanoxin), atenolol, amiodarone, Humulin insulin 70/30, propoxyphene, lorazepam, sertraline, cyclobenzaprine, diltiazem, aspirin, furosemide, K-Dur (potassium), ipratropium, albuterol, ranitidine, and azithromycin.

1. What type of medication allergy reaction is penicillin most likely to cause?
   a. Type I, anaphylactic
   b. Type II, cytotoxic
   c. Type III, serum sickness
   d. Type IV, contact dermatitis

_____

2. Which of his home medications have an effect on the autonomic nervous system?

_____

3. Which of his home medications are given by the parenteral route?

_____

4. One of his medications, Lanoxin, has a very low therapeutic index. Why is that important for you to know?

_____

5. What factors may contribute to medication noncompliance in an older adult?

_____

6. Which of his home medications could be contributing to his confusion?

_____

7. Which of his medications is a(n)

    a. Antihypertensive

    b. Antidysrhythmic (list specific class)

    c. Antiplatelet

    d. Muscle relaxant

    e. Controlled substancei

    f. Bronchodilator

    g. Analgesic

    h. H_2 receptor antagonist

    i. Antibiotic

---

8. Because the patient is unable to give you information about his medical history, you must try to determine what medical conditions he could have based on his medication list. What conditions do you suspect he suffers from?

---

9. Based on this knowledge and your physical exam of the patient, what are some possible causes for his signs and symptoms today?

CHAPTER 17 ANSWERS

REVIEW QUESTIONS

1. h   **6.** l
2. b   **7.** a
3. j   **8.** c
4. i   **9.** g
5. k
(Questions 1 to 9, Objective 5)

10. a. Chemical
    b. Generic or nonproprietary
    c. Trade or proprietary
    d. Official
    (Objective 2)

11. a. Protected the public from mislabeled drugs, prohibited the use of false and misleading claims for medications, and restricted sales of drugs with abuse potential
    b. Prevented marketing of drugs until they were tested and required names of all ingredients and directions on labels
    c. Controlled the sale of narcotics and established *narcotic* as a legal term
    (Objective 3)

12. a. Federal Trade Commission
    b. Food and Drug Administration
    c. Drug Enforcement Administration
    d. Public Health Service
    (Objective 3)

13. a. For chronic control of bronchial asthma
    b. Contraindicated in the treatment of acute episodes of asthma or status asthmaticus or if a known hypersensitivity exists (PDR)
    (Objective 12)

14. A paramedic's responsibilities relative to drug administration include the following: using correct techniques; observing and documenting effects of drugs; maintaining current knowledge regarding pharmacology; maintaining professional relationships; understanding pharmacology; evaluating drug indications and contraindications; using drug reference materials; taking a patient history; and consulting with medical direction. (Objective 4)

15. The patient is demonstrating signs and symptoms of a type I hypersensitivity allergic reaction. (Objective 4)

16. The chemicals histamine and slow-reacting substance of anaphylaxis are released during an anaphylactic reaction. Diphenhydramine and/or epinephrine are used to treat this. (Objective 4)

17. Sometimes patients may have an allergic reaction to a drug they have never taken that is chemically similar to another drug to which they are allergic. This information can be found in the drug profile. (Objective 4)

18. a. Idiosyncrasy
    b. Stimulant
    c. Drug allergy
    d. Antagonism
    e. Potentiation
    f. Side effect
    g. Synergism
    h. Drug dependence
    (Objective 12)

    i. Depressant
    j. Therapeutic action
    k. Contraindications
    l. Drug interaction
    m. Tolerance
    n. Cumulative action.

19. The nature of the absorbing surface through which the drug must travel, the blood flow to the site of administration, the solubility of the drug, the pH of the drug environment, the drug concentration, and the drug dosage form
    (Objective 7)

20. Drug-drug interactions commonly are associated with blood thinners, tricyclic antidepressants, amphetamines, digitalis glycosides, diuretics, alcohol, antihypertensives, and cigarette smoking.
    (Objective 9)

21. Rectal
    (Objective 10)

22. Subcutaneous
    (Objective 11)

23. Intravenous
    (Objective 11)

24. Intraosseous
    (Objective 11)

25. Faster
    (Objective 7)

26. Placenta and blood-brain barrier
    (Objective 7)

27. a. Less, more
    b. Decreased, more
    (Objective 10)

28. Decreased renal function, altered nutrition habits, greater consumption of nonprescription drugs, reduced gastric acid, slowed gastric motility, decreased serum albumin, congestive heart failure, and decreased blood flow to the liver
    (Objective 10)

29. Inability to pay for new drugs, forgetfulness or confusion, lack of symptoms (causing patient to become noncompliant), and other physical disabilities not mentioned
    (Objective 10)

30. a. Benzodiazepines: alprazolam (Xanax), chlordiazepoxide (Librium), clorazepate (Tranxene), diazepam (Valium), flurazepam (Dalmane), lorazepam (Ativan), midazolam (Versed), temazepam (Restoril), clonazepam (Klonopin).
    b. Fibrinolytic agents: anisoylated plasminogen streptokinase activator (Eminase), streptokinase (Streptase), reteplase (Retavase), tenecteplase (TNKase)

c. Antiemetics/antihistamines: diphenhydramine hydrochloride (Benadryl), hydroxyzine pamoate (Vistaril), meclizine hydrochloride (Antivert), promethazine hydrochloride (Phenergan)

d. Adrenergics: dobutamine (Dobutrex), dopamine (Intropin), isoproterenol (Isuprel), norepinephrine (Levophed)

e. Diuretics: furosemide (Lasix), spironolactone (Aldactone).

f. Angiotensin-converting enzyme (ACE) inhibitor: enalapril (Vasotec), benazepril (Lotensin), fosinopril (Monopril), lisinopril (Prinivil, Zestril), quinapril (Accupril)

g. Anticonvulsants, barbiturate: mephobarbital (Gemonil)

h. Narcotic analgesics: codeine, methylmorphine, meperidine (Demerol), methadone (Dolophine, Methadose), morphine sulfate (Astramorph and others), oxycodone (Percodan, Tylox, Percocet), propoxyphene (Darvon, Dolene), hydrocodone (Lortab).

i. Class IV antidysrhythmics: verapamil (Isoptin), amlodipine (Norvasc), felodipine (Plendil)

j. Antiplatelet agents: aspirin, sulfinpyrazone (Anturane), clopidogrel (Plavix), ticlopidine (Ticlid), abciximab (ReoPro)

k. Beta$_2$-selective bronchodilators: albuterol (Proventil, Ventolin), bitolterol (Tornalate), terbutaline sulfate (Brethine, Bricanyl), salmeterol (Serevent), levalbuterol (Xopenex)

l. Nonbarbiturate anesthetic agents: fentanyl (Sublimaze), sufentanil (Sufenta), alfentanil (Alfenta)

m. Anticoagulants: heparin sodium (Liquaemin)

n. Opioid agonist-antagonist agents: nalbuphine hydrochloride (Nubain)

o. Muscarinic antagonists used to treat respiratory emergencies: glycopyrrolate (Robinul)

p. Anticonvulsants (succinimides): methsuximide (Celontin), phensuximide (Milontin)

q. Selective serotonin reuptake inhibitors: sertraline (Zoloft), paroxetine (Paxil), fluvoxamine (Luvox), and citalopram (Celexa)

r. Antipsychotic agents: chlorpromazine (Thorazine), thioridazine (Mellaril), fluphenazine (Prolixin), molindone (Lidone), loxapine (Loxitane), olanzapine, resperidol

s. Tricyclic antidepressants: mirtazapine (Remeron), nortriptyline (Pamelor)

t. Proton pump inhibitors: lansoprazole (Prevacid), omeprazole (Prilosec), pantoprazole (Protonix), rabeprazole (AcipHex)

u. Antihyperlipidemic drugs: fenofibrate (Tricor), fluvastatin (Lescol), gemfibrozil (Lopid), pravastatin (Pravachol), simvastatin (Zocor)

v. Drugs that affect brain dopamine (used in treatment of Parkinson's disease): cabidopa-levodopa (Sinemet), amantadine (Symmetrel), bromocriptine (Parlodel), pergolide (Permax)

w. H$_2$-receptor antagonists: cimetidine (Tagamet), famotidine (Pepcid)

(Objective 12)

31.

Group	Drug Name	Actions
IA	Quinidine, procainamide	Decrease conduction velocity; prolong electrical potential of cardiac tissue
IB	Lidocaine, phenytoin	Increase or have no effect on conduction velocity
IC	Flecainide, encainide	Profoundly slow conduction
II	Propranolol	Beta-blockers
III	Bretylium, amiodarone	Antiadrenergic agents; positive inotropic action; terminate reentry dysrhythmias
IV	Verapamil, diltiazem	Block flow of calcium into cardiac and smooth muscle cells; decrease automaticity

(Objective 11)

32.

Classification	Generic Name	Actions
Diuretics	Furosemide, hydrochlorothiazide, spironolactone with hydrochlorothiazide (Aldactazide)	Increase renal excretion of salt and water; decrease blood volume direct effect on arterioles

Beta-blocking agents	Propranolol, acebutolol, atenolol, metoprolol, labetalol, nadolol	Decrease cardiac output; inhibit renin secretion from kidneys; beta-blockers compete with epinephrine for beta receptor sites and inhibit tissue/organ response to beta stimulation
Adrenergic inhibiting agents	Clonidine (central acting), guanethidine, reserpine (peripheral inhibitors) prazosin hydrochloride, phentolamine, phenoxy benzamine (alpha$_1$- and alpha$_2$-blocking agents, nonselective)	Block sympathetic stimulation; have multiple sites of action
Vasodilator drugs	Diazoxide, hydralazine, minoxidil (arteriolar dilator), sodium nitroprusside, amyl nitrite, isosorbide dinitrate, nitroglycerin (arteriolar and venous dilator drugs)	Act directly on smooth muscle walls of arterioles, veins, or both; lower peripheral resistance and blood pressure
Angiotensin-converting enzyme inhibitors, angiotensin II receptor antagonists	Captopril, enalapril, lisinopril, irbesartan (Avapro), losartan (Cozaar, Hyzaar), valsartan (Diovan)	Inhibit the conversion of angiotensin I to angiotensin II. Angiotensin II is a powerful vasoconstrictor that suppresses renin-angiotensin aldosterone system. Selectively inhibit angiotensin receptors that include vasoconsriction, renal tubular sodium reabsorption, aldosterone release, and stimulation of arterial and peripheral sympathetic activity.
Calcium channel blockers	Verapamil, nifedipine, diltiazem	Decrease peripheral resistance by inhibiting blockers and the contractility of vascular smooth muscle

(Objective 11)

33. b, a, e, g, f, d, c
(Objective 11)

34. b. An *antidote* is a specific drug taken to minimize the adverse effects of an ingested drug or poison. *Parenteral* refers to a drug route. A *vaccine* is an injection of drug given to prevent disease.
(Objective 1)

35. b
(Objective 3)

36. b. Only selected antibiotics pass through these barriers.
(Objective 7)

37. a. Antagonists block receptor sites and inhibit action.
(Objective 8)

38. d. Median lethal dose is the lethal dose for 50% of animals that took the drug. Median effective dose is the effective dose for 50% of animals that took the drug. Biological half-life is the time required to excrete half of the total amount of drug introduced into the body.
(Objective 7)

39. d. Atropine, lidocaine, and epinephrine also may be given by this route.
(Objective 7)

40. d. Then intramuscular, subcutaneous, and oral
(Objective 7)

41. b. All of the other routes listed give unpredictable, slow absorption because of poor perfusion in shock.
(Objective 7)

42. b. Butorphanol tartrate and pentazocine are opioid agonist-antagonists, and oxycodone hydrochloride is an opioid analgesic-agonist.
(Objective 11)

43. c. Nalbuphine is an opioid agonist-antagonist.
(Objective 11)

44. a. Methylphenidate (Ritalin) and pemoline (Cylert) are used to manage patients with attention deficit disorder and hyperactivity. Phenmetrazine is an anorexiant.
(Objective 11)

45. d. Depression usually is treated with a tricyclic antidepressant. Hypotension is treated based on the cause. Occasionally, intravenously administered dopamine will be used, but it acts in a different manner than the drugs that affect brain dopamine levels. Drugs used to treat myasthenia gravis elevate acetylcholine at the myoneural junctions.
(Objective 11)

46. d. Carbamazepine (Tegretol) is used to treat seizure disorders. Chlordiazepoxide (Librium) and chlorpromazine (Thorazine) are antipsychotic drugs. Baclofen (Lioresal) and diazepam (Valium) are also antispasmodics that may be used to manage muscle spasms.
(Objective 11)

47. c. These drugs paralyze muscles and usually are given concurrently with other drugs that decrease the intracranial pressure during intubation (lidocaine) and sedatives and/or pain relievers.
(Objective 11)

48. c. Physostigmine is used to manage poisonings. Glucagon is a pancreatic hormone that increases blood glucose, lorazepam is a minor tranquilizer, and verapamil is an antidysrhythmic drug.
(Objective 11)

49. a. Norepinephrine is the primary neurotransmitter for the sympathetic nervous system. *Adrenalin* is a trade name for epinephrine, and *Aramine* is the trade name for metaraminol.
(Objective 6)

50. c
(Objective 11)

51. c
(Objective 6)

52. d. Chronotropes increase heart rate; dromotropes increase conduction velocity. Cholinergic drugs increase parasympathetic effects.
(Objective 6)

53. a. Influenza-like symptoms and a variety of dysrhythmias are associated with digoxin toxicity. Tricyclic antidepressant or isoproterenol overdose likely would produce tachyarrhythmias. Verapamil overdose may cause bradycardias and severe hypotension.
(Objective 11)

54. d. Bretylium tosylate is a group III, lidocaine is a group IB, and procainamide is a group IA antidysrhythmic agent.
(Objective 11)

55. d. Some also decrease heart rate and contractility; however, the majority achieve their effects by decreasing vascular resistance.
(Objective 11)

56. d. All of the others prevent clot formation.
(Objective 11)

57. a. Ephedrine and isoproterenol are nonspecific beta-agonists, and aminophylline is a xanthine derivative.
(Objective 11)

58. b. Antihistamines may worsen an acute asthma attack by thickening bronchial secretions.
(Objective 11)

59. b. Antiinfective and antiinflammatory agents are used to treat conjunctivitis or keratitis. Topical anesthetic agents are used to treat pain.
(Objective 11)

60. d. Insulin is secreted continually in amounts determined by the needs of the body.
(Objective 11)

61. d. Amoxicillin and dicloxacillin are penicillin drugs. A percentage of persons who are allergic to penicillin have cross-reactivity to cephalosporins such as cefazolin.
(Objective 11)

62. d. Acyclovir (Zovirax) typically is prescribed for herpes infection (some patients infected with human immunodeficiency virus also may take this to treat opportunistic herpes infections). Pyrimethamine (Daraprim) and quinine (Qui-namm) are antimalarial drugs.
(Objective 11)

63. d
(Objective 11)

WRAP IT UP

1. a. The reaction may vary from hives to life-threatening airway compromise. Cytotoxic reactions usually involve hemolysis and result from administration of procainamide or hydralazine. Serum sickness can be caused by penicillins, iodides, sulfonamides, phenytoin, and some antitoxins and can cause a severe inflammatory reaction. Contact dermatitis results from exposure to poison ivy, sunscreens, and other topical ointments.
(Objective 6)

2. Atenolol is a beta-blocker and albuterol is a beta$_2$-selective stimulant.
(Objective 7)

3. His Humulin insulin is given by subcutaneous injection.
(Objective 7)

4. The margin between the therapeutic dose of digoxin (Lanoxin) and its lethal dose is small. Often patients experience signs and symptoms of digoxin overdose.
(Objective 8)

5. Drug cost may be too much for the older adult; confusion may cause overdosing or underdosing; visual or physical impairment can cause drug errors; or the patient may choose not to follow the prescribed medication plan. (Objective 11)

6. Propoxyphene, lorazepam, sertraline, or cyclobenzaprine could cause some confusion. If his blood sugar is low because of his Humulin insulin administration, that also could cause confusion. (Objective 12)

7. a. Atenolol, diltiazem, furosemide
  b. Digoxin (Lanoxin; cardiac glycoside), atenolol (Class II—beta-blockers); diltiazem (Class IV—calcium channel blockers); amiodarone (Class III—potassium channel blockers)
  c. Aspirin
  d. Lorazepam, cyclobenzaprine
  e. Propoxyphene, lorazepam
  f. Albuterol, ipratropium (indirectly)
  g. Propoxyphene, aspirin
  h. Ranitidine
  i. Azithromycin
  (Objective 12)

8. Based on the medication list that you have found, you can suspect that his medical history may include diabetes (Humulin), hypertension (atenolol, diltiazem, furosemide), cardiac rhythm disturbance (digoxin [Lanoxin], atenolol, amiodarone, diltiazem), risk factors for or history of myocardial infarction/stroke (aspirin); musculoskeletal pain or arthritis (propoxyphene, lorazepam, cyclobenzaprine); chronic obstructive pulmonary disease (ipratropium, albuterol); gastritis or ulcers (ranitidine); recent infection (azithromycin). (Objective 12)

9. Clues to the cause of his present illness may be found in the physical examination. He could be confused because of his drugs, sepsis, a stroke, chronic dementia, electrolyte imbalance (low sodium or potassium), hypotension and subsequent decrease in cerebral perfusion; or he could be having a stroke; he could have taken too much of his medications; or he may be hypoxic. (Objective 12)

Venous Access and Medication Administration

READING ASSIGNMENT
Chapter 18, pages 388-428, in *Mosby's Paramedic Textbook,* ed. 3

OBJECTIVES
Upon completion of this chapter, the paramedic student will be able to:
1. Convert selected units of measurement into the household, apothecary, and metric systems.
2. Identify the steps in the calculation of drug dosages.
3. Calculate the correct volume of drug to be administered in a given situation.
4. Compute the correct rate for an infusion of drugs or intravenous fluids.
5. List measures for ensuring the safe administration of medications.
6. Describe actions paramedics should take if a medication error occurs.
7. List measures for preserving asepsis during parenteral administration of a drug.
8. Explain drug administration techniques for the enteral and parenteral routes.
9. Describe the steps for safely initiating an intravenous infusion.
10. Identify complications and adverse effects associated with intravenous access.
11. Describe the steps for safely initiating an intraosseous infusion.
12. Explain drug administration techniques for percutaneous routes.
13. Identify special considerations in the administration of pharmacological agents to pediatric patients.
14. Explain the technique for obtaining a venous blood sample.
15. Describe the safe disposal of contaminated items and sharps.

SUMMARY
- Three systems for measuring drug dosage are in common use today. These are the metric system, the apothecary system, and the common household system. Each system deals with units of mass and volume. Any of these three systems may be used by a physician when ordering drugs.
- Paramedics should choose a drug calculation method that is precise. It also should be reliable. Paramedics should
- (1) Convert all units of measure to the same size and system.
- (2) Assess the computed dosage to determine whether it is reasonable.
- (3) Use one method of dose calculation consistently.

- Many drug calculations can be performed almost intuitively. Nevertheless, paramedics should never rely on intuitive calculations. Methods of calculation include the basic formula (desire over have), ratios and proportions, and dimensional analysis.
- Intravenous flow rates can be calculated using the following formula:

- Drops/min = $\dfrac{\text{Volume to be infused} \times \text{Drops/mL of infusion set}}{\text{Total time of infusion (min)}}$

- Safety procedures should be a high priority during the administration of any medication. The paramedic must make sure the *right* patient receives the *right* dose of the *right* drug via the *right* route at the *right* time.
- An incident involving a medication error may occur. In such a case, paramedics should take responsibility for their actions. They should quickly advise medical direction. They also should assess and monitor the patient for effects of the drug. They must document the error as required by local, state, and medical direction policies. In addition, they must change their personal practice to prevent a similar error in the future.
- Medical asepsis is accomplished by using clean technique, which involves hygienic measures, cleaning agents, antiseptics, disinfectants, and barrier fields.
- Enteral drugs are administered and absorbed through the gastrointestinal tract. They are given by the oral, gastric, and rectal routes. Parenteral drugs are administered outside the intestine. They are usually injected. Parenteral drugs are given by the intradermal, subcutaneous, intramuscular, intravenous, and intraosseous routes.
- In the prehospital setting, the route of choice for fluid replacement is through a peripheral vein in an extremity. The over-the-needle catheter generally is preferred in this setting.
- Several possible complications are associated with all intravenous techniques. These include local complications, systemic complications, infiltration, and air embolism.
- Cannulation of the central veins presents specific dangers. These are in addition to the complications common to all intravenous methods.
- Fluids and drugs that are infused by the intraosseous route pass from the marrow cavities into the sinusoids. Next, they pass into large venous channels and emissary veins. Then they pass into the systemic circulation. The site of choice for IO infusions in children is the tibia, one to two fingerbreadths below the tubercle on the anteromedial surface.
- Percutaneous drugs are absorbed through the mucous membranes or skin. These include topical drugs, sublingual drugs, buccal drugs, inhaled drugs, endotracheal drugs, and drugs for the eye, nose, and ear.
- Administering drugs to infants and children can be quite difficult. This often is especially true in emergency situations. Paramedics frequently calculate pediatric drug doses by using memory aids. Some of these aids include charts, tapes, and dosage books. Doses also are calculated with the advice of medical direction.
- If possible, venous blood samples should be obtained when intravenous access is established. They also should be obtained before any fluids are infused. If no IV line is to be used and a blood sample is still needed, it must be obtained with a needle and syringe (or a special vacuum needle and sleeve).
- The CDC recommends that needles not be capped, bent, or broken before disposal. Rather, they should be left on the syringe and discarded in an appropriate, clearly marked container that is puncture proof and leak proof.

MATH SKILLS

The following questions are a brief review of basic math skills necessary for drug dose calculation. The review is intended as a refresher. If the student does not understand these concepts, the student should consult references or seek tutoring before proceeding to the next section.

Fractions

A fraction is part of a whole number or one number divided by another number. A fraction consists of two parts, the numerator and the denominator:

$$\frac{a}{b} \qquad \begin{array}{l}\text{a is the numerator}\\ \text{b is the denominator}\end{array}$$

The denominator indicates the number of equal parts into which the whole is separated. The numerator tells how many parts are being considered (Fig. 18-1).

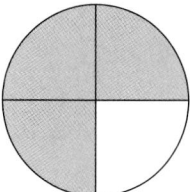

Figure 18-1

Example: $\dfrac{3}{4}$ $\dfrac{\text{Numerator is 3, so three parts are being used}}{\text{Denominator is 4 for there are four equal parts}}$

A fraction that has the same numerator and denominator equals the whole number 1 (Fig. 18-2).

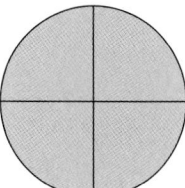

Figure 18-2

Example: $\dfrac{4}{4} = 1$

1. Identify the numerator and denominator of the following fractions.

   a. $\dfrac{7}{8}$ = ———   **b.** $\dfrac{6}{13}$ = ———

When the numerator and denominator of the fraction are multiplied by the same number, the value of the fraction remains unchanged.

Example: $\dfrac{1 \times 2}{2 \times 2} = \dfrac{2}{4} = \dfrac{1}{2}$

A fraction may be reduced to lower terms by dividing the numerator and denominator by the largest whole number that will go evenly into both of them.

Example: $\dfrac{100}{1000} \times \dfrac{100 \div 100}{1000 \div 100} = \dfrac{1}{10}$

2. Reduce the following fractions to lowest terms.
   a. $\frac{7}{28}$ **d.** $\frac{6}{36}$ **g.** $\frac{24}{120}$ **j.** $\frac{10}{25}$
   b. $\frac{9}{12}$ **e.** $\frac{25}{125}$ **h.** $\frac{9}{25}$ **k.** $\frac{17}{23}$
   c. $\frac{4}{8}$ **f.** $\frac{18}{72}$ **i.** $\frac{1000}{10,000}$ **l.** $\frac{16}{24}$

An improper fraction has a larger numerator than denominator.

Example: $\dfrac{8}{4}$

To change an improper fraction to a whole number, divide the numerator by the denominator:

Example: $\frac{8}{4} = 8 \div 4 = 2$ (Whole number)

          $\frac{7}{4} = 7 \div 4 = 1\frac{3}{4}$ (This is a mixed number because it has a whole number plus a fraction.)

3. Convert the following to whole numbers or mixed fractions.

     a. $\frac{75}{8}$ **b.** $\frac{24}{12}$ **c.** $\frac{12}{4}$ **d.** $\frac{15}{6}$

To change a mixed number into an improper fraction, multiply the whole number by the denominator of the fraction and add the numerator of the fraction to the result.

Example: $4\frac{1}{2} = \frac{(4 \times 2) + 1}{2} = \frac{9}{2}$

4. Change each of the following mixed numbers to improper fractions:

     a. $5\frac{3}{8}$ **b.** $1\frac{3}{4}$ **c.** $3\frac{1}{12}$ **d.** $15\frac{2}{3}$

To change a fraction to equivalent fractions in which both terms are larger, multiply the numerator and denominator by the same number.

Example: Enlarge $\frac{2}{5}$ to the equivalent fraction in tenths.

$$\frac{2}{5} \times \frac{2}{2} = \frac{4}{10}$$

5. Change the following fractions to the equivalent fraction indicated.

     a. $\frac{6}{8} = \frac{x}{24}$ **b.** $\frac{12}{15} = \frac{x}{60}$ **c.** $\frac{79}{100} = \frac{x}{100,000}$

To compare fractions with different denominators, find the lowest common denominator. The lowest common denominator is the smallest number that is divisible by the denominators.

Example 1: What is the lowest common denominator of $\frac{1}{2}$, $\frac{3}{5}$, and $\frac{7}{10}$?

The denominators are 2, 5, and 10. Because 10 is divisible by 2 and 5, it is the lowest common denominator.

Example 2: What is the lowest common denominator of $\frac{1}{3}$ and $\frac{2}{5}$? Because 5 is not divisible by 3, multiply the larger denominator by 2, 3, 4, and so on. Each time, determine whether the product is divisible by 3:

$5 \times 2 = 10$ 10 is not divisible by 3.
$5 \times 3 = 15$ 15 is divisible by 3, so 15 is the lowest common denominator.

6. Find the lowest common denominator.

     a. $\frac{1}{3}$ and $\frac{1}{8}$ **b.** $\frac{2}{3}$ and $\frac{1}{12}$ **c.** $\frac{1}{3}$, $\frac{2}{6}$ and $\frac{3}{8}$

7. Circle the correct response:

     a. $\frac{3}{8}$ is greater than, less than, or equal to $\frac{9}{24}$.
     b. $\frac{5}{9}$ is greater than, less than, or equal to $\frac{5}{8}$.
     c. $\frac{2}{5}$ is greater than, less than, or equal to $\frac{7}{10}$.

     To add or subtract fractions, do the following:
     1. Convert all fractions to equivalent fractions using the lowest common denominator.
     2. Add or subtract the numerator and place over the common denominator.
     3. Simplify to the lowest terms.

Example: $\dfrac{5}{9} + \dfrac{2}{6} = \dfrac{5(2)}{9(2)} + \dfrac{2(3)}{6(3)} = \dfrac{10}{18} + \dfrac{6}{18} \div \dfrac{2}{2} = \dfrac{8}{9}$

8. Add the following fractions and mixed numbers:

    a. ⅞ + ⅔ + ¹⁄₁₀   **b.** 1¼ + 2⅔

9. Subtract the following fractions and mixed numbers:

    a. 1⅗ − ⁹⁄₁₀   **b.** 2¾ − ⅚

To multiply fractions, do the following:
1. Change mixed numbers to improper fractions.
2. Multiply numerators.
3. Multiply denominators.
4. Simplify to the lowest terms.

Example: $\dfrac{3}{4} \times \dfrac{4}{5} = \dfrac{12}{20} \div \dfrac{4}{4} = \dfrac{3}{5}$

10. Multiply the following fractions and mixed numbers:

    a. ⁵⁄₁₆ × ¹¹⁄₁₃   **c.** 6⅞ × 2

    b. 8½ × 3   **d.** ⅓ × ⅞

To divide fractions, do the following:
1. Change mixed numbers to improper fractions.
2. Turn the number after the division sign (÷) upside down.
3. Follow the steps for multiplication of fractions.
4. Simplify to the lowest terms.

Example: $\dfrac{4}{5} \div \dfrac{2}{3} = \dfrac{4}{5} \times \dfrac{3}{2} = \dfrac{12}{10} \div \dfrac{2}{2} = \dfrac{6}{5} = 1\frac{1}{5}$

11. Divide the following fractions:

    a. ⅜ ÷ ³⁄₁₀   **b.** 2½ ÷ ⁷⁄₁₁

Decimals

All whole numbers are to the left of the decimal; all decimal fractions are to the right of the decimal (Fig. 18-3).

12. Write the decimal notation for the following examples:

    a. 3 and 4 tenths   **b.** 5 and 35 hundredths   **c.** 62 thousandths

To convert a fraction into a decimal, do the following:
1. Divide the numerator by the denominator.
2. Place the decimal point in the proper position.

Example: $\dfrac{3}{5} = 3 \div 5 = 5\overline{)3.0}^{\,0.6}$

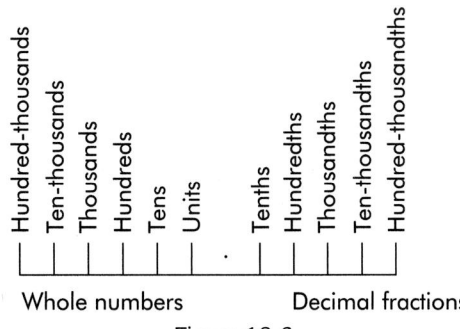

Figure 18-3

225

13. Change the following fractions to decimals:

  a. ¼   **b.** ⁷⁄₂₅   **c.** ³⁄₁₅₀

To convert a decimal to a fraction, do the following:

1. Write the numerator of the fraction as the numbers expressed in the decimal.
2. Write the denominator of the fraction as the number 1 followed by the number of zeros as there are places to the right of the decimal point.
3. Simplify the fraction to the lowest terms.

  Example: $0.234 = x$
  Numerator = 234
  Denominator = 1 + three zeros = 1000

  Simplify: $\dfrac{234}{1000} = \dfrac{234}{1000} \div \dfrac{2}{2} = \dfrac{117}{500}$

14. Change the following decimals to fractions.

  a. 0.5   **b.** 3.24   **c.** 6.007

To add or subtract decimals, do the following:

1. Line up the decimal points.
2. Add zeros to make all decimal numbers equal length.
3. Add or subtract as with whole numbers.
4. Place the decimal point in the sum.

  Example: $0.6 + 4.23 + 1.123 = x$

Line up the decimal points:	0.6
	4.23
	1.123
Add zeros:	0.600
	4.230
	1.123
Add as whole numbers:	5.953
Place the decimal point in the sum.	

15. Add the following decimals.

  a. $0.03 + 0.12 + 0.32$ **b.** $0.26 + 0.01 + 0.75$

16. Subtract the following decimals.

  a. $91.5 - 62.5$ **b.** $17 - 3.42$

To multiply decimals, do the following:
1. Multiply as with whole numbers.
2. Count the total number of decimal places in the decimals multiplied.
3. Place the decimal point in the answer to the left of the total decimal places calculated in step 2.
4. When multiplying a decimal by a power of 10, move the decimal point the same number of places to the right as there are zeros in the multiplier.

  Example: $1.25 \times 3.3 = x$
  1.25   (two decimal places)
  $\times 3.3$ (one decimal place)
  4.125   (The decimal point is placed to the left of three decimal places.)

  Example: $3.46 \times 10 = 3.4.6 = 34.6$

17. Multiply the following decimals.

  a. 3.62×0.02 **c.** 7.25×0.03 **e.** 2.9×10
  b. 27×0.04 **d.** 4.256×100 **f.** 7.052×1000

To divide decimals, do the following:
1. If the divisor (number you are dividing by) is a whole number, divide as you would with whole numbers. Place the decimal place in the answer in the same place it was in the number to be divided.
2. If the divisor (number you are dividing by) is a decimal, make it a whole number by moving the decimal place to the end of the divisor. Move the decimal in the number being divided by the same number of places.
3. If the divisor is a power of 10, move the decimal point to the left as many places as there are zeros in the divisor.

Example: $25.5 \div 5 = 5\overline{)25.5} = 5.1$

Example: $25.5 \div 0.5 = 0.5\overline{)25.5} = 5\overline{)255} = 51$

Example: $25.5 \div 10 = 2.55 (2.5.5)$

18. Divide the following.
    a. $0.25 \div 5$ **d.** $0.16 \div 0.04$
    b. $5.16 \div 2$ **e.** $14.237 \div 100$
    c. $4 \div 0.5$ **f.** $0.17 \div 10$

Rounding decimal fractions: Most drug calculations require rounding to the hundredth or greater. This depends on the individual example. To round off, consider the number in the next position to the right. If the number is greater than or equal to 5, increase the number being considered by 1. If it is less than 5, do not increase the number being considered.

Example: Round off 0.74 to the nearest tenths. Because the number in the hundredths column is less than 5, the answer will be 0.7.

Example: Round off 0.24555 to the nearest hundredths. Because the number in the thousandths column is 5, the answer will be 0.25.

19. Round off the following examples to the nearest tenth:
    a. 7.6245   **b.** 0.081   **c.** 0.851

20. Round off the following examples to the nearest hundredth:
    a. 0.10423   **b.** 5.6258   **c.** 892.02975

Ratios

Ratios indicate the relationship of one quantity to another. They indicate division and may be expressed as the following:

$\frac{a}{b}$, a to b, or a:b

Example: Five gallons of gas for $6 means the ratio of gas to dollars is as follows:

$\frac{5}{6}$, 5 to 6, or 5:6

21. Write the ratio for the following examples.
    a. The heart ejects approximately 5000 mL of blood every 60 seconds.
    b. Approximately 6000 mL of air is moved in and out of the lungs every 60 seconds.
    c. The intravenous line delivers 100 mL every 30 minutes.
    d. There are 100 mg of the drug in 10 mL of solution.

To simplify a ratio that compares two measures, divide the denominator into the numerator to calculate the unit rate.

Example: On a routine transfer, we traveled 120 miles in 2 hours.

$$\text{The unit rate} = \frac{120 \text{ miles}}{2 \text{ hours}} = 60 \text{ miles per hour}$$

The unit rate is 60 miles per hour.

22. Calculate the unit rate for each of the following (based on the examples in Question 21).
    a. How many milliliters of blood are ejected from the heart each second?
    b. How much air is moved in and out of the lungs each second?
    c. How much fluid is being delivered each minute?
    d. How many milligrams are in each milliliter?

A proportion shows the relationship between two different ratios. To determine whether a proportion is true (equivalent), do the following:
1. If the proportion is expressed as a fraction, ($\frac{1}{2}$ = $\frac{2}{4}$), multiply the cross products and then determine whether the proportion is equivalent.

Example: $\dfrac{1}{2} = \dfrac{2}{4} = \dfrac{1}{2} \bullet \dfrac{2}{4} = 1 \times 4 = 4$ and $2 \times 2 = 4$;

4 = 4; therefore the proportion is true.

2. If the proportion is expressed as a ratio (2:5::4:10), multiply the two inside numbers ($5 \times 4 = 20$) and the two outside numbers ($2 \times 10 = 20$); 20 = 20; therefore the proportion is equivalent.

23. Determine whether each of the following proportions is true:
    a. $\dfrac{5}{10} = \dfrac{1}{2}$ **b.** $\dfrac{4}{6} = \dfrac{8}{10}$ **c.** $\dfrac{25}{75} = \dfrac{1}{3}$

To solve a proportion problem when one of the numbers is unknown *(x)*, do the following:
1. Use either proportion method demonstrated previously.
2. Make x stand alone by dividing both sides of the equation by the number on the side of x.
3. Solve for x.

Example: $\dfrac{17}{20} = \dfrac{x}{100}$ $20x = 17 \times 100 = \dfrac{20x}{20} = \dfrac{17 \times 100}{20}$

$$x = \frac{17 \times 100}{20}$$

$$x = 85$$

Example: $17:20::x:100$ $20x = 17 \times 100$

$$\frac{20x}{20} = \frac{17 \times 100}{20}$$

24. Solve for x in the following problems:
    a. $\frac{2}{4} = \frac{x}{8}$ **c.** $\frac{2}{3} = \frac{x}{6}$ **e.** $3:5::x:45$ **g.** $x:35::80:100$
    b. $\frac{1}{4} = \frac{x}{16}$ **d.** $\frac{5}{4} = \frac{x}{12}$ **f.** $4:9::16:x$ **h.** $1.5:3::x:18$
    Simplifying a problem by cancelling common elements will make problem solving easier.

Example: $x = \dfrac{12 \times 10}{20} = 6$ Zeros cancel. Then 2 divides into 12 six times.

Example: $x = \dfrac{1 \text{ mg} \times 1 \text{ mL}}{1 \text{ mg}} = 1 \text{ mL}$ *mg* cancels *mg*. 1 mL is left.

25. Simplify the following problems as much as possible and then solve.

a. $x = \dfrac{10 \times 150}{50}$

b. $x = \dfrac{25 \times 2}{50}$

c. $x = \dfrac{2500 \times 500}{20,000}$

d. $x = \dfrac{1\,g \times 1\,L}{1\,g}$

e. $x = \dfrac{2\,mg \times 1\,mL}{10\,mg}$

f. $x = \dfrac{10\,mg \times 10\,mL}{100\,mg}$

Percentages

Percent (%) is a portion of a whole divided by 100.
1. To change a percent to a decimal, drop the percent sign and move the decimal two places to the left.
Example: 15.0% = 0.15
2. To change a decimal to a percent, move the decimal two places to the right and add the percent sign.
Example: 0.76 = 76%
3. To change a fraction to a percent, convert it to a decimal and follow rule 2.
Example: ⅖ = 0.2   0.2 = 20%

26. Change the following percentages to decimals.
   a. 25%   **b.** 110%   **c.** 0.5%

27. Convert the following decimals to percentages.
   a. 0.34   **b.** 2.29   **c.** 0.07

28. Express the following as percentages:
   a. ³⁴⁄₅₀   **b.** ¹⁰⁰⁄₅₀₀   **c.** ³⁄₇

29. Rewrite the following fractions as ratios, decimals, and percentages:

Fraction	Ratio	Decimal	Percentage
a. ⅚			
b. ¹⁄₂₀			
c. ⁷⁄₃₃			

30. Solve the following:
   a. 15% of 75   **b.** 0.5% of 250
This concludes the refresher.

MATHEMATICAL EQUIVALENTS AND DRUG DOSE CALCULATIONS

31. In the metric system the primary unit of volume is the (a) _____, the primary unit of mass (weight) is

the (b) _____, and the primary unit of length is the (c) _____.

32. List the four metric mass units commonly used in the prehospital environment, beginning with the largest and ending with the smallest.

   a.

   b.

   c.

   d.

33. Each of the units listed in question 32 differs in value from the next unit by _____.

34. To convert from one unit to the next smallest unit in question 32, you must move the decimal point three places to the right or left? _____

35. To convert from one unit to the previous unit (example unit 32d to unit 32c), you must move the decimal point three places to the right or left? _____

36. Convert the following units of mass to the units indicated.
   a. 2 kg = _____ g
   b. 4 mg = _____ mcg
   c. 2 g = _____ mg
   d. 600 mg = _____ kg
   e. 400 mcg = _____ mg
   f. 350 mg = _____ g
   g. 0.25 mg = _____ mcg
   h. 12.5 g = _____ mg

37. Convert the following units of volume to the units indicated.
   a. 1 cc = _____ mL
   b. 10 mL = _____ cc
   c. 250 mL = _____ L
   d. 0.33 L = _____ mL

38. The primary unit of mass in the apothecary system is the _____.

39. The primary unit of volume in the apothecary system is the _____.

40. If the physician orders acetaminophen gr *X*, how many milligrams will you give? _____

41. Your patient has chest pain, and medical direction orders nitroglycerin gr ⅟₁₅₀. How many milligrams will you administer?

   (a) _____
   When it is time for a second nitroglycerin, the patient's blood pressure is slightly low, so this time the physician orders nitroglycerin gr ⅟₂₀₀. How many milligrams will you give?

   (b) _____

42. Convert the following measures in the household system to the units indicated:
   a. 1 T = _____ tsp
   b. 1 lb = _____ oz
   c. 1 pt = _____ oz
   d. 1 gal = _____ qt
   e. 1 fl oz = _____ T
   f. 1 c = _____ fl oz

43. Convert the following measures in the household system to the appropriate metric units.
   a. 1 tsp = _____ mL
   b. 1 T = _____ mL
   c. 1 fl oz = _____ mL
   d. 1 qt = _____ mL
   e. 22 lb = _____ kg
   f. 110 lb = _____ kg

44. Convert the following measures to the appropriate units indicated.
   a. A patient's family tells you that he lost about a cup of blood from a head wound. You will relay to medical

   direction that the estimated blood loss is approximately _____ mL.

   b. A patient vomits about a quart of coffee-grounds emesis. This is equal to _____ mL.

    c. The patient took 1 oz or _____ mL of antacid. Then she drank 16 oz of milk. This is equal to _____ mL of milk.

    d. A parent reads a drug label and, instead of administering 2 mL of a drug, accidentally gives 2 oz of a drug.

       How many milliliters in excess of the prescribed dose did the parent give? _____ mL

    e. The human body normally contains about 5 L of blood, or _____ qt.

    f. A pregnant woman states that her membranes have ruptured and about a pint of amniotic fluid leaked out.

       This is equal to _____ mL.

    g. A premature newborn you have just delivered weighs 2 lb, or _____ kg (_____ g).

45. Identify the following information from the drug label or package in Fig. 18-4.
    a. Drug name: **d.** Total drug:
    b. Expiration date: **e.** Concentration of drug:
    c. Total volume:

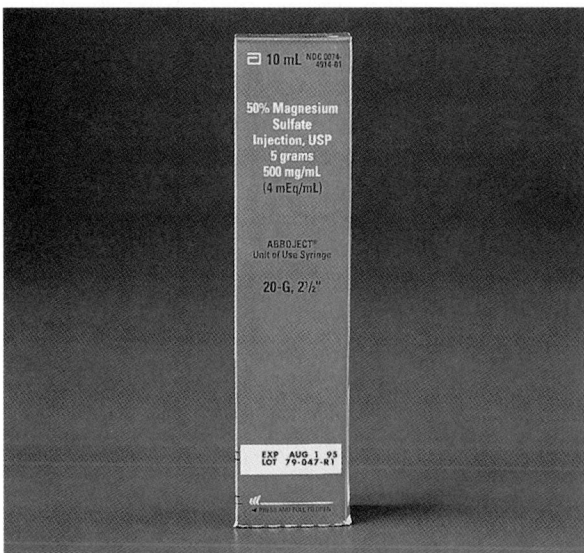

Figure 18-4

46. Convert the following drug concentrations into the total number of grams.

    a. Calcium chloride 10% solution = _____ g in 100 mL.

    b. Epinephrine 1:1000 solution = _____ g in 1000 mL.

    c. Magnesium sulfate 10% solution = _____ g in 100 mL.

    d. Epinephrine 1:10,000 solution = _____ g in 10,000 mL.

    e. Lidocaine 0.4% solution = _____ g in 100 mL.

    f. Mannitol 25% solution = _____ g in 100 mL.

    g. Dextrose 50% solution = _____ g in 100 mL.

47. Calculate the concentration per milliliter of the following drugs using the following formula: Concentration = Total dose of drug (mg) ÷ Total volume (mL). For example, a 10-mL vial of lidocaine contains 100 mg of the drug. Concentration = 100 mg ÷ 10 mL = 10 mg/ml.

  a. A 40-mg vial of furosemide is in a 4-mL vial. Concentration = _____.

  b. A 10-mL vial of epinephrine contains 1 mg of the drug. Concentration = _____.

  c. You have 25 g of D50W in 50 mL. Concentration = _____.

  d. A 2-mL vial of diphenhydramine contains 50 mg of the drug. Concentration = _____.

  e. A 250-mL bag contains 1 g of lidocaine. Concentration = _____.

48. Calculate the total dose of a drug to be administered.

  a. Lidocaine 1 mg/kg is ordered for a 100-kg patient who is having many premature ventricular contractions

   each minute. Dose = _____ mg.

  b. The maximum dose of procainamide is 17 mg/kg and the patient weighs 60 kg. Total dose = _____ mg.

  c. Push sodium bicarbonate 1 mEq/kg during a lengthy cardiac arrest. The patient weighs 80 kg. Dose =

   _____mEq.

  d. Hang a dopamine drip at 5 mcg/kg/min on a hypotensive patient who weighs 50 kg. Dose = _____ mcg/min.

  e. Give epinephrine 0.01 mg/kg to an 11-lb child who is in cardiopulmonary arrest. Dose = _____ mg.

  f. Administer mannitol 1 g/kg to a 176-lb patient with rising intracranial pressure. Dose = _____ g.

49. Solve the following problems using the following formula:

$$\text{Volume (x)} = \frac{\text{Desired dose (D)} \times \text{Volume on hand (Q)}}{\text{Dose on hand (H)}}$$

  a. You wish to give furosemide 20 mg. It is supplied in a 4-mL vial containing 40 mg of the drug.

   Volume = _____ mL.

  b. You wish to administer morphine 3 mg. You have a 1-mL Tubex containing 10 mg of the drug.

   Volume = _____ mL.

  c. You wish to give amiodarone 300 mg. You have a 3-mL vial containing 150 mg of the drug. Volume = _____ mL.

  d. You must give 2.5 mg of diazepam. It is supplied in a 2-mL vial containing 10 mg. Volume = _____ mL.

  e. You have 50 mg of meperidine in a 1-mL Tubex. You need to give 12.5 mg of the drug.

   Volume = _____ mL.

  f. Your patient needs 0.3 mg of epinephrine (1:1000). You have a 1-mL vial containing 1 mg.

   Volume = _____ mL.

  g. Your patient needs 0.5 mg of dopamine. You have a 500-mL bag containing 400 mg of the drug.

   Volume = _____ mL.

50. Solve the following drug dose problems using the following equation:
Desired dose:Desired volume::Dosage on hand:Volume on hand.

Example: Give 50 mg of procainamide. It is supplied in a 10-mL vial containing 1000 mg.

$$50 \text{ mg:x} = 1000 \text{ mg:10 mL} \quad \text{Set up the ratio.}$$

$$\frac{1000 \text{ mg} \times \text{x}}{1000 \text{ mg}} = \frac{50 \text{ mg} \times 10 \text{ mL}}{1000 \text{ mg}} \quad \text{Multiply inside (means) and then outside (extremes) numbers.}$$

$$\text{x} = \frac{50 \text{ mg} \times 10 \text{ mL}}{1000 \text{ mg}} \quad \text{Solve for } x.$$

$$\text{x} = 0.5 \text{ mL}$$

a. Administer adenosine 6 mg. It is supplied in a 2-mL vial containing 6 mg of the drug. Desired volume =

_____ mL.

b. Administer diphenhydramine 25 mg. You have a 2-mL vial containing 50 mg of the drug. Desired volume =

_____ mL.

c. Give 2.5 mg of verapamil. It is supplied in a 2-mL vial containing 5 mg of the drug. Desired volume =
_____mL.

d. Give 1000 mg of mannitol. You have a 20% solution. Desired volume = _____ mL.

51. Calculate the drops per minute needed to deliver the following volumes of fluid over the required time.
a. The physician orders an intravenous fluid to run at 30 mL/hr (drop factor, 60 drops/mL). Drops/min =

_____.

b. You want to give a fluid challenge of 200 mL over 20 minutes (drop factor, 10 drops/mL). Drops/min =

_____.

c. You need to infuse a drug mixed in 50 mL of fluid over 15 minutes (drop factor, 15 drops/mL). Drops/min =

_____.

d. Online medical direction orders 150 mL of lactated Ringer's solution to infuse in 2 hours (drop factor, 15

drops/mL). Drops/min = _____.

e. You are told to give 275 mL over 2 hours (drop factor, 10 drops/mL). Drops/min = _____.

f. The intravenous drug must run in at 0.5 mL/min (drop factor, 60 drops/mL). Drops/min = _____.

g. You have delivered a baby, and medical direction advises you to add 10 units (1 mL) of oxytocin to 1000 mL

of normal saline and infuse it at 200 mL/hr (drop factor, 10 drops/mL). Drops/min = _____.

h. You have added magnesium sulfate to D_5W for a total volume of 100 mL. You must infuse it over 2 minutes

to treat your patient's ventricular arrhythmia (drop factor, 10 drops/mL). Drops/min = _____.

i. A severely acidotic patient needs bicarbonate. You have added 50 mEq of sodium bicarbonate (50 mL) to

1000 mL of normal saline and are to infuse it over 2 hours (drop factor, 15 drops/mL). Drops/min = _____.

j. You have added 2 mg (2 mL) of epinephrine to a 250-mL bag of normal saline and wish to infuse it at 1

mL/min to your severely bradycardic patient (drop factor, 60 drops/mL). Drops/min = _____.

k. Your patient has just converted from ventricular fibrillation. You are hanging a lidocaine drip at 3 mg/min.
You have mixed 1 g of lidocaine in 250 mL normal saline. How many drops per minute will you set your IV to

deliver the 0.75 mL/min necessary for this dose of drug (drop factor, 60 drops/mL)? Drops/min = _____.

52. Calculate the following problems using any of the methods demonstrated. Ensure that all units are compatible. If the dosage is given in milligrams per kilogram, make the appropriate calculation.

    a. You wish to give lidocaine 1 mg/kg to a 75-kg man. The lidocaine is supplied in a 10-mL syringe containing 100 mg of the drug. How many milliliters will you administer?

    b. You must give amiodarone 300 mg to a 60-kg woman. You have a 2-mL vial containing 150 mg of the drug. How many mL will you give?

    c. You must give 0.5 mg of glucagon to a 90-kg patient. When you mix it up, you have 1 mg in 1 mL of solution. How much will you give?

    d. You have diluted your phenobarbital so that you have 130 mg in 10 mL. You need to give 100 mg. The patient weighs 100 kg. How much will you give?

    e. You must give 1 g/kg of mannitol. The patient weighs 70 kg. You have a 20% solution. How many milliliters will you give?

    f. You need to administer 150 mg of aminophylline. You have 500 mg in a 20-mL ampule. How many milliliters will you give?

    g. Your patient needs a dopamine drip at 5 mcg/kg/min. He weighs 100 kg. You have 400 mg of dopamine in 500 mL of D_5W. How many milliliters per minute will you administer and at how many drops per minute will you set the microdrip intravenous line?

    h. You wish to administer a lidocaine drip at 2 mg/min. You have an intravenous bag containing a 0.4% solution of lidocaine. How many milliliters will you give each minute, and how fast will you set your microdrip tubing to deliver this rate?

53. For each of the following situations, calculate the correct volume of solution to be administered using the drug package information illustrated.

    a. Give 0.5 mg of atropine (Fig. 18-5). Desired volume = _____ mL.

    b. Give 0.3 mg of epinephrine (Fig. 18-6). Desired volume = _____ mL.

    c. Give lidocaine 0.5 mg/kg to an 80-kg patient (Fig. 18-7). Desired volume = _____ mL.

54. After determining the correct volume of drug to be administered in the following examples, shade the corresponding syringe in Fig. 18-8 to illustrate the proper amount to be given.

    a. Adenosine 6 mg must be given to a patient with paroxysmal supraventricular tachycardia. You have a 2-mL vial containing 3 mg/mL of the drug. How many milliliters will you give?

    b. Your patient has had a seizure and needs phenytoin 200 mg. You have a 5-mL vial containing 250 mg of the drug. How much will you give?

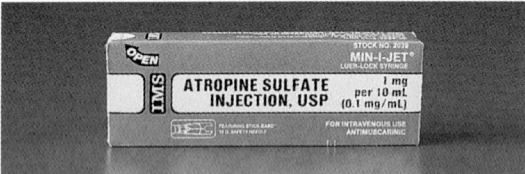

Figure 18-5

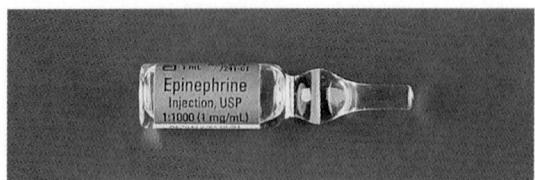

Figure 18-6

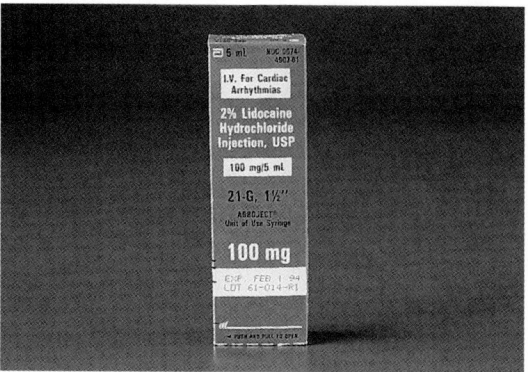

Figure 18-7

c. You have a 10-mL vial of furosemide containing 10 mg/mL of the drug. A total of 70 mg is indicated for your patient, who is in congestive heart failure. What volume will you administer?

d. You wish to administer epinephrine 0.3 mg to a patient experiencing an allergic reaction. The epinephrine is supplied in a 1-mL ampule containing 1 mg of a 1:1000 solution of the drug. How much will you give?

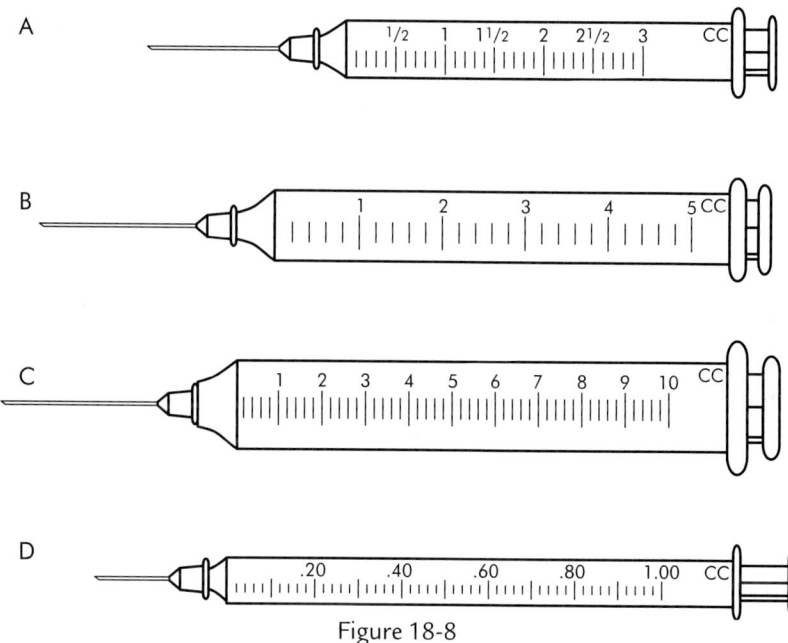

Figure 18-8

DRUG ADMINISTRATION

55. List at least 10 general steps to be taken when administering any drug to avoid errors.

a.

b.

c.

d.

e.

f.

g.

h.

i.

j.

56. You intended to deliver the lidocaine drip at 1 mL/min during your 15-minute transport, but when you look at the 250-mL bag, the roller clamp has been opened, and almost 150 mL has been infused. List five actions that you should take after this error.

a.

b.

c.

d.

e.

57. List two methods to ensure medical asepsis when you administer an intramuscular injection.

a.

b.

58. Complete the following sentences regarding drug administration routes:

Oral medications should be given with the patient in the (a) _____ position. The drug should be swallowed with (b) _____ oz of fluid to ensure that it reaches the (c) _____. Sublingual medications should be placed under the (d) _____ and allowed to (e) _____. They should not be (f) _____ because this will delay action of the drug. Parenteral drug administration may cause (g) _____, (h) _____, or (i) _____. The correct needle length and size are important. For subcutaneous injections a (j) _____-inch, (k) _____-gauge needle should be used. When administering an intramuscular shot, you should select a (l) _____-inch, (m) _____-gauge needle. To minimize the risk of needle stick injury, you should understand that the use of two-handed needle recapping is (n) _____. Also, all sharp items, including needles, should be placed in (o) _____. When withdrawing medication from a multidose vial, you should cleanse the stopper with alcohol and then inject the same amount of (p) _____ as drug to be withdrawn before aspirating the appropriate amount of medicine into the syringe. To minimize the risk of glass particles entering the injection when aspirating from a glass ampule, use a (q) _____ needle. Subcutaneous injections should be administered at a (r) _____-degree angle. Sites of administration for this route include (s) _____, _____, and _____. Intramuscular injections should be administered at a (t) _____-degree angle. Administration sites for this route include the (u) _____ and

_____. To prevent drug effects on the rescuer, you should always wear (v) _____ when administering transdermal medicines. Dilution with at least (w) _____ mL of fluid is recommended to ensure maximum absorption of drugs administered by the endotracheal route. Two advantages of drugs administered by inhalation are (x) _____ and fewer _____.

59. List three complications of intravenous line placement for each of the following approaches:
   a. Peripheral site:

_____

   b. Internal jugular and subclavian sites:

_____

   c. Femoral site:

_____

60. You respond to care for a 3-year-old child who is in cardiac arrest. Attempts to intubate and secure intravenous access are unsuccessful, so you elect to attempt intraosseous infusion. After applying gloves and preparing your equipment, you select the preferred site, located (a) _____ _____. You then insert the needle using a (b) _____ motion and advance it until (c) _____. The next step involves aspirating marrow into a syringe. Then you use a syringe filled with (d) _____ to ensure that free flow occurs without resistance. If you detect correct placement, you connect the (e) _____ and infuse the drug at the appropriate rate. To prevent the needle from being dislodged, you should (f) _____ the needle.

STUDENT SELF-ASSESSMENT

61. Your patient's mother states that her child's temperature is 38.5° C. What is her temperature in degrees Fahrenheit?
   a. 69.9　　　　　　　　**c.** 101.3
   b. 99.6　　　　　　　　**d.** 103.6

62. You must administer a drug that is calculated based on milligrams per kilogram. The patient tells you that he weighs 144 lb. How many kilograms does that convert to (rounded to the nearest kilogram)?
   a. 65　　　　　　　　**c.** 80
   b. 72　　　　　　　　**d.** 86

63. You wish to administer mannitol 500 mg/kg to a 100-kg woman. You have a 10% solution of the drug. How many milliliters will you give?
   a. 2　　　　　　　　**c.** 20
   b. 5　　　　　　　　**d.** 500

64. You are going to give epinephrine 0.01 mg/kg to a 6-kg child. The epinephrine is supplied as 1 mg in a 10-mL syringe. How many milliliters will you administer?
   a. 0.006　　　　　　　　**c.** 0.6
   b. 0.06　　　　　　　　**d.** 6.0

65. Which syringe will you use to withdraw the drug volume that you calculated in question 64?
   a. 1 mL　　　　　　　　**c.** 5 mL
   b. 3 mL　　　　　　　　**d.** 10 mL

66. Which measure should be taken to ensure safe administration of drugs?
  a. Learn a rapid dose calculation method that you can always perform in your head.
  b. Set unlabeled syringes in a consistent place so that you will know what is in them.
  c. Verify the label of the drug selected once before administration.
  d. Monitor the patient closely for drug effects for the first 5 minutes after you give them.

67. Your patient suddenly vomits and has chest pain after you administer epinephrine intravenously instead of subcutaneously as ordered for his anaphylaxis. How should this be recorded in the patient care report?
  a. Document the correct route only.
  b. Document the route ordered and the incorrect route.
  c. Document the incorrect route only.
  d. Omit the route in the report.

68. What parenteral route would you use to test for allergies?
  a. Intradermal   **c.** Intravenous
  b. Intramuscular   **d.** Subcutaneous

69. Which muscle is appropriate for an intramuscular injection in a 2-year-old child?
  a. Deltoid   **c.** Ventrogluteal site
  b. Dorsogluteal site   **d.** Vastus lateralis

70. You suspect that your patient has a ruptured ectopic pregnancy. She is in profound shock. Which intravenous catheter will you select?
  a. 14 gauge, 1½ inch   **c.** 18 gauge, 1½ inch
  b. 14 gauge, 3 inch   **d.** 18 gauge, 3 inch

71. You are transferring a patient with a jugular central line. Suddenly, the patient becomes unconscious, cyanotic, and tachycardic. You note that the intravenous tubing has been disconnected from the central line catheter. The patient should be positioned immediately on his
  a. Left side with his head down   **c.** Right side with his head down
  b. Left side with his head up   **d.** Right side with his head up

72. You wish to administer normal saline intravenously at 30 mL/hr. The infusion set delivers 60 drops/mL. How fast will you run it?
  a. 1 drop/min   **c.** 100 drops/min
  b. 30 drops/min   **d.** 400 drops/min

73. A 200-mL fluid challenge is to be infused over 15 minutes. The drop factor is 10 drops/mL. How fast will you run it?
  a. 35 drops/min   **c.** 133 drops/min
  b. 75 drops/min   **d.** 150 drops/min

74. Which of the following statements is true regarding intraosseous infusion?
  a. It generally is recommended for children between 1 and 3 years of age.
  b. It is associated with a risk of air embolism if the tubing is disconnected.
  c. Absorption of drugs is irregular and slow through this route.
  d. The procedure should be considered only in critically ill patients.

75. Which of the following is true regarding sublingual drug administration?
  a. The patient may have a sip of water after administration.
  b. This route should not be used if the patient is nauseated.
  c. The drug should be permitted to dissolve under the tongue.
  d. Swallowing the drug will increase its effects.

76. When administering medication into a 2-year old child's ear, you should pull the ear
  a. Down and back   **c.** Up and back
  b. Down and forward   **d.** Up and forward

77. Which is true regarding administration of medication to young children?
  a. Tell the child to cry and make noise.
  b. Avoid any physical restraint.
  c. Give injections slowly and firmly.
  d. Be honest about painful techniques.

78. Which of the following describes an appropriate procedure for obtaining a blood sample for glucose on an adult patient?

    a. Disconnect the intravenous infusion, insert the vacutainer into the hub of the intravenous catheter, and withdraw.

    b. Insert the intraosseoous needle, flush with normal saline, attach a syringe, and pull back.

    c. Enter the vein with a 24-gauge needle attached to a syringe and withdraw.

    d. Push blood collection tubes into the barrel of the vacutainer and allow to fill.

WRAP IT UP

Case Study: Venous Access and Medication Administration

You are dispatched to a school for an allergic reaction. On arrival you find a 66-lb 7-year-old who was stung by a bee and is having an anaphylactic reaction. She has hives, her eyes are swollen, and she is wheezing. You and your partner apply oxygen, and you draw up and administer epinephrine 0.5 mg subcutaneously; give diphenhydramine (1.25 mg/kg) intramuscularly (you carry 50 mg/mL vials); and albuterol by nebulizer treatment. You initiate an IV and reevaluate her vital signs. Her wheezing has cleared almost completely, and the hives are beginning to dissipate, but she is anxious and tachycardic. Your partner asks how much epinephrine you gave, and you realize that you administered a dose in excess of the 0.01 mL/kg (1:1000) maximum 0.3 mL indicated in your protocol.

1. Convert this child's weight to the metric system. _____

2. **a.** Compute the correct dose of epinephrine that should have been given. _____

    b. How much did you overdose or underdose this patient? _____

3. **a.** Compute the correct dose of diphenhydramine. _____

    b. How many milliliters should be administered? _____

    c. In what location should the intramuscular injection of diphenhydramine be given? _____

4. What steps should have been taken before giving the drugs to ensure safe administration? (Five rights of drug administration)

_____

5. Now that you recognize an error has been made, what should you do?

_____

6. Fill in the information missing in the table:

Injection Site	Angle of Administration	Volume to Be Given
Intradermal		
Subcutaneous		
Intramuscular		

7. Which of the following is true regarding vascular access on this child?

    a. Aseptic technique should be followed.

    b. External jugular would be the initial site of choice.

    c. Intraosseous infusion should be used.

    d. Vascular access is not needed in this situation.

8. Describe the procedure for administration of nebulized albuterol by aerosol mask.

CHAPTER 18 ANSWERS

VENOUS ACCESS AND MEDICATION ADMINISTRATION

1. a. 7 is the numerator, 8 is the denominator.
b. 6 is the numerator, 13 is the denominator.

2. a. 1/4; b. 3/4; c. 1/2; d. 1/6; e. 1/5; f. 1/4; g. 1/5; h. 9/25; i. 1/10; j. 2/5; k. 17/23; l. 2/3

3. a. 15; b. 2; c. 3; d. 2 1/2

4. a. 43/8; b. 7/4; c. 37/12; d. 47/3

5. a. 18/24; b. 48/60; c. 79,000/100,000

6. a. 45; b. 12; c. 24

7. a. Equal to; b. Greater than; c. Less than

8. a. 1 3/8; b. 3 11/12

9. a. 1; b. 1 11/12

10. a. 55/208; b. 25 1/2; c. 13 3/4; d. 7/24

11. a. 1 1/4; b. 3 13/14

12. a. 3.4; b. 5.35; c. 0.062

13. a. 0.25; b. 0.28; c. 0.02

14. a. 1/2; b. 3 6/25; c. 6 7/1000

15. a. 0.47; b. 1.02

16. a. 29; b. 13.58

17. a. 0.0724; b. 1.08; c. 0.2175; d. 425.6; e. 29; f. 7052

18. a. 0.05; b. 2.58; c. 8; d. 4.0; e. 0.14237; f. 0.017

19. a. 7.6; b. 0.1; c. 0.9

20. a. 0.10; b. 5.63; c. 892.03

21. a. 5000:60 (5000 mL:60 seconds); b. 6000:60 (6000 mL:60 seconds); c. 100:30 (100 mL:30 minutes); d. 100:10 (100 mg:10 mL)

22. a. 83 mL/sec; b. 100 mL/sec; c. 3 mL/min; d. 10 mg/mL

23. a. True; b. Not true; c. True

24. a. x = 3; b. x = 4; c. x = 10.5; d. x = 15; e. x = 27; f. x = 36; g. x = 28; h. x = 9

25. a. $x = \dfrac{10 \times 150}{50} = \dfrac{10 \times \cancel{150}^{30}}{50} = 30$

b. $x = \dfrac{25 \times 2}{50} = \dfrac{^1\cancel{25} \times \cancel{2}^1}{50^1} = 1$

c. $x = \dfrac{2500 \times 500}{20{,}000} = \dfrac{\cancel{2500} \times \cancel{500}}{\cancel{20{,}000}} = \dfrac{125}{2} = 62.5$

d. $x = \dfrac{1\,g \times 1\,L}{1\,g} = \dfrac{\cancel{1\,g} \times 1\,L}{\cancel{1\,g}} = 1\,L$

e. $x = \dfrac{2\,mg \times 1\,mL}{10\,mg} = \dfrac{\cancel{2\,mg} \times 1\,mL}{^5\cancel{10\,mg}} = \dfrac{1\,mL}{5} = 0.2\,mL$

f. $x = \dfrac{10\,mg \times 10\,mL}{100\,mg} = \dfrac{\cancel{10\,mg} \times \cancel{10\,mL}}{\cancel{100\,mg}} = 1\,mL$

26. a. 0.25; b. 1.1; c. 0.005

27. a. 34%; b. 229%; c. 7%

28. a. 68%; b. 20%; c. 43%

29.

Fraction	Ratio	Decimal	Percentage
a. $\frac{5}{6}$	5:6 or 5 to 6	0.83	83%
b. $\frac{1}{20}$	1:20 or 1 to 20	0.05	5%
c. $\frac{7}{33}$	7:33 or 7 to 33	0.21	21%

30. a. 11.25; b. 1.25

31. a. Liter; b. Gram; c. Meter
(Objective 1)

32. Kilogram (kg), gram (g), milligram (mg), and microgram (mcg)
(Objective 1)

33. 1000
(Objective 1)

34. Right
(Objective 1)

35. Left
(Objective 1)

36. a. 2000 g; b. 4000 mcg; c. 2000 mg; d. 0.0006 kg; e. 0.4 mg; f. 0.35 g; g. 250 mcg; h. 12,500 mg
(Objective 1)

37. a. 1; b. 10; c. 0.25; d. 330
(Objective 1)

38. Grain (gr)
(Objective 1)

39. Minim
(Objective 1)

40. 600 mg
(Objective 1)

41. a. 0.4 mg; b. 0.3 mg
(Objective 1)

42. a. 3; b. 16; c. 16; d. 4; e. 2; f. 8
(Objective 1)

43. a. 5; b. 15: c. 30; d. 960; e. 10; f. 50
(Objective 1)

44. a. 240; b. 960; c. 30; 480; d. 58; e. 5.2; f. 480; g. 0.9 and 900
(Objective 1)

45. a. Magnesium sulfate; b. Aug. 1, 1995; c. 10 mL; d. 5g; e. 500 mg/mL (4 mEq/mL)
(Objective 2)

46. a. 10; b. 1; c. 10; d. 1; e. 0.4; f. 25; g. 50
(Objective 2)

47. a. 40 mg/4 mL = 10 mg/mL; b. 1 mg/10 mL = 0.1 mg/mL; c. 25 g/50 mL = 25,000 mg/50 mL = 500 mg/mL; d. 50 mg/2 mL = 25 mg/mL; e. 1 g/250 mL = 1000 mg/250 mL = 4 mg/mL
(Objective 2)

48. a. 100; b. 1020; c. 80; d. 250; e. 0.05 (Do not forget to convert to kilograms.); f. 80
(Objective 2)

49. a. $x = \dfrac{20 \text{ mg} \times 4 \text{ mL}}{40 \text{ mg}} = 2 \text{ mL}$

b. $x = \dfrac{3 \text{ mg} \times 1 \text{ mL}}{10 \text{ mg}} = 0.3 \text{ mL}$

c. $x = \dfrac{300 \text{ mg} \times 3 \text{ mL}}{150 \text{ mg}} = 6 \text{ mL}$

d. $x = \dfrac{2.5 \text{ mg} \times 2 \text{ mL}}{10 \text{ mg}} = 0.5 \text{ mL}$

e. $x = \dfrac{12.5 \text{ mg} \times 1 \text{ mL}}{50 \text{ mg}} = 0.25 \text{ mL}$

f. $x = \dfrac{0.3 \text{ mg} \times 1 \text{ mL}}{1 \text{ mg}} = 0.3 \text{ mL}$

g. $x = \dfrac{0.5 \text{ mg} \times 500 \text{ mL}}{400 \text{ mg}} = 0.625 \text{ mL}$
(Objective 3)

50. a. 6 mg:x::6 mg:2 mL

$$x \times 6 \text{ mg} = 6 \text{ mg} \times 2 \text{ mL}$$

$$\frac{x \times 6 \text{ mg}}{6 \text{ mg}} = \frac{6 \text{ mg} \times 2 \text{ mL}}{6 \text{ mg}}$$

$$x = 2 \text{ mL}$$

b. 1 mL

c. 1 mL

d. 1 g:x::20 g:100 mL, x = 5 mL

(Objective 3)

51. a. 30; b. 100; c. 50; d. 19; e. 23; f. 30 g. 33; h. 500; i. 130; j. 60; k. 45

(Objective 4)

52. a. 7.5 mL; b. 4.0 mL; c. 0.5 mL; d. 7.7 mL; e. 350 mL; f. 0.5 mL; g. 0.625 mL and 38 gtt/min; h. 0.5 mL and 30 gtt/min

(Objectives 3, 4)

53. a. 5; b. 0.3; c. 2.0

(Objective 3)

54.

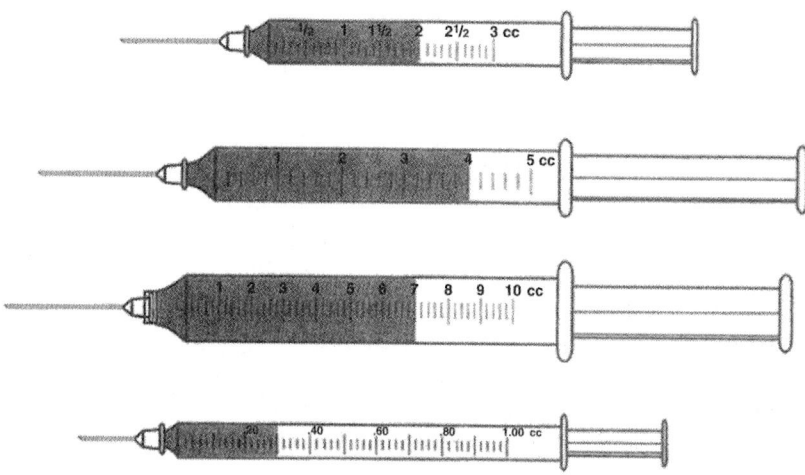

(Objective 3)

55. Avoid distractions; repeat orders to medical direction; verify that you are giving the right patient the right dose of the right drug at the right time by the right route; verify the correct drug on the label at least 3 times; verify the route of administration; ensure that the labeling information is correct for the drug you want to give; never give drugs from an unlabeled container; verify difficult calculations on paper, with a co-worker, or both; label the syringe immediately after withdrawing a drug that will not be completely administered immediately; do not give unlabeled drugs prepared by another person; do not give medications that are outdated or appear discolored, cloudy, or unusual; if the patient or a co-worker questions the drug or dose, double-check it; monitor the patient for adverse effects after administration; and document carefully.

(Objective 5)

56. a. Stop the infusion.

b. Evaluate the patient's response to the drug. Perform an assessment that includes level of consciousness, vital signs, and electrocardiogram rhythm.

c. Advise medical direction and the receiving physician of the amount of drug infused and ask for their treatment advice if you have not yet arrived at the receiving facility.

d. Document the amount of drug administered on the patient care report objectively. Document all facts surrounding the error on the appropriate confidential departmental quality improvement (incident) form.

e. Critique the situation with your crew (if appropriate), and identify measures that can be taken to prevent a similar error in the future.

(Objective 6)

57. a. Wash hands before initiating the procedure.

b. Cleanse the area with an antiseptic solution before puncturing the skin.

(Objective 7)

58. a. Upright (sitting)
  b. 4 to 8 oz
  c. Stomach
  d. Tongue
  e. Dissolve
  f. Swallowed
  g., h., and i. Infection, lipodystrophy, abscesses, necrosis, skin slough, nerve injuries, prolonged pain, and periostitis
  j. ½ or ⅝
  k. 23 or 25
  l. 1½ to 2
  m. 19 or 21
  n. Prohibited
  o. An appropriate sharps container
  p. Air
  q. Filter
  r. 45
  s. Upper arm, abdomen, thigh, and back
  t. 90
  u. Deltoid muscle, dorsogluteal site, vastus lateralis muscle, rectus femoris muscle, and ventrogluteal muscle
  v. Gloves
  w. 10
  x. Rapid onset and side effects
  (Objectives 8, 12, and 15)

59. a. Hematoma, cellulitis, thrombosis, phlebitis, sepsis, pulmonary thromboembolism, catheter embolism, fiber embolism, infiltration
  b. All complications in (a), plus air embolism, hematoma, damage to arteries or nerves, pneumothorax, hemothorax, and infiltration of fluid into the pleural space or mediastinum
  c. All complications in (a), plus hematoma, thrombosis extending to deep veins, and an inability to use the saphenous vein
  (Objective 10)

60. a. One to two fingerbreadths below the tubercle on the anteromedial surface of the tibia
  b. Boring or screwing
  c. Decreased resistance is felt (trapdoor effect)
  d. Saline
  e. Intravenous fluid infusion
  f. Secure
  (Objective 11)

61. c. To convert degrees Celsius to degrees Fahrenheit: $\dfrac{38.5 \times 9}{5} + 32 = 101.3°$ F.

  (Objective 1)

62. a. Multiply pounds by 0.45 to convert to kilograms. $144 \times 0.45 = 64.8$. Round to 65 kg.
  (Objective 1)

63. d. $\dfrac{50\ g \times 100\ mL}{10\ g} = 500$ mL
  (Objective 3)

64. c. $\dfrac{0.06 \times 10}{1} = 0.6$
  (Objective 3)

65. a. The 1-mL syringe will permit the most accurate measurements.
(Objective 8)

66. d. Many dose calculations can be done in your head; however, you should always write down any calculation that is difficult or that you question. Do not set down an unlabeled syringe with drug in it. Label the syringe or tape the medicine vial to it. The drug label should be verified at least 3 times before administration.
(Objective 5)

67. c. On the patient care report, only the actual action taken (the incorrect route) should be documented. The circumstances surrounding the error, including the actual correct route ordered, should be recorded in the appropriate confidential incident (quality improvement) reports.
(Objective 6)

68. a. Slower absorption and fewer systemic effects are achieved in this manner.
(Objective 8)

69. d. The other muscles are not developed adequately in the young child.
(Objective 13)

70. a. The 14-gauge, 1½-inch needle has the widest diameter and is the shortest. Both of these properties will allow rapid fluid administration.
(Objective 9)

71. a. The goal is to cause the air to stay in the right side of the heart and away from the cardiac valves.
(Objective 10)

72. b.
(Objective 4)

73. c.
(Objective 4)

74. d. Intraosseous infusion generally is recommended for children who are 6 years of age or younger. Complications include infiltration of fluid, fat embolism, osteomyelitis, periostitis at the site, infection, or fracture. Absorption of drugs and fluids from a properly placed intraosseous needle is rapid.
(Objective 11)

75. c. Swallowing a sublingual medicine will decrease its effectiveness; therefore water should not be given.
(Objective 8)

76. a. The angle of the ear canal will promote faster absorption if this technique is used.
(Objectives 12 and 13)

77. d. Recognize the child's fear and allow them to express it in appropriate ways such as crying or yelling. Use mild restraint if necessary and firmly stabilize injection sites. Give injections quickly.
(Objective 13)

78. d. Blood should not be drawn from an intravenous catheter if fluids already have been infusing (except under special circumstances and with the authorization of medical direction). Typically, a large 19- or 21-gauge needle should be used; however, in neonates a smaller needle should be used.
(Objective 14)

WRAP IT UP

1. $66 \div 2.2 = 30$ kg
   (Objective 1)

2. a. 0.01 mL/kg $\times 30$ kg $= 0.3$ mL
   b. 0.5 mL given $- 0.3$ mL indicated $= 0.2$ mL overdose
   (Objective 3)

3. a. 1.25 mg/kg $\times 30$ kg $= 37.5$ mg total dose
   b. 37.5 mg $\div 50$ mg $\times 1$ mL $= 0.75$ mL
   c. Diphenhydramine should be given by deep intramuscular injection into the dorsogluteal or vastus lateralis injection sites.
   (Objectives 3 and 8)

4. Ensure that the right patient gets the right dose of the right drug at the right time by the right route.
   (Objective 5)

5. After a medication error, advise medical direction and the person receiving the patient; monitor the patient; document the error according to state and local policy; determine how to prevent errors in the future.
   (Objective 6)

6. Intradermal: 15 degrees; less than 0.5 mL
   Subcutaneous: 45 degrees; less than 0.5 mL
   Intramuscular: 90 degrees; up to 5 mL (less in small children)
   (Objective 12)

7. a. Intraosseous infusion could be performed on a child in critical condition if no venous access site was readily available. A peripheral intravenous site on the arm would be preferred because of its easier access, ability to secure, and complication potential. An intravenous line is indicated to permit drug administration should the child's condition worsen.
   (Objective 9)

8. Add prescribed drug to nebulizer; attached to oxygen and mask; adjust flow meter to 6 to 10 L/min; place mask on patient; instruct patient to inhale slowly and deeply and hold breath 3 to 5 seconds before exhaling.
   (Objective 8)

PART FIVE

Airway Management and Ventilation

READING ASSIGNMENT
Chapter 19, pages 430-498, in *Mosby's Paramedic Textbook,* ed. 3

OBJECTIVES
Upon completion of this chapter, the paramedic student will be able to:
1. Distinguish between respiration, pulmonary ventilation, and external and internal respiration.
2. Explain the mechanics of respiration.
3. Explain the relationship of the partial pressures of gases in the blood and lungs to atmospheric gas pressures.
4. Describe pulmonary circulation.
5. Explain the process of exchange and transport of gases in the body.
6. Describe voluntary, chemical, and nervous regulation of respiration.
7. Discuss the assessment and management of medical or traumatic obstruction of the airway.
8. Outline the causes and effects of and preventive measures for pulmonary aspiration.
9. Outline the essential parameters for evaluating the effectiveness of the airway and breathing.
10. Describe the indications, contraindications, and techniques for delivery of supplemental oxygen.
11. Discuss methods of patient ventilation based on the indications, contraindications, potential complications, and use of each method.
12. Describe the use of manual airway maneuvers and mechanical airway adjuncts based on the indications, contraindications, potential complications, and techniques for each.
13. Describe assessment techniques and devices used to ensure adequate oxygenation, correct placement of the endotracheal tube, and elimination of carbon dioxide.
14. Explain variations in assessment and management of airway and ventilation problems in pediatric patients.
15. Given a patient scenario, identify possible alterations in oxygenation and ventilation based on a knowledge of gas exchange and the mechanics of breathing.

SUMMARY
- A key aspect of emergency care is a full understanding of the respiratory system. Another is mastery of airway management and ventilation techniques.
- The two phases of respiration are external respiration and internal respiration. External respiration is the transfer of oxygen and carbon dioxide between the inspired air and pulmonary capillaries. Internal respiration is the transfer of oxygen and carbon dioxide between the peripheral blood capillaries and the tissue cells.

- The mixture of gases that compose the atmosphere exerts a combined partial pressure of 100%, or 760 mm Hg at sea level. The composition of atmospheric gas is 21% oxygen, 0.03% carbon dioxide, and 78% nitrogen.
- The respiratory system delivers oxygen from inspired air to the blood and removes carbon dioxide.
- The 200 mL of oxygen that crosses the alveoli each minute is added to the oxygen already in the pulmonary capillaries. It is then transported to the body tissues by the circulatory system. After the body cells use the oxygen, the oxygen remaining in the blood returns to the heart and lungs. This exchange of oxygen and carbon dioxide is carried out by the passive process of diffusion.
- Respiration is controlled at any instant by a number of factors. Breathing is mainly an involuntary process. Within limits, however, the pattern of respiration can be consciously changed. The inspiratory muscles are made up of skeletal muscle. They cannot contract unless they are stimulated by nerve impulses. The activities of the respiratory centers are determined by changes in oxygen and carbon dioxide concentrations. They are also determined by the pH of the body fluids.
- The elderly cannot effectively make up for changes in airway and ventilation. Pulmonary changes that occur as a result of aging reduce vital capacity and increase physiological dead space. Po_2 also tends to decline gradually as a person ages.
- Causes of inadequate ventilation include upper airway obstruction and aspiration by inhalation. The most crucial lifesaving action for any patient who has respiratory problems from any cause is establishing and maintaining an open airway. This should always be the first priority of patient care.
- Essential parameters of airway evaluation include rate, regularity, effort, and recognition of airway problems that might indicate respiratory distress.
- The most common form of oxygen used in the prehospital setting is pure oxygen gas. This is delivered in liters per minute (LPM). Therapy regulators are used to deliver a safe pressure of oxygen to patients. Flowmeters control the amount of oxygen delivered to the patient. Several oxygen delivery devices provide supplemental oxygen to patients who have spontaneous respirations. They are the nasal cannula, simple face mask, partial rebreather mask, nonrebreather mask, and Venturi mask.
- In the prehospital setting, ventilation can be provided in several ways. These methods include rescue breathing (mouth-to-mouth, mouth-to-nose, mouth-to-stoma), mouth-to-mask breathing, use of bag-valve devices, and automatic transport ventilators.
- Emergency airway management should progress rapidly from the least to the most invasive techniques. Manual techniques for airway management include the head-tilt chin-lift method, the jaw-thrust, and the jaw-thrust without head-tilt.
- Suction catheters are used to clear the air passages of secretions and debris.
- Relief of gastric distention and/or emesis control can be accomplished through nasogastric or orogastric decompression.
- Mechanical devices for airway management include the nasal airway, oral airway, endotracheal intubation, digital intubation, nasotracheal intubation, laryngeal mask airway, multilumen airways, translaryngeal cannula ventilation, and cricothyrotomy.
- Rapid sequence intubation (RSI) involves administration of a potent sedative and a neuromuscular blocking drug at the same time. These are administered for the purpose of ET intubation.
- In the management of a child's airway, the differences in the pediatric airway must be considered. Compared to the adult airway, the child's upper airway structures have very different proportions. Their orientation to each other also differs. Smaller bag-valve devices are needed for infants and children. These reduce the chance of overinflation and barotrauma.
- End-tidal carbon dioxide detectors, pulse oximeters, and esophageal detectors can help the paramedic determine whether an ET tube has been placed correctly.

REVIEW QUESTIONS

Match the lung volume in Column II with its description in Column I. Use each answer only once.

Column I

1. _____ The air inhaled and exhaled during a normal respiratory cycle (500 to 600 mL)
2. _____ Quantity of air moved on deepest inspiration and expiration
3. _____ Tidal volume multiplied by respiratory rate
4. _____ Air remaining in respiratory passages after a forceful exhalation
5. _____ Amount of air that can be exhaled forcefully after a normal breath is exhaled

Column II

a. Expiratory reserve volume
b. Inspiratory reserve volume
c. Minute volume
d. Residual volume
e. Tidal volume
f. Vital capacity

6. Pulmonary ventilation is the movement of oxygen and carbon dioxide into and out of the lungs. True/false. If this is false, why is it false?

_____

7. pH is a measurement that reflects hydrogen ion concentration. True/false. If this is false, why is it false?

_____

8. The pressure regulator attached to an oxygen cylinder permits administration of a specific amount of oxygen. True/false. If this is false, why is it false?

_____

9. Describe the *mechanical* process by which air is moved into and out of the lungs.

_____

_____

_____

10. Complete the sentences in the following paragraph: At sea level, atmospheric pressure is (a) _____.

    The pressure in the alveoli is known as the (b) _____ pressure. Changes in this pressure are caused by

    changes in the (c) _____ size. During inspiration the pressure in the alveoli will (d) _____

    approximately 1 mm Hg relative to atmospheric pressure, whereas during exhalation the pressure will

    (e) _____ by 1 mm Hg. The ability of the lungs to expand during changes in pressure is known as

    (f) _____. This ability can be impaired by diseases such as (g)_____, _____,

    and _____.

11. The major blood vessels that carry deoxygenated blood to the lungs are the (a) _____. Oxygenated

    blood is carried away from the lungs by the (b) _____.

12. Your patient is a 70-year-old man with chronic bronchitis and emphysema who experienced an acute onset of shortness of breath while at the grocery store. Describe your ongoing assessment of this patient's head, neck,

chest, and abdomen. Be specific when describing the muscle groups that you will inspect to help determine his degree of distress.

_____

_____

13. The partial pressure of nitrogen = (a) _____ % × atmospheric pressure (b) _____ mm Hg =

(c) _____ mm Hg. The partial pressure of oxygen (Po_2) = (d) _____ % × atmospheric pres-

sure (e) _____ mm Hg = (f) _____ mm Hg.

14. List three physiological factors that can increase the work of breathing.

a. _____

b. _____

c. _____

15. Describe the *structural* aspects of the lung that explain the following:

a. Normal lung expansion:

_____

b. Alveolar collapse that occurs because of decreased surfactant in a premature infant:

_____

c. Poor ventilation during an asthma attack:

_____

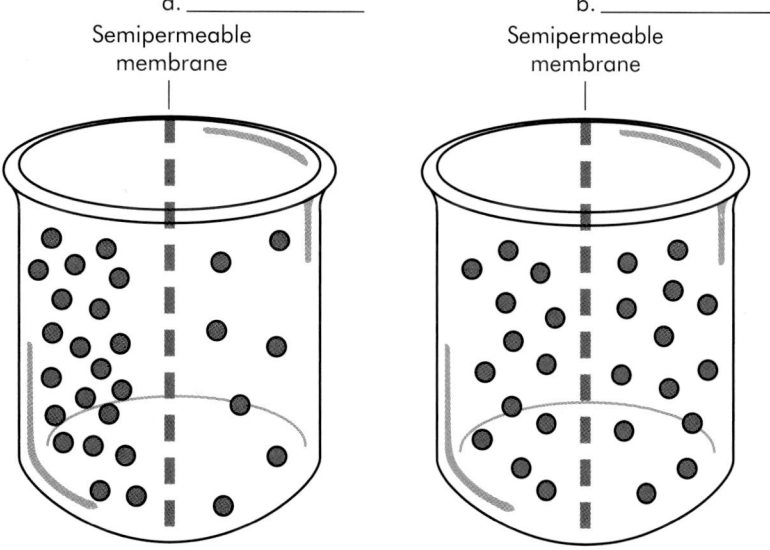

Figure 19-1

16. Each of the diagrams in Fig. 19-1 represents solutions separated by a semipermeable membrane. In each illustration, indicate whether the process of diffusion will cause a net movement of solute particles to the *left*, *right*, or *not at all*.

17. Complete the missing values for P_{CO_2} and P_{O_2} in the following. Then draw an arrow indicating the direction of movement of each of the gases across the respiratory membrane.

Alveolar Gas	**Direction of Movement of Gas**	**Venous Blood (Pulmonary Capillaries)**
P_{CO_2} _____ torr	P_{CO_2} _____ torr	
P_{O_2} _____ torr	P_{O_2} _____ torr	

18. Complete the following sentences.

  a. The primary way that oxygen is transported in the blood is by a chemical bond to _____.

  b. P_{O_2} describes the oxygen level dissolved in blood _____.

  c. The amount of carbon dioxide present in the venous blood is influenced by the rate and type of

  _____.

  d. Carbon dioxide is transported in the blood in three forms: _____, _____

  _____, and _____.

19. In one sentence describe the physiological basis for poor blood oxygenation in the following patients:

  a. A 23-year-old woman who is paralyzed completely from Guillain-Barré syndrome:

  _____

  b. A 52-year-old patient with pneumonia:

  _____

  c. An 8-year-old who is having an acute asthma attack:

  _____

  d. A 42-year-old with massive head trauma caused by a motor vehicle crash:

  _____

20. Briefly explain the origin or site of stimulation, location of effect, and action of each of the following mechanisms that control respiration:

Mechanism	**Origin or Stimulus**	**Location of Effect**	**Action**
Inspiratory centers			
Expiratory centers			
Hering-Breuer reflex			
Pneumotaxic center			
Apneustic center			

21. For each of the following scenarios, briefly explain why the patient's respirations will increase or decrease or be unchanged.

   a. A 3-year-old who loses consciousness from breath-holding following a temper tantrum:

   _____

   b. A 34-year-old with a morphine overdose:

   _____

   c. A 17-year-old football player with a dislocated shoulder:

   _____

   d. A hostage with no apparent injuries who has just been freed:

   _____

   e. A student who is sleeping in class:

   _____

   f. An individual who suffers from chronic obstructive pulmonary disease who has fallen and for whom an oxygen level of 10 L/min is being administered by nonrebreather mask:

   _____

   g. A lost snow skier who has a core temperature of 84° F (28.9° C):

   _____

22. Briefly describe the benefit of the following modified forms of respiration:

   a. Cough:

   _____

   b. Sneeze:

   _____

   c. Hiccup:

   _____

   d. Sigh:

   _____

23. For each of the following scenarios, identify the pathological condition or injury you would suspect, and list the signs and symptoms the patient may develop.

   a. A 50-year-old man unable to speak after choking on a piece of steak:

   _____

   b. A nursing home patient with shortness of breath after "inhaling" some food:

   _____

   c. A 17-year-old hockey player who has difficulty speaking after being struck across the neck by a stick:

   _____

d. A 2-year-old with croup:

_____

e. A 23-year-old who reportedly overdosed, is unconscious, and has vomitus draining from the side of her mouth.

_____

24. You are transporting a patient with severe asthma to a medical center 40 minutes away. What are the advantages of using a pulse oximeter in this scenario?

_____

25. For each of the following scenarios, circle the best oxygen-delivery device and explain why you made that selection.

a. A 76-year-old patient with chronic obstructive pulmonary disease complains of chest pain on the right side and a nosebleed after a fall. Vital signs are normal. Nasal cannula at 2 L/min oxygen or Venturi mask at 24% oxygen?

_____

b. A 25-year-old patient involved in a motor vehicle crash has ineffective respirations, cyanosis, and signs of a flail chest segment. Simple face mask at 8 L/min oxygen or bag-valve-mask with reservoir device at 15 L/min oxygen?

_____

c. A 45-year-old patient with slight chest pain (SaO_2 on room air is 98%). Simple face mask at 4 L/min oxygen or nasal cannula at 4 L/min oxygen?

_____

d. A 17-year-old patient who sustained a crush injury to the abdomen in a farming accident is pale, with cyanosis around the lips and decreased blood pressure. Simple mask at 6 L/min oxygen or complete non-rebreather mask at 10 L/min oxygen?

_____

26. For each of the following scenarios, choose the airway adjunct from the list that is most appropriate after initial manual airway maneuvers have been used. Explain why you selected your answer.

Oral airway	Nasal airway
Oral endotracheal intubation	Nasal endotracheal intubation
Percutaneous tracheal ventilation	Esophageal obturator airway

a. Your patient is a 17-year-old victim of a snowmobiling accident who struck a concealed barbed wire fence, injuring his neck. The airway is not patent. All attempts to secure the airway, including oral and nasal intubation, are unsuccessful.

_____

b. You are called to evaluate a 34-year-old patient who is postictal after a single grand mal seizure. He has snoring respirations and no gag reflex.

_____

c. Your patient was pulled from a swimming pool after an unsuccessful dive into the shallow end. He has ineffective shallow respirations and flaccid paralysis of all limbs.

_____

d. A 32-year-old woman with a history of diabetes has taken her insulin but has not eaten. She has snoring respirations and can be aroused with painful stimulus.

_____

e. A 19-year-old ejected from his all-terrain vehicle has an obviously severe head injury and shallow agonal respirations.

_____

f. A 79-year-old is in cardiac arrest of medical origin.

_____

27. Describe your actions if you discover the following physical findings after endotracheal intubation of a patient:

a. The carbon dioxide detector fades from purple to yellow as the patient exhales.

_____

b. Breath sounds are present bilaterally.

_____

c. Gurgling is auscultated over the epigastric region during ventilation.

_____

d. Breath sounds are diminished significantly over the left lung.

_____

e. The patient's color deteriorates, and the abdomen becomes distended.

_____

f. The bulb of the esophageal detector device fills in 8 seconds after placement on the end of the endotracheal tube.

_____

28. Fill in the blanks with the appropriate airway adjunct(s) from the following list:

Esophageal obturator airway (EOA)   Esophageal gastric tube airway (EGTA)

Pharyngeal tracheal lumen (PtL) airway   None

a. _____ Permits direct gastric suction

b. _____ May be used if placed in trachea or esophagus

c. _____ May cause regurgitation on removal

d. _____ Permits ventilation that is as effective as with an endotracheal tube

e. _____ Requires 5 to 8 mL of air to inflate a balloon

f. _____ Requires a tight mask seal for effective use

29. Briefly describe each step of the orotracheal intubation procedure illustrated in Fig. 19-2.

a.

b.

c.

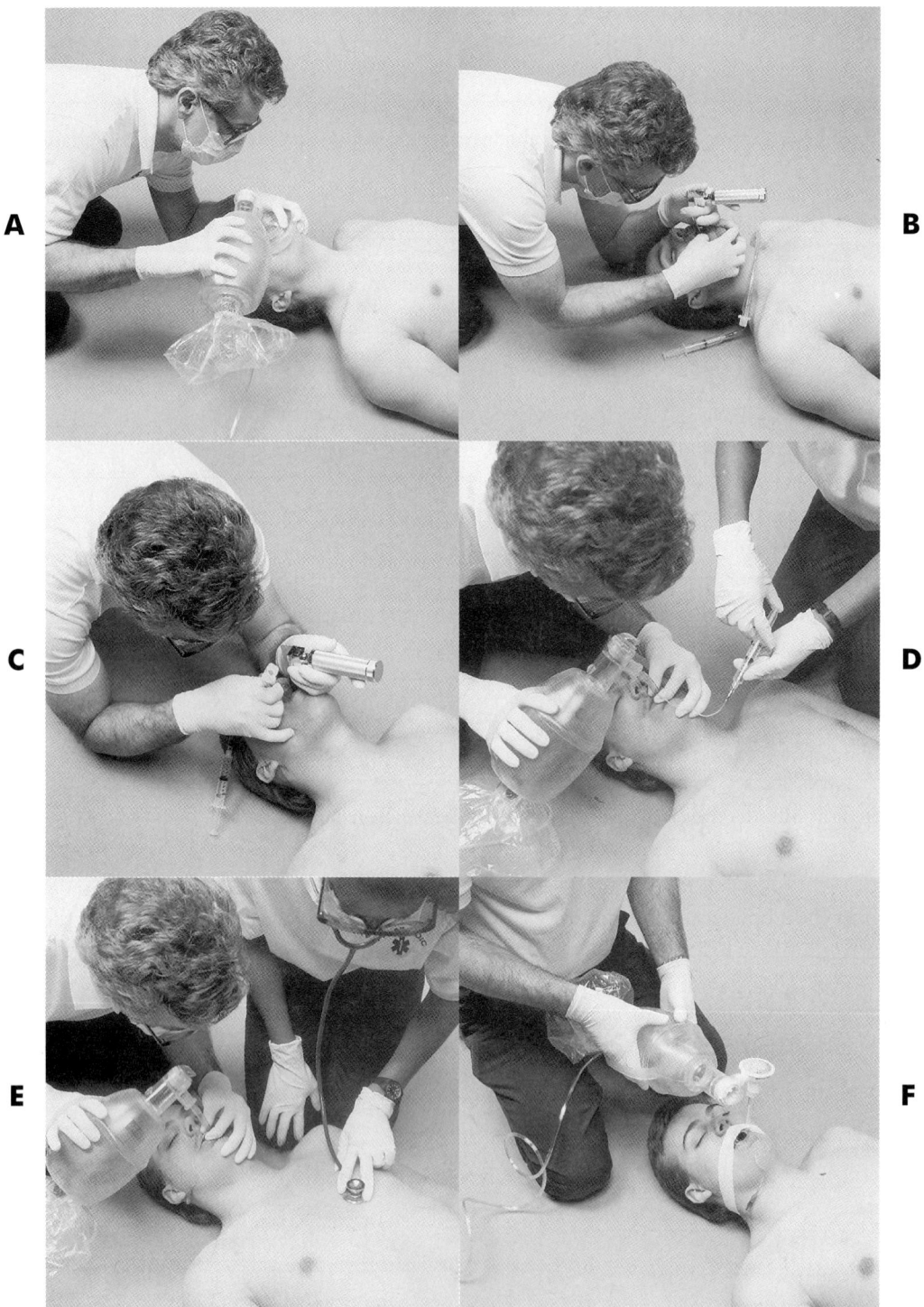

Figure 19-2

d.

e.

f.

30. List one advantage and one disadvantage for each of the following ventilation adjuncts:

Adjunct	Advantage	Disadvantage
a. Mouth to mouth		
b. Mouth to mask		
c. Bag-valve-mask		

31. List three patient situations in which use of tonsil-tip suction is indicated:

a.

b.

c.

32. What precautions should be taken to prevent complications when using a whistle-tip suction device for tracheal suctioning?

_____

33. Explain the anatomical basis for the following variations in pediatric airway management:

a. The oral airway should be inserted only with direct visualization with a tongue blade, never upside down and then rotated:

_____

b. Uncuffed endotracheal tubes should be used for children under 8 years of age:

_____

c. The endotracheal tube may "hang up" in the newborn, necessitating use of the Sellick maneuver to attain successful placement:

_____

34. You are called to the home of an 86-year-old patient who fell down 12 steps. Her chief complaint is rib pain and shortness of breath. On physical examination, you note crepitus and bruising on the lower rib cage. Why is it important to provide rapid, aggressive intervention for this older patient?

_____

_____

STUDENT SELF-ASSESSMENT

35. What is the term for the transfer of oxygen and carbon dioxide between the peripheral blood capillaries and tissue cells?
- **a.** External respiration
- **b.** Internal respiration
- **c.** Pulmonary ventilation
- **d.** Respiration

36. In what structure must continuous negative pressure be maintained to maintain lung expansion?
- **a.** Alveoli
- **b.** Mediastinum
- **c.** Pleural space
- **d.** Thoracic cage

37. When you arrive at the hospital, blood gasses on your 18-year-old patient indicate that the P_{O_2} is 70 mm Hg. What does this mean?
   a. Seventy percent of the hemoglobin is filled with oxygen.
   b. The patient is oxygenated adequately.
   c. Less than 3 mL of oxygen is dissolved in 1 L of blood.
   d. The blood sample must have been venous.

38. Which of the following factors will result in an *increased* energy requirement for breathing?
   a. Loss of pulmonary surfactant
   b. A decrease in airway resistance
   c. An increase in lung compliance
   d. Bronchodilation

39. Which of the following patients is most likely to have a decreased minute volume?
   a. A 17-year-old with deep respirations and signs of hyperventilation
   b. A 20-year-old patient with a head injury with shallow, slow respirations
   c. An alert 45-year-old with a possible myocardial infarction
   d. A 30-year-old in early shock with an increased respiratory rate

40. Your patient is on a pulse oximeter, and the reading is 100% saturation. What does this mean?
   a. The patient is on 100% oxygen by mask.
   b. The partial pressure of oxygen is 100.
   c. All hemoglobin has converted to oxyhemoglobin.
   d. The blood will not carry any more oxygen.

41. Which of the following conditions causes decreased oxygenation because of increased resistance in the airways?
   a. Asbestosis
   b. Asthma
   c. Poliomyelitis
   d. Tuberculosis

42. Why might the tissues of a patient with anemia not be well oxygenated?
   a. The blood does not reach all tissue to off-load oxygen.
   b. The respiratory drive in the brain is depressed.
   c. The number of red blood cells is insufficient to carry oxygen.
   d. The pulmonary vessels are not well perfused with blood.

43. Respiratory chemoreceptors in the medulla, aortic bodies, and carotid bodies are stimulated by changes in all of the following except which one?
   a. Blood pressure
   b. Carbon dioxide
   c. Oxygen
   d. pH

44. If a person appears to be choking but still can speak and cough, what should the rescuer do?
   a. Deliver five back blows.
   b. Perform the Heimlich maneuver.
   c. Administer five chest thrusts.
   d. Not intervene but just observe.

45. What is the most frequent cause of airway obstruction in the unconscious adult?
   a. Hot dogs
   b. Steak
   c. Tongue
   d. Vomitus

46. You arrive at a private residence, where you find an unconscious 52-year-old man. You open his airway and determine that he is not breathing. You attempt to ventilate his lungs, but the airflow is blocked. What is your next step?
   a. Assess the pulse.
   b. Reposition the head.
   c. Administer five abdominal thrusts.
   d. Perform a cricothyrotomy.

47. Which of the following represents the *most* effective measure to prevent aspiration of stomach contents?
   a. Applying cricoid pressure during bag-valve-mask ventilation
   b. Frequent suctioning of the mouth using a tonsil-tip suction
   c. Inserting an oropharyngeal airway and nasogastric tube
   d. Positioning the patient in the modified Trendelenberg's position

48. Your patient attempted suicide by hanging. She is hoarse and has hemoptysis and stridor. What do you suspect?
   a. Laryngeal fracture
   b. Laryngeal spasm
   c. Foreign body obstruction
   d. Tracheal injury

49. All of the following are potential complications of nasopharyngeal airway insertion except which one?
  a. It is poorly tolerated by sedated patients with gag reflexes.
  b. It may enter the esophagus if it is of excessive length.
  c. It may cause injury and bleeding to the nasal mucosa.
  d. It may become obstructed with blood or mucus.

50. To ensure adequate ventilation when combitube airway is used, you must be certain that
  a. The tube passes into the trachea.
  b. The mask seal is tight.
  c. The patient is less than 5 feet tall.
  d. Breath sounds are audible over the gastric area.

51. The pharyngeal tracheal lumen airway may be used successfully if the tube is placed in which structure?
  a. The esophagus
  b. The trachea
  c. The right main stem bronchus
  d. The esophagus or trachea

52. If 30 seconds have elapsed from the last ventilation and tracheal intubation has not been accomplished, what should you do?
  a. Remove the tube, hyperventilate, and try again.
  b. Continue if intubation can be done in a few more seconds.
  c. Insert an esophageal obturator airway.
  d. Have another paramedic attempt the skill.

53. Which of the following statements is true regarding percutaneous transtracheal ventilation?
  a. Demand valves may be used to provide adequate ventilations.
  b. It is a good long-term airway management device.
  c. It minimizes the risk of aspiration.
  d. The high pressures generated may cause pneumothorax.

54. Which of the following is *not* an advantage of the bag-valve-mask device?
  a. It allows delivery of high oxygen concentrations.
  b. It can give the rescuer a sense of the patient's lung compliance.
  c. It is used easily by one rescuer to deliver ventilations.
  d. It can provide a wide range of inspiratory pressures.

55. Which of the following indicates a properly placed endotracheal tube?
  a. End tidal CO_2 shows purple during ventilation.
  b. Gurgling is heard during auscultation over the stomach.
  c. Esophageal detection bulb refills in 10 seconds.
  d. Oxygen saturation changes from 79% to 94%.

56. Which of the following statements is true regarding suctioning of fluids from a patient?
  a. Hyperventilation for 2 minutes should precede suctioning.
  b. Suction should be applied for a maximum of 30 seconds.
  c. Coughing may cause decreased intracranial pressure.
  d. Suction should be set between 200 and 300 mm Hg.

57. The patient who is on a nasal cannula at 5 L/min is receiving approximately how much oxygen?
  a. 36%
  b. 40%
  c. 44%
  d. 50%

58. Your patient has been removed from a smoky building and is confused and tachycardic. What is the appropriate oxygen delivery device for this person?
  a. Nasal cannula
  b. Nonrebreather mask
  c. Simple face mask
  d. Venturi mask

59. Why might lidocaine be administered during rapid sequence induction for intubation?
  a. To minimize the potential for ventricular dysrhythmias
  b. To reduce the incidence of vomiting during the procedure
  c. To minimize the increase in intracranial pressure and prevent laryngospasm
  d. To anesthetize the airway structures and minimize the cough reflex

60. Which of the following complications related to cricothyrotomy will result in the absence of breath sounds when ventilation begins?
  a. Aspiration
  b. False passage
  c. Injury to the vocal cords
  d. Perforation of a great vessel

WRAP IT UP

You are dispatched to a school playground for an unconscious person. You arrive simultaneously with an ALS pumper crew and find a drowsy male who appears to be in his early 20s, lying across the playground equipment. He is arousable to voice, but very drowsy and snores when not stimulated. You open his airway using the head-tilt–chin-lift method, and as you insert a nasal airway, you note some vomitus has dried partially around his mouth. Oxygen saturation readings on room air are 93%, and his lung sounds reveal sonorous wheezes (rhonchi) throughout. His pupils are midpoint and 3 mm and sluggishly react to light. Vital signs are BP 94/58 mm Hg, P 148, R 28 and shallow. Oxygen by nonrebreather mask is applied, and the patient quickly is packaged onto the stretcher and placed in the ambulance. Your partner shows you some empty pill bottles nearby, and you recognize that he likely has taken some sedatives and antipsychotic drugs. In the ambulance the patient is attached quickly to the ECG monitor, a nasogastric tube is inserted, automatic BP monitoring is set up, an IV is established, and blood glucose is checked. As you prepare to depart the scene, the patient's respirations become irregular and slow with apneic pauses. When you attempt to stimulate him, there is no response, and a glance at the monitor reveals a rapidly slowing heart rate and oxygen saturation level. You instruct your partner to set up the intubation equipment as you insert an oral airway and begin to hyperventilate with a bag-mask device. When ready, you orally intubate the patient and then verify the correct placement of the tube, secure it, and begin to ventilate using an automatic transport ventilator. His heart rate increases, oxygen saturation levels rise, and his condition remains unchanged for the 10-minute transport to the medical center.

1. Would pulmonary aspiration interfere with internal or external respiration?
2. What was the likely explanation for this patient's slow irregular respirations?
   a. Anatomical dead space increase
   b. Central nervous system depression
   c. Decreased intrapulmonary pressure
   d. Increased atmospheric pressure
3. What actions were taken to reduce the risk of further aspiration?

---

4. Which of the following irregular patterns of breathing was this patient displaying?
   a. Air trapping
   b. Bradypnea
   c. Cheyne-Stokes
   d. Kussmaul's
5. Why was the nonrebreather mask chosen as the first oxygen delivery device?

---

6. When the patient's respirations became irregular and slow, what acid-base disturbance most likely was occurring?
   a. Metabolic acidosis
   b. Metabolic alkalosis
   c. Respiratory acidosis
   d. Respiratory alkalosis
7. What measure was taken to correct the acid-base disturbance?

---

8. How should the correct size of oral airway have been selected?

---

9. a. Why was suctioning indicated before intubation?
   b. Should suctioning be performed after intubation? Yes/No. If you answered yes, describe why it would be indicated.

10. For this patient's situation, describe the finding that suggests tracheal intubation.

Method	Finding

a. Auscultation over the epigastrium

_____

_____

b. Bilateral auscultation of the lungs

_____

_____

c. Esophageal detector device—syringe

_____

_____

d. Esophageal detector device—bulb

_____

_____

e. Colorimetric end-tidal CO_2 detector

_____

_____

f. Digital end-tidal CO_2 detector

_____

_____

g. Oxygen saturation

_____

_____

h. Direct laryngoscopic visualization

_____

_____

11. What settings should be selected on the automatic transport ventilator?

Rate: _____/min Volume: _____mL

CHAPTER 19 ANSWERS

REVIEW QUESTIONS

1. e
   (Objective 5)

2. f
   (Objective 5)

3. c
   (Objective 5)

4. d
   (Objective 5)

5. a
   (Objective 5)

6. True
   (Objective 1)

7. True
   (Objective 3)

8. False. The pressure regulator reduces the pressure in the oxygen cylinder to 30 to 70 psi to permit safe administration. The flow meter regulates the amount of oxygen delivered.
   (Objective 10)

9. During inspiration, the dome of the diaphragm is flattened when it contracts. This causes an increase in the superior-inferior distance of the chest cavity. The intercostal muscles contract, resulting in an increase in the anteroposterior and lateral diameter of the chest cavity. This increase in the size of the chest cavity results in a pressure drop in the chest approximately 1 mm Hg below atmospheric pressure. This negative pressure causes gas to move into the lungs. During expiration the relaxation of the diaphragm and other breathing muscles results in a decrease in the size of the chest wall and an increase in pressure in the chest approximately 1mm Hg above atmospheric pressure. This positive pressure in the chest forces the gas out of the lungs.
   (Objective 2)

10. a. 760 mm Hg; b. intrapulmonic; c. thoracic; d. decrease; e. increase; f. compliance; g. asthma, emphysema, bronchitis, pulmonary edema, and lung cancer.
    (Objectives 2 and 3)

11. a. Pulmonary arteries; b. pulmonary veins
    (Objective 4)

12. Head: Inspect for cyanosis around lips and "puffing" of the cheeks; neck: inspect for the use of accessory muscles or tracheal tugging; chest: inspect for intercostal muscle use and an increased anteroposterior diameter of the chest, auscultate lung sounds; abdomen: inspect for the use of abdominal muscles when breathing.
    (Objective 9)

13. a. 79; b. 760; c. 600.2; d. 21; e. 760; f. 160
    (Objective 3)

14. Loss of pulmonary surfactant, increase in airway resistance, and decrease in pulmonary compliance
    (Objective 2)

15. a. The lungs are coated with visceral pleura that adhere to the parietal pleura that line the chest wall. In the potential space between these two membranes, negative pressure "holds" the lungs to the chest wall. Disruption of this potential space causes collapse of the lung.

b. Surfactant reduces the surface tension in the alveoli. In other words, surfactant reduces the tendency of the alveolar walls to "stick" together. In the newborn with insufficient surfactant production, extremely high airway pressures must be used to maintain inflation of the alveoli so that effective ventilation can occur.

c. The bronchioles are surrounded by smooth muscle. During an asthma attack, the smooth muscle contracts forcefully and decreases the diameter of the bronchioles, which impairs the exchange of gases.
(Objectives 2 and 15)

16. a. Right; b. not at all
(Objective 5)

17.

Alveolar Gas	Direction Movement of Gas	Venous Blood (Pulmonary Capillaries)
P_{CO_2} *0* torr	$\leftarrow$	P_{CO_2} *46* torr
P_{O_2} *100* torr	$\rightarrow$	P_{O_2} *40* torr

(Objectives 3 and 5)

18. a. Hemoglobin; b. plasma; c. metabolism; d. plasma, blood proteins, and bicarbonate ions.
(Objective 5)

19. a. Loss of function of respiratory muscles prevents ventilation from occurring without mechanical assistance.

b. Compliance of the lungs and surface area for gas exchange will decrease.

c. Resistance in the airways will increase, which will decrease the flow of gases to and from the lungs.

d. The respiratory centers may be damaged, resulting in abnormal or absent breathing. The airway may not be patent.
(Objective 15)

20.

Mechanism	Origin or Stimulus	Location of Effect	Action
Inspiratory centers	Medulla to spinal cord to phrenic and intercostal nerves	Send impulses of respiration	Stimulates muscles
Expiratory centers	Medulla	Send impulses to spinal cord to phrenic and intercostal nerves	Stimulates muscles of respiration to increase force of exhalation
Hering-Breuer reflex	Vagus nerve	Medulla discharges inhibitory impulses	Causes inspiration to cease so lungs do not overinflate
Pneumotaxic center	Pons	Inspiratory center	Inhibits inspiratory center during labored breathing
Apneustic center	Lower pons	Inspiratory center	Baseline stimulation of inspiratory neurons

(Objective 6)

21. a. The respirations increase or resume because of the increased P_{CO_2}, which stimulates the respiratory centers.
b. The respiratory rate decreases as the respiratory centers of the brain are depressed by the morphine.
c. Pain causes an increased respiratory rate.
d. The fear involved in such a situation causes an increased respiratory rate.
e. The respiratory rate slows because of the decreased metabolic rate during sleep.
f. The history of chronic lung disease may mean that the patient is operating on a hypoxic drive. If this is the case, the chemoreceptors will sense an increase in the P_{O_2} and respond by decreasing the respiratory rate.
g. During hypothermia the metabolic rate decreases, as does the respiratory rate.
(Objective 15)

22. a. The cough reflex is designed to expel foreign matter from the respiratory passages.
b. Sneezing is caused by nasal irritation and also rids the respiratory tract of unwanted irritants.
c. Hiccups serve no known useful purpose but may signal pathological conditions.
d. Sighing provides intermittent hyperinflation of the lungs to help maintain expansion of the alveoli.
(Objective 2)

23. a. Obstructed airway: The patient initially will be apneic, will lose consciousness, and finally will suffer cardiac arrest if untreated.
b. Aspiration of food and possibly gastric juices: Initially the patient may experience a cough, mucus production, decreased breath sounds, or wheezes.
c. Fractured larynx: The patient may experience localized pain, edema, or hemoptysis. Dysphagia and subcutaneous emphysema may be present if airway obstruction is imminent.
d. Croup with potential for laryngeal spasm: The patient may be anxious and have crowing respirations (stridor) because of airway tissue swelling.
e. Decreased level of consciousness may result in partial airway obstruction and aspiration of vomit.
(Objective 7)

24. The pulse oximeter permits monitoring of the effectiveness of interventions by observing the oxygen saturation and pulse rate. If the oxygen saturation does not improve, additional interventions may be needed.
(Objective 13)

25. a. Venturi mask at 24% oxygen: A nasal cannula would be ineffective because the patient has a nosebleed.
b. Bag-valve-mask with reservoir device at 15 L/min oxygen: The patient clearly is not ventilating properly and needs ventilatory assistance in addition to the highest flow of oxygen possible.
c. Nasal cannula at 4 L/min oxygen: The simple face mask should never be used with an oxygen flow set at less than 6 L/min.
d. Complete nonrebreather mask at 10 L/min oxygen: The patient is demonstrating signs of shock and decreased oxygenation, so the highest amount of oxygen possible should be administered.
(Objective 10)

26. a. Percutaneous tracheal ventilation: All other less invasive airway maneuvers have been unsuccessful, possibly because of a laryngeal injury. The patient's airway is not patent, so needle access should be attempted.
b. Oral airway: If this is an isolated seizure, the patient's level of consciousness should be improving gradually, and a more invasive airway maneuver probably can be avoided.
c. Nasal intubation: Because of the patient's spontaneous respirations, this would be selected over oral intubation because of the high probability of cervical spine injury.
d. Nasal airway: This should secure the airway quickly while glucose is administered, which should arouse the patient.
e. Oral endotracheal intubation (using manual in-line stabilization of the cervical spine): This would be chosen because of the possibility of cervical spine injury. Nasal intubation would not be an option until basilar skull fracture could be ruled out.
f. Oral intubation: This is the airway of choice in the unconscious apneic patient with no potential for cervical spine injury.
(Objective 12)

27. a. This indicates that the tube is in the correct position. The tube should be secured.
b. The endotracheal tube is in the correct position, so the tube may be secured.
c. If breath sounds are absent, the cuff should be deflated and the tube quickly removed. After hyperventilation of the patient's lungs with a bag-valve-mask and 100% oxygen, another attempt at intubation may be made.
d. The cuff should be deflated and the tube withdrawn 1 to 2 cm. The cuff should be reinflated and correct placement verified by auscultation of breath sounds bilaterally.
e. The tube is probably in the esophagus. Auscultate for breath sounds, and if they are absent or diminished, deflate the cuff and remove the tube immediately. Hyperventilate the patient's lungs with a bag-valve-mask with a reservoir at 100% oxygen.
f. The tube is probably not in the trachea. Placement should be confirmed by auscultation of lung and epigastric sounds and by direct visualization of the vocal cords and use of an end-tidal CO_2 detector.
(Objective 13)

28. a. EGTA; b. PtL; c. EOA, EGTA, and PtL; d. none; e. none; f. EOA and EGTA
(Objective 12)

29. a. Hyperventilate the patient's lungs with 100% oxygen for at least 2 minutes.
b. With the laryngoscope in the left hand, insert the blade in the right corner of the mouth, displacing the tongue to the left.
c. Advance the endotracheal tube through the right corner of the mouth and, under direct vision, through the vocal cords.
d. Inflate the cuff with 5 to 8 mL of air, and ventilate the patient's lungs with a mechanical airway device.
e. Confirm endotracheal tube placement by auscultation of the abdomen and chest during ventilation.
f. Secure the endotracheal tube to the patient's head and face, and provide ventilatory support with supplemental oxygen. Continue to monitor correct placement of endotracheal tube using end-tidal CO_2 detection and other methods.
(Objective 12)

30.

Adjunct	Advantage	Disadvantage
a. Mouth to mouth	Easy to perform No equipment necessary	Risk of infectious disease No supplemental oxygen
b. Mouth to mask	Easy to apply Can give supplemental oxygen	Not possible to deliver 100% oxygen
c. Bag-valve-mask	Can give 100% oxygen Can vary volume	Mask seal difficult to maintain Frequently requires two persons

(Objective 11)

31. Vomiting with inadequate ability to expel emesis, facial trauma with bleeding in mouth, and epistaxis (nosebleed) where blood is accumulating in the oral cavity.
(Objectives 8 and 12)

32. Place the patient on a cardiac monitor, hyperoxygenate the lungs with 100% oxygen for 5 minutes before the procedure, and apply suction for no longer than 10 seconds.
(Objective 12)

33. a. The tongue is disproportionately large in a child, and the oral airway easily can occlude the airway if it is inserted by rotation.
b. A child younger than 8 years has a circular narrowing at the level of the cricoid cartilage that serves as a functional cuff.
c. The vocal cords slope from front to back, necessitating rotation of the tube or performance of the Sellick maneuver to facilitate intubation.
(Objective 14)

34. In many older patients there is increased thoracic rigidity, decreased elastic recoil of the lungs, and diminished P_{O_2}. In addition, the chemoreceptors do not function as well, which results in a decreased ventilatory response because of compromise of the respiratory system. Therefore the patient who experiences a significant chest injury may lack the physiological capability to compensate for the injury and will need aggressive intervention by the paramedic.
(Objective 15)

35. b. External respiration is the transfer of O_2 and CO_2 between the inspired air and pulmonary capillaries. Pulmonary ventilation refers to the movement of air into and out of the lungs. Respiration is the exchange of O_2 and CO_2 between an organism and the environment.
(Objective 1)

36. c. Pressure within the lungs (including the alveolar sacs) drops approximately 1 mm Hg during inspiration to permit the entry of air but is equal to atmospheric pressure at the end of quiet exhalation. The mediastinum does not maintain inflation of the lungs. Integrity of the thoracic cage is necessary to maintain negative pressure within the pleural space.
(Objective 2)

37. c. Only 3 mL of oxgyen can be dissolved in 1 L of blood at the normal arterial P_{O_2} of 100 mm Hg. Oxygen saturation measures the amount of hemoglobin that is saturated with oxygen. Normal oxygenation for a healthy 18-year-old is indicated by a P_{O_2} of 80 to 100 or greater. Venous P_{O_2} is typically about 40 mm Hg.
(Objective 3)

38. a. Without pulmonary surfactant, alveoli tend to collapse, making the work of breathing more difficult. All other factors listed decrease the work of breathing.
(Objective 15)

39. b. Minute volume = tidal volume × respiratory rate. Anything that decreases one of these variables without a reciprocal increase in the other decreases the minute volume.
(Objective 15)

40. c. It means that all hemoglobin is saturated with oxygen. When oxygen saturation is 100%, the oxygen is typically between 80% and 100% but may vary under certain pathological conditions.
(Objective 13)

41. b. Oxygenation is impaired in all these examples by different mechanisms.
(Objective 15)

42. c.
(Objectives 5 and 15)

43. a. Only if the changes in respiratory rate alter the oxygen or carbon dioxide level or the pH will chemical receptors be triggered.
(Objective 6)

44. d. If the patient's physiological signs deteriorate, the rescuer should intervene.
(Objective 7)

45. c.
(Objective 7)

46. b. Because the tongue is the most frequent cause of airway obstruction, repositioning the airway may be the only maneuver necessary to permit air exchange.
(Objective 7)

47. a. Cricoid pressure (Sellick maneuver), if done properly, can greatly minimize the risk of aspiration during artificial ventilation until the airway is secured with an endotracheal tube. Suctioning will reduce but not eliminate the risk of aspiration. A nasogastric tube will decrease the risk of aspiration by minimizing the gastric content, but an oropharyngeal airway may stimulate the gag reflex and cause aspiration. The most appropriate position to minimize the risk of aspiration is the left lateral recumbent position.
(Objective 8)

48. a. The mechanism of injury and signs are consistent with this life-threatening emergency, which necessitates aggressive airway management.
(Objective 7)

49. a. It is a frequently underused adjunct usually well tolerated by a semiconscious patient with a gag reflex.
(Objective 12)

50. b. The tube should be in the esophagus of a patient more than 5 feet tall, and no sounds should be audible over the gastric area when the patient's lungs are ventilated.
(Objective 12)

51. d. The tube is designed to function correctly in the trachea or esophagus.
(Objective 12)

52. a. Repeat attempts should be performed after hyperventilation.
(Objective 12)

53. d. Percutaneous transtracheal ventilation is a short-term (less than 45 minutes) airway device used when other measures to secure the airway are unsuccessful. The demand valve does not provide sufficient pressure to ventilate by this method. It offers no protection from aspiration. (Objective 11)

54. c.
(Objective 11)

55. d.
(Objective 11)

56. a. Suction should be applied for no longer than 10 seconds. A cough is stimulated frequently and may increase intracranial pressure. Suction should be set between 80 and 120 mm Hg.
(Objective 12)

57. d.
(Objective 10)

58. b. A patient with this mechanism and symptoms of hypoxia clearly needs the highest percentage of oxygen available.
(Objective 10)

59. c. Ideally this should be done 3 minutes before intubation.
(Objective 12)

60. b. If the tube passes into tissue outside of the trachea, ventilation will not be possible. Aspiration, vocal cord injury, and perforation of great vessels also are complications but still may allow delivery of ventilation.
(Objective 12)

WRAP IT UP

1. External respiration is interrupted because the substance aspirated and resulting inflammation of the alveoli impair the passage of oxygen to the pulmonary capillaries.
   (Objective 1)

2. b. The drugs the patient ingested are central nervous system depressants that will inhibit the respiratory center in the brain and also impair the protective airway reflexes.
   (Objective 6)

3. Suctioning secretions from the airway, nasogastric tube insertion with suction of gastric contents, and endotracheal intubation will help to prevent further aspiration.
   (Objective 8)

4. c. Air trapping occurs from chronic obstructive pulmonary disease; bradypnea is a slow regular respiratory pattern; Kussmaul's respirations are rapid and deep and occur in diabetic ketoacidosis.
   (Objective 9)

5. A nonrebreather mask delivers the highest amount of oxygen.
   (Objective 10)

6. c. Respiratory acidosis occurs when ventilation is impaired, resulting in decreased oxygen and increased CO_2.
   (Objectives 9 and 15)

7. Hyperventilation helps to reverse respiratory acidosis.
   (Objective 15)

8. Measure the oropharyngeal airway from the tragus of the ear to the corner of the mouth or the angle of the jaw.
   (Objective 12)

9. a. Suctioning vomit from the oropharynx before intubation reduces the risk of aspiration and improves visualization of the vocal cords.
   b. After intubation suctioning with a soft whistle-tipped catheter would help to eliminate vomit that previously was aspirated.
   (Objectives 8 and 12)

10. a. No sounds heard over epigastrium
    b. Breath sounds clearly audible bilaterally
    c. Syringe fills freely with air and no stomach contents aspirated
    d. Bulb fills with air within 2 seconds and no stomach contents are aspirated
    e. Yellow color
    f. CO_2 reads 35 to 45 mm Hg
    g. Oxygen saturation increases or reads from 93% to 100%
    h. Tube directly observed to be passing through vocal cords
    (Objective 13)

11. Rate, 12; volume, 6 to 7 mL/kg
    (Objective 11)

PART SIX

Trauma Systems and Mechanism of Injury

READING ASSIGNMENT

Chapter 20, pages 499-519, in *Mosby's Paramedic Textbook*, ed. 3

OBJECTIVES

Upon completion of this chapter, the paramedic student will be able to:

1. Describe the incidence and scope of traumatic injuries and deaths.
2. Identify the role of each component of the trauma system.
3. Predict injury patterns based on knowledge of the laws of physics related to forces involved in trauma.
4. Describe injury patterns that should be suspected when injury occurs related to a specific type of blunt trauma.
5. Describe the role of restraints in injury prevention and injury patterns.
6. Discuss how organ motion can contribute to injury in each body region depending on the forces applied.
7. Identify selected injury patterns associated with motorcycle and all-terrain vehicle collisions.
8. Describe injury patterns associated with pedestrian collisions.
9. Identify injury patterns associated with sports injuries, blast injuries, and vertical falls.
10. Describe factors that influence tissue damage related to penetrating injury.

SUMMARY

- Trauma is the leading cause of death among persons 1 to 34 years of age and is the fifth leading cause of death among all Americans.
- Trauma care is divided into three phases: preincident, incident, and postincident.
- Components of the trauma system include injury prevention, prehospital care, emergency department care, interfacility transportation (if needed), definitive care, trauma critical care, rehabilitation, data collection, and trauma registry.
- Injuries are caused by a transfer of energy from some external source to the human body. The extent of injury is determined by the type of energy applied, by how quickly it is applied, and by the part of the body to which the energy is applied.
- Blunt trauma is an injury produced by the wounding forces of compression and change of speed, which can disrupt tissues.
- Four restraining systems are available in the United States. These are lap belts, diagonal shoulder straps, child safety seats, and air bags. All of these significantly reduce injuries. However, if they are used inappropriately, these protective devices also can produce injuries.

- Organ injuries can result from sudden movement caused by deceleration and compression forces. The recognition of these injuries requires a high degree of suspicion. The paramedic must use the principles of kinematics.
- Small motorized vehicles such as motorcycles, all-terrain vehicles, snowmobiles, motorboats, water bikes, and farm machinery are considered to be more dangerous than other motor vehicles. They are more dangerous because they offer little protection to the rider. They offer minimal protection from the transfer of energy associated with collisions.
- All auto-pedestrian collisions can produce serious injuries. They require a high degree of suspicion for multiple-system trauma.
- Sports provide a variety of health benefits. However, they also can produce severe injury.
- Blast injury is damage to a patient exposed to a pressure field that is produced by an explosion of volatile substances. Blasts release large amounts of energy in the form of pressure and heat.
- Falls from greater than 3 times the height of a person (15 to 20 feet) are associated with an increased incidence of severe injuries. In predicting injuries associated with falls, the paramedic should evaluate three things: the distance fallen, the body position of the patient on impact, and the type of landing surface struck.
- All penetrating objects, regardless of velocity, cause tissue disruption. The character of the penetrating object, its speed of penetration, and the type of body tissue it passes through or into determine whether crushing or stretching forces will cause injury.

REVIEW QUESTIONS

Match the appropriate energy law listed in Column II with its description in Column I.

Column I

1. _____ Force is equal to mass times acceleration or deceleration.
2. _____ Equal to ½ mass × velocity².
3. _____ An object at rest or in motion remains in that state unless force is applied.
4. _____ Energy can neither be created nor destroyed; it can only change form.

Column II

a. Newton's first law of motion
b. Newton's second law of motion
c. Conservation of energy law
d. Joule's law
e. Kinetic energy law

5. Identify three causes of death for each of the periods of the trimodal distribution of traumatic death; for each period, identify prehospital interventions that may increase patient survival.
   a. Immediate:

   _____

   b. Early:

   _____

   c. Late:

   _____

6. A 17-year-old female falls asleep at the wheel, rides the median for 50 feet, and then strikes a concrete bridge abutment head-on.
   a. Identify the three collisions that occur in this situation.

   _____

   _____

   _____

   b. Assuming that this driver took the down-and-under pathway during the collision, what injuries should you anticipate?

   _____

7. Aside from speed and size, what factor affects the injury pattern found in a lateral impact collision?

8. In which of the following rear-end collisions will damage be greater, assuming that mass and other factors are equal? Why?
   a. A vehicle traveling 50 mph is struck by a vehicle traveling 70 mph.
   b. A vehicle traveling 5 mph is struck by a vehicle traveling 40 mph.

9. For each of the body regions, list the injury or injuries that may occur during sudden, rapid deceleration.
   a. Head and neck injuries:

   b. Thoracic injuries:

   c. Abdominal injuries:

10. You are called to the scene of a high-speed frontal crash caused by a crossover accident. The driver of one of the vehicles complains of severe dyspnea and has a large circular bruise on her chest. You note greatly decreased lung sounds on the right side of the chest and suspect a pneumothorax.
   a. What traumatic mechanism can cause a pneumothorax in this example?

   b. The driver of the other vehicle has severe abdominal pain and is exhibiting signs of hypovolemic shock. Which abdominal organs or structures can be injured from sudden compression of the abdomen?

11. Identify the type of motorcycle collision most frequently associated with the pattern of injuries listed.
   a. A seasoned biker has a severely angulated fracture of the right forearm and extensive abrasions to the right side of the body.

   b. A 47-year-old executive has bilateral fractured femurs and facial injuries.

   c. A traffic officer has a severe crush injury to the left lower leg.

12. Identify the injuries to be anticipated in the following situations:
   a. A motorist swerves across the highway and is struck by an oncoming vehicle.

   b. As a young child hurries to avoid being late to school, he is struck by a full-size automobile.

13. When evaluating a sports injury, what principles of kinematics must be considered to determine probable areas of injury?

14. A suitcase filled with plastic explosives detonates in a locker at a busy urban airport. Describe the type of injuries the paramedic should anticipate in each of the following categories:
   a. Primary blast injuries:

   b. Secondary blast injuries:

   c. Tertiary blast injuries:

15. You are called to a home to care for a person who has fallen.
   a. List three things you must determine to predict injuries associated with this fall.

   b. What age of patient is most likely to fall?

   c. If the person who fell is an adult, how is she likely to land?

16. Briefly describe the way each of the following ballistic properties influences injury patterns in penetrating trauma.
   a. Character of the penetrating object:

   b. Speed of penetration:

   c. Distance from patient that a bullet is fired:

STUDENT SELF-ASSESSMENT
17. Trauma is the leading cause of death in persons of which of the following ages?
   a. Less than 1 year
   b. 1 to 34 years
   c. 35 to 65 years
   d. More than 65 years
18. What actions can a paramedic take to intervene at the incident phase of trauma?
   a. Educate the community
   b. Decrease scene time
   c. Promote safety legislation
   d. Wear personal restraint systems

19. Which of the following is a component of a trauma system as defined in the National Standard Paramedic Curriculum?
    a. Emergency medical services education
    b. Fire suppression
    c. Pain management
    d. Rehabilitation
20. What factor influences trauma triage guidelines?
    a. Mechanism of injury
    b. Patient's ability to pay
    c. Paramedic preference
    d. Patient preference
21. What is the process of predicting injury patterns that may result from the forces and motions of energy known as?
    a. Force of energy applied
    b. Index of suspicion
    c. Kinematics
    d. Mechanism of injury
22. Injury resulting from blunt trauma most often is caused by which of the following forces?
    a. Compression
    b. Deceleration
    c. Distraction
    d. Torsion
23. Your patient was restrained when her car was struck on the right side on her door at a high rate of speed. What injuries do you predict?
    a. Aortic injury
    b. Liver injury
    c. Pancreatic injury
    d. Splenic injury
24. Which injuries are more likely if the lap belt is applied improperly?
    a. Duodenal injuries
    b. Maxillofacial injuries
    c. Pelvic fractures
    d. Sternal fractures
25. Which of the following is true regarding ejection from a vehicle?
    a. It will not happen if the person is restrained.
    b. It usually happens before impact.
    c. Spinal injuries are common.
    d. There is little risk of death.
26. Steering wheel/dash air bags are designed to reduce injuries in which of the following collisions?
    a. Frontal collisions
    b. Lateral collisions
    c. Rollover collisions
    d. All of the above
27. Which of the following are predictable injuries from all-terrain vehicle crashes?
    a. Abdominal injuries
    b. Kidney injuries
    c. Thoracic injuries
    d. Upper extremity injuries
28. Which of the following is more likely to occur when a child is struck by a car, compared with an adult?
    a. The child may strike the hood of the vehicle.
    b. The child may be dragged under the vehicle.
    c. The child may land on the ground.
    d. The child may strike the bumper of the vehicle.
29. A roofer falls from the top of a two-story residence. What type of injuries do you anticipate?
    a. Minor injuries to the feet and spine
    b. Severe injuries to the feet and spine
    c. Minor injuries to the head and neck
    d. Major injuries to the head and neck
30. A 2-year-old child falls from a second-story window. What area of the body is most likely to be injured?
    a. Head and neck
    b. Arm
    c. Leg
    d. Pelvis
31. Which of the following is a high-energy weapon with the potential to cause the greatest injury to tissues?
    a. M-16
    b. .357 magnum
    c. 12-gauge shotgun
    d. Knife
32. Which organ is likely to experience the most severe injury from tissue crushing caused by cavitation after a gunshot wound?
    a. Bowel
    b. Liver
    c. Lung
    d. Muscle

WRAP IT UP

You are checking your ambulance at shift change on a foggy September morning when you are dispatched to the interstate highway for a chain reaction collision involving multiple vehicles. You and your supervisor arrive on the scene simultaneously, and she sends you to begin triage. As you move from vehicle to vehicle, you note the following. The first two cars appear to have struck each other head on—there is major damage. In vehicle #1 there are two front seat passengers, both restrained with air bags that now are deflated. They are conscious, but the passenger has abdominal and low back pain and lifts his shirt to show you the abrasion over his abdomen. In vehicle #2 the passengers were not restrained. The driver was thrown up and over the steering wheel and into the now starred windshield. He is dyspneic, pale, and anxious. His passenger was ejected and lies motionless at the side of the road; there is no breathing, even after you open his airway, so you move on. Vehicle #3, a small sedan, struck vehicle #2 on the right rear fender in a glancing blow and then swerved into the ditch and rolled several times. The front seat passenger, who is belted with her lap and shoulder belt, and her child, appropriately secured in a child seat in the middle rear seat, are crying, are alert, and have normal skin color. As vehicle #3 swerved, it struck a sport utility vehicle (vehicle #4) that spun and came to rest sideways in the highway. The SUV was then struck laterally on the driver door by a national express delivery truck (vehicle #5). There were no side air bags, and the restrained SUV driver has chest pain and severe arm and hip pain. The truck driver was restrained and is ambulatory with no complaints. A motorcyclist (vehicle #6), seeing an imminent collision with vehicle #5, laid his bike down and slid on his side 30 feet before striking the rear dual wheels of the truck. The protective coating on his helmet has been worn away on the lateral side, as has his jacket, and he is conscious, alert and complaining of severe pain from his deep skin abrasions. A police officer, struck by a car as he set up traffic cones, is unconscious on the ground. You report to command a brief synopsis of patient condition so that appropriate transport decisions can be made; the closest level I or II trauma center is 75 miles away.

1. Which phase of trauma care will you be involved with on this scene?
   a. Preincident
   b. Incident
   c. Postincident
   d. Preventive
2. Place a check mark beside the components of a sophisticated trauma system that could (or did) benefit any of the patients on this call.
   a. _____ Injury prevention
   b. _____ Prehospital care
   c. _____ Emergency department care
   d. _____ Interfacility transportation if needed
   e. _____ Definitive care
   f. _____ Trauma critical care
   g. _____ Rehabilitation
   h. _____ Data collection and trauma registry
3. List injuries that you would anticipate based on the mechanism of injury for each of the following patients.

   Patient   **Injuries Predicted**
   a. Passenger vehicle #1 (restrained with air bag)

   _____

   b. Driver vehicle #2 (up and over)

   _____

   c. Passenger car #2 (ejected)

   _____

   d. Passenger vehicle #3 (child in car seat)

   _____

   e. Driver vehicle #4 (SUV)

   _____

   f. Rider vehicle #6 (motorcycle)

   _____

   g. Police officer

   _____

CHAPTER 20 ANSWERS

REVIEW QUESTIONS

1. b
   (Objective 3)

2. e
   (Objective 3)

3. a
   (Objective 3)

4. c
   (Objective 3)

5. a. Lacerations of the brain, brainstem, upper spinal cord, heart, aorta, and other large vessels; injury prevention programs
   b. Subdural or epidural hematoma, hemopneumothorax, ruptured spleen, lacerated liver, pelvic fracture, and numerous injuries associated with significant blood loss; decreasing time from injury to definitive care, which must be brief
   c. Sepsis, infection, and multiple organ failure; early recognition and treatment of life-threatening injury in the field, with adequate fluid resuscitation and aseptic technique
   (Objective 1)

6. a. The vehicle strikes the abutment, the passenger strikes the inside of the vehicle, and the internal organs pull forward rapidly and strike the bony structures inside the body.
   b. Dislocated knees, patellar fractures, fractured femurs, posterior fracture or dislocation of the acetabulum, vascular injury, and hemorrhage
   (Objective 1)

7. Whether the car struck remains stationary (injuries likely on the side of the impact) or moves away from the point of impact (injuries likely on the side opposite the impact)
   (Objective 4)

8. b. The velocity that produces damage is determined by calculating the difference between the speed of the two vehicles. In example a it is $70 - 50 = 20$, and in example b it is $40 - 5 = 35$.
   (Objective 3)

9. a. Intracerebral hemorrhage and cervical fracture; b. ruptured aorta; c. kidney, liver, and spleen lacerations
   (Objective 4)

10. a. Pneumothorax could be caused by displaced rib fractures that puncture a lung or by a paper bag injury, in which impact occurs after the patient has inhaled against a closed glottis.
    b. Lacerated spleen, liver, or kidney; rupture of the bladder, diaphragm, gallbladder, duodenum, colon, stomach, and small bowel
    (Objective 4)

11. a. Laying the bike down; b. head-on (up and over the handle bars); c. angular
    (Objective 7)

12. a. Fractures of the lower legs, femur, pelvis, thorax, and spine; injuries to the intraabdominal or intrathoracic contents; and head and spinal injuries

b. Fractures of the femur and pelvis; abdominopelvic and thoracic trauma; and head and neck injuries

(Objective 8)

13. Energy forces involved, body part to which energy is transferred, speed of acceleration and deceleration, forces involved (compression, twisting, hyperextension, hyperflexion), protective gear

(Objective 9)

14. a. Hearing loss, pulmonary hemorrhage, cerebral air embolism, thermal injuries, abdominal hemorrhage, and bowel perforation

b. Lacerations, contusions, fractures, and impaled objects

c. Fractures and abdominopelvic, thoracic, head, and spine injuries

(Objective 9)

15. a. The paramedic should evaluate: the distance fallen; the body position of the patient on impact; and the type of landing surface.

b. Children and elderly are more likely to fall.

c. An adult is more likely to land on her feet.

(Objective 9)

16. a. Length and width of knives determine the depth and extent of the injury. With bullets, missile damage increases if the bullet is designed to rotate, flatten, or fragment during or after impact.

b. Kinetic injury increases with increased speed, and tissue damage increases with increased energy applied.

c. As the range increases, the damage decreases because of decreased velocity. Close-range injuries produce more damage because of the direct injury of gases from combustion and the explosion of powder.

(Objective 10)

17. b. Trauma is the fifth leading cause of death overall.

(Objective 1)

18. d. Community education and legislation are preincident interventions, and decreasing scene time is a postinjury intervention.

(Objective 1)

19. d. The other components are injury prevention, prehospital care, emergency department care, interfacility transportation, definitive care, trauma critical care, data collection, and trauma registry.

(Objective 2)

20. a. Other factors include patient condition, injury severity indices, and available patient care resources.

(Objective 2)

21. c. Kinematics is based on mechanism of injury and force of energy applied. Index of suspicion for certain types of injuries is related to kinematics, the age of the patient, and preexisting illness.

(Objective 3)

22. a. Direct compression or pressure on a structure is the most common type of force applied in blunt trauma.

(Objective 4)

23. b. Because she was struck on the right side, injury to the liver is more likely than injury to the spleen.

(Objective 4)

24. a. All the other injuries can occur in high-speed crashes in which the lap belt is applied properly.

(Objective 5)

25. c. A small number of restrained persons are ejected. Risk of death is 6 times greater than the risk for those who are not ejected. Ejection typically happens after impact.
(Objective 5)

26. a. The air bag inflates and then rapidly deflates after the first frontal collision.
(Objective 5)

27. d. Head and neck injuries also are common.
(Objective 7)

28. b. This may compound other injuries and cause traumatic amputation.
(Objective 8)

29. b. Falls from more than 3 times the height of the individual are likely to produce serious injury. Adults who fall from a height greater than 15 feet usually land on their feet.
(Objective 9)

30. a. Children tend to fall head first because their heads are proportionately larger.
(Objective 9)

31. a.
(Objective 10)

32. b. Nonelastic organs do not stretch.
(Objective 10)

WRAP IT UP

1. b.
(Objective 1)

2. a. Injury prevention (seat belt education, passive restraint [air bags] systems; prehospital care (triage, treatment, transport); emergency department care (examination, diagnostics, interventions); interfacility transport if needed (to higher-level trauma centers); definitive care (surgery for intraabdominal injuries); trauma critical care (early postresuscitation care); rehabilitation (physical, head injury); data collection and trauma registry (to monitor trauma quality, track demographics)
(Objective 2)

3. a. If lap belt was improperly worn too high, injury to T12, L1, and L2 could occur. If compressed, injury could be provided to the liver, spleen, duodenum, or pancreas could be present.
(Objectives 3, 4, and 5)

   b. Rib fractures, ruptured diaphragm, hemopneumothorax, pulmonary contusion, cardiac contusion, myocardial rupture, or aortic rupture are possible if thorax absorbed impact. If abdomen absorbed impact, tears to liver, spleen, or blood vessels are possible. Head and neck injuries are also common.
(Objectives 3 and 4)

   c. Spinal fracture, death
(Objectives 3 and 4)

   d. Rollover: difficult to categorize injuries—None may be present if proper restraints were used.
(Objectives 3 and 4)

e. Lateral impact: fractured ribs, pulmonary contusion, ruptured liver or spleen, fractured clavicle, fractured pelvis, and head and neck injury
(Objectives 3 and 4)

f. Motorcyclist laying the bike down: abrasions, fractures to the affected side
(Objective 7)

g. Pedestrian struck: lower extremity fractures; femur, pelvis, spine fractures; head injuries, internal hemorrhage
(Objective 8)

CHAPTER 21

Hemorrhage and Shock

READING ASSIGNMENT
Chapter 21, pages 520-537, in *Mosby's Paramedic Textbook,* ed. 3

OBJECTIVES
Upon completion of this chapter, the paramedic student will be able to:
1. Describe how to recognize signs and symptoms of internal or external hemorrhage.
2. Define shock.
3. Outline the factors necessary to achieve adequate tissue oxygenation.
4. Describe how the diameter of resistance vessels influences preload.
5. Describe the function of the components of blood.
6. Outline the changes in the microcirculation during the progression of shock.
7. List the causes of hypovolemic, cardiogenic, neurogenic, anaphylactic, and septic shock.
8. Describe pathophysiology as a basis for signs and symptoms associated with the progression through the stages of shock.
9. Describe key assessment findings to distinguish the etiology of the shock state.
10. Outline the prehospital management of the patient in shock based on knowledge of the pathophysiology associated with each type of shock.
11. Discuss how to integrate the assessment and management of the patient in shock.

SUMMARY
- The seriousness of external hemorrhage depends on the anatomical source of the hemorrhage, the degree of vascular disruption, and the amount of blood loss that can be tolerated by the patient. Internal bleeding that causes the patient to be unstable usually occurs in one of three body cavities: the chest, abdomen, or retroperitoneum.
- Shock is not a single entity. Shock does not have one specific cause and treatment. Rather, shock is a complex group of physiological abnormalities. Moreover, shock can result from a variety of disease states and injuries.
- To achieve adequate oxygenation of tissue cells (perfusion), three distinct components of the cardiovascular system must function properly: the heart, vasculature, and lungs.
- The healthy body is a smooth-flowing fluid delivery system inside a container. The volume of the container is related directly to the diameter of the resistance vessels. This diameter can change rapidly.
- Normal adult blood volume is 4.5 to 5 L.

- The progression of shock affects the microcirculation. This progression follows a sequence of stages related to changes in capillary perfusion and cellular necrosis. These stages include vasoconstriction, capillary and venule opening, disseminated intravascular coagulation, and multiple organ failure.
- In emergency care, shock commonly is classified based on the cause. (For example, the cause may be hypovolemic, cardiogenic, neurogenic, anaphylactic, or septic.)
- The response of the body to the shock syndrome (hypoperfusion and its associated anaerobic metabolism) can be categorized into stages: compensated shock, uncompensated (or decompensated) shock, and irreversible shock.
- Variations in the physiological response to shock can occur based on a number of factors. The patient's age and health are factors. The patient's ability to activate compensatory mechanisms plays a role. The specific organ affected is a factor as well.
- The management and treatment plan for the patient in shock focuses on assessment. The paramedic must assess oxygenation and perfusion of the body organs. The goals of the treatment plan are to ensure a patent airway, to provide adequate oxygenation and ventilation, and to restore perfusion. The initial survey can help to identify the adequacy of cellular perfusion.

REVIEW QUESTIONS

Match the blood component in Column II with its definition in Column I. Use each answer only once.

	Column I	**Column II**
1. _____	Provides oxygen to and removes carbon dioxide from cells	**a.** Albumin
2. _____	Forms sticky plugs and initiates clotting	**b.** Erythrocytes
3. _____	Destroys red blood cells and bacteria	**c.** Fibrinogen
4. _____	Large protein that moves water from tissues into the blood	**d.** Gamma globulin
5. _____	Important in human immune response	**e.** Leukocyte
6. _____	Solvent of blood through which salts, minerals, and fats travel	**f.** Plasma
		g. Platelet

7. You are called to evaluate a 20-year-old butcher who sustained a stab wound to the femoral artery. Evaluation of the patient reveals a large amount of blood loss from an inguinal wound that is spurting bright red blood. The patient is anxious and confused. Vital signs are as follows: blood pressure, 86/70 mm Hg; pulse, 136; respirations, 28; and lungs, clear. The patient's lips and nail beds are pale and cyanotic, and capillary refill is greater than 2 seconds. List the three physiological components necessary for normal cellular oxygenation as measured by the Fick principle and determine whether each has been met.

    a.

    b.

    c.

8. Describe the structural elements of the vascular system that enable it to adjust its size and adapt to pressure changes.

_____

_____

9. Complete the following sentences: The pressure that blood exerts against the vessel walls is known as

    (a) _____ pressure. Pressure that results from contraction of the ventricles is

    (b) _____ pressure, whereas the residual pressure

    between contractions is (c) _____ pressure. The pulse felt in an artery resulting from the difference in (b) and (c) pressure is known as (d) _____ pressure.

Pressure in the vessels is greatest at the (e) _____ and least at the

(f) _____.

10. State the effect that each of the following patient situations has on the size of the patient's vascular container and on preload.
    a. A patient with a cervical spine injury from a motor vehicle collision has the following vital signs: blood pressure, 80/60 mm Hg; pulse, 60; and respirations, 28. His skin is cool and pale above the level of the injury and warm and dry below it.

    _____

    b. A 55-year-old woman with heavy vaginal bleeding has been dizzy. Vital signs are as follows: blood pressure, 106/92 mm Hg; pulse, 116; and respirations, 20.

    _____

11. For each of the following intravenous fluids, indicate whether the solution is isotonic, hypotonic, or hypertonic. Indicate whether there will be immediate net movement of fluid into or out of the intravascular space if this fluid is given, or whether no movement is observed.

Intravenous Fluid	Isotonic, Hypotonic, or Hypertonic	Fluid Movement
D50W		
Lactated Ringer's		
Normal saline		
0.45% normal saline		
D_5W		

12. A 65-year-old complains of severe abdominal pain that radiates to the back. A large pulsatile mass is evident in the abdomen. Vital signs are as follows: blood pressure, 80/70 mm Hg; pulse, 128; and respirations, 28. Predict the pathophysiological changes and associated signs and symptoms that will occur during the stages of shock for this patient.
    a. Stage 1: Vasoconstriction

    _____

    b. Stage 2: Capillary and venule opening

    _____

    _____

    c. Stage 3: Disseminated intravascular coagulation

    _____

    _____

    d. Stage 4: Multiple organ failure

    _____

    _____

13. For each of the following situations, list the type of shock and briefly describe interventions necessary for patient management.

a. You are called to evaluate a 72-year-old man whose wife states that he had chest pain all day yesterday and earlier today. He has no pain when you arrive, but he is confused, pale, and diaphoretic. No bleeding is evident. Lung sounds reveal crackles in the bases. Vital signs are as follows: blood pressure, 86/76 mm Hg; pulse, 128 and irregular; and respirations, 28.

Classification:

Interventions:

_____

_____

b. Your 17-year-old patient was unrestrained in a motor vehicle collision. He has no sensation below the nipple line and is confused. He has a large laceration on the parietal area and complains of neck pain. No other injuries are evident. His skin is pale and cool above the nipple line and warm and dry below. Vital signs are as follows: blood pressure, 84 mm Hg by palpation; pulse, 56; and respirations, 28 and very shallow.

Classification:

Interventions:

_____

_____

c. A 26-year-old woman who states that her last menstrual period was 8 weeks ago is complaining of severe right lower quadrant abdominal pain. She is pale, cool, and diaphoretic. Vital signs are as follows: blood pressure, 106/78 mm Hg; pulse, 120; and respirations, 20 while supine; blood pressure, 88/76 mm Hg; pulse, 136; and respirations, 28 while standing.

Classification:

Interventions:

_____

_____

d. A 42-year-old woman experiences acute shortness of breath, urticaria, nausea, and dizziness after ingesting a penicillin tablet prescribed by her dentist. Vital signs are as follows: blood pressure, 80 mm Hg by palpation; pulse, 140; and respirations, 40 and labored.

Classification:

Interventions:

_____

_____

e. A 72-year-old resident of a nursing home has a fever and is restless and agitated. The urine in the indwelling catheter collection bag is milky and green. Vital signs are as follows: blood pressure, 94/60 mm Hg; pulse, 132; and respirations, 30.

Classification:

Interventions:

---

f. A 55-year-old office worker has complained of a pounding sensation in his chest and has fallen from his chair, striking his head on the desk. You note a 5-cm laceration on the frontal area that is freely oozing dark red blood (about 20 mL on the floor). The patient is unconscious, and vital signs are as follows: blood pressure, 60 mm Hg by palpation; pulse, 180; and respirations, 28.

Classification:

Interventions:

---

14. For each of the following situations, identify whether the patient is in compensated or uncompensated shock and explain why.
   a. A 48-year-old has sustained second- and third-degree burns to 70% of his body. He is pale, cool, and diaphoretic. His nail beds are cyanotic, and his vital signs are as follows: blood pressure, 84/76 mm Hg; pulse, 136; and respirations, 32.

---

   b. A 22-year-old passenger in a high-speed motor vehicle crash was restrained with a lap belt. She complains of severe abdominal pain. Her skin is cool and pale. Vital signs are as follows: blood pressure, 110/86 mm Hg; pulse, 128; and respirations, 28.

---

15. Describe the characteristics of irreversible shock.

---

16. List three conditions, situations, or characteristics that decrease a patient's ability to compensate in shock.

---

17. For each of the following scenarios, select the appropriate intervention(s) from the following list. Briefly justify your answer.

Pneumatic antishock garment Drug therapy
Rapid fluid replacement Blood transfusions
Intraosseous infusion

a. A 72-year-old after experiencing a myocardial infarction with pulmonary edema and vital signs as follows: blood pressure, 86/60 mm Hg; pulse, 124; and respirations, 28.

_____

_____

b. A 2-year-old was struck by an automobile, and you suspect that he has numerous pelvic and abdominal injuries. Vital signs are as follows: blood pressure, unobtainable; pulse, 170 carotid and weak; and respirations, 40 and shallow.

_____

_____

c. A 44-year-old with a sudden onset of dizziness followed by syncope and vital signs as follows: blood pressure, 86/68 mm Hg; pulse, 44; and respirations, 20.

_____

_____

d. An 18-year-old stung by a bee at a park has generalized redness and hives and is acutely short of breath. Vital signs are as follows: blood pressure, 70 mm Hg by palpation; pulse, 132; and respirations, 36.

_____

_____

e. A 53-year-old woman with heavy abdominal bleeding for 1 week became lethargic and confused. Vital signs are as follows: blood pressure, 66 mm Hg by palpation; pulse, 136; and respirations, 32.

_____

_____

f. A 19-year-old sustained a gunshot wound to the chest. Vital signs are as follows: blood pressure, 106/88 mm Hg; pulse, 128; and respirations, 24.

_____

_____

STUDENT SELF-ASSESSMENT

18. Your patient is passing bright red blood through the rectum. What is this called?
  a. Coffee-ground emesis
  b. Epistaxis
  c. Hematochezia
  d. Melena

19. Which of the following is the best definition of shock?
  a. Systolic blood pressure less than 90 mm Hg
  b. Greater than 25% loss of circulating blood
  c. Inadequate perfusion of the capillaries
  d. Blood flow deficit to the myocardium

20. Which of the following is true according to the Fick principle?
  a. Glucose must be available for cellular oxygenation.
  b. Precapillary and postcapillary sphincters must be open for adequate flow.
  c. Red blood cells must be able to load and unload oxygen.
  d. The pH should be at least 6.5 for adequate perfusion to occur.
21. Which of the following blood characteristics is the greatest determinant of afterload (peripheral vascular resistance)?
  a. Vessel diameter
  b. Vessel length
  c. Viscosity
  d. Volume
22. A decrease in peripheral vascular resistance will cause the container size of the body to _____ and the blood pressure to _____.
  a. decrease, decrease
  b. decrease, increase
  c. increase, increase
  d. increase, decrease
23. Which blood vessels act as collecting channels and storage (capacitance) vessels?
  a. Arterioles
  b. Arteries
  c. Capillaries
  d. Venules/veins
24. Which of the following blood cells are responsible for transporting about 99% of the oxygen carried to body tissues?
  a. Erythrocytes
  b. Leukocytes
  c. Plasma proteins
  d. Platelets
25. In what phase of shock does the microcirculation develop the leaky capillary syndrome?
  a. Capillary and venule opening
  b. Disseminated intravascular coagulation
  c. Multiple organ failure
  d. Vasoconstriction
26. What happens to fluid in stage 2 of the progression of shock?
  a. It is pulled into the intravascular space because of vasoconstriction.
  b. It leaks out of the intravascular space because of vasoconstriction.
  c. It is pulled into the intravascular space because of increased hydrostatic pressure.
  d. It leaks out of the intravascular space because of decreased hydrostatic pressure.
27. What occurs when there is dilation of the precapillary sphincter while the postcapillary sphincter remains constricted during lactic acidosis?
  a. No net movement of fluid between the fluid compartments
  b. Loss of vascular fluid into the interstitial spaces
  c. Movement of fluid from the interstitial spaces to the intravascular spaces
  d. Fluid shunting around the capillaries through the arterioles
28. What is shock caused by heart (pump) failure known as?
  a. Anaphylactic shock
  b. Cardiogenic shock
  c. Hypovolemic shock
  d. Neurogenic shock
29. Which of the following shock states does not produce vasodilation?
  a. Anaphylactic
  b. Cardiogenic
  c. Neurogenic
  d. Septic
30. Your patient was stabbed in the abdomen 20 minutes ago. Vital signs are as follows: blood pressure, 80/50 mm Hg; pulse, 136; and respirations, 26. He is anxious and pale. He is probably in which stage of shock?
  a. Compensated
  b. Irreversible
  c. Transitional
  d. Uncompensated
31. Increases in peripheral vascular resistance can be measured indirectly by noting which of the following?
  a. Diastolic blood pressure
  b. Jugular distention
  c. Pulse rate
  d. Systolic blood pressure
32. For which of the following conditions is the pneumatic antishock garment considered helpful?
  a. Cardiogenic shock
  b. Pelvic fractures
  c. Penetrating chest injuries
  d. Pulmonary edema
33. Which of the following fluids is a colloid solution?
  a. Dextran
  b. 0.45% sodium chloride
  c. Lactated Ringer's solution
  d. Normal saline

34. Which of the following blood products has the greatest oxygen-carrying capacity per volume?
    a. Fibrinogen
    b. Packed red blood cells
    c. Plasma
    d. Whole blood

35. You arrive at the emergency department with a patient who has been vomiting bright red blood and is exhibiting signs and symptoms of shock. Which fluid is most beneficial to him at this time?
    a. Blood plasma
    b. Dextran
    c. Packed red blood cells
    d. Plasmanate

36. Your patient has fallen 30 feet from scaffolding and is anxious, confused, and in obvious shock. Which of the following is your priority of care, in the proper order?
    a. Rapid transport, oxygen, intravenous therapy
    b. Oxygen, intravenous therapy, rapid transport
    c. Intravenous therapy, rapid transport, oxygen
    d. Oxygen, rapid transport, intravenous therapy

37. In the absence of spinal or head injury, in what position should the hypovolemic patient in shock be placed?
    a. Lateral recumbent
    b. Modified Trendelenberg's
    c. Supine hypotension
    d. Trendelenberg's

38. Which of the following is not an appropriate initial prehospital management technique for the patient in hypovolemic shock?
    a. Crystalloid fluid replacement
    b. External hemorrhage control
    c. Pneumatic antishock garment
    d. Treatment with dopamine

39. Fluid therapy in cardiogenic shock should be slowed to the keep-open rate in which of the following cases?
    a. If lung crackles (rales) increase.
    b. If jugular vein distention decreases.
    c. If heart rate decreases.
    d. If peripheral edema increases.

40. Which of the following is the treatment of choice for the patient in severe anaphylactic shock?
    a. Antihistamines
    b. Epinephrine
    c. Fluid challenge
    d. Pneumatic antishock garments

41. You suspect that your patient has a ruptured ectopic pregnancy. She is in profound shock. Which intravenous catheter will you select?
    a. 14 gauge, 1½ inch
    b. 14 gauge, 3 inch
    c. 18 gauge, 1½ inch
    d. 18 gauge, 3 inch

42. A 200-mL fluid challenge is to be infused over 20 minutes. The drop factor is 10 drops/mL. How fast will you run it?
    a. 1 drop/min
    b. 33 drops/min
    c. 100 drops/min
    d. 400 drops/min

43. Which of the following is not a goal of prehospital care for the patient with severe hemorrhage and shock?
    a. Definitive care for internal hemorrhage
    b. Initiation of treatment
    c. Rapid recognition of the event
    d. Rapid transport to the appropriate hospital

WRAP IT UP

You are dispatched to a construction site for a fall. When you arrive, you are directed to the rear of an apartment building under construction. A 35-year-old worker has fallen about 30 feet onto a pile of dirt and rock. She is conscious but confused and is bleeding from a large head laceration. You immediately apply direct pressure to the laceration with a 5 × 9 inch dressing as you hold in-line immobilization of her head and continue your assessment. Her airway is patent, breathing is rapid, skin is pale and cool, and heart rate is rapid. The bleeding from her head laceration appears to have been controlled from direct pressure, so your partner wraps it with a gauze roller bandage as you continue your assessments. Her trachea is midline, neck veins are flat, and breath sounds are clear and equal bilaterally. A large reddened area begins on her lateral chest and extends down across her upper abdomen. There is tenderness to palpation over the left lateral ribs and diffuse tenderness over her abdomen. Both lower legs are swollen, tender, and deformed, with weak pedal pulses noted. She is rolled onto the backboard with spinal precautions and support of her legs and is moved to the ambulance. Vital signs are BP 84/66 mm Hg, P 136, R 28, SaO_2 not obtainable. Oxygen is delivered by non-rebreather mask at 15 L/min, transport is initiated, and the trauma center is notified that you are en route with an unstable patient who has fallen. En route to the hospital, an IV of normal saline is initiated in the left antecubital space and administered wide open; ECG monitoring is performed, and serial blood pressures obtained by an automatic BP cuff show a slight improvement in blood pressure, although her heart rate does not come down. Her head bandage is reinforced when blood soaks through the first one. The trauma team is awaiting you in the resuscitation room. Immediately, cross-table cervical spine, and chest radiographs are performed. Uncrossmatched blood is transfused, and as the patient's condition rapidly deteriorates, she is rushed to the surgical suite where her severely injured spleen is removed.

1. Were this patient's signs and symptoms of shock a result of external or internal hemorrhage? Explain your answer.

_____

2. Which of the following factors needed for adequate tissue perfusion was impaired in this patient?
   a. Adequate oxygen must be available in the lungs.
   b. Oxygen must be able to move freely across the alveolar walls.
   c. Normal hemoglobin levels must exist to carry oxygen.
   d. Tissue cells must close to capillaries so oxygen can off-load.
3. Circle the appropriate answer. The pale color of the patient's skin reflected a narrowing/widening of the blood vessels, which would cause a(n) decrease/increase in cardiac preload.
4. Which blood component most urgently needs replacement in this patient?
   a. Erythrocytes
   b. Fibrinogen
   c. Leukocytes
   d. Plasma
5. Your initial assessment of this patient reveals that she is in what stage of shock?
   a. Compensated
   b. Irreversible
   c. Multiple organ dysfunction syndrome
   d. Uncompensated
6. What sites (injuries) were possible causes for her shock?

_____

7. Pick the compensatory responses in shock that would be responsible for the following signs or symptoms present in this patient.
   a. Sympathetic response   b. Hormonal response   c. Adrenal response

Sign or Symptom	Compensatory Mechanism
Narrowed pulse pressure	
Pale, cool skin	
Tachycardia	

8. Which of the following represents definitive care for this patient?
   a. Isotonic fluid administration
   b. High-concentration oxygen delivery
   c. Surgical intervention
   d. Uncrossmatched blood transfusion

CHAPTER 21 ANSWERS

REVIEW QUESTIONS

1. b
(Objective 5)

2. g
(Objective 5)

3. e
(Objective 5)

4. a
(Objective 5)

5. d
(Objective 5)

6. f
(Objective 5)

7. a. An adequate amount of oxygen is available to red blood cells. There is a sufficient F_{IO_2}, his airway is patent, and his lungs are clear.
b. Red blood cells must be circulated to all tissue cells. Based on the history of significant blood loss and the physical findings that indicate decreased cerebral perfusion (anxiety and confusion) and peripheral perfusion (pale, cyanotic lips and nail beds), it is evident that red blood cell transport is inadequate.
c. Red blood cells must be able to off-load oxygen adequately. This seems to be occurring in this situation, although acid-base abnormalities can impair this ability, and insufficient information is available to determine this accurately.
(Objective 3)

8. All blood vessels larger than capillaries are surrounded by layers of connective tissue that counter the pressure of blood in the vascular system, have elastic properties to dampen pressure pulsations and minimize flow variations throughout the cardiac cycle, and contain muscle fibers to control vessel diameter.
(Objective 4)

9. a. systemic; b. systolic; c. diastolic; d. pulse; e. heart (or aorta); f. vena cava
(Objective 4)

10. a. Spinal cord injury results in a loss of sympathetic tone and therefore impairs the ability of the blood vessels to constrict below the level of the injury. This increases the container size, decreasing the effective circulating volume and preload.
b. When blood loss occurs, a situation potentially exists in which the container is the same size but the volume has decreased, reducing the preload. Body compensatory mechanisms attempt to decrease the size of the container by vasoconstriction in an effort to match the container to the volume.
(Objective 4)

11.

Intravenous Fluid	Isotonic, Hypotonic, or Hypertonic	Fluid Movement
D50W	Hypertonic	Into intravascular space
Lactated Ringer's	Isotonic	No net movement
Normal saline	Isotonic	No net movement
0.45% normal saline	Hypotonic	Out of intravascular space
D_5W	Isotonic initially but rapidly hypotonic because of glucose metabolism	Out of intravascular space

(Objective 10)

12. a. Oxygen to cells in vasoconstricted areas decreases. Anaerobic metabolism occurs. Leaky capillary syndrome evolves. Pale, sweaty skin; rapid, thready pulse; elevation in blood glucose; and dilation of coronary, cerebral, and skeletal muscle arterioles occur.

b. Precapillary sphincters open. Blood pools and vascular space is expanded greatly, resulting in increased container size. Decreased preload and congestion of the viscera occur. Increased anaerobic metabolism results in increased respiratory rate. Rouleaux formation inhibits perfusion in visceral capillaries and impedes flow. Hypercoagulability develops.

c. Blood coagulates in microcirculation, clogging capillaries and causing congestion; fibrinolytic mechanisms then are overstimulated, causing pulmonary edema and hemorrhage. Cell membrane function is lost, and anaerobic metabolism increases. Water and sodium leak into cells and potassium leaks out. Cells swell and die. Oxygen absorption and carbon dioxide elimination are impaired in the lungs, and acute respiratory distress syndrome may result.

d. After 1 to 2 hours a dramatic decrease in blood pressure occurs. Cellular metabolism stops. Organ failure occurs and may include liver, kidney, and heart failure; gastrointestinal bleeding; pancreatitis; and pulmonary thrombosis.

(Objective 6)

13. a. Cardiogenic shock: Administer high-flow oxygen, continue assessment, initiate intravenous normal saline to keep the vein open, consider a fluid challenge of 100 to 200 mL of lactated Ringer's solution or normal saline, monitor lung sounds and patient response carefully, and consider vasopressor drug therapy.

b. Neurogenic shock: Apply cervical spine immobilization, assess the need to assist ventilations, administer high-flow oxygen, initiate intravenous lactated Ringer's solution or normal saline (avoiding excessive amounts), monitor lung sounds frequently, apply and inflate pneumatic antishock garments if local protocol advises, continue assessment, and consider vasopressor drug therapy.

c. Hypovolemic shock: Administer high-flow oxygen, place patient in modified Trendelenberg's position, transport rapidly, initiate two large-bore (14- or 16-gauge) intravenous lines with lactated Ringer's solution or normal saline and infuse rapidly, apply pneumatic antishock garment if local protocol advises, and prepare to inflate it if patient's condition deteriorates.

d. Anaphylactic shock: Ensure a patent airway, administer high-flow oxygen (administer subcutaneous epinephrine), initiate intravenous lactated Ringer's solution or normal saline with a 14- or 16-gauge catheter, consider administration of diphenhydramine (Benadryl).

e. Septic shock: Administer high-flow oxygen, determine whether the patient has preexisting obstructive pulmonary disease, initiate intravenous therapy with a 14- or 16-gauge catheter, and obtain an accurate patient history.

f. Cardiogenic shock: Assess for a patent airway, administer high-flow oxygen, initiate a 16- or 18-gauge intravenous line with normal saline to keep the vein open, institute electrocardiographic monitoring, initiate maneuvers to decrease heart rate based on the electrocardiographic tracing and patient symptoms (drugs, cardioversion), and apply dressing to head wound.

(Objectives 7 and 10)

14. a. Uncompensated shock: The compensatory mechanisms can no longer sustain a normal systolic blood pressure. The pulse pressure is narrowed. Blood oxygenation is decreased as evidenced by cyanosis.

b. Compensated shock: Systolic blood pressure is adequate, but other signs of shock are evident (cool, pale skin and increased pulse and respiratory rate).

(Objective 8)

15. Irreversible shock may occur suddenly or 1 to 3 weeks after the event. Clinical signs include bradycardia; pale, cold, clammy skin; and cardiac arrest.
(Objective 8)

16. Preexisting disease, medication, older or young age
(Objective 8)

17. a. Drug therapy: Neither pneumatic antishock garments nor rapid fluid infusion is considered because this patient is already in heart failure. Therapy should be directed at improving the function of the heart with drugs.
b. Pediatric pneumatic antishock garments (if indicated by local medical direction), rapid fluid replacement, blood transfusions, and intraosseous infusion: The patient has a mechanism of injury for significant blood loss and is exhibiting signs of uncompensated shock. Pneumatic antishock garments may decrease the container size and maximize flow to the vital organs. Rapid fluid infusion may restore circulating volume. Blood transfusion may be necessary on arrival to emergency department to enhance oxygen-carrying capability and restore the vascular volume. Rapid peripheral intravenous therapy may be impossible in this situation, making intraosseous infusion the vascular access method of choice. Rapid transport is essential.
c. Drug therapy: The heart rate is slow and is likely the reason why this person is exhibiting signs of shock. None of the other interventions increases heart rate.
d. Drug therapy and rapid fluid replacement: The primary cause of the shock state in this patient is probably histamine release. Drug therapy is the only intervention that can arrest and reverse these symptoms. Rapid fluid replacement also may help restore circulating volume until drug therapy is effective.
e. Pneumatic antishock garments, rapid fluid replacement, and blood transfusions: The primary cause of the shock symptoms according to the patient history is loss of blood. Rapid fluid replacement can restore circulating volume. At the emergency department the blood transfusion helps restore oxygen-carrying capacity and circulating volume.
f. Rapid fluid replacement if indicated by local medical direction: At this time the patient is maintaining a normal blood pressure. The pulse and respiratory rate are elevated somewhat, so as assessment continues, the effects of a rapid fluid bolus can be monitored to determine whether the patient has lost a significant amount of blood. Other interventions may be necessary if the patient's condition deteriorates.
(Objective 10)

18. c. Coffee-ground emesis indicates gastrointestinal bleeding. Epistaxis is bleeding from the nose. Melena is dark, black, tarry stools.
(Objective 1)

19. c. A systolic blood pressure less than 90 mm Hg may be normal in certain individuals. Loss of blood volume may lead to shock but does not define it. Shock leads to decreased myocardial blood flow.
(Objective 2)

20. c. The Fick principle states that adequate oxygen must be available to red blood cells through the alveolar cells of the lungs. So that hemoglobin can be oxygenated, red blood cells must be circulated to the tissue cells, and red blood cells must be able to load oxygen at the lungs and unload oxygen at the peripheral cells.
(Objective 3)

21. a. Vessel length and viscosity are relatively constant. Blood volume may influence pressure but not resistance.
(Objective 4)

22. d. As peripheral vascular resistance decreases, vessel capacitance increases and the container size increases. This makes the existing blood volume insufficient to maintain an adequate preload.
(Objective 4)

23. d
(Objective 4)

24. a
(Objective 5)

25. d. Leaky capillary syndrome develops after lactate and hydrogen ions build up in the capillaries and their linings lose their ability to retain large molecular structures within their walls.
(Objective 6)

26. b. This fluid loss is caused by the increased hydrostatic pressure created in this situation.
(Objective 6)

27. b. The precapillary sphincter opens, whereas the postcapillary sphincter remains closed, increasing the pressure inside the capillary and forcing fluid out through the already compromised capillary walls.
(Objective 6)

28. b. Anaphylactic shock is caused by the release of chemicals after an antigen-antibody reaction. Hypovolemic shock results from a loss of body fluid (water, plasma, blood). Neurogenic shock is a loss of vasomotor tone.
(Objective 7)

29. b. Loss of vasomotor tone is a contributing factor to shock in each of the other types of shock.
(Objective 9)

30. d. The compensatory mechanisms of vasoconstriction, increased heart rate, and increased contractility are no longer sufficient to maintain adequate blood pressure.
(Objective 8)

31. a. As peripheral vascular resistance increases, diastolic blood pressure also increases.
(Objective 8)

32. b. Use of pneumatic antishock garments generally is not recommended for any of the other situations.
(Objective 10)

33. a. All the others are crystalloid solutions.
(Objective 10)

34. b. Whole blood and packed red blood cells have red cells and therefore the greatest ability to carry oxygen. Packed cells do not contain plasma and therefore have a greater concentration of red blood cells per unit volume. Only a small amount of oxygen is carried dissolved in plasma.
(Objective 10)

35. c. This is the only fluid that contains red blood cells.
(Objective 10)

36. d. Priorities of care always follow the ABCs; therefore oxygen should be first and intravenous therapy should be initiated en route unless a transportation delay exists; in this case, definitive care may be expedited.
(Objective 10)

37. b. This position permits better perfusion without compromising respiratory status.
(Objective 10)

38. d. Vasoactive drugs are not indicated for use in the patient with hypovolemic shock until adequate fluid volume has been replaced at the hospital. Pneumatic antishock garments occasionally may be used to treat hypovolemic shock associated with pelvic fractures.
(Objective 10)

39. a. Increased lung congestion indicates that the failing heart cannot deal with the existing fluid volume. Jugular venous distention should increase with fluid overload. Peripheral edema has a slow onset and is not an acute sign evident in the prehospital phase of care. A moderate decrease in heart rate indicates patient improvement. (Objective 10)

40. b. Epinephrine is the only treatment that rapidly improves all the life-threatening effects of anaphylaxis. Other adjunct therapy may be used after epinephrine has been given. (Objective 10)

41. a. The shortest catheter with the widest diameter should be selected. (Objective 10)

42. c. Drops/minute $= \dfrac{200 \times 10}{20} = 100$ (Objective 10)

43. a. Control of internal hemorrhage often requires surgical intervention or other definitive care measures available only in the hospital. (Objective 11)

WRAP IT UP

1. This patient had internal bleeding and external bleeding. The internal bleeding was most likely responsible for her shock. (Objective 1)

2. c. Most of the oxygen in the body is carried on hemoglobin. This patient's blood loss has caused a decrease in hemoglobin. (Objective 2)

3. The blood vessels narrow in an attempt to increase the preload. (Objective 4)

4. a. The red blood cells contain hemoglobin, which carry oxygen and are critical for normal tissue oxygenation. (Objective 5)

5. d. Because the blood pressure has decreased, the patient is no longer compensating adequately for the shock. (Objective 6)

6. Bleeding from head, concealed intraabdominal bleeding, or long bone fractures of lower legs (Objective 7)

7. Narrow pulse pressure: a, b, c
Pale, cool, skin: a, b, c
Tachycardia: a, b, c
(Objective 8)

8. c. If the patient had uncontrolled bleeding from the spleen, the only definitive intervention would be surgical. Prehospital care includes oxygenation, monitoring, fluid replacement, and transport to the closest appropriate hospital (trauma center preferred). (Objective 10)

CHAPTER
22

Soft Tissue Trauma

READING ASSIGNMENT
Chapter 22, pages 538-557, in *Mosby's Paramedic Textbook,* ed. 3

OBJECTIVES
Upon completion of this chapter, the paramedic student will be able to:
1. Describe the normal structure and function of the skin.
2. Describe the pathophysiological responses to soft tissue injury.
3. Discuss pathophysiology as a basis for key signs and symptoms, and describe the mechanism of injury and signs and symptoms of specific soft tissue injuries.
4. Outline management principles for prehospital care of soft tissue injuries.
5. Describe, in the correct sequence, patient management techniques for control of hemorrhage.
6. Identify the characteristics of general categories of dressings and bandages.
7. Describe prehospital management of specific soft tissue injuries not requiring closure.
8. Discuss factors that increase the potential for wound infection.
9. Describe the prehospital management of selected soft tissue injuries.

SUMMARY
- The skin and its accessory organs are the main cosmetic structures of the body. These structures perform many functions that are critical to survival. The skin is composed of two distinct layers of tissue: the outer layer (epidermis) and the inner layer (dermis).
- Surface trauma can disrupt the normal distribution of body fluids and electrolytes. Surface trauma also can interfere with the maintenance of body temperature. The two physiological responses to surface trauma are vascular and inflammatory reactions. These can lead to healing, scar formation, or both. Many factors can affect or alter wound healing.
- Soft tissue injuries are classified as closed or open. Classification is determined by the absence or presence of a break in the continuity of the epidermis. Closed wounds include contusions, hematoma, and crush injury. Open wounds are classified as abrasions, lacerations, punctures, avulsions, amputations, and bites.
- Assessment of life-threatening injuries and resuscitation precedes evaluation and intervention of non–life-threatening soft tissue injuries. General wound assessment should include a history of the event that caused the wound and a careful examination of the injury.
- Methods of hemorrhage control include direct pressure, elevation, pressure point, immobilization by splinting, and pneumatic pressure devices.
- The general categories of dressings used in trauma care are sterile, nonsterile, occlusive, nonocclusive, adherent, and nonadherent. The general categories of bandages are absorbent, nonabsorbent, adherent, and nonadherent.
- Depending on the nature and location of the patient's injury, dressings, bandages, and immobilization may be indicated to care for a wound properly.

- The goals of wound care are to prevent infection and protect from infection. Factors that influence the likelihood of infection include unclean wounds and wound mechanisms and a patient's poor state of health.
- Special considerations for specific wounds include penetrating chest or abdominal injury, avulsion, amputation, and crush syndrome.

REVIEW QUESTIONS

Match the type of dressing listed in Column II with its description in Column I. Use each answer only once.

Column I	Column II
1. _____ Air does not pass through this dressing.	a. Adherent dressing
2. _____ Bacteria have been eliminated from this dressing.	b. Nonadherent
3. _____ This dressing can be used when infection is not a concern.	c. Nonocclusive dressing
4. _____ This dressing sticks to the wound surface.	d. Nonsterile dressing
5. _____ This dressing allows air to pass through to the wound.	e. Occlusive dressing
6. _____ This dressing does not stick to the wound.	f. Sterile dressing

7. List at least six structures or tissues located in the dermis.

   a.

   b.

   c.

   d.

   e.

   f.

8. Identify at least three functions of the integumentary system.

   a.

   b.

   c.

9. Identify the three crucial steps in the clotting mechanism.

   a.

   b.

   c.

10. Why are redness, swelling, warmth, and pain found at the site of an inflammatory response?

   _____

   _____

11. List six types of drugs that can impair normal wound healing.

   a.

   b.

   c.

   d.

   e.

   f.

12. List six types of wounds that are likely to require closure.

a.

b.

c.

d.

e.

f.

13. For each of the following scenarios, list the soft tissue injury described and key prehospital interventions to manage the trauma.

a. A 45-year-old woman is being transported for care after her husband repeatedly struck her head and face with his fist. You note numerous swollen, ecchymotic areas on the face and head.
Injury:
Interventions:

_____

_____

b. Rescuers have just removed a victim who had been trapped in a concrete structure for 2 days. The patient's lower torso had been pinned under a concrete piling. During the rescue phase, the patient was alert but somewhat confused. Vital signs were within normal limits. Shortly after extrication the patient's physiological status begins to deteriorate.
Injury:
Interventions:

_____

_____

c. A wallpaper hanger has sustained a deep linear wound after cutting himself with an Exacto knife. The wound is oozing dark red blood, and fatty tissue is visible at the edges of the injury.
Injury:
Interventions:

_____

_____

d. A motorcyclist wearing only her swimsuit had to lay the bike down to avoid a collision. The patient states that the bike slid about 100 feet along the asphalt road. She has huge scrape-type injuries on her entire left side. She denies pain or tenderness anywhere else.
Injury:
Interventions:

_____

_____

e. Neighbors direct you to a yard where a young child has been attacked by a large dog. No one is sure of the dog's present location. The child is screaming, and his left arm has many puncture wounds and lacerations.

Injury:

Interventions:

_____

_____

f. A hunter has been impaled with an arrow. The arrow has penetrated the right upper quadrant of the abdomen. She is pale and cool.

Injury:

Interventions:

_____

_____

g. A mechanic reports an injury to her right hand while working with a high-pressure grease gun. You note a small puncture wound with a drop of grease on it at the distal end of the left thumb.

Injury:

Interventions:

_____

_____

h. A butcher slices off the distal tip of his index finger.

Injury:

Interventions:

_____

_____

i. A factory employee catches his hair in some large machinery and avulses a large portion of the posterior aspect of his scalp.

Injury:

Interventions:

_____

_____

j. A weekend handyman severs his right index finger with a skill saw. He drives himself to a nearby firehouse but does not have the digit with him.

Injury:

Interventions:

_____

_____

Questions 14 and 15 pertain to the following case study:

> Your patient was treated and released from the emergency department with a diagnosis of tibial fracture after a fall. He has a plaster splint that was applied there and is complaining of pain so severe, "I just can't take it anymore."

14. What further assessments should you perform on this patient's leg to look for compartment syndrome?

_____

15. If he has compartment syndrome, what could a delay in treatment cause?

_____

Questions 16 and 17 pertain to the following case study:

    You are called to the scene of a construction site, where a 57-year-old workman has lacerated his left hand.

16. What questions should you ask to obtain the wound history on this patient?

_____

_____

17. Outline the physical examination of the wound and hand.

_____

_____

18. You are called to a rural farm, where a 17-year-old has sustained a partial amputation of his left lower arm after tangling it in a corn picker. There is extensive soft tissue damage and deformity of the extremity, which is squirting bright red blood. Your estimated time of arrival to the nearest hospital is 30 minutes. Describe in the proper sequence six measures you can use to control the bleeding in this patient and briefly describe the proper technique for using each skill.

    a. _____

_____

    b. _____

_____

    c. _____

_____

    d. _____

_____

    e. _____

_____

    f. _____

_____

    For questions 19 to 23, circle (a) or (b) to indicate the wound that is at _greater risk_ for infection. Explain why you chose your answer in (c).

19. a. A farmer lacerates his hand on a combine.
    b. A chef cuts his hand on a butcher knife.
    c.

20. a. A 25-year-old athlete is stabbed.
    b. A 79-year-old nursing home resident is stabbed.
    c.

21. a. The patient cut his abdomen.
    b. The patient's laceration is on his hand.
    c.

22. a. Your patient reports to the emergency department for sutures 18 hours after the injury.
    b. The patient drives to the emergency department 2 hours after injury.
    c.

23. a. His finger was split open after he jammed it in a door.
    b. He sliced his finger on a piece of metal on the door.
    c.

STUDENT SELF-ASSESSMENT

24. What is the avascular layer of the skin called?
    a. Dermis   **c.** Sebaceous
    b. Epidermis   **d.** Subcutaneous tissue

25. Which of the following does *not* play a role in normal hemostasis?
    a. Activation of platelets   **c.** Thrombin formation
    b. Aldosterone synthesis   **d.** Vasoconstriction

26. Which medications can interfere with hemostasis?
    a. Acetaminophen   **c.** Decongestants
    b. Aspirin   **d.** Insulin

27. Which of the following medical conditions is associated with delayed healing?
    a. Alcoholism   **c.** Cardiac dysrhythmias
    b. Asthma   **d.** Stroke

28. Which of the following wound forces is least likely to be associated with a high risk for infection?
    a. Foreign bodies   **c.** Injection injuries
    b. Human and animal bites   **d.** Paring knife wounds

29. Which of the following is considered a closed injury?
    a. Avulsion   **c.** Hematoma
    b. Bite   **d.** Puncture

30. High-pressure injection injuries can be limb-threatening. Why is the severity of this wound difficult to assess in the prehospital environment?
    a. The light is too poor to evaluate the wound adequately.
    b. The location of the wound is difficult to visualize.
    c. The equipment needed for assessment is not available.
    d. The wound is small with minimal external signs.

31. What is the appropriate prehospital care for avulsed body tissue?
    a. Placing it directly on ice
    b. Sealing it in a plastic bag
    c. Soaking it in a cup of lactated Ringer's solution
    d. Débriding it of all dirt

32. Which type of soft tissue injury may result in abscesses, lymphangitis, cellulitis, osteomyelitis, tenosynovitis, tuberculosis, hepatitis B, and tetanus?
    a. Amputation   **c.** Bites
    b. Avulsion   **d.** Crush injury

33. Which of the following is an early finding in crush injury?
    a. Paralysis   **c.** Paresthesia
    b. Paresis   **d.** Pulselessness

34. Where is compartment syndrome most likely to be found?
    a. Abdomen   **c.** Head
    b. Upper arm   **d.** Thorax

35. What causes life-threatening symptoms in patients with crush syndrome after being released from entrapment?
   a. Circulatory overload when blood rushes back to the central circulation
   b. Hypokalemia, hypouricemia, hypercalcemia, and hypophosphatemia
   c. Myoglobin is released and filtered through the liver, causing liver failure.
   d. Toxic substances from anaerobic metabolism are released into the blood.

36. Blast injuries can cause rupture in air-filled organs such as which of the following?
   a. Bladder
   b. Heart
   c. Lungs
   d. Pancreas

37. Which wound is least likely to require physician evaluation if tetanus immunization is up to date?
   a. A needle fragment imbedded in the wound.
   b. Weakness in the finger distal to the laceration.
   c. Laceration extending over the border of the lip.
   d. A painful abrasion on the leg that is oozing slightly.

38. Who would *not* be a candidate for tetanus toxoid if the person reports not having had a booster in more than 10 years?
   a. A patient who takes insulin for diabetes
   b. A patient whose baby is due in 3 weeks
   c. A patient whose arm was sore the last time he had one
   d. A patient whose home medicines include digoxin (Lanoxin)

WRAP IT UP

You are dispatched to a ranger's cabin deep in a rugged national park for "traumatic injuries." A 20-year-old climber initially injured when he fell about 12 feet, sliding down a steep rock face a day ago, lost his way, was bitten by a wild dog, and then cut his forearm in a desperate attempt to enter the cabin when there was no response to his initial knocks at the door. He has numerous swollen, painful blunt injuries because of small collections of blood under the skin; several puncture wounds to the left forearm from the bite around which the skin is now tender, red, warm, and swollen; several areas on his hands, arms, and legs where the skin was scraped off and is oozing clear liquid; and a deep wound on the right forearm from the glass injury that is bleeding freely and in which fatty tissue is visible. You easily control the bleeding and complete your assessment of this patient, finding no additional injuries, and assess his vital signs, which are BP 126/72 mm Hg, P 98, R 16, SaO$_2$ 98%. You transport him to the local hospital where he is treated and released 8 hours later.

1. Which of the skin layers were injured?

_____

2. What signs and symptoms of inflammation are present from his wounds?

_____

3. Place a check mark beside the soft tissue injuries present in this patient.
   a. _____ Closed wounds
   b. _____ Contusions
   c. _____ Crush injury
   d. _____ Open wounds
   e. _____ Abrasion
   f. _____ Laceration
   g. _____ Puncture
   h. _____ Avulsion
   i. _____ Amputation
   j. _____ Bites

4. Describe appropriate steps in management of this patient's bleeding.

_____

5. How will you treat his other wounds? _____

6. What risk factors are present in this patient for the development of infection?

_____

CHAPTER 22 ANSWERS

REVIEW QUESTIONS

1. e
(Objective 6)

2. f
(Objective 6)

3. d
(Objective 6)

4. a
(Objective 6)

5. c
(Objective 6)

6. b
(Objective 6)

7. Connective tissue, elastic fibers, blood vessels, lymphatic vessels, motor and sensory fibers, hair, nails, and glands
(Objective 1)

8. Protection and cushioning against injury, barrier against infection, temperature regulation, and preservation of body fluids
(Objective 1)

9. a. Release of platelet factors at injury site
   b. Formation of thrombin
   c. Trapping of red blood cells in fibrin to form a clot
(Objective 2)

10. The warmth and redness are caused by vasodilation and enhanced blood supply to the affected area. Swelling is caused by increased capillary permeability, which allows plasma, plasma proteins, and electrolytes to leak into extracellular space. Pain is caused by chemicals and increased pressure resulting from fluid buildup.
(Objective 2)

11. a. Corticosteroids; b. nonsteroidal antiinflammatory drugs; c. penicillin; d. colchicine; e. anticoagulants; f. antineoplastic agents
(Objective 2)

12. a. Wounds to cosmetic regions; b. gaping wounds; c. wounds over tension areas; d. degloving injuries; e. ring finger injuries; f. skin tearing
(Objective 2)

13. a. Contusion or hematoma: Apply ice or cold packs and compression with manual pressure or compression bandage. Assess for underlying injury.
   b. Crush syndrome: Provide airway and ventilation support, administer high-flow oxygen, maintain body temperature, rehydrate with expanding intravenous fluids (1 to 1.5 L initial bolus), and administer pharmacological agents such as sodium bicarbonate (to help control hyperkalemia and acidosis), glucose and insulin (to decrease serum potassium), and mannitol (to promote diuresis).

c. Laceration: Control hemorrhage and monitor for signs of hypovolemic shock.

d. Abrasions: Clean gross contaminants from injured surface and lightly cover with sterile dressing.

e. Dog bite: Ensure that animal is contained, control bleeding, rinse off gross contaminants, splint extremity, and obtain a medical history from the pet owner.

f. Penetrating or impaled object: Leave object in place, do not manipulate object unless it is necessary for patient extrication or transport, control bleeding with direct pressure around the impaling object, stabilize the object with bulky dressings, and immobilize the patient. Treat shock if present.

g. Puncture wound: Evaluate wound, elevate affected extremity, immobilize, and transport.

h. Avulsion: Control bleeding, retrieve the avulsed tissue, wrap tissue in gauze that is dry or moistened with lactated Ringer's or saline solution (per local protocol), seal in plastic bag, and place sealed bag on crushed ice.

i. Degloving: Control bleeding, evaluate for hypovolemia, elevate head of stretcher after you rule out mechanism for cervical spine injury.

j. Amputation: Control bleeding, retrieve amputated tissue, and treat as for avulsion.

(Objectives 3 and 9)

14. Assess for pain, paresis, paresthesia, pallor, and pulselessness in the affected extremity. Determine whether there is swelling or tightness of the compartment, tenderness to palpation, weakness in the leg, or pain on passive stretch (early sign).
(Objective 3)

15. A delay in treatment of compartment syndrome can cause nerve death, muscle necrosis, and crush syndrome.
(Objective 3)

16. When did you cut yourself? Was it a dirty place where you got the cut? How did the injury happen? Does anything else hurt? How much blood did you lose? Rate your pain on a scale of 1 to 10 with 1 being no pain and 10 the worst pain you have ever had. Do you take any medicines? Do you have any major illnesses? When was your last tetanus shot?
(Objective 4)

17. Inspect the wound for bleeding, size, depth, presence of foreign bodies, amount of tissue lost, edema, and deformity. Inspect the surrounding area for damage to arteries, nerves, tendons, and muscle. Assess the sensory and motor function of his hand. Evaluate the perfusion of the wound and of the tissues of the hand distal to the wound. Assess capillary refill, distal pulse, tenderness, temperature, edema, and crepitus (if underlying bone injury is suspected).
(Objective 4)

18. a. Apply direct pressure to the wound with a gloved hand or handheld dressing (4 to 6 minutes), and then secure a pressure dressing firmly if bleeding is controlled.

b. Elevate the affected area above the level of the heart.

c. Apply pressure point control if other measures have failed. Select the appropriate pressure point proximal to the wound and compress the artery against the underlying bone for at least 10 minutes.

d. Immobilize by splinting. (Immobilization is used as an adjunct to other control devices.) Select the appropriate splint for the body area and apply it to minimize blood flow.

e. Use pneumatic pressure devices. (Devices such as air splints or pneumatic antishock garments serve as adjuncts for pressure control after the bleeding is controlled by other methods.)

f. Use a tourniquet only when other methods are unsuccessful in controlling bleeding and when preservation of life is selected over preservation of the limb. Notify medical control and select a site 2 inches proximal to the wound over the brachial or femoral artery. Place a tourniquet over the artery and a pad over the artery to be compressed. Wind tourniquet twice around the extremity and tie it in a half knot over the pad. Place a windlass on the half knot and secure it with a square knot. Tighten the windlass until the hemorrhage stops and secure it. Note the time of application and mark "TK" on the patient's forehead and notify the receiving hospital.
(Objective 5)

19. a. This wound is likely much more contaminated than one that occurred in a clean indoor setting.
(Objective 8)

20. b. The risk of infection increases in older patients and in those who have preexisting medical conditions.
(Objective 8)

21. b. Injuries of the hand, foot, lower extremity, scalp, and face have a higher than normal risk of infection.
(Objective 8)

22. a. The risk of infection is greater in wounds that are not cleaned and repaired for longer than 8 to 12 hours after the injury.
(Objective 8)

23. a. Injuries associated with a crushing mechanism are more susceptible to infection than those caused by fine cutting forces.
(Objective 8)

24. b. The dermis provides the vascular supply to the epidermis. The sebaceous glands are in the dermis. The subcutaneous tissue lies under the dermis.
(Objective 1)

25. b. Aldosterone aids in body fluid regulation.
(Objective 2)

26. b. Aspirin decreases platelet activity.
(Objective 2)

27. a. Other conditions associated with impaired healing are advanced age, uremia, diabetes, hypoxia, peripheral vascular disease, malnutrition, advanced cancer, hepatic failure, and cardiovascular disease.
(Objective 2)

28. d. A knife wound would be considered high risk if it were contaminated with organic material or if the patient were immunocompromised or had poor circulation.
(Objective 2)

29. c. All the others are open wounds.
(Objective 3)

30. d. The wound site may only have minimal bleeding, numbness, and blanching. Surgical intervention is often necessary.
(Objective 3)

31. b. All other interventions could cause further damage.
(Objective 9)

32. c. Bites may be a combination of puncture, laceration, avulsion, and crush injuries heavily laden with infectious organisms.
(Objective 3)

33. c. All others are late findings.
(Objective 3)

34. b. The most common sites are below the knee and above the elbow.
(Objective 3)

35. d. Blood pools in the injured extremity, causing hypovolemia. Elevated blood potassium, phosphate and uric acid levels, and low blood calcium levels occur. Myoglobin is filtered in the kidneys, resulting in acute renal failure.
(Objective 3)

36. c. Other air-filled structures that may be affected are the eardrum, sinuses, stomach, and intestines.
(Objective 3)

37. d. All the other injuries have a high potential for impaired wound healing or infection if not treated by a physician.
(Objective 7)

38. b. Tetanus toxoid should not be given to pregnant patients or children younger than 6 weeks.
(Objective 7)

WRAP IT UP

1. Epidermis and dermis (puncture wounds may be deeper)
(Objective 1)

2. Pain, warmth, redness, swelling
(Objective 2)

3. Closed wounds, contusions, crush injury is possible (from dog bite), open wounds, abrasions, lacerations, punctures (bites), bites
(Objective 3)

4. Direct pressure may be all that is necessary to control bleeding. If not, elevation of the extremity and reinforcement of the bandage may be helpful. For severe and persistent bleeding, arterial pressure point control, and when life is threatened, a tourniquet may be applied.
(Objective 5)

5. The wounds should be cleansed of gross decontamination. If transport time will be prolonged, wounds may be covered with nonadherent dressings to prevent further contamination.
(Objectives 7 and 9)

6. Wounds were sustained in a dirty environment; bite wounds are highly susceptible to infection; no wound care was provided for a prolonged period of time.
(Objective 8)

Burns

READING ASSIGNMENT
Chapter 23, pages 558-579, in *Mosby's Paramedic Textbook*, ed. 3

OBJECTIVES
Upon completion of this chapter, the paramedic student will be able to:
1. Describe the incidence, patterns, and sources of burn injury.
2. Describe the pathophysiology of local and systemic responses to burn injury.
3. Classify burn injury according to depth, extent, and severity based on established standards.
4. Discuss the pathophysiology of burn shock as a basis for key signs and symptoms.
5. Outline the physical examination of the burned patient.
6. Describe the prehospital management of the patient who has sustained a burn injury.
7. Discuss pathophysiology as a basis for key signs, symptoms, and management of the patient with an inhalation injury.
8. Outline the general assessment and management of the patient who has a chemical injury.
9. Describe specific complications and management techniques for selected chemical injuries.
10. Describe the physiological effects of electrical injuries as they relate to each body system based on an understanding of key principles of electricity.
11. Outline assessment and management of the patient with electrical injury.
12. Describe the distinguishing features of radiation injury and considerations in the prehospital management of these patients.

SUMMARY
- Each year more than 2 million Americans seek medical attention for burns. Morbidity and mortality rates from burn injury follow significant patterns regarding gender, age, and socioeconomic status. A burn injury is caused by an interaction between thermal, chemical, electrical, or radiation energy and biological matter.
- Tissue damage from burns depends on the degree of the heat and on the duration of exposure to the thermal source. As local events occur at the injury site, other organ systems become involved in a general response to the stress caused by the burn.
- Burns are classified in terms of depth as superficial, partial-thickness, and full-thickness. The rule of nines provides a rough estimate of burn injury size (extent) and is most accurate for adults and for children older than age 10. The Lund and Browder chart is a more accurate method of determining the area of burn injury. Severity of burn injury and burn center referral guidelines are based on standards that take into account the depth, extent, and severity of the burn wound; the source of injury; patient age; presence of concurrent medical or surgical problems; and the body region that is burned.
- Shock after thermal injury results from edema and accumulation of vascular fluid. These tissue changes occur in the area of injury and can produce systemic hypovolemia if the burn area is large.

- Emergency care for a burn patient begins with the initial assessment. The goal is to recognize and treat life-threatening injuries.
- Goals for prehospital management of the severely burned patient include preventing further tissue injury, maintaining the airway, administering oxygen and ventilatory support, providing fluid resuscitation, providing rapid transport to an appropriate medical facility, using aseptic (clean) technique to minimize the patient's exposure to infectious agents, managing pain, and providing psychological and emotional support.
- Prehospital considerations in caring for patients with inhalation injury include recognition of the dangers inherent in the fire environment, pathophysiology of inhalation injury, and early detection and treatment of impending airway or respiratory problems.
- The severity of chemical injury is related to three things: the chemical agent, the concentration and volume of the chemical, and the duration of contact. Treatment is directed at stopping the burning process by using copious irrigation.
- Three types of injury may occur as a result of contact with electrical current: direct contact burns, arc injuries, and flash burns. Once the scene is safe, patient intervention may begin. Internal damage from electrical current may be much more significant than external wounds.
- Persons who are injured by radiation rarely require emergency care. Radioactive particles are classified into three types: alpha, beta, and gamma. The Federal Emergency Management Agency recommends that basic radiation protection for the rescuer and the patient include four factors: minimize time in the radiation field; maintain a safe distance from the source; place shielding between the rescuers and the source; and limit the amount of radioactive material in a specific area.

REVIEW QUESTIONS

Match the chemicals listed in Column II with the appropriate description in Column I.

Column I	Column II
1. _____ Chemical used to clean fabric and metal, can cause hypocalcemia and severe burns	a. Alkali
2. _____ Noxious gas that, when in solution, can cause blindness if it contaminates the eye	b. Ammonia
3. _____ Chemical that causes burns after prolonged exposure and also may result in lead poisoning	c. Hydrofluoric acid
4. _____ Chemical that produces heat if exposed to water and should be removed or covered with oil	d. Petroleum
5. _____ Exposure to this chemical may be painless and result in dysrhythmias and central nervous system depression	e. Phenol

6. Identify the four major sources of burn injury.

   a.

   b.

   c.

   d.

7. Label the three zones of burn injury on Fig. 23-1 and briefly describe the characteristics of the tissue in each.

   A. _____

   _____

   B. _____

   _____

C. _____

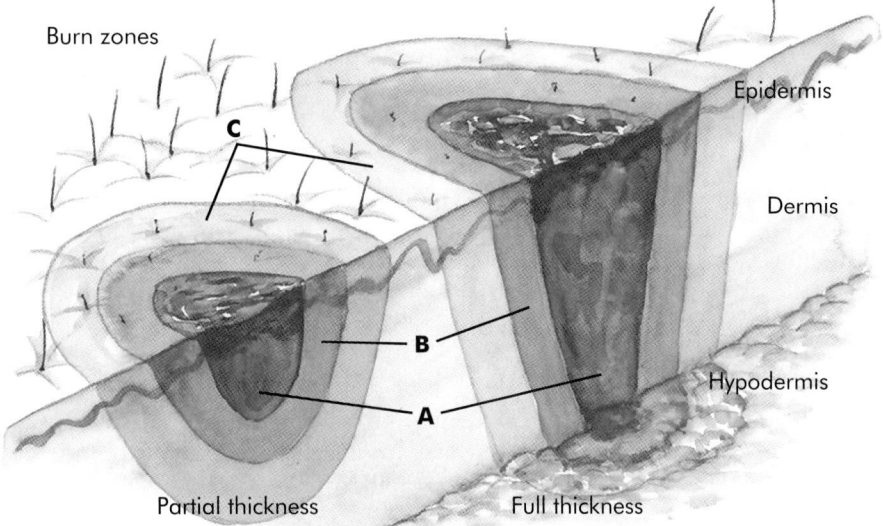

Figure 23-1

8. Explain two mechanisms that cause swelling in the burned tissue.

   a.

   b.

9. Describe the response in each of the following body systems to a major burn injury:

   a. Cardiovascular:

_____

   b. Pulmonary:

_____

   c. Gastrointestinal:

_____

   d. Musculoskeletal:

_____

   e. Neuroendocrine:

_____

   f. Metabolic:

_____

   g. Immune:

_____

   h. Emotional:

_____

10. For each of the following situations, classify the burn according to depth (first-, second-, or third-degree), extent (body surface area), and severity (according to the American Burn Association). Identify those patients who meet the American Burn Association criteria for referral to a burn center.

   a. A chef at a local restaurant has spilled hot grease down the anterior surface of his body. The wound is extremely painful, moist, and red, with many blisters. The burns cover the anterior surface of his chest, abdomen, arms, and left leg.
      Depth:
      Extent:
      Severity:
      Referral:

   b. On a hot summer day a young motorist opens his radiator cap and sprays hot steam and fluid over the upper half of his torso. The wounds are painful, moist, and red, with some blistering, and they blanch to the touch. The burns cover his face, anterior chest, and abdomen.
      Depth:
      Extent:
      Severity:
      Referral:

   c. An 80-year-old woman steps into a tub of extremely hot water. Because of her severe arthritis, she takes a long time to get out. She has circumferential burns around the right lower extremity up to the knee. The burn wound appears white and leathery and has no capillary refill.
      Depth:
      Extent:
      Severity:
      Referral:

11. As you arrive at the scene of a residential fire, rescue workers carry out an approximately 40-year-old, 80-kg man who is unconscious and has white, leathery burns. The burns cover the entire body surface except the posterior surface of both legs. He has shallow respirations at a rate of 24/min, and his blood pressure is 106/70 mm Hg. Patchy pieces of his smoldering clothing remain.

   a. Describe your initial assessment of this patient, including depth, extent, and severity of burns.

   _____

   _____

   b. Describe the prehospital care, including airway and fluid resuscitation, with type of fluid and rate.

   _____

   _____

12. Describe the specific interventions to be used when the following third-degree burns are present:

   a. Burns to the face:

   _____

   b. Extremity burns:

   _____

   c. Circumferential burns:

   _____

Questions 13 to 16 pertain to the following case study:

   A 13-year-old boy uses gasoline to start a bonfire and ignites his clothing. As he attempts to pull his flaming jacket over his head, it gets stuck while continuing to burn. On your arrival, he is alert after an initial brief loss of consciousness. He has extensive burns on his face, neck, and chest. The burns are white and dry, with charred patches. They do not blanch when touched. His nasal hair is singed, and he is coughing up black, sooty sputum.

13. What aspects of the mechanism of injury and history of the event lead you to believe that this patient may have an inhalation injury?

_____

14. What physical findings suggest inhalation injury?

_____

15. At what point would you consider intubation?

_____

16. Do you suspect an inhalation injury above or below the glottis, and why?

_____

17. You are responding to a call for a person who has a chemical burn. En route to the industrial complex, you review the questions you will ask to determine the potential seriousness of the burn.

   a. Provide two examples of these questions.

_____

_____

   b. You find your patient covered with a powder known to cause chemical burns to the skin. Describe patient decontamination techniques.

_____

_____

18. Identify two examples of chemicals that can cause burn injury in each of the following categories:

   a. Acids:

_____

   b. Alkalis:

_____

   c. Organic compounds:

_____

19. The amount of tissue damage caused by an electrical current depends on six factors: (a) _____,

_____, _____, _____ _____, and _____. Amperage is

the measure of current (b) _____ per unit time. Voltage is a continuous (c) _____ applied to any electrical circuit causing a flow of electricity. High-voltage electrical injuries result from contact with an

electrical source of (d) _____ or greater. Resistance to electricity depends on four factors:

(e) _____ _____, _____, _____, and _____. Resistance to

electrical flow in the body is greatest in the (f) _____ tissue. The two types of current commonly used

are (g) _____ and _____. Direct current flows in (h) _____ direction. It is used

in (i) _____. Alternating current periodically reverses (j) _____ of flow. This reversal may

cause muscle contractions that may (k) _____ the patient to the source. In general, the current

pathway in low-voltage current follows the path of (l) _____ _____, and high-voltage

current follows the (m) _____ path. As the duration of contact with the patient increases, tissue

damage (n) _____.

20. Name the three burn patterns that can result from electrical current.

   a.

   b.

   c.

21. Briefly describe the potential effects of electrical injury on each of the following body regions.

   a. Cutaneous:

_____

   b. Cardiovascular:

_____

   c. Neurological:

_____

   d. Vascular:

_____

   e. Muscular:

_____

   f. Renal:

_____

   g. Pulmonary:

_____

   h. Orthopedic:

_____

   i. Ocular and otic:

_____

22. A home owner was trimming his trees when he came into contact with overhead electrical wires. On your arrival, he is still in contact with the electrical source.

    a. What must be done before treatment commences?

_____

    The patient falls 10 feet from the tree to the ground. The scene is now safe. He is conscious and alert. You note multiple small, round, white burns on his right hand. When his clothing is removed, you discover significant burns and tissue injury to both feet.

    b. Describe your history and physical examination of this patient.

_____

_____

_____

    c. Describe treatment, including fluid resuscitation (rate and type).

_____

_____

23. Describe the appearance of wounds characteristically associated with lightning burns.

_____

24. For each of the following classes of lightning injury, list two physical signs:

    a. Minor:

_____

    b. Moderate:

_____

    c. Severe:

_____

25. Describe the characteristics of the following three types of radiation particles:

    a. Alpha:

_____

    b. Beta:

_____

    c. Gamma:

_____

26. Describe the physical effects that can be expected at the following levels of radiation exposure:

    a. Less than 100 rem:

_____

b. 100 to 200 rem:

_____

c. Greater than 450 rem:

_____

Questions 27 to 29 pertain to the following case study:

You arrive at a clinical laboratory, where a significant amount of radioactive material reportedly was released when a worker fell 1 foot from a platform.

27. Describe your approach to the emergency scene.

_____

_____

28. The victim must be accessed. Describe how the crew members designated to perform the rescue can minimize their radiation exposure.

_____

_____

_____

29. Describe any special measures that you should use to care for this patient after you reach him or her.

_____

_____

STUDENT SELF-ASSESSMENT

30. Which is an example of a thermal mechanism of injury?
   a. Arcing
   b. Alkali agents
   c. Ionizing agents
   d. Scalding
31. Which of the following risk factors is associated with a high incidence of burn fatality?
   a. Female gender
   b. Child
   c. Industrial setting
   d. High-income family
32. The most common source of burn injury is
   a. Chemical
   b. Electrical
   c. Radiation
   d. Thermal
33. Which of the following is a systemic response to burn injury?
   a. Hypoventilation
   b. Hyperactive gastrointestinal tract
   c. Decreased metabolic rate
   d. Depressed inflammatory response
34. A burn characterized by a moist, red appearance with blisters is probably what degree?
   a. First
   b. Second
   c. Third
   d. Fourth
35. A 5-year-old patient with third-degree burns of the anterior and posterior surfaces of both legs would be estimated to have a(n) _____ burn.
   a. 18%
   b. 24%
   c. 28%
   d. 36%

36. Hypovolemia in burn injury occurs because of which of the following?
    a. Blood loss
    b. Condensation of tissue fluid
    c. Increased capillary permeability
    d. Decrease in fluid intake

37. When calculating the extent of burn injury to ensure accurate fluid resuscitation, the paramedic should do which of the following?
    a. Calculate the burn size after arriving at the hospital.
    b. Estimate size before cooling the burn.
    c. Not include first-degree burns.
    d. Use the Lund and Browder chart.

38. To cool the burn of a patient burned on 50% of the body surface area, the paramedic should do which of the following?
    a. Apply ice intermittently in 15-minute cycles.
    b. Leave the patient exposed to air and apply a fan.
    c. Apply cool water and then cover the patient with sheets and blankets.
    d. Continuously apply cool water while en route to the hospital.

39. Using the consensus burn formula, calculate the minimum fluid requirement during the first hour for a 100-kg patient who has 60% third-degree burns covering his body.
    a. 250 mL
    b. 500 mL
    c. 750 mL
    d. 6000 mL

40. Which of the following is *not* a reason to suspect inhalation injury?
    a. Burns involving petroleum products
    b. Documented loss of consciousness
    c. Hoarseness or stridor
    d. Burns in an enclosed space

41. Which of the following statements is true regarding carbon monoxide poisoning?
    a. Oxygen saturation on the pulse oximeter is 80 or less.
    b. Skin color is cyanotic and often mottled.
    c. Respiratory rate is depressed in the early stages.
    d. Oxygen administration reduces the half-life of carbon monoxide.

42. What is the treatment of choice for almost all chemical injuries?
    a. Vigorous drying of the chemical
    b. Application of a chemical antidote
    c. Copious irrigation with water
    d. Delayed treatment until arrival at the hospital

43. Severity of chemical injury is related to all of the following except which one?
    a. Chemical concentration
    b. Duration of contact
    c. Environmental temperature
    d. Type of chemical agent

44. Calcium gluconate gel and solution are used to treat which of the following chemical injuries?
    a. Ammonia
    b. Hydrofluoric acid
    c. Petroleum
    d. Phenol

45. Electrical burns that result when the heat of the electrical current ignites the patient's clothing are what type of burns?
    a. Alternating
    b. Arc
    c. Direct
    d. Flame

46. Which tissue does electrical current flow through most easily?
    a. Bone
    b. Blood
    c. Muscle
    d. Nerve

47. Death in lightning injury most frequently results from which of the following?
    a. Cardiac or respiratory arrest
    b. Central nervous system injury
    c. Coagulation of the blood
    d. Severe burn shock

48. Which type of radiation requires a lead shield to stop penetration?
    a. Alpha
    b. Beta
    c. Gamma
    d. Nonionizing

WRAP IT UP

You are dispatched to a refinery for an explosion. When you arrive, you are directed into a dock area where you find a 37-year-old worker who was touching a forklift when it contacted a high-voltage electrical line, breaking it. He was thrown into some packing material that ignited because of the arcing. It took several minutes for the power to be interrupted so the fire could be extinguished. When you arrive, he is conscious, alert, and complaining of severe pain of his right arm. You provide cervical spine immobilization and continue your assessment as your partner applies high-concentration oxygen. You note a brown leathery wound on his left hand, and a charred wound on his right foot. He has moist, painful, partially blistered burns on his abdomen, and waxy, pale, tan-colored burns on his back from his shoulders to his buttocks. His vital signs are BP 170/100 mm Hg, P 124 irregular, R 20, SaO_2 on room air of 95%. You cool the burns with sterile saline, apply a clean sheet over the long spine board, secure him, cover his burns with clean sheets and warm blankets, and move him into the ambulance where you initiate an IV of LR at a rate prescribed by medical direction. An ECG monitor is applied, and morphine is administered for his increasing pain. Medical direction advises you to transport him to the burn center. En route, you monitor vital signs, peripheral pulses, which are diminished in the right foot, and continue to administer pain medication. When the urinary catheter is inserted in the ED, you note that it is a dark red wine color. The patient is hospitalized for 3 months, has his right lower leg amputated, and requires numerous skin grafts.

1. What source(s) caused this patient's burns?
   a. Chemical
   b. Electrical
   c. Thermal
   d. Electrical and thermal

2. Why did this patient have no signs of burn shock? _____

   _____

3. What was the burn depth? _____ Extent? _____ Severity? _____

4. Why was it necessary to monitor peripheral pulses? _____

   _____

5. Explain the following treatment decisions.

   a. Application of cool saline to the wound _____

   b. Administration of oxygen despite normal SaO_2 _____

   _____

   c. Initiating the IV in the left arm _____

   d. Giving morphine intravenously instead of intramuscularly _____

   _____

6. What should you specifically assess to determine whether this patient has any indication of inhalation injury?

   _____

   _____

7. His electrical wounds were on the hand and on the foot. Explain why you did not find electrical burns in other places.

   _____

8. Place a check mark beside each of the signs or symptoms this patient had that indicate electrical injury.

a. _____ Hypertension

b. _____ Tachycardia

c. _____ Dysrhythmias

d. _____ Seizures

e. _____ Coma

f. _____ Motor/sensory deficits

g. _____ Respiratory depression

h. _____ Peripheral circulation impaired

i. _____ Myoglobinuria

CHAPTER 23 ANSWERS

REVIEW QUESTIONS

1. c
(Objective 8)

2. b
(Objective 8)

3. d
(Objective 8)

4. a
(Objective 8)

5. e
(Objective 8)

6. a. Thermal
   b. Electrical
   c. Chemical
   d. Radiation
   (Objective 1)

7. A. Zone of coagulation: nonviable tissue
   B. Zone of stasis: seriously injured but potentially viable (Cells will die if no supportive measures are taken within 24 hours.)
   C. Zone of hyperemia: increased blood flow caused by inflammatory response (Cells will recover in 7 to 10 days if no shock or infection develops.)
   (Objective 2)

8. a. Chemical mediators cause increased capillary permeability and a fluid shift from the intravascular space to burned tissues.
   b. The sodium pump in cell walls is damaged, and sodium moves into injured cells and increases swelling.
   (Objective 2)

9. a. Decreased venous return, decreased cardiac output, increased vascular resistance (except in zone of hyperemia), hemolysis, and rhabdomyolysis that may lead to renal failure
   b. Increased respiratory rate to meet increased metabolic demands
   c. Adynamic ileus, vomiting, and stress ulcer
   d. Decreased range of motion resulting from edema and immobilization; osteoporosis and demineralization later
   e. Increased circulating levels of epinephrine, norepinephrine, and aldosterone
   f. Increased basal metabolic rate
   g. Increased susceptibility to infection and depressed inflammatory response
   h. Pain, isolation, and fear of disfigurement
   (Objectives 2 and 4)

10.

Depth	Extent	Severity	Referral
a. Second degree (partial thickness)	36%	Major	Yes
b. Second degree (partial thickness)	22.5%	Moderate	Yes
c. Third degree (full thickness)	9%	Major	Yes (involves feet)

(Objective 3)

11. a. Simultaneously put out the fire and cool the burn while performing initial assessment; monitor vital signs; assess burn depth (third degree), extent (82%), and severity (major); perform a head-to-toe survey; assess lung sounds and distal pulse, movement, sensation, and capillary refill in all extremities.

b. Cool the burn with clean water; open the airway; intubate as necessary; ventilate with 100% oxygen; prepare to intubate; remove remaining clothing and jewelry; cover the patient to maintain warmth; initiate lactated Ringer's solution intravenously at 820 mL/hr (2 mL/kg per percent body surface area burned 24 hours [half of daily fluid to be given in first 8 hours]) up to 1640 mL/hr (4 mL/kg per percent body surface area burned, over 24 hours) in an unburned extremity; and rapidly transport patient.
(Objectives 5 and 6)

12. a. Realize that the burns may swell and be associated with airway problems. Raise the head of the stretcher 30 degrees if spinal injury is not suspected. If the ears are burned, do not use a pillow.

b. Remove jewelry, assess neurovascular status frequently, and elevate extremities.

c. Monitor distal pulse, movement, sensation, and respirations and rapidly transport the patient to the nearest appropriate facility.
(Objective 6)

13. His jacket created an enclosed space, and he experienced a loss of consciousness.
(Objective 7)

14. Facial burns, singed nasal hair, and carbonaceous sputum suggest inhalation injury.
(Objective 7)

15. Increased dyspnea, decreased level of consciousness, hoarseness, and stridor indicate the need for intubation.
(Objective 7)

16. Above the glottis is the most likely area of injury. The mechanism of injury does not suggest injury below the glottis.
(Objective 7)

17. a. What type, concentration, and volume of chemical was involved? How did the injury occur? When did the injury occur? Was any first aid given? Does the patient feel any pain?

b. With appropriate protective clothing, brush most of the powder off and then irrigate profusely (using a shower if available).
(Objective 7)

18. a. Rust removers, bathroom cleaners, and swimming pool acidifiers

b. Drain cleaners, fertilizers, heavy industrial cleaners, and cement and concrete

c. Phenols, creosote, and gasoline
(Objective 8)

19. a. Amperage, voltage, resistance, type of current, current pathway, duration of current flow

b. Flow (intensity)

c. Force (tension)

d. 1000 volts

e. Resistivity, size of object pathway, length of object pathway, and temperature

f. Bone

g. Alternating, direct

h. One

i. Industry

j. Direction

k. Freeze

l. Least resistance

m. Shortest

n. Increases
(Objective 10)

20. a. Direct contact
   b. Arc
   c. Flash
   (Objective 10)

21. a. Direct contact can create large areas of coagulation necrosis. The entry wound is often a characteristic bull's-eye (dry and leathery), and the exit is ulcerated and explosive.
   b. Dysrhythmias and damage to the myocardium may occur. Cardiac arrest is the most common cause of death after electrical injury. Hypertension caused by increased catecholamine levels is common.
   c. Central nervous system injury may result in coma, seizures, and peripheral nerve injury and may lead to sensory or motor deficits. Brainstem injury may cause respiratory depression or arrest or cerebral edema or hemorrhage, which can lead to death.
   d. Blood vessel necrosis may cause immediate or delayed hemorrhage or thrombosis.
   e. Muscle injury may result in release of myoglobin, which can cause renal failure.
   f. Acute renal failure occurs in 10% of significant electrical injuries.
   g. The patient may have decreased ventilation or respiratory arrest because of central nervous system injury or chest wall dysfunction.
   h. Fractures and dislocations can result from direct electrical injury or from injury caused by fall or electrocution.
   i. Burns to conjunctiva or cornea and ruptured tympanic membrane are common.
   (Objective 10)

22. a. The electrical source must be removed safely from the patient, preferably by interruption of power by the electric company.
   b. Perform cervical spine immobilization and ABCDEs. Determine the patient's chief complaint, source of electricity, duration of exposure, level of consciousness before and after injury, and medical history. Perform a head-to-toe survey, looking for entry and exit burn wounds or trauma associated with the fall. Assess distal pulse, movement, sensation, and capillary refill in all extremities and document them. Monitor electrocardiographic rhythm.
   c. Immobilize the cervical spine, open the airway, apply 100% oxygen, assess the need to assist ventilations, remove all jewelry, initiate lactated Ringer's solution intravenously at 20 to 40 mL/kg, monitor the vital signs and electrocardiogram, and maintain body warmth.
   (Objective 11)

23. Linear, feathery, pinpoint appearance
   (Objective 10)

24. a. The patient is usually conscious and may be confused and amnesic, with stable vital signs.
   b. The patient may be combative or comatose, with associated injuries from lightning strike, first- and second-degree burns, tympanic membrane rupture (common), and possible internal injuries.
   c. The patient may have immediate brain damage, seizures, respiratory paralysis, and cardiac arrest.
   (Objective 10)

25. a. Alpha particles are positively charged atoms with minimal penetrability; however, they are dangerous when internal exposure occurs.
   b. Beta particles are positively or negatively charged electrons that have more penetrating power than alpha particles and can permeate subcutaneous tissue.
   c. Gamma particles have a much higher penetrating power than alpha or beta rays and require lead shielding to stop penetration. (Protective clothing does not stop these rays.) Exposure may produce local skin burns and extensive internal damage.
   (Objective 12)

26. a. Less than 100 rem usually causes no significant acute problems.
   b. A total of 100 to 200 rem can cause symptoms such as nausea and vomiting but is not life threatening.
   c. Exposure of greater than 450 rem has a 50% mortality rate within 30 days.
   (Objective 12)

27. The rescuers and emergency vehicle initially should be positioned 200 to 300 feet upwind of the site. No eating, smoking, or drinking should be permitted at the site. The appropriate local authorities and medical control should be notified of the situation.
(Objective 12)

28. Protective clothing should be worn, if available. The victim should be approached quickly by trained rescue teams. Rescue personnel should trade off frequently until the victim is stabilized sufficiently to remove him or her a safe distance from the contaminated area. If possible, the crew members should position themselves behind any protective barrier available.
(Objective 12)

29. If ventilation is required for the radiation-contaminated victim, an airway adjunct should be used. The patient should be moved away from the radiation source as soon as possible, but lifesaving care should not be delayed if the patient cannot be moved immediately. Intravenous lines should be initiated only if absolutely necessary, and good aseptic technique should be used to minimize the risk of introducing contaminants into the patient's body.
(Objective 12)

30. d. Alkali agents cause chemical burns, ionizing agents cause radiation burns, and arcing is caused by electrical energy.
(Objective 1)

31. b. Men die more frequently than women from burns. Three fourths of burn fatalities occur in the home. Deaths are also common in low-income homes.
(Objective 1)

32. d. This source includes flames, scalds, or contact with hot substances.
(Objective 1)

33. d. The patient hyperventilates to adapt to the increased metabolic rate. The gastrointestinal tract slows and, with large burns, adynamic ileus is a frequent complication.
(Objective 2)

34. b. First-degree burns are usually red, dry, and painful without blisters. Third-degree burns are white, yellow, tan, brown, or black; leathery; and often painless.
(Objective 3)

35. c. Each leg is between 13.5% and 14% body surface area.
(Objective 3)

36. c. Evaporation of fluid from the injured area also accounts for significant fluid loss.
(Objective 4)

37. c. The presence of first-degree burns should be noted in the narrative; however, these burns should not be included in the estimate of percent body surface area burned.
(Objective 3)

38. c. The burn should be cooled rapidly, and then body temperature should be maintained with sheets and blankets.
(Objective 6)

39. c. $2 \text{ mL} \times 60 \times 100 = 12,000 \text{ mL}$ in the first 24 hours
One half in the first 8 hours = 6,000 mL
$6,000 \text{ mL} \div 8 = 750 \text{ mL}$
The formula states that 2 to 4 mL/kg per percent body surface area burned is given in 24 hours, so the range would be 750 to 1500 mL.
(Objective 6)

40. a. Petroleum products are not associated with inhalation burns unless they occur in an enclosed space or meet one of the other criteria.
(Objective 6)

41. d. Oxygen saturation levels may be normal because the hemoglobin still is saturated (with carbon monoxide, not oxygen), and the oximeter may not differentiate between the two. Intravenous fluid therapy is not helpful in these patients.
(Objective 7)

42. c. Drying the chemical or delaying treatment only prolongs contact with the skin and increases the burn injury. Application of a chemical antidote is recommended only for a few chemicals.
(Objective 8)

43. c. Each other factor has a direct effect on the severity of the injury.
(Objective 7)

44. b. Subcutaneous injection of the calcium gluconate gel under the burn eschar is the most effective method.
(Objective 9)

45. d. An arc occurs when electrical energy "jumps" from its source through the air to another conductive medium. Direct burns result when the current passes through a person. *Alternating* is a description of a type of electrical current.
(Objective 10)

46. d. Bone provides the most resistance to electrical energy.
(Objective 10)

47. a. All the other pathological conditions can occur following lightning injury but cause death less frequently than cardiac or respiratory arrest.
(Objective 10)

48. c. Gamma rays have 10,000 times the penetrating power of alpha particles and 100 times the penetrating power of beta particles.
(Objective 12)

WRAP IT UP

1. d. Direct contact electrical and flame burns.
(Objective 1)

2. Burn shock evolves over 8 to 24 hours after injury and often is not seen immediately after injury.
(Objective 2)

3. Depth: Second- and third-degree (partial and full thickness)
Extent: ~24% (rule of nines); ~28% (Lund and Browder chart)
Severity: Major burn (>25%; electrical injury; significant involvement of hands/feet)
(Objective 3)

4. Damage from direct electrical current is often greatest in the tissues between the entrance and exit wounds. If the swelling occurs in the tissue compartments, severe circulatory compromise to the extremities can occur, causing progressive loss of pulses.
(Objective 5)

5. a. Cools the wound to minimize tissue damage.

b. Progressive burn shock should be anticipated, and oxygen should be delivered despite an initially normal SaO_2. Additionally, if the possibility of carbon monoxide exposure exists, SaO_2 will be normal despite tissue hypoxia.

c. Electrical burns were present in the right hand and right foot. The current had to travel through the right arm to reach the foot so that arm should be avoided because of the potential for impaired circulation.

d. As burn shock progresses, blood flow to the muscles will decline, resulting in ineffective management of pain.

(Objective 6)

6. Did the burns occur in an enclosed space? Does the patient have any stridor, facial burns, soot in the nose or mouth, facial burns, singed facial or nasal hair, edema of the lips or oral cavity, coughing, difficulty swallowing, hoarse voice, or circumferential neck burns?
(Objective 7)

7. Electrical current usually follows the path of least resistance to ground. Body tissues with the least resistance include the nerves and the blood vessels, not external skin structures.
(Objective 10)

8. a, b, c, h, i
(Objective 10)

CHAPTER
24

Head and Facial Trauma

READING ASSIGNMENT
Chapter 24, pages 580-605, in *Mosby's Paramedic Textbook*, ed. 3

OBJECTIVES
Upon completion of this chapter, the paramedic student will be able to:
1. Describe the mechanisms of injury, assessment, and management of maxillofacial injuries.
2. Describe the mechanisms of injury, assessment, and management of ear, eye, and dental injuries.
3. Describe the mechanisms of injury, assessment, and management of anterior neck trauma.
4. Describe the mechanisms of injury, assessment, and management of injuries to the scalp, cranial vault, or cranial nerves.
5. Distinguish between types of traumatic brain injury based on an understanding of pathophysiology and assessment findings.
6. Outline the prehospital management of the patient with cerebral injury.
7. Calculate a Glasgow Coma Scale, trauma score, Revised Trauma Score, and pediatric trauma score when given appropriate patient information.

SUMMARY
- Major causes of maxillofacial trauma are motor vehicle crashes, home accidents, athletic injuries, animal bites, intentional violent acts, and industrial injuries.
- With the exception of compromised airway and the potential for significant bleeding, damage to the tissues of the maxillofacial area is seldom life threatening. Blunt trauma injuries may be classified as fractures to the mandible, midface, zygoma, orbit, and nose.
- Injury to the ears, eyes, or teeth may be minor or may result in permanent sensory function loss and disfigurement. Trauma to the ear may include lacerations and contusions, thermal injuries, chemical injuries, traumatic perforation, and barotitis. Evaluation of the eye should include a thorough history. Assessment also should include measurement of visual acuity, pupillary reaction, and extraocular movements.
- Anterior neck injuries may result in damage to the skeletal structures, vascular structures, nerves, muscles, and glands of the neck.
- Injuries to the skull may be classified as soft tissue injuries to the scalp and skull fractures. Skull fractures may be classified as linear fractures, basilar fractures, depressed fractures, and open vault fractures.

- The categories of brain injury include DAI and focal injury. Diffuse axonal injury may be mild (concussion), moderate, or severe. Focal injuries are specific, grossly observable brain lesions. Included in this category are lesions that result from skull fracture, contusion, edema with associated increased ICP, ischemia, and hemorrhage.
- The prehospital management of a patient with head injuries is determined by a number of factors. One factor is the mechanism of injury. A second factor is the severity of injury. A third factor is the patient's level of consciousness. Associated injuries affect the priorities of care.
- Several injury rating systems are used to triage, guide patient care, predict patient outcome, identify changes in patient status, and evaluate trauma care. Rating systems commonly used in emergency care include the Glasgow Coma Scale, trauma score/Revised Trauma Score, and pediatric trauma score.

REVIEW QUESTIONS

Match the type of skull fracture listed in Column II with the appropriate description in Column I. Use each answer only once.

Column I	Column II
1. _____ Associated with Battle's sign and raccoon's eyes	a. Basilar
2. _____ Most common skull fracture; has low complication rate	b. Depressed
3. _____ Direct communication between scalp laceration and brain tissue	c. Linear
4. _____ Fracture when bone is pushed downward; often associated with scalp laceration	d. Open vault

Match the cranial nerve in Column II with the abnormal sign or symptom associated with it in Column I. Use each cranial nerve only once.

Column I	Column II
5. _____ Hearing loss	a. Olfactory
6. _____ Loss of vision in one eye	b. Optic
7. _____ Weakness of one side of the face	c. Oculomotor
8. _____ Double vision	d. Facial
9. _____ Loss of sense of smell	e. Acoustic
	f. Glossopharyngeal

10. A 6-year-old unrestrained child strikes his face on the stick shift of a truck in a head-on collision. On arrival, you find him seated in the cab of the truck, alert, crying, and complaining of pain in his face. Blood is oozing from his mouth.

   a. Describe your focused assessment of his head and face.

   _____

   _____

   b. On physical examination, you note the child's difficulty closing his mouth and an apparent space between the two lower front teeth, as well as a laceration that extends down through the gums. The bleeding continues, and you note excessive oral secretions. Vital signs are stable. Describe how you would transport and manage this child.

   _____

   _____

11. Briefly describe the evaluation of a suspected eye injury on a patient with no life threats.

_____

_____

12. For each of the following patients, identify the injury you suspect and list prehospital management techniques:

   a. A 10-year-old complains of severe pain in the right eye after he was struck in the face with a handful of sand. The right eye is reddened and tearing.

_____

_____

   b. A 35-year-old has sustained a partially avulsed right upper lid.

_____

_____

   c. A fish hook is embedded in the eye of a 42-year-old woman.

_____

_____

   d. A handball player is struck directly in the eye by the ball. He is having difficulty seeing from the injured eye. You note blood in the anterior chamber of the eye.

_____

_____

   e. During hockey playoffs, a high stick strikes a player in the eye. You note an irregular pupil on the affected side. A jellylike substance extrudes from an apparent laceration to the globe.

_____

_____

Questions 13 and 14 pertain to the following case study:

You are en route to a domestic disturbance in which a 45-year-old man reportedly has been stabbed in the neck with an ice pick.

13. Identify possible signs and symptoms of penetrating neck trauma that you should anticipate.

_____

On arrival, you note an ashen-colored unconscious patient who is breathing and has a weak pulse. A large pool of blood surrounds him, and a large amount of blood is coming from his neck.

14. List the steps in management of this patient with respect to the neck wound.

_____

_____

15. Briefly list the signs and symptoms associated with the following brain injuries, and state whether the injury is a diffuse axonal injury or focal brain injury:

   a. Concussion:

   _____

   b. Contusion:

   _____

   c. Subdural hematoma:

   _____

   d. Epidural hematoma:

   _____

   e. Severe diffuse axonal injury:

   _____

16. A man has been struck on the head with a baseball bat during a barroom brawl. He is alert and oriented, with an obvious depression and laceration at the right temporal area. Describe the signs and symptoms you will see if his intracranial pressure progressively rises en route to the hospital.

   _____

17. You are transporting by air a patient who has sustained an isolated head injury in a motorcycle accident. Initially, he was awake and talking, but over the past 10 minutes, his condition has deteriorated rapidly. He now has a fixed, dilated right pupil; irregular respirations; a blood pressure of 170/100 mm Hg; and a pulse of 64. Identify treatment modalities you would provide for this patient.

   _____

   _____

18. Calculate the score indicated (Glasgow Coma scale [GCS], Revised Trauma Score [RTS], pediatric trauma score [PTS]) for each of the following patient examples:

   a. Your patient opens her eyes to voice, is confused, and pulls her hand away when you start intravenous therapy. Her vital signs are blood pressure, 90/70 mm Hg; pulse, 120; and respirations, 24 and unlabored. Capillary refill is 1 second. GCS_____ RTS_____

   b. Your patient opens his eyes to deep pain, moans some unrecognizable sounds, and withdraws slightly from pain. His vital signs are blood pressure, 70 mm Hg by palpation; pulse, 136; and respirations, 30 and shallow. His capillary refill is 4 seconds.
   GCS_____ RTS _____

   c. Your 10-day-old, 4-kg patient fell to the floor. She is crying vigorously. You note a small abrasion on her head, with a slight amount of swelling but no palpable crepitus. No other injuries are noted. Her blood pressure is 80 mm Hg. PTS _____

19. Which of the following is a sign of midface fracture?

    a. Diplopia

    b. Lengthening of the face

    c. Mastoid ecchymosis

    d. Numbness of the forehead

20. Your patient has signs and symptoms of midface fractures with a Glasgow Coma Scale score of 6. Which of the following is an appropriate prehospital intervention?

    a. Elevation of the head of the cot

    b. Nasogastric intubation

    c. Orotracheal intubation

    d. Pressure dressing over the nares

21. What is the name of the bone that, when fractured, often is associated with signs and symptoms similar to orbital fractures?

    a. Frontal

    b. Mandible

    c. Maxilla

    d. Zygoma

22. Your patient has been struck in the eye with a ball. She has diplopia, subconjunctival ecchymosis, enophthalmos, and numbness in the cheek. Which of the following bone fractures is consistent with these findings?

    a. Mandible

    b. Maxilla

    c. Orbit

    d. Zygoma

23. Displaced nasal fractures are most significant when they

    a. Are displaced to one side.

    b. Are associated with bleeding.

    c. Depress the dorsum of the nose.

    d. Occur in children.

24. The upper segment of the patient's pinna was avulsed in a motor vehicle collision. Which of the following treatments is appropriate for this patient?

    a. Approximate the edges of the avulsed tissue to the ear and apply a pressure dressing.

    b. Care for the remaining ear only. No chance exists to reimplant avulsed ear tissue.

    c. Scrub the avulsed tissue before wrapping it for transport to prevent infection.

    d. Wrap the avulsed tissue in moist gauze, seal it in a plastic bag, and place the bag on ice.

25. Prehospital management of ear pain following barotrauma may include which of the following?

    a. Administration of nitrous oxide by inhalation

    b. A request that the patient perform the Valsalva maneuver

    c. Oxygen delivery to increase the absorption of trapped air

    d. Placement of the patient in the lateral recumbent position

26. Which of the following is an acceptable way to transport an avulsed tooth?

    a. In a mild soap solution

    b. In sterile water

    c. In a dry gauze dressing

    d. In fresh whole milk

27. Why are zone I neck injuries associated with the highest mortality? It contains which of the following?

    a. Brainstem, carotid artery, and nasopharynx

    b. Carotid artery, jugular vein, trachea, larynx, esophagus, and cervical spine

    c. Distal carotid arteries, salivary glands, and pharynx

    d. Subclavian and jugular vessels, lung, esophagus, trachea, cervical spine, cervical nerve roots

28. Which sign or symptom may indicate compromise of the upper airway associated with a hematoma in the neck?

    a. Cough

    b. Dysphagia

    c. Stridor

    d. Wheezing

29. Intubation of the patient with laryngeal or tracheal trauma may be difficult because of which of the following?

    a. Absence of spontaneous respirations

    b. Collapse of the trachea and bronchial tubes

    c. The presence of acute hypoxia

    d. Distorted and invisible vocal cords

30. Which of the following is an injury associated with focal brain injury?

    a. Concussion

    b. Contusion

    c. Minute petechial bruising of brain tissue in several areas

    d. Mechanical disruption of axons in both cerebral hemispheres

31. Which of the following is the most reliable indicator of increasing intracranial pressure?
    a. Deteriorating level of consciousness
    b. Nausea and vomiting
    c. Increased blood pressure and decreased pulse
    d. Unilateral dilated pupil
32. Which of the following breathing patterns is *not* likely to be exhibited by the patient with a brain injury?
    a. Ataxic breathing
    b. Cheyne-Stokes respirations
    c. Hypoventilation
    d. Kussmaul's respirations
33. Characteristic signs and symptoms of subarachnoid hemorrhage include which of the following?
    a. Clinical signs of unexplained hypovolemia
    b. Gradual onset of unilateral weakness of the arms
    c. Intermittent pain and double vision in both eyes
    d. Sudden onset of "the worst headache I've ever had"
34. Which is the most rapid and effective intervention to decrease intracranial pressure in a patient with a severe head injury and a Glasgow Coma Scale score of 6?
    a. Elevation of the head of the bed
    b. Intravenous administration of mannitol
    c. Intubation and adequate ventilation
    d. Massive doses of steroids
35. You wish to give 40 g of mannitol to a patient who has a head injury. You have a 20% solution of the drug. How many milliliters do you give?
    a. 8
    b. 50
    c. 80
    d. 200
36. Which drug may be administered before intubation to prevent a sudden increase in intracranial pressure?
    a. Atropine
    b. Lidocaine
    c. Mannitol
    d. Midazolam

WRAP IT UP

You are working at an amusement park, when a call comes over your walkie-talkie for a person who has fallen off a ride. You respond in a motorized golf cart and find a 17-year-old who has fallen about 20 feet from a ride onto the concrete. Bystanders found her prone and rolled her onto her back. Your direct a security officer to maintain spinal immobilization while you assess that her only response to painful stimulation is flexion of her arms. She is making no sounds and her eyes remain closed; pupils are midline, 5 mm, and reactive. She has multiple contusions and lacerations to her face, her nose is flattened, and there is thin bloody drainage from it. You insert an oral airway, and because her respirations are shallow and only about eight per minute, you begin to ventilate her with a bag-valve-mask resuscitator and oxygen as the local ambulance crew arrives. Her radial pulse is 60 per minute, her skin is pale and cool, and her blood pressure is 80/50 mm Hg. She is logrolled with spinal precautions, her back is examined quickly, and after she is secured to the long spine board and stretcher, she is moved into the ambulance where the paramedic crew leader intubates her trachea. An ECG and noninvasive blood pressure monitor are attached, and an IV of normal saline is initiated. After a bolus of 200 mL is given, her pressure rises to 100/70 mm Hg. Physical exam shows no crepitus or deformity anywhere except her face. Moments before arrival at the ED, her right pupil dilates to 7 mm and becomes nonreactive, BP is 130/50 mm Hg, P 50, and she has no motor response to painful stimulus and no spontaneous respirations when bagging is paused. You begin hyperventilation at 20 per minute. She is diagnosed with a severe diffuse axonal injury and dies during the flight to the regional trauma center.

1. If this patient had a gag reflex, should you have considered nasal instead of oral intubation?
    a. No, there is a possibility of midface fracture and penetration of the cranial vault.
    b. No, there would not have been a need to intubate if that patient had a gag reflex.
    c. Yes, nasal intubation would have been less likely to raise intracranial pressure.
    d. Yes, nasal intubation would have tamponaded the nasal bleeding when in place.
2. Based on the information given, which type of skull fractures would you anticipate?
    a. Basilar
    b. Depressed
    c. Linear

d. a and b

e. a and c

3. What type of brain hemorrhage is present in diffuse axonal injury?

    a. Cerebral hematoma

    b. Epidural hematoma

    c. Subarachnoid hemorrhage

    d. Subdural hematoma

    e. None of the above

4. Explain your rationale for providing the following treatment:

    a. Tracheal intubation:_____

    b. Fluid bolus with normal saline:_____

    c. Hyperventilation after the pupil dilated_____

_____

5. Calculate the following scores for this patient:

	Glasgow Coma Scale	Revised Trauma Score
Initial		
During transport		

6. Place a check mark beside the indicators of increasing intracranial pressure that were present in this patient.

a. _____ Headache		**g.** _____ Widening pulse pressure	
b. _____ Nausea/vomiting		**h.** _____ Fixed, dilated pupil	
c. _____ Altered level of consciousness		**i.** _____ Central neurogenic hyperventilation	
d. _____ Blood pressure rises		**j.** _____ Abnormal posturing	
e. _____ Pulse slows		**k.** _____ Ataxic respirations	
f. _____ Cheyne-Stokes respirations		**l.** _____ Irregular pulse rate	

CHAPTER 24 ANSWERS

REVIEW QUESTIONS

1. a
   (Objective 4)

2. c
   (Objective 4)

3. d
   (Objective 4)

4. b
   (Objective 4)

5. e. This nerve is associated with basilar skull fracture.
   (Objective 4)

6. b. Injury to the brain affecting the optic nerve may cause blindness in one or both eyes or visual field defects.
   (Objective 4)

7. d. Damage involving the facial nerve may cause immediate or delayed facial paralysis and is associated with basilar skull fracture.
   (Objective 4)

8. c. Injury affecting the oculomotor nerve can result in double vision because of the inability of the eye to move medially and down and out. Ptosis and pupil dilation or unresponsiveness to light also may occur.
   (Objective 4)

9. a. Loss or alteration of sense of smell associated with injury affecting the olfactory nerve is a common finding associated with basilar skull fracture.
   (Objective 4)

10. a. Inspect and palpate the head for lacerations, contusions, and deformities. Inspect the face for asymmetry and soft tissue injury. Evaluate the child's vision by holding up fingers and assessing pupil response. Assess for EOMs by asking the child to look up and down and side to side. Look for deformity of the nose and any drainage of blood or cerebrospinal fluid. Inspect the oral cavity for bleeding, soft tissue injury, and missing teeth. Palpate the face for crepitus, and question the child about tenderness or numbness. Ask the child to open and close the mouth and move the lower jaw from side to side. Gently palpate for loose teeth.
    b. Immobilize the cervical spine, and secure the child to the backboard while frequently suctioning the oral cavity. Tilt the backboard to the side and secure it firmly with straps. Suction the oral cavity frequently, and instruct the child to signal when he needs additional suctioning or if he has difficulty breathing. Continually reevaluate for life threats.
    (Objective 1)

11. Obtain a history to include the exact mode of injury; previous ocular, medical, and drug history, including cataracts, glaucoma, and presence of hepatitis or human immunodeficiency virus; use of eye medications; use of corrective glasses or contact lenses; presence of ocular prostheses; and symptoms and treatment interventions that may have been attempted before emergency medical services arrival. Observe the patient for signs of external trauma, discoloration, injury to the lid, fluid or jelly extruding from the eye, bleeding, blood in the anterior chamber, and the presence of contact lenses. Measure visual acuity with a handheld acuity chart or any printed material with small, medium, and large point sizes. Record the distance at which the visual material was held. Measure each eye separately and assess vision with and without corrective lenses. Evaluate pupil reaction

to ensure that they constrict in concert when light is applied and dilate in response to darkness. Assess extraocular muscles by asking the patient to track an object with the eyes (without head movement) up, down, right, and left.
(Objective 2)

12. a. Injury: foreign body (or corneal abrasion); management: irrigate with normal saline.
    b. Injury: lid avulsion; management: assess for underlying injury to the eye; control bleeding with gentle pressure; for transport, cover with a dressing moistened with normal saline and an eye shield.
    c. Injury: embedded foreign body; management: patch uninjured eye; stabilize hook and cover with cardboard cup secured with tape.
    d. Injury: traumatic hyphema; management: elevate head of ambulance cot or spine board 40 to 45 degrees; instruct patient to avoid straining.
    e. Injury: ruptured globe; management: cover affected eye with damp, sterile dressings and an eye shield.
    (Objective 2)

13. Bleeding, shock, hematoma, pulse deficit, neurological deficit, dyspnea, hoarseness, stridor, subcutaneous emphysema, hemoptysis, dysphagia, and hematemesis
    (Objective 3)

14. Secure airway and breathing. Maintain spinal immobilization. Apply firm, direct pressure to the affected vessels, and tamponade the vessel by direct pressure with a gloved finger only to the affected vessel(s). If venous injury is suspected, keep the patient supine or in Trendelenberg's position to prevent an air embolism. If air embolism is suspected, turn the immobilized patient on the left side, head lower than feet, to attempt to trap the air embolus in the right ventricle.
    (Objective 3)

15. a. Diffuse axonal injury; loss of consciousness (usually less than 5 minutes), retrograde or antegrade amnesia, vomiting, combativeness, transient visual disturbances, and problems with coordination; should all improve, not deteriorate
    b. Focal injury; seizures, hemiparesis, aphasia, personality changes, and loss of consciousness (lasting hours, days, or longer)
    c. Focal injury; headache, nausea, vomiting, decreasing level of consciousness, coma, abnormal posturing, paralysis, and bulging fontanelles in infants
    d. Focal injury; transient loss of consciousness followed by a lucid interval (6 to 18 hours) and a subsequent decreasing level of consciousness, headache, and contralateral hemiparesis (opposite the side of the bleeding); 50% unconscious without improvement
    e. Diffuse axonal injury; patients being usually unconscious for prolonged periods; may have posturing and signs of increased intracranial pressure
    (Objective 5)

16. Headache, nausea, vomiting, altered level of consciousness, increased systolic blood pressure, widened pulse pressure, decreased pulse rate, abnormally slow respiratory pattern, unilateral dilated pupil, and abnormal posturing
    (Objective 5)

17. Intubate tracheally (possibly nasally if signs of basilar skull fracture are not present) using spinal precautions. Hyperventilate the lungs with 100% oxygen at a rate of 24 per minute. Consider gastric tube insertion if available. Maintain fluids to keep the vein open unless signs of shock develop. Consider pharmacological agents, such as mannitol and furosemide, in consultation with medical direction. Notify medical direction, and transport the patient to the closest appropriate trauma center.
    (Objective 6)

18. a. GCS is 12, and RTS is 11.
    b. GCS is 8, and RTS is 7.
    c. PTS is 7.
    (Objective 7)

19. b. "Donkey face" is associated with this injury. Edema, unstable maxilla, epistaxis, numb upper teeth, nasal flattening, and cerebrospinal fluid rhinorrhea are also signs of midface fracture.
(Objective 1)

20. c. Neither an endotracheal tube nor a gastric tube should be placed nasally in the patient with midface fracture because they may pass into the cranial vault. Elevation of the head of the cot would be appropriate only after the cervical spine is cleared by radiographs in the emergency department. Cerebrospinal fluid drainage often accompanies these injuries and should be allowed to drain freely.
(Objective 1)

21. d. The zygoma commonly is called the *cheek bone*.
(Objective 1)

22. c. Orbital fractures often are associated with other fractures, such as Le Fort II and III and zygomatic fractures.
(Objective 1)

23. d. In children, minimal displacement may result in growth changes and ultimate deformity.
(Objective 1)

24. d. A chance to reimplant does exist, so if possible, the ear should be transported as described. However, ear injuries that involve cartilage often heal poorly and are infected easily.
(Objective 2)

25. b. Nitrous oxide is contraindicated and may increase the pain. Other measures that may help include requests that the patient yawn, swallow, and move the lower jaw.
(Objective 2)

26. d. Milk may be used if a commercial tooth solution, such as Hank's solution, is not available.
(Objective 2)

27. d. Zone II injuries (b) occur more often but are associated with lower mortality.
(Objective 3)

28. c. Stridor indicates that the upper airway is compromised significantly.
(Objective 3)

29. d. Attempting intubation actually may increase the damage associated with the injury and, if unsuccessful, cause partial airway obstruction to become complete.
(Objective 3)

30. b. Contusion is bruising of a specific area of the brain. All other answers reflect injuries that represent diffuse axonal injury.
(Objective 5)

31. a. This is the earliest sign and is consistent with all patients who have increased intracranial pressure.
(Objective 5)

32. d. The patient in diabetic ketoacidosis demonstrates Kussmaul's respirations in an attempt to correct acidosis.
(Objective 5)

33. d. Other common signs and symptoms include dizziness, neck stiffness, unequal pupils, vomiting, seizures, and loss of consciousness.
(Objective 5)

34. c. All other interventions are indicated (depending on medical control) to decrease intracranial pressure; however, ventilation at a rate not to exceed 24 per minute is the fastest method with the least risk to the patient. (Objective 6)

35. d. $\dfrac{40 \text{ g} \times 100 \text{ mL}}{20 \text{ g}} = 200 \text{ mL}$

or 20 g:100 mL = 40 g:x mL

4000 = 20x

200 mL = x

36. b. Atropine may be given to children before intubation to counteract the vagal stimulation. Mannitol is an osmotic diuretic given to decrease intracranial pressure but usually is not given for this purpose. Midazolam (Versed) is often given during rapid sequence induction procedures to sedate the patient. (Objective 6)

WRAP IT UP

1. a. The nasal bleeding, massive facial trauma, and flattened nose are indicators of midface fractures. Nasal intubation of this patient is associated with the risk of perforation of the cranial vault. (Objective 1)

2. e. Midface fractures are associated with basilar skull fractures. There is no indication of depression of the skull bones. (Objective 1)

3. e. Diffuse axonal injury is associated with severe shearing, stretching, or tearing of the nerve fibers of the brain rather than a large collection of blood in an area of the brain. (Objective 4)

4. a. Intubation will protect the airway of a patient with a severe head injury with altered level of consciousness as evidenced by a Glasgow Coma Scale score of less than 8. (Objective 6)

b. Fluid bolus is given to raise the blood pressure. Because the cerebral perfusion pressure (pressure needed to deliver oxygenated blood to the brain tissue) is equal to the mean arterial pressure less the intracranial pressure, if the blood pressure falls too low, the blood delivery to the brain is severely compromised. Fluid bolus may be needed to increase the blood pressure. (Objective 6)

c. Hyperventilation is indicated when the pupil dilates and the Glasgow Coma Scale score is less than 9. This will cause constriction of the blood vessels in the brain and a resulting decrease in the intracranial pressure, which will decrease the risk of brain herniation. (Objective 6)

5. Initial Glasgow Coma Scale score: 5; initial Revised Trauma Score: 6
Transport Glasgow Coma Scale score: 3; transport Revised Trauma Score: 4
(Objective 7)

6. c, d, e, g, h, j. There is insufficient information given to determine whether the patient had ataxic or Cheyne-Stokes respirations. (Objective 5)

CHAPTER

25

Spinal Trauma

READING ASSIGNMENT
Chapter 25, pages 606-629, in *Mosby's Paramedic Textbook,* ed. 3

OBJECTIVES
Upon completion of this chapter, the paramedic student will be able to:
1. Describe the incidence, morbidity, and mortality related to spinal injury.
2. Predict mechanisms of injury that are likely to cause spinal injury.
3. Describe the anatomy and physiology of the spine and spinal cord.
4. Outline the general assessment of a patient with suspected spinal injury.
5. Distinguish between types of spinal injury.
6. Describe prehospital evaluation and assessment of spinal cord injury.
7. Identify prehospital management of the patient with spinal injuries.
8. Distinguish between spinal shock, neurogenic shock, and autonomic hyperreflexia syndrome.
9. Describe selected nontraumatic spinal conditions and the prehospital assessment and treatment of them.

SUMMARY
- Most SCIs are the result of motor vehicle crashes. Other causes are falls, penetrating injuries from acts of human violence, and sport injuries.
- The paramedic can classify the MOI as positive, negative, or uncertain. This classification is combined with the clinical guidelines for evaluating SCI, which include the following signs and symptoms: pain, tenderness, painful movement, deformity, cuts/bruises over spinal area, paralysis, paresthesias, and weakness. This system can help to identify cases in which spinal immobilization is appropriate.
- The spinal column is composed of 33 vertebrae. These are divided into five sections. The sections are 7 cervical, 12 thoracic, 5 lumbar, 5 sacral (fused), and 4 coccygeal (fused).
- The specific mechanisms of injury that frequently cause spinal trauma are axial loading; extremes of flexion, hyperextension, or hyperrotation; excessive lateral bending; and distraction.
- Spinal injuries may be classified as sprains and strains, fractures and dislocations, sacral and coccygeal fractures, and cord injuries. The spinal cord may sustain a primary or a secondary injury. Lesions (transections) of the spinal cord are classified as complete or incomplete.
- With spinal injuries, the first priority is to evaluate and manage any threats to life. The second priority is to preserve spinal cord function. This includes avoiding secondary injury to the spinal cord. These goals are best met by maintaining a high degree of suspicion for the presence of spinal trauma, by providing early spinal immobilization, by rapidly correcting any volume deficit, and by administering oxygen.
- General principles of spinal immobilization include prevention of further injury; treating the spine as a long bone with a joint at either end (the head and pelvis); always using complete spinal immobilization; beginning spinal

333

immobilization in the initial assessment and maintaining it until the spine is immobilized completely on the long spine board; and placing the patient's head in a neutral, in-line position, unless contraindicated.

- Spinal shock refers to a temporary loss of all types of spinal cord function distal to the injury.
- Neurogenic shock produces a loss of sympathetic tone to the vessels. This causes relative hypotension; warm, dry, and pink skin; and relative bradycardia.
- Autonomic hyperreflexia syndrome results from a massive, uncompensated cardiovascular response that stimulates the sympathetic nervous system. This response in turn causes an increase in blood pressure and other symptoms.
- Some nontraumatic spinal conditions include low back pain, degenerative disk disease, spondylolysis, herniated intervertebral disk, and spinal cord tumors. The management of patients with nontraumatic back pain in the prehospital setting is mainly supportive. The goal is to help patients decrease their pain and discomfort.

REVIEW QUESTIONS

Match the spinal illness/injury in Column II with the description in Column I. Use each term only once.

Column I	Column II
1. _____ A tear in the capsule that encloses the center of the disk	**a.** Anterior cord syndrome
2. _____ Nontraumatic structural defect that involves the lamina or vertebral joint	**b.** Autonomic hyperreflexia syndrome
3. _____ Paralysis and decreased pain and temperature sensation below a flexion injury	**c.** Brown-Séquard syndrome
4. _____ Sprain causing partial dislocation of intervertebral joints	**d.** Central cord syndrome
5. _____ Hemitransection of cord with weakness on the injured side	**e.** Herniated nucleus pulposus
6. _____ Whiplash from a low-speed, rear-end collision	**f.** Hyperextension strain
7. _____ Sudden rapid increase in blood pressure, relieved by emptying of the bladder	**g.** Neurogenic hypotension
8. _____ Bradycardia, warm skin, and low blood pressure	**h.** Spinal cord tumors
9. _____ Abnormal tissue growth in the spine that may cause spasticity	**i.** Spinal shock
10. _____ Injury characterized by paralysis of the arms with sacral sparing	**j.** Spondylosis
	k. Subluxation

11. In each of the following situations, state whether the mechanism of injury is negative, positive, or uncertain related to your assessment of the spine.

   a. A soccer player falls and twists her knee._____

   b. A patient is ejected during a rollover crash._____

   c. A patient has a gunshot wound lateral to the spine._____

   d. A young man falls 3 feet off a porch._____

   e. A patient is the restrained driver in a motor vehicle crash, and the rear hood is buckled.

   _____

   f. A child dives off the high board and strikes the bottom of the pool with his head.

   _____

   g. A woman who was running slips and falls, striking her head on a ceramic tile floor.

   _____

12. List five preexisting conditions that can increase the risk of spine injury or complicate the injury.

    a.

    b.

    c.

    d.

    e.

13. Spinal sprains and strains usually result from (a) _____ and (b) _____ forces. A hyperflexion sprain occurs when a tear is present in the posterior (c) _____ and _____, which allows partial (d) _____ of the intervertebral joints. Hyperextension strains are common with low-velocity, rear-end automobile collisions and are known commonly as (e) _____. The most frequently injured spinal regions, in descending order, are (f) _____ to _____, (g) _____ to _____, and (h) _____ to _____. The most common are wedge-shaped (i) _____ fractures. (j) _____ and (k) _____ are extremely unstable injuries caused by a combination of severe hyperflexion and compression forces.

14. A cyclist was thrown from his bike and has severe pain in the back between his scapulae. List signs and symptoms that can indicate a complete cord lesion as a result of this injury.

    _____

    _____

Questions 15 to 17 pertain to the following case study:

   A 35-year-old was involved in a motor vehicle crash with moderate damage, which you classify as an uncertain mechanism for spine injury. She says she is fine and just wants to be "checked out" at the hospital.

15. Which conditions or situations would make her unreliable to perform spinal examination for clinical criteria?

    _____

    _____

16. Describe your examination for motor findings suggestive of spine injury.

    _____

    _____

17. Describe how to perform the sensory exam to evaluate for spine injury on this patient.

    _____

18. Identify five situations involving suspected cervical spine injury when the head should *not* be moved to a neutral inline position with manual immobilization.

    a.

    b.

c.

d.

e.

19. Identify the steps involved in rolling of a supine patient (Fig. 25-1), including positioning of rescuers.

A.

B.

C.

D.

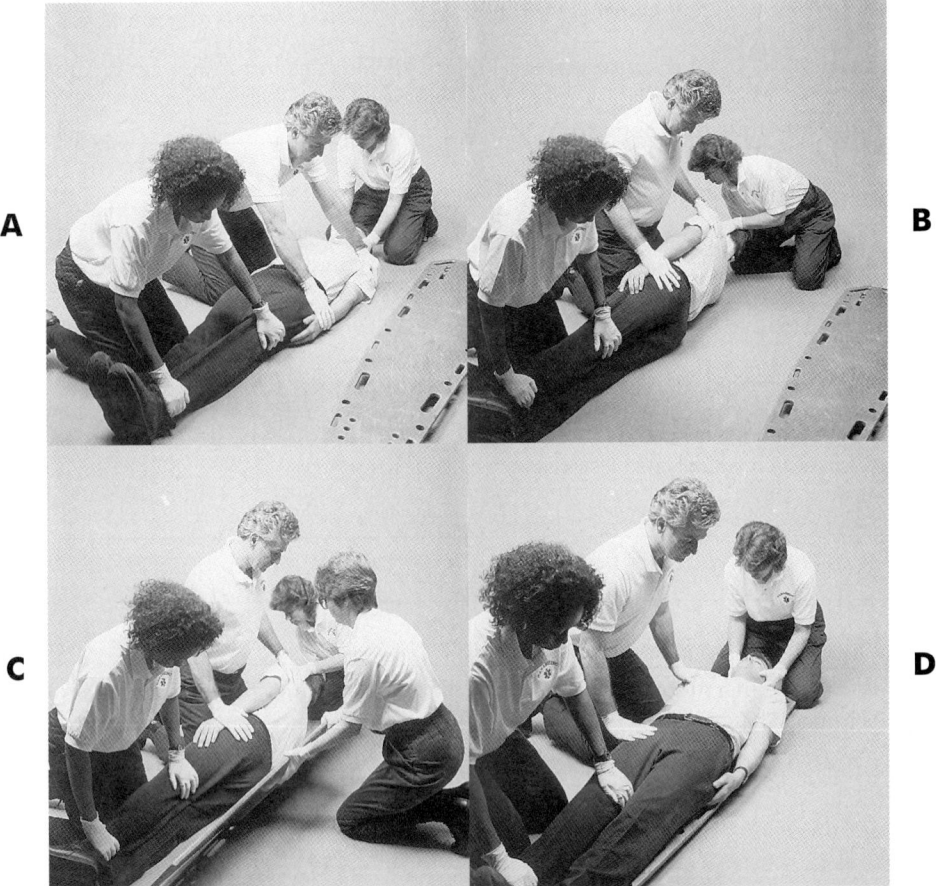

Figure 25-1

20. Identify drugs that may be used for each of the following spinal cord emergencies:

a. Spinal cord injury with paralysis:

_____

b. Spinal cord injury with hypotension and bradycardia:

_____

STUDENT SELF-ASSESSMENT

21. Most spinal injuries occur as a result of which of the following?
    a. Falls
    b. Motor vehicle crashes
    c. Sports-related injuries
    d. Penetrating injuries from acts of violence
22. Which of the following classifications of mechanism of injury would be given to a fall from the roof of a single-story residence?
    a. Alternative mechanism of injury
    b. Negative mechanism of injury
    c. Positive mechanism of injury
    d. Uncertain mechanism of injury
23. Which of the following patients would be considered reliable to assess for spinal cord injury?
    a. A patient who witnessed the death of his or her child in crash.
    b. A patient with a severely angulated, partially amputated foot.
    c. A patient who cannot communicate in a language you understand.
    d. A patient who is complaining of knee and hip pain with no deformity.
24. Which is the most flexible area of the spine?
    a. Cervical spine   c. Sacral spine
    b. Lumbar spine   d. Thoracic spine
25. A side-impact motor vehicle collision is most likely to produce spinal injury from extremes in which motion?
    a. Axial loading   c. Flexion
    b. Distraction   d. Lateral bending
26. Which finding on a patient with uncertain mechanism of injury should cause you to suspect spine trauma and to immobilize the spine?
    a. High blood pressure
    b. History of Parkinson's disease
    c. Laceration on the scalp
    d. Pain or tenderness of the neck
27. Hyperflexion sprains can cause partial dislocation of the intervertebral joints. This condition is known as which of the following?
    a. Axial loading   c. Subluxation
    b. Herniated disks   d. Whiplash
28. Fractures at the level of S1 and S2 may lead to which of the following?
    a. Loss of bowel and bladder function
    b. Neurogenic shock
    c. Paralysis of the legs
    d. Transection of the spinal cord
29. Paralysis and loss of sensation below the umbilicus indicate an injury at the level of which of the following?
    a. C4   c. T10
    b. T4   d. S1
30. Which of the following is a sign of autonomic dysfunction resulting from spinal cord injury?
    a. Bradycardia   c. Profuse sweating
    b. Hypertension   d. Polyuria
31. Which of the following signs or symptoms is associated with central cord syndrome?
    a. Intact light touch and position sensation
    b. Greater motor weakness or paralysis in the arms than legs
    c. Loss of pain and temperature sensation on the side of injury
    d. Weakness in the upper and lower extremities on the side opposite the injury
32. Respiratory distress should be anticipated in the patient with which of the following?
    a. Brown-Séquard syndrome
    b. Herniated thoracic disk
    c. Hyperextension strain
    d. Spinal cord transection above C5 to C6

33. The purpose of immobilizing the patient suspected to have spinal injury in the prehospital setting is which of the following?
   a. To apply traction to pull apart injured bones
   b. To minimize neurogenic shock
   c. To prevent primary injury
   d. To prevent additional cord hypoxia or edema
34. When a patient on a long spine board is immobilized, which of the following body regions should be secured first?
   a. Arms
   b. Head
   c. Legs
   d. Torso
35. Which of the following cord injury presentations involves flaccid paralysis that usually resolves within 24 hours?
   a. Autonomic hyperreflexia syndrome
   b. Neurogenic hypotension
   c. Spinal shock
   d. Spondylosis
36. Which of the following medical conditions of the spine can increase the risk of spinal fractures?
   a. Degenerative disk disease
   b. Herniated intervertebral disk
   c. Spinal cord tumors
   d. Spondylolysis

WRAP IT UP

You are dispatched to a call to "assist the invalid." As per protocol, you respond "on the quiet" with no lights or sirens. When you arrive at the home of the 87-year-old patient, his wife tells you that he tripped over a videotape in the living room and fell forward, striking his forehead on the coffee table. As you approach him, he apologizes profusely for calling you to help him up off the floor. He is conscious, alert, and oriented, and you can see a small abrasion on his mid-forehead. When you ask him if anything hurts, he reaches around to his neck, rubs it vigorously, and says that his neck is sore. You palpate his neck, and he says the cervical spine area is tender, but you feel no crepitus and note no deformity. Your partner begins cervical-spine immobilization as you continue your exam. You can see that his breathing is normal, and palpation of his radial pulse reveals a normal, regular rate with warm, dry skin. A quick head-to-toe exam is unremarkable except for his persistent complaint of an "electric shock" sensation in his extremities. You explain to the patient your concern that he may have a spine injury, and he consents to transport. After application of the cervical collar, you logroll him and secure him to the long backboard. Vital signs are BP 134/78 mm Hg, P 60, R 20, SaO$_2$ 96%. You initiate an IV and contact medical direction, who advises no further. The patient's condition remains stable, and you give report to the charge nurse in the ED. Later, the charge nurse calls you to let you know that the patient has an unstable fracture of C2 and C3. A halo vest has been applied, and his condition remains stable.

1. Which is the most common mechanism of injury for spinal injuries?
   a. Falls
   b. Motor vehicle crashes
   c. Penetrating injuries
   d. Sport injuries
2. Which mechanism of injury occurred in this case?
   a. Negative
   b. Positive
   c. Uncertain
3. Place a check mark beside the signs or symptoms that made you determine that spinal immobilization was indicated for this patient.
   a. _____ Trauma with use of intoxicating substances
   b. _____ Seizure activity
   c. _____ Complaints of pain in neck or arms
   d. _____ Tender neck on examination
   e. _____ Unconscious after head injury
   f. _____ Significant injury above clavicle
   g. _____ Fall greater than 3 times patient's height
   h. _____ Fall and bilateral heel fracture
   i. _____ Injury from high-speed motor vehicle collision

4. Which forces likely injured the spine in this case?
   a. Axial loading
   b. Distraction
   c. Lateral bending
   d. Hyperextension and/or hyperflexion

5. If you had merely assisted the patient to his feet without performing a history or examination on him, what could have happened to his spinal cord?

_____

6. List some signs or symptoms that would indicate that this patient had a spinal cord injury.

_____

7. Place a check mark beside the signs or symptoms you would anticipate if the spinal cord were injured and the patient were developing neurogenic shock.
   a. _____ Bradycardia   **e.** _____ Hypotension
   b. _____ Cool skin   **f.** _____ Moist skin
   c. _____ Dry skin   **g.** _____ Tachycardia
   d. _____ Hypertension   **h.** _____ Warm skin

CHAPTER 25 ANSWERS

REVIEW QUESTIONS

1. e
(Objective 9)

2. j
(Objective 9)

3. a
(Objective 5)

4. k
(Objective 5)

5. c
(Objective 5)

6. f
(Objective 5)

7. b
(Objective 8)

8. g
(Objective 8)

9. h
(Objective 9)

10. d
(Objective 5)

11. a. Negative
  b. Positive
  c. Positive
  d. Uncertain
  e. Uncertain
  f. Positive
  g. Uncertain
  (Objective 2)

12. Damage from spinal injury can occur more easily or be complicated by one or more of the following:
  a. Increased age
  b. Osteoporosis
  c. Spondylosis
  d. Rheumatoid arthritis
  e. Paget's disease
  f. Congenital cord anomalies (fusion, narrow spinal canal)
  (Objective 4)

13. a. Hyperflexion
   b. Hyperextension
   c. Ligamentous complex and joint capsule
   d. Dislocation (subluxation)
   e. Whiplash
   f. C5 to C7
   g. C1 to C2
   h. T12 to L2
   i. Compression
   j. Teardrop fractures
   k. Dislocations
   (Objective 5)

14. Absence of motor and sensory function below the nipple, relative bradycardia, hypotension, priapism, unstable body temperature, loss of bowel and bladder control, and decreased depth of respiration (loss of inervation of most intercostal muscles)
   (Objective 6)

15. To be reliable, she must be calm, cooperative, sober, alert, and oriented. If she exhibits any of the following, she should be considered unreliable: acute stress reaction, brain injury, intoxication, abnormal mental status, distracting injuries, or problems in communication.
   (Objective 4)

16. Motor evaluation: Ask the patient to move her arms and legs. Ask her to flex her elbow, grab and squeeze your fingers, and extend her elbows. Have the patient spread the fingers of both hands and keep them apart while you squeeze the second and fourth fingers. A normal exam produces springlike resistance. Support the patient's lower arm and ask her to hold her wrists or fingers out straight while you press down on her fingers. Moderate resistance should be felt. Place your hands at the sole of each foot and ask the patient to push against your hands. Both sides should feel equal and strong. Then, hold the patient's feet (with fingers on her toes) and instruct her to pull them back to her nose. Both sides should feel equal and strong.
   (Objectives 4 and 6)

17. Sensory evaluation: Question the patient about pain in the neck or back and any feelings of numbness or tingling in the body. Assess light touch on each hand and each foot (with the patient's eyes closed) and then, if necessary, prick the hands and feet with a sharp object (without breaking the skin).
   (Objectives 4 and 6)

18. a. Increasing pain or neurological deficits during movement
   b. Resistance to movement
   c. Muscle spasm
   d. Airway compromise caused by repositioning
   e. Severe misalignment of head from midline
   (Objective 7)

19. a. Rescuer 1 is positioned at the patient's head, providing in-line manual stabilization. Rescuers 2 and 3 are positioned at the patient's midthorax and knees.
   b. While maintaining immobilization, the rescuers, in one organized move, slowly logroll the patient onto his or her side, perpendicular to the ground.
   c. Rescuer 4 positions the long spine board by placing the device flat on the ground or at a 30- to 40-degree angle against the patient's back.
   d. In one organized move, the rescuers slowly logroll and center the patient onto the long spine board.
   (Objective 7)

20. a. Methylprednisolone 30 mg/kg bolus, followed by 5.4 mg/kg/hr for 23 hours
   Other experimental treatments include naloxone and calcium channel blockers (consult medical direction).
   b. Dopamine

21. b. In order of frequency of occurrence, they are motor vehicle crashes, falls, penetrating injuries, and sports injuries.
(Objective 1)

22. c. Most single-story homes are more than 3 times a person's height, which is classified as positive mechanism of injury.

23. d. The patient in (a) may be experiencing a stress reaction. The patient in (b) has a distracting injury. You cannot examine the patient in (c) well enough to rule out spinal injury by clinical criteria because of the language barrier.
(Objective 2)

24. a. The cervical spine allows the head to rotate with an almost 180-degree range of motion, 60 degrees of flexion, and 70 degrees of extension.
(Objective 3)

25. d. Axial loading occurs when the spine is compressed vertically. Distraction results from excessive "pulling" on the spinal cord. Flexion is a bending motion that decreases the angle between two joints, which more often results from anterior/posterior-type motion.
(Objective 2)

26. d. Pain or tenderness of the neck with or without palpation always should indicate immobilization of the spine.
(Objective 4)

27. c. Axial loading is a vertical loading mechanism of injury. A herniated disk occurs when the cartilage surrounding an intervertebral disk ruptures and releases the pulpy elastic substance that cushions the vertebrae above and below, causing pain and damage to nerve roots.[1]
(Objective 5)

28. a. The spinal cord terminates at L2.
(Objective 5)

29. c. C3 and C4 would involve sensory loss at the top of the shoulder; T4 at the nipple; and S1 on the lateral foot.
(Objectives 4 and 6)

30. a. Hypotension, priapism, loss of sweating and shivering, poikilothermy, and loss of bowel and bladder control are also signs.
(Objective 6)

31. b. This weakness usually results from hyperextension or hyperflexion injuries.
(Objective 5)

32. d. Transection of the cord above C3 usually results in respiratory arrest. Lesions that occur at C4 may result in diaphragmatic paralysis. Lesions at C5-C6 spare the diaphragm but result in loss of significant intercostal muscle function.
(Objective 6)

33. d. Traction should not be applied on the spine in the field. Primary injury occurs at the time the initial forces are applied.
(Objective 7)

34. d. Immobilize the torso first to prevent angulation of the cervical spine.
(Objective 7)

---

[1] Anderson KN, Anderson LE: *Mosby's medical, nursing, & allied health dictionary,* ed 3, St Louis, 1990, Mosby.

35. c. Spinal shock results from a temporary loss of all spinal cord function distal to the injury.
(Objective 8)

36. d. Rotational stress fractures are common at the affected site of spondylosis.
(Objective 9)

WRAP IT UP

1. b. Motor vehicle collisions, falls, and then penetrating trauma and sports injuries.
(Objective 1)

2. c. This was a single-level fall.
(Objective 2)

3. c, d. Neck pain is the most important predictor of cervical spine injury.
(Objective 4)

4. d. The mechanism of injury and abrasion to his forehead lead us to believe that his head was flexed or extended forcefully.
(Objective 2)

5. It could have caused a partial or complete cord injury (causing paralysis) if the unstable cervical spine impinged on the delicate spinal cord.
(Objective 2)

6. The patient was complaining of radicular (electrical shock) pain, a symptom of cord injury. Additional signs or symptoms could include paralysis, paresthesias, weakness, neurological deficit, priapism, loss of sweating/shivering, poikilothermy, and loss of bowel and bladder control.
(Objective 6)

7. a, c, e, h
(Objective 8)

CHAPTER

26

Thoracic Trauma

READING ASSIGNMENT
Chapter 26, pages 630-643, in *Mosby's Paramedic Textbook*, ed. 3

OBJECTIVES
Upon completion of this chapter, the paramedic student will be able to:
1. Discuss the factor and mechanism of injury associated with thoracic trauma.
2. Describe the mechanism of injury, signs and symptoms, and management of skeletal injuries to the chest.
3. Describe the mechanism of injury, signs and symptoms, and prehospital management of pulmonary trauma.
4. Describe the mechanism of injury, signs and symptoms, and prehospital management of injuries to the heart and great vessels.
5. Outline the mechanism of injury, signs and symptoms, and prehospital care of the patient with esophageal and tracheobronchial injury and diaphragmatic rupture.

SUMMARY
- Thoracic trauma injuries are caused by blunt or penetrating trauma. Such trauma often results from motor vehicle crashes, falls from heights, blast injuries, blows to the chest, chest compression, gunshot wounds, and stab wounds.
- Fractures of the clavicle, ribs, or sternum, and as well as flail chest, may be caused by blunt or penetrating trauma. Complications of skeletal trauma of the chest may include cardiac, vascular, or pulmonary injuries.
- Closed pneumothorax may be life-threatening if (1) it is a tension pneumothorax, (2) it occupies more than 40% of the hemithorax, or (3) it occurs in a patient in shock or a preexisting pulmonary or cardiovascular disease. Open pneumothorax may result in severe ventilatory dysfunction, hypoxemia, and death unless it is quickly recognized and corrected. Tension pneumothorax is a true emergency. It results in profound hypoventilation. It may result in death if it is not quickly recognized and managed. Hemothorax may result in massive blood loss. These patients often have hypovolemia and hypoxemia. Pulmonary contusion results when trauma to the lung causes alveolar and capillary damage. Severe hypoxemia may develop. The degree of hypoxemia is directly related to the size of the contused area. Traumatic asphyxia results from forces that cause an increase in intrathoracic pressure. When it occurs alone, it is often not lethal. However, brain hemorrhages, seizures, coma, and death have been reported after these injuries.
- The extent of injury from myocardial contusion may vary. The injury may be only a localized bruise. However, it also may be a full-thickness injury to the wall of the heart. The full-thickness injury may result in cardiac rupture, ventricular aneurysm, or a traumatic myocardial infarction. Pericardial tamponade occurs if 150 to 200 mL of blood enters the pericardial space suddenly. This results in a decrease in stroke volume and cardiac output. *Myocardial rupture* refers to an acute traumatic perforation of the ventricles or atria. It is nearly always immediately fatal. However, death may be delayed for several weeks after blunt trauma. Aortic rupture is a severe injury. There is

an 80% to 90% mortality rate in the first hour. The paramedic should consider the possibility of aortic rupture in any trauma patient who has unexplained shock after a rapid deceleration injury.

- Esophageal injuries most frequently often are caused by penetrating trauma (e.g., missile projectile and knife wounds). Tracheobronchial injuries are rare. (They occur in fewer than 3% of victims of blunt or penetrating chest trauma, but the mortality rate is over 30%.) A tension pneumothorax that does not improve following needle decompression or the absence of a continuous flow of air from the needle following decompression should alert the paramedic to the possibility of a tracheobronchial injury.

- Diaphragmatic ruptures may allow abdominal organs to enter the thoracic cavity. There they may cause compression of the lung, resulting in a reduction in ventilation, a decrease in venous return, a decrease in cardiac output, and shock.

REVIEW QUESTIONS

Questions 1 to 3 pertain to the following case study:

> You are transferring a 26-year-old woman who was a passenger in a car struck laterally on her door. She has a fractured right humerus and multiple fractures of ribs 3 to 8. En route to the trauma center, you note paradoxical movement of her chest.

1. What chest injury do you suspect?

_____

2. Why is the patient likely to become hypoxic following this injury?

_____

3. What patient care measures should you use to improve ventilation?

_____

4. Identify three symptoms common to all types of pneumothorax.
   a.
   b.
   c.

5. A deer hunter is shot accidentally with a 30-30 caliber rifle. The hunter has an open wound inferior to the right nipple, and you cannot find an exit wound.

   a. Why is this patient likely to become hypoxic?

_____

_____

   b. What interventions must be taken immediately to correct the hypoxia?

_____

_____

6. A patient from a motor vehicle crash has sustained severe blunt chest trauma. He has diminished breath sounds on the right side of the chest. He is anxious and dyspneic.

   a. What additional signs and symptoms would indicate that he has developed a tension pneumothorax?

_____

b. Describe the prehospital intervention for tension pneumothorax.

_____

_____

7. What two life-threatening conditions may be caused by hemothorax?

   a.

   b.

8. You are called to care for a worker who was crushed momentarily between a truck and a loading dock. His face and head are a bright, reddish purple, and his jugular veins are greatly distended.

   a. What injury do you suspect?

_____

   b. What treatment would you provide?

_____

9. A 28-year-old woman was involved in a frontal collision, during which her chest struck the steering wheel. She complains of crushing substernal chest pain and palpitations. Her blood pressure is normal, her pulse is 110 and irregular, and her lungs are clear.

   a. What injury do you suspect?

_____

   b. What treatment measures should be instituted for this patient?

_____

10. A 27-year-old was splitting wood when a metal splinter flew off the ax and penetrated his chest. On your arrival, he is confused, with a systolic blood pressure of 80 mm Hg, a narrow pulse pressure, muffled heart sounds, and distended neck veins. You notice bulging veins on his forearm when you prepare to start an IV.

   a. What chest injury do you suspect?

_____

   b. What prehospital care should be rendered?

_____

11. What signs should be anticipated in a patient with an aortic rupture caused by a rapid deceleration injury?

_____

STUDENT SELF-ASSESSMENT

12. Which of the following is true regarding chest trauma?
    a. It is associated with a small number of deaths each year.
    b. It only occurs with motor vehicle crashes and penetrating injury.
    c. It only includes soft tissue injuries to the chest.
    d. The use of seat belts decreases the mortality associated with it.

13. Which of the following is true regarding clavicle fractures?
    a. Clavicle fractures are unusual injuries.
    b. They are never serious injuries.
    c. They usually occur when the arm is twisted.
    d. They can be treated with a sling and swath.
14. Which of the following is true regarding rib fractures?
    a. They are more common in children.
    b. The first rib frequently is fractured.
    c. They are associated with pancreatic injury.
    d. Ribs 3 to 8 are most commonly fractured.
15. Respiratory distress in a patient with flail chest most often is associated with which of the following?
    a. Impaired mechanics of respiration
    b. Open chest wounds
    c. Severe pain that increases with respiration
    d. Underlying pulmonary contusion
16. Sternal injuries frequently are associated with which of the following?
    a. Airway compromise
    b. Flail chest
    c. Myocardial injury
    d. Spleen injury
17. Which is the most common cause of pneumothorax?
    a. Excessive pressure on the chest wall
    b. Penetration from a gun or knife
    c. Penetration from a rib fracture
    d. Spontaneous pneumothorax
18. When is a pneumothorax least likely to cause a life threat?
    a. It is closed.
    b. It is a tension pneumothorax.
    c. It occupies more than 40% of the hemithorax.
    d. It occurs in a patient with shock.
19. Your patient has a pneumothorax and may be developing a hemothorax. What signs or symptoms will you anticipate?
    a. Bradypnea
    b. Hypotension
    c. Tracheal deviation away from the affected side
    d. Widened pulse pressure
20. Injury to the lung tissue may occur when overexpansion of air in the lungs occurs after the primary energy wave has passed. This is known as which of the following?
    a. Implosion effect
    b. Inertial effect
    c. Paper-bag effect
    d. Spalding effect
21. What often occurs as a result of pulmonary contusion?
    a. Hypovolemia
    b. Hypoxia
    c. Pericardial tamponade
    d. Pneumothorax
22. Which of the following is *not* a sign associated with Beck's triad (found in pericardial tamponade)?
    a. Jugular vein distention
    b. Muffled heart sounds
    c. Narrowing pulse pressure
    d. Tracheal deviation
23. Which of the following is a complication of pericardiocentesis?
    a. Cardiac dysrhythmias
    b. Increased tamponade
    c. Laceration of a coronary artery
    d. Laceration of the ventricle
    e. All of the above
24. Your patient was involved in a high-speed motor vehicle crash. Which of the following signs may signal aortic rupture?
    a. Congestive heart failure
    b. Decreased breath sounds
    c. Hypertension
    d. Jugular venous distention
25. Your patient was in a motorcycle crash and has dyspnea and bowel sounds at the nipple line on the left side of the chest. You suspect which of the following?
    a. Pericardial tamponade
    b. Liver rupture
    c. Diaphragmatic rupture
    d. Kidney injury

WRAP IT UP

You respond to a "vehicle accident" with possible rescue. When you arrive, you see a single car that has struck a light standard, knocking it to the ground. The safety officer verifies that you can approach the vehicle after he determines that it is not in contact with the pole, and he ensures that the scene is blocked from oncoming traffic. You are able to open the driver door to access your only patient, an 18-year-old man who was not restrained and was driving an older car with no air bags. He is conscious and alert, with a laceration on his forehead. He is moaning loudly and complaining of pain in his legs. Your partner takes spinal precautions while you quickly assess his condition. He has a weak, rapid radial and carotid pulse with pale, cool skin and rapid respirations, and you think that his breath sounds are diminished slightly on the left. He has tenderness and redness over his anterior chest and both lower legs. You and the fire crew on the scene apply oxygen and a cervical collar and perform a rapid extrication, moving him quickly to the ambulance after he is secured onto the stretcher. In the ambulance your team moves quickly to assess vital signs: BP 130/80 mm Hg, P 128, R 24, and SaO_2 on non-rebreather mask is 95%. His breath sounds are difficult to hear, but it seems they are still decreased on the left. The rest of your exam shows bilateral tenderness, deformity, and swelling in the lower legs with weak pedal pulses palpable. You ask your partner to get en route to the trauma center quickly and initiate two IVs and call a report en route. Repeat vital signs remain unchanged during transport. Your medical officer calls back an hour later and is told that the patient was diagnosed with concussion, left pneumothorax, fractured second left rib, and bilateral closed fractures of the tibia and fibula and that they are monitoring the patient for an aortic tear because the initial films show some widening in the mediastinum. He is presently stable with a chest tube in the left side of his chest.

1. Circle the classifications of chest trauma with which the patient has been diagnosed or for which he is being evaluated.
    a. Diaphragmatic injury
    b. Heart and great vessel injury
    c. Pulmonary injury
    d. Skeletal injury
2. What signs or symptoms were present that indicated possible bony chest injury?

_____

3. i. Place a check mark beside the signs or symptoms of pneumothorax that this patient displayed.
   ii. Place a *t* beside additional signs or symptoms that would have indicated this patient was developing a tension pneumothorax.

   a. _____ Chest pain   f. _____ Hypotension
   b. _____ Cyanosis   g. _____ Subcutaneous emphysema
   c. _____ Decreased breath sounds on affected side   h. _____ Tachycardia
   d. _____ Distended neck veins   i. _____ Tachypnea
   e. _____ Dyspnea   j. _____ Tracheal deviation

4. How did you treat the pneumothorax in the field?

_____

5. Which of the following is true regarding aortic rupture?
    a. Fracture of the second rib is associated with this injury.
    b. Hypotension will always be seen.
    c. Immediate death rarely is seen with aortic tears.
    d. Quadriplegia can be associated with this injury.

CHAPTER 26 ANSWERS

REVIEW QUESTIONS

1. Flail chest
   (Objective 2)

2. The pulmonary contusion and injured segment of the chest will not expand; therefore insufficient negative pressure is generated in the chest to draw in a normal amount of air.
   (Objective 2)

3. Intubate if the Glasgow Coma Scale score is less than 8 or if the patient has severe hypoxia and assist ventilations with positive pressure (demand valve, bag-valve) with 100% oxygen. Monitor vital signs, electrocardiogram, and oxygen saturation.
   (Objective 2)

4. Dyspnea, tachypnea, diminished breath sounds on the affected side, and chest pain on inspiration
   (Objective 3)

5. a. During inspiration, some air will enter the wound instead of the trachea, which decreases air entering the lung for ventilation
   b. Seal wound on three sides with occlusive dressing. Administer high-flow oxygen by non-rebreather mask.
   (Objective 3)

6. a. Cyanosis, tracheal deviation, tachycardia, hypotension, and distended neck veins
   b. Insert a 14-gauge catheter in the midclavicular line of the second or third intercostal space on the side of the pneumothorax. Listen for a rush of air, consider a flutter valve, reevaluate the patient, and repeat these steps en route if the needle clots.
   (Objective 3)

7. Hypoxia and hypovolemic shock
   (Objective 3)

8. a. Traumatic asphyxia
   b. Oxygenate and maintain airway and ventilation and evaluate for associated injuries.
   (Objective 3)

9. a. Myocardial contusion
   b. Oxygen administration, electrocardiographic monitoring, and treatment of dysrhythmias per protocol
   (Objective 4)

10. a. Pericardial tamponade
    b. Oxygen administration, fluid replacement, rapid transport, consideration of pericardiocentesis (only with authorization and specialized training)
    (Objective 4)

11. Upper extremity or generalized hypertension, systolic murmur, paraplegia (rare), and severe shock
    (Objective 4)

12. d. At least 25% of trauma deaths are associated with chest trauma. Falls, crush injuries, blast injuries, and blows to the chest also can cause significant thoracic trauma.
    (Objective 1)

13. d. The clavicle is one of the most commonly fractured bones. Rarely, clavicle fracture can be complicated by injury to the subclavian vein or artery from bony fragment penetration. The mechanism typically involves a fall on outstretched arms or the shoulder.
(Objective 2)

14. d. Children have more elastic chests and are less likely to have rib fractures. The first rib is rarely fractured. The pancreas lies protected behind other abdominal organs and is unlikely to be affected by rib fractures.
(Objective 2)

15. d. The damaged tissue often results in significant hypoxia.
(Objective 2)

16. c. The heart lies under the sternum and may be compressed if it is injured.
(Objective 2)

17. c. Excessive pressure on the chest wall can cause pneumothorax (paper-bag effect). Spontaneous pneumothorax occurs when a rupture or tear develops in the lung parenchyma for no apparent reason.
(Objective 3)

18. a. Pneumothorax in a patient with preexisting lung or heart disease also can be lethal.
(Objective 3)

19. b. Hypotension will develop as a result of hypovolemic shock. Tachypnea, deviation to the affected side (rare), and narrowed pulse pressure also may occur.
(Objective 3)

20. c. Inertial effect is a stretching and shearing of alveoli and intravascular structures. When the kinetic wave of energy is reflected partially at the alveolar membrane surface and the remainder causes a localized release of energy, it is referred to as the *Spalding effect*.
(Objective 3)

21. b. Profound hypoxia can result from abnormal lung function.
(Objective 3)

22. d. Tracheal deviation may be found in some patients with tension pneumothorax.
(Objective 4)

23. e. Laceration of the liver also may occur.
(Objective 4)

24. c. Pulses may be decreased in the lower extremities.
(Objective 5)

25. c. When the bowel moves into the chest, severe respiratory compromise occurs.
(Objective 5)

WRAP IT UP

1. b, c, d
(Objective 1)

2. Pain, redness of the skin over the area, tenderness on palpation
(Objective 2)

3. i. a, c, e, h, i
ii. b, d, f, g, j
(Objective 3)

4. High-concentration oxygen
(Objective 3)

5. a. Hypertension can be seen initially if vessel tamponade has occurred. There is an 80% to 90% chance of immediate death. Paraplegia is possible.
(Objective 4)

Abdominal Trauma

READING ASSIGNMENT
Chapter 27, pages 644-651, in *Mosby's Paramedic Textbook,* ed. 3

OBJECTIVES
Upon completion of this chapter, the paramedic student will be able to:
1. Identify mechanisms of injury associated with abdominal trauma.
2. Describe mechanisms of injury, signs and symptoms, and complications associated with abdominal solid organ, hollow organ, retroperitoneal organ, and pelvic organ injuries.
3. Outline the significance of injury to intraabdominal vascular structures.
4. Describe the prehospital assessment priorities for the patient suspected of having an abdominal injury.
5. Outline the prehospital care of the patient with abdominal trauma.

SUMMARY
- Blunt trauma to abdominal organs usually results from compression or shearing forces.
- Penetrating injury may result from stab wounds, gunshot wounds, or impaled objects.
- The two solid organs most commonly injured are the liver and the spleen. Both of these organs are primary sources of death from hemorrhage. Injuries to the hollow abdominal organs may result in sepsis, wound infection, and abscess formation.
- Injury to the retroperitoneal organs (kidneys, ureters, pancreas, duodenum) may cause massive hemorrhage.
- Injury to the pelvic organs (bladder, urethra) usually results from motor vehicle crashes that produce pelvic fractures.
- Injuries to abdominal vascular structures may be life threatening. This is due to their potential for massive hemorrhage.
- The most significant sign of severe abdominal trauma is the presence of unexplained shock.
- Emergency care of patients with abdominal trauma usually is limited to two courses of action. One is to stabilize the patient. The other is to rapidly transport the patient to a hospital for surgery to repair the injury.

REVIEW QUESTIONS
1. A 12-year-old boy recovering from mononucleosis has been hit on the left side by another child. He complains of severe left upper quadrant abdominal pain and left shoulder pain. He has signs of shock.

    a. What solid organ has most likely been injured in this situation?

b. Why would the boy complain of shoulder pain?

_____

c. What care should you provide for him?

_____

2. Describe complications that may result when hollow organs of the abdomen are injured.

_____

_____

3. List nine signs or symptoms associated with abdominal trauma.

a.

b.

c.

d.

e.

f.

g.

h.

i.

STUDENT SELF-ASSESSMENT

4. Which of the following is true of abdominal trauma?
  a. Blunt injuries do not occur when personal restraints are used.
  b. Complications of penetrating abdominal trauma appear immediately.
  c. Penetrating injury is associated with higher mortality than blunt trauma.
  d. Shearing forces may produce a tear or rupture of solid organs or blood vessels.

5. Which one of the following is the most commonly injured solid organ?
  a. Adrenal gland   **c.** Liver
  b. Kidney   **d.** Pancreas

6. After injury to the liver, patients often experience which of the following?
  a. Bowel obstruction   **c.** Peritoneal irritation
  b. Gastrointestinal bleeding **d.** Renal failure

7. Which of the following is true about renal trauma?
  a. Bleeding is usually minimal.
  b. Fractures often need surgical repair.
  c. It occurs only as a result of posterior trauma.
  d. Urine output stops.

8. Which of the following mechanisms of blunt trauma is most often associated with pancreatic injury?
  a. Bicycle handlebar impalement
  b. Falls from higher than 20 feet
  c. Punch injuries from abuse
  d. Restrained passenger in head-on crash

9. What sign or symptom is a contraindication to insertion of an indwelling Foley catheter?
  a. Blood at the urinary meatus   **c.** Burning during urination
  b. Bruising over the flank   **d.** Microscopic hematuria

10. Intraabdominal arterial and venous injuries
    a. Always present with a palpable mass
    b. Have the potential for massive hemorrhage
    c. Involve only the aorta or vena cava
    d. Occur only with penetrating trauma
11. The patient was involved in a high-speed motor vehicle crash. He refuses care. When he stands to leave, he becomes pale and states that he feels nauseated and dizzy. For which condition should you first assess as a possible cause of these signs and symptoms?
    a. Hyperventilation
    b. Preexisting medical problem
    c. Severe abdominal injury
    d. Vagal reaction to pain
12. Scene care of the patient who has signs of shock from abdominal injury should include which of the following?
    a. Comprehensive physical examination
    b. Initiation of IV fluid therapy
    c. Ongoing assessment
    d. Oxygen administration

Questions 13 to 15 pertain to the following case study:

> Your patient is a 30-year-old woman who was stabbed in the right upper quadrant of the abdomen. She is pale and restless and has cool, clammy skin. Vital signs are blood pressure, 76/58 mm Hg; pulse, 128/min; and respirations, 28/min.

13. You would suspect injury to the (1) chest, (2) liver, (3) spleen, (4) urinary bladder?
    a. (1) and (2)
    b. (1) and (3)
    c. (2) and (4)
    d. (3) and (4)
14. Interventions for this patient include which of the following?
    a. Oxygen (4 L/min via nasal cannula) and intravenous lactated Ringer solution to keep the vein open
    b. Oxygen (10 L/min via mask) and intravenous lactated Ringer solution to keep the vein open
    c. Oxygen (4 L/min via nasal cannula) and intravenous lactated Ringer solution via rapid infusion
    d. Oxygen (10 L/min via mask) and intravenous lactated Ringer solution via rapid infusion
15. Your *first* priority on arrival at this call would be
    a. Airway maintenance
    b. Administration of oxygen
    c. Scene safety
    d. Stopping the bleeding

WRAP IT UP

Dispatch radios you to respond to a call for a "cutting," stating that the scene is not safe and police are en route. You stage in the area and notify dispatch, waiting to proceed in when police notify you that the scene has been secured. Your patient is a 55-year-old obese male who was stabbed in the abdomen with a 6-inch kitchen knife by an "unknown" assailant. He is awake and alert but very anxious, and he wants to get up and walk around despite his blood-soaked shirt. You note his pale, cool skin; feel a thready, rapid, radial pulse; and then quickly pull off his shirt and pants. One stab wound is visible in the right upper quadrant on his abdomen, just below his rib cage. He denies being short of breath when you question him, and you hear clear and equal breath sounds bilaterally, but his abdomen is rigid and very tender to palpation. No other wounds are visible on your quick head to toe assessment. You quickly administer oxygen and move him to the ambulance, where you assess his vital signs: BP, 78/50 mm Hg; P, 136/min; R, 28/min; Sao$_2$ is unobtainable. You realize that the patient is a critical trauma case, but your rural location is too far from the trauma center, and no helicopter is available. You tell your partner to head for the nearest hospital. Then you continue care; you insert one IV of normal saline, wide open on blood tubing, and another in the other arm of lactated Ringer solution. By the time you have established the second line, you have arrived at the hospital, where the patient is transfused with uncrossmatched blood. Luckily the surgeon is available in-house; she determines that immediate surgery is indicated. The patient is rushed to the operating room, where his lacerated liver is repaired. He is discharged home in 10 days.

1. What other mechanisms can cause injuries to the abdominal organs?

2. Which of the following is true regarding his injury?
    a. Liver contents spilling into the peritoneal cavity cause no signs or symptoms.
    b. The liver is a solid organ, therefore the chief concern after injury is bleeding.
    c. The liver is very vascular and can be removed to prevent death from uncontrolled hemorrhage.
    d. Retroperitoneal bleeding can be severe and is hard to control after liver injury.
3. Place a ✔ beside the signs or symptoms of peritoneal irritation that this patient displayed.
    a. _____ Distention   d. _____ Pain
    b. _____ Fever   e. _____ Tenderness to palpation
    c. _____ Guarding/rigidity
4. What major artery that supplies the liver could have been injured by this penetrating wound?
    a. Celiac artery
    b. Iliac artery
    c. Inferior mesenteric artery
    d. Hepatic artery
5. What three critical interventions needed to enhance the chance of survival for patients with abdominal trauma were performed on this patient?

    a.

    b.

    c.

CHAPTER 27 ANSWERS

REVIEW QUESTIONS

1. a. Spleen; b. referred pain caused by irritation of the diaphragm by a splenic hematoma or blood in the peritoneum (Kehr sign); c. This child should have a rapid assessment. Oxygen should be administered, and rapid transport to the closest appropriate trauma center should begin immediately. Intravenous therapy using an isotonic solution should be administered at 20 mL/kg during transport. Repeat IV bolus may be indicated based on the reevaluation.
(Objective 2)

2. Sepsis, infection, abscess formation, and peritonitis (resulting from leakage of the contents of hollow organs).
(Objective 2)

3. a. Unexplained shock; b. bruising and discoloration of the abdomen; c. abrasions; d. obvious bleeding; e. pain, abdominal tenderness, or guarding; f. abdominal rigidity, distention; g. evisceration; h. rib fractures; i. pelvic fractures.
(Objective 4)

STUDENT SELF-ASSESSMENT

4. d. This injury is caused by stretching of organs and blood vessels.
(Objective 1)

5. c. The other organ most often injured is the spleen.
(Objective 2)

6. c. Shock also occurs often.
(Objective 2)

7. b. Bleeding can be severe and difficult to detect. Injury can result from anterior or posterior trauma. Urine output may contain blood.
(Objective 2)

8. a. Steering wheel trauma and penetrating trauma are also associated with pancreatic injury.
(Objective 2)

9. a. This may indicate urethral injury, which could be complicated by insertion of a catheter.
(Objective 2)

10. b. The patient often presents with signs and symptoms of shock.
(Objective 3)

11. c. With unexplained shock in a trauma patient, abdominal injury should always be at the top of your "rule out" list.
(Objective 4)

12. d. The initial exam can be done on the scene. Further examination and IV therapy may be performed en route to the hospital.
(Objective 5)

13. a. The liver is located in the right upper quadrant. The diaphragm extends low, therefore the chest cavity is easily penetrated in these types of injuries.
(Objective 1)

14. d. Administration of high-concentration oxygen and fluid resuscitation are indicated.
(Objective 5)

15. c. Scene safety should always be the first priority on every call, especially when a crime has been committed.
(Objective 5)

WRAP IT UP

1. Blunt: assault, motor vehicle collisions, falls, industrial injuries, pedestrian injuries, blast injuries. Penetrating: impaled objects, gunshot wounds.
(Objective 1)

2. b. When bile and blood spill into the peritoneal cavity after liver injury, signs and symptoms of peritoneal irritation occur. The liver is necessary for life; it can be partially removed, but complete removal results in death.
(Objective 2)

3. c, d, e
(Objective 2)

4. a. The iliac and inferior mesenteric arteries are lower in the abdomen. The portal vessel is a vein, not an artery.
(Objective 3)

5. a. Rapid transport for definitive care (surgery)
b. Oxygenation
c. Fluid resuscitation
(Objective 5)

Musculoskeletal Trauma

READING ASSIGNMENT

Chapter 28, pages 652-672, in *Mosby's Paramedic Textbook,* ed. 3

OBJECTIVES

Upon completion of this chapter, the paramedic student will be able to do the following:
1. Describe the features of each class of musculoskeletal injury.
2. Describe the features of bursitis, tendonitis, and arthritis.
3. Given a specific patient scenario, outline the prehospital assessment of the musculoskeletal system.
4. Outline general principles of splinting.
5. Describe the significance and prehospital management principles for selected upper extremity injuries.
6. Describe the significance and prehospital management principles for selected lower extremity injuries.
7. Identify prehospital management priorities for open fractures.
8. Describe the principles of realignment of angular fractures and dislocations.
9. Outline the process for referral of patients with a minor musculoskeletal injury.

SUMMARY

- Injuries that can result from traumatic force on the musculoskeletal system include fractures, sprains, strains, and joint dislocations. Problems associated with musculoskeletal injuries include hemorrhage, instability, loss of tissue, simple laceration and contamination, interruption of blood supply, and long-term disability.
- Several inflammatory and degenerative conditions may manifest as or may be complicated by extremity injury. These include bursitis, tendonitis, and arthritis.
- Common signs and symptoms of extremity trauma include pain on palpation or movement, swelling or deformity, crepitus, decreased range of motion, false movement, and decreased or absent sensory perception or circulation distal to the injury.
- Once the paramedic has assessed for life-threatening conditions, the extremity injury should be examined for pain, pallor, paresthesia, pulses, paralysis, and pressure. In addition, DCAP-BTLS should be evaluated for the injured extremity.
- Immobilization by splinting helps alleviate pain; reduces tissue injury, bleeding, and contamination of an open wound; and simplifies and facilitates transport of the patient. Splints can be categorized as rigid, soft or formable, and traction splints.
- Upper extremity injuries can be classified as fractures or dislocations of the shoulder, humerus, elbow, radius and ulna, wrist, hand, and finger. Most upper extremity injuries can be adequately immobilized by application of a sling and swathe.

- Lower extremity injuries include fractures of the pelvis and fractures or dislocations of the hip, femur, knee and patella, tibia and fibula, ankle and foot, and toes.
- Most open fractures are obvious because of associated hemorrhage. However, a small puncture wound may not be initially apparent. In addition, bleeding may be minimal. Therefore the paramedic must consider any soft tissue wound in the area of a suspected fracture to be evidence of an open fracture. Open fractures are considered a true surgical emergency. This is due to the potential for infection.
- Only *one* attempt at realignment should be made. This should be done *only* if severe neurovascular compromise is present (e.g., extremely weak or absent distal pulses). Moreover, it should be done *only* after consultation with medical direction.
- The paramedic should evaluate the need for emergency department assessment versus having the patient see his or her private physician. This need is determined by the patient's condition and the mechanism of injury.

REVIEW QUESTIONS

Match the type of fracture in column II with the description in column I. Use each answer only once.

Column I

1. _____ A cancer patient sustains a fracture despite no apparent trauma.
2. _____ A fracture is incomplete, and the bone is bent.
3. _____ Bone is sticking out of a laceration.
4. _____ A runner feels increased pain in the foot and is found to have a fracture.
5. _____ A patient's arm is broken after having been twisted in an auger.
6. _____ The skin over a deformed ankle is intact.
7. _____ The fracture extends through the growth plate.
8. _____ The x-ray reveals a shattered bone.
9. _____ The fracture appears to be at a 45-degree angle across the bone.

Column II

a. Closed
b. Comminuted
c. Epiphyseal
d. Greenstick
e. Oblique
f. Open
g. Pathological
h. Spiral
i. Stress
j. Transverse

Select *all* the appropriate immobilization devices from column II that would be used to treat the fractures in column I. You may use each term *more* than once.

Column I

10. _____ Shoulder
11. _____ Humerus
12. _____ Elbow
13. _____ Forearm
14. _____ Wrist
15. _____ Hand
16. _____ Finger
17. _____ Pelvis
18. _____ Hip
19. _____ Femur
20. _____ Knee or patella
21. _____ Tibia or fibula
22. _____ Ankle or foot
23. _____ Toes

Column II

a. Buddy splint
b. Formable splint
c. Long spine board
d. Rigid splint
e. Pneumatic antishock garment
f. Sling
g. Swathe
h. Traction splint

Questions 24 to 26 pertain to the following case study:

A 16-year-old injured his wrist after falling during a hockey game.

24. What is your primary objective when performing the initial assessment on this patient?

_____

25. What are the six *P*s of assessment for this injury?

P

P

P

P

P

P

26. As you examine this patient, you inspect and palpate the extremity to identify

D

C

A

P

B

T

L

S

27. Identify at least 11 general principles of splinting.

a.

b.

c.

d.

e.

f.

g.

h.

i.

j.

k.

Questions 28 and 29 pertain to the following case study:

A 55-year-old patient has a shortened and externally rotated hip with no pedal pulse distal to the injury. You antici-pate a 45-minute transport to the nearest medical center.

28. Why is it appropriate to attempt to realign this dislocation?

_____

29. Explain the procedure for attempting to realign the hip in this situation.

_____

STUDENT SELF-ASSESSMENT

30. Which of the following is true about a sprain?
   a. It means injury to a tendon.
   b. No tissue disruption occurs, but bruising does occur.
   c. Severe hemorrhage can occur.
   d. Joint instability and dislocation may result.

31. A _subluxation_ is another name for which of the following?
   a. Complete dislocation
   b. Incomplete dislocation
   c. Open fracture
   d. Strain

32. What is the cause of the pain associated with bursitis, tendonitis, and arthritis?
   a. Aging
   b. Degeneration
   c. Infection
   d. Inflammation

33. What group of drugs is often used to treat arthritis?
   a. Antibiotics
   b. Antipyretics
   c. Muscle relaxants
   d. NSAIDs

34. Signs or symptoms of extremity trauma that have a high urgency include which of the following?
   a. Absent distal pulses
   b. Crepitus
   c. Decreased range of motion
   d. Swelling and deformity

35. Your patient has been intubated and has signs of severe shock. His right wrist is swollen and deformed, and crepitus is present. How will you manage this extremity injury during your 7-minute transport time to the hospital?
   a. Elevation and application of ice
   b. Forearm splint
   c. Long spine board
   d. Sling and swathe

36. Boxer's fracture is the most common fracture of which bone(s)?
   a. Carpals
   b. Metacarpal
   c. Phalanges
   d. Radius

37. When a patient has a dislocation of the hip, the affected leg is usually which of the following?
   a. Lengthened and externally rotated
   b. Lengthened and internally rotated
   c. Shortened and externally rotated
   d. Shortened and internally rotated

38. A traction splint may be helpful for a patient with which of the following fractures?
   a. Femoral fracture
   b. Humeral fracture
   c. Tibial fracture
   d. Pelvic fracture

39. Your patient has severe deformity of the knee and a diminished pulse in the foot on the affected leg. This may be an indication of injury to which of the following?
   a. Femoral artery
   b. Dorsalis pedis artery
   c. Popliteal artery
   d. Posterior tibial artery

40. A bone is protruding through a wound on the lower leg. When you immobilize the fracture, the bone end slips back into the wound. What action should you take?
   a. Cover the wound with a dry sterile dressing.
   b. Irrigate the wound with sterile normal saline.
   c. Move the leg gently until the bone reappears.
   d. Soak the wound with Betadine solution.

41. Your patient fell and has a grossly deformed shoulder. Which of the following is a contraindication to realignment?
   a. Absent radial pulse
   b. Paresthesias
   c. Severe pain
   d. Thoracic spine injury

42. A woman injured her ankle during a skating activity. She has refused care and transport by EMS. What should you do before leaving the scene?
  a. Administer morphine intramuscularly for the pain.
  b. Instruct her to elevate the leg and apply ice.
  c. Have her try to bear weight and walk.
  d. Tell her to see a physician if pain persists for 2 days.

WRAP IT UP

At 0230 your pager beeps you to respond to a vehicle collision in your township. You know that you are the closest volunteer, so you respond in your truck, knowing that the ambulance will be about 10 minutes behind you. Your patient is a 45-year-old nurse whom you recognize from the ED. She was heading home from her shift when she apparently dozed off and her car ran off the road, striking a tree. Major damage was done to the front of her car, and her airbags deployed. She is conscious and crying. She says the only thing she remembers is looking up, seeing the tree, and holding on to the steering wheel. As you speak with her, you unbuckle her belt. Her skin is pink and warm, and her heart rate is increased. She tells you she thinks she has broken her arms and legs. She denies any other pain or difficulty breathing. She has bilaterally equal breath sounds and no obvious chest or abdominal trauma. Her wrists are both tender and deformed but have good pulses. Her right femur is swollen and very tender; her left lower leg is deformed, and a laceration is slowly oozing blood over the painful area. She has good sensation and movement distal to all her extremity injuries. You and another volunteer administer oxygen, assess her vital signs (BP, 110/70 mm Hg; P, 124/min; R, 20/min), initiate an IV of normal saline in the left antecubital space, and splint her left lower leg. As the ambulance arrives, she vomits and says she is feeling faint. A repeat set of vital signs shows BP, 106/70 mm Hg; P, 128/min; and R, 20/min. Even though the patient denies neck pain or tenderness, a collar is applied and she is rapidly extricated to the long spine board. A traction splint is applied to her right leg, and she is secured to the stretcher and moved to the ambulance. Under the guidance of medical direction, IV morphine is given in 2 mg doses to relieve her pain. Her forearms are splinted and elevated on pillows, and ice is applied to all injured extremities. Continuous monitoring of vital signs and extremity pulses, movement, and sensation shows no change during transport. After a total of 6 mg of morphine, the patient reports that the pain has dulled from a "10" to a "7," so you give an additional 2 mg, knowing that the movement on arrival at the ED will be painful. You apply a sterile 4 × 4 gauze to the wound on her left lower leg. You note fat globules in the oozing dark blood.

On your next trip to the hospital, you visit the patient. She will miss at least 3 months of work because of her multiple fractures. She thanks you repeatedly for giving her the pain medicine; she says her attitude toward patients who are in pain has been changed forever.

  1. List six things you should assess each time you think a patient has fractured an extremity.

  2. Describe how you would have changed your treatment if you suspected a fracture in her lower right leg as well.

  3. Identify which splint (or splints) would be appropriate for each of the patient's injuries on this call.
  a. Sling and swathe   **d.** Traction splint
  b. Rigid splint   **e.** Pillow splint
  c. Formable splint
      _____ Right and left upper extremity injuries
      _____ Right upper leg injury
      _____ Left lower leg injury

  4. Explain the principles that should be followed in applying the splints to both arms and the left lower leg.

5. What was the significance of the wound over the patient's painful leg deformity?
   a. It could greatly increase the risk of blood loss.
   b. It could signify an open fracture, which poses a high risk of infection.
   c. Unless bone can be seen sticking out, it is not significant.
   d. Unless the bleeding is uncontrolled, the wound should not be covered.

6. Explain the rationale for administering oxygen and initiating an IV in this patient.

CHAPTER 28 ANSWERS

REVIEW QUESTIONS

1. g
2. d
3. f
4. i
5. h
6. a
7. c
8. b
9. e
   (Questions 1-9: Objective 1)

10. f and g
11. b, d, f, and g
12. b, d, f, and g
13. b, d, and f
14. b, d, and f
15. b and d
16. a, b, and d
    (Questions 10-16: Objective 5)

17. c and e
18. c
19. c and h
20. b and d
21. b and d
22. b
23. a
    (Questions 17-23: Objective 6)

24. With every patient you must assess for the presence of life threats in the initial assessment.
    (Objective 3)

25. The six *P*s are pain, pallor, paresthesia, pulses, paralysis, and pressure.
    (Objective 3)

26. The initials *DCAP-BTLS* refer to deformity, contusions, abrasions, penetrations or punctures, burns, tenderness, lacerations, and swelling.
    (Objective 3)

27. The general principles of splinting are: splint joints above and below, as well as bone ends; immobilize open and closed fractures in the same manner; cover open fractures to minimize contamination; check pulses, sensation, and motor function before and after splinting; stabilize the extremity with gentle, in-line traction to the position of normal alignment; immobilize a long bone extremity in a straight position that can easily be splinted; immobilize dislocations in a position of comfort; ensure good vascular supply; immobilize joints as found; joint injuries are aligned only if no distal pulse is detected; apply cold to reduce swelling and pain; apply compression to reduce swelling; and elevate the extremity if possible.
    (Objective 4)

28. No pulse is present distal to the injury; this is an indication to attempt realignment in the prehospital setting.
    (Objective 8)

29. Administer an analgesic and/or benzodiazepine (with appropriate monitoring) if not contraindicated by other injuries. Apply in-line traction along the shaft of the femur with the hip and knee flexed at 90 degrees. Apply slow and steady traction to relax the muscle spasm. Listen for a "pop," with accompanying sudden relief of pain and easy manipulation of the leg to full extension. Immobilize the leg in full extension with the patient supine on a long spine board; reevaluate pulses and neurovascular status. If attempt is unsuccessful, place the patient supine and use pillows or blankets to immobilize the leg at a flexion not exceeding 90 degrees. (Objective 8)

STUDENT SELF-ASSESSMENT

30. d. Sprains represent injuries to ligaments. (Objective 1)

31. b. A complete dislocation is a *luxation*. (Objective 1)

32. d. Bursitis involves inflammation of the bursa; tendonitis is inflammation of a tendon caused by injury; and arthritis is inflammation of the joint. (Objective 2)

33. d. The traditional drugs in this group cause gastrointestinal complications and are being replaced by newer agents with fewer side effects. (Objective 2)

34. a. Treatment is needed for all the other signs; however, emergent interventions are needed to preserve the limb when distal pulses are absent. (Objective 3)

35. c. Because of the life threats present in this patient, time would not be taken to treat this isolated injury except to provide full-body immobilization on a spine board. (Objective 3)

36. b. The fifth metacarpal is broken in a boxer's fracture. (Objective 5)

37. d. After a hip fracture, the extremity is usually shortened and externally rotated. (Objective 6)

38. a. It is not indicated for other types of fractures. (Objective 6)

39. c. Injury to the popliteal artery is associated with knee trauma. (Objective 6)

40. a. Make sure that this is reported to the receiving medical personnel and documented in the patient care report. Assess distal pulse and sensation. (Objective 7)

41. d. The movement necessary to realign the arm could cause further injury to the back. (Objective 8)

42. b. Instructions about care of the injury should be given to the patient (preferably in writing) before you depart. (Objective 9)

WRAP IT UP

1. Assess for pain, tenderness, deformity, swelling, crepitus, any soft tissue wounds in the area of a suspected fracture, as well as distal pulses, sensation, and movement before and after splinting
   (Objective 3)

2. A traction splint would not have been appropriate if the lower leg also had been fractured. The patient could have been splinted on the spine board, using blankets or pillows to stabilize the extremity or perhaps long board splints.
   (Objective 4)

3. Upper extremity injuries: b or c. Although a sling may be helpful for immobilizing and elevating the splinted isolated upper extremity, in this case, because the patient was supine on the spine board, it wouldn't have been indicated.
   (Objectives 4, 5)

   Right upper leg injury: d
   (Objectives 4, 6)

   Left lower leg injury: b or c
   (Objectives 4, 6)

4. The distal pulse, movement, and sensation should be assessed before and after splinting. The splint should be applied to include the joints above and below the injury and should be secured firmly. The extremity should be elevated if possible and ice applied.
   (Objective 4)

5. b. Although significant open fractures pose an increased risk of bleeding, the chief concern is infection of the bone, which is very difficult and time-consuming to treat.
   (Objective 7)

6. Aside from the potential for chest and abdominal injuries based on the mechanism of injury, there is significant risk of internal bleeding from long bone fractures. This is particularly true for the femur and secondarily for the tibia and fibula.
   (Objective 3)

PART SEVEN

PART SEVEN

Cardiology

READING ASSIGNMENT

Chapter 29, pages 673-815, in *Mosby's Paramedic Textbook*, ed. 3

OBJECTIVES

Upon completion of this chapter, the paramedic student will be able to do the following:

1. Identify risk factors and prevention strategies associated with cardiovascular disease.
2. Describe the normal physiology of the heart.
3. Discuss electrophysiology as it relates to the normal electrical and mechanical events in the cardiac cycle.
4. Outline the activity of each component of the electrical conduction system of the heart.
5. Outline the appropriate assessment of a patient who may be experiencing a cardiovascular disorder.
6. Describe basic monitoring techniques that permit electrocardiogram interpretation.
7. Explain the relationship of the electrocardiogram tracing to the electrical activity of the heart.
8. Describe in sequence the steps in electrocardiogram interpretation.
9. Identify the characteristics of normal sinus rhythm.
10. When shown an electrocardiogram tracing, identify the rhythm, site of origin, possible causes, clinical significance, and prehospital management that is indicated.
11. Describe prehospital assessment and management of patients with selected cardiovascular disorders based on knowledge of the pathophysiology of the illness.
12. List indications, contraindications, and prehospital considerations when using selected cardiac interventions, including basic life support, monitor-defibrillators, defibrillation, implantable cardioverter defibrillators, synchronized cardioversion, and transcutaneous cardiac pacing.
13. List indications, contraindications, dose, and mechanism of action for pharmacological agents used to manage cardiovascular disorders.
14. Identify appropriate actions to take in the prehospital setting to terminate resuscitation.

SUMMARY

- Persons at high risk for cardiovascular disease include those with diabetes, a family history of premature cardiovascular disease, and prior myocardial infarction. Prevention strategies include community educational programs in nutrition, cessation of smoking (smoking prevention for children), and screening for hypertension and high cholesterol.
- The left coronary artery carries about 85% of the blood supply to the myocardium. The right coronary artery carries the rest. The pumping action of the heart is a product of rhythmic, alternate contraction and relaxation of the atria and ventricles. The stroke volume is the amount of blood ejected from each ventricle with one contraction. Stroke volume depends on preload, afterload, and myocardial contractility. Cardiac output is the amount of blood pumped by each ventricle per minute.

- In addition to the intrinsic control of the body in regulating the heart, extrinsic control by the parasympathetic and sympathetic nerves of the autonomic nervous system is a major factor influencing the heart rate, conductivity, and contractility. Sympathetic impulses cause the adrenal medulla to secrete epinephrine and norepinephrine into the blood.
- The major electrolytes that influence cardiac function are calcium, potassium, sodium, and magnesium. The electrical charge (potential difference) between the inside and outside of cells is expressed in millivolts. When the cell is in a resting state, the electrical charge difference is referred to as a resting membrane potential. The specialized sodium-potassium exchange pump actively pumps sodium ions out of the cell. It also pumps potassium ions into the cell. The cell membrane appears to have individual protein-lined channels. These channels allow for passage of a specific ion or group of ions.
- Nerve and muscle cells are capable of producing action potentials. This property is known as *excitability*. An action potential at any point on the cell membrane stimulates an excitation process. This process is spread down the length of the cell and is conducted across synapses from cell to cell.
- The contraction of cardiac and skeletal muscle is believed to be activated by calcium ions. This results in a binding between myosin and actin myofilaments.
- The conduction system of the heart is composed of two nodes and a conducting bundle. One of the nodes is the sinoatrial node. The other is the atrioventricular node.
- Common chief complaints of the patient with cardiovascular disease include chest pain or discomfort, including shoulder, arm, neck, or jaw pain or discomfort; dyspnea; syncope; and abnormal heartbeat or palpitations. Paramedics should ask patients suspected of having a cardiovascular disorder whether they take prescription medications, especially cardiac drugs. Paramedics should ask whether patients are being treated for any serious illness as well. They also should ask whether patients have a history of myocardial infarction, angina, heart failure, hypertension, diabetes, or chronic lung disease. In addition, paramedics should ask whether patients have any allergies or have other risk factors for heart disease.
- After performing the initial assessment of the patient with cardiovascular disease, the paramedic should look for skin color, jugular venous distention, and the presence of edema or other signs of heart disease. The paramedic should listen for lung sounds, heart sounds, and carotid artery bruit. The paramedic should feel for edema, pulses, skin temperature, and moisture.
- The electrocardiogram represents the electrical activity of the heart. The electrocardiogram is generated by depolarization and repolarization of the atria and ventricles.
- Routine monitoring of cardiac rhythm in the prehospital setting usually is obtained in lead II or MCL$_1$. These are the best leads to monitor for dysrhythmias because they allow visualization of P waves. A 12-lead electrocardiogram can be used to help identify changes relative to myocardial ischemia, injury, and infarction; distinguish ventricular tachycardia from supraventricular tachycardia; determine the electrical axis and the presence of fascicular blocks; and determine the presence of bundle branch blocks.
- The paper used to record electrocardiograms is standardized. This allows comparative analysis of an electrocardiogram wave.
- The normal electrocardiogram consists of a P wave, QRS complex, and T wave. The P wave is the first positive deflection on the electrocardiogram. The P wave represents atrial depolarization. The P-R interval is the time it takes for an electrical impulse to be conducted through the atria and the atrioventricular node up to the instant of ventricular depolarization. The QRS complex represents ventricular depolarization. The ST segment represents the early part of repolarization of the right and left ventricles. The T wave represents repolarization of the ventricular myocardial cells. Repolarization occurs during the last part of ventricular systole. The Q-T interval is the period from the beginning of ventricular depolarization (onset of the QRS complex) until the end of ventricular repolarization or the end of the T wave.
- The steps in electrocardiogram analysis include analyzing the QRS complex, P waves, rate, rhythm, and P-R interval.
- Dysrhythmias originating in the sinoatrial node include sinus bradycardia, sinus tachycardia, sinus dysrhythmia, and sinus arrest. Most sinus dysrhythmias are the result of increases or decreases in vagal tone.
- Dysrhythmias originating in the atria include wandering pacemaker, premature atrial complexes, paroxysmal supraventricular tachycardia, atrial flutter, and atrial fibrillation. Common causes of atrial dysrhythmias are ischemia, hypoxia, and atrial dilation caused by congestive heart failure or mitral valve abnormalities.
- When the sinoatrial node and the atria cannot generate the electrical impulses needed to begin depolarization because of factors such as hypoxia, ischemia, myocardial infarction, and drug toxicity, the atrioventricular node or the area surrounding the atrioventricular node may assume the role of the secondary pacemaker. Dysrhythmias

originating in the atrioventricular junction include premature junctional contractions, junctional escape complexes or rhythms, and accelerated junctional rhythm.

- Ventricular dysrhythmias pose a threat to life. Ventricular rhythm disturbances generally result from failure of the atria, atrioventricular junction, or both to initiate an electrical impulse. They also may result from enhanced automaticity or reentry phenomena in the ventricles. Dysrhythmias originating in the ventricles include ventricular escape complexes or rhythms, premature ventricular complexes, ventricular tachycardia, ventricular fibrillation, asystole, and artificial pacemaker rhythm.

- Partial delays or full interruptions in cardiac electrical conduction are called *heart blocks*. Causes of heart blocks include atrioventricular junctional ischemia, atrioventricular junctional necrosis, degenerative disease of the conduction system, and drug toxicity. Dysrhythmias that are disorders of conduction are first-degree atrioventricular block, type I second-degree atrioventricular block (Wenckebach), type II second-degree atrioventricular block, third-degree atrioventricular block, disturbances of ventricular conduction, pulseless electrical activity, and preexcitation (Wolff-Parkinson-White) syndrome.

- Atherosclerosis is a disease process characterized by progressive narrowing of the lumen of medium and large arteries. Atherosclerosis has two major effects on blood vessels. First, the disease disrupts the intimal surface. This causes a loss of vessel elasticity and an increase in thrombogenesis. Second, the atheroma reduces the diameter of the vessel lumen. Thus this decreases the blood supply to tissues.

- Angina pectoris is a symptom of myocardial ischemia. Angina is caused by an imbalance between myocardial oxygen supply and demand. Prehospital management includes placing the patient at rest, administering oxygen, initiating intravenous therapy, administering nitroglycerin and possibly morphine, monitoring the patient for dysrhythmias, and transporting the patient for physician evaluation.

- Acute myocardial infarction occurs when a coronary artery is blocked and blood does not reach an area of heart muscle. This results in ischemia, injury, and necrosis to the area of myocardium supplied by the affected artery. Death caused by myocardial infarction usually results from lethal dysrhythmias (ventricular tachycardia, ventricular fibrillation, and cardiac standstill), pump failure (cardiogenic shock and congestive heart failure), or myocardial tissue rupture (rupture of the ventricle, septum, or papillary muscle). Some patients with acute myocardial infarction, particularly those in the older age groups, have only symptoms of dyspnea, syncope, or confusion. However, substernal chest pain is usually present in patients with acute myocardial infarction (70% to 90% of patients). ST segment elevation greater than or equal to 0.5 mV in at least two side-by-side electrocardiogram leads indicates an acute myocardial infarction. However, some patients infarct without ST segment elevation changes. Other conditions also can produce ST segment elevation. Prehospital management of the patient with a suspected myocardial infarction should include placing the patient at rest; administering oxygen at 3 to 4 L per minute via nasal cannula; frequently assessing vital signs and breath sounds; initiating an intravenous line with normal saline or lactated Ringer's solution to keep the vein open; monitoring for dysrhythmias; administering medications such as nitroglycerin, morphine, and aspirin; and screening for risk factors for fibrinolytic therapy.

- Left ventricular failure occurs when the left ventricle fails to function as an effective forward pump. This causes a back-pressure of blood into the pulmonary circulation. This in turn may lead to pulmonary edema. Emergency management is directed at decreasing the venous return to the heart, improving myocardial contractility, decreasing myocardial oxygen demand, improving ventilation and oxygenation, and rapidly transporting the patient to a medical facility.

- Right ventricular failure occurs when the right ventricle fails as a pump. This causes back-pressure of blood into the systemic venous circulation. Right ventricular failure is not usually a medical emergency in itself; that is, unless it is associated with pulmonary edema or hypotension.

- Cardiogenic shock is the most extreme form of pump failure. It usually is caused by extensive myocardial infarction. Even with aggressive therapy, cardiogenic shock has a mortality rate of 70% or higher. Patients in cardiogenic shock need rapid transport to a medical facility.

- *Cardiac tamponade* is defined as impaired filling of the heart caused by increased pressure in the pericardial sac.

- Abdominal aortic aneurysms are usually asymptomatic. However, signs and symptoms will signal impending or active rupture. If the vessel tears, bleeding initially may be stopped by the retroperitoneal tissues. The patient may be normotensive on the arrival of emergency medical services. If the rupture opens into the peritoneal cavity, however, massive fatal hemorrhage may follow.

- Acute dissection is the most common aortic catastrophe. Any area of the aorta may be involved. However, in 60% to 70% of cases the site of a dissecting aneurysm is in the ascending aorta, just beyond the takeoff of the left subclavian artery. The signs and symptoms depend on the site of the intimal tear. They also depend on the extent of dissection. The goals of managing suspected aortic dissection in the prehospital setting are relief of pain and immediate transport to a medical facility.

- Acute arterial occlusion is a sudden blockage of arterial flow. Occlusion most commonly is caused by trauma, an embolus, or thrombosis. The most common sites of embolic occlusion are the abdominal aorta, common femoral artery, popliteal artery, carotid artery, brachial artery, and mesenteric artery. The location of ischemic pain is related to the site of occlusion.

- Noncritical peripheral vascular conditions include varicose veins, superficial thrombophlebitis, and acute deep vein thrombosis. Of these conditions, deep vein thrombosis is the only one that can cause a life-threatening problem. This problem is pulmonary embolus.

- Hypertension often is defined by a resting blood pressure that is consistently greater than 140/90 mm Hg. Chronic hypertension has an adverse effect on the heart and blood vessels. It requires the heart to perform more work than normal. This leads to hypertrophy of the cardiac muscle and left ventricular failure. Conditions associated with chronic, uncontrolled hypertension are cerebral hemorrhage and stroke, myocardial infarction, and renal failure.

- Hypertensive emergencies are conditions in which a blood pressure increase leads to significant, irreversible end-organ damage within hours if not treated. The organs most likely to be at risk are the brain, heart, and kidneys. As a rule, the diagnosis is based on altered end-organ function and the rate of the rise in blood pressure, not on the level of blood pressure.

- Basic cardiac life support helps to maintain the circulation and respiration of a victim of cardiac arrest. Basic life support is continued until advanced cardiac life support is available. Two mechanisms are thought to be responsible for blood flow during cardiopulmonary resuscitation. One is direct compression of the heart between the sternum and the spine. This increases pressure within the ventricles to provide blood flow to the lungs and body organs. The second one is increased intrathoracic pressure transmitted to all intrathoracic vascular structures. This creates an intrathoracic-to-extrathoracic pressure gradient. This gradient causes blood to flow out of the thorax. A number of mechanical devices provide external chest compression. Others provide chest compression with ventilation in the cardiac arrest patient.

- Cardiac monitor-defibrillators are classified as manual or automated external defibrillators. Defibrillation is the delivery of electrical current through the chest wall. Its purpose is to terminate ventricular fibrillation and certain other nonperfusing rhythms.

- Implantable cardioverter defibrillators work by monitoring the patient's cardiac rhythm. When a monitored ventricular rate exceeds the preprogrammed rate, the implantable cardioverter defibrillator delivers a shock of about 6 to 30 J through the patches. This is an attempt to restore a normal sinus rhythm.

- Synchronized cardioversion is designed to deliver a shock about 10 milliseconds after the peak of the R wave of the cardiac cycle. (Thus the device avoids the relative refractory period.) Synchronization may reduce the amount of energy needed to end the dysrhythmia. It also may decrease the chances of causing another dysrhythmia.

- Transcutaneous cardiac pacing is an effective emergency therapy for bradycardia, complete heart block, asystole, and suppression of some malignant ventricular dysrhythmias. Proper electrode placement is important for effective external pacing.

- What is becoming more and more evident is that patients who cannot be resuscitated in the prehospital setting rarely survive. This is the case even if they are resuscitated temporarily in the emergency department. Cessation of resuscitative efforts in the prehospital setting should follow system-specific criteria established by medical direction

REVIEW QUESTIONS

Match each term in Column II with its definition in Column I. Use each answer only once.

Column I	Column II
1. _____ Heart rate × stroke volume	**a.** Afterload
2. _____ Volume available for ventricles to pump each contraction	**b.** Blood pressure
3. _____ Peripheral vascular resistance produces this pressure	**c.** Cardiac output
4. _____ Ventricular relaxation	**d.** Contractility
5. _____ Cardiac output × peripheral vascular resistance	**e.** Diastole
6. _____ Increased myocardial contractility in response to increased preload	**f.** Preload
	g. Starling's law
7. _____ Ventricular ejection per heartbeat	**h.** Stroke volume
	i. Systole

8. Identify a prevention strategy for each of the following risk factors for cardiovascular disease and a community resource where you can refer the patient to assist with modification of this risk factor.

Risk Factor	Prevention Strategy	Resource
a. Smoking		
b. Hypercholesterolemia		
c. Obesity		
d. Sedentary lifestyle		

9. Explain how the sympathetic and parasympathetic divisions of the autonomic nervous system influence cardiac function in the following areas.

	Sympathetic	Parasympathetic
a. Heart rate		
b. Myocardial contractility		
c. Lungs		
d. Blood vessels (peripheral)		

10. Name the two adrenal hormones and describe the effects of each on the cardiovascular system.

	Name	Function
a.		
b.		

11. Fill in the blanks in the following sentences about electrophysiology: Within the body, separated charged particles

with opposite charges have a (a) _____ force of attraction that gives them (b) _____

energy. This energy is released when the cell membrane becomes (c) _____ to the charged particles

and allows the charges to come together. The electrical charge between the inside and outside of cells is the

(d) _____ difference and is measured in (e) _____. Although there is a relatively equal number of positively and negatively charged ions inside and outside the cell, the intracellular area has a

(f) _____ charge because of the (g) _____ charged proteins that cannot move outside the cell. The electrical charge difference in the resting state has the potential to do work and is known as the

resting membrane (h) _____ (RMP). During this phase, the inside of the cell is electrically

(i) _____ relative to the outside of the cell (approximately [j] _____ mV). The RMP results

primarily from the difference between the intracellular and extracellular (k) _____ ion level.

Because of the chemical gradient (more of these ions inside than outside of the cell), the (l) _____ would move out of the cell in an attempt to achieve equilibrium. However, these ions remain in the cell because

of the negtive intracellular charge generated by the (m). _____ In the RMP, sodium will not rush

into the cell because the cell membrane is not (n) _____ to sodium. The ability of nerve and muscle

cells to produce action potentials is known as (o) _____. If this action potential results in a decreased charge difference across the cell membrane, the RMP becomes less negative, and this is called

(p) _____. If a stimulus is strong enough to cause depolarization of a cell membrane to a level

called the (q) _____, a chain reaction of permeability changes cause an (r) _____ to

spread over the entire cell membrane. Action potentials have two phases: a (s) _____ phase and a

(t) _____ phase. During an action potential, the sodium ions rush into the cell, and RMP becomes

(u) _____ on the inside and (v) _____ on the outside of the cell membrane. This occurs

during the (w) _____ phase. The repolarization phase results from potassium leakage outside the

cell and the return of the cell membrane to its normal resting (x) _____ state.

12. Answer the following questions regarding the five phases of the cardiac action potential:

a. During phase 0 (rapid depolarization), what causes the inside of the cell to become positive?

_____

b. What is the membrane potential during phase 1 (early rapid repolarization)?

_____

c. How is the membrane potential held at 0 during phase 2 (plateau phase)?

_____

d. What happens to the membrane potential of the cell during phase 3 (terminal phase of rapid repolarization)?

_____

e. How is the balance of sodium and potassium restored during phase 4?

_____

f. Why can cardiac pacemaker cells depolarize without an external stimulus to initiate an action potential?

_____

INTRODUCTION TO ELECTROCARDIOGRAM MONITORING

13. Circle the correct response in each of the following statements:

The electrocardiogram tracing represents an amplified view of the myocardial (**a**) action potentials/contractions. If the voltage displayed is positive, the electrocardiogram tracing will display a(n) (**b**) upward/downward/isoelectric deflection. Cardiac pacemaker cells spontaneously can generate impulses, a property known as (**c**) automaticity/conductivity. This rhythmic activity occurs because these cells do not have a stable (**d**) action potential/resting membrane potential.

14. Label Fig. 29-1 illustrating the cardiac conduction system.

A.

B.

C.

D.

E.

F.

G.

H.

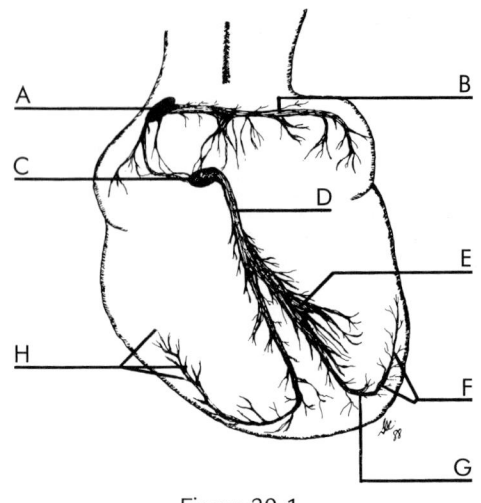

Figure 29-1

15. The sinoatrial node is the dominant pacemaker. If it fails to fire, what will happen?

_____

16. Briefly describe the mechanism for ectopic impulse formation by each of the following mechanisms:

    a. Enhanced automaticity:

_____

    b. Reentry:

_____

ASSESSMENT OF THE PATIENT WITH CARDIAC DISEASE

17. A 62-year-old woman complains of chest pain. What questions should you ask using the OPQRST mnemonic to determine the nature and severity of her pain?

    O

    P

    Q

    R

    S

    T

18. List three chief complaints that may lead you to believe a patient has a cardiovascular problem.

    a.

    b.

    c.

19. An older man experiences a syncopal episode at a local gym. List at least two questions you should ask in an attempt to determine the nature of his syncopal episode.

a.

b.

20. A 34-year-old woman walks into your ambulance base complaining of a fluttering sensation in her chest. What will your history and physical examination include to determine the cause of this sensation?

_____

_____

Questions 21 to 23 pertain to the following case study:

An 87-year-old woman calls you to her home and complains of weakness and nausea. On arrival, you find her seated on the commode. She is pale, cool, and diaphoretic. Her blood pressure is 70 mm Hg by palpation, and her electrocardiogram is shown in Fig. 29-2.

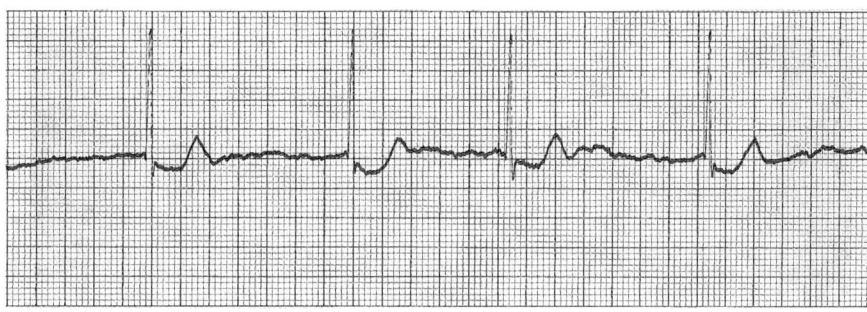

Figure 29-2

21. What information from this patient's medical history will be important to elicit at this time?

_____

22. What is your interpretation of her electrocardiogram?

_____

23. She tells you that she is taking digoxin, diltiazem, potassium, and furosemide. Could any of her home medicines be playing a role in her problem? If yes, which ones and why?

_____

_____

24. An older man is found unresponsive and bradycardic in a local park. A caretaker states that he complained of chest pain before collapsing. No one is available to give you any information regarding his history. Briefly outline specific findings you may encounter in your patient assessment if he has a history of cardiac problems.

_____

_____

ELECTROCARDIOGRAM MONITORING

25. Place the positive (+) and negative (–) and electrodes for the four leads shown in Fig. 29-3.

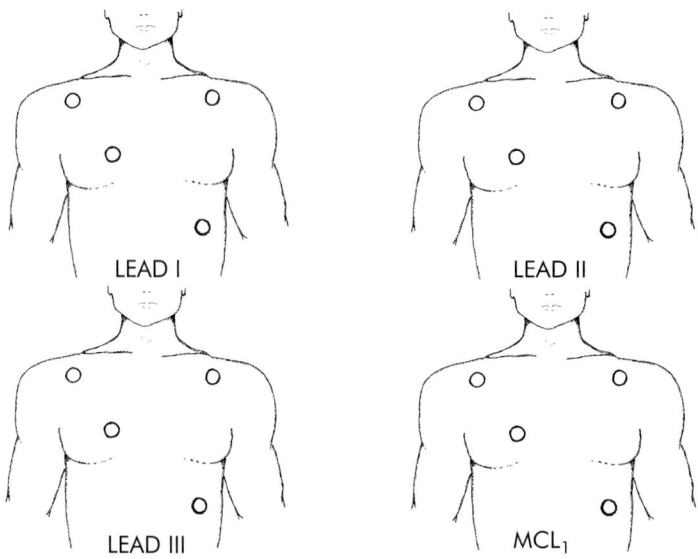

Figure 29-3

26. Describe the location of each of the 10 electrodes needed to record a 12-lead electrocardiogram.

a.   f.

b.   g.

c.   h.

d.   i.

e.   j.

27. List six problems that may interfere with a clear electrocardiogram recording. For each problem, discuss a possible solution.

a.   d.

b.   e.

c.   f.

28. Label Fig. 29-4 with the appropriate measurement intervals

a. _____ mm

b. _____ second

c. _____ second

d. _____ second

e. _____ second

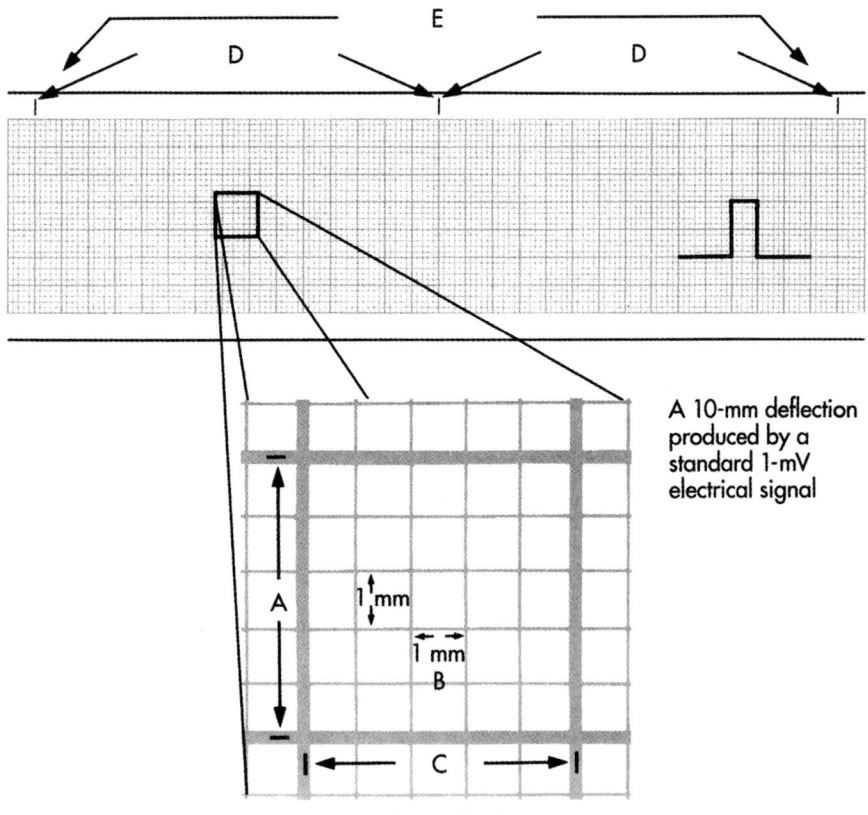

A 10-mm deflection produced by a standard 1-mV electrical signal

Figure 29-4

29. Label the sample electrocardiogram tracing in Fig. 29-5.

a.

b.

c.

d.

e.

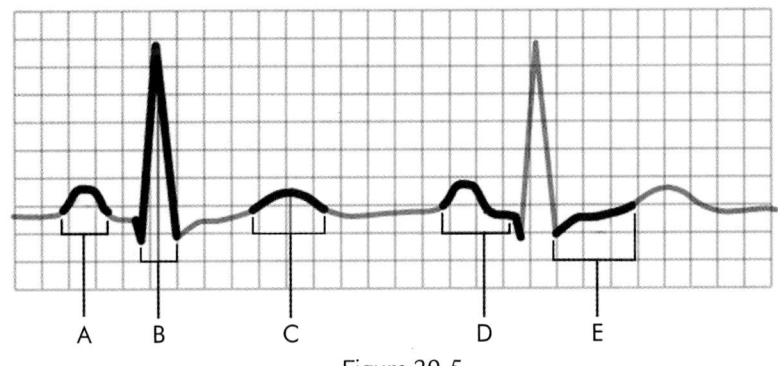

Figure 29-5

30. List five causes of artifact.

a.

b.

c.

d.

e.

ELECTROCARDIOGRAM INTERPRETATION

31. List the five steps in electrocardiogram analysis.

a.

b.

c.

d.

e.

32. Calculate the rate of the electrocardiogram in Fig. 29-6 using four different methods, describing the steps you use in each method.

a. _____

_____

b. _____

_____

c. _____

_____

d. _____

_____

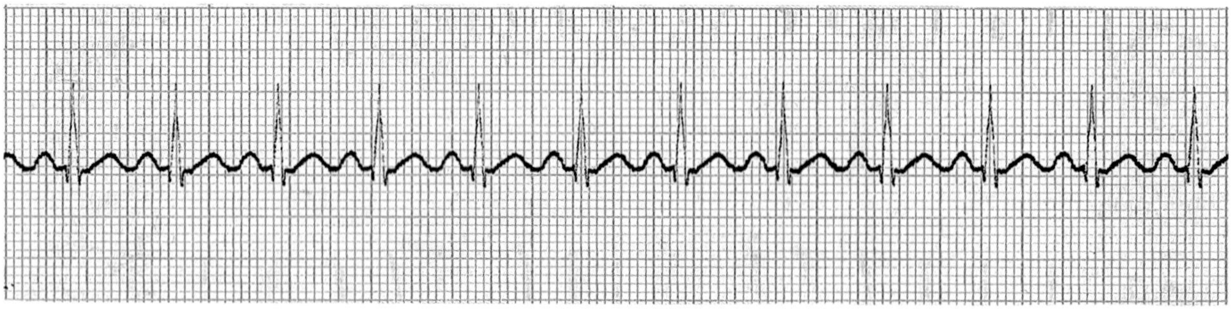

Figure 29-6

33. If the rate in question 32 is within normal limits, can we assume the patient is stable in this situation?

_____

34. Which method of calculation would be *most* accurate if the rhythm in question 32 was

    a. Regular?

_____

    b. Irregularly irregular?

_____

35. What criterion must be met when analyzing the electrocardiogram rhythm to determine that the rhythm is regular?

_____

36. What analysis can be made about conduction in each of the following examples?

    a. The QRS complex width is less than or equal to 0.12 second.

_____

    b. The QRS complex width is greater than 0.12 second.

_____

37. List the four criteria that must be evaluated when analyzing the P waves.

    a.

    b.

    c.

    d.

38. Briefly describe the significance of each of the following P-R interval findings.

    a. P-R interval 0.08 second:

_____

    b. P-R interval 0.16 second:

_____

_____

    c. P-R interval 0.24 second:

_____

39. Analyze the electrocardiogram rhythm strip in Fig. 29-7 using the five steps described in question 31, and give your interpretation.

    a. Step 1:

_____

    b. Step 2:

_____

c. Step 3:

_____

d. Step 4:

_____

e. Step 5:

_____

Interpretation:

_____

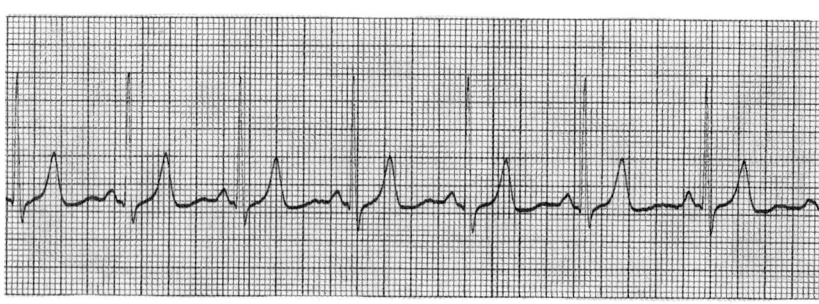

Figure 29-7

INTRODUCTION TO DYSRHYTHMIAS

40. When a dysrhythmia is noted on the monitor, what factors must be considered to determine whether any intervention is necessary?

_____

41. Dysrhythmias originating in the sinoatrial node frequently result from increases or decreases in

a. _____. Electrocardiogram features common to all sinoatrial node dysrhythmias are

b. QRS complex.

_____

c. P waves (lead II).

_____

d. P-R interval.

_____

42. List two causes of each bradycardic and tachycardic dysrhythmia that originates in the sinus node.

a. Sinus bradycardia:

_____

b. Sinus tachycardia:

Complete the missing information on Flashcards 1 to 4 at the end of the text.

43. Complete Flashcard 1 (Fig. 29-8): sinus bradycardia.

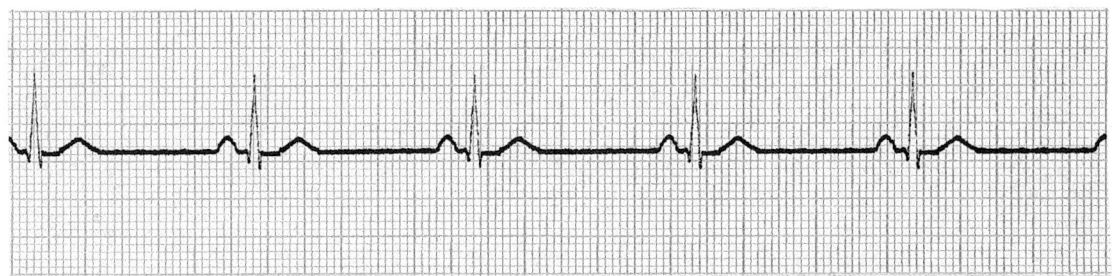

Figure 29-8

44. Complete Flashcard 2 (Fig. 29-9): sinus tachycardia.

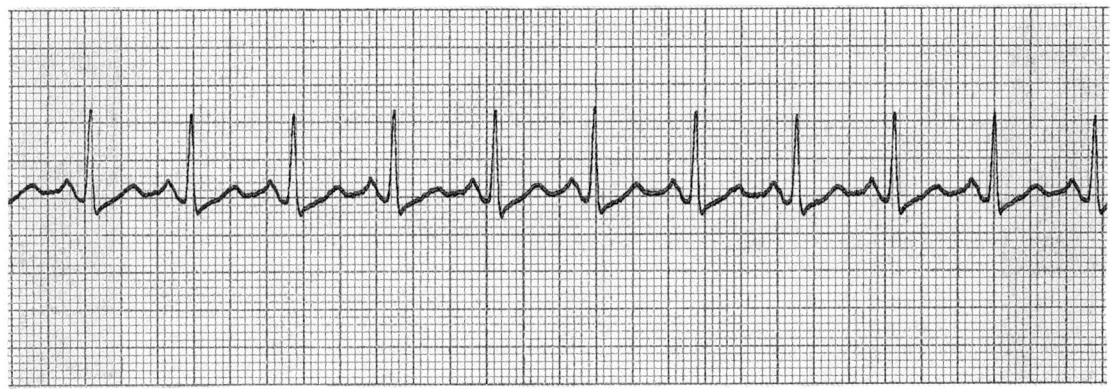

Figure 29-9

45. Complete Flashcard 3 (Fig. 29-10): sinus dysrhythmia.

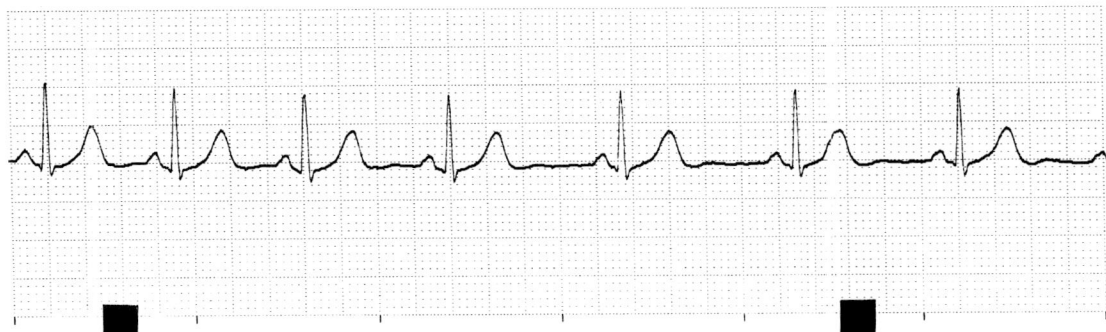

Figure 29-10

46. Complete Flashcard 4 (Fig. 29-11): sinus arrest.

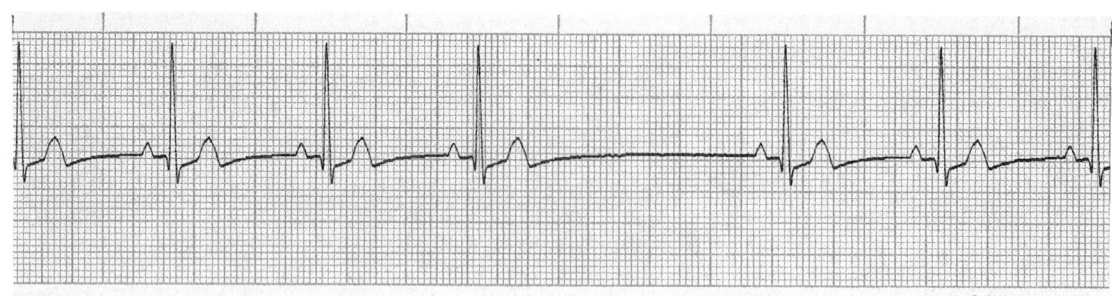

Figure 29-11

47. Atrial dysrhythmias originate in the (a) _____ of the (b) _____

or in the (c) _____ pathways.

48. Common features of atrial dysrhythmias are

    a. QRS complex.

_____

    b. P waves (if present).

_____

    c. P-R intervals.

_____

49. List four causes of dysrhythmias that originate in the atria.

    a.

    b.

    c.

    d.

Complete the missing information on Flashcards 5 to 9 showing dysrhythmias originating in the atria.

50. Complete Flashcard 5 (Fig. 29-12): wandering atrial pacemaker.

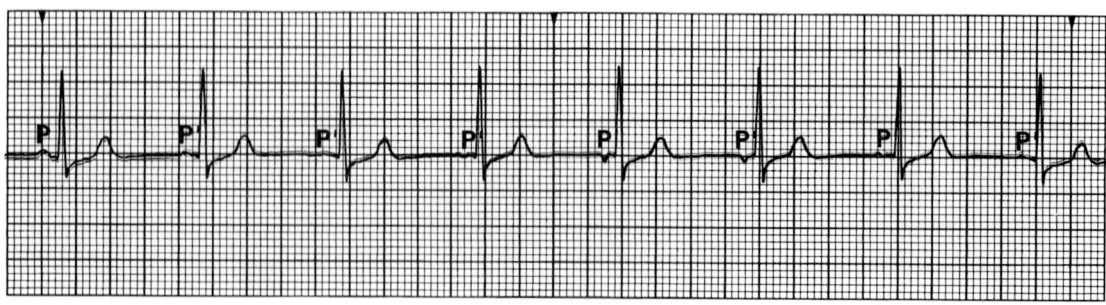

Figure 29-12

51. Complete Flashcard 6 (Fig. 29-13): premature atrial contraction.

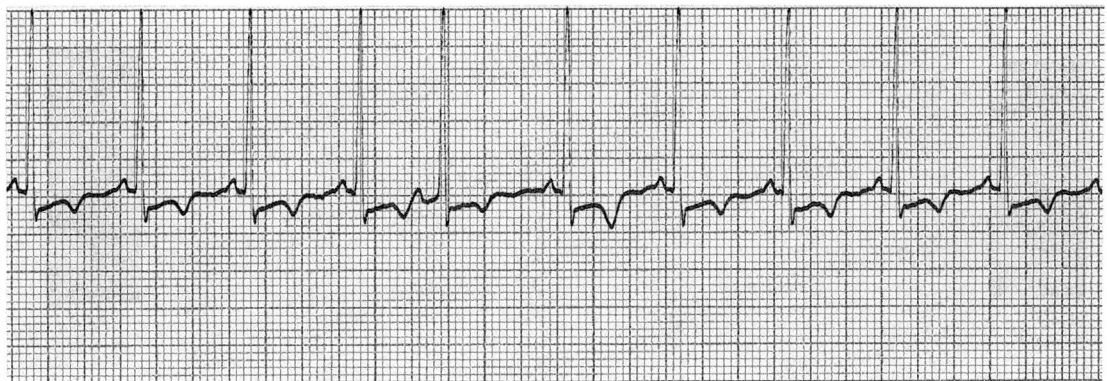

Figure 29-13

52. Complete Flashcard 7 (Fig. 29-14): supraventricular tachycardia.

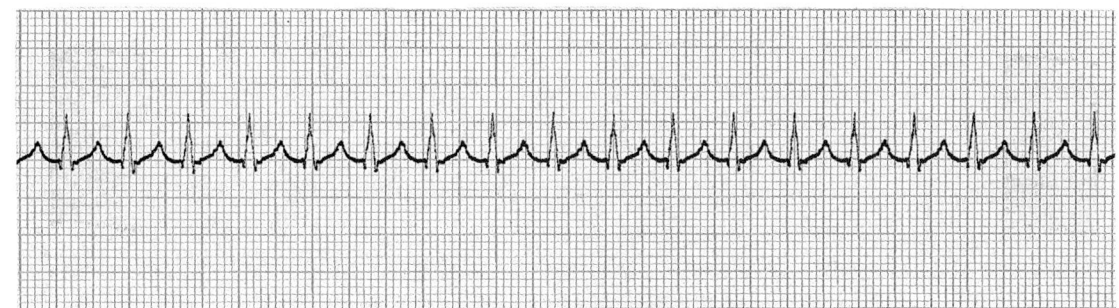

Figure 29-14

53. Complete Flashcard 8 (Fig. 29-15): atrial flutter with 3:1 conduction.

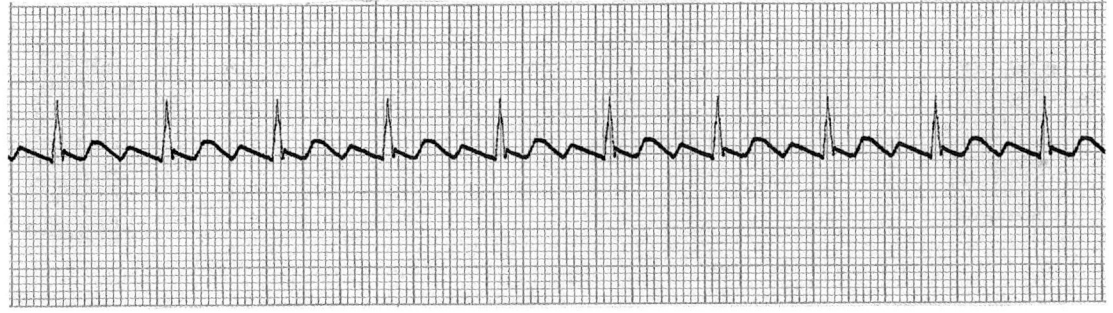

Figure 29-15

54. Complete Flashcard 9 (Fig. 29-16): atrial fibrillation.

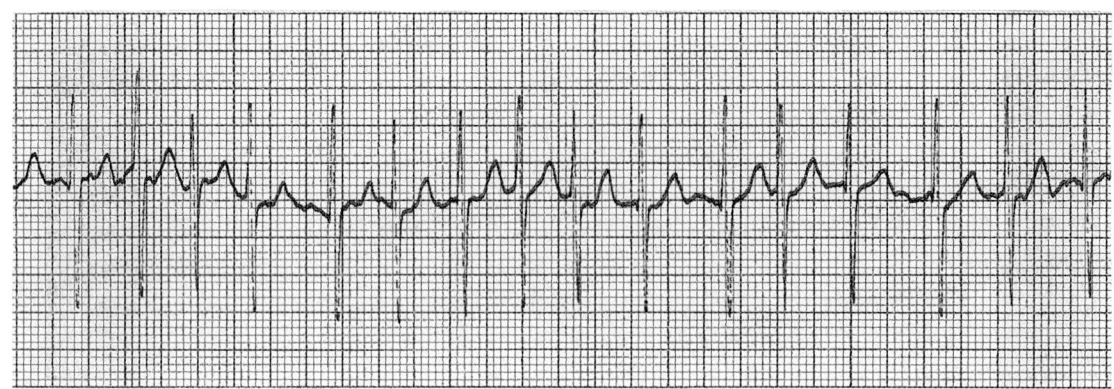

Figure 29-16

55. Rhythms that start in the atrioventricular node or junction are called (a) _____ rhythms. These rhythms share the following common features:

    b. QRS complex:

_____

    c. P waves:

_____

    d. P-R interval:

_____

56. List four causes of dysrhythmias that start in the atrioventricular junction.

    a.

    b.

    c.

    d.

Complete the missing information on Flashcards 10 to 12 showing dysrhythmias originating in the atrioventricular junction.

57. Complete Flashcard 10 (Fig. 29-17): sinus rhythm (borderline bradycardia) with two premature junctional contractions.

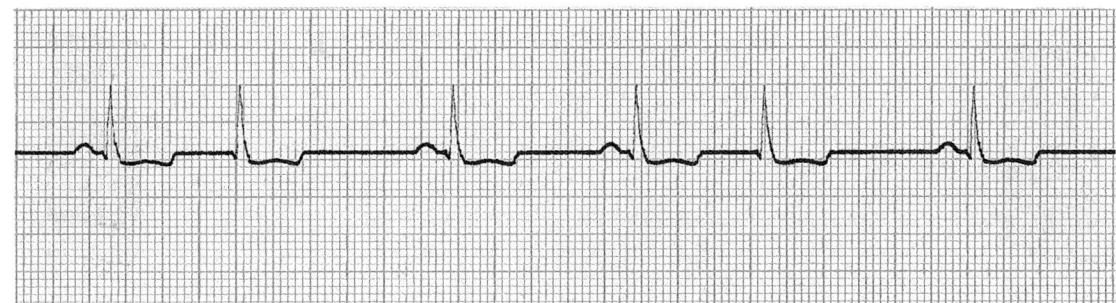

Figure 29-17

58. Complete Flashcard 11 (Fig. 29-18): junctional escape rhythm.

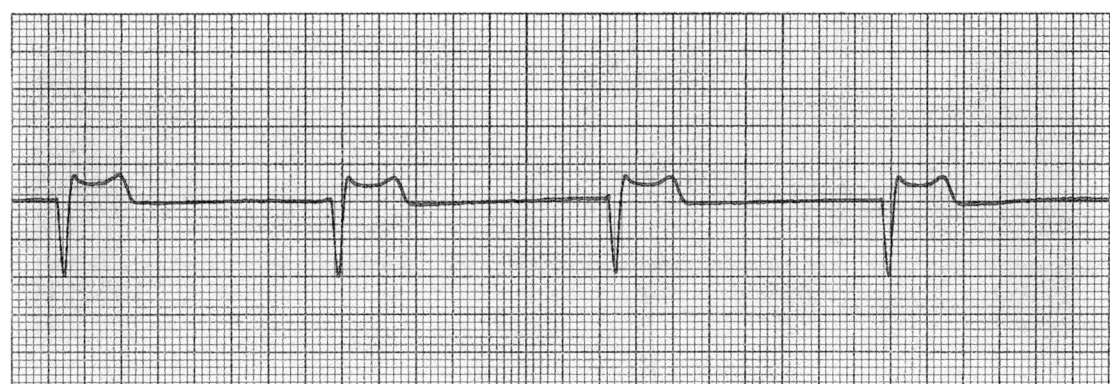

Figure 29-18

59. Complete Flashcard 12 (Fig. 29-19): accelerated junctional rhythm.

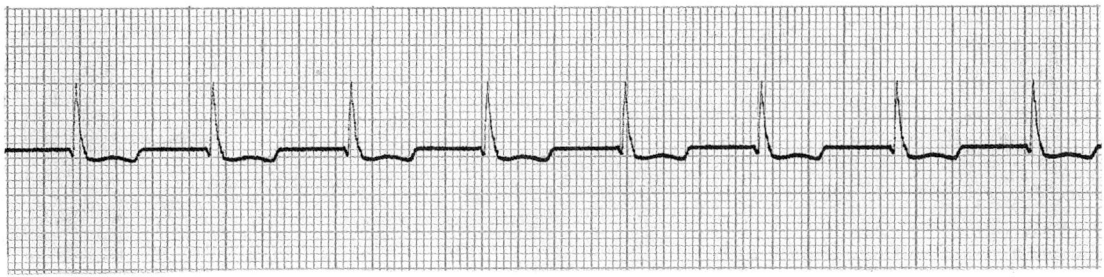

Figure 29-19

60. Rhythms originating from the ventricle have an intrinsic rate of (a) _____ to _____ but can be accelerated at rates up to (b) _____ or tachycardic at rates greater than (c)_____.

61. List five causes of dysrhythmias that originate in the ventricles.

   a.

   b.

   c.

   d.

   e.

62. Identify five steps that can be used when evaluating a 12-lead electrocardiogram to distinguish between wide-complex tachycardias of ventricular versus supraventricular origin.

   a.

   b.

   c.

   d.

   e.

Complete the missing information on Flashcards 13 to 18 showing dysrhythmias originating in the ventricles.

63. Complete Flashcard 13 (Fig. 29-20): ventricular escape rhythm.

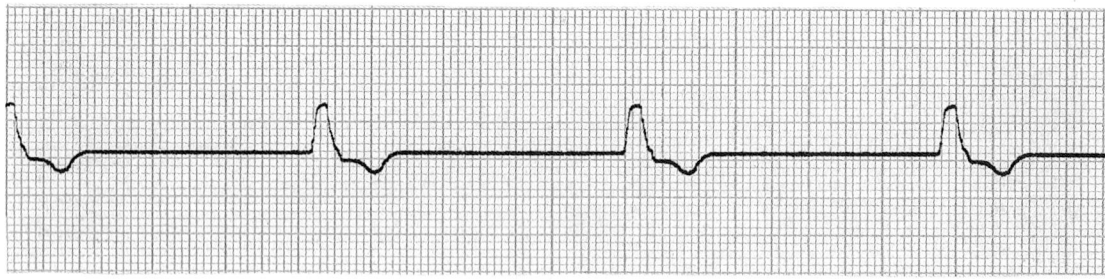

Figure 29-20

64. Complete Flashcard 14 (Fig. 29-21): normal sinus rhythm with one premature ventricular contraction.

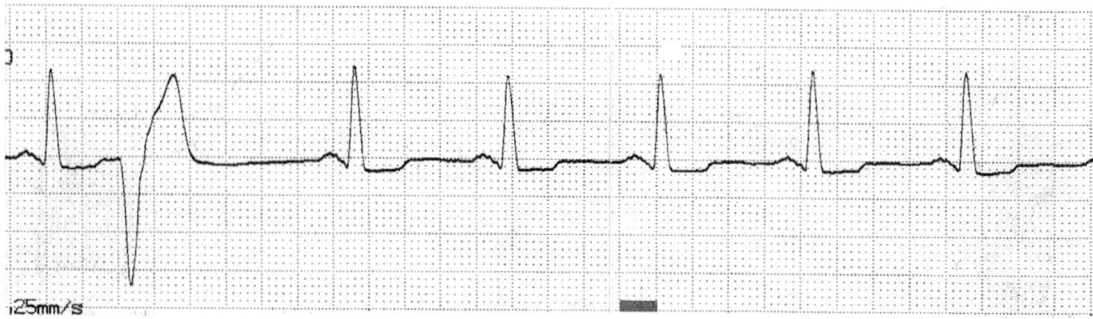

Figure 29-21

65. Complete Flashcard 15 (Fig. 29-22): monomorphic ventricular tachycardia.

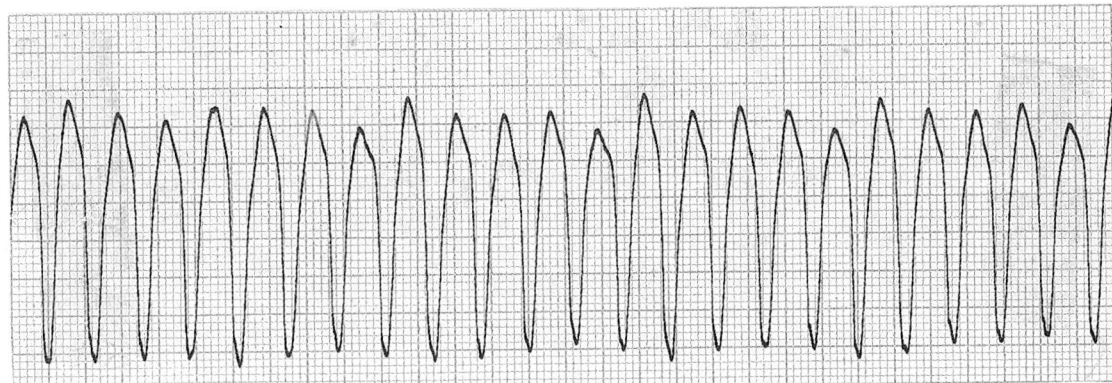

Figure 29-22

66. Complete Flashcard 16 (Fig. 29-23): ventricular fibrillation.

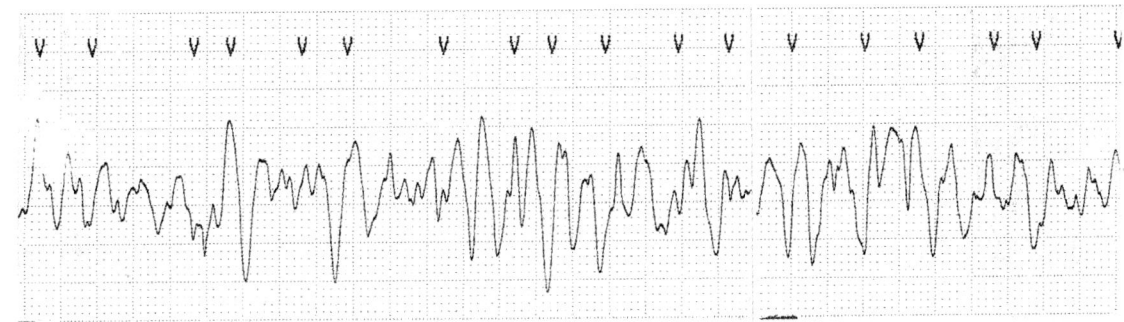

Figure 29-23

67. Complete Flashcard 17 (Fig. 29-24): asystole.

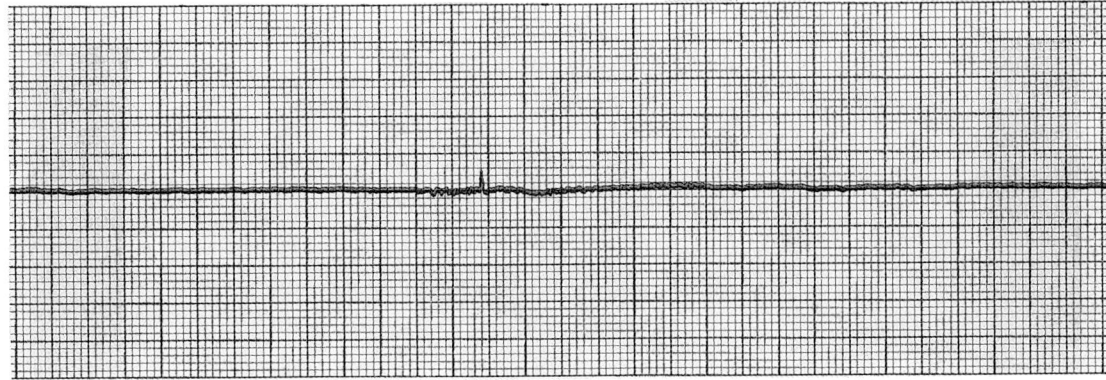

Figure 29-24

68. Complete Flashcard 18 (Fig. 29-25): ventricular paced rhythm.

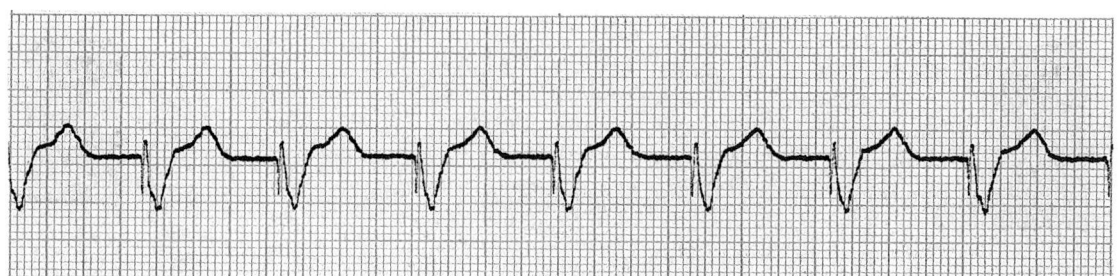

Figure 29-25

69. Delays or interruptions in cardiac electrical conduction are called (a) _____. They may be caused by disease of the (b) _____.

70. List five causes of dysrhythmias caused by delays in cardiac electrical conduction.

a.

b.

c.

d.

e.

Complete the missing information on Flashcards 19 to 22 showing dysrhythmias originating from conduction disorders.

71. Complete Flashcard 19 (Fig. 29-26): sinus rhythm with first-degree atrioventricular block.

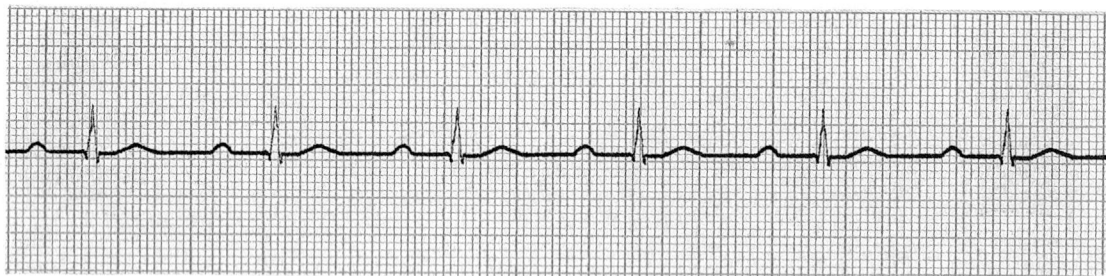

Figure 29-26

72. Complete Flashcard 20 (Fig. 29-27): second-degree atrioventricular block (Mobitz type I or Wenckebach).

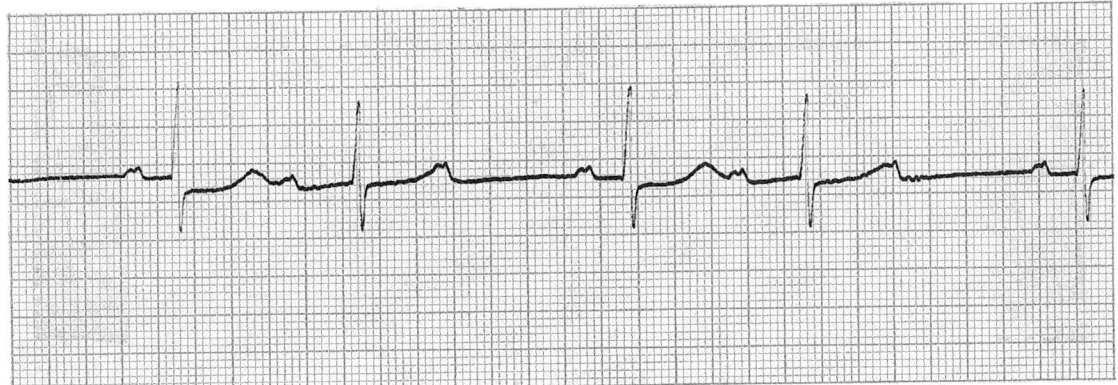

Figure 29-27

73. Complete Flashcard 21 (Fig. 29-28): second-degree atrioventricular block (Mobitz type II).

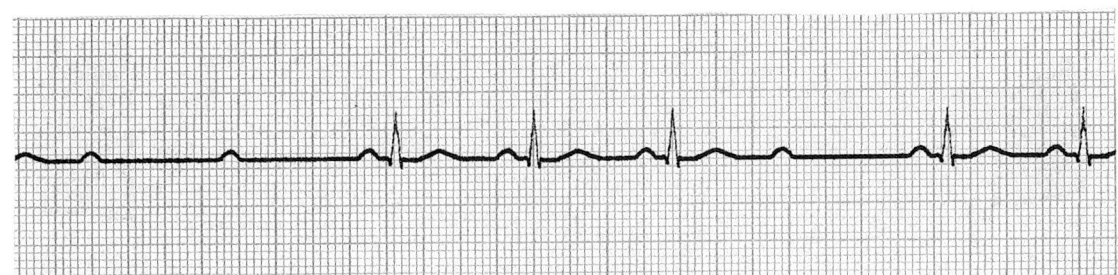

Figure 29-28

74. Complete Flashcard 22 (Fig. 29-29): third-degree (complete) atrioventricular block.

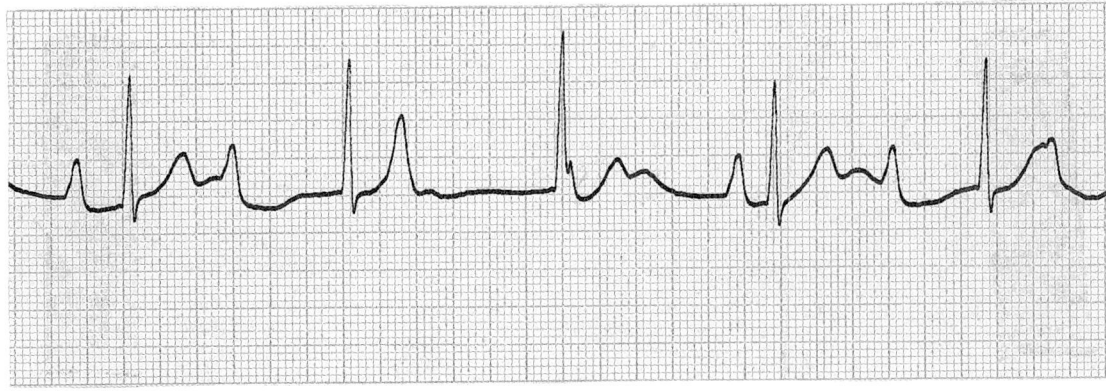

Figure 29-29

75. List the characteristics to identify the following:

    a. Right bundle branch block _____

    b. Left bundle branch block _____

    c. Anterior hemiblock _____

    d. Posterior hemiblock _____

76. Identify patients at risk for developing complete heart block if they are given procainamide, digoxin, verapamil, or diltiazem:

    a.

    b.

    c.

77. An approximately 50-year-old man is found unconscious in a parking lot downtown. He is pulseless and apneic. The attendant is certain he has been there less than 5 minutes but does not know what happened. The patient's electrocardiogram is shown in Fig. 29-30.

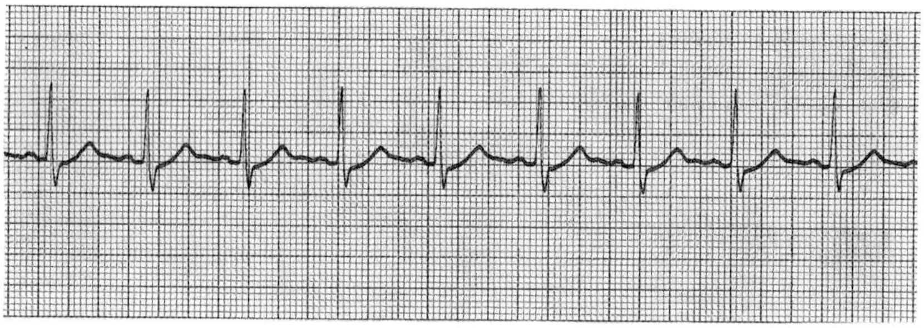

Figure 29-30

    a. You identify the rhythm as

_____

    b. Outline the appropriate interventions for this patient based on current treatment guidelines by the American Heart Association.

_____

78. Outline the electrocardiogram features that may allow detection of a patient with Wolff-Parkinson-White syndrome.

    a. QRS complex:

_____

    b. P-R interval:

_____

79. Why is it clinically important to recognize a patient with a history of Wolff-Parkinson-White syndrome?

_____

_____

SPECIFIC CARDIOVASCULAR DISEASES

80. Explain the pathophysiology of atherosclerotic effects on blood vessels.

_____

_____

81. List two triggers that may initiate an anginal attack in a susceptible patient:

   a.

   b.

82. Describe the following features of angina:

   a. Duration:

   _____

   b. Relieved by:

   _____

83. How can a paramedic distinguish between unstable angina and myocardial infarction in the prehospital environment?

   _____

84. Briefly outline the sequence of pathophysiological events that occur from the time that a clot forms until cardiac tissue dies in acute myocardial infarction.

   _____

   _____

85. Complete the information regarding myocardial infarction that is missing in the following table:

Area of Heart Injured or Infarcted	Coronary Vessel Involved Most Often	Leads with Visible ST Segment Changes
Anterior		
Lateral		
Septal		
Inferior		

86. How much ST segment elevation must be present to be clinically significant?

   _____

87. List six conditions other than myocardial infarction that can cause ST segment elevation.

   a.

   b.

   c.

   d.

   e.

   f.

88. List the five-step analysis described in this text for infarct recognition.

a.

b.

c.

d.

e.

89. Identify four complications resulting from myocardial infarction.

a.

b.

c.

d.

Questions 90 to 94 pertain to the following case study:

A 57-year-old, 80-kg man with a history of untreated hypertension complains of crushing midsternal chest pain that began 2 hours ago. He takes no medicines but admits to smoking two packs of cigarettes per day. His blood pressure is 162/102 mm Hg. His electrocardiogram strip is shown in Fig. 29-31.

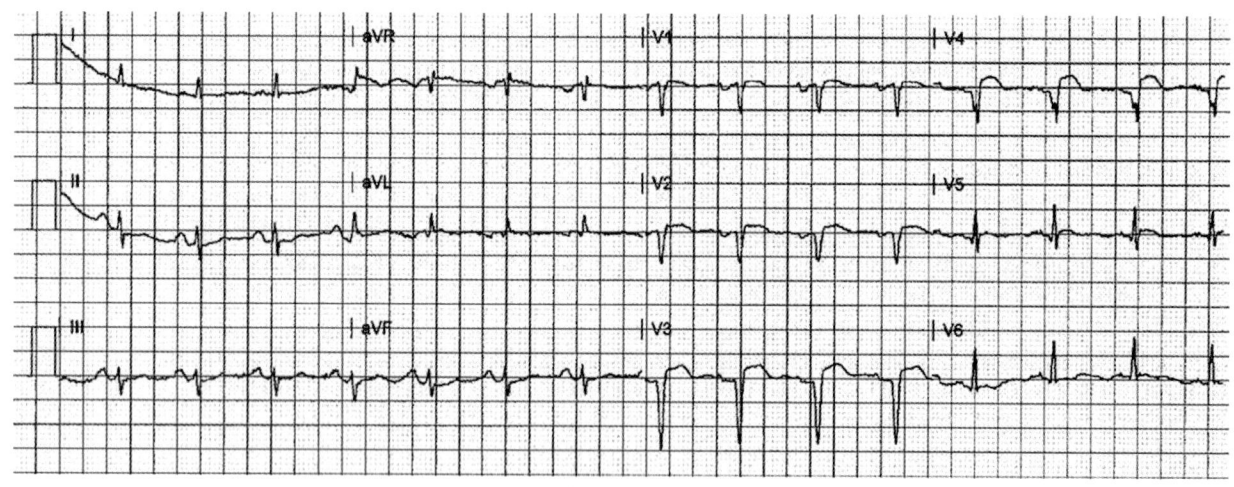

Figure 29-31

90. What other associated signs or symptoms may be present if the patient is experiencing a myocardial infarction?

_____

91. What is your interpretation of his electrocardiogram?

_____

92. Describe general treatment measures you will use for this patient.

_____

_____

93. List three drugs (excluding oxygen) with the appropriate dosage to administer to this patient.

   a.

   b.

   c.

94. You transmit the 12-lead to the hospital and are asked to determine whether the patient meets inclusion or exclusion criteria for thrombolytic therapy.

   a. List 5 inclusion criteria:

_____

   b. List 11 exclusion criteria:

_____

_____

_____

95. Interpret each of the following 12-lead electrocardiograms.

   a. Fig. 29-32:

_____

_____

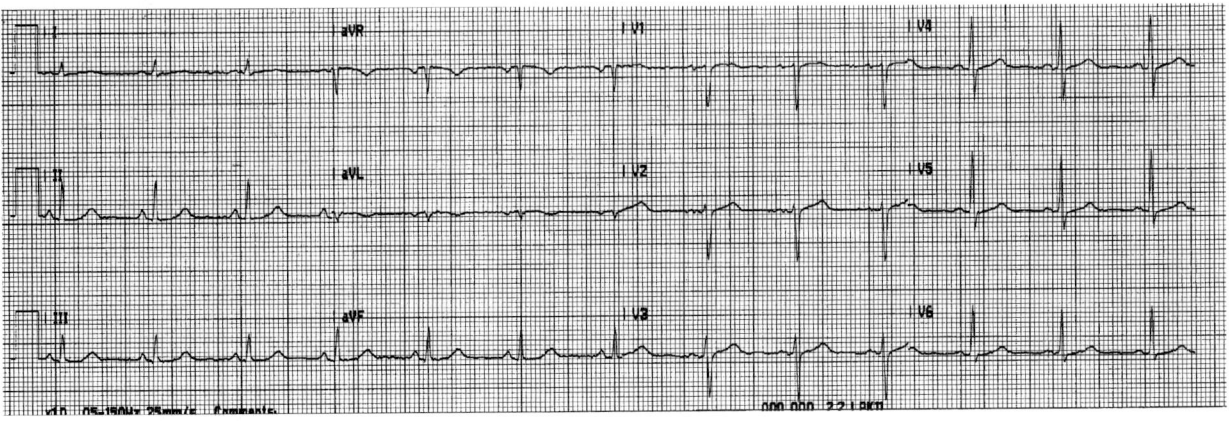

Figure 29-32

b. Fig. 29-33:

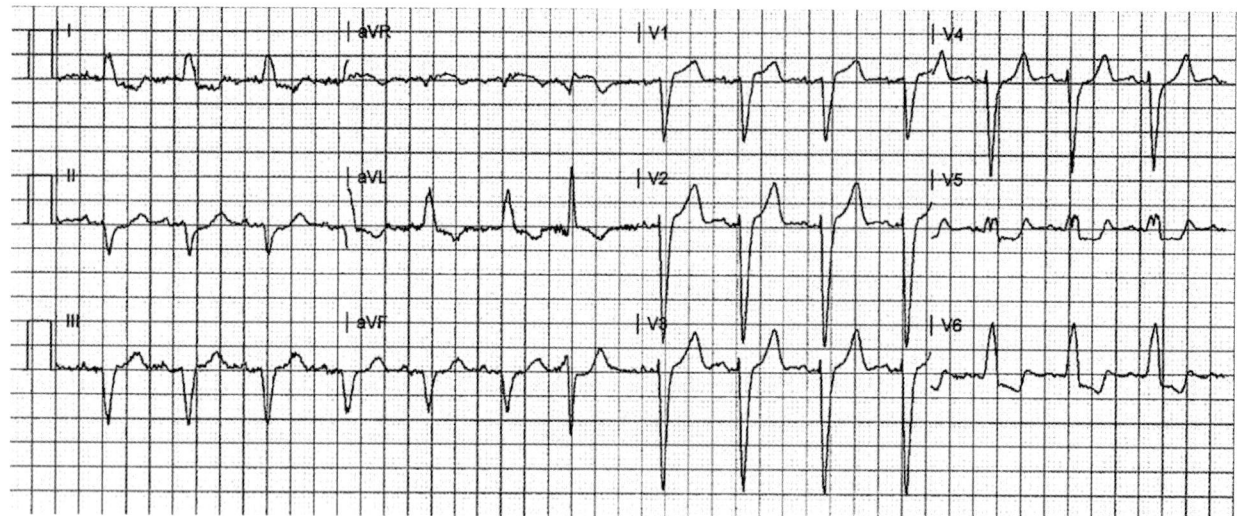

Figure 29-33

c. Fig. 29-34:

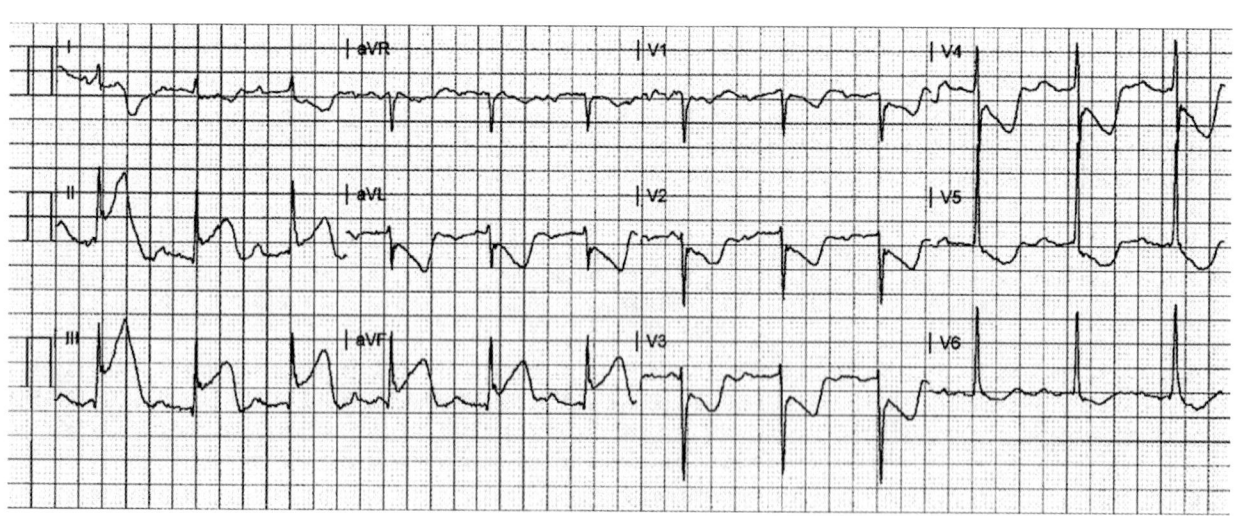

Figure 29-34

d. Fig. 29-35:

_____

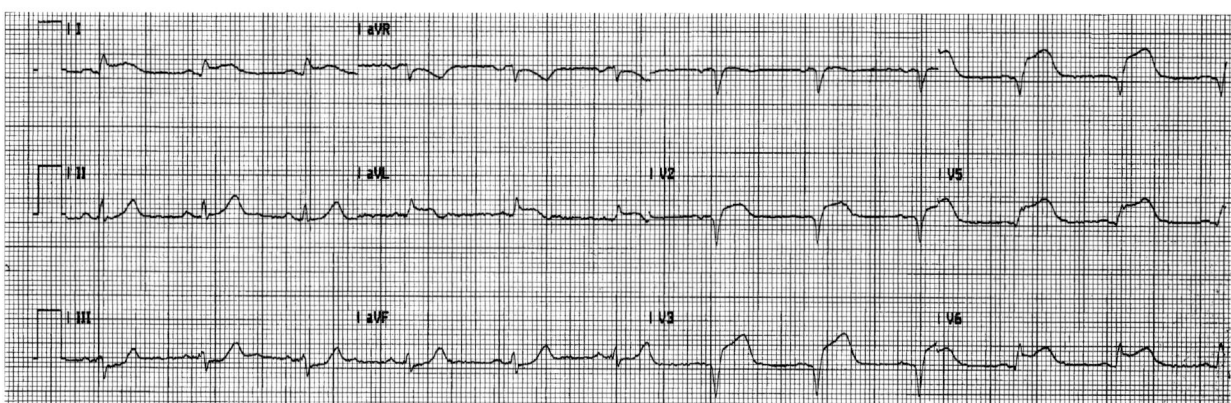

Figure 29-35

Questions 96 to 100 pertain to the following case study:

An 80-kg patient who had a syncopal episode and chest pain has the following electrocardiogram (Fig. 29-36).

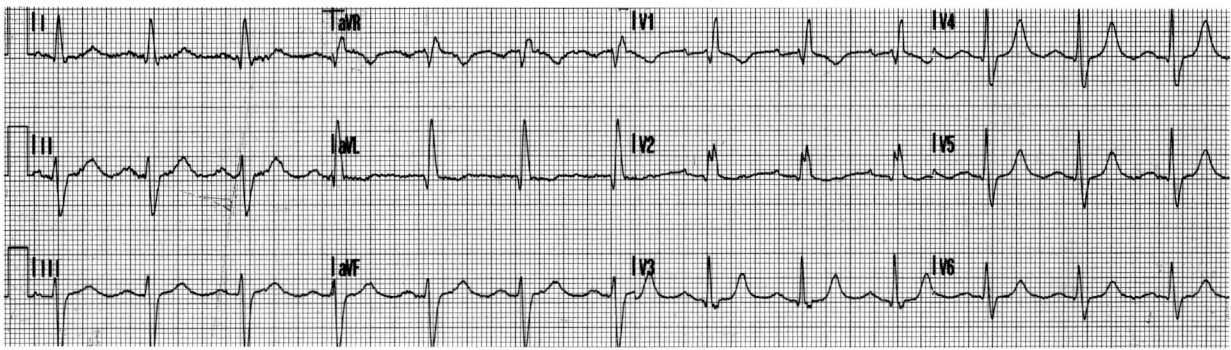

Figure 29-36

96. What is the axis of this electrocardiogram? _____

97. The QRS complex duration is 0.134 second. Draw a triangle that begins at the J point in lead V_1 and, working backward, ends at the first QRS deflection that is encountered. Does the triangle point up or down?

_____

98. Based on your determination of axis, the QRS duration, and the triangle you drew, identify the two blocks that are present in this electrocardiogram.

_____

99. What is the significance of these blocks?

_____

100. Based on the patient's chief complaint and your electrocardiogram findings, what interventions do you perform in addition to routine cardiac care?

_____

Questions 101 to 105 pertain to the following case study:

A 72-year-old, 70-kg woman calls you to her home and complains of a sudden onset of severe dyspnea without chest pain. You find her anxious, sitting upright, with diaphoretic skin and circumoral cyanosis. Her only home medicine is a diuretic. Vital signs are blood pressure, 170/106 mm Hg; pulse, 124; and respirations, 28 and labored. Rales are audible to the level of the scapulae. SaO_2 is 86%. Her electrocardiogram is shown in Fig. 29-37.

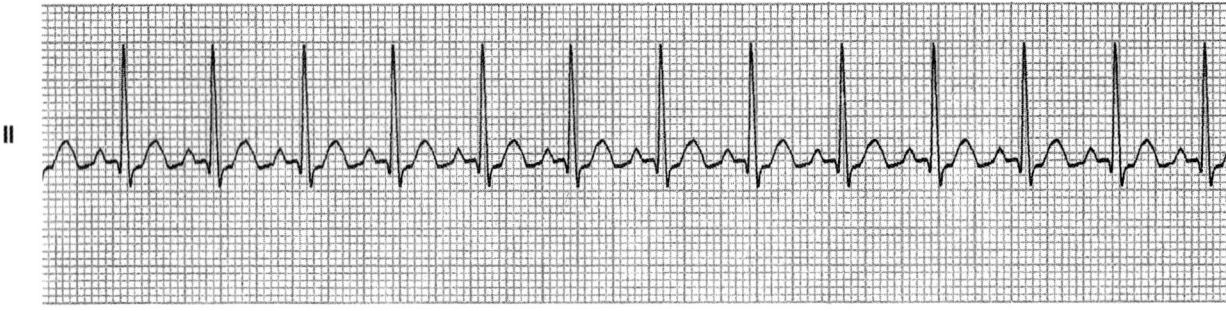

Figure 29-37

101. What medical condition or conditions do you suspect?

_____

102. What other physical findings would help confirm this diagnosis?

_____

103. What is your interpretation of her electrocardiogram?

_____

104. You have placed the patient on oxygen and wish to administer other pharmacological agents to improve her oxygenation. List three drugs that you would consider, and give the correct dose and desired effect of each.

a._____

b._____

c._____

105. You decide to administer furosemide 0.5 mg/kg. It is supplied in a 4-mL ampule that contains 40 mg of the drug. How many milliliters will you give? _____ mL

106. List causes and signs and symptoms of right ventricular failure.

a. Causes:

_____

b. Signs and symptoms:

Questions 107 to 110 pertain to the following case study:

You are evaluating a 67-year-old man who has a history of two myocardial infarctions. His wife states he had chest pain that began 4 hours ago but that he refused to let her call emergency medical services and then passed out. He is conscious but confused and is pale and diaphoretic. His blood pressure is 80/50 mm Hg, his respiratory rate is 20, his SaO_2 is 90%, and his breath sounds are clear. His only home medicine is nitroglycerin paste, which he has on his left chest. This patient's electrocardiogram is shown in Fig. 29-38.

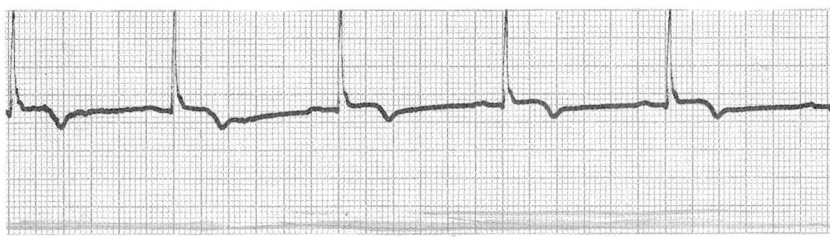

Figure 29-38

107. What is your interpretation of his electrocardiogram?

---

108. What drug and dosage will you administer in consultation with medical direction to correct this dysrhythmia?

After administering the first dose of this drug, the heart rate accelerates to 70 beats/min; however, the patient's other physical findings remain unchanged.

109. What do you suspect this patient is suffering from?

---

110. List critical interventions, including drug therapy, that you should use, assuming that your estimated time of arrival to the hospital is 30 minutes.

Questions 111 to 114 pertain to the following case study:

A 70-year-old man experiences a sudden onset of a "tearing" abdominal pain at the area of the umbilicus that radiates to his back. He is pale and complains of the urge to defecate. His only history is hypertension, for which he takes captopril. Vital signs are blood pressure, 106/70 mm Hg; pulse, 100; and respirations, 20. On physical examination, you auscultate a bruit over the periumbilical area.

111. What illness do you suspect?

---

112. Should you palpate this patient's abdomen?

---

113. Should you allow this patient to go to the toilet and defecate?

_____

114. Briefly outline your management of this patient.

_____

_____

Questions 115 to 117 pertain to the following case study:

An older man complains of a severe "ripping" pain between his scapulae that extends down to his legs. He is pale and diaphoretic and has the following vital signs: blood pressure 170/110 mm Hg in the right arm and 130/80 mm Hg in the left arm.

115. What medical emergency do you suspect?

_____

116. Describe other physical findings that may confirm your suspicions.

_____

117. Outline your management of this patient in the prehospital phase.

_____

_____

118. Differentiate between the following characteristics of embolic arterial occlusion and thrombotic arterial occlusion.

	Embolic	**Thrombotic**
Causes:		
Onset:		
Signs and symptoms:		

119. An older woman calls you to her home because she bumped her leg and a varicose vein is bleeding. What care should be rendered to this patient?

_____

120. List three signs or symptoms of acute deep vein thrombosis.

    a.

    b.

    c.

Questions 121 to 124 pertain to the following case study:

A 60-year-old man complains of a severe headache, blurred vision, and vomiting. He states that he has a history of hypertension but has not been taking his medicine because the cost is too high. His vital signs are blood pressure, 190/128 mm Hg; pulse, 88; and respirations, 20.

121. What medical emergency do you suspect?

_____

122. If this man is not treated promptly, what other signs and/or symptoms may result?

_____

123. Outline general management principles for this patient.

_____

124. If your transport time is delayed, list one drug (with the appropriate dose) that medical direction may order to lower this patient's blood pressure.

_____

TECHNIQUES OF MANAGING CARDIAC EMERGENCIES

125. You are at a friend's home playing tennis. After retrieving the ball, you turn around see that your friend has collapsed on the court. Outline the steps you must take from this moment until emergency medical services arrives if he has had a cardiac arrest. (Assume that no one else is nearby to help.)

_____

_____

_____

126. A basic life support unit is caring for a patient who is in cardiac arrest when your advanced life support unit arrives on the scene. An automated external defibrillator without a display is attached to the patient, and five shocks already have been delivered.

   a. When should you defibrillate this patient if you determine that ventricular fibrillation is present?

_____

   b. If a rescuer is in contact with the patient when the automated external defibrillator fires, will an injury occur?

_____

Questions 127 to 129 pertain to the following case study:

You arrive on the scene to care for a patient who is pulseless and apneic. The monitor displays the rhythm shown in Fig. 29-39.

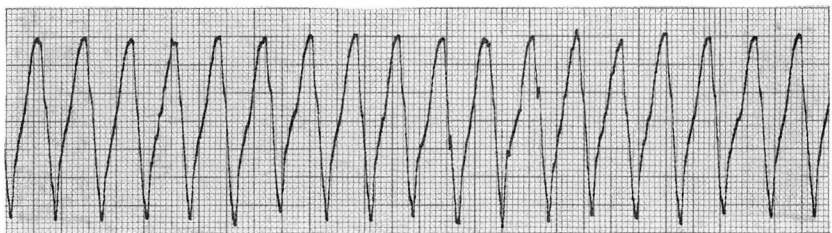

Figure 29-39

127. What is your interpretation of the electrocardiogram?

_____

128. What is your first intervention after rhythm determination and verification of pulselessness?

_____

129. List two factors that will improve the success rate of this treatment.

    a.

    b.

130. List the steps in performing this intervention.

_____

_____

_____

_____

131. You are at the home of a patient whose wife states that he was experiencing severe chest pain. Moments after you hook up the patient to your monitor, he loses consciousness, and the rhythm shown in Fig. 29-40 is displayed. Blood pressure is 60 mm Hg by palpation, and ventilations are adequate. Another paramedic applies oxygen by non-rebreather mask at 12 L/min. State the appropriate therapy for this patient up to and including administration of the first drug.

_____

_____

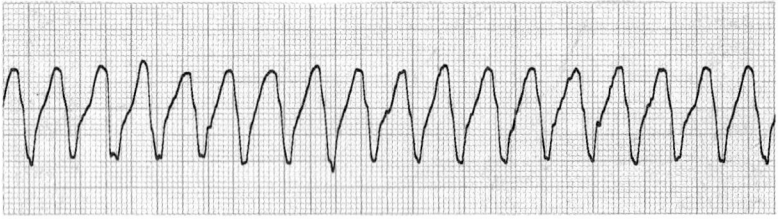

Figure 29-40

132. What is the advantage of synchronized cardioversion?

_____

133. Briefly outline the steps in synchronized cardioversion that are different from unsynchronized cardioversion.

_____

_____

134. A 69-year-old patient has a blood pressure of 76/50 mm Hg and the electrocardiogram shown in Fig. 29-41.

    a. What is your interpretation of the electrocardiogram?

_____

b. Assuming that no drugs are readily available, list the steps you would take to initiate transcutaneous pacing on this patient.

_____

_____

_____

_____

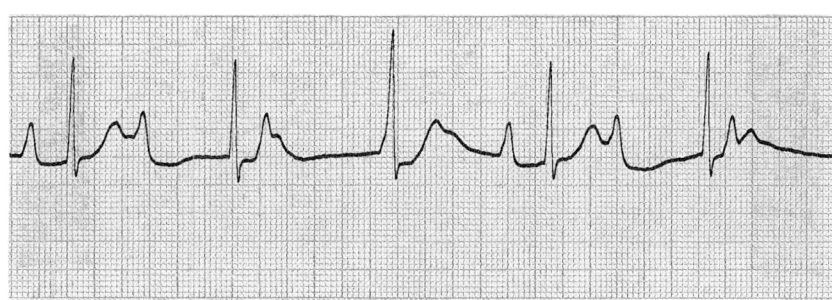

Figure 29-41

135. An older man is found unresponsive, apneic, and pulseless in the busy bathroom of a shopping mall. A quick examination reveals the monitor pattern shown in Fig. 29-42.

a. What is your interpretation of the rhythm?

_____

b. What drugs (with appropriate doses) should be administered?

_____

c. What electrical therapy would be appropriate for this patient?

_____

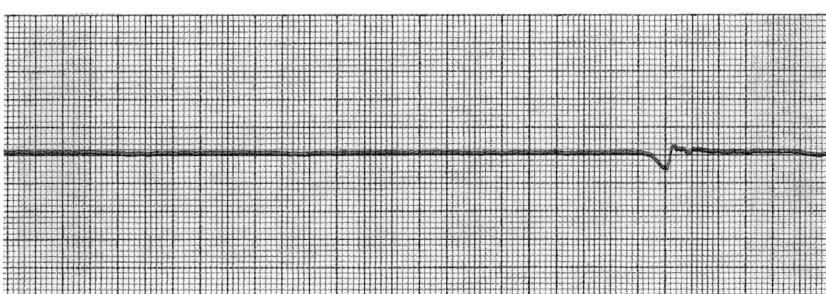

Figure 29-42

136. You are en route to the hospital with a 55-year-old man whom you suspect is having an acute myocardial infarction. Suddenly, the patient gasps and becomes pulseless and apneic. As you look at the monitor, you note the electrocardiogram shown in Fig. 29-43.

    a. What is the rhythm?

    b. What single treatment modality is most likely to restore circulation in this patient?

    c. List the appropriate drugs (in the proper order) with correct doses that may be given to this patient if the answer in (b) is unsuccessful.

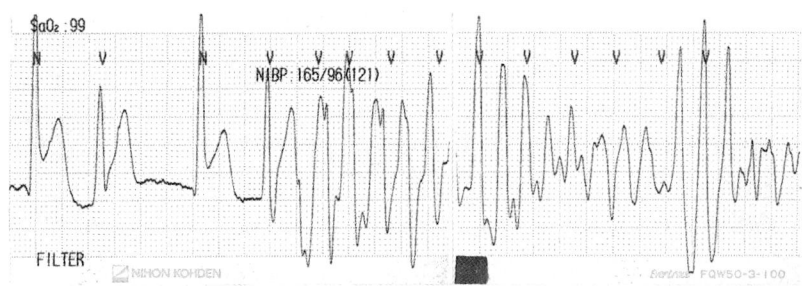

Figure 29-43

137. For each of the following situations, state whether criteria to stop resuscitation have been met. Explain your decision. Assume the patient is now in asystole.

    a. The patient is 94 years old and was found in full arrest, having last been seen 30 minutes previously. You have intubated the patient, given epinephrine, and attempted pacing.

    b. A 65-year-old patient collapses in a mall. You have been resuscitating for 20 minutes, although you have not been able to intubate. You have administered epinephrine (three doses), attempted pacing (unsuccessfully), and administered atropine sulfate (two doses).

c. A 16-year-old is in full arrest after falling from a fourth-floor balcony. You initially got back a sinus rhythm with a pulse, but now asystole is on the monitor. The patient is intubated, and you have two large-bore intravenous lines infusing wide open and have given three doses of epinephrine, attempted pacing, and given two doses of atropine.

_____

_____

d. A 70-year-old is in asystole. You have intubated and given epinephrine (three doses), attempted pacing (unsuccessfully), and administered the maximum dose of atropine with no success. You elect to terminate resuscitation, but the family is objecting strongly.

_____

_____

STUDENT SELF-ASSESSMENT

138. Your patient is experiencing chest pain. He is 75 years of age, says his last cholesterol test result was 300 mg/dL, and takes Diabinese (chlorpropamide), Accupril, and indapamide. How many risk factors for cardiovascular disease did you identify in this patient?
   a. Two   **c.** Four
   b. Three   **d.** Five

139. Blood pressure is equal to which of the following?
   a. Heart rate × Stroke volume × Cardiac output
   b. Stroke volume × Peripheral vascular resistance
   c. Heart rate × Stroke volume × Peripheral vascular resistance
   d. Heart rate × Contractility × Stroke volume

140. Your patient is experiencing signs of a large infarct affecting the anterior portion of the left ventricle. Which coronary vessel most likely is involved?
   a. Circumflex artery   **c.** Left anterior descending
   b. Coronary sinus   **d.** Right coronary artery

141. Which valve separates the left atrium from the left ventricle?
   a. Aortic   **c.** Pulmonic
   b. Mitral   **d.** Tricuspid

142. The magnetic force that occurs when particles with opposite charges are separated across the cell membrane is known as which of the following?
   a. Action potential   **c.** Millivolts
   b. Depolarization   **d.** Potential energy

143. Which ions are critical to maintain the normal resting membrane potential?
   a. Chloride   **c.** Sodium
   b. Phosphate   **d.** Sulfate

144. Which drugs may affect the threshold level of cardiac conduction cells?
   a. Atropine   **c.** Nitroglycerin
   b. Morphine   **d.** Verapamil

145. Which phase of the cardiac action potential represents depolarization?
   a. Phase 1   **c.** Phase 3
   b. Phase 2   **d.** Phase 4

146. What is the purpose of the absolute refractory period in the heart?
   a. To allow electrolyte balance to be restored
   b. To initiate the next action potential
   c. To permit the muscle to relax so the heart can fill
   d. To stretch the cardiac fibers for more forceful contraction

147. Which are the smallest divisions of the His bundles?
  a. Anterior-superior fascicles
  b. Posterior-inferior fascicles
  c. Right and left bundle branches
  d. Purkinje fibers

148. Why do pacemaker cells fire repeatedly without external stimulation?
  a. Cerebral biorhythms cause intrinsic stimulation.
  b. Epinephrine initiates the action potential in regular cycles.
  c. Sympathetic nervous system causes hormonal stimulation.
  d. They have an unstable resting membrane potential.

149. Why is there a conduction delay in the atrioventricular node of the normal cardiac cycle?
  a. So ectopic rhythms do not have a chance to enter the cycle
  b. So simultaneous contraction of the atria can occur
  c. To allow for contraction of the atria before ventricular contraction
  d. To permit refilling of the coronary arteries before atrial systole

150. Which of the following may cause a decrease in sinoatrial node discharge, resulting in decreased heart rate?
  a. Acetylcholine
  c. Norepinephrine
  b. Epinephrine
  d. Parasympatholytic effects

151. Mechanisms that produce dysrhythmias following reentry include which of the following?
  a. Atropine administration
  c. Hypercapnia
  b. Digitalis toxicity
  d. Hyperkalemia

152. Which of the following signs or symptoms would be atypical for a coronary event?
  a. Abdominal discomfort
  c. Jaw pain
  b. Dyspnea
  d. Syncope

153. Dyspnea associated with myocardial infarction usually is related to which of the following?
  a. Chronic obstructive pulmonary disease
  b. Drug administration
  c. Hypercarbia
  d. Pulmonary congestion

154. Syncope should be assumed to be caused by a dysrhythmia if which of the following is associated with it?
  a. Nausea preceded the event.
  b. The patient is older.
  c. The patient has a history of diabetes.
  d. It occurred when the patient was standing.

155. When evaluating a patient for jugular venous distention, the paramedic should do which of the following?
  a. Raise the head of the bed 90 degrees.
  b. Raise the head of the bed 45 degrees.
  c. Lay the patient in the supine position.
  d. Have the patient stand with assistance.

156. Why may it be helpful to find the point of maximum impulse on the patient's chest?
  a. For appropriate defibrillation or pacing patch placement
  b. For assessment of strength of myocardial contractions
  c. To identify a point to auscultate the mitral valve
  d. To place electrodes for monitoring a 12-lead electrocardiogram

157. What does the electrocardiogram tracing assess?
  a. Cardiac output
  c. Myocardial contractility
  b. Electrical conduction
  d. Stroke volume

158. Which of the following represents a bipolar lead?
  a. aV_F
  c. Lead II
  b. aV_R
  d. V_1

159. In lead II the positive electrode is located on the left lower extremity. During normal conduction, which way should the QRS complex deflect?
  a. Biphasic
  c. Isoelectric
  b. Downward
  d. Upward

160. You are looking at leads II, III, and aV$_F$. What part of the heart can you "view" in those leads?
   a. Anterior
   c. Lateral
   b. Inferior
   d. Septum
161. Modified chest leads mimic the view that can be obtained by looking at which of the following?
   a. Augmented leads
   c. Posterior leads
   b. Limb leads
   d. V leads
162. Where should the positive electrode be placed for MCL$_1$?
   a. Below the lateral end of the left clavicle
   b. Below the lateral end of the right clavicle
   c. Fourth intercostal space to the right of the sternum
   d. Left axillary line at the level of the fifth intercostal space
163. Why are leads II and MCL$_1$ preferred for routine monitoring for dysrhythmias?
   a. P waves can be visualized easily.
   b. The tallest QRS complex can be seen.
   c. Rates are calculated more easily.
   d. ST segment elevation or depression can be viewed.
164. Which precordial leads are septal leads?
   a. aV$_L$
   c. V$_3$ and V$_4$
   b. V$_1$ and V$_2$
   d. V$_5$ and V$_6$
165. What represents the absence of electrical activity in the heart on the electrocardiogram strip?
   a. Isoelectric line
   c. QRS complex
   b. P wave
   d. ST segment
166. What is the normal duration of the QRS complex?
   a. 0.04 to 0.08 second
   c. 0.12 to 0.14 second
   b. 0.08 to 0.10 second
   d. 0.14 to 0.16 second
167. During what point does the absolute refractory period occur in the heart?
   a. P wave
   c. Q-T interval
   b. P-R interval
   d. T wave
168. To assess abnormal QRS width accurately, the paramedic should do which of the following?
   a. Determine the J point and measure back from it.
   b. Identify the lead with the widest QRS complex and then measure it.
   c. Measure from the end of the P wave to the end of the S wave.
   d. Measure from R-R wave from left to right.
169. There are 10 small boxes between the R waves on the electrocardiogram tracing. What is the heart rate?
   a. 6 beats/min
   c. 60 beats/min
   b. 30 beats/min
   d. 150 beats/min
170. Identify the electrocardiogram tracing in Fig. 29-44.
   a. Normal sinus rhythm
   b. Sinus rhythm with first-degree atrioventricular block
   c. Second-degree heart block type II
   d. Ventricular demand pacer with capture

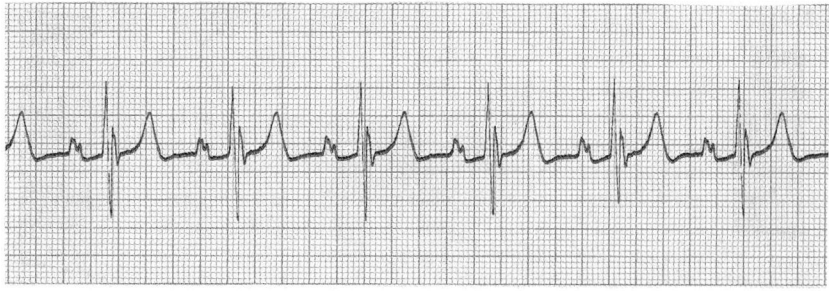

Figure 29-44

171. Identify the electrocardiogram tracing in Fig. 29-45.
   a. Accelerated idioventricular rhythm
   b. Junctional tachycardia
   c. Ventricular pacemaker
   d. Ventricular tachycardia

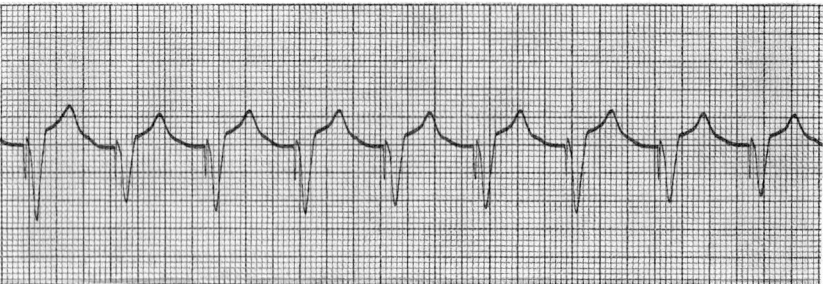

Figure 29-45

172. Identify the electrocardiogram tracing in Fig. 29-46.
   a. Multifocal premature ventricular contractions
   b. Couplet of premature ventricular contractions
   c. Ventricular bigeminy
   d. Ventricular escape rhythm

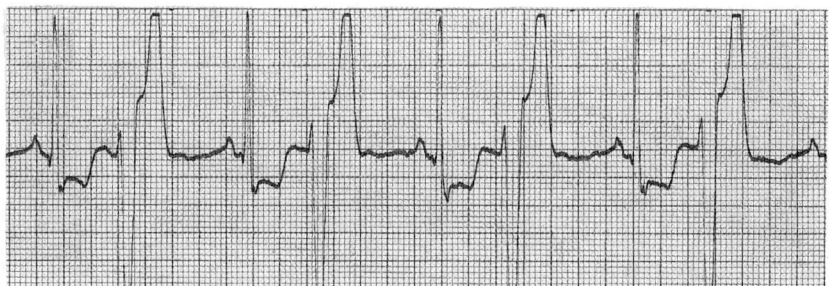

Figure 29-46

173. Identify the electrocardiogram tracing in Fig. 29-47.
   a. Second-degree atrioventricular block type I
   b. Second-degree atrioventricular block type II
   c. Sinus arrest
   d. Sinus arrhythmia

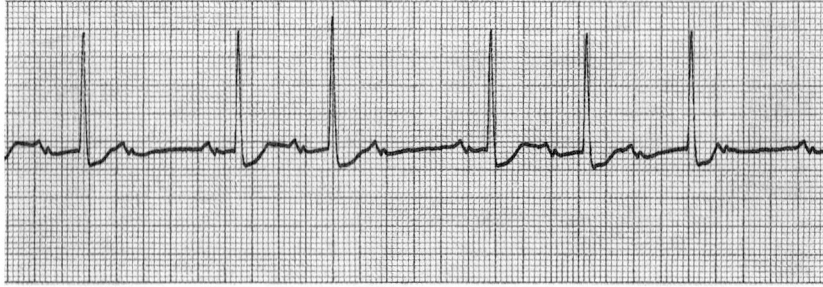

Figure 29-47

174. Identify the electrocardiogram tracing in Fig. 29-48.
- **a.** Atrial fibrillation
- **b.** Atrial flutter
- **c.** Junctional tachycardia
- **d.** Third-degree atrioventricular block

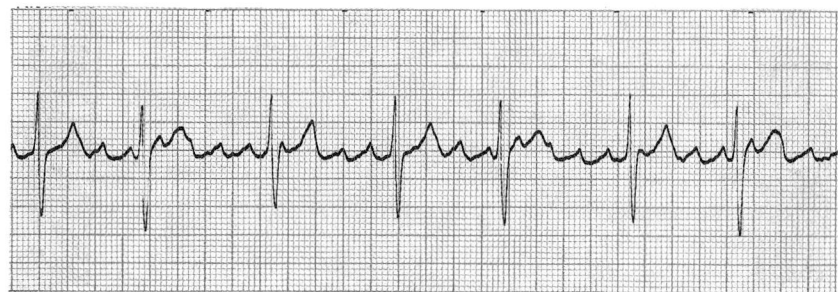

Figure 29-48

175. Identify the electrocardiogram tracing in Fig. 29-49.
- **a.** Atrial fibrillation
- **b.** Atrial flutter
- **c.** Atrial tachycardia
- **d.** Sinus tachycardia

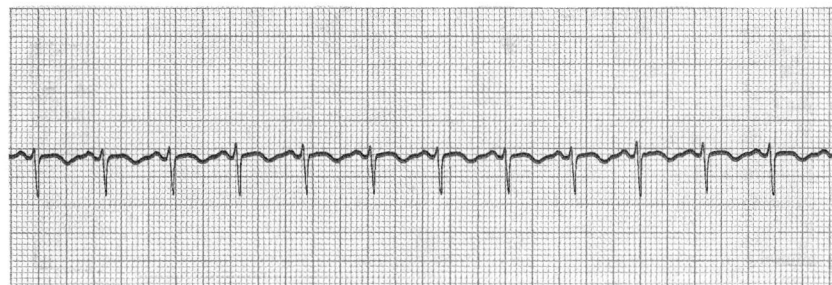

Figure 29-49

176. Identify the electrocardiogram tracing in Fig. 29-50.
- **a.** Accelerated junctional rhythm followed by pacemaker
- **b.** Junctional rhythm followed by pacemaker
- **c.** Junctional rhythm followed by idioventricular
- **d.** Second-degree atrioventricular block type II followed by idioventricular

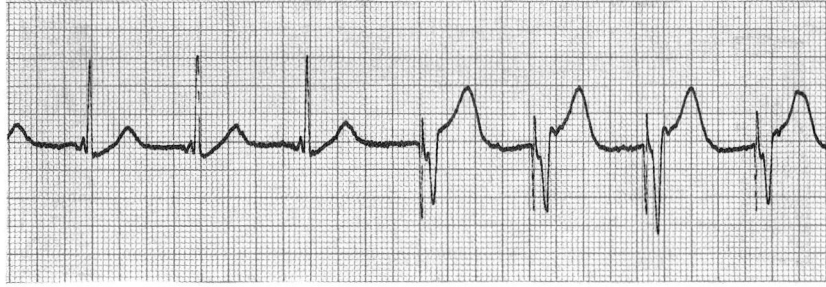

Figure 29-50

177. You are treating a 60-year-old woman with atrial fibrillation at a rate of 168 beats/min. Her blood pressure is 80 mm Hg by palpation, and she feels faint. The appropriate intervention would be which of the following?
    a. Adenosine 6 mg via rapid intravenous administration
    b. Verapamil 2.5 mg intravenously over 2 minutes
    c. Procainamide 30 mg/min intravenously
    d. Synchronized cardioversion at 100 J

178. Which of the following is an ectopic rhythm?
    a. Atrial tachycardia   c. Normal sinus rhythm
    b. Junctional tachycardia   d. Sinus bradycardia

179. Which of the following will *not* cause sinus bradycardia?
    a. Digoxin   c. Isoproterenol
    b. Increased vagal tone   d. Sleep

180. What is the most common cause of decreased cardiac output in atrial fibrillation or atrial flutter?
    a. Decreased ventricular contractility
    b. Development of blood clots
    c. Inadequate atrial filling
    d. Loss of atrial kick

181. What can result from atrial fibrillation?
    a. Congestive heart failure c. Rheumatic heart disease
    b. Pericarditis   d. Vagal stimulation

182. If your patient has accelerated junctional rhythm, what medical history should you inquire about that is associated specifically with this rhythm?
    a. Chronic obstructive pulmonary disease
    b. Diabetes
    c. Marijuana use
    d. Treatment with digoxin

183. Which of the following mechanisms may cause ventricular dysrhythmias?
    a. Enhanced automaticity
    b. Reentry phenomena
    c. Enhanced automaticity and reentry phenomena
    d. Neither enhanced automaticity nor reentry phenomena

184. Premature ventricular contractions that occur every second complex are known as which of the following?
    a. Bigeminy   c. Idioventricular
    b. Couplets   d. Multifocal

185. Your patient has a wide-complex tachycardia. Which of the following electrocardiogram findings would indicate ventricular tachycardia?
    a. All precordial leads (V leads) have a positive deflection.
    b. Negative QRS deflection with a single peak in MCL_1 and MCL_6.
    c. Positive QRS complex in leads I, II, and III.
    d. RS interval is less than 0.10 second in any V lead.

186. What type of pacemaker fires only when the patient's own heart rate drops below a predetermined rate?
    a. Asynchronous   c. Dual chamber
    b. Demand   d. Fixed rate

187. What rhythm occurs when a complete block develops at or below the atrioventricular node?
    a. Bundle branch block
    b. Fascicular block
    c. Second-degree atrioventricular block type II
    d. Third-degree atrioventricular block

188. Which of the following is true regarding left bundle branch block?
    a. It produces an initial R wave in MCL_1 instead of the normal small Q wave.
    b. There is a shallow, narrow QS pattern, and the QRS complex is less than 0.12 second.
    c. There is an RSR prime pattern seen in MCL_1 with a QRS complex greater than 0.12 second.
    d. The fibers that usually fire the interventricular septum are blocked.

189. Which of the following has the greatest potential to deteriorate into complete heart block?
    a. Anterior hemiblock
    c. Posterior hemiblock
    b. Bifascicular block
    d. Right bundle branch block
190. Your patient has a history of Wolff-Parkinson-White syndrome. You note a wide-complex supraventricular tachycardia. Which drug is not appropriate for this patient?
    a. Adenosine
    c. Procainamide
    b. Lidocaine
    d. Verapamil
191. What distinguishes unstable angina from stable angina?
    a. It is caused by atherosclerotic disease of the coronary arteries.
    b. The pain lasts 1 to 5 minutes and is relieved by oxygen or nitroglycerin.
    c. The pain changes in its onset, frequency, duration, or quality.
    d. It is precipitated by physical exertion or emotional stress.
192. Death from myocardial infarction is *most commonly* the result of which of the following?
    a. Dysrhythmias
    c. Pulmonary embolism
    b. Low blood pressure
    d. Cardiac rupture
193. Appropriate care for a stable patient with acute myocardial infarction would include all of the following except which one?
    a. Placing the patient in a semi-Fowler position
    b. Administering lactated Ringer's solution at 500 mL/hr intravenously
    c. Administering oxygen by nasal cannula
    d. Documenting and reporting all intravenous sticks
194. Which of the following is *not* diagnostic of an acute myocardial infarction?
    a. Pathological Q waves
    c. ST segment depression
    b. Peaked tented T waves
    d. ST segment elevation
195. Medications that may help in the management of a patient with cardiac pulmonary edema include all of the following *except* which one?
    a. Epinephrine
    c. Morphine
    b. Furosemide
    d. Nitroglycerin
196. When a patient suffers from right ventricular heart failure, blood backs up into which of the following?
    a. Aorta
    c. Pulmonary veins
    b. Pulmonary arteries
    d. Venae cavae
197. Cardiogenic shock is
    a. Fatal in only 10% to 15% of patients.
    b. Caused by extensive myocardial damage.
    c. The result of an intravascular electrolyte imbalance.
    d. Caused by obstruction of the renal vessels.
198. Your patient has a history of cancer and is having chest pain and tachycardia. What is an early sign that may indicate the development of cardiac tamponade?
    a. Decreased systolic pressure
    c. Pericardial friction rub
    b. Jugular venous distention
    d. Tracheal deviation
199. Which is the most common presentation of dissection of the thoracic aorta?
    a. Chest heaviness of slow onset
    b. Intense back pain with sudden onset
    c. Neck pain that began suddenly
    d. Substernal dull pain that increased gradually
200. Acute arterial occlusion may result in which of the following?
    a. Absent distal pulses
    c. Pulmonary congestion
    b. Hypertension
    d. Torsades de pointes
201. You suspect that your patient has an arterial occlusion affecting the lower leg. Which of the following treatment measures would be appropriate?
    a. Initiate intravenous fluid therapy and administer a fluid challenge.
    b. Massage the affected extremity to encourage circulation.
    c. Immobilize the affected extremity and protect it from injury.
    d. Administer furosemide 40 mg intravenously to flush out the embolus.

202. Chronic, uncontrolled hypertension puts a patient at risk for all *except* which of the following?
  a. Cerebral hemorrhage   **c.** Myocardial infarction
  b. Diabetes mellitus   **d.** Renal failure

203. According to the American Heart Association, how soon should basic cardiac life support be initiated in the patient in cardiac arrest?
  a. 4 minutes   **c.** 8 minutes
  b. 6 minutes   **d.** 12 minutes

204. You work at a service that uses biphasic defibrillation. Which of the following is true regarding this device?
  a. It compensates for chest impedence.
  b. The batteries are larger.
  c. The energy flows in one direction.
  d. Three patches are needed.

205. What principle should be followed when placing paddles or patches on the chest for defibrillation?
  a. Anterior-posterior placement may be used for patches.
  b. Never reverse the polarity, or defibrillation will not occur.
  c. Place one paddle over the sternum directly over the heart.
  d. Use pediatric paddles for children up to 8 years of age.

206. What should you consider when caring for a patient who has an implantable cardioverter defibrillator?
  a. Apply a magnet to the chest to activate these devices if the patient is unresponsive.
  b. If defibrillation at 360 J is unsuccessful, paddle placement should be changed.
  c. The complete sequence of up to three shocks may take as long as 1 minute.
  d. Touching the patient during implantable cardioverter defibrillator defibrillation is dangerous and should be avoided.

207. Which of the following statements is true regarding synchronized cardioversion?
  a. It is faster than unsynchronized cardioversion.
  b. It is not as safe as unsynchronized cardioversion.
  c. It is indicated for pulseless ventricular tachycardia.
  d. It is indicated for unstable paroxysmal supraventricular tachycardia.

208. When attempting to initiate transcutaneous pacing on a conscious patient, set the current at which of the following?
  a. 70 to 80 per minute and increased until the patient is stable
  b. 50 mA and increased until capture occurs
  c. 70 to 80 per minute and decreased until the patient becomes unstable
  d. Maximum mA and decreased until capture is lost

209. Which of the following drugs is used to treat asystole?
  a. Atropine   **c.** Calcium chloride
  b. Bretylium   **d.** Lidocaine

210. Which of the following is a side effect from bretylium tosylate?
  a. Drowsiness   **c.** Hypotension
  b. Headache   **d.** Hypothermia

211. Which of the following is an action of morphine sulfate?
  a. Dilation of peripheral vasculature
  b. Increase in cardiac preload
  c. Calming of the patient with a head injury
  d. Bronchodilation

212. Which of the following is true of digoxin?
  a. It increases the force of ventricular contraction.
  b. It is a first-line drug in the management of bradycardia.
  c. It causes decreased cardiac output.
  d. It increases impulse conduction through the atrioventricular node.

213. Which of the following drugs stimulates the beta receptors?
  a. Amyl nitrite   **c.** Epinephrine
  b. Atropine   **d.** Propranolol

214. A 60-year-old, 100-kg woman has a blood pressure of 80/50 mm Hg. The electrocardiogram is shown in Fig. 29-51. Which of the following is not appropriate to correct this?
  a. Atropine 0.5 to 1.0 mg intravenously
  b. Dopamine 5 to 20 mcg/kg/min
  c. Epinephrine 2 to 10 mcg/kg/min
  d. Isoproterenol 2 to 10 mcg/min

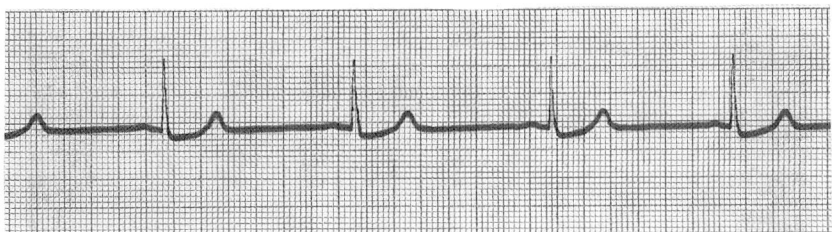

Figure 29-51

215. Which of the following criteria should be considered to determine whether to terminate resuscitation of a patient?
  a. Family who objects to termination
  b. Presence of a nonofficial do not resuscitate order
  c. Quality of life judgments
  d. Time of collapse before emergency medical services arrival

WRAP IT UP

"4027 respond to a cardiac arrest, 1425 Humes, 4027 . . .": the dispatcher's familiar voice jolts you awake from a nap. As you respond, you are updated that CPR instructions are in progress. You hear the local fire department announce their arrival at the scene when you are about 10 blocks away, and as you walk into the house you can hear a mechanical voice say, "Deliver shock now." As the firefighter presses the button on the AED, the patient's lifeless body jolts, and then the AED commands, "Assessing rhythm, do not touch the patient," followed what seems like an eternity later by, "No shock advised, check breathing and pulse." You quickly check breathing and pulse and are surprised to feel weak slow pulsations under your fingers at the carotid artery. "Begin ventilations," you instruct the firefighter at the patient's head, and she begins to ventilate the patient with a bag. By now your partner has disconnected the defibrillation pads from the AED and reconnected them to your monitor/defibrillator. You note a bradycardia rhythm that appears to be increasing at a fairly rapid rate. "He's breathing!" the firefighter ventilating the patient exclaims. The patient begins to cough and push away the bag from his face. Vital signs are BP 100/70 mm Hg, P 88, R 18, SaO_2 95%. You calm the patient, apply oxygen, and initiate an IV. The hospital advises you to administer an antidysrhythmic drug to prevent a recurrence of his lethal rhythm. The patient's wife says her 55-year-old husband was complaining of indigestion for about an hour before he collapsed. He is normally healthy and takes no medications, and so he would not let her take him to the ER. After the patient is secured in the ambulance, you perform a 12-lead electrocardiogram. You note 4-mm ST segment elevation in leads V_1 to V_4. The patient is awake but slightly confused and rubbing his chest. You give him aspirin and nitroglycerin after obtaining another BP at 116/84 mm Hg. His ER stay is brief; the cardiologist whisks him to the cardiac catheter lab where balloon angiography is performed. As you enter your times in the computer, you note that the initial fire department unit arrived 4 minutes after the 911 call was placed. They delivered the shock 1½ minutes later. You meet the patient a month later at the grocery store with his four children; he is ready to return to work and is emotional as he gives you his thanks.

1. Place a check mark beside the elements of the chain of survival that were present on this call.
  a. _____ Early recognition of the emergency
  b. _____ Activation of 911
  c. _____ Early cardiopulmonary resuscitation
  d. _____ Early defibrillation
  e. _____ Early advanced care
  f. _____ Rapid interventional cardiology

2. What rhythm(s) was the patient in when the fire department arrived?

_____

3. What antidysrhythmic drug(s) could you administer?

_____

4. What is the significance of your 12-lead electrocardiogram findings?

_____

5. Which element of this patient's situation would be a relative contraindication to fibrinolytic therapy?
   a. Cardiopulmonary resuscitation less than 10 minutes
   b. Suspected aortic dissection
   c. Terminal illness
   d. Uncontrolled hypertension

CHAPTER 29 ANSWERS

REVIEW QUESTIONS

1. c
(Objective 2)

2. f
(Objective 2)

3. a
(Objective 2)

4. e
(Objective 2)

5. b
(Objective 2)

6. g
(Objective 2)

7. h
(Objective 2)

8.

Risk Factor	Prevention Strategy	Resource
a. Smoking	Quit smoking with use of medications, hypnosis, behavior modification, health clinic	Private physician, heart association, cancer association, alternative nicotine products
b. Hypercholesterolemia	Diet modification, drugs	Private physician, health clinic, heart association
c. Obesity	Diet, exercise	Private physician, exercise, community health clinic, dietitian, American Heart Association
d. Sedentary lifestyle	Exercise program, leisure activities	Private physician, local hospital

(Objective 1)

9.

	Sympathetic	Parasympathetic
a. Heart rate	Increase	Decrease
b. Myocardial	Increase	No effect contractility
c. Lungs	Beta-bronchiolar dilation	Constriction
d. Blood vessels (peripheral)	Constriction	No effect

(Objective 2)

10. a. Epinephrine: increased heart rate, contractility, bronchiolar dilation, and blood vessel constriction in skin, kidneys, gastrointestinal tract, and viscera
b. Norepinephrine: peripheral vasoconstriction
(Objective 2)

11. a. Magnetic
   b. Potential
   c. Permeable
   d. Potential
   e. Millivolts
   f. Negative
   g. Negatively
   h. Potential
   i. Negative
   j. −70 to −90
   k. Potassium
   l. Potassium
   m. Proteins
   n. Permeable
   o. Excitability
   p. Depolarization
   q. Threshold potential
   r. Action potential
   s. Depolarization
   t. Repolarization
   u. Positive
   v. Negative
   w. Depolarization
   x. Membrane potential
   (Objective 3)

12. a. Sodium rushes into the cell through the fast sodium channels.
   b. The membrane potential drops to approximately 0.
   c. The slow calcium channels allow calcium to enter the cell while potassium continues to leave, maintaining the membrane potential of 0.
   d. The membrane potential returns to −90 mV.
   e. The sodium pump allows the exchange of sodium and potassium to their proper compartments.
   f. During phase 4, cardiac pacemaker cells slowly depolarize from their most negative membrane potential to a level at which threshold is reached and phase 0 begins. Nonpacemaker cells maintain a stable resting membrane potential and do not depolarize unless stimulated by a sufficiently strong stimulus.
   (Objective 3)

13. a. Action potentials; b. upward; c. automaticity; d. resting membrane potential
   (Objective 3)

14. a. Sinoatrial node; b. intranodal pathways; c. atrioventricular node; d. common bundle of His; e. left posterior bundle branch; f. Purkinje fibers; g. left anterior bundle branch; h. right bundle branch
   (Objective 4)

15. The next pacemaker (atrioventricular node) should take over and fire.
   (Objective 4)

16. a. Acceleration of phase 4 depolarization so cells reach their threshold prematurely (may result from digoxin toxicity, increased catecholamine levels, hypoxia, hypercapnia, myocardial ischemia, infarction, increased venous return, hypokalemia, hypocalcemia, heating or cooling of the heart, or atropine administration)
   b. Reactivation of tissue by a returning impulse
   (Objective 4)

17. O—Onset. What were you doing when the pain began?
P—Is there anything that makes the pain better or worse?
Q—What does the pain feel like? (Is it sharp, dull, crushing, squeezing?)
R—Where is the pain? Does it go anywhere else?
S—On a scale of 1 to 10, with 1 being no pain and 10 being the worst pain you have ever had, describe your pain.
T—When did you first feel the pain?
(Objective 5)

18. Chest pain, dyspnea, syncope, and palpitations
(Objective 5)

19. How did you feel before you passed out? What were you doing when you passed out? What position were you in before you passed out (i.e., laying down, sitting, or standing)? How long were you unconscious? Do you have a history of heart disease or other significant medical history? What medicines do you take? Do you feel unusual in any other way? How has your health been over the past several days?
(Objective 5)

20. Pulse rate and regularity, electrocardiogram, vital signs, circumstances of occurrence, duration, associated symptoms, previous history of palpitations, medical history, and daily medicines
(Objective 5)

21. Major medical illnesses, home medicines, and similar previous episodes
(Objective 5)

22. Atrial fibrillation with a slow ventricular response
(Objective 10)

23. Yes. Digoxin (Lanoxin) or calcium channel blocker (Cardizem) toxicity can cause this presentation. Digitalis toxicity is more likely in the patient who also is taking a diuretic (furosemide).
(Objective 5)

24. Neck: jugular venous distention. Chest: implanted pacemaker generator, median sternotomy scar, lung sounds (crackles), heart sounds (S_3 gallop), and pulse deficit. Abdomen: generator for automatic implantable cardioverter defibrillator visible. Extremities: edema and ulceration. Back: sacral edema. Medical alert tags or medical information in wallet
(Objective 5)

25.

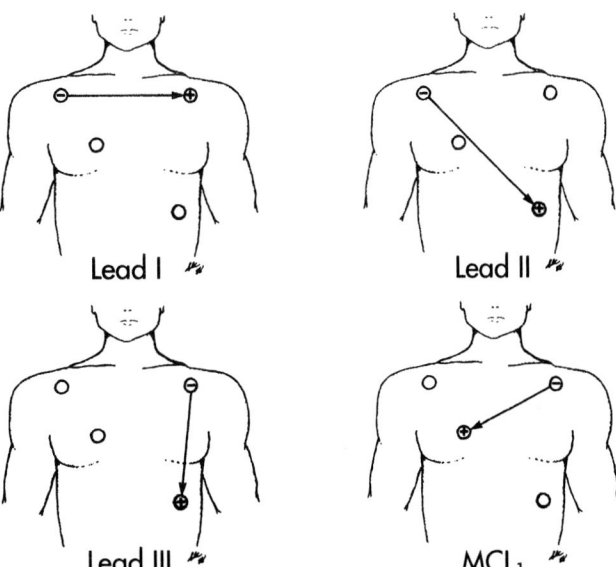

(Objective 6)

26. a. Right arm (right anterior forearm)
   b. Left arm (left anterior forearm)
   c. Right leg (right lower leg)
   d. Left lower leg (left leg)
   e. V_1, fourth intercostal space to the right of the sternum
   f. V_2, fourth intercostal space to the left of the sternum
   g. V_4, fifth intercostal space, midclavicular line
   h. V_3, between V_2 and V_4
   i. V_5, anterior axillary line in a straight line with V_4
   j. V_6, midaxillary line, level with V_4 and V_5 (In women, V_4 to V_6 should be placed under the left breast.)
   (Objective 6)

27. a. Excessive body hair: Shave.
   b. Diaphoresis: Dry area and apply tincture of benzoin.
   c. Poor electrode placement: Reapply correctly.
   d. 60-cycle interference: Run monitor on batteries.
   e. Poor cable connections: Recheck all connections.
   f. Close proximity to electrical motors
   (Objective 6)

28. a. 5; b. 0.04; c. 0.20; d. d3; e. 6
   (Objective 6)

29. a. P wave; b. QRS complex; c. T wave; d. P-R interval; e. ST segment
   (Objective 7)

30. Muscle tremor, AC (60-cycle interference), loose electrodes, patient movement, loss of electrode contact, and external chest compression
   (Objective 7)

31. Analyze the QRS complex; analyze the P waves; analyze the rate; analyze the rhythm; analyze the P-R interval.
   (Objective 8)

32. a. Triplicate method (120 beats/min.): Find the R wave on the dark line, count 300-150-100-75 for each next dark line until the next R wave. The R wave falls between 100 and 150. Estimate rate to be 120 beats/min.
   b. R-R method: $300 \div$ Number of large boxes between R waves $= 300 \div$ (almost) $3 = 100$ beats/min
   c. R-R method: $1500 \div$ Number of small boxes between R waves $= 1500 \div 13 = 115$ beats/min
   d. 6-second method: Number of R waves in a 6-second strip $\times 10 = 12 \times 10 = 120$ beats/min
   (Objective 8)

33. No, this reveals only the rate, not the perfusion status (and the rate is faster than normal for an adult).
   (Objective 7)

34. a. R-R method ($1500 \div$ Number of small boxes between the R waves) or triplicate method (but only if R waves both fall on dark lines)
   b. The 6-second method is the most accurate and quick estimate for irregular rhythm.
   (Objective 8)

35. The R-R distance should be equal when measured left to right across an electrocardiogram strip (it can vary no greater than 0.16 second).
   (Objective 8)

36. a. Through the ventricles is normal.
   b. Conduction through the ventricles is delayed and may follow an abnormal pathway.
   (Objective 7)

37. Are they regular? Is there a P wave in front of each QRS complex? Are they upright or inverted? Do they all look the same?
(Objective 8)

38. a. Electrical impulse that progressed from the atria to the ventricles through pathways other than the atrioventricular node of the bundle of His
b. Normal conduction from the sinoatrial node through the atrioventricular node
c. Delay in conduction of impulse through the atrioventricular node or bundle of His
(Objective 7)

39. a. QRS complex: 0.08 sec (normal is less than 0.12 second)
b. P waves: regular, one for each QRS complex, upright, all the same
c. Rate: 75 beats/min (triplicate method)
d. Rhythm: regular (R-R intervals equal)
e. P-R interval: 0.14 second. Interpretation: normal sinus rhythm
(Objectives 8 and 9)

40. Patient history, chief complaint, and physical findings
(Objective 10)

41. a. Parasympathetic stimulation
b. QRS complex less than 0.12 second (unless a conduction delay is present)
c. P waves (regular, preceding each QRS complex, upright, similar)
d. P-R interval: 0.12 to 0.20 second
(Objective 10)

42. a. Sinus node disease, increased parasympathetic vagal tone, hypothermia, hypoxia, and drug effects (digitalis, propranolol, verapamil)
b. Exercise, fever, anxiety, ingestion of stimulants, smoking, hypovolemia, anemia, congestive heart failure, and excessive administration of atropine or vagolytic or sympathomimetic drugs (cocaine, phencyclidine, epinephrine, isoproterenol)
(Objective 10)

43. QRS complex: 0.08 second. P waves: present, upright, similar. Rate: 50 beats/min. Rhythm: regular. P-R interval: 0.16 second. Interpretation: sinus bradycardia. Distinguishing features: all features of normal sinus rhythm except that rate is less than 60 beats/min. Treatment: stable—observe; unstable—atropine 0.5 to 1.0 mg every 3 to 5 minutes to a maximum dose of less than 2.5 mg (0.03 to 0.04 mg/kg), transcutaneous pacing, dopamine 5 to 20 mcg/kg/min, epinephrine 2 to 10 mcg/min, isoproterenol 2 to 10 mcg/min
(Objective 10)

44. QRS complex: 0.06 second. P waves: present, upright, similar. Rate: 110 beats/min. Rhythm: regular. P-R interval: 0.16 second. Interpretation: sinus tachycardia. Distinguishing features: all features of normal sinus rhythm except that rate is greater than 100 beats/min. Treatment: stable—none; unstable—seek and treat underlying cause
(Objective 10)

45. QRS complex: 0.08 second; P waves: present, upright, similar. Rate: 70 beats/min. Rhythm: irregular. P-R interval: 0.12 second. Interpretation: sinus dysrhythmia. Distinguishing features: all features of normal sinus rhythm but irregular rhythm that varies in cycles. Treatment: none
(Objective 10)

46. QRS complex: 0.08 second. P waves: normal, upright. Rate: 50 beats/min. Rhythm: irregular. P-R interval: 0.16 second. Interpretation: sinus arrest. Distinguishing features: normal sinus rhythm until the sinoatrial node fails to fire. Treatment: stable—observe; unstable—atropine and transcutaneous pacing
(Objective 10)

47. a. Tissues; b. atria; c. internodal
(Objective 10)

48. a. QRS complex: normal
b. P waves (if present): different from normal sinus P waves
c. P-R interval: abnormal, shortened, or prolonged
(Objective 10)

49. Stress, overexertion, tobacco, caffeine, Wolff-Parkinson-White syndrome, digoxin toxicity, hypoxia, chronic obstructive pulmonary disease, congestive heart failure, damage to sinoatrial node, rheumatic heart disease, and atherosclerotic heart disease
(Objective 10)

50. QRS complex: 0.06 second. P waves: changes from beat to beat. Rate: 75 beats/min. Rhythm: regular. P-R interval: variable. Interpretation: wandering atrial pacemaker. Distinguishing features: typically slightly irregular P wave shapes and variable P-R interval. Treatment: stable—monitor; unstable following bradycardia—treat as bradycardia
(Objective 10)

51. QRS complex: 0.06 second. P waves: present, upright. Rate: 100 beats/min. Rhythm: regular interrupted by premature beats. P-R interval: 0.10 second (premature atrial contraction 0.16 second). Interpretation: normal sinus rhythm with one premature atrial contraction. Distinguishing features: extra beat occurring earlier than next expected sinus beat; premature atrial contraction has features of sinus beat except that P-R interval may be different. Treatment: none
(Objective 10)

52. QRS complex: 0.06 second. P waves: unable to determine, may be hidden in T wave. Rate: 180 beats/min. Rhythm: regular. P-R interval: unable to determine. Interpretation: supraventricular tachycardia. Distinguishing features: rate greater than 150 beats/min, with complexes originating in atria (QRS complex is <0.12 second unless a conduction defect is present.) Treatment: stable—oxygen, intravenous line, 12-lead electrocardiogram, consideration of vagal maneuvers, adenosine (6 mg, 12 mg, 12 mg rapid intravenous push at 1- to 2-minute intervals), diltiazem or verapamil or beta-blockers, consider digoxin (Class IIb); unstable—synchronized cardioversion at 50, 100, 200, 300, and 360 J
(Objective 10)

53. QRS complex: 0.06 second. P waves: f-R waves. Rate: 100 beats/min. Rhythm: regular. P-R interval: none. F-R interval: may vary. Interpretation: atrial flutter with 3:1 conduction. Distinguishing features: flutter waves. Treatment: stable—(usually no treatment prehospital); with tachycardic rate—diltiazem or verapamil or beta-blockers or digoxin to control rate; if impaired cardiac function is present—diltiazem or amiodarone or digoxin; unstable—synchronized cardioversion at 50, 100, 200, 300, and 360 J
(Objective 10)

54. QRS complex: 0.06 second. P waves: none. Rate: 160 beats/min. Rhythm: irregularly irregular. P-R interval: none. Interpretation: atrial fibrillation. Distinguishing features: irregularly irregular, no P waves, fibrillation waves. Treatment: calcium channel or beta-blocker; impaired cardiac function—diltiazem or amiodarone; acute and associated with serious signs or symptoms—synchronized cardioversion at 100, 200, 300, and 360 J
(Objective 10)

55. a. junctional (nodal); b. normal; c. may occur before, during, or after QRS complex or may be absent; inverted in lead II; d. often less than 0.12 second
(Objective 10)

56. Increased vagal tone on sinoatrial node, pathological slowing of sinoatrial discharge, complete atrioventricular block, digitalis toxicity, damage to the atrioventricular junction, inferior wall myocardial infarction, and rheumatic fever
(Objective 10)

57. QRS complex: 0.08 second. P waves: present, upright, similar in underlying rhythm, absent in premature beats. Rate: 60 beats/min. Rhythm: irregular. P-R interval: 0.16 second (underlying rhythm), none in premature beats. Interpretation: sinus rhythm (borderline bradycardia) with two premature junctional contractions. Distinguishing features: premature beats occurring earlier than next expected sinus beat, lack of P waves, QRS complex within normal limits. Treatment: monitor patient and treat bradycardia if present and symptomatic. (Objective 10)

58. QRS complex: 0.08 second. P waves: absent. Rate: 40 beats/min. Rhythm: regular. P-R interval: none. Interpretation: junctional escape rhythm. Distinguishing features: rate 40 to 60 beats/min, inverted P waves if present (may occur before, during [absent], or after QRS complex). Treatment: stable—monitor; unstable—atropine 0.5 to 1.0 mg every 5 minutes to total dose of 2.5 mg (0.03 to 0.04 mg/kg), transcutaneous pacing, dopamine 5 to 20 mcg/kg/min, epinephrine 2 to 10 mcg/min, and isoproterenol 2 to 10 mcg/min (Objective 10)

59. QRS complex: 0.08 second. P waves: absent. Rate: 80 beats/min. Rhythm: regular. P-R interval: none. Interpretation: accelerated junctional rhythm. Distinguishing features: rate 60 to 100 beats/min, inverted P waves in lead II if present (may be absent or occur before, during, or after QRS complex). Treatment: monitor. (Objective 10)

60. a. 20, 40; b. 100 beats/min; c. 100 beats/min (Objective 10)

61. Failure of higher pacemakers, heart block, myocardial ischemia, hypoxia, acid-base or electrolyte imbalance, congestive heart failure, increased catecholamine levels, use of stimulants, medicine toxicity (digitalis, tricyclic antidepressant overdose), sympathomimetic drugs, cardiac trauma, and electrical injury (Objective 10)

62. If unstable, all rhythms need cardioversion. If stable, the following:
a. Assess leads I, II, III, MCL_1 (V_1), and MCL_6 (V_6) to determine axis deviation. If the QRS complex is negative in leads I, II, and III (extreme right axis or "no-man's land") and positive in MCL_1 (V_1), the rhythm is ventricular tachycardia; if not,
b. Assess the QRS deflection in MCL_1 (V_1) and MCL_6 (V_6). Positive QRS deflections with a single peak, a taller left rabbit ear, or an RS complex with a fat r wave or slurred s wave in MCL_1 (V_1) indicates ventricular tachycardia. A negative QS complex, a negative rS complex, or any wide Q wave in MCL_6 (V_6) also indicates ventricular tachycardia.
c. If right axis deviation is present (negative QRS complex in lead I; positive QRS complex in leads II and III) and the QRS complex is negative in MCL_1 (V_1), it indicates ventricular tachycardia.
d. If all precordial (V) leads are positive or negative (precordial concordance), it indicates ventricular tachycardia.
e. If the RS interval is greater than 0.10 second in any V lead, it indicates ventricular tachycardia.
(Objective 10)

63. QRS complex: 0.16 second. P waves: absent. Rate: 40 beats/min. Rhythm: regular. P-R interval: none. Interpretation: ventricular escape rhythm. Distinguishing features: rate 20 to 40 beats/min, absent P waves, QRS complex greater than 0.12 second. Treatment: oxygen, transcutaneous pacing, dopamine 5 to 20 mcg/kg/min, epinephrine 2 to 10 mcg/min, and isoproterenol 2 to 10 mcg/min (Objective 10)

64. QRS complex: underlying rhythm 0.10 second. Premature beat: 0.16 second. P wave: present, upright (except premature beat). Rate: 75 beats/min. Rhythm: regular interrupted by premature beats. P-R interval: 0.16 second (underlying rhythm). None: premature beat. Interpretation: normal sinus rhythm with one premature ventricular contraction. Distinguishing features: ectopic beat occurs earlier than next expected sinus beat, wide bizarre QRS complex with T wave deflection opposite QRS complex, no P waves, compensatory pause. Treatment: in presence of hemodynamically compromising premature ventricular contractions—oxygen, lidocaine 1.0 to 1.5 mg/kg repeated at 0.5- to 0.75-mg/kg doses to a maximum of 3 mg/kg (Objective 10)

65. QRS complex: 0.20 second. P waves: absent. Rate: 230 beats/min. Rhythm: regular. P-R interval: none. Interpretation: monomorphic ventricular tachycardia. Distinguishing features: rate greater than 100 beats/min (usually greater than 150 beats/min), regular, no P waves, QRS complex equal to or greater than 0.12 second. Treatment: stable—oxygen, procainamide or sotalol or amiodarone or lidocaine; impaired cardiac function—amiodarone or lidocaine; unstable—synchronized cardioversion at 100, 200, 300, and 360 J; or unconsciousness, hypotension, or pulmonary edema—defibrillate at 100, 200, 300, and 360 J or equivalent biphasic energy; pulseless—treat as ventricular fibrillation
(Objective 10)

66. QRS complex: none. P waves: none. Rate: none. Rhythm: none, chaotic. P-R interval: none. Interpretation: ventricular fibrillation. Distinguishing features: no organized rhythm, chaotic fibrillatory waves. Treatment: rapid defibrillation at 200, 300, and 360 J or equivalent biphasic energy, cardiopulmonary resuscitation, intubation, epinephrine or vasopressin, amiodarone or lidocaine, magnesium sulfate, and procainamide; consider sodium bicarbonate
(Objective 10)

67. QRS complex: none. P waves: none. Rate: none. Rhythm: none. P-R interval: none. Interpretation: asystole. Distinguishing features: isoelectric rhythm. Treatment: cardiopulmonary resuscitation, transcutaneous pacing, epinephrine, atropine, and consideration of underlying cause
(Objective 10)

68. QRS complex: 0.16 second. P waves: absent. Rate: 80 beats/min. Rhythm: regular. P-R interval: none. Interpretation: ventricular paced rhythm. Distinguishing features: pacemaker spike followed by wide-complex ventricular beat. Treatment: none
(Objective 10)

69. a. Heart blocks; b. conduction system
(Objective 10)

70. Myocardial ischemia, acute myocardial infarction, increased parasympathetic tone, drug toxicity (digitalis, propranolol, verapamil), and electrolyte imbalance
(Objective 10)

71. QRS complex: 0.06 second. P waves: present, upright. Rate: 60 beats/min. Rhythm: regular. P-R interval: 0.32 second. Interpretation: sinus rhythm with first-degree atrioventricular block. Distinguishing features: P-R interval greater than 0.20 second. Treatment: observe.
(Objective 10)

72. QRS complex: 0.08 second. P waves: present, upright, more P waves than QRS complexes. Rate: 60 beats/min. Rhythm: irregular. P-R interval: progressively longer until one is not conducted. Distinguishing features: more P waves than QRS complexes, progressively lengthens P-R interval until a QRS complex is dropped. Interpretation: second-degree atrioventricular block (Mobitz type I or Wenckebach). Treatment: asymptomatic—observe; if bradycardic with hemodynamic compromise—oxygen, atropine, transcutaneous pacing, dopamine, epinephrine, and isoproterenol
(Objective 10)

73. QRS complex: 0.06 second. P waves: present, upright, more P waves than QRS complexes. Rate: 50 beats/min. Rhythm: irregular. P-R interval: 0.16 second for conducted P waves. Interpretation: second-degree atrioventricular block (Mobitz type II). Treatment: stable—transport for transvenous pacemaker insertion; unstable—oxygen, transcutaneous pacing, dopamine, epinephrine, and isoproterenol
(Objective 10)

74. QRS complex: 0.08 second. P waves: present, upright. Rate: 50 beats/min. Rhythm: regular. P-R interval: no relationship between P waves and QRS complexes. Interpretation: third-degree (complete) atrioventricular block. Distinguishing features: R-R interval usually regular, more P waves than QRS complexes, no relationship between P waves and QRS complex. Treatment: stable—monitor and transport for transvenous pacemaker insertion; unstable—oxygen, transcutaneous pacing, atropine 0.5 to 1.0 mg (maximum dose 0.04 mg/kg), dopamine 5 to 20 mcg/kg/min, epinephrine 2 to 10 mcg/min, and isoproterenol 2 to 10 mcg/min (Objective 10)

75. a. QRS complex equal to or greater than 0.12 second. QRS complexes produced by supraventricular activity. RSR prime pattern. In V_1, line drawn backward from the J point into the QRS makes a triangle pointing up.
b. QRS complex less than 0.12 second. QRS complexes produced by supraventricular activity. QS pattern. In V_1, line drawn backward from J point into the QRS makes a triangle pointing down
c. QRS complex less than 0.12 second. QRS complexes produced by supraventricular activity and pathological left axis deviation. A small Q wave followed by a tall R wave in lead I, and a small R wave followed by a deep S wave in lead III
d. Right axis deviation with a normal QRS complex
(Objective 10)

76. a. Any patient with type II atrioventricular block
b. Any patient with evidence of disease of both bundle branches
c. Any patient with two or more blocks of any kind
(Objective 10)

77. a. Pulseless electrical activity (the patient has a rhythm but no perfusing pulse.)
b. Cardiopulmonary resuscitation, intubation, intravenous therapy, epinephrine 1.0 mg every 3 to 5 minutes; consideration of causes (hypovolemia, pulmonary embolus, acidosis, tension pneumothorax, cardiac tamponade, hypoxia, hypothermia, hyperthermia, hyperkalemia, massive myocardial infarction, drug overdose) and treatment if causes are found; if rate is slow, administer atropine 1 mg every 3 to 5 minutes to a maximum dose of 0.04 mg/kg.
(Objective 10)

78. a. QRS normal or wide. Delta wave and onset of QRS complex are slurred or notched
b. P-R interval is usually less than 0.12 second.
(Objective 10)

79. Patients with Wolff-Parkinson-White syndrome are susceptible to paroxysmal supraventricular tachycardias. Verapamil is contraindicated because it may cause rapid atrial to ventricular conduction and lead to ventricular fibrillation and sudden death.
(Objective 10)

80. Atherosclerosis is a process that progressively narrows the lumen of medium and large arteries. Thick, hard atherosclerotic plaques called *atheromata* form especially in areas of turbulent blood flow. The plaques are thought to be an endothelial cell response to chronic mechanical or chemical injury. The response includes platelet adhesion and aggregation and proliferation and migration of smooth muscle cells from the media into the intima. Eventually the atheromata become fibrotic and calcified and partially or totally obstruct the involved arteries. The two major effects are (1) disruption of the intimal surface causing a loss of vessel elasticity and an increase in thrombogenesis and (2) a reduction in the diameter of the vessel lumen with resulting decreased blood supply to tissues.
(Objective 11)

81. a. Physical exertion; b. emotional stress
(Objective 11)

82. a. Angina typically lasts 1 to 5 minutes but may last as long as 15 minutes.
b. Relieved by rest, nitroglycerin, or oxygen
(Objective 11)

83. Unless 12-lead electrocardiogram interpretation is available, it is impossible to distinguish between these two conditions in the field. Even a negative 12-lead electrocardiogram does not exclude acute myocardial infarction. Serial cardiac enzyme tests and electrocardiograms and other tests such as echocardiograms and stress tests may be needed. Both patients should be managed as though they are having a myocardial infarction (excluding thrombolytic therapy).
(Objective 11)

84. Atherosclerotic plaque forms in coronary artery; plaque ruptures; platelets adhere to it, and then thrombus forms on the plaque; as thrombus enlarges, it occludes the coronary artery. (Other causes are coronary vasospasm, coronary embolism, severe hypoxia, hemorrhage into diseased arterial wall, and shock.)
(Objective 11)

85.

Area of Heart Injured or Infarcted	Coronary Vessel Involved Most Often	Leads with Visible ST Segment Changes
Anterior	Left coronary	V_3, V_4
Lateral	Left coronary	V_5, V_6, I, aV_L
Septal	Left coronary	V_1, V_2
Inferior	Right coronary	II, III, aV_F

(Objective 11)

86. a. 0.1 mV in at least two contiguous leads
(Objective 11)

87. Left bundle branch block, some ventricular rhythms, left ventricular hypertrophy, pericarditis, ventricular aneurysm, and early repolarization
(Objective 11)

88. a. Identify rate and rhythm; b. Identify the area of infarct; c. Consider miscellaneous conditions; d. Assess the patient's clinical presentation; e. Recognize the infarction and initiate treatment.
(Objective 11)

89. Lethal dysrhythmias, congestive heart failure, pulmonary edema, cardiogenic shock, and myocardial tissue rupture.
(Objective 11)

90. Nausea; vomiting; diaphoresis; radiation of pain to the neck, jaw, arm, or back; palpitations; dyspnea; and a sense of impending doom
(Objective 11)

91. ST segment elevation in leads V_2, V_3, and V_4. Possible acute anterior myocardial infarction.
(Objective 11)

92. Administer oxygen via nasal cannula, minimize physical activity, monitor electrocardiogram and oxygen saturation (if pulse oximetry is available), assess vital signs frequently (including lung sounds for crackles), and establish an intravenous line to keep the vein open with normal saline or lactated Ringer's solution.
(Objective 11)

93. Aspirin 162 to 325 mg; nitroglycerin 0.4 mg sublingually, repeated 2 times; morphine sulfate 2 to 4 mg intravenously titrated to relieve pain
(Objective 11)

94. a. Patient is alert and able to give informed consent; chest pain or symptoms of acute myocardial infarction for at least 30 minutes and less than 6 hours; less than 75 years of age; electrocardiogram changes consistent with an acute anterior or inferior myocardial infarction; chest pain and electrocardiogram changes that persist after the administration of sublingual nitroglycerin.

b. History of intracranial bleeding, stroke, ulcer or gastrointestinal bleeding, pregnancy or postpartum state, uncontrolled hypertension, recent surgery, intravenous catheters at noncompressible sites, intracranial tumor, thoracic aortic aneurysm, cardiopulmonary resuscitation in progress more than 10 minutes, and trauma or any condition that would result in a significant bleeding hazard

(Objective 11)

95. a. Normal axis; no ST segment elevation, depression. Normal 12-lead electrocardiogram

b. QRS 0.14 second. Pathologic left axis deviation. Left bundle branch block. Cannot detect ST segment elevation in the presence of left bundle branch block

c. Normal axis; ST segment elevation leads II, III, aV_F. ST segment depression in leads aV_L, V_2, V_3, V_4, V_5. Possible inferior myocardial infarction

d. Normal axis; ST segment elevation leads I, aV_L, V_2, V_3, V_4, V_5, V_6. Extensive anterior myocardial infarction

96. There is a pathological left axis deviation. QRS is upright in lead I and down in leads II and III.
(Objective 10)

97. The triangle should point upward.
(Objective 8)

98. The patient has a left anterior hemiblock (pathological left axis deviation) and a right bundle branch block (QRS >0.12 second and upward triangle).
(Objective 10)

99. The presence of more than one block is known as *bifascicular block* and is associated with a high risk of advancement to complete heart block and increased mortality in the presence of myocardial infarction. This patient's symptoms suggest the potential for myocardial infarction.
(Objective 10)

100. The potential for serious rhythm deterioration should be anticipated. Prophylactic application of defibrillation or pacing pads in this setting may be indicated based on local protocol.
(Objective 10)

101. Left ventricular failure leading to pulmonary edema and possible myocardial infarction
(Objective 11)

102. Pulmonary edema: orthopnea and frothy, blood-tinged sputum. Myocardial infarction: chest pain, radiation of pain, nausea, and vomiting
(Objective 11)

103. Sinus tachycardia
(Objective 10)

104.

Drug	Dose	Desired Effect
a. Furosemide	0.5 to 1.0 mg/kg intravenously	Venodilation and diuresis
b. Morphine	2 to 4 mg intravenously	Venodilation, decreased myocardial work, and decreased anxiety
c. Nitroglycerin	0.4 mg sublingually	Peripheral vasodilation and decreased preload and afterload

(Objectives 11 and 13)

105. 3.5
(Objective 13)

106. a. Left ventricular failure, pulmonary embolism, right ventricle infarct, chronic hypertension, chronic obstructive pulmonary disease, and valvular disease
b. Jugular venous distention, tachycardia, enlarged liver or spleen, peripheral and sacral edema, and ascites
(Objective 11)

107. Sinus bradycardia
(Objective 10)

108. Administer oxygen by non-rebreather mask, and give atropine 0.5 mg intravenously.
(Objectives 10 and 13)

109. Cardiogenic shock
(Objective 11)

110. High-flow oxygen by non-rebreather mask; supine position (if tolerated); intravenous therapy with normal saline—consider fluid challenge (250 to 500 mL); dopamine infusion via intravenous piggyback 5 to 15 mcg/kg/min; remove nitroglycerin paste and wipe chest with gauze; and monitor electrocardiogram for dysrhythmias.
(Objective 11)

111. Expanding or ruptured abdominal aortic aneurysm
(Objective 11)

112. Palpation in this situation could cause a bulging aneurysm to rupture. If medical direction advises palpation, it should be done gently.
(Objective 11)

113. No. Increased intraabdominal pressure could cause rupture of the aneurysm.
(Objective 11)

114. Administer oxygen, transport rapidly, apply pneumatic antishock garments (if indicated by protocol) but do not inflate unless the patient's condition deteriorates, initiate two large-bore intravenous lines en route and infuse normal saline or lactated Ringer's solution to keep the vein open unless the patient's condition deteriorates.
(Objective 11)

115. Dissecting thoracic aortic aneurysm
(Objective 11)

116. Unequal peripheral pulses, neurological deficit, or signs of pericardial tamponade
(Objective 11)

117. Minimize movement and anxiety, administer high-concentration oxygen, initiate a 14- or 16-gauge intravenous line in arm with good pulses (higher blood pressure) to keep the vein open, and monitor vital signs and the electrocardiogram frequently.
(Objective 11)

118.

	Embolic	**Thrombotic**
Causes	Clot breaks loose and travels to narrow area in blood vessel	Clot develops at narrow spot in blood vessel
Onset	Rapid	Gradual

	Embolic	**Thrombotic**
Signs and symptoms	Pulseless extremity pain; decreased motor and sensory function; pallor; cool skin temperature distal to the occlusion; decreased capillary refill; possible shock	Pain in hips, lower limbs, buttocks, leg, and abdomen (depends on affected artery); pain; delayed motor and sensory function; pallor; decreased skin temperature distal to the occlusion; decreased CR; possible shock

(Objective 11)

119. Control bleeding with direct pressure and elevation. The bleeding may be persistent and require hospital management.
(Objective 11)

120. Pain, edema, warmth, erythema, tenderness, and a palpable cord
(Objective 11)

121. Hypertensive encephalopathy
(Objective 11)

122. Aphasia, hemiparesis, transient blindness, seizures, stupor, coma, and death
(Objective 11)

123. Calm patient, apply oxygen, and insert intravenous line to keep the vein open; monitor electrocardiogram; and transport rapidly.

124. Nitroglycerin 0.4 mg sublingually or nitroglycerin paste. Labetalol 10 to 20 mg intravenously over 1 to 2 minutes
(Objective 13)

125. Determine unresponsiveness; call for help if no one else is available; open the airway; look, listen, and feel for breathing; if there is none, deliver two slow rescue breaths; assess carotid pulse; if there is none, begin cardiopulmonary resuscitation until help arrives.
(Objective 12)

126. a. After intubation, intravenous therapy, and the first dose of epinephrine
   b. Yes. Electric shock resulting in injury or death can occur.
   (Objective 12)

127. Ventricular tachycardia
(Objective 10)

128. Defibrillate with 200 J (then 300 and 360 J if the rhythm is the same) and then reassess the rhythm and pulse.
(Objective 12)

129. Amount of time patient has been in pulseless ventricular tachycardia (success decreases over time with bystander cardiopulmonary resuscitation), conductive gel applied to paddles, and proper paddle placement
(Objective 12)

130. Apply conductive gel on the patient's chest (or hands-off defibrillation patches); turn on power (there is a separate power source for the defibrillator and monitor with some monitors); select correct energy level; place paddles (or patches) in an appropriate position on the patient's chest; charge the defibrillator; call "clear" and visually check to ensure that no one is in contact with the patient or cot; lean firmly on paddles (if used) with 20 to 25 lb of pressure; discharge both paddle buttons simultaneously (or depress discharge button on monitor for hands-off defibrillator); and reassess pulse and rhythm.
(Objective 12)

131. Defibrillate at 100, 200, 300, and 360 J.
(Objective 12)

132. It is synchronized with the patient's heartbeat so there is less risk of firing on the relative refractory period and causing ventricular fibrillation.
(Objective 12)

133. Depress the synchronize button before each synchronized shock, and hold the paddles firmly on the chest after activation until they discharge.
(Objective 12)

134. a. Third-degree atrioventricular block
b. Inform the patient that he may feel some discomfort; apply the pacing and monitoring pads; ensure adequate upright R wave on monitor; select pacing mode; select pacing rate (70 to 80 beats/min); set current at 50 mA and slowly increase until capture is observed; reassess patient's vital signs (use right arm for blood pressure); and document and obtain rhythm strips.
(Objective 12)

135. a. Asystole; b. epinephrine 1.0 mg every 3 to 5 minutes and atropine 1 mg every 5 minutes until a maximum dose of 0.04 mg/kg is reached; c. transcutaneous pacing
(Objectives 10 and 12)

136. a. Ventricular fibrillation; b. defibrillation; c. epinephrine 1.0 mg every 3 to 5 minutes or vasopressin 40 U intravenous bolus, amiodarone 300 mg intravenous bolus diluted in 20 to 30 mL of NS or D_5W, or lidocaine 1 to 1.5 mg/kg intravenously
(Objectives 10 and 13)

137. a. Do not stop resuscitation. Patient is older than 18 years, successfully intubated, last seen 30 minutes (cannot consider for termination). Resuscitation should be considered after four rounds of resuscitation drugs.
b. Do not stop resuscitation. Patient is older than 18 years, five drugs have been given, but intubation was unsuccessful.
c. Do not stop resuscitation. Patient is younger than 18 years and has sustained trauma, and you were able to get back a perfusing pulse during the resuscitation.
d. Do not stop resuscitation. The patient has met criteria for resuscitation; however, the family objects strongly, so efforts should continue.
(Objective 14)

138. d. His identified risk factors are male sex, age, hypercholesterolemia, diabetes, and hypertension (Acupril is an angiotensin-converting enzyme inhibitor, and indapamide is a diuretic).
(Objective 1)

139. c. Blood pressure = Cardiac output × Peripheral vascular resistance.
(Objective 1)

140. c. The circumflex supplies the lateral and posterior portions of the left ventricle and part of the right ventricle. The right coronary artery and the left anterior descending supply most of the right atrium and ventricle and the inferior aspect of the left ventricle.
(Objective 2)

141. b. The aortic valve separates the aorta and left ventricle, the pulmonic valve separates the pulmonary arteries and right ventricle, and the tricuspid valve separates the right atrium and right ventricle.
(Objective 2)

142. d. The electrical charge is the potential difference and is measured in millivolts. Depolarization (electrical conduction) occurs when sodium rushes into the cell, altering the electrical balance.
(Objective 3)

143. c. Potassium is also essential.
(Objective 3)

144. d. Calcium channel blockers selectively block the slow channel and alter the threshold level.
(Objective 3)

145. a. Phase 0 is the rapid depolarization phase; phase 1 is the early rapid depolarization phase; phase 2 is the plateau phase; phase 3 is the terminal phase of rapid repolarization; and phase 4 is the period between action potentials.
(Objective 3)

146. c. This allows complete relaxation of the cardiac muscle before another contraction can be initiated.
(Objective 3)

147. d. The His bundle divides into the right and left bundle branches. The left bundle divides into the anterior and posterior fascicles. A third fascicle of the left bundle branch that innervates the interventricular septum and the base of the heart also has been identified. The bundle branches subdivide and become Purkinje fibers.
(Objective 4)

148. d. The resting membrane potential gradually decreases with time until it reaches a critical threshold, at which time depolarization results.
(Objective 4)

149. c. This pause allows the atria to finish contraction and empty before ventricular contraction occurs.
(Objective 4)

150. a. Acetylcholine causes the cell membrane of the sinoatrial node to become hyperpolarized, causing a delay in reaching threshold, and therefore it decreases the heart rate. All other answers increase heart rate.
(Objective 4)

151. d. The other answers represent causes of dysrhythmias that result from enhanced automaticity.
(Objective 4)

152. a. Mental status change, abdominal or gastrointestinal complaints, or vague complaints of ill-being may be presenting symptoms in an older adult patient with a coronary event.
(Objective 5)

153. d. If the heart is unable to pump effectively, blood will back up into the lungs, causing decreased diffusion of gases in the lungs and dyspnea.
(Objective 5)

154. b. Younger patients may experience syncope because of increased vagal tone. Nausea or syncope when standing does not predict the incidence of dysrhythmias.
(Objective 5)

155. b
(Objective 5)

156. c. Peripheral pulses and perfusion would be used to assess strength of myocardial contractions. Placement of patches usually is performed using ribs and gross anatomy.
(Objective 5)

157. b. The electrocardiogram does not measure mechanical events.
(Objective 7)

158. c. The others are unipolar leads (a single positive electrode and a reference point).
(Objective 6)

159. d. If the depolarization moves toward a positive electrode, the tracing should show an upward deflection.
(Objective 6)

160. b. These leads all look up onto the inferior portion of the heart.
(Objective 6)

161. d. These leads may help distinguish between supraventricular tachycardia with aberration and ventricular tachycardia and can help diagnose bundle branch blocks.
(Objective 6)

162. c. The negative lead is placed at the lateral end of the left clavicle. The positive lead for MCL_6 is placed on the left axillary line at the level of the fifth intercostal space.
(Objective 6)

163. a. Many dysrhythmias involve abnormalities of the P wave.
(Objective 6)

164. b. V_3 and V_4 are anterior leads, and V_5 and V_6 are lateral precordial leads.
(Objective 6)

165. a. This is used as the baseline.
(Objective 7)

166. b
(Objective 4)

167. c. The relative refractory period is from the peak of the T wave onward.
(Objective 7)

168. b. In some leads, part of the QRS complex is blended with the baseline and is difficult to measure.
(Objective 8)

169. d. $1500 \div 10 = 150$ beats/min
(Objective 8)

170. b
(Objective 10)

171. c
(Objective 10)

172. c
(Objective 10)

173. a
(Objective 10)

174. b
(Objective 10)

175. d
(Objective 10)

176. a
(Objective 10)

177. d. Adenosine is not indicated for atrial fibrillation, and verapamil is not indicated when a patient is hypotensive. The patient needs electrical cardioversion because her condition is unstable. Procainamide is indicated for ventricular dysrhythmias.
(Objective 10)

178. a. It originates from tissue other than an intrinsic pacemaker.
(Objective 10)

179. c. Isoproterenol is a beta stimulant, so it will increase the heart rate.
(Objective 10)

180. d. The atria cannot contract to empty. This decreases the blood flow to the ventricles and the cardiac output.
(Objective 10)

181. a
(Objective 10)

182. d. It also is associated with excessive catecholamine administration, damage to the atrioventricular junction, inferior wall myocardial infarction, and rheumatic fever.
(Objective 10)

183. c. Other causes include failure of higher pacemakers to initiate impulses.
(Objective 10)

184. a. Couplets are two premature ventricular contractions in a row. An idioventricular rhythm originates in the ventricles and supersedes the underlying rhythm. Multifocal premature ventricular contractions have varied appearance depending on their site of origination.
(Objective 10)

185. a. Precordial concordance with all positive or all negative deflection in the V leads indicates ventricular tachycardia.
(Objective 10)

186. b. Asynchronous (fixed rate) pacemakers stimulate the heart at a set rate regardless of the action of the heart. A dual chamber pacemaker stimulates the atria and the ventricles.
(Objective 10)

187. d. Bundle branch block occurs when one of the bundles of His is blocked. Second-degree atrioventricular block type II is an intermittent block.
(Objective 10)

188. d. It yields an initial Q wave in MCL_1 (V_1) instead of the normal small R wave. There will be a deep QS pattern that is at least 0.12 second.
(Objective 10)

189. b. The blockage of two of the three pathways for ventricular consduction (right bundle branch block with anterior or posterior hemiblock, and left bundle branch block) poses the greatest risk.
(Objective 10)

190. d. Verapamil may cause rapid atrial to ventricular conduction down the accessory pathway and may lead to ventricular fibrillation and sudden death.
(Objective 10)

191. c. Both have the same cause.
(Objective 11)

192. a. Hypotension caused by pump failure and cardiac rupture can occur but is much less common than lethal dysrhythmias.
(Objective 11)

193. b. A small fluid challenge (250 mL) may be given to a patient with cardiac disease who is hypotensive; however, in the normotensive patient, intravenous fluids should be infused to keep the vein open.
(Objective 11)

194. b. Deep inverted T waves may be present in acute myocardial infarction.
(Objective 11)

195. a. Epinephrine will increase the work, and oxygen demands on the heart precipitate lethal dysrhythmias in this patient.
(Objectives 11 and 13)

196. d. Signs include jugular venous distention and peripheral edema.
(Objective 11)

197. b. Cardiogenic shock is fatal in up to 70% to 80% of patients.
(Objective 11)

198. b. Decreased systolic pressure is a later sign. Muffled heart sounds are associated with this. Tracheal deviation is seen in tension pneumothorax.
(Objective 11)

199. b. The pain often is described as ripping or tearing and is high intensity.
(Objective 11)

200. a
(Objective 11)

201. c
(Objective 11)

202. b. The patient with diabetes is at higher risk for heart disease; however, hypertension does not precipitate diabetes.
(Objective 11)

203. a. The goal is for cardiopulmonary resuscitation within 4 minutes and advanced cardiac life support treatment within 8 minutes.
(Objective 12)

204. a. Lower energy levels may be used. Energy flow is bidirectional. Two patches are used.
(Objective 12)

205. b. Anterior-posterior placement is not practical for paddle use. Avoid placing the patch or paddle over the sternum because bone is a poor conductor of electricity. Pediatric paddles are indicated for children under 1 year of age.
(Objective 12)

206. b. The implantable cardioverter defibrillator sequence includes up to five shocks in 2 minutes. There is no danger in touching the patients. Strong magnets may inactivate the device.
(Objective 12)

207. d
(Objective 14)

208. b
(Objective 14)

209. a
(Objective 13)

210. c
(Objective 13)

211. a. Morphine will decrease the preload. It is contraindicated in the patient with head injury. It does not cause bronchodilation.
(Objective 13)

212. a
(Objective 13)

213. c
(Objective 13)

214. c. The correct dose is 2 to 10 mcg/2 to 10 mcg/min.
(Objective 13)

215. a. None of the other criteria should be used to evaluate whether resuscitation should be stopped.
(Objective 14)

WRAP IT UP

1. a, b, c, d, e, f
(Objective 11)

2. Ventricular fibrillation and ventricular tachycardia are the only two rhythms that will advise a shock on an automated external defibrillator.
(Objective 12)

3. Lidocaine or amiodarone
(Objective 13)

4. ST segment elevation in leads V_1 to V_4 would indicate septal and anterior myocardial infarction.
(Objective 10)

5. a. The other risk factors mentioned would be absolute contraindications.
(Objective 13)

PART EIGHT

IN THIS PART

Pulmonary Emergencies

READING ASSIGNMENT
Chapter 30, pages 816-835, in *Mosby's Paramedic Textbook,* ed. 3

OBJECTIVES
Upon completion of this chapter, the paramedic student will be able to:
1. Distinguish the pathophysiology of respiratory emergencies related to ventilation, diffusion, and perfusion.
2. Describe the causes, complications, signs and symptoms, and prehospital management of patients diagnosed with obstructive airway disease, pneumonia, adult respiratory distress syndrome, pulmonary thromboembolism, upper respiratory infection, spontaneous pneumothorax, hyperventilation syndrome, and lung cancer.

SUMMARY
- Diseases responsible for respiratory emergencies include those related to ventilation, diffusion, and perfusion.
- Obstructive airway disease is a triad of distinct diseases that often coexist. These are chronic bronchitis, emphysema, and asthma. The patient with chronic obstructive pulmonary disease usually has an acute episode of worsening dyspnea that is manifested even at rest, an increase or change in sputum production, or an increase in the malaise that accompanies the disease. The main goal of prehospital care for these patients is the correction of hypoxemia through improved air flow.
- Asthma, or reactive airway disease, is characterized by reversible airflow obstruction caused by bronchial smooth muscle contraction; hypersecretion of mucus, resulting in bronchial plugging; and inflammatory changes in the bronchial walls. The typical patient with asthma is in obvious distress. Respirations are rapid and loud. Initial medications in the prehospital setting probably will have a short onset of action.
- Pneumonia is a group of specific infections (bacterial, viral, or fungal). These infections cause an acute inflammatory process of the respiratory bronchioles and the alveoli. Pneumonia usually manifests with classic signs and symptoms. These include a productive cough and associated fever that produces "shaking chills." Prehospital care of patients with pneumonia includes airway support, oxygen administration, ventilatory assistance as needed, IV fluids, cardiac monitoring, and transport.
- Adult respiratory distress syndrome is a fulminant form of respiratory failure. It is characterized by acute lung inflammation and diffuse alveolar-capillary injury. It develops as a complication of illness or injury. In ARDS, the lungs are wet and heavy, congested, hemorrhagic, and stiff, with decreased perfusion capacity across alveolar membranes and includes airway and ventilatory support.
- Pulmonary thromboembolism is a blockage of a pulmonary artery by a clot or other foreign material. When one or more pulmonary arteries are blocked by an embolism, a section of lung is ventilated but hypoperfused.

Prehospital care is mainly supportive and includes oxygen administration, IV access, and transport for definitive care.

- Upper respiratory infections affect the nose, throat, sinuses, and larynx. Signs and symptoms of a URI include sore throat, fever, chills, headache, cervical adenopathy, and an erythematous pharynx. Prehospital care is based on the patient's symptoms.
- A primary spontaneous pneumothorax usually results when a subpleural bleb ruptures. This allows air to enter the pleural space from within the lung. Signs and symptoms include shortness of breath and chest pain that often are sudden in onset, pallor, diaphoresis, and tachypnea. Prehospital care is based on the patient's symptoms and degree of distress.
- Hyperventilation syndrome is abnormally deep or rapid breathing. This type of breathing results in an excessive loss of carbon dioxide. If the syndrome clearly is caused by anxiety, prehospital care is mainly supportive (i.e., calming measures and reassurance). The paramedic may suspect that the syndrome is a result of illness or drug ingestion. If this is the case, care may include oxygen administration and airway and ventilatory support.
- Lung cancer is an expression of the uncontrolled growth of abnormal cells. As the disease progresses, signs and symptoms may include cough, hemoptysis, dyspnea, hoarseness, and dysphagia. Prehospital management includes airway, ventilatory, and circulatory support.

REVIEW QUESTIONS

Match the description in column I with the correct noninfectious pulmonary disease in column II. Use each answer only once.

Column I		Column II
1. _____	Chronic production of excessive mucus, hypoxia, and inflammation of bronchi	**a.** Adult respiratory distress syndrome
2. _____	Pulmonary edema secondary to trauma, inhaled toxins, or metabolic disorders	**b.** Asthma **c.** Chronic bronchitis
3. _____	Condition caused by a rupture of a bleb in the lung	**d.** Emphysema
4. _____	Impaired oxygenation resulting from blockage of a pulmonary artery by a clot	**e.** Lung cancer **f.** Hyperventilation syndrome
5. _____	Bronchiolar smooth muscle spasm and excess mucus production caused by allergy	**g.** Pneumonia **h.** Pulmonary thromboembolism
6. _____	Bacterial, viral, or fungal lung infection	**i.** Spontaneous pneumothorax
7. _____	Uncontrolled abnormal cell growth in the lung	
8. _____	Chronic disease that results in a decrease in the alveolar membrane surface area and polycythemia	

9. For each case below, identify whether the respiratory problem is related to ventilation, diffusion, or perfusion or is a combination of two or more of these factors.
   a. Your patient is found unconscious with a plastic bag over her head.
   b. A 26-year-old is found semiconscious with a respiratory rate of 8/min. Track marks are found on the arms, legs, and under the tongue.
   c. An elderly woman with a history of congestive heart failure is acutely dyspneic and cyanotic. She has crackles throughout her lungs and coughs up frothy, bloody sputum.
   d. A woman has experienced vaginal bleeding for 2 weeks. She has profound fatigue and shortness of breath.
   e. A 56-year-old is choking in a restaurant.
   f. Your patient delivered a baby yesterday and has severe chest pain and dyspnea and an Sao_2 of 89% on room air.
   g. An 88-year-old has a large flail segment of the right chest and is hypoxic.

Questions 10 to 12 pertain to the following case study:

You are dispatched to a call for "difficulty breathing." Dispatch tells you en route that the first responders report that the patient is in moderate respiratory distress.

10. What conditions come to mind en route to this call?

_____

11. What findings in your initial assessment would indicate life-threatening respiratory distress?

_____

12. What information should be gathered during the focused history and physical examination of this patient?

_____

_____

13. Differentiate the signs and symptoms of chronic bronchitis and emphysema.
   a. Chronic bronchitis:

_____

   b. Emphysema:

_____

Questions 14 to 16 pertain to the following case study:

> Your 65-year-old patient has a history of chronic bronchitis and emphysema. She states that she has become acutely short of breath today and cannot complete a sentence without gasping for air. Loud wheezing is audible without a stethoscope.

14. How much oxygen should you administer to this patient?_____

15. Name a drug other than oxygen that may be administered to alleviate this patient's dyspnea, if not contraindicated by the history or physical findings.

_____

16. Describe any additional patient care to be given en route to the hospital.

_____

_____

Questions 17 to 22 pertain to the following case study:

> You are called to a junior college to evaluate a 19-year-old who became acutely short of breath during a soccer game. He states that he has a history of asthma. On examination, you note inspiratory and expiratory wheezes throughout the lung fields. Vital signs are: BP, 130/80 mm Hg; pulse, 136/min; and respirations, 30/min. You also note a pulsus paradoxus of 30 mm Hg.

17. Describe the pathophysiological changes in the lungs that cause the patient's signs and symptoms.

_____

18. Why would you perform a peak expiratory flow rate measurement on this patient?

_____

19. Other than oxygen, what drug can be administered to treat this patient? Include the correct dose and route.

_____

20. Describe how you will reassess the patient after the medication has been administered and what you will find if the patient's condition is improving.

_____

21. If therapy is unsuccessful and the patient continues to deteriorate despite aggressive medication therapy, what condition might exist?

_____

22. What additional treatment measures will you use?

_____

23. You respond to a call for difficulty breathing. Your assessment reveals that the patient is wheezing. List one pathological cause of wheezes for each of the following:

    a. Upper airway obstruction:

_____

    b. Lower airway obstruction:

_____

    c. Trauma:

_____

    d. Alveolar pathology:

_____

    e. Interstitial space pathology:

_____

Questions 24 to 26 pertain to the following case study:

    A physician calls 9-1-1 to have you transport a patient with a diagnosis of pneumonia from her office to the hospital.

24. List four types of pneumonia.

    a.

    b.

    c.

    d.

25. List the signs and symptoms that may be present if this patient has bacterial pneumonia.

_____

26. Describe the prehospital care of patients with known or suspected pneumonia.

_____

_____

27. You are transporting a 56-year-old man from a small rural hospital to a trauma center 70 miles away. Approximately 24 hours ago, he was involved in a head-on motor vehicle collision. He has been diagnosed with bilateral pulmonary contusions and two fractured ribs. Early in his care, he received a large volume of normal saline intravenously. He has been increasingly short of breath, was intubated before your arrival, and is very difficult to ventilate. Paralytic drugs and sedatives were administered immediately before your departure.

    a. What problem do you suspect?

_____

    b. Describe the measures you will use during transport to assess and care for this patient.

_____

28. List eight factors that increase the risk of pulmonary emboli.

    a.

    b.

    c.

    d.

    e.

    f.

    g.

    h.

29. List the signs and symptoms of pulmonary embolism.

_____

_____

30. List common characteristics of the patient who develops spontaneous pneumothorax.

_____

STUDENT SELF-ASSESSMENT

31. Which of the following is an extrinsic factor associated with the development or exacerbation of respiratory disease?
    a. Cardiac or circulatory pathologies
    b. Smoking
    c. Genetic predisposition
    d. Stress
32. Which of the following is essential for normal ventilation to occur?
    a. Adequate blood volume
    b. Functional diaphragm and intercostal muscles
    c. Interstitial space that is not filled with fluid
    d. Pulmonary capillaries that are not occluded
33. Your patient has a chronic respiratory illness; she called you complaining of difficulty breathing. What is usually the most reliable indicator of the severity of the patient's present condition?
    a. One- or two-word dyspnea   c. Patient's description of severity
    b. Pallor and diaphoresis   d. Tachycardia
34. Which physical finding indicates chronic hypoxemia?
    a. Accessory muscle use   c. Clubbing
    b. Carpopedal spasm   d. Pursed-lip breathing

35. Which of the following distinguishes chronic bronchitis from both emphysema and asthma?
    a. Cough
    b. Excessive mucus production
    c. Resistance to air flow
    d. Wheezing
36. Which of the following is evidence of chronic emphysema on physical examination?
    a. Decreased anterior-posterior chest diameter
    b. Decreased capillary refill in the nail beds
    c. Diminished breath sounds throughout the lungs
    d. Decreased diastolic blood pressure
37. Pulmonary hypertension can lead to which of the following?
    a. Pulmonary edema
    b. Pulmonary embolism
    c. Renal failure
    d. Right heart failure
38. Signs and symptoms of an acute asthma attack result from all of the following except which one?
    a. Bronchial muscle contraction
    b. Bronchial inflammation
    c. Mucus hypersecretion
    d. Pulmonary hypertension
39. Which physical finding is the most serious when found in an asthma patient who appears to be having acute respiratory distress?
    a. Expiratory wheezing
    b. Inspiratory wheezing
    c. Silent chest (no wheezing)
    d. Wheezing audible with a stethoscope
40. Pharmacological therapy to treat wheezing in patients with bronchitis or asthma usually includes which of the following?
    a. Albuterol
    b. Aminophylline
    c. Epinephrine
    d. Isoproterenol
41. Which pulmonary function test may be used in the prehospital setting to evaluate the effectiveness of patient ventilation?
    a. Peak expiratory flow rate (PEFR)
    b. Residual capacity
    c. Tidal volume
    d. Vital capacity
42. The most effective preventive measure for bacterial pneumonia is
    a. Antibiotic therapy
    b. Patient positioning
    c. Strict isolation measures
    d. Vaccination
43. What is the most common factor associated with aspiration pneumonia?
    a. Age
    b. Airway pathology
    c. Decreased level of consciousness
    d. Drowning
44. Which of the following is true about adult respiratory distress syndrome regardless of the cause?
    a. Death always occurs as a result of this complication.
    b. Disseminated intravascular coagulation always occurs.
    c. Pneumonia will be a secondary complication.
    d. Pulmonary edema will result.
45. Which ventilation adjunct provides continuous positive airway pressure and may prevent the need for intubation if used successfully?
    a. Venturi mask
    b. BVM
    c. CPAP
    d. PEEP
46. The signs and symptoms of pulmonary embolus vary and are related primarily to
    a. The patient's age
    b. The cause of the embolus
    c. The origin of the embolus
    d. The size of the embolus
47. What is the most important action the paramedic can take to prevent the spread of upper respiratory infections?
    a. Obtain the appropriate immunizations
    b. Place a mask on the patient during transport
    c. Practice good hand washing techniques
    d. Wear a mask and goggles during patient care
48. Which of the following is associated with the development of spontaneous pneumothorax?
    a. Asthma
    b. Free-base cocaine use
    c. IV drug abuse
    d. Thromboembolus

49. Which of the following is *not* a cause of hyperventilation?
    a. Fever
    c. Hyperglycemia
    b. Narcotic overdose
    d. Hypoxia

50. What is the most common risk factor for lung cancer?
    a. Cigarette smoking
    c. Exposure to coal products
    b. Exposure to asbestos
    d. Exposure to ionizing radiation

WRAP IT UP

You know as you respond to a call for "difficulty breathing" that your patient is likely quite ill because the dispatcher has a pumper running the call with you. Your patient is a 74-year-old male with a history of asthma and chronic bronchitis. He is seated leaning forward in a tripod position, using pursed-lip breathing; his neck muscles strain with each breath; and he is able to say only two or three words at a time. His son tells you that his dad hasn't been feeling too good all week, and today he became much worse, developing a fever and coughing up green sputum flecked with blood. His home medicines include ipratropium (Atrovent), beclomethasone (Beclovent), Advair, Singulair, and albuterol.

The patient's skin is gray and wet, the radial pulse is rapid, and an initial oxygen saturation reading is 84% on room air. You pull up his shirt and listen to his lungs; they sound wet and noisy, with wheezes throughout but somewhat diminished in the left base, so you apply a nebulizer mask with albuterol 2.5 mg and set the oxygen at 7 L/min. In the ambulance, the ECG monitor shows sinus tachycardia at 120/min; the Sao_2 is 94% and BP is 164/90 mm Hg; his skin is now dry, and he is speaking a bit more clearly. You start an IV, administer methylprednisolone (125 mg IV), and administer oxygen by nasal cannula at 4 L/min. The patient is admitted with a diagnosis of left lower R lobe pneumonia. He returns home in 4 days.

1. Which of the following was likely the primary problem for this patient's acute hypoxia?
    a. Inadequate diffusion between alveoli and pulmonary capillaries
    b. Inadequate perfusion of blood through the pulmonary capillary bed
    c. Inadequate ventilation in and out of the lungs
    d. a and b
    e. a and c

2. Put a ✔ beside the signs or symptoms of life-threatening respiratory distress that this patient displayed.
    a. _____ Altered mental status
    e. _____ One- or two-word dyspnea
    b. _____ Severe cyanosis
    f. _____ Tachycardia
    c. _____ Absent breath sounds
    g. _____ Pallor or diaphoresis
    d. _____ Audible stridor
    h. _____ Accessory muscle use

3. Based on this patient's reported history, what would you anticipate?
    a. He normally produces very little sputum.
    b. A thin, pink appearance would be normal for him.
    c. Lung tissue is scarred and susceptible to infection.
    d. In the absence of disease, the Po_2 is normal.

4. Explain your rationale for administration of
    a. Albuterol

_____

_____

    b. Methylprednisolone

_____

_____

5. Which is true about pneumonia?
    a. It is always caused by a bacterial infection.
    b. Fever is always present.
    c. Antibiotic treatment always cures it.
    d. Inflammation of the alveoli interferes with gas exchange.

CHAPTER 30 ANSWERS

REVIEW QUESTIONS

1. c
2. a
3. i
4. h
5. b
6. g
7. e
8. d
(Questions 1-8: Objective 3)

9. a. This is a problem with diffusion, because insufficient oxygen is available to diffuse across the alveolar membrane into the capillaries.
b. This represents a problem with ventilation. The drugs may have depressed the central nervous system causing slower, shallower breathing.
c. This is likely to be related to a problem with diffusion from the fluid that has leaked into the interstitial spaces and with perfusion because the left side of the heart is not functioning well.
d. These symptoms are likely related to anemia, which causes a problem with perfusion such that oxygen cannot be carried to the tissues.
e. Airway obstruction creates a problem with ventilation.
f. These signs and symptoms suggest pulmonary embolism, which creates a problem with perfusion.
g. Flail chest is often accompanied by pulmonary contusion. This would create a problem with ventilation because of the mechanical disruption and diffusion related to the fluid in the pulmonary spaces.
(Objective 1)

10. Asthma, chronic obstructive pulmonary disease, heart failure, pulmonary edema, pulmonary embolism, bronchiolitis (infants), foreign body aspiration, toxic inhalation, pneumonia, spontaneous pneumothorax, hyperventilation syndrome, or lung cancer are some of the conditions that may present with this chief complaint.
(Objective 2)

11. Signs and symptoms that indicate a life threat include alterations in mental status, severe cyanosis, absent breath sounds, audible stridor, one- or two-word dyspnea, tachycardia, pallor and diaphoresis, cardiac dysrhythmias, a pulse rate over 130/min, poor, floppy muscle tone, and the presence of retractions and/or the use of accessory muscles.
(Objective 2)

12. You should ask about the patient's chief complaint and determine whether he or she has any chest pain, productive or nonproductive cough, hemoptysis, wheezing, or signs of respiratory infection (e.g., fever or increased sputum production). Inquire about the patient's past history, especially with regard to similar problems and the individual's perceived severity of this episode. Obtain a medication history and ask whether the patient has ever needed intubation to manage this type of illness. The physical examination should begin by noting your general impression of the patient. Note the patient's position, mentation, ability to speak, respiratory effort, and skin color. Observe the heart rate for tachycardia or bradycardia. Note any abnormal respiratory patterns. Assess the face and neck for pursed-lip breathing and use of accessory muscles. Evaluate the neck for jugular venous distention. Inspect the chest for injury, indicators of chronic disease, accessory muscle use, and chest symmetry. Auscultate the lungs for abnormal breath sounds. Assess the extremities for peripheral cyanosis, clubbing of the fingers, and carpopedal spasm.
(Objective 2)

13. a. "Blue bloater," chronic cough with production of a large amount of sputum, hypercapnia, hypoxemia, cyanosis, pulmonary hypertension, and cor pulmonale; b. "pink puffer," hyperexpansion of the lungs, barrel chest, resistance to airflow (especially on expiration), pursed-lip breathing, and thinness.
(Objective 2)

14. Oxygen should be administered initially at 2 L/min if the patient is not in respiratory failure. If rapid improvement does not occur, the flow of oxygen should be increased while the paramedic carefully monitors the patient. If the patient's condition is critical, intubation and assisted ventilation may be necessary.
(Objective 2)

15. Albuterol, metaproterenol
(Objective 2)

16. Transport the patient in a position of comfort; instruct the patient to use pursed-lip breathing and to minimize physical activity to conserve energy for breathing; calmly reassure and care for the patient and provide a cool environment for transport.
(Objective 2)

17. An acute asthma attack is marked by reversible airflow obstruction caused by bronchial smooth muscle contraction; hypersecretion of mucus, causing bronchial plugging; and inflammatory changes in the bronchial walls.
(Objective 2)

18. Measurement of the peak expiratory flow rate can aid in the determination of the severity of an asthma attack, as well as the evaluation of the effectiveness of treatment in reversing airway obstruction.
(Objective 2)

19. Albuterol, 0.5 mL (2.5 mg) in 2.5 mL normal saline by nebulizer at 6 to 7 L/min O_2.
(Objective 2)

20. Ask the patient if his breathing is easier. Observe the patient for decreased anxiety, changes in level of consciousness, and ability to converse more easily. Note the degree of respiratory distress by observing the patient's position, use of accessory muscles, and respiratory rate. Monitor vital signs (the pulse and respiratory rate should decrease, and pulsus paradoxus should drop below 20 mm Hg). As the patient improves, the inspiratory and then expiratory wheezes should disappear.
(Objective 2)

21. Status asthmaticus
(Objective 2)

22. Make sure that oxygen is at 100% and humidified; increase the fluid rate to hydrate the patient; administer other medications (e.g., methylprednisolone, hydrocortisone) as ordered by medical direction; expedite transport; monitor the patient closely for signs of respiratory failure and prepare to intubate if necessary. If intubation is indicated, follow local medical protocols, which may include sedation (ketamine, benzodiazepine, or barbiturates); paralyze the patient; intubate; administer 2.5 to 5 mg of albuterol directly into the endotracheal (ET) tube; confirm ET tube placement; and ventilate at 8 to 10 breaths/min.
(Objective 2)

23. a. Upper airway obstruction: foreign body, epiglottitis; b. lower airway obstruction: asthma, airway edema; c. trauma: inhalation injury, adult respiratory distress syndrome (ARDS) secondary to pulmonary contusion; d. alveolar pathology: chronic obstructive pulmonary disease (COPD), lung cancer, inhalation injury; e. interstitial space pathology: pulmonary edema, near drowning.
(Objective 2)

24. Viral, bacterial, mycoplasmal, and aspiration
(Objective 2)

25. Signs and symptoms of bacterial pneumonia include shaking chills, tachypnea, tachycardia, cough with sputum (rust colored, hemoptysis, yellow, green, or gray), malaise, anorexia, flank or back pain, vomiting, fever, wheezing, fine crackles, dyspnea, and sore throat.
(Objective 2)

26. Care includes airway support, oxygen administration, ventilatory assistance, IV fluids, cardiac and oxygen saturation monitoring, and transportation. If wheezing is present, bronchodilator therapy may be used.
(Objective 2)

27. a. Adult respiratory distress syndrome; b. Monitor the rise and fall of the chest to determine the effectiveness of ventilation; note any difficulty or increasing pressure necessary to ventilate the patient; frequently assess vital signs, observing for an increased heart rate; monitor the electrocardiogram, end-tidal CO_2, and oxygen saturation by pulse oximetry; observe for cyanosis. Ventilate with high-flow oxygen; ventilate with positive end-expiratory pressure, using Boehringer valve if trained and authorized by medical direction; and administer steroids and diuretics if ordered by medical direction.
(Objective 2)

28. Extended travel; prolonged bed rest; obesity; older adulthood; burns; varicose veins; surgery of the thorax, abdomen, pelvis, and legs; pelvic or leg fractures; malignancy; use of birth control pills; congenital or acquired coagulopathies; pregnancy; chronic obstructive pulmonary disease; congestive heart failure; sickle cell anemia; cancer; atrial fibrillation; myocardial infarction; previous pulmonary embolism; deep vein thrombosis; infection; diabetes mellitus; and multiple trauma.
(Objective 2)

29. Dyspnea, cough, hemoptysis, pain, anxiety, syncope, hypotension, diaphoresis, increased respiratory rate, increased heart rate, fever, distended neck veins, chest splinting, pleuritic chest pain, pleural friction rub, crackles, and wheezes (localized).
(Objective 3)

30. This typically occurs in tall, thin males between the ages of 20 and 40. It may also be found in patients with COPD, patients with acquired immunodeficiency syndrome (AIDS) who have pneumonia, and drug abusers who deeply inhale free-base cocaine, marijuana, or inhalants such as glue or solvents.
(Objective 2)

STUDENT SELF-ASSESSMENT

31. b. Cardiac, genetic, and stress factors are all intrinsic factors.
(Objective 1)

32. b. Adequate blood volume and patent pulmonary capillaries are related to perfusion. Normal interstitial space affects diffusion.
(Objective 1)

33. c. All the answers represent findings that indicate respiratory distress; however, in the patient with chronic respiratory illness, the patient's reported level of distress is often the best indication of the severity of the condition.
(Objective 2)

34. c. This sign takes a long time to develop. Acutely hypoxic patients may use accessory muscles or pursed-lip breathing in an attempt to improve ventilation. Carpopedal spasm is seen secondary to hypocapnia.
(Objective 2)

35. b. All will have wheezing and cough when acutely ill. Resistance to airflow is seen in all three conditions, although less so in emphysema.
(Objective 2)

36. c. The patient is more likely to be tachycardic than bradycardic. Capillary refill is an indicator of perfusion (flow) rather than oxygenation.
(Objective 2)

37. d. Right-heart failure can develop secondary to pulmonary hypertension (cor pulmonale). The right side of the heart increasingly is forced to pump harder to overcome the excess pressure in the pulmonary arteries. Eventually it cannot force the blood through, and fluid backs up to the venous side of the system.
(Objective 2)

38. d
(Objective 2)

39. c. Expiratory wheezing indicates narrowing of the smaller airways. As the larger airways become obstructed, inspiratory wheezing becomes audible. When the obstruction becomes so severe that almost no airflow is present, the chest is silent, with diminished breath sounds and no wheezes.
(Objective 2)

40. a. Albuterol is a beta-2 agonist that causes relatively few side effects. Although all the other drugs also cause bronchodilation, they are rarely used because of their high incidence of side effects.
(Objective 2)

41. a. The PEFR is most helpful when the patient's normal baseline peak flow is known.
(Objective 2)

42. d. The vaccine is 80% to 90% effective in the prevention of pneumonia caused by the *pneumococcus* bacillus.
(Objective 2)

43. c. Altered level of consciousness may impair the gag reflex or the patient's ability to handle secretions.
(Objective 2)

44. d. Not all patients die, although the mortality rate is high (over 65%). Disseminated coagulation may occur in some but not all patients.
(Objective 2)

45. a.
(Objective 2)

46. d. The size and location of the embolus determine whether mild signs and symptoms or sudden death occurs.
(Objective 2)

47. c. Most upper respiratory infections have no identifiable cause. Good hand washing is an important action for preventing their spread.
(Objective 2)

48. b. Other risk factors for spontaneous pneumothorax include patients with emphysema, people with AIDS who develop pneumonia, and healthy tall, thin men between the ages of 20 and 40.
(Objective 2)

49. b. Narcotic overdose is associated with respiratory depression.
(Objective 2)

50. a. Heavy smokers have a 25 times greater risk of developing lung cancer than nonsmokers.
(Objective 2)

WRAP IT UP

1. e. Mucus production and inflammation of the alveoli impair ventilation and diffusion.
(Objective 1)

2. b, e, f, g, h
(Objective 2)

3. c. Patients with chronic bronchitis tend to be overweight and have persistent hypoxia and chronic excessive mucus production.
(Objective 2)

4. a. Albuterol is a bronchodilator that relaxes bronchiolar smooth muscle, enlarging the airway passages and allowing better exchange of gases in the lungs.
b. Methylprednisolone is a steroid that reduces swelling and inflammation in the lung tissues, permitting better airflow and diffusion.
(Objective 2)

5. d. Pneumonia can be caused by bacterial, viral, or fungal infections. Not all these organisms are susceptible to antibiotics. Fever may not be present, especially in immunocompromised patients.
(Objective 2)

Neurology

READING ASSIGNMENT
Chapter 31, pages 836-863, in *Mosby's Paramedic Textbook,* ed. 3

OBJECTIVES
Upon completion of this chapter, the paramedic student will be able to do the following:
1. Describe the anatomy and physiology of the nervous system.
2. Outline pathophysiological changes in the nervous system that may alter the cerebral perfusion pressure.
3. Describe the assessment of a patient with a nervous system disorder.
4. Describe the pathophysiology, signs and symptoms, and specific management techniques for each of the following neurological disorders: coma, stroke and intracranial hemorrhage, seizure disorders, headaches, brain neoplasm and brain abscess, and degenerative neurological diseases.

SUMMARY
- The human body's ability to maintain a state of balance, or *homeostasis,* results from the nervous system's regulatory and coordinating activities. The blood supply to the brain comes from the vertebral arteries and the internal carotid arteries.
- Some neurological emergencies are a consequence of structural changes or damage, circulatory changes, or alterations in intracranial pressure that affect cerebral blood flow.
- The initial survey should begin by determining the patient's level of consciousness and by ensuring an open and patent airway. Key elements of the physical examination that may provide clues to the nature of the neurological emergency include the patient history and the history of the event, vital signs, and respiratory patterns.
- *Coma* is an abnormally deep state of unconsciousness. The patient cannot be aroused from this state by external stimuli. In general, two mechanisms produce coma: structural lesions and toxic-metabolic states.
- *Stroke* is a sudden interruption in blood flow to the brain that results in a neurological deficit. Strokes can be classified as ischemic strokes or hemorrhagic strokes.
- A *seizure* is a brief alteration in behavior or consciousness. It is caused by abnormal electrical activity of one or more groups of neurons in the brain. In the prehospital setting, determining the cause of a seizure is not as important as other measures. These include managing the complications and recognizing whether the seizure is reversible with therapy (e.g., it is caused by hypoglycemia).
- The four fairly common types of headaches are tension headaches, migraines, cluster headaches, and sinus headaches.
- A brain tumor, or *neoplasm,* is a mass in the cranial cavity. This mass can be either malignant or benign. Heredity may play a role in the development of brain tumors. They also are associated with several risk factors. These include exposure to radiation, tobacco use, dietary habits, some viruses, and the use of some medications.
- A *brain abscess* is a buildup of purulent material (pus) surrounded by a capsule within the brain. It develops from a bacterial infection. The infection often starts in the nasal cavity, middle ear, or mastoid bone.

- Muscular dystrophy is an inherited muscle disorder. The cause is unknown. The disease is marked by a slow but progressive degeneration of muscle fibers.
- Damage to the white matter of the brain in multiple sclerosis may lead to fatigue, vertigo, clumsiness, unsteady gait, slurred speech, blurred or double vision, and facial numbness or pain.
- The term *dystonia* refers to local or diffuse changes in muscle tone. These may cause painful muscle spasms, unusually fixed postures, and strange movement patterns.
- Parkinson disease usually begins as a slight tremor in one hand, arm, or leg. In the later stages, the disease affects both sides of the body, causing stiffness, weakness, and trembling of the muscles.
- The term *central pain syndrome* refers to infection or disease of the trigeminal nerve.
- *Bell palsy* is paralysis of the facial muscles. It is caused by inflammation of the seventh cranial nerve. The condition is usually one sided and temporary. It often develops suddenly.
- Amyotrophic lateral sclerosis is also called *Lou Gehrig disease*. It is one of a group of rare nervous system disorders. In these disorders, the nerves that control muscular activity degenerate in the brain and spinal cord.
- Peripheral neuropathies usually arise from damage to or irritation of either the axons or their myelin sheaths. This slows or fully blocks the passage of electrical signals.
- The term *myoclonus* refers to rapid and uncontrollable muscle contractions or spasms. These occur at rest or during movement.
- *Spina bifida* is a congenital defect in which part of one or more vertebrae fails to develop completely. This leaves a portion of the spinal cord exposed.
- Polio is caused by a virus. The severity of the disease can range from unapparent infection, to a febrile illness without neurological aftereffects, to aseptic meningitis, and finally to paralytic disease and possibly death.

REVIEW QUESTIONS

For each of the etiologies in column I, identify the appropriate general cause of coma in column II. Each answer may be used *more* than once.

Column I	Column II
1. _____ The patient's blood pressure rose suddenly to 240/140 mm Hg.	**a.** Cardiovascular system
2. _____ The patient's chronic bronchitis is much worse.	**b.** Drugs
3. _____ The patient has missed dialysis for a week.	**c.** Infectious
4. _____ The patient's blood alcohol level is 400 mg/dL.	**d.** Metabolic system
5. _____ The patient's glucose level is 30 mg/dL.	**e.** Respiratory system
6. _____ The teenage patient has meningitis.	**f.** Structural cause

Match the illness in column II with the description in column I. Use each illness only once.

Column I	Column II
7. _____ Blurred vision and unsteady gait	**a.** Amyotrophic lateral sclerosis
8. _____ Severe muscle spasms because of torticollis	**b.** Bell palsy
9. _____ Burning sensation in the feet because of diabetes	**c.** Central pain syndrome
10. _____ Viral illness causing respiratory paralysis	**d.** Dystonia
11. _____ Muscle trembling because of a decrease in dopamine	**e.** Multiple sclerosis
12. _____ Male genetic disorder that causes muscle wasting	**f.** Muscular dystrophy
13. _____ Intense facial pain activated by a trigger point	**g.** Myoclonus
14. _____ Central nervous system degeneration in patients over age 50 that leads to severe muscle deterioration	**h.** Parkinson disease
15. _____ Temporary facial paralysis caused by inflammation	**i.** Peripheral neuropathy
	j. Polio
	k. Spina bifida

16. _____ Genetic defect that leaves the spinal cord exposed

17. Complete the following sentences.

The cells of the nervous system that protect the neurons are called **(a)** _____ _____

_____. Each neuron has three main parts. The area that contains the nucleus is the

(b) _____; one or more branching projections that receive impulses are known as

the **(c)** _____; and a single, elongated projection that transmits impulses is called the

(d) _____. In the peripheral nervous system, bundles of axons and their sheaths are called

(e) _____. Neurons are classified by the direction in which they transmit impulses. The neurons that

transmit impulses to the spinal cord and brain from the body are **(f)** _____ neurons. Neurons that

transmit impulses away from the brain to muscle and glandular tissue are **(g)** _____ neurons.

Neurons that conduct impulses from sensory neurons directly to motor neurons are **(h)** _____. In its

resting state the charge inside the neuron is **(i)** _____, and the charge outside the neuron is

(j) _____. When the neuron is stimulated while the outside is positively charged,

(k) _____ ions rush into the cell and begin a wave of **(l)** _____ that travels down the cell.

Myelinated axons have interruptions in the myelin sheaths, called **(m)** _____, _____

that cause the action potential to be conducted more **(n)** _____than unmyelinated axons. The space

between the nerve endings of two adjacent neurons is known as a **(o)** _____. Impulses are trans-

mitted across these spaces by neurotransmitters such as **(p)** _____, _____, and

_____.

18. List the basic anatomical components of a reflex.

_____

19. Name the two paired arteries that supply blood to the brain.
   a.
   b.

20. State whether the following factors will _increase, decrease,_ or _not change_ the cerebral blood flow.
   a. Intracranial pressure of 30 mm Hg:
   b. Mean arterial pressure of 40 mm Hg:
   c. Expanding tumor in the brain:
   d. Hypovolemic shock:

21. List at least two causes of coma for each of the following six general classifications.

   a. Structural:

_____

448

b. Metabolic:

_____

c. Drug induced:

_____

d. Cardiovascular:

_____

e. Respiratory:

_____

f. Infectious:

_____

22. You have been called to care for a patient who is suspected of suffering from a neurological disorder. He opens his eyes when you call his name but does not know what day it is. He is moving all extremities normally.

    a. List six specific questions you should ask the family to elicit the nature of the neurological problem.

_____

_____

    b. What vital sign findings would suggest increased intracranial pressure?

_____

    c. Using the AVPU assessment, describe the patient's level of consciousness.

_____

    d. What is his score on the Glasgow Coma Scale?

_____

    e. Describe your assessment of this patient's eyes.

_____

23. State whether the following symptoms of coma are most likely to be found in structural or toxic-metabolic coma.
    a. Asymmetrical neurological findings:
    b. Slow onset:
    c. Unilateral fixed and dilated pupil:

24. You arrive at a private residence to evaluate a 65-year-old woman whose neighbors found her unresponsive. She has snoring respirations at a rate of 8/min, and an oral airway is easily placed. Carotid and radial pulses are present and rapid. Blood pressure is 110/70 mm Hg. She flexes to painful stimuli, no history is available, and her blood glucose level is 60 mg/dL. Outline your assessment and management of this patient, including the appropriate dose and route of administration of any drugs you would give.

_____

_____

_____

Questions 25 to 29 refer to the following case study:

You respond to a private residence, where you find an elderly African-American man lying on the sofa. His family states, "He hasn't been acting right." On exam you find him awake and confused, with slurred speech. He follows commands appropriately. When you ask him to smile, he has an apparent facial droop on the right. Ongoing assessment reveals weakness in the left arm and leg. His vital signs are BP, 160/108 mm Hg; P, 72/min; and R, 16/min and regular. His Sao_2 is 95%, and his blood glucose level is 94 mg/dL. History reveals no allergies, and his medications include hydrochlorothiazide, nitroglycerin, and insulin. His family states that a similar incident occurred yesterday and lasted about 5 minutes after he took a walk. He smokes one pack of cigarettes a day.

25. List eight risk factors for stroke that you can identify for this patient and note whether each is modifiable or nonmodifiable.

	Risk Factor	**Modifiable (Yes or No)**
a.		
b.		
c.		
d.		
e.		
f.		
g.		
h.		

26. List at least six signs or symptoms of cerebrovascular accident that are common to embolic and thrombotic strokes. (Place a star beside the ones experienced by this patient.)

_____

_____

27. List the physical findings that would indicate the probability of stroke for this patient based on

  a. The Cincinnati stroke scale_____

_____

  b. The Los Angeles Prehospital Stroke Screen_____

_____

28. List the seven *D*s of stroke management.

  D

  D

  D

  D

  D

  D

  D

450

29. Outline your prehospital care of this patient.

_____

_____

_____

30. Although patients may have diverse presentations, describe the typical progression of signs and symptoms of hemorrhagic stroke.

_____

_____

31. List five causes of seizures:

   a.

   b.

   c.

   d.

   e.

32. State the type of seizure for each of the following signs and symptoms.

   a. Numbness of the body or unusual visual, auditory, or taste symptoms:

_____

   b. Brief loss of consciousness in a child (without loss of posture) that lasts less than 15 seconds:

_____

   c. Partial seizure activity that spreads in an orderly fashion to surrounding areas:

_____

   d. Preceding aura, followed by loss of consciousness and tonic-clonic motor activity, followed by a postictal state:

_____

   e. Aura followed by automatisms such as lip smacking and chewing, during which time the patient is amnesic:

_____

33. What history should be obtained from the family of a patient who has had a grand mal seizure?

_____

34. List two findings that suggest that the seizure is hysterical rather than grand mal.

   a.

   b.

35. State whether each of the following characteristics is more suggestive of seizure or syncope:

   a. It starts in a standing position:

_____

b. It is preceded by lightheadedness:

_____

c. The patient remains unconscious for minutes to hours:

_____

d. Tachycardia occurs:

_____

36. List two anticonvulsants (with the appropriate doses) that may be given to an adult patient having a seizure.

   a.

   b.

37. Identify the type of headache (tension, migraine, cluster, or sinus) typically associated with each of the following case presentations.

   a. You are dispatched at 0100 to care for a patient who is complaining of a severe headache that woke him. He says the pain is most intense around his left eye, and you note that his eyes are tearing and his nose is

   running._____

   b. Your partner is recovering from an upper respiratory infection and complaining of a headache that affects her forehead and upper face. She describes an intense pressure sensation that increases when she bends over.

   _____

   c. Your patient is complaining of a dull, throbbing headache that started a week ago and will not stop.

   _____

   d. A 24-year-old woman is complaining of a severe headache that began as an intense throbbing on the right side of her head and is now generalized. She has vomited three times. She indicates a history of this and

   takes a beta blocker._____

STUDENT SELF-ASSESSMENT

38. Which blood vessel or vessels supply the front lobes of the brain?
   a. Anterior cerebral arteries
   b. Midline basilar artery
   c. Posterior cerebral arteries
   d. Right and left vertebral arteries

39. An important function of the circle of Willis is to maintain blood supply to the brain if which of the following occurs?
   a. The patient becomes hypoxic because of shock.
   b. The patient has a large hemorrhagic stroke.
   c. Intracranial pressure increases suddenly.
   d. The vertebral or internal carotid arteries are blocked.

40. Which of the following will cause a decrease in the cerebral blood flow?
   a. Blood pressure of 70/50 mm Hg
   b. Intracranial pressure of 15 mm Hg
   c. Decreased levels of intraocular fluid
   d. Body temperature of 102° F (38.9° C)

41. Respiratory patterns associated with neurological disorders include all of the following *except* which symptom?
   a. Ataxic respirations
   b. Cheyne-Stokes respirations
   c. Diaphragmatic breathing
   d. Kussmaul respirations

42. Posturing caused by structural impairment of the subcortical regions of the brain is known as which of the following?
  a. Extension rigidity
  b. Flexion rigidity
  c. Dysconjugate gaze
  d. Flaccidity

43. Your comatose patient's pupils are 2 mm and round and reactive to light. What does this suggest?
  a. Barbiturate overdose
  b. Medullary injury
  c. Opiate overdose
  d. Temporal herniation

44. Management of the postictal patient with a known seizure disorder who initially aroused to pain and then begins to moan and move spontaneously includes which of the following?
  a. Administration of naloxone (2 mg IV)
  b. Administration of diazepam (5 mg IV)
  c. Intravenous fluid therapy with normal saline (100 mL/hr)
  d. Recumbent positioning of the patient

45. Significant findings in the medical history of a patient you suspect is having a stroke include all of the following *except* which characteristic?
  a. Cigarette smoking
  b. Obesity
  c. Oral contraceptive use
  d. Sickle cell disease

46. Which of the following findings would indicate a high probability of stroke based on the Cincinnati prehospital stroke scale?
  a. The patient has the worst headache ever felt.
  b. The patient cannot speak clearly to you.
  c. The patient experiences a new onset of seizures.
  d. The patient complains of double vision.

47. Your patient has continuous, rapid muscle jerking that the family says is related to his neuromuscular disease. What are these movements called?
  a. Dystonia
  b. Inanition
  c. Myoclonus
  d. Palsy

WRAP IT UP

You respond to a call for "seizures." When you arrive, you find a 72-year-old male who opens his eyes to pain, pushes your hand away when you apply nail bed pressure, and calls out cuss words, then quickly appears to sleep again and has snoring respirations. You insert a nasal airway and administer oxygen by mask while you continue your examination. His wife explains that he was in the bathroom having a bowel movement when she heard a noise, and when she got to him, his limbs jerked rhythmically for several minutes and then he "passed out." She says that he had been complaining of a headache this morning. He takes furosemide and enalapril. As you continue your examination, the patient becomes progressively more awake. His vital signs are BP, 192/98 mm Hg; P, 96/min; R, 20/min; Sao_2, 99% (on oxygen); blood glucose, 99 mg/dL; pupils 4 mm, equal, and reactive to light. You initiate an IV of normal saline TKO and, seeing no traumatic injury on your exam, move the patient to your stretcher. In the ambulance you place the patient on an ECG monitor and observe a normal sinus rhythm. You transport him 4 minutes to the closest hospital, continuously monitoring his neurological status and vital signs, which have not changed. As you move him to the ED cot, he experiences another seizure with tonic-clonic movements; his breathing then becomes ataxic, his pupils become fixed and dilated, he is unresponsive to painful stimulus, and his heart rate drops quickly until his ventilations are assisted. CT scan reveals a large hemorrhagic stroke, and the patient dies within 6 hours of arrival at the hospital.

1. What were the patient's Glasgow Coma Scale values
  a. Initially
  b. After his seizure in the ED

2. Were any signs of increased intracranial pressure present
  a. When you arrived
  b. After the patient had his second seizure

3. If the patient had continued to have a seizure, list two drugs (and their appropriate dose) that could have been administered.

  a.

  b.

4. Explain some possible causes of the patient's condition that you tried to rule out as you initially assessed the patient.

5. Identify at least four risk factors for stroke that you have determined this patient had.

_____

6. Place a ✔ beside the signs or symptoms of stroke that this patient showed.

a. _____ Aphasia		**h.** _____ Headache
b. _____ Ataxia		**i.** _____ Hemiparesis
c. _____ Confusion		**j.** _____ Incontinence
d. _____ Coma		**k.** _____ Monocular blindness
e. _____ Diplopia		**l.** _____ Numbness
f. _____ Dizziness		**m.** _____ Seizure
g. _____ Dysarthria			

7. What leads you to believe that this patient had a hemorrhagic rather than an ischemic stroke?

_____

8. Which is true of this patient's Cincinnati or Los Angeles Prehospital Stroke Screen:
   a. Both demonstrate a high probability of stroke.
   b. Both confirm the presence of stoke.
   c. Neither can be performed on this patient.
   d. Only the LAPSS demonstrates stroke in this case.

CHAPTER 31 ANSWERS

REVIEW QUESTIONS

1. a
2. e
3. d
4. b
5. d
6. c
7. e
8. d
9. i
10. j
11. h
12. f
13. c
14. a
15. b
16. k
    (Questions 1-16: Objective 4)

17. a. Neuroglia; b. cell body; c. dendrites; d. axon; e. white matter; f. sensory; g. motor; h. interneurons; i. negative; j. positive; k. sodium; l. depolarization; m. nodes of Ranvier; n. quickly; o. synapse; p. norepinephrine, epinephrine, and dopamine.
    (Objective 1)

18. Sensory receptor, sensory neuron, interneurons, motor neuron, and effector organ.
    (Objective 1)

19. Vertebral arteries and internal carotid arteries.
    (Objective 1)

20. a. Decrease; b. decrease; c. decrease; d. decrease
    (Objective 2)

21. a. Intracranial bleeding, head trauma, brain tumor, or another space-occupying lesion; b. anoxia, hypoglycemia, diabetic ketoacidosis, thiamine deficiency, kidney and liver failure, and postictal phase of a seizure; c. barbiturates, narcotics, hallucinogenics, depressants, and alcohol; d. hypertensive encephalopathy, shock, dysrhythmias, and stroke; e. chronic obstructive pulmonary disease and toxic inhalation; f. meningitis and sepsis.
    (Objective 4)

22. a. Why did you call EMS? What happened during the course of this situation? Does the patient have any medical problems, such as heart or lung disease, neurological illness, diabetes, or high blood pressure? Does the patient have a history of drug or alcohol abuse or stroke? Has this ever happened to him before? Do you know if he has had any injuries recently?
    b. Increased blood pressure, decreased pulse, widened pulse pressure, slow or irregular respiratory rate.
    c. He is responsive to verbal stimuli.
    d. GCS = 13
    e. Assess the pupils for shape, size, equality, and response to light. Assess the patient's extraocular movements by asking him to follow your finger movements with his eyes (to the extreme left, up and down, to the extreme right, up and down).
    (Objective 3)

23. a. Structural; b. toxic-metabolic; c. structural
(Objective 4)

24. Secure the airway and ventilate with 100% oxygen (with in-line immobilization of the spine). Assess the carotid and radial pulses. Assess vital signs, oxygen saturation, breath sounds, ECG, and pupil response. Scan the body for obvious trauma. Draw a blood sample while initiating an IV with 0.9% normal saline. Because the blood glucose level is less than 80 mg/dL, administer thiamine (100 mg IV), reassess, administer 25 g of $D_{50}W$ IV, and reassess. (If the blood glucose level had been normal, you would have administered naloxone [Narcan] [2 mg IV] and reassessed.) If no improvement occurs and patient has no gag reflex, she should be intubated (and tube placement verified). Perform ongoing assessment and transport.
(Objectives 3, 4)

25.

Risk Factor	Modifiable (Yes or No)
a. Age (elderly)	No
b. Race (African-American)	No
c. Gender (male)	No
d. Hypertension	Yes
e. Heart disease (nitroglycerin)	Yes
f. Diabetes (insulin)	Yes
g. Transient ischemic attacks	Yes
h. Cigarette smoking	Yes

(Objective 4)

26. Confusion[*] or coma, dysarthria[*], aphasia, facial droop[*] or facial numbness, hemiparesis[*] or hemiplegia, convulsions, incontinence, diplopia, headache, dizziness, ataxia, monocular blindness, or vertigo.
(Objective 4)

27. a. Facial droop, arm drift, and slurred speech; b. Patient is over age 45, has no history of seizures, symptom duration is longer than 24 hours, patient is not wheelchair bound, blood glucose is normal, and patient has obvious asymmetry of smile and arm strength.
(Objective 4)

28. Detection, dispatch, delivery (to a stroke center), door (appropriate hospital for rapid treatment of stroke), data (include CT scan), decision (to identify appropriateness of fibrinolytic therapy), drug.
(Objective 4)

29. Make sure that his airway remains patent, administer supplemental oxygen if his Sao_2 drops below 90% or his condition worsens, monitor vital signs and ECG, elevate head of stretcher 15 degrees, initiate IV LR or NS at 50 mL/hour; protect affected extremities, maintain normal temperature, rapid transport to closest stroke center, control seizures, if present, with benzodiazepines; comfort and reassure the patient and family.
(Objective 4)

30. Hemorrhagic stroke commonly occurs during stress or exertion. It starts abruptly and often begins with a headache, nausea, vomiting, and progressive deterioration of neurological status. The patient may rapidly lose consciousness or have a seizure.
(Objective 4)

31. Stroke, head trauma, toxins, hypoxia, hypoglycemia, infection, metabolic abnormalities, brain tumor, vascular disorders, eclampsia, and drug overdose.
(Objective 4)

32. a. Simple sensory seizure (partial seizure); b. petit mal (generalized seizure); c. jacksonian seizure (partial seizure); d. grand mal seizure (generalized seizure); e. complex partial seizures (partial seizure).
(Objective 4)

33. History of seizures, including frequency and medication compliance; description of seizure (length, features, incontinence, tongue biting); history of head trauma; fever, headache, or nuchal rigidity before seizure; medical history, including diabetes, cardiovascular disease, and stroke.
(Objective 4)

34. With a hysterical seizure, the following do not occur: trauma to the tongue, incontinence, and response to conventional therapy. A hysterical seizure may stop with a sharp command or sternal rub.
(Objective 4)

35. a. Syncope; b. syncope; c. seizure; d. seizure
(Objective 4)

36. Lorazepam (1 to 2 mg IV); or diazepam (5 to 10 mg IV) every 15 minutes as necessary.
(Objective 4)

37. a. Cluster headache; b. sinus headache; c. tension headache; d. migraine headache.
(Objective 4)

STUDENT SELF-ASSESSMENT

38. a. The internal carotid arteries give rise to the anterior cerebral arteries. The vertebral arteries supply the cerebellum and unite to form the basilar artery.
(Objective 1)

39. d. The circle of Willis would not protect against a large cerebral bleed, systemic hypoxia, or increased ICP. It can help to maintain blood flow if a clot exists in the vertebral or carotid arteries.
(Objective 1)

40. a. This will decrease cerebral perfusion pressure. CPP does not usually decrease until the ICP exceeds 22 mm Hg (the body compensates to that level). Fluid in the eye has no influence on CPP. Metabolic rate will increase, but CPP is not affected by a temperature of $102°$ F ($38.9°$ C).
(Objective 2)

41. d. Kussmaul respirations occur secondary to the metabolic acidosis that occurs in diabetic ketoacidosis. Each of the other breathing patterns may be encountered in a patient who has a neurological problem.
(Objective 3)

42. a. Flexion posturing occurs with impairment of the cortical regions of the brain. Flaccidity is usually caused by brain stem or cord dysfunction. Dysconjugate gaze is not a posture but an abnormal eye movement.
(Objective 3)

43. c. Barbiturate overdose and medullary injury are more likely to present with dilated pupils. Temporal herniation causes a unilateral dilated pupil.
(Objective 3)

44. d. Airway maintenance is critical. Drug administration would be indicated only if the seizure recurs.
(Objective 4)

45. b. All other choices are risk factors for stroke.
(Objective 4)

46. b. The three components of the stroke scale are facial droop, arm drift, and speech disturbances. All other choices are possible signs or symptoms of stroke but are not included in the stroke scale.
(Objective 4)

47. c. *Dystonia* refers to an alteration in muscle tone that can cause painful spasms, fixed postures, or strange movement patterns. *Inanition* refers to starvation or failure to thrive. *Palsy* is weakness.
(Objective 4)

WRAP IT UP

1. a. 10; b. 3 (no response to pain)
(Objective 3)

2. Altered level of consciousness; hospital: decreasing level of consciousness, bradycardia, fixed and dilated pupils, ataxic breathing
(Objective 3)

3. Lorazepam (Ativan), 1 to 4 mg IV given slowly; or diazepam (Valium), 5 mg over 2 minutes.
(Objective 4)

4. Intracranial bleeding, head trauma, brain tumor, anoxia, hypoglycemia, seizure disorder, drug overdose, poisoning, hypertensive encephalopathy, dysrhythmia, stroke, meningitis
(Objective 3)

5. High blood pressure, age, male gender
(Objective 4)

6. d, h, m
(Objective 4)

7. Symptoms developed abruptly, occurred during exertion (using the toilet), seizure ensued, as did progressive and rapid deterioration
(Objective 4)

8. c. The patient is unconscious and unable to be evaluated using either scale.
(Objective 3)

32

Endocrinology

READING ASSIGNMENT
Chapter 32, pages 864-881, in *Mosby's Paramedic Textbook,* ed. 3

OBJECTIVES
Upon completion of this chapter, the paramedic student will be able to:
1. Describe how hormones secreted from endocrine glands help the body to maintain homeostasis.
2. Describe the anatomy and physiology of the pancreas and how its hormones work to maintain normal glucose metabolism.
3. Discuss pathophysiology as a basis for key signs and symptoms, patient assessment, and patient management for diabetes and diabetic emergencies of hypoglycemia, diabetic ketoacidosis, and hyperosmolar hyperglycemic nonketotic coma.
4. Discuss pathophysiology as a basis for key signs and symptoms, patient assessment, and patient management for disorders of the thyroid gland.
5. Discuss pathophysiology as a basis for key signs and symptoms, patient assessment, and patient management of Cushing syndrome and Addison disease.

SUMMARY
- The endocrine system consists of ductless glands and tissues. These glands and tissues produce and secrete hormones. Endocrine glands secrete their hormones directly into the bloodstream. They exert a regulatory effect on various metabolic functions. All hormones operate within feedback systems. (These are either positive or negative.) These systems work to maintain an optimal internal environment.
- The pancreatic islets are composed of beta cells, alpha cells, and other cells. The beta cells secrete insulin. The alpha cells secrete glucagon. The other cells are of questionable function. The chief functions of insulin are to increase glucose transport into cells, increase glucose metabolism by cells, increase the liver glycogen level, and decrease the blood glucose concentration toward normal. Glucagon has two major effects: (1) increase blood glucose levels by stimulating the liver to release glucose stores from glycogen and other glucose storage sites (glycogenolysis) and (2) stimulate gluconeogenesis through the breakdown of fats and fatty acids, thereby maintaining a normal blood glucose level.
- Diabetes mellitus is characterized by a deficiency of insulin or an inability of the body to respond to insulin. Diabetes generally is classified as type 1 or type 2. Type 1 is insulin dependent. Type 2 is non-insulin dependent. Type 1 diabetes requires lifelong treatment. This consists of insulin injections, exercise, and diet regulation. Most patients with type 2 diabetes require oral hypoglycemic medications, exercise, and dietary regulation to control the illness.
- Hypoglycemia is a syndrome related to blood glucose levels below 80 mg/dL. Any diabetic patient with behavioral changes or unconsciousness should be treated for hypoglycemia. This condition is a true emergency. It requires immediate administration of glucose to prevent permanent brain damage or death.

- Diabetic ketoacidosis results from an absence of or a resistance to insulin. The signs and symptoms of DKA are related to diuresis and acidosis. They usually are slow in onset.
- Hyperosmolar hyperglycemic nonketotic coma is a life-threatening emergency. It often occurs in older patients with type 2 diabetes. It also frequently occurs in undiagnosed diabetics. The hyperglycemia produces a hyperosmolar state. This is followed by an osmotic diuresis, dehydration, and electrolyte losses.
- Important components of the patient history in the assessment of diabetic patients include the onset of symptoms, food intake, insulin or oral hypoglycemic use, alcohol or other drug consumption, predisposing factors, and any associated symptoms.
- Any patient with a glucose reading below 80 mg/dL and signs and symptoms consistent with hypoglycemia should be given dextrose.
- Thyrotoxicosis is any toxic condition that results from overactivity of the thyroid gland.
- Thyroid storm is a life-threatening condition resulting from an overactive thyroid gland. Thyroid hormones play a key role in controlling body metabolism. They are essential in children for normal physical growth and development.
- Myxedema is a condition that results from a thyroid hormone deficiency. Myxedema coma is a rare illness. In addition to myxedema, it is characterized by hypothermia and mental obtundation. It is a medical emergency.
- Cushing syndrome is caused by an abnormally high circulating level of corticosteroid hormones. These are produced naturally by the adrenal glands.
- Addison disease is a rare but life-threatening disorder. It is caused by a deficiency of the corticosteroid hormones cortisol and aldosterone. These are normally produced by the adrenal cortex.

REVIEW QUESTIONS

Match the signs or symptoms in column II with the appropriate diabetic emergencies in column I. Each answer may be used *more* than once.

Column I	Column II
1. _____ Diabetic ketoacidosis	a. Abdominal pain
2. _____ Hyperosmolar hyperglycemic nonketotic coma	b. Coma
3. _____ Hypoglycemia	c. Cool, clammy skin
	d. Fruity breath odor
	e. Kussmaul respirations
	f. Polyuria
	g. Psychotic behavior
	h. Seizures
	i. Tachycardia
	j. Warm, dry skin
	k. Vomiting

4. Name the hormone secreted from each of these cells in the pancreas.
   a. Alpha cells:
   b. Beta cells:
   c. Delta cells:

5. When food is ingested, it is broken down into smaller units and used or stored. Name the breakdown products and storage sites for the following food types.

Food	Breakdown Products	Storage
a. Carbohydrates		
b. Proteins		
c. Fats		

6. a. How is excess glucose stored in the liver?

_____

b. How are glucose stores released from the liver?

_____

7. Briefly explain the role of glucagon in the metabolism of food.

_____

8. Why does a patient develop cerebral signs and symptoms of hypoglycemia rapidly?

_____

9. List at least three signs or symptoms that might lead you to suspect that a patient has undetected type 1 diabetes.

_____

_____

_____

10. List at least three medical illnesses associated with long-term diabetes.

_____

_____

_____

11. You arrive on the scene of a suspected diabetic emergency. You find a 35-year-old man whose wife says he took his insulin 2 hours ago and has not eaten. He arouses only to pain and has noisy, snoring respirations. He has no other medical history. Outline the steps in your patient management.

_____

_____

_____

_____

Questions 12 to 16 refer to the following case study:

A 20-year-old diabetic patient calls you complaining of difficulty breathing. On arrival, the patient states that he has had the flu for 2 days. You note that his respiratory rate is 40/min and his breath has a very sweet odor. You auscultate his lungs, and his breath sounds are clear bilaterally.

12. What do you suspect?

_____

13. What other specific questions will you ask about the history of this patient's illness?

_____

_____

14. What specific findings will you be looking for during your physical assessment of the patient?

_____

You perform a blood glucose analysis, and your machine reads "high." The patient appears dehydrated.

15. What interventions should you perform for this patient in the prehospital setting?

_____

16. Should you be concerned about rapid transport for this patient? Why?

_____

17. List six factors that predispose a patient to the development of hyperosmolar hyperglycemic nonketotic coma.

a.

b.

c.

d.

e.

f.

18. Complete the missing information for each endocrine disorder in the table below.

Disorder	Endocrine Gland and Hormone Affected	Hormone Excess or Shortage?	Signs and Symptoms	Potentially Life Threatening?
Graves disease				
Thyroid storm				
Myxedema				
Cushing syndrome				
Addison disease				

STUDENT SELF-ASSESSMENT

19. How do hormones achieve their desired actions?
   a. They travel by ducts to the specific organ to be stimulated.
   b. They stimulate nerves to send messages to their target tissue.
   c. They trigger cell-specific receptors to initiate specific functions.
   d. They activate the organ adjacent to the gland that produces them.
20. What is the primary action of insulin?
   a. To reduce the glucose needs of the cells
   b. To increase blood glucose levels
   c. To transport glucose into the cells
   d. To manufacture amino acids
21. Oral hypoglycemic agents include all of the following _except_ which drug?
   a. Diabinese   **c.** Insulin
   b. Dymelor   **d.** Orinase

22. Type 2 diabetes mellitus most likely does which of the following?
    a. Requires insulin injections
    b. Develops after age 40
    c. Has a sudden onset of symptoms
    d. Results in life-threatening emergencies
23. What is the breakdown of glucose stores in the liver called?
    a. Glucagon
    b. Glucosuria
    c. Gluconeogenesis
    d. Glycogenolysis
24. Before administration of $D_{50}W$ in a lethargic patient with diabetes, you should do all of the following *except* which procedure?
    a. Initiate intravenous fluids
    b. Administer glucagon
    c. Draw a blood sample
    d. Determine the blood glucose level
25. Before giving $D_{50}W$ to a diabetic who is also a known alcoholic, what should you administer?
    a. Glucagon
    b. Half the usual dose
    c. Insulin
    d. Thiamine
26. An advantage of glucagon over $D_{50}W$ is that it is
    a. Faster acting
    b. Less expensive
    c. Given IM
    d. More effective
27. What is the correct dose of glucagon for an adult?
    a. 0.5 to 1 mg IM
    b. 1 to 2 mg IM
    c. 12.5 g IV
    d. 25 g IV
28. Which of the following signs or symptoms would be *unlikely* in a patient who is in a hyperosmolar hyperglycemic nonketotic coma?
    a. Altered level of consciousness
    b. Dry mucous membranes
    c. Fruity breath odor
    d. Thirst
29. Your patient is very anxious and is complaining of abdominal pain and difficulty breathing. Her vital signs are BP, 80/50 mm Hg; P, 136/min; and R, 24/min. You note basilar rales in her lungs. What endocrine condition may cause this presentation?
    a. Cushing syndrome
    b. Graves disease
    c. Myxedema
    d. Thyroid storm

WRAP IT UP

At 1400 on a warm summer day, you respond for a "diabetic sick case." When you arrive, you find a 21-year-old patient with type 1 diabetes who is pale, cool, and diaphoretic; she responds to painful stimuli only by telling you to go away. Her husband tells you that she is 8 weeks pregnant, and she hasn't been feeling well for a couple of days because of her "morning sickness." He says her insulin is off schedule, and her sugars have been "all over the place." Her vital signs are BP, 100/70 mm Hg; P, 120/min; and R, 20/min. You start an IV and simultaneously obtain a blood glucose level, which is 34 mg/dL. Minutes after 25 g of $D_{50}W$ has been administered IV, the patient awakens and is embarrassed about the situation. She refuses further treatment and transport; you contact medical direction, which recommends that she call her endocrinologist for an appointment immediately.

1. Which is true about type 1 diabetes?
    a. It results from a pituitary abnormality.
    b. Its symptoms occur when glucagon production decreases.
    c. It occurs when the cells lose their ability to absorb glucose.
    d. It results from inadequate pancreatic production of insulin.

2. Which hormone is responsible for the initial shakiness, tachycardia, and dry mouth felt by diabetics who are hypoglycemic?

   a. Adrenocorticotrophic hormone

   b. Epinephrine

   c. Glucagon

   d. Vasopressin

3. Put a ✔ beside the signs or symptoms this patient had that could indicate hypoglycemia. Put an 8 beside those that could indicate diabetic ketoacidosis (hyperglycemia).

   a. _____ Altered level of consciousness   **d.** _____ Tachycardia

   b. _____ Cool skin   **e.** _____ Sweaty

   c. _____ Hypotension

4. How would your patient care have changed if

   a. The patient had been alert, and oriented.

   _____

   _____

   b. Her blood glucose had been 434 mg/dL.

   _____

   _____

   c. Your blood glucose monitor had not functioned.

   _____

   _____

CHAPTER 32 ANSWERS

REVIEW QUESTIONS

1. a, b, d, e, f, i, j, k
2. b, f, h, i, j
3. b, c, g, i, j
   (Questions 1-3: Objective 3)

4. a. Glucagon; b. insulin; c. somatostatin
   (Objective 2)

5.

Food	Breakdown Products	Storage
a. Carbohydrates	Glucose	Liver and muscles (excess converted to fat)
b. Proteins	Amino acids	Small amounts in cytoplasm of all cells
c. Fats		Fatty acids, glycerol Liver and fat cells

   (Objective 2)

6. a. Glucose is stored in the liver as glycogen. b. As the blood sugar begins to drop, glucagon is released from the pancreas and stimulates the breakdown of glycogen to glucose.
   (Objective 2)

7. Glucagon breaks down glycogen and stimulates gluconeogenesis (the formation of glucose from amino acids).
   (Objective 2)

8. Glucose cannot be stored in the brain; therefore when blood sugar drops, no reserves exist. The brain cannot use fats or proteins for energy.
   (Objective 3)

9. New onset of diabetes is associated with increased fluid intake (polydipsia), increased urine output (polyuria), dizziness, blurred vision, and rapid weight loss.
   (Objective 3)

10. Long-term complications of diabetes include blindness, kidney disease, peripheral neuropathy, autonomic neuropathy, peripheral vascular disease, heart disease, and stroke.
    (Objective 3)

11. Assess and protect the airway; place a nasal or oral airway and suction if necessary; evaluate breathing, assist if necessary, and administer oxygen; assess pulse; evaluate vital signs; determine blood glucose level; start an IV in the antecubital space; if the blood glucose is less than 80 mg/dL, administer $D_{50}W$ (25 g IV) and reassess the patient.
    (Objective 3)

12. Diabetic ketoacidosis or a pulmonary problem.
    (Objective 3)

13. Have you had any vomiting or diarrhea? If yes, how much? When did you last eat? What medications do you take and when did you last take them (especially insulin)? How much have you been urinating? Do you feel dizzy when you stand up? Have you lost any weight? Are you thirsty and have you been drinking a lot of fluids? Do you have any abdominal pain?
    (Objective 3)

14. As you perform your total patient assessment, you should check to see if the patient has warm, dry skin; dry mucous membranes; tachycardia; postural hypotension; fruity breath odor; or a decreased level of consciousness. (Objective 3)

15. Oxygen should be administered and the patient monitored for dysrhythmias. An IV of 0.9% normal saline should be initiated. Medical direction likely will advise infusion at a rapid rate, often 250 mL/hour or more. (Objective 3)

16. Transport rapidly because definitive treatment includes administration of insulin, which is not usually available on EMS units. (Objective 3)

17. Type 2 diabetes; advanced age; preexisting cardiac or renal disease; inadequate insulin secretion or action; increased insulin requirements (stress, infection, trauma, burns, myocardial infarction); medications such as thiazide diuretics, glucocorticoids, phenytoin, sympathomimetics, propranolol, and immunosuppressants; and parenteral or enteral feedings. (Objective 17)

18.

Disorder	Endocrine Gland and Hormone Affected	Hormone Excess or Shortage?	Signs and Symptoms	Potentially Life Threatening?
Graves disease	Thyroid hormone	Excess	Enlarged thyroid, swollen neck, protruding eyes	Yes if it progresses to to thyroid storm
Thyroid storm	Thyroid hormone	Excess	Tachycardia, heart failure, dysrhythmias, shock, hyperthermia, restlessness, agitation, abdominal pain, coma	Yes
Myxedema	Thyroid hormone	Shortage	Hoarse voice, fatigue, weight gain, cold intolerance, depression, dry skin, hair loss, infertility, constipation, heavy menses	Not unless it progresses to myxedema coma
Cushing syndrome	Adrenal cortex (corticosteroid hormones)	Excess	Round red face, obese trunk, wasted limbs, acne, purple stretch marks, increased facial and body hair, hump on neck, weight gain, hypertension, psychiatric disturbance, insomnia, diabetes	No
Addison disease	Adrenal cortex (cortisol, aldosterone)	Shortage	Weakness, weight loss, anorexia, hyperpigmented skin, hypotension, hyponatremia, hyperkalemia, gastrointestinal disturbances	Usually not unless a rapid, acute onset occurs

(Objectives 4, 5)

19. c. Hormones travel through the blood and may trigger a receptor site in only one organ or throughout the body, depending on the hormone.
(Objective 1)

20. c. Insulin increases glucose transport into cells, increases glucose metabolism by cells, increases liver glycogen levels, and decreases the blood glucose concentration.
(Objective 2)

21. c. Insulin is administered by parenteral injection.
(Objection 3)

22. b. Most type 2 diabetics can control the disease with diet and oral hypoglycemic agents. This disease has a slow onset and does not often cause life-threatening emergencies.
(Objective 3)

23. d. *Glucagon* is a pancreatic hormone. *Glucosuria* is urine that contains glucose. *Gluconeogenesis* is the formation of glucose from the breakdown of fats and fatty acids.
(Objective 2)

24. b. If IV access can be established, intravenous $D_{50}W$ should be administered.
(Objective 3)

25. d. Thiamine promotes the uptake of glucose in the brain.
(Objective 3)

26. c. When an IV cannot be established in a patient with hypoglycemia, glucagon may be given IM. Glucagon is slower, more expensive, and less effective than $D_{50}W$.
(Objective 3)

27. a. 0.5 to 1 mg IM
(Objective 3)

28. c. No ketogenesis occurs with HHNK, therefore no acetone (fruity) breath odor is noted, as it is in hyperglycemia.
(Objective 3)

29. d. These conditions are caused by adrenergic hyperactivity.
(Objective 4)

WRAP IT UP

1. d. Type 1 diabetes is characterized by inadequate production of insulin by the pancreas.
(Objective 3)

2. b. The body releases epinephrine in an attempt to stimulate the release of sugar stored in the liver.
(Objective 3)

3. Hypoglycemia: a, b, c, d, e; hyperglycemia: a, c, d
(Objective 3)

4. a. Oral glucose or foods high in simple sugars (e.g., sweetened orange juice) could have been given.

b. A high blood glucose level would have indicated diabetic ketoacidosis. Oxygenation and rapid administration of normal saline would have been indicated, along with careful monitoring of the patient (including ECG).

c. If no blood glucose value could be obtained, then based on the patient history and presenting signs and symptoms, $D_{50}W$ would be given and the patient's response monitored. (If the EMS blood glucose monitor is not working, the patient's monitor could be used.)

(Objective 3)

CHAPTER 33

Allergies and Anaphylaxis

READING ASSIGNMENT
Chapter 33, pages 882-891, in *Mosby's Paramedic Textbook,* ed. 3

OBJECTIVES
Upon completion of this chapter, the paramedic student will be able to do the following:
1. Describe the antigen-antibody response.
2. Differentiate between an allergic reaction and a normal immune response.
3. Describe signs and symptoms and management of local allergic reactions based on an understanding of the pathophysiology associated with this condition.
4. Identify allergens associated with anaphylaxis.
5. Describe the pathophysiology, signs and symptoms, and management of anaphylaxis.

SUMMARY
- Antibodies bind to the antigen that produced them. Antibodies aid in neutralizing the antigen and removing it from the body.
- Allergic reaction is an increased physiological response to an antigen after a previous exposure to the same antigen. Localized allergic reactions do not affect the entire body.
- Anaphylaxis is the most extreme form of allergic reaction. Rapid recognition and aggressive therapy are needed for patient survival.
- Almost any substance can cause anaphylaxis. The risk of anaphylaxis increases with the frequency of exposure.
- Symptoms of anaphylaxis may include sneezing and coughing; airway obstruction; wheezing; hypotension or vascular collapse; chest pain; nausea, vomiting, or diarrhea; and weakness, headache, syncope, seizures, or coma.

REVIEW QUESTIONS
1. Complete the following sentences.

   Antigens can enter the body by four routes: **(a)** _____, **(b)** _____,

   (c) _____ or **(d)** _____. The allergic reaction is initiated when a circulating

   (e) _____

combines with a specific antigen, causing a **(f)** _____ reaction or to antibodies bound to

(g) _____ _____ or **(h)** _____.

2. List agents in each of the following groups that can cause anaphylaxis.

   a. Drugs:_____

   _____

   b. Insects:_____

   _____

   c. Foods:_____

   _____

   d. Other:_____

   _____

3. List the signs and symptoms associated with each of the following chemical mediators released from basophils and mast cells in an anaphylactic reaction.
   a. Histamines:
   b. Leukotrienes:
   c. Eosinophil chemotactic factor:

4. You are called to a church picnic to care for a 30-year-old woman with wheezing and dyspnea. After a careful assessment, you determine that she is having an anaphylactic reaction.
   a. What other illness or injury may produce these symptoms?
   b. List two home medicines that may influence your care of this patient.

Questions 5 to 7 refer to the following case study:

> You are at a Chinese restaurant caring for a 25-year-old patient experiencing an anaphylactic reaction. He is in acute respiratory distress with wheezing and has a blood pressure of 90/70 mm Hg.

5. What are some causative agents that may be found at this restaurant that could trigger this man's anaphylaxis?

6. After a rapid primary survey and vital sign assessment, you determine that immediate pharmacological therapy is indicated. Identify two drugs, with the appropriate dose and route, that may be indicated for this patient.

   a.

   b.

7. Describe other signs or symptoms that this patient may have.

8. You arrive at a dental office, where you find a 35-year-old woman who rapidly developed hives, angioedema, and stridor after an injection of a local anesthetic. She is unconscious and has labored, stridorous respirations, no radial pulse, and a rapid, irregular, barely palpable carotid pulse. No medicines have been administered to treat her. Describe your priorities of care for this patient, including the appropriate drugs, doses, and routes.

_____

_____

_____

STUDENT SELF-ASSESSMENT

9. What is the term used for any substance that causes the formation of antibodies in the body?
   a. Anaphylactic
   b. Antigen
   c. Basophil
   d. Mast cell

10. Which immunoglobulin (antibody) is responsible for anaphylaxis?
   a. IgA
   b. IgE
   c. IgG
   d. IgM

11. Which of the following is a sign or symptom of a type IV (localized) allergic reaction?
   a. Angioedema
   b. Hoarseness
   c. Vomiting
   d. Wheezing

12. Your 20-year-old patient has hives, normal vital signs, and clear breath sounds. He complains of severe itching. Which of the following drugs would be indicated in this situation?
   a. Diphenhydramine (Benadryl), 5 mg IV
   b. Diphenhydramine (Benadryl), 25 mg IM
   c. Epinephrine (Adrenalin), 0.1 mg (1:1000) IV
   d. Epinephrine (Adrenalin), 0.3 mg (1:1000) SQ

13. What term is used for mediators that cause blood vessels to dilate?
   a. Chemotactic substances
   b. Leukotactic substances
   c. Opsonins
   d. Vasoactive substances

14. Which of the following agents is *not* commonly associated with anaphylaxis?
   a. Acetaminophen
   b. Aspirin
   c. Fire ants
   d. Peanuts

15. What is the most likely cause of death in anaphylaxis?
   a. Upper airway obstruction
   b. Hypoxia resulting from bronchospasm
   c. Hypotension resulting from fluid leakage
   d. Vasogenic shock caused by histamines

16. Which of the following signs or symptoms is *not* associated with anaphylaxis?
   a. Abdominal cramps
   b. Cool, pale skin
   c. Rhinorrhea
   d. Urticaria

17. Diphenhydramine is considered which of the following?
   a. Anticholinergic
   b. Antihistamine
   c. Bronchodilator
   d. Sedative-hypnotic

18. Which of the following is a potential complication of IV epinephrine?
   a. Dysrhythmias
   b. Myocardial ischemia
   c. Seizures
   d. Vomiting
   e. All of the above

WRAP IT UP

You are dispatched for a "person down" at a local business. You find your patient in the cafeteria, lying unconscious on the floor. Co-workers tell you that she complained of itching and said, "That bee just stung me" She then complained of difficulty breathing, and after a 9-1-1 call was made, she became unconscious. You ask about any known allergies, and no one seems to know. They tell you she was at her doctor's office this morning for a vaccination, and when the police officer on the scene looks through her purse, he shows you aspirin, ibuprofen, and penicillin tablets. The remnants of her partly eaten lunch are on the table: fried shrimp; deviled eggs; fruit salad with strawberries, mangoes, and a sesame honey dressing; peanut butter crackers; and a glass of milk. Her skin is flushed red, and she has raised welts on her arm; her eyes and lips appear swollen; and her breathing is very stridorous. Her vital signs are BP, 76 by palpation; P, 134/min; R, 24/min; and Sao$_2$, 88%. You administer oxygen by nonrebreather mask and set up an IV; at the same time, your partner draws up 0.3 mg of epinephrine and administers it IM. You start an IV of normal saline and give a fluid bolus; you then administer diphenhydramine (25 mg IV), followed by methylprednisolone (125 mg IV). The stridor has now subsided, but you hear some persistent wheezing in the lungs, and the woman's vital signs are now BP, 104/60 mm Hg; P, 120/min; R, 20/min; and Sao$_2$, 98%. You administer an albuterol updraft for the persistent wheezing and continue to monitor her condition, which has improved dramatically by the time you arrive at the hospital. She is discharged with a prescription and instructions for an EpiPen and is told to purchase a bracelet or necklace to alert first responders to her severe allergic condition.

1. Which of the following describes the internal mechanisms responsible for this patient's life-threatening condition?
    a. IgE antibodies react to a foreign antigen, triggering the release of histamines, leukotrienes, and other chemicals
    b. IgM antibodies initiate a type IV allergic reaction, which triggers a life-threatening release of kinins
    c. IgG antibodies trigger the release of antigens, which stimulate the eosinophil chemotactic factor of anaphylaxis
    d. Immunoglobulins begin a process of cellular destruction in the lymphatic system that causes anaphylaxis
2. List the possible causes of anaphylaxis that you observed on this patient call.
3. Put a ✔ beside the signs or symptoms of anaphylaxis that were observed in this patient.

a. _____ Hoarseness	k. _____ Hypotension	u. _____ Weakness
b. _____ Stridor	l. _____ Dysrhythmia	v. _____ Headache
c. _____ Laryngeal edema	m. _____ Chest tightness	w. _____ Seizure
d. _____ Rhinorrhea	n. _____ Nausea	x. _____ Coma
e. _____ Bronchospasm	o. _____ Vomiting	y. _____ Angioedema
f. _____ Increased mucus production	p. _____ Abdominal cramps	z. _____ Urticaria
g. _____ Accessory muscle use	q. _____ Diarrhea	aa. _____ Pruritus
h. _____ Wheezing	r. _____ Anxiety	bb. _____ Erythema
i. _____ Decreased breath sounds	s. _____ Dizziness	cc. _____ Edema
j. _____ Tachycardia	t. _____ Syncope	dd. _____ Tearing of the eyes

4. Explain your rationale for each of the following interventions that were performed for this patient.

    a. Oxygen administration:

    _____

    b. Epinephrine administration:

    _____

    c. Normal saline fluid bolus:

    _____

    d. Diphenhydramine administration:

    _____

    e. Steroid administration:

    _____

    f. Albuterol administration:

    _____

CHAPTER 33 ANSWERS

REVIEW QUESTIONS

1. a. Injection; b. ingestion; c. inhalation; d. absorption; e. antibody; f. hypersensitivity; g. mast cells; h. basophils
(Objective 1)

2. a. Antibiotics (especially penicillin), local anesthetics, cephalosporins, chemotherapeutics, aspirin, nonsteroidal antiinflammatory agents, opiates, muscle relaxants, vaccines, and insulin; b. wasps, bees, and fire ants; c. peanuts, soybeans, cod, halibut, shellfish, egg white, strawberries, food additives, wheat and buckwheat, sesame and sunflower seeds, cotton seed, milk, and mango; d. latex.
(Objective 3)

3. a. Histamine release may result in decreased blood pressure, increased gastrointestinal secretions, rhinorrhea, tearing, flushing, urticaria, and angioedema. b. Leukotrienes cause wheezing, which may precipitate chest pain (resulting from coronary vasoconstriction) and enhance the hypotensive effects of histamine. c. Eosinophil chemotactic factor can produce fever, chills, bronchospasm, and pulmonary vasoconstriction.
(Objective 3)

4. a. These same signs and symptoms could be caused by asthma, upper airway obstruction, pulmonary edema, or toxic inhalation. b. If the patient takes a beta blocker (e.g., atenolol, propranolol), it could interfere with the action of epinephrine. If the patient has already self-administered epinephrine (EpiPen, AnaPen), determine the time it was administered and whether symptoms have improved or worsened since administration.
(Objective 4)

5. Foods such as crab, shrimp, nuts, egg, and food additives are known to cause anaphylaxis.
(Objective 3)

6. a. Epinephrine, 0.3 to 0.5 mg (1:1000) IM or subcutaneously; b. diphenhydramine (Benadryl), 25 to 50 mg IM or IV, and then albuterol (Proventil, Ventolin) updraft.
(Objective 4)

7. He may also have stridor, hoarseness, tachypnea, tachycardia, agitation, headache, seizures, decreasing level of consciousness, angioedema, tearing, swelling of the tongue, urticaria, pruritus, sneezing, coughing, tracheal tugging, intercostal retractions, decreased breath sounds, dysrhythmias, chest tightness, nausea, vomiting, and diarrhea.
(Objective 4)

8. Secure the airway, ventilate with 100% oxygen, and intubate. Initiate IV therapy with a large-bore catheter into the antecubital space, infuse fluid rapidly, and administer epinephrine (0.1 to 0.5 mg [1:10,000] IV) over 5 minutes (try to do this simultaneously with airway management if resources permit). If necessary, administer diphenhydramine (25 to 50 mg IM or IV) as a second-line drug. Reevaluate the need to administer a second dose of epinephrine if the patient has not responded. Consider giving methylprednisolone.
(Objective 4)

STUDENT SELF-ASSESSMENT

9. b. An anaphylactic response is a type of life-threatening allergic response. Basophils and mast cells are white blood cells that are involved in the immune response.
(Objective 1)

10. b. IgA immunoglobulins are antibodies found in blood, secretions such as tears, and the respiratory system. IgG antibodies are the most common antibodies involved in the immune response. Production of IgM antibodies precedes IgG production in acute infections.
(Objective 1)

11. a. Angioedema may be found in local or systemic allergic reactions. All of the other signs or symptoms, if present during an allergic reaction, would be most often associated with a systemic (anaphylactic) reaction.
(Objective 2)

12. b. Because no systemic signs or symptoms exist, intramuscular diphenhydramine is indicated. Epinephrine 1:1000 should never be given IVP to treat anaphylaxis.
(Objective 2)

13. d. Chemotactic substances cause the attraction of phagocytic cells toward or away from the antigen; leukotactic substances attract leukocytes to the pathogenic agent; and opsonins bind phagocytes to the invading microorganism.
(Objective 1)

14. a. All the other agents are known to cause anaphylaxis.
(Objective 3)

15. a. Each of the other problems could cause death, but upper airway obstruction is associated with the most deaths from anaphylaxis.
(Objective 4)

16. b. The skin is usually flushed and warm because of the profound vasodilation.
(Objective 4)

17. b
(Objective 2)

18. e
(Objective 4)

WRAP IT UP

1. a. IgE antibodies are the primary mediators in anaphylaxis. Additional chemicals that are triggered include eosinophil chemotactic factor of anaphylaxis, heparin, kinins, prostaglandins, and thromboxanes.
(Objective 1)

2. Antibiotic (penicillin), aspirin, nonsteroidal antiinflammatory agent (ibuprofen), vaccine, possible insect sting, peanuts (peanut butter crackers), shellfish (fried shrimp), egg white (deviled eggs), strawberries, mangoes, sesame seeds (salad), and milk.
(Objective 4)

3. b, c, e, h, j, k, x, y, z, aa, bb, cc
(Objective 5)

4. a. The patient is hypoxic and in shock. Oxygen administration is indicated for both conditions.
b. Epinephrine antagonizes the effects of histamine, and exerts beta-2 effects, which dilate bronchioles; beta-1 effects, which improve myocardial contractility; and alpha effects, which provide vasoconstriction to counteract the effects of anaphylaxis.
c. Normal saline bolus is given as an adjunct to epinephrine in the treatment of the shock associated with anaphylaxis.

d. Diphenhydramine is an antihistamine that can help to reverse some of the symptoms (especially cutaneous) of anaphylaxis.

e. Steroids such as methylprednisolone and dexamethasone suppress acute inflammatory responses that accompany anaphylaxis; they also potentiate smooth muscle relaxation by beta-adrenergic agonists (epinephrine, albuterol) and may alter airway hyperreactivity.

f. Albuterol can aid the management of some of the bronchospasm that is unresolved by epinephrine. However, if signs and symptoms of upper airway edema, severe bronchospasm, or shock persist, an additional dose of epinephrine would be indicated instead of albuterol.

(Objective 5)

CHAPTER
34

Gastroenterology

READING ASSIGNMENT
Chapter 34, pages 892-907 in *Mosby's Paramedic Textbook,* ed. 3

OBJECTIVES
Upon completion of this chapter, the paramedic student will be able to:
1. Label a diagram of the abdominal organs.
2. Outline prehospital assessment of a patient who has abdominal pain.
3. Describe general prehospital management techniques for the patient with abdominal pain.
4. Describe signs and symptoms, complications, and prehospital management for the following gastrointestinal disorders: gastroenteritis, gastritis, colitis, diverticulosis, appendicitis, peptic ulcer disease, bowel obstruction, Crohn's disease, pancreatitis, esophagogastric varices, hemorrhoids, cholecystitis, and acute hepatitis.

SUMMARY
- The major organs most commonly associated with the gastrointestinal system include the esophagus, stomach, small and large intestine, liver, gallbladder, and pancreas.
- After the initial survey, assessment of abdominal pain should begin with a thorough history. The physical examination may help to determine if the pain is visceral, somatic, or referred.
- The most common treatment for abdominal pain will occur at the hospital. The paramedic should provide supportive treatment, manage life threats, and transport the patient to an appropriate facility.
- Gastroenteritis is inflammation of the stomach and intestines secondary to infectious agents, chemicals, or other conditions.
- Gastritis is acute or chronic inflammation of the gastric mucosa. It commonly results from hyperacidity, alcohol or other drug ingestion, bile reflux, and *Helicobacter pylori* infection.
- Colitis is an inflammatory condition of the large intestine. It is characterized by severe diarrhea and ulceration of the mucosa of the intestine (ulcerative colitis).
- Diverticulosis may result in bright red rectal bleeding if perforation occurs.
- Diverticulitis results when a diverticulum becomes obstructed with fecal matter.
- Appendicitis occurs when the passageway between the appendix and cecum is obstructed by fecal material or by inflammation due to infection.
- Peptic ulcer disease occurs when open wounds or sores develop in the stomach or duodenum.
- Bowel obstruction is an occlusion of the intestinal lumen. It results in blockage of the normal flow of intestinal contents.
- Crohn's disease is a chronic, inflammatory bowel disease. It is of unknown origin.
- Inflammation of the pancreas is called pancreatitis. It causes severe abdominal pain.
- Esophagogastric varices result from obstruction of blood flow to the liver as a result of liver disease.

476

- Hemorrhoids are distended veins in the rectoanal area.
- Cholecystitis is inflammation of the gallbladder. It most often is associated with the presence of gallstones.
- Hepatitis is characterized by the sudden onset of malaise, weakness, anorexia, intermittent nausea and vomiting, and dull right upper quadrant pain. This is usually followed within 1 week by the onset of jaundice, dark urine, or both.

REVIEW QUESTIONS

Match the gastrointestinal disorder in column II with its description in column I. Use each disorder only once.

Column I

1. _____ Occlusion of the intestinal lumen
2. _____ Increased pain after ethyl alcohol ingestion; fever and signs of sepsis and shock also possible
3. _____ Protrusion of viscus from normal position through opening in groin or abdominal wall
4. _____ Pain that is most intense at McBurney point
5. _____ Most common cause of massive rectal bleeding in older adults
6. _____ Open erosion wound in digestive system that may bleed
7. _____ Characterized by blood dripping into the toilet after a normal bowel movement
8. _____ Left lower quadrant abdominal pain resulting from a pouch in the colon wall
9. _____ Painless bleeding resulting from a vascular abnormality in the gastrointestinal tract
10. _____ Bright red hematemesis caused by rupture of vessels distended by portal hypertension
11. _____ Inflammation of the gallbladder
12. _____ Inflammation of the gastric mucosa

Column II

a. Appendicitis
b. Arteriovenous malformation
c. Cholecystitis
d. Diverticulitis
e. Diverticulosis
f. Esophageal varices
g. Esophagitis
h. Gastritis
i. Hemorrhoids
j. Hernia
k. Intestinal obstruction
l. Pancreatitis
m. Peptic ulcer

13. Label the abdominal organs in Fig. 34-1.

a. _____   f. _____

b. _____   g. _____

c. _____   h. _____

d. _____   i. _____

e. _____

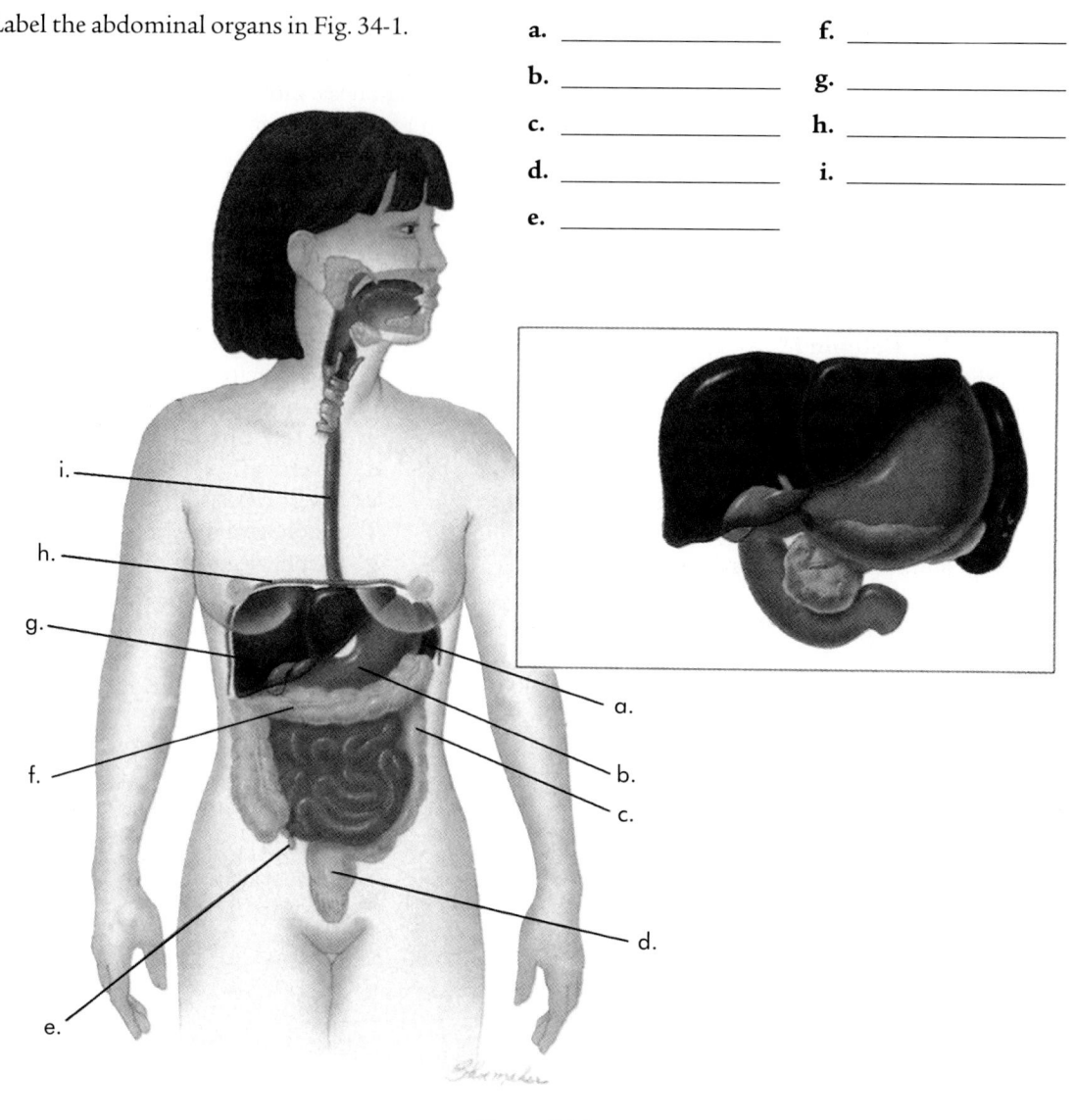

Figure 34-1

14. Your patient is a 72-year-old man complaining of left lower quadrant abdominal pain. State why you would or would not suspect each of the following illnesses as a cause of his pain.

a. Pancreatitis:

_____

b. Cholecystitis:

_____

c. Diverticulitis:

_____

d. Peptic ulcer:

_____

15. A 65-year-old man complains of severe epigastric pain.

    a. List specific questions you must ask this patient to obtain a complete medical history and to determine whether this is a gastrointestinal problem.

_____

_____

_____

    b. What other significant medical problems must you try to rule out by asking these questions?

_____

_____

16. Name the type of pain described in each of the following statements.

    a. Your patient is supine with his legs flexed and complains of a constant, sharp, stabbing pain.

_____

    b. A 40-year-old woman complains of a severe cramping pain at the umbilicus that peaks and then subsides. She is nauseated and has vomited twice.

_____

    c. An obese 47-year-old female complains of right upper quadrant abdominal pain that travels to her right shoulder blade.

_____

17. A 17-year-old boy states that he had severe right lower quadrant pain that diminished several hours ago and is now generalized.

    a. What signs and symptoms would indicate that this patient has an acute abdominal condition and may be developing peritonitis?

_____

    b. Describe the prehospital treatment for this patient.

_____

_____

_____

STUDENT SELF-ASSESSMENT

18. Which of the following abdominal organs is located in the retroperitoneal space?
    a. Liver
    b. Pancreas
    c. Spleen
    d. Stomach

19. A 78-year-old man states that he has been unable to have a bowel movement for a week and has been vomiting profusely. What do you suspect?
    a. Appendicitis
    b. Bowel obstruction
    c. Diverticulosis
    d. Peptic ulcer

20. You are called at 1900 to care for a 40-year-old woman who is complaining of intermittent severe right upper quadrant abdominal pain. She is vomiting and has a low-grade fever. What do you suspect?
   a. Colitis
   b. Cholecystitis
   c. Esophagitis
   d. Hepatitis

21. Which of the following is most likely to cause life-threatening hemorrhage?
   a. Arteriovenous malformations
   b. Diverticulitis
   c. Esophagogastric varices
   d. Hemorrhoids

22. The cause of acute abdominal pain is most accurately assessed in the prehospital setting by which of the following?
   a. Abdominal examination
   b. Patient history
   c. Secondary survey
   d. Vital sign assessment

23. Which of the following is most suggestive of a hemorrhagic gastrointestinal problem?
   a. Anorexia
   b. Fever
   c. Melena
   d. Tachycardia

Questions 24 and 25 refer to the following case study:

A pale, elderly man has had severe vomiting and diarrhea for 3 days. His only history is high blood pressure controlled by an ACE inhibitor and a diuretic. He has severe lower abdominal cramping and is in a fetal position. His wife has a similar illness, but it is not as severe. His blood pressure is 92/50 mm Hg; P, 128/min; and R, 20/min.

24. What is a likely cause of the man's pain?
   a. Appendicitis
   b. Cholecystitis
   c. Diverticulosis
   d. Gastroenteritis

25. Which is a priority in your care of this patient at this time?
   a. Administer pain medicine to relieve his pain.
   b. Give him some medicine to relieve his nausea.
   c. Position him to allow for maximum comfort.
   d. Start an IV and administer fluids to treat shock.

26. Which of the following conditions may cause jaundice?
   a. Colitis
   b. Gastritis
   c. Hepatitis
   d. Peptic ulcer disease

Questions 27 and 28 pertain to the following case study:

A 57-year-old alcoholic male is complaining of nausea and vomiting. He has abdominal pain that starts in the area of the umbilicus and goes to both shoulders. He is hot to the touch. Vital signs are BP, 94/58 mm Hg; P, 132/min; and R, 28/min.

27. Which intervention is indicated first for this man?
   a. Morphine (4 mg IV push)
   b. Normal saline (200 mL bolus)
   c. Oxygen (15 L/min by mask)
   d. Promethazine (Phenergan), 25 mg IV

28. What abdominal illness is a probable diagnosis for this man?
   a. Crohn disease
   b. Esophageal varices
   c. Pancreatitis
   d. Ulcerative colitis

WRAP IT UP

You have just fallen asleep after your third call of the night when the horn sounds and the speaker blares, "4017, respond to an EMS call, abdominal pains, Haven Golden Rest Home, 222 Main, cross street Elm." Your patient is an 80-year-old man who has a history of dementia. The nurse gives you a medication sheet that lists a number of anti-hypertensives, aspirin, some antiarthritic drugs, and some laxatives and stool softeners. She states that he had a shaking chill, vomited twice, seems agitated, and has been moaning and holding his lower abdomen. She thinks his last bowel movement was 4 days ago, and a note in his record states that it was very dark in color. His skin is very warm, moist, and pale, and he is very restless. Vital signs are BP, 100/70 mm Hg; P, 116/min; R, 20/min; Sao$_2$, 93% on room air; and T (axilla), 100.4° F (38° C). His skin is dry and tents slightly, and his mucous membranes are dry. The rest of his physical examination is unremarkable, except that his abdomen is tender to palpation and he is guarding it. Because of his dementia, it is difficult to communicate well enough with him to have him localize the pain. You administer oxygen by nasal cannula at 6 L/min; you then start an IV of normal saline and infuse a bolus of 100 mL, reassessing his breath sounds and vital signs after it has been infused. Medical direction asks you to hold off on pain medicine administration until he can be assessed more thoroughly.

You transport the patient and later find out that free air was present in his abdomen secondary to a ruptured diverticulum. In consultation with his family, after his status deteriorated, the decision was made not to operate.

1. Which abdominal organs could cause pain in the following regions?

   a. Left upper quadrant:

   _____

   b. Right upper quadrant:

   _____

   c. Left lower quadrant:

   _____

   d. Right lower quadrant:

   _____

2. Which of the following describes the correct procedure for an abdominal examination?
   a. Percuss carefully so that painful stimulus can be evaluated.
   b. Auscultate after palpation so that you can focus on tender areas.
   c. Begin palpation in an area of no reported pain and move to the painful area last.
   d. Inspection can often reveal the source of the abdominal pain.

3. Put a ✔ beside any illnesses that could be responsible for this patient's signs and symptoms.

   a. _____ Appendicitis   e. _____ Diverticulosis
   b. _____ Bacterial infection   f. _____ Hepatitis B
   c. _____ Cholecystitis   g. _____ Intestinal obstruction
   d. _____ Crohn disease   h. _____ Pancreatitis

4. What additional interventions could have been provided for this patient?

   _____

CHAPTER 34 ANSWERS

REVIEW QUESTIONS

1. k
2. l
3. j
4. a
5. e
6. m
7. i
   (Questions 1-7: Objective 2)

8. d
   (Objective 2 or 3)

9. b
   (Objective 3)

10. f
    (Objective 3)

11. c
    (Objective 2)

12. h
    (Objective 2)

13. a. Spleen; b. stomach; c. descending colon; d. rectum; e. appendix; f. transverse colon; g. liver; h. diaphragm; i. esophagus
    (Objective 1)

14. a. No. The pain of pancreatitis is located in the epigastric region or right or left upper quadrant. b. No. The pain of cholecystitis is located in the epigastric region or right upper quadrant. It is more common in women under age 50. c. Yes. Diverticulitis is one possibility. It is common in older adults, and the pain is often in the left lower quadrant. d. No. Pain from a peptic ulcer would typically be in the epigastric area.
    (Objective 2)

15. a. Does anything make the pain better or worse? What does the pain feel like (sharp, stabbing, cramping, dull)? Can you show me where the pain is? Does the pain go anywhere else? On a scale of 0 to 10, with 0 being no pain and 10 being the worst pain you have ever had, rate the pain. When did the pain begin? Associated signs and symptoms—Do you have or have you had any nausea, vomiting, diarrhea, constipation, unusual-colored stools, chills, fever, or shortness of breath? Medical history and medications.
    b. Myocardial infarction and abdominal aneurysm.
    (Objective 4)

16. a. Somatic; b. visceral; c. referred
    (Objective 4)

17. a. Fever, chills, tachycardia, tachypnea, position (lying on side with knees flexed and pulled in toward the chest), reluctance to move, skin pallor, absent bowel sounds, generalized involuntary guarding, and rigidity of the abdomen.
    (Objective 4)

b. Oxygen by nonrebreather mask; IV by 16-gauge catheter with normal saline or lactated Ringer solution (rate at least 100 mL/hour, determined by patient's vital signs).
(Objective 4)

STUDENT SELF-ASSESSMENT

18. b. All of the other organs are in the abdominal cavity. (Objective 1)

19. b. Appendicitis would be unusual at this age and typically would not cause the symptoms listed. Diverticulosis and peptic ulcer would not typically produce the symptoms described.
(Objective 2)

20. b. Her age, the time of day, and the description of the pain are characteristics of cholecystitis.
(Objective 2)

21. c. All the disorders listed cause bleeding, but rupture of the esophagogastric varices usually produces rapid, life-threatening bleeding. Bleeding from AV malformations may be minor or severe. Bleeding from diverticulitis may be serious but is not typically an acute life-threatening emergency at onset. Hemorrhoidal bleeding is usually not severe.
(Objective 3)

22. b. The patient's age and gender and the description of the medical history often disclose more about the cause of the abdominal illness than a physical examination. The severity of the patient's present condition is determined by the physical examination.
(Objective 4)

23. c. Melena (black or maroon stool) indicates the presence of bleeding. Tachycardia can be caused by bleeding, fever, pain, or other fluid loss.
(Objective 4)

24. d. The signs and symptoms, as well as the fact that the man's wife had the same illness, point to this as a probable cause.
(Objective 2)

25. d. The most pressing problem is the shock from fluid loss. IV fluid replacement is needed as soon as possible.
(Objective 5)

26. c
(Objective 2)

27. c. A normal saline bolus is given next, as soon as an IV line has been established.
(Objective 5)

28. c. Esophageal varices present with life-threatening bleeding. Crohn disease and ulcerative colitis would be unusual in someone of this age without a prior history.
(Objective 2)

WRAP IT UP

1. Left upper quadrant: Liver, bowel, gallbladder
Right upper quadrant: Stomach, bowel, pancreas, spleen
Left lower quadrant: Bowel
Right lower quadrant: Bowel, appendix
(Objective 1)

2. c. Palpate from an area of no pain (if possible) to the area of greatest pain to facilitate the best exam. The exam should be performed in the following order: inspection, auscultation, palpation, percussion
(Objective 2)

3. a, b, c, e, f, g, h
(Objective 4)

4. If the patient's vomiting had persisted, medical direction might have ordered an antiemetic. It's also possible that some pain medicine could have been ordered (a small dose) to relieve his obvious discomfort. This would have had to be done in consultation with medical direction because of the patient's complex history.
(Objective 3)

Urology/Renal

READING ASSIGNMENT

Chapter 35, pages 908-918, in *Mosby's Paramedic Textbook,* ed. 3

OBJECTIVES

Upon completion of this chapter, the paramedic student will be able to:
1. Label a diagram of the urinary system.
2. Describe pathophysiology, signs and symptoms, assessment, and prehospital management of the patient with urinary retention, urinary tract infection, pyelonephritis, urinary calculus, epididymitis, and testicular torsion.
3. Outline the physical examination for patients with genitourinary disorders.
4. Discuss general prehospital management for the patient with a genitourinary disorder.
5. Distinguish between acute and chronic renal failure.
6. Describe the signs and symptoms of renal failure.
7. Describe dialysis and emergent conditions associated with it, including prehospital management.

SUMMARY

- The urinary system removes waste products from the blood. It helps to maintain a constant body fluid volume and composition as well.
- Urinary retention is the inability to urinate.
- Urinary tract infections can involve the upper or lower urinary tract.
- Pyelonephritis is inflammation of the kidney parenchyma.
- Urinary calculi are stones that originate in the kidney.
- Epididymitis is inflammation of the epididymis. The epididymis is the tube that carries sperm from the testicle to the seminal vesicles.
- Testicular torsion is a true emergency. In this condition a testicle twists on its spermatic cord. This disrupts the blood supply to the testicle.
- The physical examination for a patient with a urinary tract problem is similar to that performed for abdominal pain. Patients with genitourinary pain should be managed as any other patient with acute pain.
- Renal failure may result in uremia, hyperkalemia, acidosis, hypertension, and volume overload with congestive heart failure. Renal failure can be classified as acute or chronic. Classification depends on the duration and on the potential for reversibility.
- Dialysis is a technique used to normalize blood chemistry. Dialysis is used in patients who have acute or chronic renal failure. Dialysis also is used to remove blood toxins. The two dialysis techniques are hemodialysis and peritoneal dialysis. Dialysis emergencies may include problems with vascular access, hemorrhage, hypotension, chest pain, severe hyperkalemia, disequilibrium syndrome, and air embolism.

REVIEW QUESTIONS

Match the genitourinary problem in column II with the description in column I. Use each disorder only once.

Column I

1. _____ Can cause vascular infarction and loss of function
2. _____ Inflammation of part of the male reproductive system
3. _____ Systemic disease linked with diabetes and hypertension
4. _____ Infectious process that causes dysuria and hematuria
5. _____ Causes include enlarged prostate and CNS dysfunction
6. _____ Caused by an excess of insoluble salts in the urine
7. _____ Upper urinary infection treated with IV antibiotics

Column II

a. Acute renal failure
b. Chronic renal failure
c. Epididymitis
d. Pyelonephritis
e. Testicular torsion
f. Urinary calculus
g. Urinary retention
h. Urinary tract infection

8. Label the parts of the urinary system shown in Fig. 35-1.

a.

b.

c.

d.

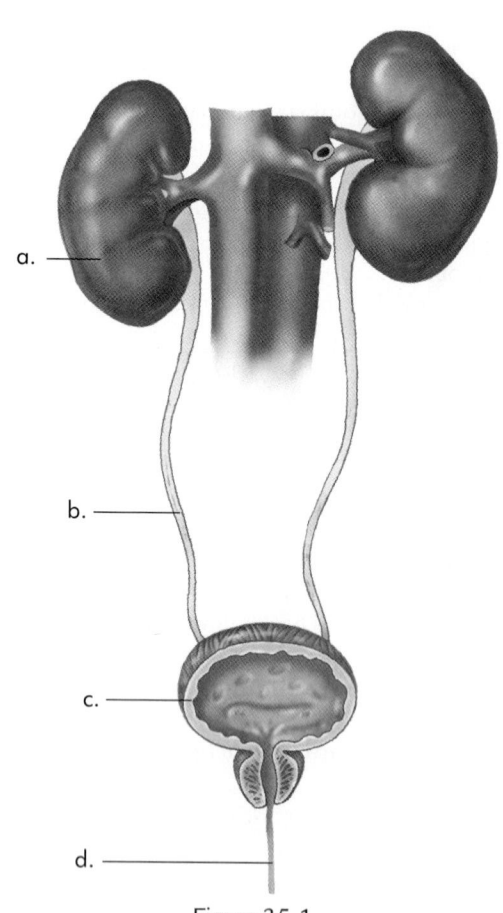

Figure 35-1

9. Identify the genitourinary disorder suspected and the prehospital care needed in each of the following situations.

    a. A 35-year-old afebrile man complains of a sudden onset of severe flank pain that radiates into his testicle.

Condition:

_____

Care:

_____

    b. Your 21-year-old patient complains of painful swelling in the scrotal sac that is unrelieved by elevation. He is in acute distress and has vomited twice.

Condition:

_____

Care:

_____

    c. A 35-year-old woman with a recent history of recurrent urinary infections complains of fever, chills, and severe flank pain.

Condition:

_____

Care:

_____

    d. A 27-year-old woman complains of burning on urination and of feeling as if she must urinate every 20 minutes.

Condition:

_____

Care:

_____

10. How can you minimize psychological discomfort for a patient with a urology problem when performing the physical examination?

_____

11. Identify three causes of each of the following disorders.

    a. Acute renal failure:

_____

    b. Chronic renal failure:

_____

12. You are called to a dialysis center for a person in shock.

a. What types of patient problems should you anticipate en route to this call?

_____

b. If the patient is hypotensive and needs fluid resuscitation, describe how you will initiate fluid therapy and indicate the volume you will infuse.

_____

13. Complete the information in the following table regarding dialysis emergencies.

Disorder	Cause	Effect on Patient	Interventions
Hemorrhage			
Hypotension			
Chest pain			
Hyperkalemia			
Disequilibrium syndrome			
Air embolism			

14. You are dispatched to a private residence for a patient in full arrest. On arrival, you find a 55-year-old man in asystolic cardiac arrest. The family reports that he lost consciousness about 5 minutes before your arrival. The patient's history includes renal failure. He missed hemodialysis this week and was feeling bad before cardiac arrest.

a. You begin CPR and prepare to initiate transcutaneous pacing. List the first three drugs you should consider administering to this patient, including dose and route.

_____

_____

b. How will the drug therapy help to correct some of the problems that may have caused the patient's cardiac arrest?

_____

c. What problem may occur if this combination of drugs is administered improperly?

_____

STUDENT SELF-ASSESSMENT

15. Which genitourinary emergency requires treatment within 4 hours to prevent irreversible damage?
   a. Epididymitis   **c.** Testicular torsion
   b. Pyelonephritis   **d.** Urinary calculus

16. Which of the following is a prerenal cause of acute renal failure?
   a. Kidney infection   **c.** Shock
   b. Prostatic enlargement   **d.** Ureteral strictures

17. How is prehospital care affected if the patient has a dialysis fistula or shunt?
   a. Blood pressure should be checked in the arm opposite the shunt.
   b. The arm in which the shunt is placed should be elevated.

c. Vascular access should be initiated in the fistula or shunt.

d. No special consideration is required.

18. You are caring for a patient with a temperature of 102.5° F (39.2° C) who is on continuous peritoneal dialysis. What is a common cause of fever in patients undergoing this treatment?
    a. Dehydration
    b. Infected fistula
    c. Peritonitis
    d. Pneumonia

19. You are called to the home of an unconscious person in chronic renal failure. The ECG tracing is shown in Fig. 35-2. Which electrolyte imbalance do you suspect?
    a. Hyperkalemia
    b. Hypokalemia
    c. Hypercalcemia
    d. Hypocalcemia

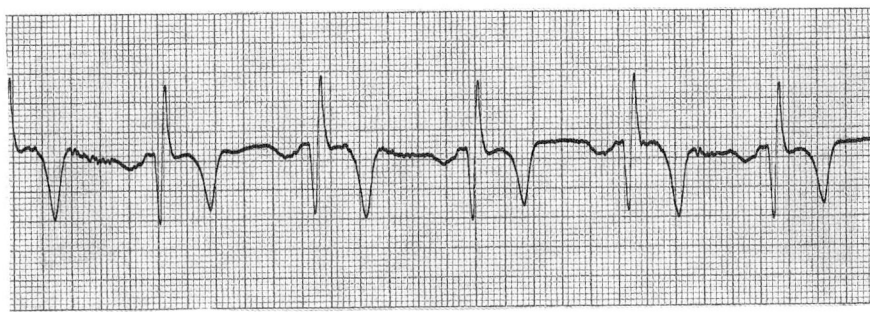

Figure 35-2

20. What drug may be ordered by medical direction to correct the underlying electrolyte imbalance in question 19?
    a. Atropine sulfate (1 mg IV)
    b. Sodium bicarbonate (1 mEq/kg IV)
    c. Magnesium sulfate (1 to 2 g IV)
    d. Verapamil (2.5 mg IV)

21. What physiological problem makes patients in renal failure more susceptible to hypoxia?
    a. Anemia
    b. Glucose intolerance
    c. Pericarditis
    d. Uremia

WRAP IT UP

At 1400 you are dispatched to a dialysis center for a patient who has chest pain. On arrival you find a 59-year-old man who is anxious, pale, and diaphoretic. He missed dialysis for a week because of a severe snowstorm in the area. He came in today very fatigued and twitching. About 10 minutes into his dialysis session, he had several episodes of hypotension and then began complaining of chest pain and nausea. He has a history of type 1 diabetes, hypertension, and renal failure. He is pale, sweaty, and complains of midsternal chest pain. His oxygen saturation is 94% on room air. You administer oxygen at 4 L/min, which quickly improves his Sao_2 to 98%. The nurse is keeping pressure on the dialysis fistula site in his left arm, so you go to the right arm to assess vital signs. Your findings are BP, 198/106 mm Hg; P, 110/min; R, 20/min; and blood glucose, 170 mg/dL. The patient has generalized edema, and you can hear bibasilar crackles in his lungs. You start an IV in the right forearm, administer one spray (0.4 mg) of nitroglycerin, apply the ECG monitor, and then move him by stretcher into the ambulance. You note tall, tented T waves on his ECG. Just as you are attaching the electrodes to perform a 12-lead ECG, his eyes roll back and his body goes limp, and you note a very wide, slow ventricular complex on the monitor. You immediately determine that he is not breathing and begin to ventilate with a bag-valve-mask; you assess a carotid pulse but find none. Your partner immediately radios for additional help and then takes over CPR. You administer epinephrine IV and set up for intubation. You intubate the patient orally with an 8.0 endotracheal tube and verify its placement by listening to the epigastric area and the lungs and by applying the end-tidal CO_2 monitor, which reads 46.

Because the wide complex rhythm on the monitor is only about 30/min, epinephrine is repeated and atropine is given after absence of a carotid pulse is confirmed. You go en route when the pumper unit arrives; you have one firefighter perform chest compressions while your partner ventilates and another firefighter drives the ambulance. En route, you consider possible causes of arrest in this patient and then administer sodium bicarbonate. As you are giving the bicarbonate, the patient's rhythm changes to asystole; you attempt pacing but can't get capture. The ED staff works for another 10 minutes to resuscitate the patient but are unsuccessful, and the man is pronounced dead.

1. What risk factors does the patient have for chronic renal failure?

_____

2. Put a ✔ beside any of the following signs or symptoms of chronic renal failure that you observed in this patient.

   a. ____ Anorexia   i. ____ Mental dullness   q. ____ Seizures
   b. ____ Anemia   j. ____ Muscle twitching   r. ____ Uremic front
   c. ____ Anxiety   k. ____ Nausea   s. ____ Vomiting
   d. ____ Delirium   l. ____ Pericarditis
   e. ____ Electrolyte disturbances m. ____ Peripheral edema
   f. ____ Fatigue   n. ____ Progressive obtundation
   g. ____ Glucose intolerance   o. ____ Pasty, yellow, skin
   h. ____ Hallucinations   p. ____ Pulmonary edema

3. Which is true regarding the dialysis fistula?
   a. Blood pressures can be obtained in that arm without harm to the fistula.
   b. Patency should be verified by using a Doppler to auscultate pulsation.
   c. Drug administration by this route is contraindicated.
   d. Venous access by this site should be avoided in almost all cases.

4. Explain some possible causes for the following conditions this patient had:
   a. Hypotension:

_____

_____

   b. Chest pain:

_____

_____

   c. Cardiac arrest:

_____

_____

5. Discuss your rationale for the following interventions used in this patient:
   a. Nitroglycerin:

_____

_____

   b. Atropine:

_____

_____

   c. Sodium bicarbonate:

_____

_____

CHAPTER 35 ANSWERS

REVIEW QUESTIONS

1. e
(Objective 2)

2. c
(Objective 2)

3. b
(Objective 5)

4. h
5. g
6. f
7. d
(Questions 4-7: Objective 2)

8. a. Kidney
b. Ureter
c. Bladder
d. Urethra
(Objective 1)

9. a. Urinary calculus: Initiate intravenous line; consult with medical direction regarding administration of analgesics such as ketorolac or morphine. b. Testicular torsion: Initiate intravenous line; apply ice pack to scrotum and transport rapidly. c. Pyelonephritis: Initiate intravenous line; transport. d. Urinary tract infection: transport.
(Objective 2)

10. Protect the patient's privacy with drapes. Have a paramedic who is the same gender as the patient perform the examination if possible. Have a chaperone present during a physical exam of the genitalia (if indicated). Explain all actions to the patient and proceed in a calm, caring manner.
(Objective 3)

11. a. Trauma, shock, infection, urinary obstruction, and multisystem diseases; b. hypertension, diabetes, congenital condition, and pyelonephritis.
(Objective 5)

12. a. Too much fluid taken off in dialysis and bleeding at the fistula caused by a pseudoaneurysm (any cause of bleeding is serious because the patient has decreased platelets and is heparinized during dialysis); sepsis; acute myocardial infarction. b. Initiate large-bore intravenous line in the arm without the arteriovenous fistula; infuse a small volume initially (200 to 300 mL) and reevaluate the patient for signs of fluid overload (crackles, engorged neck veins, pulmonary edema).
(Objective 7)

13.

Disorder	Cause	Effect on Patient	Interventions
Hemorrhage	Decrease in platelet function; anticoagulant use; anemia; bleeding from fistula or graft	Signs and symptoms of shock; dyspnea, angina	Control external bleeding; treat for shock; rapid transport
Hypotension	Hemodialysis because of decreased volume; changes in electrolyte concentration; vascular instability	Decreased blood pressure; signs and symptoms of shock	Small fluid challenge (200 to 300 mL); monitor for signs and symptoms of congestive heart failure
Chest pain	Hypotension and hypoxemia during dialysis	Chest pain, headache, dizziness	Oxygen, fluid replacement, antianginal drugs
Hyperkalemia	Poor diet regulation; missed dialysis	Weakness; may have no symptoms; tall, tented T wave; prolonged PRI (K >6 to 6.5 mmol/L); depressed ST segments and loss of P waves (K >7 mmol/L); wide QRS	Suspect if renal patient in arrest; medical direction may order CaCl and NaHCO3 during arrest
Disequilibrium syndrome	Increased osmolality of the ECF compared with ICF in the brain or with the cerebrospinal fluid	HA, nausea, fatigue; confusion, seizures, coma	Transport; treat seizures with diazepam or lorazepam
Air embolism	Negative pressure in dialysis tubing; malfunction in dialysis machine	Dyspnea, cyanosis, hypotension, respiratory distress	Oxygen, rapid transport; position patient on left side with head down

(Objective 7)

14. a. Epinephrine (1 mg IV), $NaHCO_3$ (1 mEq/kg IV), and atropine (1 mg IV)
(Objective 7)

b. Epinephrine can increase peripheral vascular resistance and is a sympathomimetic. Sodium bicarbonate should be given because the patient likely has hyperkalemia and severe acidosis related to his chronic renal failure and missed dialysis sessions. Atropine is a parasympatholytic and theoretically may help to initiate sinus activity.
(Objective 7)

c. Bicarbonate may inactivate epinephrine, therefore tubing should be flushed between drugs.
(Objective 7)

STUDENT SELF-ASSESSMENT

15. c. Because a twisted testicle causes blockage of the blood supply to the testis, intervention within 4 to 6 hours is essential.
(Objective 2)

16. c. Kidney infection is a renal cause, and prostatic enlargement and ureteral strictures are postrenal causes.
(Objective 6)

17. a. Do not assess blood pressure or start an IV on the side where the fistula or shunt is placed. Vascular access should not routinely be obtained through the shunt. In rare cases, because of an arrest situation, medical direction may authorize vascular access through the shunt.
(Objective 5)

18. c. Infection at the site of catheter insertion is common and may lead to peritonitis.
(Objective 7)

19. a. Peaked, tented T waves are associated with hyperkalemia, a common electrolyte imbalance.
(Objective 7)

20. b. Sodium bicarbonate may temporarily cause movement of potassium out of the vascular space and may relieve the cardiac effects until definitive care (dialysis) can be given.
(Objective 7)

21. a. Anemia secondary to lack of a substance needed for red blood cell production reduces the oxygen-carrying capacity of the blood.
(Objective 6)

WRAP IT UP

1. Hypertension, diabetes
(Objective 5)

2. b, c, e, j, k, m
(Objective 6)

3. d. If the fistula is damaged during the attempt to access it, the patient's emergency dialysis will be delayed. After venous access has been established, drugs can be given by this route. Patency can be verified by palpation of a bruit over the fistula. Blood pressure assessment and vascular access should not be performed in the arm with the fistula to avoid damaging the fistula.
(Objective 7)

4. a. During dialysis, hypotension can be caused by a rapid reduction in vascular volume, fast changes in electrolytes, or vascular instability.
b. Hypotension and mild hypoxia, in addition to the patient's high risk factors, can result in chest pain during dialysis.
c. Cardiac arrest could be a result of myocardial irritability related to occlusion of blood vessels or of acidosis and electrolyte imbalance related to the patient's week without dialysis.
(Objective 7)

5. a. Nitroglycerin was given to dilate his coronary blood vessels, improving blood flow to the heart, and to decrease preload and afterload, thereby reducing the work the heart must do.
b. Atropine was given to block parasympathetic stimulation because the patient had a pulseless arrest with a rate of less than 60/min.
c. Sodium bicarbonate was given because of the possibility that acidosis or hyperkalemia (or both) related to the renal failure caused the cardiac arrest.
(Objective 7)

CHAPTER
36

Toxicology

READING ASSIGNMENT
Chapter 36, pages 920-969, in *Mosby's Paramedic Textbook,* ed. 3

OBJECTIVES
Upon completion of this chapter, the paramedic student will be able to do the following:
1. Define poisoning.
2. Describe general principles for assessment and management of the patient who has ingested poison.
3. Describe the causative agents and pathophysiology of selected ingested poisons and management of patients who have taken them.
4. Describe how physical and chemical properties influence the effects of inhaled toxins.
5. Distinguish among the three categories of inhaled toxins: simple asphyxiants, chemical asphyxiants and systemic poisons, and irritants or corrosives.
6. Describe general principles of managing the patient who has inhaled poison.
7. Describe the signs, symptoms, and management of patients who have inhaled cyanide, ammonia, or hydrocarbon.
8. Describe the signs, symptoms, and management of patients injected with poison by insects, reptiles, and hazardous aquatic creatures.
9. Describe the signs, symptoms, and management of patients with organophosphate or carbamate poisoning.
10. Outline the general principles of managing patients with drug overdose.
11. Describe the effects, signs and symptoms, and specific management for selected drug overdose.
12. Describe the short- and long-term physiological effects of ethanol ingestion.
13. Describe signs, symptoms, and management of alcohol-related emergencies.
14. Identify general management principles for the most common toxic syndromes based on a knowledge of the characteristic physical findings associated with each syndrome.

SUMMARY
- A poison is any substance that produces harmful physiological or psychological effects.
- The toxic effects of ingested poisons may be immediate or delayed. This depends on the substance that is ingested. The main goal is to identify effects on the three vital organ systems most likely to produce immediate morbidity and mortality. These are the respiratory system, the cardiovascular system, and the central nervous system. The goal of managing serious poisonings by ingestion is to prevent the toxic substance from reaching the small intestine. This limits its absorption.
- Strong acids and alkalis may cause burns to the mouth, pharynx, esophagus, and sometimes the upper respiratory and GI tracts. Prehospital care is usually limited to airway and ventilatory support, IV fluid replacement, and rapid transport to the appropriate medical facility.

- The most important physical characteristic in the potential toxicity of ingested hydrocarbons is its viscosity. The lower the viscosity, the higher the risk of aspiration and associated complications. Hydrocarbon ingestion may involve the patient's respiratory, gastrointestinal, and neurological systems. The clinical features may be immediate or delayed in onset.
- Methanol is a poisonous alcohol. It is found in a number of products. Methanol itself is no more toxic than ethanol. Yet its metabolites (formaldehyde and formic acid) are very toxic. Ingestion can affect the central nervous system, the gastrointestinal tract, and the eyes. It also can cause the development of metabolic acidosis.
- Ethylene glycol toxicity is caused by the buildup of toxic metabolites, especially glycolic and oxalic acids after metabolism. This occurs mainly in the liver and kidneys. This toxicity may affect the central nervous system and cardiopulmonary and renal systems. It may result in hypocalcemia as well.
- The majority of isopropanol (isopropyl alcohol) is metabolized to acetone after ingestion. Isopropanol poisoning affects several body systems, including the central nervous, gastrointestinal, and renal systems.
- Infants and children are high-risk groups for accidental iron, lead, and mercury poisoning. This is due to their immature immune systems or increased absorption as a function of age. Ingested iron is corrosive to gastrointestinal tract mucosa. It may produce lethal GI hemorrhage, bloody vomitus, painless bloody diarrhea, and dark stools.
- Food poisoning is a term used for any illness of sudden onset (usually associated with stomach pain, vomiting, and diarrhea) suspected of being caused by food eaten within the previous 48 hours. Food poisoning can be classified as infectious. This results from a bacterium or virus. It also can be classified as noninfectious. This results from toxins and pollutants.
- The toxic effects of major poisonous plant ingestions are predictable. They are categorized by the chemical and physical properties of the plant. Most responses are consistent with the type of major toxic chemical component in the plant.
- The concentration of a chemical in the air helps to determine the severity of an inhalation injury. The duration of exposure helps to determine this as well. Solubility also influences the extent of an inhalation injury. Highly reactive chemicals cause more severe and rapid injury than less-reactive chemicals. Properties that determine chemical reactivity are chemical pH; direct-acting potential of chemicals; indirect-acting potential of chemicals; and allergic potential of chemicals.
- Cyanide refers to any of a number of highly toxic substances that contain the cyanogen chemical group. Regardless of the route of entry, cyanide is a rapidly acting poison. It combines and reacts with ferric ions of the respiratory enzyme cytochrome oxidase. This inhibits cellular oxygenation. This produces a rapid progression from dyspnea to paralysis, unconsciousness, and death.
- Ammonia is a toxic irritant. It causes local pulmonary complications after inhalation. In severe cases, bronchospasm and pulmonary edema may develop.
- Hydrocarbon inhalation may cause aspiration pneumonitis. It also has the potential for systemic effects such as CNS depression and liver, kidney, or bone marrow toxicity.
- Simple asphyxiants cause toxicity by lowering ambient oxygen concentration. Chemical asphyxiants possess intrinsic systemic toxicity. This toxicity occurs after absorption into the circulation. Irritants or corrosives cause cellular destruction and inflammation as they come into contact with moisture in the respiratory tract.
- The general principles of managing inhaled poisons are the same as for any other hazardous materials incident.
- Hymenoptera and arachnida cause the highest incidence of need for emergency care. Arthropod venoms are complex and diverse in their chemistry and pharmacology. They may produce major toxic reactions in sensitized persons. Such reactions include anaphylaxis and upper airway obstruction.
- The two main families of venomous snakes indigenous to the United States are pit vipers and coral snakes. Pit viper venom can produce various toxic effects on blood and other tissues. These effects include hemolysis, intravascular coagulation, convulsions, and acute renal failure. The venom of the coral snake is mainly neurotoxic. Signs and symptoms range from slurred speech, dilated pupils, and dysphagia to flaccid paralysis and death.
- The marine animals most likely to be involved in human poisonings in U.S. coastal waters are coelenterates, echinoderms, and stingrays. Coelenterate envenomation ranges in severity from irritant dermatitis to excruciating pain, respiratory depression, and life-threatening cardiovascular collapse. Echinoderm toxins may cause immediate intense pain, swelling, redness, aching in the affected extremity, and nausea. Delayed effects may include respiratory distress, paresthesia of the lips and face, and in severe cases, respiratory paralysis and complete atonia. Locally, stingray venom produces a painful traumatic injury. It may cause bleeding and necrosis. Systemic manifestations range from weakness and nausea to seizures, paralysis, hypotension, and death.

- Organophosphates and carbamates inhibit the effects of acetylcholinesterase. A mnemonic aid that may help the paramedic to recognize this type of poisoning is *SLUDGE*. (This stands for *s*alivation, *l*acrimation, *u*rination, *defe*cation, *g*astrointestinal upset, and *e*mesis.) The most specific findings, however, are miosis, rapidly changing pupils, and muscle fasciculation.
- General principles for managing drug abuse and overdose include scene safety; ensuring adequate airway, breathing, and circulation; history; substance identification; focused physical exam; initiation of an IV; administration of an antidote if needed; prevention of further absorption; and rapid transport.
- Narcotics are CNS depressants. They can cause life-threatening respiratory depression. In severe intoxication, hypotension, profound shock, and pulmonary edema may be present. Naloxone is a pure narcotic antagonist effective for virtually all narcotic and narcotic-like substances.
- Sedative-hypnotic agents include benzodiazepines and barbiturates. Signs and symptoms of sedative-hypnotic overdose are chiefly related to the central nervous and cardiovascular symptoms. Flumazenil (Romazicon) is a benzodiazepine antagonist. It is useful in reversing the effects of these agents.
- Commonly used stimulant drugs are those of the amphetamine family. Adverse effects include tachycardia, increased blood pressure, tachypnea, agitation, dilated pupils, tremors, and disorganized behavior. With sudden withdrawal, the patient becomes depressed, suicidal, incoherent, or near coma.
- Phencyclidine (PCP) is a dissociative analgesic with sympathomimetic and CNS stimulant and depressant effects. In low doses, PCP intoxication produces an unpredictable state that can resemble drunkenness (and rage). High-dose intoxication may cause coma. This may last from several hours to days. Respiratory depression, hypertension, and tachycardia may be present. PCP psychosis is a psychiatric emergency. It may mimic schizophrenia.
- Hallucinogens are substances that cause distortions of perceptions. Depending on the agent, overdose may range from visual hallucinations and anticholinergic syndromes, to more serious complications, including psychosis, flashbacks, and respiratory and CNS depression.
- Tricyclic antidepressant toxicity is thought to result from central and peripheral, atropine-like anticholinergic effects and direct depressant effects on myocardial function. A prolonged QRS complex, a GCS score less than 8, or both, should alert the paramedic to a major TCA toxicity.
- Lithium is a mood-stabilizing drug. Toxic ingestion can include CNS effects that can range from blurred vision and confusion to seizure and coma.
- Cardiac drugs are a common cause of poisoning deaths in children and adults. The drugs responsible for the majority of these fatalities are digitalis, beta blockers, and calcium channel blockers.
- MAO inhibitors block or diminish the activity of the monoamines (norepinephrine, dopamine, serotonin). Toxic effects include CNS depression and various neuromuscular and cardiovascular system manifestations.
- Nonsteroidal antiinflammatory drugs (NSAIDs) work by blocking the production of prostaglandins. The effects of overdose of ibuprofen are usually reversible, are seldom life-threatening, and include mild GI and CNS effects. Salicylate poisoning may cause CNS stimulation, GI irritation, glucose metabolism, fluid and electrolyte imbalance, and coagulation defects.
- Acetaminophen overdose may cause life-threatening liver damage. This results from formation of a hepatotoxic intermediate metabolite if it is not managed within 16 to 24 hours of ingestion.
- Some drugs are abused for sexual purposes or for sexual gratification. These are commonly classified by users as "uppers," "downers," and those that have more than one primary effect ("all-arounders"). Problems associated with their use vary widely.
- Alcohol dependence is a disorder characterized by chronic, excessive consumption of alcohol that results in injury to health or in inadequate social function and the development of withdrawal symptoms when the patient stops drinking suddenly. Alcohol causes multiple systemic effects. These include neurological disorders, nutritional deficiencies, fluid and electrolyte imbalances, gastrointestinal disorders, cardiac and skeletal muscle myopathy, and immune suppression. Several conditions caused by consumption or abstinence from alcohol that may require emergency care are acute alcohol intoxication, alcohol withdrawal syndromes, and disulfiram-ethanol reaction.
- The most common toxic syndromes are cholinergic, anticholinergic, hallucinogenic, opiate, and sympathomimetic. Using these classifications allows the paramedic to group similar toxic agents together. It allows him or her to more easily remember how to assess and treat the poisoned patient.

REVIEW QUESTIONS

Match the illnesses in Column II with the toxic syndromes in Column I. You may use the signs and symptoms more than once.

Column I

1. _____ Anticholinergic syndrome
2. _____ Cholinergic syndrome
3. _____ Opiate/sedative/ethanol syndrome
4. _____ Sympathomimetic syndrome

Column II

a. Bradycardia
b. Cardiac dysrhythmias
c. Dry mouth
d. Hypertension
e. Respiratory depression
f. Salivation
g. Tachycardia
h. Urination

Match the poisons in Column II with their descriptions in Column I. Use each poison only once.

Column I

5. _____ Metabolizes to formic acid and causes toxic visual effects
6. _____ Ingestion of odorless, sweet liquid in antifreeze causes central nervous system depression
7. _____ Inhalation, ingestion, and absorption prevents oxygen from reaching cells
8. _____ Inhalation produces lacrimation, dyspnea, and inflammation of the airway
9. _____ Vomiting should not be induced for phenol and others in this group
10. _____ These chemicals include lye and cause immediate damage to the mucosa
11. _____ The long duration of action requires treatment with atropine and pralidoxime

Column II

a. Acid
b. Alkali
c. Ammonia
d. Carbamate
e. Cyanide
f. Ethylene glycol
g. Hydrocarbon
h. Isopropanol
i. Methanol
j. Organophosphate

12. You are called to the home of a young child whose family states that he ingested some liquid from a bottle in the garage. He is arousable only to painful stimulation. After a rapid assessment of the patient, you contact the regional poison control center.

    a. What information should you be prepared to give the center?

    _____

    b. What general care measures should you take when caring for this patient if the source of the poisoning is unknown?

    _____

    _____

13. You insert a 36 to 40 French orogastric tube into a patient.

    a. What position should the patient be in?

    _____

    b. What precaution should be taken for the unconscious patient?

    _____

c. How should irrigation be performed?

_____

_____

14. Complete the information missing in the following table.

Ingested Poison	Charcoal (Yes/No)	Other Interventions
a. Bleach		
b. Ammonia		
c. Gasoline		
d. Methanol		
e. Ethylene glycol		
f. Isopropanol		
g. Cyanide		

15. A 65-year-old woman complains of food poisoning after eating at a local seafood restaurant 2 hours earlier.

a. What is the typical time onset for signs of food poisoning?

_____

b. What treatment should be provided for the patient with food poisoning?

_____

_____

Questions 16 to 18 refer to the following case study:

A 21-year-old man calls 911 after becoming extremely ill from eating some wild mushrooms. The patient is awake and complaining of nausea, vomiting, and diarrhea. He has pinpoint pupils and the following vital signs: BP 90/50 mm Hg, P 48, and R 24. His electrocardiogram rhythm shows a sinus bradycardia with occasional ventricular escape beats.

16. What type of toxic syndrome does this patient appear to be exhibiting?

_____

17. How can you find out more about the specific poison involved in this case?

_____

18. What treatment measures may be indicated for this patient in consultation with medical direction?

_____

19. Complete the information missing in the following table.

Toxic Chemical	Class of Toxin	Signs and Symptoms	Treatment
Copper welding fumes			
Hydrogen sulfide			
Methane gas			
Chlorine gas			

20. A worker in a chemical plant is exposed to ammonia gas and is dyspneic, choking, and wheezing. What treatment should be provided for this patient?

_____

_____

Questions 21 to 24 refer to the following case study:

A farmer calls you to his ranch after spraying pesticide on a windy day. On your arrival, he is coming out of the bathroom complaining of severe diarrhea and says he cannot stop urinating. Tears are running down his face, and he is coughing up large amounts of phlegm. His electrocardiogram is shown in Fig. 36-1.

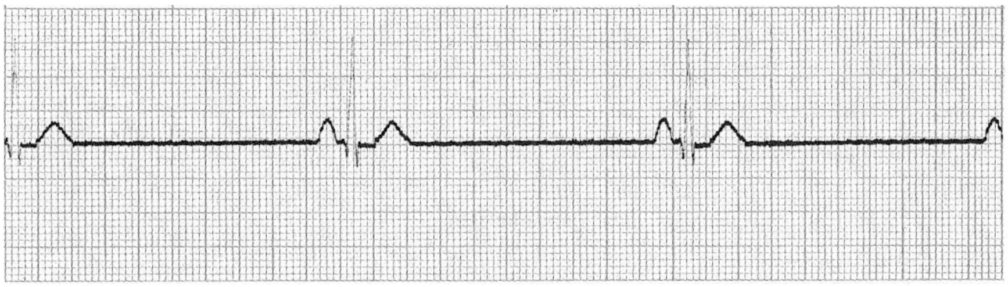

Figure 36-1

21. What poisoning do you suspect?

_____

22. What other signs or symptoms might be present?

_____

23. What is your interpretation of the electrocardiogram?

_____

24. List specific interventions to be used in his care.

_____

_____

_____

25. Interpret the following historical information presented to you at the scene of a potential drug overdose.

    a. "He mainlined some China white."

_____

    b. "She was space-basing angel dust and candy."

_____

    c. "They were freebasing a rock."

_____

d. "He was skin-popping some M."

_____

e. "She snorted some PCP before she went crazy."

_____

Match the drugs in Column II with the appropriate overdose description in Column I. Use each drug only once.

Column I	Column II
26. _____ Central nervous system stimulant and depressant properties can produce violent, unpredictable behavior.	**a.** Acetaminophen
27. _____ It causes visual disturbances, dry mouth, seizures, and tachycardia with a wide QRS complex.	**b.** Cocaine **c.** Heroin
28. _____ It causes tachypnea, central nervous system depression, gastrointestinal irritation, and tinnitus.	**d.** Iron **e.** Phencyclidine
29. _____ Mild, influenza-like symptoms are followed by latent liver failure.	**f.** Salicylate **g.** Tricyclic antidepressant
30. _____ This stimulant can cause dysrhythmias, myocardial infarction, and hyperthermia.	

Questions 31 and 32 refer to the following case study:

A 32-year-old woman has overdosed on sleeping pills. She is awake but drowsy.

31. What information regarding the poisoning is critical to the care of this patient?

_____

_____

32. What dose of activated charcoal should be given?

_____

33. Complete the information missing in the following table.

Ingested Poison	Charcoal (Yes/No)	Other Interventions
a. Aspirin		
b. Acetaminophen		
c. Iron		

34. Give two examples of drugs commonly abused in each of the following categories.

a. Narcotics: _____

b. Central nervous system depressants: _____

c. Central nervous system stimulants: _____

d. Hallucinogens: _____

Questions 35 to 37 refer to the following case study:

Your patient injected heroin intravenously and arouses only to pain. He has pinpoint pupils and slow, snoring respirations.

35. What is the primary life threat that must be managed immediately in this patient?

_____

36. List the appropriate drug and dose used to improve this patient's condition.

_____

37. If this man is a chronic heroin abuser and the drug listed previously is administered, what signs and symptoms of narcotic withdrawal will you anticipate?

_____

Questions 38 to 40 refer to the following case study:

> A 17-year-old has taken about 50 tablets of chlordiazepoxide and is comatose, with slow, irregular respirations.

38. What is the pupil response likely to be in this patient?

_____

39. What drug may be given to this patient on arrival to the emergency department to antagonize the effects of this ingestion?

_____

40. Before you administer an antidote, careful history and scene assessment must be done to ensure that the patient has not taken which additional medication?

_____

41. Local college students call you to a party, where participants have been freebasing cocaine. One of the participants has lost consciousness. What life-threatening effects of this drug may have caused loss of consciousness in this patient?

_____

Questions 42 to 44 refer to the following case study:

> A popular group is playing at a local club. Security calls you to the parking lot to care for a patient who has reportedly taken PCP (phencyclidine).

42. What should be your primary concern when caring for this patient?

_____

43. Describe the appropriate initial approach to this patient, who is alert and quiet.

_____

44. List signs and symptoms that may be displayed by this patient.

_____

Questions 45 to 48 refer to the following case study:

An 18-year-old woman took about 20 tablets of amitriptyline about 1 hour before your arrival at her home. She is drowsy and confused, has a dry mouth, and complains of blurred vision. Her electrocardiogram is shown in Fig. 36-2.

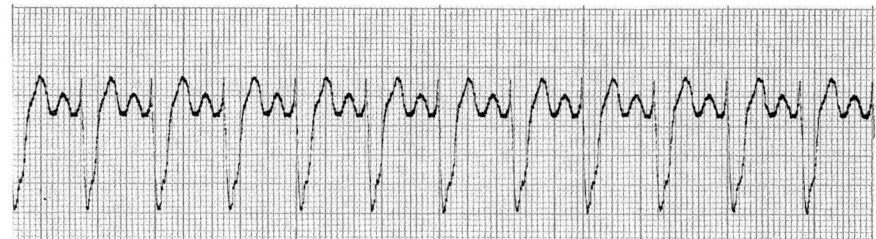

Figure 36-2

45. Should you administer syrup of ipecac to this patient? Why or why not?

_____

_____

46. What is your interpretation of the electrocardiogram?

_____

47. What drug and appropriate dose may be given to prevent deterioration of this patient's cardiac status?

_____

48. What additional signs and symptoms do you anticipate as this patient's condition deteriorates?

_____

Questions 49 and 50 refer to the following case study:

Your unit is on the scene of a two-car accident. You are caring for a 47-year-old man who appears to be intoxicated. His friend says that he is an alcoholic. The patient states that he drank three beers in the past 5 hours.

49. Should you accept this history of the number of drinks as reliable?

_____

50. If the patient is an alcoholic, what *chronic* physiological changes in the following areas will make it more difficult to assess his condition and more likely for severe injury to occur?

   a. Neurological changes:

_____

   b. Nutritional problems:

_____

   c. Fluid and electrolyte imbalances:

_____

   d. Coagulation disorders:

_____

51. Describe the management of a comatose patient suspected to be severely intoxicated by alcohol.

_____

_____

_____

52. Describe the management of a patient experiencing alcohol withdrawal accompanied by severe seizures.

_____

_____

_____

53. List signs and symptoms of delirium tremens.

_____

_____

54. You are at the first aid station for a church picnic. A 16-year-old boy comes to the station complaining of a bee sting. No signs of anaphylaxis are present.

a. List general care measures for this person.

_____

b. Describe the method for removing the stinger.

_____

55. List two diseases produced by ticks and possible signs and symptoms for each.

a.

b.

56. Describe the proper technique for removing a tick.

_____

57. A hysterical 20-year-old man states that he has just been bitten by a copperhead snake while camping.

a. List signs and symptoms that would be present if a moderate envenomation had occurred.

_____

b. Describe the appropriate prehospital management of this patient.

_____

_____

58. For each of the following marine animal classifications, list one example and outline general management principles for envenomation:

a. Coelenterates:

_____

b. Echinoderms:

_____

c. Stingrays:

_____

STUDENT SELF-ASSESSMENT

59. Any substance that produces harmful physiological or psychological effects is known as a(n):
  a. Overdose
  b. Poison
  c. Toxin
  d. Venom
60. Which toxic syndrome would present for the patient who has ingested cocaine?
  a. Anticholinergic syndrome
  b. Cholinergic syndrome
  c. Opiate/sedative/ethanol syndrome
  d. Sympathomimetic syndrome
61. What is the primary goal when assessing a poisoned patient?
  a. Begin decontamination of the poison as quickly as possible with activated charcoal.
  b. Determine the exact nature of the poison so that appropriate treatment can be given.
  c. Obtain a history to determine the exact time that the poisoning occurred.
  d. Identify the effects on the respiratory, cardiovascular, and central nervous systems.
62. Charcoal is effective in treating specific overdoses because it does which of the following?
  a. Reverses the effects of the ingested drug
  b. Binds the drug and prevents absorption
  c. Causes severe nausea and vomiting
  d. Makes the drug speed through the intestine
63. Which is true regarding syrup of ipecac?
  a. It is indicated for use in petroleum distillate ingestion.
  b. It is not associated with life-threatening complications.
  c. It may interfere with other methods of decontamination.
  d. It should be given within the first 2 hours after ingestion.
64. What should be your primary concern when caring for a patient who has ingested hydrocarbon?
  a. Aspiration
  b. Central nervous system effects
  c. Dysrhythmias
  d. Hypotension
65. Medical direction may advise administration of sodium bicarbonate in all of the following *except* which poisoning and overdose situation?
  a. Ethylene glycol
  b. Methanol
  c. Isopropanol
  d. Tricyclic antidepressant
66. Which of the following is true regarding poison plant ingestions?
  a. Dialysis is an effective treatment for most plant poisons.
  b. Ingestion of poisonous plants is common in the United States.
  c. Most signs and symptoms are delayed several days.
  d. Specific treatment should not begin until the plant is identified.
67. Symptoms commonly associated with poisonous mushroom ingestion are likely to include which of the following?
  a. Bradycardia
  b. Dry mouth
  c. Hypertension
  d. Hyperthermiaj

68. Which of the following hydrocarbon properties is associated with the greatest risk?
   a. Low adhesion of molecules along a surface
   b. Low surface tension
   c. High viscosity
   d. High volatility

69. Toxic hydrocarbon inhalation most often is associated with which of the following?
   a. Childhood ingestions
   b. Industrial exposures
   c. Mixing chemicals
   d. Recreational huffing

70. Which of the following overdose or poisoning typically will lead to bradycardia?
   a. Carbamates
   b. Cocaine
   c. Isopropanol
   d. Methanol

71. What should your first priority be when evaluating a patient contaminated with organophosphates?
   a. Administer atropine.
   b. Establish intravenous therapy.
   c. Put on protective gear.
   d. Suction excess secretions.

72. Atropine is supplied in a 10-mL syringe that contains 1 mg of the drug. You wish to administer 2 mg to a patient who has organophosphate poisoning. How many milliliters will you give?
   a. 1 mL
   b. 2 mL
   c. 10 mL
   d. 20 mL

73. Naloxone will antagonize the effects of all of the following except which drug?
   a. Diazepam
   b. Meperidine
   c. Morphine
   d. Propoxyphene

74. What should your highest priority be when caring for a patient at a methamphetamine lab?
   a. Administration of diazepam to control tremors
   b. Decontamination of the patient
   c. Maintaining scene safety
   d. Talking down the paranoid patient

75. The patient who has taken an overdose of oil of wintergreen most likely will have which of the following?
   a. Bradycardia, hyperglycemia, and nystagmus
   b. Seizures, hyperglycemia, and ventricular tachycardia
   c. Hypoglycemia, tachypnea, and tinnitus
   d. Hematemesis, metabolic alkalosis, and coma

76. What are the typical findings in patients within the first 24 hours of an overdose of acetaminophen?
   a. Dysrhythmias
   b. Hypoglycemia
   c. No symptoms
   d. Right upper quadrant abdominal pain

77. When ingestion of multivitamins is suspected in a child, it is critical to determine whether the preparation contains
   a. Ascorbic acid.
   b. Folic acid.
   c. Iron.
   d. Thiamine.

78. Which of the following drugs most likely will produce tachycardia if a patient overdoses?
   a. Digoxin (Lanoxin)
   b. Propranolol (Inderal)
   c. Sertraline (Zoloft)
   d. Verapamil (Calan)

79. An alert 4-year-old child ingested about 10 of his grandmother's blood pressure tablets 20 minutes ago. He is awake and alert. What drug should be administered in this situation?
   a. Activated charcoal
   b. Atropine
   c. Calcium chloride
   d. Dopamine

80. Intravenous therapy in the alcoholic with depleted thiamine stores may lead to which of the following?
   a. Disulfiram-ethanol reaction
   b. Guillain-Barré syndrome
   c. Mallory-Weiss tears
   d. Wernicke-Korsakoff syndrome

81. Which of the following is true regarding delirium tremens?
   a. It affects almost all alcoholics going through alcohol withdrawal.
   b. It is associated with a high mortality rate if untreated.
   c. It is characterized by bradycardia, hypotension, and hypothermia.
   d. It usually occurs 12 to 24 hours following cessation of alcohol ingestion.

82. Alcohol withdrawal seizures should be treated with which of the following?
    a. Dextrose 50%
    b. Diazepam
    c. Magnesium sulfate
    d. Thiamine

83. An 18-year-old man who attempts to extract honey from a beehive on a dare sustains 20 to 30 stings. He has a headache, fever, and involuntary muscle spasms and reports a syncopal episode. What type of reaction do you suspect?
    a. Anaphylactic
    b. Delayed
    c. Local
    d. Toxic

84. A 52-year-old man states that he was bitten by a spider at a woodpile. He now is complaining of back, chest, and abdominal pain and has a severe headache. What type of spider envenomation would produce these symptoms?
    a. Black widow
    b. Brown recluse
    c. Tarantula
    d. Wolf

85. A hiker states that he was bitten by a red and yellow snake and is now complaining of slurred speech and dysphagia. His pupils are dilated. You suspect envenomation by what kind of snake?
    a. Copperhead
    b. Cottonmouth moccasin
    c. Coral
    d. Massasauga

86. Which treatment may be harmful for the patient who has sustained a venomous snake bite?
    a. Applying ice to wound on affected extremity
    b. Initiating an intravenous line in an unaffected extremity
    c. Positioning extremity in dependent position
    d. Splinting the affected extremity in neutral position

87. For which overdose would isoproterenol be indicated to treat symptomatic bradycardia?
    a. Digoxin
    b. Nortriptyline
    c. Propranolol
    d. Verapamil

Questions 88 and 89 relate to the following scenario.

> Your patient is a 42-year-old found "asleep" in the park. Rangers were unable to wake him. He is unresponsive to pain and has snoring respirations at about 2 per minute. His pupils are pinpoint. He has track marks on his arms.

88. What type of overdose would be a likely cause of his decreased level of consciousness?
    a. Cocaine
    b. Heroin
    c. Methamphetamine
    d. Phencyclidine

89. Which intervention will be your first priority in his care?
    a. Assist ventilations with bag-mask device.
    b. Check his blood glucose level.
    c. Deliver a fluid bolus of 200 mL normal saline.
    d. Give naloxone (Narcan) 0.4 to 2.0 mg intravenously.

WRAP IT UP

You are dispatched to a home for a "possible overdose." On arrival, you find your 22-year-old male patient in the bathtub. He moans and flexes slightly in response to painful stimulus. Emesis is sprayed around the toilet, and a pile of pill bottles is in the sink. The pill bottles are prescribed to several persons and you find Tylenol, aspirin, Vicodin, Glucophage, vitamins with iron, Elavil, Ativan, Ritalin, metoprolol, and empty bottles of rubbing alcohol and vodka. You assess him and find his vital signs are BP 100/70 mm Hg, P 104, R 6, SaO$_2$ 65%. You assist his respirations with a bag-valve-mask, and he gags when you try to place an oral airway, so you insert a nasopharyngeal airway. You find his skin to be pale and dry, and his pupils are 2 mm. An IV is started, and his blood glucose reading is 25 mg/dL. You administer naloxone (Narcan) followed by D50W. An electrocardiogram tracing shows sinus tachycardia with occasional PVCs. His level of consciousness improves slightly, and he is somewhat combative on arrival to the ED.

1. Which of the substance(s) that he ingested can cause the following:
    a. Hypoglycemia
    b. Acidosis
    c. Tachycardia
    d. Respiratory depression

e. Decreased level of consciousness
   f. Pupil constriction
   g. Bradycardia
   h. Cardiac dysrhythmias
   i. Seizures

2. Place a check mark beside the drugs, or classifications of drugs, that this patient may have taken.

   a. _____ Acetaminophen   **g.** _____ Isopropanol
   b. _____ Benzodiazepine   **h.** _____ Mineral
   c. _____ Beta-blocker   **i.** _____ Opioid/narcotic
   d. _____ Ethanol alcohol   **j.** _____ Organophosphate
   e. _____ Hypoglycemic   **k.** _____ Stimulant
   f. _____ Salicylate   **l.** _____ Tricyclic antidepressant

3. For each of the following drugs this patient has taken, describe the action that is most likely to cause death.
   a. Acetaminophen
   b. Metoprolol
   c. Vodka
   d. Metformin (Glucophage)
   e. Aspirin
   f. Iron
   g. Hydrocodone/acetaminophen (Vicodin)
   h. Tricyclic antidepressant

4. Explain your rationale for the interventions that you performed.
   a. Bag-valve-mask
   b. Naloxone
   c. D50W

5. Would other antidotes or therapeutic interventions be indicated for this patient if these drugs were taken individually?

---

6. Which of the following is true regarding the care of the overdosed patient?
   a. The most important goal for prehospital treatment is gastric emptying.
   b. Gathering of information from the scene is critical in toxicology emergencies.
   c. Administration of antidotes, when indicated, takes priority over all interventions.
   d. Syrup of ipecac should be given to all overdose patients if not contraindicated.

7. Which of the drugs he ingested, when taken individually, could cause the following toxidromes:
   a. Cholinergic
   b. Anticholinergic
   c. Hallucinogen
   d. Opioid
   e. Sympathomimetic

CHAPTER 36 ANSWERS

REVIEW QUESTIONS

1. c, g
2. a, b, f, h
3. b, e, g
4. b, d, g
   (Questions 1 to 4, Objective 2)

5. i
   (Objective 4)

6. f
   (Objective 4)

7. e
   (Objectives 4 and 6)

8. c
   (Objective 8)

9. g
   (Objective 4)

10. b
    (Objective 4)

11. j
    (Objective 9)

12. a. You should be prepared to tell the poison control center the specific agent ingested, amount of agent ingested, time ingested, age, patient weight, medical condition, and treatment rendered before arrival of emergency medical services personnel.
    (Objective 3)

    b. Ensure adequate airway, ventilation, and circulation. Obtain a history (especially specific to substance ingested), and perform a physical exam. Assess for hypoglycemia. Consult with medical direction for further treatment guidelines. Monitor vital signs and electrocardiogram. Transport rapidly for definitive treatment.
    (Objective 3)

13. a. Position the patient in the left lateral Trendelenberg's (swimmer's) position
    b. Peform rapid sequence endotracheal intubation before orogastric tube intubation if patient has a decreased level of consciousness with an absent gag reflex
    c. After assessment for proper tube placement, normal saline (preferably warmed) should be infused into the orogastric tube in 200- to 300-mL boluses, and the tube should be allowed to drain after each bolus. Continue this process until the gastric drainage returns clear.
    (Objective 3)

14.

Ingested Poison	Charcoal (Yes/No)	Other Interventions
a. Bleach	No	Dilution with milk or water (200 to 300 mL for an adult or 15 mL/kg for a child)
b. Ammonia	No	Dilution with milk or water
c. Gasoline	No	Initiation of intravenous line, monitoring of airway, and electrocardiogram
d. Methanol	Controversial	Lavage, sodium bicarbonate intravenously (30 to 60 mL), and 80-proof ethanol by mouth
e. Ethylene glycol	Yes	Lavage, sodium bicarbonate intravenously (30 to 60 mL), 80-proof ethanol by mouth, and (rarely) furosemide, thiamine, and calcium gluconate
f. Isopropanol	Yes	Lavage
g. Cyanide	No	Amyl nitrite pearls, 3% sodium nitrite, and 25% sodium thiosulfate

(Objective 4)

15. a. Time varies: chemical, 1 to 2 hours; bacterial toxins, 1 to 12 hours; viral or bacterial, 12 to 48 hours.

b. Take universal precautions, maintain airway and breathing, and initiate intravenous therapy with crystalloid solution to treat dehydration and fluid and electrolyte imbalance.
(Objective 4)

16. Cholinergic syndrome
(Objective 2)

17. Ask the patient if he still has a sample of the mushroom and what time he took it. If he does not have a sample, have him describe the mushroom. Contact poison control and medical direction (per protocol) for help with identification and treatment information. Prehospital treatment likely will be guided by signs and symptoms rather than specific identification information.
(Objective 2)

18. Maintain airway and prepare to suction secretions if needed; administer high-concentration oxygen; monitor electrocardiogram and vital signs frequently; initiate an intravenous line and infuse fluids as ordered by medical direction; and prepare to administer atropine sulfate as ordered by medical direction.
(Objective 4)

19. Rescuers should wear appropriate personal protective equipment.

Toxic Chemical	Class of Toxin	Sign and Symptoms	Treatment
Copper welding fumes	Metal fumes	Chills, fever, myalgias; headache, cough, leukocytosis	Remove patient from source, treat symptoms.
Hydrogen sulfide	Chemical asphyxiant	Sudden collapse, rotten egg smell, rapid fatigue	Remove patient from source, oxygenate.
Chlorine gas	Irritant	Lacrimation, sore throat, stridor, tracheobronchitis, pulmonary edema	Remove patient from source, give humidified oxygen and bronchodilators, manage airway.

(Objective 6)

20. Ensure personal protection; open airway; administer high-flow oxygen; initiate an intravenous line to keep the vein open; and if pulmonary edema develops, consider administration of diuretics and bronchodilators.
(Objective 8)

21. Carbamate or organophosphate
(Objective 9)

22. Pupil constriction, muscle fasciculation, headache, weakness, dizziness, hypotension, bronchoconstriction, anxiety, seizures, and convulsions
(Objective 9)

23. Sinus bradycardia
(Objective 9)

24. Wear protective gear; decontaminate as appropriate; suction oral secretions as necessary; prepare to intubate if patient's condition deteriorates; initiate intravenous therapy with crystalloid to keep the vein open; administer atropine 2 to 4 mg intravenously every 5 to 15 minutes as necessary to induce relative tachycardia, flushing, and decreased secretions; monitor for dysrhythmias; administer pralidoxime; administer diazepam as necessary for seizures.
(Objective 9)

25. a. He took fentanyl or heroin intravenously.
   b. She was smoking PCP and crack (cocaine).
   c. They were smoking purified crack cocaine.
   d. He injected morphine subcutaneously.
   e. She ingested PCP nasally.
   (Objective 10)

26. e
27. g
28. f
29. a
30. b
(Questions 26 to 30, Objective 11)

31. What was taken? Where is the container? How much was in it and how much is left (may need to estimate based on date prescription issued, amount prescribed daily, and amount left in bottle)? When was the drug taken? Has the patient vomited or taken anything to induce vomiting since the drug was taken? Has any antidote been given to the patient? Ask the patient the following: Why did you do this? Were you trying to hurt or kill yourself?
(Objective 10)

32. 30 to 100 g activated charcoal
(Objective 10)

33.

Ingested Poison	Charcoal (Yes/No)	Other Interventions
a. Aspirin	Yes	D50W if patient is hypoglycemic
b. Acetaminophen	Usually not (varies by medical direction)	Acetylcysteine (Mucomyst; varies by medical direction)
c. Iron	No	Monitor airway, initiate intravenous line

34. a. Heroin, morphine, and methadone; b. barbiturates (secobarbital, phenobarbital) and benzodiazepines (diazepam, chlordiazepoxide); c. amphetamines and cocaine; d. lysergic acid diethylamide (LSD) and phencyclidine (PCP).
(Objective 10)

35. Respiratory depression (partial airway obstruction and decreased minute volume)
(Objective 11)

36. Naloxone (Narcan) 2.0 mg intravenously. (Administer enough to ensure adequate airway reflexes and ventilation.)
(Objective 11)

37. Gooseflesh (piloerection), tachycardia, diaphoresis, irritability, insomnia, abdominal cramps, tremors, nausea, vomiting, cold sweats and chills, fever, and diarrhea
(Objective 11)

38. Bilaterally dilated and slow to react to light
(Objective 11)

39. Flumazenil (Romazicon)
(Objective 11)

40. Tricyclic antidepressants
(Objective 11)

41. Cardiac dysrhythmias, seizures, or cerebrovascular accident (following intracranial hemorrhage)
(Objective 11)

42. Personal safety
(Objective 11)

43. Quiet, calm approach. Interview the patient while minimizing external sensory stimuli (for example, bright lights, noise).
(Objective 11)

44. Euphoria, disorientation, seizures, hypertensive crisis, dysrhythmias, catatonia, unresponsiveness, and bizarre and violent behavior. These patients are extremely difficult to manage and dangerous if found in or provoked into violent behavior.
(Objective 11)

45. No. She is drowsy and her level of consciousness could deteriorate further. Also, more than 20 minutes has passed since ingestion of the drug.
(Objective 11)

46. Sinus tachycardia with delayed ventricular conduction (wide QRS complex)
(Objective 11)

47. Sodium bicarbonate 1 to 2 mEq/kg intravenously
(Objective 11)

48. Delirium, depressed respirations, hypertension or hypotension, hyperthermia or hypothermia, seizures, coma, and dysrhythmias
(Objective 11)

49. No. Alcoholics frequently underestimate the number of drinks they have had.
(Objective 13)

50. a. Short-term memory deficit, problems with coordination, and difficulty with concentration can mimic signs and symptoms of head injury
b. Nutritional deficiencies can cause muscle cramps, paresthesias, seizures, tremor or ataxia, and poor wound healing.
c. Chronic dehydration may be difficult to distinguish from a new onset of fluid loss. Patient will decompensate faster if acute fluid loss occurs resulting from trauma.
d. Clotting factors are suppressed by chronic alcohol abuse, resulting in increased risk of bleeding, especially subdural hematoma, with minor trauma.
(Objective 12)

51. Protect airway (high risk of aspiration); ventilate as necessary; initiate intravenous therapy; draw blood samples per protocol; determine blood glucose levels and if low, administer thiamine 100 mg intravenously and D50W 25 g intravenously; if opiate overdose is suspected or unknown, administer naloxone 2 mg intravenously; monitor airway, breathing, vital signs, and electrocardiogram.
(Objective 13)

52. Manage as in answer 51 and protect from injury; administer diazepam 2.5 to 5.0 mg or lorazepam 1 to 2 mg intravenously if additional seizures occur; examine for signs or symptoms of traumatic injury.
(Objective 13)

53. Hyperactive motor, speech, and autonomic activity; confusion; disorientation; delusion; hallucinations; tremor; agitation; insomnia; tachycardia; fever; hypertension; dilated pupils; profuse diaphoresis; and in severe cases, cardiovascular collapse
(Objective 13)

54. a. Assess for anaphylaxis, apply ice packs, and immobilize and elevate affected extremity.
b. Scrape or brush off. Do not squeeze because doing so will inject additional venom.
(Objective 14)

55. a. Lyme disease. Early signs are fever, lethargy, muscle pain, and general malaise; late signs are cardiac abnormalities, cranial nerve palsies, and arthritis
b. Tick paralysis. Signs include restlessness and paresthesia in hands and feet progressing to ascending symmetrical flaccid paralysis, which may include respiratory muscles.
(Objective 14)

56. Apply gloves and grasp tick as close to skin surface as possible (may use tweezers or forceps if available), pull out with steady pressure (avoid squeezing tick), and cleanse wound and observe for any remnants of tick.
(Objective 14)

57. a. Fang marks, pain and edema, weakness, diaphoresis, nausea, vomiting, and paresthesias

b. Ensure personal safety from another bite; monitor airway, breathing, and circulation; initiate intravenous therapy in unaffected extremity; immobilize affected extremity in dependent position; and keep patient at rest.
(Objective 14)

58. a. Jellyfish, fire corals, and sea anemones. Rinse wound with seawater; apply vinegar, baking soda, isopropanol, ammonia, meat tenderizer (for 5 to 10 minutes only); remove visible tentacles with forceps; apply shaving cream, gently shave affected area or use knife or spatula to gently scrape remaining tentacles; and rinse again

b. Sea urchins, starfish, and sea cucumbers. Remove embedded spines with forceps and immerse affected extremity (and unaffected extremity to prevent thermal injury) in hot water during transport

c. Stingrays. Irrigate wound with saltwater or freshwater; remove venom apparatus if it is visible; and immerse the affected part in hot water.
(Objective 14)

59. b
(Objective 1)

60. d
(Objective 2)

61. d. Life threats that will need immediate management usually are identified by assessing these areas.
(Objective 3)

62. b. Charcoal binds the drug by adsorption. It often is given with a cathartic that speeds the bound drug through the gastrointestinal tract.
(Objective 3)

63. c. Gastric lavage and charcoal generally are considered superior. Ipecac is contraindicated in petroleum distillate ingestions. Ipecac is associated with aspiration, Mallory-Weiss tear of the esophagus, pneumomediastinum, and fatal diaphragmatic or gastric rupture. If indicated, it should be given within 20 minutes after ingestion.
(Objective 2)

64. a. Inducing emesis usually is contraindicated for these patients, unless the toxicity of the specific hydrocarbon is so great that the risks of absorption in the gastrointestinal tract outweigh the risks of aspiration.
(Objective 4)

65. c. Methanol and ethylene glycol produce metabolic acidosis, so $NaHCO_3$ is indicated. In a tricyclic antidepressant overdose, $NaHCO_3$ will decrease the toxic cardiac side effects. No metabolic acidosis usually is associated with isopropanol ingestion.
(Objective 4)

66. b. The second most common reported category of poisonings is from plants. Dialysis is not effective for most plant poisonings. Most signs and symptoms occur within several hours after ingestion. Treatment should be based on symptoms and not be delayed until the identity of the plant can be determined.
(Objective 4)

67. a. Salivation and hypotension are likely to accompany the bradycardia. Symptoms vary according to the specific variety of mushroom ingested.
(Objective 4)

68. d. The lower the viscosity, the higher the risk of aspiration.
(Objective 5)

69. d. Huffing or sniffing substances such as carbon tetrachloride, methylene chloride, or aromatic hydrocarbons such as benzene and toluene is the most common method.
(Objective 8)

70. a. All of the other chemicals are more likely to cause tachycardia.
(Objective 9)

71. c. All other interventions are critical; however, rescuer safety should precede treatment because these poisons are absorbed readily through the skin, by ingestion, or by inhalation.
(Objective 9)

72. d
(Objective 9)

73. a. All of the others are narcotics.
(Objective 11)

74. c. Methamphetamine labs may produce hazards because of booby traps, explosive chemicals, a violent patient, or hazardous material contamination. Scene safety should be the highest priority.
(Objective 11)

75. c. Oil of wintergreen contains a large amount of salicylate and has produced many fatal ingestions.
(Objective 11)

76. c. Unless patients volunteer information regarding an overdose of acetaminophen, they may be asymptomatic or complain of only mild influenza-like symptoms for the first 24 hours after ingestion.
(Objective 11)

77. c. Ingestion of an overdose of iron is often lethal
(Objective 11)

78. c. All of the other drugs are more likely to produce bradycardia, although digoxin can produce bradycardia or tachycardia.
(Objective 11)

79. a. The immediate goal is to adsorb the drug and prevent its passage into the small intestine where it can be absorbed into the blood. Later, if signs and symptoms develop, they will be treated.
(Objective 11)

80. d. Wernicke-Korsakoff syndrome can lead to irreversible neurological problems and may be avoided by giving thiamine before administration of D50W.
(Objective 12)

81. b. The mortality rate has been reported as high as 15% for delirium tremens. It affects about 5% of hospitalized alcoholics undergoing withdrawal and usually occurs 72 to 96 hours after withdrawal of alcohol. Symptoms are associated with autonomic hyperactivity.
(Objective 13)

82. b. Diazepam in doses of 5 mg every 5 minutes up to a total of 30 mg may be needed. Lorazepam 1 to 2 mg intravenously is an alternative.
(Objective 13)

83. d. Anaphylaxis likely would include respiratory distress and urticaria. His reaction was immediate and generalized and involved a large exposure to venom.
(Objective 14)

84. a. The brown recluse spider produces a local reaction leading to delayed skin necrosis. Envenomation from most other spiders typically causes local versus systemic reactions.
(Objective 14)

85. c. This description matches a coral snake, which is the only neurotoxic snake listed.
(Objective 14)

86. a. Ice or cold packs may increase tissue damage and are not indicated.
(Objective 14)

87. c. Isoproterenol may induce or aggravate hypotension and ventricular dysrhythmias and should not be given unless massive beta-blocker poisoning has occurred.
(Objective 11)

88. b. The other three are stimulants and the patient has pinpoint pupils, so an opiate overdose is more likely.
(Objective 11)

89. a. The most likely cause of death in an opiate overdose is respiratory arrest, and this patient appears to be close.
(Objective 10)

WRAP IT UP

1. a. Hypoglycemia: aspirin, Glucophage, acetaminophen (72 to 96 hours), ethanol (Vodka)
   b. Acidosis: aspirin
   c. Tachycardia: Ritalin, Elavil
   d. Respiratory depression: Vicodin, Ativan, Elavil, aspirin (late), ethanol alcohol
   e. Decreased level of conciousness: Glucophage (from hypoglycemia), Vicodin, Elavil, Ativan, rubbing alcohol, ethanol (Vodka)
   f. Pupil constriction: Vicodin, Ritalin
   g. Bradycardia: metoprolol
   h. Cardiac dysrhythmias: Elavil, metoprolol, Tylenol (4 to 14 days)
   (Objectives 2 and 11)
   i. Seizures: aspirin, Glucophage (hypoglycemia), Elavil, metoprolol

2. a, b, c, d, e, f, g, h, i, k, l
   (Objective 3)

3. a. Acetaminophen: respiratory depression or cardiac dysrhythmias
   b. Metoprolol: bradycardia, ventricular dysrhythmias
   c. Vodka (ethanol): airway obstruction
   d. Glucophage: hypoglycemic coma
   e. Aspirin: acidosis, convulsions, respiratory arrest, brain death
   f. Iron: gastrointestinal bleeding
   g. Vicodin: respiratory depression
   h. Tricyclic antidepressant: cardiac dysrhythmias, CNS depression
   (Objective 2, 10, and 11)

4. a. Support depressed, slow respirations.
   b. Naloxone is an antidote for narcotic (Vicodin) overdose and its accompanying respiratory depression.
   c. Blood glucose tests revealed hypoglycemia, which occurred as a result of his ingestions.
   (Objectives 10 and 11)

5. Flumazenil (Romazicon) is indicated if there is a benzodiazepine overdose. However, it should be used with caution in multiple-drug overdoses because life-threatening side effects can occur in patients who have taken certain other drugs, including tricyclic antidepressants.

Sodium bicarbonate is indicated in cases of tricyclic antidepressant overdose, and medical control may or may not have ordered it in this polydrug situation.

Glucagon can be administered in beta-blocker overdose.

Activated charcoal sometimes is indicated to adsorb drugs that are ingested; however, with the airway not yet secured, this could increase the risk of aspiration.

(Objective 11)

6. b. Gathering information related to the toxic ingestion is a key element in the prehospital care of the poisoned patient. Ipecac rarely is indicated and is contraindicated in many ingestions. Antidotes are available for few poisonings.

(Objective 10)

7. a. None
b. Elavil
c. None
d. Vicodin
e. Ritalin
(Objective 14)

CHAPTER
37

Hematology

READING ASSIGNMENT
Chapter 37, pages 970-982, in *Mosby's Paramedic Textbook,* ed. 3

OBJECTIVES
Upon completion of this chapter, the paramedic student will be able to:
1. Describe the physiology of blood and its components.
2. Discuss pathophysiology and signs and symptoms of specific hematological disorders.
3. Outline general assessment and management of patients with hematological disorders.

SUMMARY
- Blood is composed of cells and formed elements surrounded by plasma. About 95% of the volume of formed elements consists of RBCs (erythrocytes). The remaining 5% consists of WBCs (leukocytes) and cell fragments (platelets).
- Anemia is a condition in which the amount of hemoglobin or erythrocytes in the blood is below normal. Two common forms of anemia are iron deficiency anemia and hemolytic anemia. All forms of anemia share signs and symptoms. These signs and symptoms include fatigue and headaches, sometimes a sore mouth or tongue, brittle nails, and in severe cases, breathlessness and chest pain. Diagnosis is made by history and from blood tests and bone marrow biopsy.
- *Leukemia* refers to any of several types of cancer in which an abnormal proliferation of WBCs usually occurs in the bone marrow. The proliferation of leukemic cells crowds and impairs the normal production of RBCs, WBCs, and platelets. Leukemia is classified as acute or chronic. The proliferation of leukemic cells makes the patient highly susceptible to serious infections, anemia, and bleeding episodes. The diagnosis is confirmed by bone marrow biopsy.
- *Lymphoma* refers to a group of diseases that range from slowly growing chronic disorders to rapidly evolving acute conditions. Hodgkin's disease is one type; all others are called *non-Hodgkin's lymphomas.*
- Polycythemia is characterized by an unusually large number of RBCs in the blood as a result of their increased production by the bone marrow. Polycythemia may be a natural response to hypoxia. (This is known as secondary polycythemia.) Polycythemia also may occur for unknown reasons. (This is known as primary polycythemia.)
- Disseminated intravascular coagulopathy is a complication of severe injury, trauma, or disease. It disrupts the balance among procoagulants, thrombin formation, inhibitors, and lysis. Signs and symptoms of disseminated intravascular coagulation include dyspnea, bleeding, and those associated with hypotension and hypoperfusion. The treatment is aimed at reversing the underlying illness or injury that triggered the event.
- Hemophilia A is caused by a deficiency of a blood protein called *factor VIII.* Hemophilia B is caused by a deficiency of factor IX. Bleeding from hemophilia can occur spontaneously, after even minor injury, or during some medical procedures.

- Sickle cell disease is a debilitating and unpredictable recessive genetic illness. It affects persons of African descent. Less often, it affects persons of Mediterranean origin. Sickle cell anemia produces an abnormal type of hemoglobin. This is called *hemoglobin S*. This abnormal type has an inferior oxygen-carrying capacity. Complications of sickle cell disease include episodes of severe pain, fatigue, pallor, jaundice, stroke, delayed growth, hematuria, priapism, and splenomegaly.
- Multiple myeloma is a malignant neoplasm of the bone marrow. The tumor destroys bone tissue (especially flat bones). This causes pain, fractures, hypercalcemia, and skeletal deformities.
- In many cases of hematological disorders, the prehospital treatment is supportive. Treatment includes ensuring adequate airway, ventilatory, and circulatory support.

REVIEW QUESTIONS

Match the hematology terms in Column II with the description in Column I. Use each term only once.

Column I	Column II
1. _____ Include eosinophils, basophils, and neutrophils	**a.** Basophils
2. _____ Destroy red blood cells	**b.** Bilirubin
3. _____ Destroy invading organisms and include monophils	**c.** Erythrocytes
4. _____ Waste product after destruction of hemoglobin	**d.** Macrophages
5. _____ Activate chemicals that trigger inflammation	**e.** Phagocytes
6. _____ Contains albumin, globulins, and fibrinogen	**f.** Plasma of hemoglobin
7. _____ Composed of water and hemoglobin	**g.** Platelets
	h. White blood cell inflammation

8. Complete the information in the following table.

Condition	Cause	Signs and Symptoms
Anemia		
Leukemia		
Lymphomas		
Polycythemia		
Disseminated intravascular coagulation		
Hemophilia		
Sickle cell disease		
Multiple myeloma		

9. You respond to a private residence and find a 21-year-old black woman who is complaining of pain in her abdomen, hands, and feet. She said she had the flu and vomited 3 times yesterday. She tells you that she suffers from sickle cell disease.

   a. What type of sickle cell crisis may present in this manner?

b. What event may have triggered a crisis in this patient?

_____

c. What specific organ should you try to palpate on your physical examination of this patient?

_____

d. Outline the prehospital care of this patient.

_____

STUDENT SELF-ASSESSMENT

10. Which is true regarding red bone marrow?
  a. Only white blood cells are formed here.
  b. It is formed in the liver.
  c. It is composed mainly of connective tissue and fat.
  d. It is found in the vertebrae, pelvis, sternum, and ribs.
11. Which of the following is a normal value for hemoglobin?
  a. 10 g/100 mL   **c.** 35%
  b. 15 g/100 mL   **d.** 50%
12. Which type of anemia may be cured by splenectomy?
  a. Aplastic   **c.** Iron deficiency
  b. Hemolytic   **d.** Sickle cell
13. Which is true of acute myeloblastic leukemia?
  a. It affects mostly young children.
  b. Reed-Sternberg cells are present.
  c. Generalized itching may be present.
  d. It is difficult to cure.
14. Which hematological disorder is diagnosed using bone marrow biopsy?
  a. Disseminated intravascular coagulation
  b. Leukemia
  c. Hodgkin's disease
  d. Sickle cell anemia
15. Which of the following is a target organ in Hodgkin's lymphoma?
  a. Kidney   **c.** Spleen
  b. Liver   **d.** Testes
16. What can trigger secondary polycythemia?
  a. Blood loss   **c.** Hypoxia
  b. Hypothermia   **d.** Infection
17. Which of the following occurs when disseminated intravascular coagulation is present?
  a. Coagulation inhibition levels are increased.
  b. Fibrin is deposited in small vessels in multiple organs.
  c. Platelets and fibrinogen V, VIII, and XIII increase.
  d. Thrombin is destroyed.
18. What is needed to stop the bleeding that occurs during hemophilia?
  a. Factor VIII   **c.** Oxygen administration
  b. Intravenous fluids   **d.** Topical thrombin
19. Although all sickle cell disease emergencies can cause death, which one represents an immediate life-threatening situation?
  a. Aplastic crisis   **c.** Splenic sequestration
  b. Hemolytic crisis   **d.** Vasoocclusive crisis
20. In which hematological disorder of the bone marrow does the tumor destroy bone tissue?
  a. Hodgkin's disease   **c.** Lymphoma
  b. Leukemia   **d.** Multiple myeloma

21. Prehospital care for a conscious patient with a hematological problem should always include which of the following?

   a. Analgesics
   b. Antidysrhythmics
   c. Blood transfusion
   d. Emotional support

WRAP IT UP

You are dispatched to respond to a call for a person with difficulty breathing. Your patient is a 45-year-old white male who is the soccer coach at a local high school. He experienced shortness of breath and sweating during a practice drill with his team, and a player called 911. On arrival you note a pale man in moderate distress. He is alert and oriented and says he was fine until he started running. His initial SaO_2 is 89%, and his breath sounds are clear and equal bilaterally. You mention to him that he appears to have an unusual number of bruises on various areas of his body—ranging from old yellow or gray ones to purplish red newer ones. He appears nervous when you ask about his medical history and denies any significant illness, injury, or medications. His vital signs are BP 108/66 mm Hg, P 124, and R 24. You administer oxygen by non-rebreather mask and move him by stretcher into the ambulance. In the privacy of the ambulance, he confides to you that he has been ill and just this week saw his doctor because he has never had any medical problems but has been feeling tired all the time; has generalized bone pain, night sweats, and swollen "glands" in his neck; and has lost 25 lb in the last 8 weeks. This afternoon, his doctor called and said that his blood tests were grossly abnormal and he wanted to hospitalize him to run more tests to rule out leukemia. The coach confesses that he could not believe it and decided to go ahead with practice because he did not know what to tell the kids. His oxygen saturation is now 98%, and you initiate an IV and transport him, completing your physical exam en route. He subsequently is diagnosed with acute myeloblastic leukemia, and 6 months later you read of his death in the obituaries.

1. Which of the following blood cells increase or decrease in leukemia?

   a. Red blood cells   Increase/decrease
   b. White blood cells   Increase/decrease
   c. Platelets   Increase/decrease

2. What explains the following signs/symptoms that this patient experienced?

   a. Fatigue
   b. Swollen lymph nodes
   c. Difficulty breathing
   d. Bruising

3. What additional findings might you encounter when you assess the abdomen?

4. Place a check mark beside other hematological conditions you might have suspected, based on his history and presenting condition, if the patient had not confessed his presumed diagnosis.

   a. _____ Anemia
   b. _____ Hemophilia
   c. _____ Hodgkin's disease
   d. _____ Lymphoma
   e. _____ Multiple myeloma
   f. _____ Polycythemia
   g. _____ Sickle cell disease

CHAPTER 37 ANSWERS

REVIEW QUESTIONS

1. h
2. d
3. e
4. b
5. a
6. f
7. c
(Questions 1 to 7, Objective 1)

8.

Condition	Cause	Signs and Symptoms
Anemia	Iron deficiency; decreased production and survival of red blood cells	Fatigue headaches, sore mouth or tongue, brittle nails, breathlessness, or chest pain
Leukemia	Abnormal chromosomes; disorganized proliferation of white blood cells in bone marrow	Bleeding, bone pain, frequent bruising, sternal tenderness, fatigue, headache, weight loss, height sweets; enlarged lymph nodes, liver, spleen; anemia, infections
Lymphomata	Proliferation of cells in lymph tissues (may be genetic link)	Swollen lymph nodes in neck, armpits, groin; fatigue, chills, and night sweats; severe itching, cough, weight loss, dyspnea, chest discomfort
Polycythemia	Unusually large number of red blood cells	Headache, dizziness, blurred vision, generalized itching; hypertension, splenomegaly, platelet disorders, red hands and feet, purple complexion, stroke and development of leukemias
Disseminated intra-vascular coagulation	Complication of severe injury, trauma, disease; imbalance of clotting mechanisms	Dyspnea, bleeding, hypotension, hypoper-fusion
Hemophilia	Inherited bleeding disorder; deficiency of factor VIII or less often factor IX	Spontaneous bleeding (joints, deep muscles, urinary tract, and intracranial sites most common) after injury or during medical procedures
Sickle cell disease	Genetic illness; red blood cells are distorted into sickle shape that is easily destroyed and can clog blood vessels	Episodes of severe pain, fatigue, pallor, jaundice, stroke; delayed growth, development, and sexual maturation; hematuria, priapism, splenomegaly
Multiple myeloma	Malignant neoplasm of bone marrow	Pain, fractures, hypercalcemia, skeletal deformities, kidney failure, anemia, weight loss, rib fractures, recurrent infections

(Objective 2)

9. a. Possibly a vasoocclusive sickle cell crisis
   b. Dehydration or stress from her illness the day before may have triggered her crisis.
   c. The spleen may enlarge during a sickle cell crisis, so it should be evaluated.
   d. You should administer oxygen by non-rebreather mask at 12 to 15 L/min. You should initiate an intravenous line and administer a fluid bolus under medical direction. Although analgesia will be a high priority for this patient, medical direction may not order it until the abdomen can be examined to ensure that an urgent surgical condition does not exist.
   (Objective 2)

10. d. All types of blood cells are formed here. Yellow marrow is composed of connective tissue and fat.
    (Objective 1)

11. b. Normal hemoglobin ranges from 13.5 to 18 g/100 mL. Normal hematocrit ranges from 38% to 54%.
    (Objective 1)

12. b. Treatment for aplastic anemia may include blood transfusion, folic acid, and bone marrow transplantation. Iron deficiency anemia is treated with supplemental iron and folic acid.
    (Objective 2)

13. d. Acute myeloblastic anemia affects middle-aged adults. Reed-Sternberg cells are characteristic of Hodgkin's lymphoma. Itching is not a classic symptom.
    (Objective 2)

14. b. Disseminated intravascular coagulation is diagnosed based on clinical history and laboratory values that include clotting studies, platelet count, and fibrin degradation products. Sickle cell anemia is confirmed by laboratory testing.
    (Objective 2)

15. c. Hodgkin's lymphoma primarily affects lymphoid tissues.
    (Objective 2)

16. c. The body produces more red cells in an attempt to improve oxygenation in conditions such as high altitude and chronic lung disease.
    (Objective 2)

17. b. Coagulation inhibition levels are decreased. Platelets and coagulation factors are consumed, and thrombin is formed.
    (Objective 2)

18. a. Factor VIII is needed to reestablish a normal clotting cascade and stop bleeding.
    (Objective 2)

19. c. Splenic sequestration occurs in childhood and is caused by blood trapped in the spleen. Aplastic crisis occurs when the bone marrow temporarily stops making red blood cells. In hemolytic crisis, red blood cell breakdown exceeds production. Vasoocclusive sickle cell crisis occurs when the sickle-shaped cells block blood flow to organs and tissues.
    (Objective 2)

20. d. Hodgkin's disease is a type of lymphoma and affects the lymph tissue. Leukemia is similar to multiple myeloma, but in multiple myeloma, the primary target is bone.
    (Objective 2)

21. d. Acute or chronic hematological disorders produce tremendous emotional stress on patients and families. You should be empathetic and provide calm support during care and transport. Analgesics and antidysrhythmics occasionally may be indicated. Prehospital blood transfusion usually is done only during interfacility transfers.
(Objective 2)

WRAP IT UP

1. a. Decrease; b. increase; c. decrease
(Objective 2)

2. a. A decrease in red blood cells causes a decrease in oxygen delivery to the cells that could affect adenosine triphosphate (energy) production.
b. Lymph nodes help to rid the body of excess or damaged white blood cells, which are characteristic of leukemia.
c. The patient's decrease in red blood cells did not permit his body to transport enough oxygen to meet the increased demand during exertion at practice.
d. Platelets are essential to control bleeding in the body and are greatly decreased in leukemia.
(Objectives 1 and 2)

3. The liver and spleen likely will be greatly enlarged.
(Objective 3)

4. a. Because of his pallor and dyspnea
c and d. Although he is somewhat young, other signs and symptoms would not exclude Hodgkin's and other lymphomata.
e. His age and bone pain are consistent with multiple myeloma.
His history does not include hemophilia, which is present at birth; polycythemia is a problem of excess red cells and typically would produce red-purple skin, not pallor as in this patient (and this patient does not seem to have risk factors for polycythemia); this patient is white, so sickle cell anemia would be unlikely, and he has no known history of sickle cell disease that would be diagnosed early in life.
(Objective 2)

Environmental Conditions

READING ASSIGNMENT
Chapter 38, pages 984-1003, in *Mosby's Paramedic Textbook,* ed. 3

OBJECTIVES
Upon completion of this chapter, the paramedic student will be able to:
1. Describe the physiology of thermoregulation.
2. Discuss the risk factors, pathophysiology, assessment findings, and management of specific hyperthermic conditions.
3. Discuss the risk factors, pathophysiology, assessment findings, and management of specific hypothermic conditions and frostbite.
4. Discuss the risk factors, pathophysiology, assessment findings, and management of submersion and drowning.
5. Identify the mechanical effects on the body based on a knowledge of the basic properties of gases.
6. Discuss the risk factors, pathophysiology, assessment findings, and management of diving emergencies and high-altitude illness.

SUMMARY
- Body temperature is regulated by a thermoregulatory center in the posterior hypothalamus. The body temperature can be increased or decreased in two ways. One of these ways is through the regulation of heat production. (This is known as thermogenesis.) The other way is through the regulation of heat loss. (This is known as thermolysis.).
- Heat illness results from one of two basic causes. First, the normal temperature-regulating functions can be overwhelmed by conditions in the environment. These conditions can include heat stress. More often, though, they involve excessive exercise in moderate to extreme environmental conditions. The other cause is the failure of the body's thermoregulatory mechanism. This may occur in older adults or ill or debilitated individuals. Heat cramps are brief, intermittent, and often severe. They are muscular cramps that occur in muscles fatigued by heavy work or exercise. Heat exhaustion is characterized by minor aberrations in mental status, dizziness, nausea, headache, and a mild to moderate rise in the core body temperature (CBT) (up to less than 103° F [39° C]). Heat stroke occurs when the temperature-regulating functions break down entirely. This failure results in body temperature rises to 105.8° F (41° C) or higher. Temperatures this high damage all tissues and lead to collapse.
- Hypothermia (a CBT lower than 95° F [35° C]) can result from a decrease in heat production, an increase in heat loss, or a combination of these two factors. The progression of clinical signs and symptoms of hypothermia is divided into three classes based on the CBT: mild (CBT between 93.2° and 96.8° F [34° and to 36° C]), moderate

(CBT between 86° and 93° F [30° and 34° C]), and severe (CBT below 86° F [30° C]). Severely hypothermic patients have no vital signs, including respiratory effort, pulse, and blood pressure.

- Frostbite is a localized injury. It results from environmentally induced freezing of body tissues. This freezing leads to the damage to blood vessels. Ischemia often produces the most damaging effects of frostbite. In deep frostbite this can include mummification and sloughing of nonviable skin and deep structures.
- Drowning is an event in which a submersion victim is pronounced dead at the scene of the attempted resuscitation, or within 24 hours after arrival in the emergency department (ED) or hospital. Near drowning is submersion with survival for a period of time. Regardless of the type of water aspirated, the pathophysiology of drowning is characterized by hypoxia, hypercapnia, and acidosis, which result in cardiac arrest.
- The three laws pertaining to the basic properties of gases that are involved in all pressure-related diving emergencies are Boyle's law, Dalton's law, and Henry's law. Increased pressure dissolves gases into blood; oxygen metabolizes, and nitrogen dissolves.
- Barotrauma is tissue damage. It results from compression or expansion of gas spaces when the gas pressure in the body differs from the ambient pressure. The type of barotrauma depends on whether the diver is in descent or ascent. Air embolism is the most serious complication of pulmonary barotrauma. It is a major cause of death and disability among sport divers.
- High-altitude illness results from exposure to reduced atmospheric pressure, which results in hypoxia. Forms of high-altitude illness include acute mountain sickness, high-altitude pulmonary edema, and high-altitude cerebral edema.

REVIEW QUESTIONS

Match the terms related to environmental conditions in Column II with the appropriate description in Column I. Use each term only once.

Column I	Column II
1. _____ Goose bumps	a. Afterdrop phenomenon
2. _____ Dissipation of heat in the body by various mechanisms	b. Boyle's law
	c. Cold diuresis
3. _____ Sudden return of cold blood and wastes to the core	d. Dalton's law
	e. Dysbarism
4. _____ Temperature difference between body and environment	f. Henry's law
	g. Piloerection
5. _____ Gas volume inversely related to its pressure	h. Rewarming shock
	i. Thermal gradient
6. _____ Decompression sickness	j. Thermogenesis
7. _____ Heat immersion causing hypotension from vasodilation	k. Thermolysis
8. _____ Total pressure of gases equaling the sum of partial pressure of component gases	
9. _____ Regulation of heat production in the body	
10. _____ Amount of gas dissolved in fluid volume is proportional to pressure of gas with which it is in equilibrium	

11. Briefly describe how each of the following contributes to heat production in the body.

a. Chemical control:

_____

b. Musculoskeletal system:

_____

c. Endocrine system:

_____

12. For each of the following situations, select the mechanisms of heat loss that apply (conduction, convection, evaporation, and radiation). You may use each answer more than once.

   a. On a windy autumn evening, you remove the clothing of a trauma patient to assess his injuries more accurately. On arrival to the emergency department, his temperature is 94° F (34.4° C). _____.

   b. During a multiple patient situation, you extricate a partially clothed patient onto a cold metal backboard. On arrival to the emergency department, her temperature is 96° F (35.6° C). _____.

   c. On a dry, cool spring evening you transport a wet patient who injured her neck after diving into a swimming pool. On arrival to the emergency department, her temperature is 94.6° F (34.8° C). _____.

   d. A patient with a 40% body surface area burn is cooled continuously with normal saline en route to the hospital. On arrival to the emergency department, his temperature is 93.5° F (34.2° C). _____.

13. You are on the scene of a multiple-car collision on a hot July day. List four ways your body will compensate to prevent your temperature from rising.

   a.

   b.

   c.

   d.

14. You are assisting with a search-and-rescue effort after a hurricane. It is cold, wet, and windy. List four ways your body will attempt to maintain a normal temperature.

   a.

   b.

   c.

   d.

15. For each of the following examples, identify the type of heat illness and briefly describe the appropriate prehospital patient care.

   a. You are working at an amusement park on a 95° F (35° C) humid day. A hot, sweaty 45-year-old woman comes to your aid station complaining of severe cramping in her calves. Her vital signs are BP 116/72 mm Hg, P 116, and temperature 98.6° F (37° C).

   Illness:

_____

   Management:

_____

b. A 55-year-old man is complaining of dizziness, nausea, and vomiting while participating in a long-distance walk fund-raiser. His vital signs while lying down are BP 104/70 mm Hg and P 108. His vital signs while standing are BP 86/50 mm Hg and P 128, and his temperature is 101° F (38.3° C).

Illness:

_____

Management:

_____

c. On a 100° F (37.8° C) day, an 80-year-old woman becomes confused and agitated and has a seizure in her apartment, which does not have air-conditioning. She is responsive to pain, has jugular venous distention, and is sweating profusely. Her vital signs are BP 92/70 mm Hg, P 120, R 24, and temperature 106° F (41.1° C).

Illness:

_____

Management:

_____

16. Why is the increased metabolic rate that is produced in mild hypothermia undesirable for a patient who already has an injury or medical illness?

_____

_____

Questions 17 to 19 refer to the following case study:

You are caring for a snowmobiler whose rig broke through the ice 30 minutes ago. He pulled himself out of the water and collapsed before rescuers reached him 20 minutes later. He has been moved to a safe area.

17. Describe general measures of care to begin immediately on this patient.

_____

_____

18. You determine that he is apneic and pulseless. His electrocardiogram displays the rhythm shown in Fig. 38-1. What actions should be taken if the following occur?

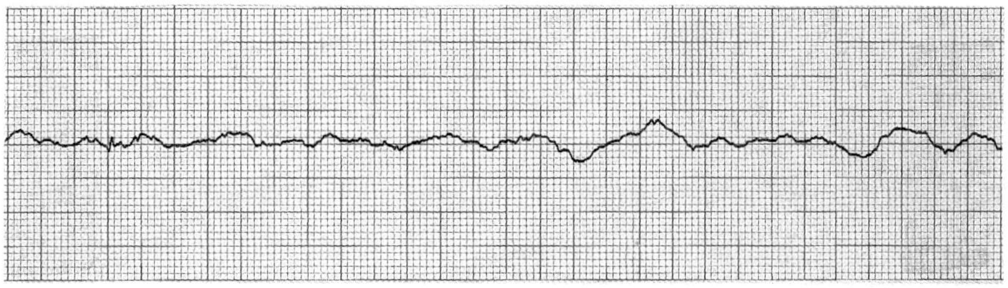

Figure 38-1

a. His core temperature is less than 86° F (30° C).

_____

_____

b. His core temperature is greater than 86° F (30° C).

_____

_____

19. When should resuscitation efforts be terminated?

_____

20. You are transporting a hiker who became lost on a trail. He is shivering and hungry and has a temperature of 97° F (36.1° C). How would you treat this patient?

_____

_____

21. A firefighter dives into an ice-covered pond to rescue a child who has fallen through the ice on a windy, cold January evening. On the 10-minute walk back to the firetruck, the firefighter develops slurred speech and ataxia and complains that his heart is pounding. At the ambulance, his temperature is 89.5° F (31.9° C). His electrocardiogram is shown in Fig. 38-2.

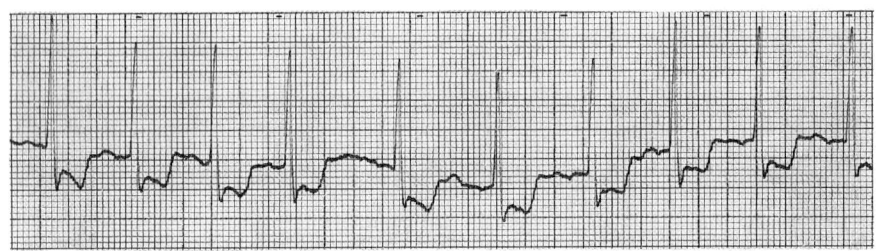

Figure 38-2

a. What is your interpretation of the electrocardiogram tracing?

_____

b. Describe your management of this patient.

_____

_____

_____

Questions 22 to 24 refer to the following case study:

During a cross-country ski meet, a participant complains of coldness, numbness, and extreme pain in the fingers of his right hand.

22. Differentiate between the findings you would anticipate for superficial frostbite and deep frostbite.

_____

_____

23. List four factors that increase susceptibility to frostbite that you should look for in this patient.

   a.

   b.

   c.

   d.

24. How would you treat frostbite in this patient?

_____

_____

Questions 25 to 27 refer to the following case study:

   A 2-year-old child pulled from a backyard pool is apneic and pulseless.

25. Identify four factors that will influence this patient's clinical outcome.

   a.

   b.

   c.

   d.

26. What complications do you anticipate if the patient is resuscitated?

_____

_____

_____

27. Describe prehospital management of this child.

_____

_____

28. List five body areas on the patient where pain may occur resulting from SQUEEZE.

   a.   **d.**

   b.   **e.**

   c.

29. A diver experiences acute distress immediately after rapidly surfacing from a deep dive.

   a. List five signs or symptoms of air embolism.

      a.   **d.**

      b.   **e.**

      c.

   b. Describe special considerations necessary for care of this patient while you are providing advanced life support and transport.

_____

_____

30. A tourist at a local resort complains of severe joint pain, fatigue, vertigo, and paraesthesia 12 hours after returning from his first dive.

    a. What diving injury do you suspect?

_____

    b. Describe prehospital management of this patient.

_____

_____

31. You respond to a mountain resort where a participant in a cycling event has become ill.

    a. List the three types of high-altitude illness.

        a.

        b.

        c.

    b. What single intervention is most critical to long-term improvement of the patient suffering from high-altitude illness after the ABCs have been managed?

_____

STUDENT SELF-ASSESSMENT

32. What is the most important organ that regulates body temperature?
    a. Heart
    b. Lungs
    c. Pituitary gland
    d. Skin

33. You are assessing firefighters in the rehab area of a major fire on a summer day. Your patient is dizzy and nauseated and has orthostatic hypotension. What should you do?
    a. Administer medication for his nausea.
    b. Ask him to rest for 15 minutes before returning to the fire.
    c. Have him drink a fluid-replacement beverage.
    d. Initiate an intravenous line and administer a fluid bolus.

34. What causes shock to develop in the patient with heat stroke?
    a. Fluid loss
    b. Myocardial depression
    c. Peripheral vasodilation
    d. All of the above

35. What is the most critical intervention for heat stroke?
    a. Fluid resuscitation
    b. Medication administration
    c. Rapid cooling in transit
    d. Rapid transport to a hospital

36. When does shivering stop in a hypothermic patient?
    a. The body temperature drops to 90° F (32.2° C).
    b. Glucose or glycogen is depleted.
    c. Excessive amounts of insulin are excreted.
    d. P_{CO_2} increases to more than 50 mm Hg.

37. Prehospital care of a frostbitten extremity should include which of the following?
    a. Application of a tourniquet
    b. Elevation of the affected extremity
    c. Rapid rewarming in hot water
    d. Refreezing of the injured extremity

38. All drownings are characterized by which of the following?
    a. Hypovolemia, hypoxia, and acidosis
    b. Hypoxia, acidosis, and hypothermia
    c. Hypoxia, acidosis, and hypercapnia
    d. Hypovolemia, acidosis, and hypercapnia
39. Which of the following best describes the term *drowning*?
    a. Death from submersion up to 24 hours after arrival in the emergency department
    b. Death related to submersion that occurs at any time after the incident
    c. Swimming-related distress sufficient to require care in the emergency department
    d. Swimming-related distress sufficient to require support in the prehospital setting
40. What is the single most important factor in determining survival after submersion injury?
    a. Age of the patient   c. Duration of submersion
    b. Contaminants in the water   d. Water temperature
41. Which law of physics states that the volume of gas is related inversely to its pressure at a constant temperature?
    a. Boyle's law   c. Henry's law
    b. Dalton's law   d. Newton's law
42. A diver is in respiratory distress after ascent. You palpate subcutaneous emphysema. He is probably suffering from which of the following?
    a. Barotrauma of descent
    b. Decompression sickness
    c. Pulmonary air embolus
    d. Pulmonary overpressurization syndrome
43. What is the primary danger of nitrogen narcosis?
    a. Hypoxemia   c. Respiratory acidosis
    b. Impaired judgment   d. Shock resulting from hypovolemia
44. What is the critical sign or symptom that indicates deterioration in a patient with acute mountain sickness?
    a. Ataxia   c. Irritability
    b. Headache   d. Vomiting

WRAP IT UP

You are standing by with searchers who are trying to find a 50-year-old hunter who is evidently lost in a marshy area and has not been heard from in 18 hours. The weather is cold and windy, with temperatures the night before dropping to 40° F (4° C) and winds of up to 20 mph. An excited transmission on the radio lets you know that he has been found alive. Crews are going to bring him out to your staging area. He arrives in the bed of a pickup truck, conscious but confused. Rescuers tell you they found him staggering in the swamp. His overalls are soaked and his boots are full of water. You move him in the warm ambulance and quickly but gently remove his clothes and cover him with warm, dry blankets. Your partner puts a warm pack on his antecubital space to try to expose a vein to start an IV. Warmed, humidified oxygen is administered by mask, and his vital signs are taken. Because of the large number of exposure incidents in your area, you have a hypothermia thermometer and obtain a core temperature of 87° F (30.5° C), BP 100/60 mm Hg, P 56, R 16, SaO_2 unobtainable; and his skin is cool and pale. You initiate an IV of warmed normal saline and obtain a blood glucose, which is 78 mg/dL; electrocardiogram rhythm is sinus bradycardia. As you go en route to the hospital, medical direction asks you to infuse a fluid challenge of 250 mL and reassess the patient. You are sweating because of the heat in the patient compartment and check the heat packs you have placed in his armpits and groin to ensure they are still warm. While you perform your comprehensive exam, you note that his feet have a waxy, white appearance and that he appears to have severe pain when you palpate them. On arrival to the ED his vital signs are BP 110/64 mm Hg, P 58, R 20, and temperature 90° F (32° C).

1. What was the equivalent chill factor at the coldest part of the night?
2. Which of the following mechanisms of heat loss played a role in this situation?
    a. Conduction
    b. Convection
    c. Evaporation
    d. Radiation

3. Place a check mark sign beside symptoms that demonstrate moderate hypothermia that are found in this patient.
   a. ____ Atrial fibrillation
   b. ____ Ataxia
   c. ____ Bradycardia
   d. ____ Cardiac instability
   e. ____ Confusion
   f. ____ Fixed, dilated pupils
   g. ____ Loss of deep tendon reflexes
   h. ____ Shivering
4. Explain why the following interventions could be harmful in this patient.
   a. Vigorous movement

   b. Lactated Ringer's solution intravenously

   c. Placing the patient in a high Fowler's position

5. Which is true regarding the assessment findings of his feet?

   a. They are likely just cold and will rewarm last because of the distal circulation.

   b. This is evidence of extensive frostbite, and he will probably need amputations.

   c. Rewarming should not be attempted because of possible tissue damage.

   d. Trench foot is possible, and blisters may begin to form as he rewarms.

CHAPTER 38 ANSWERS

REVIEW QUESTIONS

1. g
   (Objective 1)

2. k
   (Objective 1)

3. a
   (Objective 3)

4. i
   (Objective 1)

5. b
   (Objective 5)

6. e
   (Objective 6)

7. h
   (Objective 3)

8. d
   (Objective 5)

9. j
   (Objective 1)

10. f
    (Objective 5)

11. a. Oxidation of energy sources; b. shivering can increase heat production by 400%; c. increased basal metabolic rate and vasoconstriction
    (Objective 1)

12. a. Conduction, convection, and radiation; b. conduction and radiation; c. conduction, radiation, convection, and evaporation; d. conduction, radiation, convection, and evaporation
    (Objective 1)

13. Skin vasodilation (becomes warm and flushed), sweating, decreased hormone secretion, and decreased muscle tone
    (Objective 1)

14. Peripheral vasoconstriction (cool, pale skin), goose bumps, shivering, increased voluntary activity, increased hormone secretion, and increased appetite
    (Objective 1)

15. a. Heat cramps. Remove patient from hot environment, replace sodium and water, and intravenously infuse saline solution if condition is severe.
    b. Heat exhaustion. Remove patient from hot environment and intravenously infuse saline solution.

c. Heat stroke. Secure airway, assess breathing, ventilate if indicated, administer high-flow oxygen, move patient to a cool environment, remove all clothing, wet the skin with cool fluid, fan the patient, initiate intravenous fluid therapy with normal saline, consult with medical direction regarding a fluid challenge, and monitor for signs of fluid overload. If seizures recur, administer diazepam, assess for hypoglycemia, and administer D50W if indicated.
(Objective 2)

16. Increasing the metabolic rate increases the heart rate and contractility and increases the body's use of oxygen and other nutrients. The patient with preexisting trauma or illness will not tolerate these extra demands, which may compromise organ response to illness or injury.
(Objective 3)

17. Assess and secure the airway, assess breathing, and assist with 100% oxygen (warmed and humidified if available); if indicated, assess circulation and begin cardiopulmonary resuscitation only after carefully verifying that no pulse is present. Move the patient to a warm environment and remove all clothing.
(Objective 3)

18. a. Cardiopulmonary resuscitation; defibrillation at 200, 300, and 360 J; intubation; ventilation with warm humid oxygen; intravenous infusion of warm normal saline; and transport to the hospital
    b. Cardiopulmonary resuscitation, defibrillation at 200, 300, and 360 J; intubation; ventilation with warm, humid oxygen; intravenous infusion of warm normal saline; intravenous administration of medications as indicated for ventricular fibrillation with a delay between doses; and another defibrillation as core temperature rises
(Objective 3)

19. Resuscitation may be withheld if there are obvious lethal injuries or if the body is frozen, preventing chest compression or airway management. Resuscitation could stop when the patient's core temperature has reached 94° to 95° F (34° to 35° C) and all resuscitation efforts are still unsuccessful.
(Objective 3)

20. Move patient to warm area, remove any wet clothing, and wrap patient in warm blanket. If he is awake and alert, administer warm, sugar-sweetened drinks (no alcohol, coffee, or tea). If necessary, apply hot packs wrapped in towels to the neck, armpits, and groin.
(Objective 3)

21. a. Atrial fibrillation
    b. Put the patient at rest and move to a warm environment after ensuring adequate airway, breathing, and circulation. Carefully remove all wet clothing and wrap patient in a blanket. Administer 100% oxygen (heated and humidified if possible) by non-rebreather mask. Initiate intravenous therapy of normal saline (initial fluid challenge of 250 to 500 mL may be ordered by medical direction, and use warmed fluids if available). Transport gently, and monitor the patient carefully en route.
(Objective 3)

22. In deep frostbite the underlying tissue is hard and not compressible, whereas in superficial frostbite the underlying tissue springs back when palpated.
(Objective 3)

23. Lack of protective clothing; preexisting illness or injury (diabetes or vascular insufficiency); fatigue; tobacco; tight, constrictive clothing; alcohol ingestion; and medications that cause vasodilation (some antihypertensives)
(Objective 3)

24. Elevate and protect the affected extremity, provide rapid transport to a medical facility, and assess for hypothermia.
(Objective 3)

25. Temperature of water, length of submersion, cleanliness of water, and age of patient
(Objective 4)

26. Acute respiratory failure, dysrhythmias, decreased cardiac output, cerebral edema leading to central nervous system dysfunction, and renal dysfunction (rare)
(Objective 4)

27. Ensure scene safety, initiate cardiopulmonary resuscitation, secure the airway with an endotracheal tube and ventilate with 100% oxygen, assess cardiac rhythm and follow advanced life support protocols to manage appropriately, assess for hypothermia, and transport to appropriate medical facility.
(Objective 4)

28. Ears, sinuses, lungs and airways, gastrointestinal tract, thorax, and teeth
(Objective 6)

29. a. Focal paralysis or sensory changes, aphasia, confusion, blindness or another visual disturbance, convulsion, loss of consciousness, dizziness, vertigo, abdominal pain, and cardiac arrest
b. If the patient's trachea is intubated, fill the balloon with normal saline instead of air; evaluate for pulmonary over pressurization syndrome (POPS); and transport in the left lateral recumbent position with a 15-degree elevation of the thorax.
(Objective 6)

30. a. Decompression sickness
b. Administer high-flow oxygen, initiate intravenous therapy, and rapidly transport for recompression (follow local protocol so that patient can reach hyperbaric chamber as quickly as possible).
(Objective 6)

31. a. Acute mountain sickness, high-altitude pulmonary edema, and high altitude cerebral edema; b. descent to a lower altitude
(Objective 6)

32. d. Vasoconstriction and vasodilation of the blood vessels in the skin are the major ways the body releases or conserves heat.
(Objective 1)

33. d. Based on his symptoms, you suspect heat exhaustion. Because he is nauseated and has orthostatic hypotension, he needs intravenous rather than oral rehydration. He should be moved to a cool environment and not returned to the fire.
(Objective 2)

34. d
(Objective 2)

35. c. Damage to the body continues as long as the temperature remains elevated.
(Objective 2)

36. b. Shivering should continue until the core temperature reaches 86° F (30° C). A tremendous amount of energy is needed for shivering, so glucose and glycogen must be available to fuel this increased muscle activity.
(Objective 3)

37. b. Rapid rewarming in warm water is indicated only when sanctioned by medical direction if no chance of refreezing exists. Refreezing is damaging to the tissues.
(Objective 3)

38. c. The lack of ventilation causes a buildup of carbon dioxide, which coupled with the lack of oxygen intake (hypoxia) leads to acidosis.
(Objective 4)

39. a. Deaths that occur after 24 hours are referred to as *drowning-related deaths*. Submersion is swimming-related distress that is sufficient to require support in the prehospital setting and transportation to a medical facility for further assessment and care.
(Objective 4)

40. c. Although each factor listed influences patient outcome after submersion, duration of submersion and degree of hypoxia are the critical elements that determine odds of survival.
(Objective 4)

41. a. Dalton's law states that the total pressure of a mixture of gases is equal to the sum of the partial pressures of the component gases. Henry's law states that the amount of gas dissolved in a given volume of fluid is proportional to the pressure of the gas with which it is in equilibrium. Newton's law states that a body at rest will remain at rest until acted on by an outside force, and a body in motion will remain in motion until acted on by an outside force.
(Objective 5)

42. d. As trapped air in the lungs expands on rapid ascent, it ruptures alveoli and allows gas to leak into the subcutaneous tissues.
(Objective 6)

43. b. The neurodepressant effects of nitrogen narcosis may lead to diving accidents resulting from impaired judgment.
(Objective 6)

44. a. Ataxia signals progression of the illness, and coma may result within 24 hours of its onset.
(Objective 6)

WRAP IT UP

1. 18° F (−8° C)
(Objective 1)

2. a, b, d. Conduction causes heat loss from warm skin to cold air or water; convection causes heat loss from the 20 mph wind blowing over; radiation is the heat radiating off his skin.
(Objective 1)

3. b, c, e. Loss of deep tendon reflexes and dilated pupils are signs of severe hypothermia. Shivering typically has stopped by when the patient has moderate hypothermia.
(Objective 3)

4. a. The heart become irritable in hypothermia, and vigorous movement can trigger ventricular fibrillation.
b. The cold liver is unable to metabolize the lactate.
c. Orthostatic hypotension may result if the patient is moved to a sitting position.
(Objective 3)

5. d. Prolonged exposure to very cold water can cause trench foot. He will likely develop signs and symptoms similar to frostbite as he rewarms.
(Objective 3)

Infectious and Communicable Diseases

READING ASSIGNMENT
Chapter 39, pages 1004-1041, in *Mosby's Paramedic Textbook*, ed. 3

OBJECTIVES
Upon completion of this chapter, the paramedic student will be able to:
1. Identify general public health principles related to infectious diseases.
2. Describe the chain of elements necessary for an infectious disease to occur.
3. Explain how internal and external barriers affect susceptibility to infection.
4. Differentiate the four stages of infectious disease: the latent period, the incubation period, the communicability period, and the disease period.
5. Describe the mode of transmission, pathophysiology, prehospital considerations, and personal protective measures to be taken for the human immunodeficiency virus (HIV), hepatitis, tuberculosis, meningococcal meningitis, and pneumonia.
6. Describe the mode of transmission, pathophysiology, signs and symptoms, and prehospital considerations for patients who have rabies or tetanus.
7. List the signs, symptoms, and possible secondary complications of selected childhood viral diseases.
8. List the signs, symptoms, and possible secondary complications of influenza, severe acute respiratory syndrome (SARS), and mononucleosis.
9. Describe the mode of transmission, pathophysiology, prehospital considerations, and personal protective measures for sexually transmitted diseases.
10. Identify the signs and symptoms and prehospital considerations for lice and scabies.
11. Outline the reporting process for exposure to infectious or communicable diseases.
12. Discuss the paramedic's role in preventing disease transmission.

SUMMARY
- National concerns regarding communicable disease and infection control have resulted in public law, standards, guidelines, and recommendations to protect health care providers and emergency responders against infectious diseases. The paramedic must be familiar with these guidelines. He or she also must take personal protective measures against exposure to these pathogens.

- The chain of elements needed to transmit an infectious disease includes the pathogenic agent, a reservoir, a portal of exit from the reservoir, an environment conducive to transmission of the pathogenic agent, a portal of entry into the new host, and susceptibility of the new host to the infectious disease.
- The human body is protected from infectious disease by external and internal barriers. These serve as lines of defense against infection. External barriers include the skin, GI system, upper respiratory tract, and genitourinary tract. Internal barriers include the inflammatory response and the immune response.
- The progression of infectious disease from exposure to the onset of symptoms follows four stages. These are the latent period, the incubation period, the communicability period, and the disease period.
- The human immunodeficiency virus is directly transmitted person to person. This occurs through anal or vaginal intercourse, across the placenta, by contact with infected blood or body fluids on mucous membranes or open wounds, through blood transfusion or tissue transplant, or by the use of contaminated needles or syringes. The virus affects the CD4 T cells. Secondary complications are usually related to opportunistic infections that arise as the immune system deteriorates. The disease progression can be categorized into category A (acute retroviral infection, seroconversion, and asymptomatic infection); category B (early symptomatic HIV); and category C (late symptomatic HIV and advanced HIV). Paramedics should observe strict compliance with universal precautions for protection against HIV. Patient care should include helping these patients feel that they can obtain acceptance and compassion from health care workers.
- Hepatitis is a viral disease. It produces pathologic changes in the liver. The three main classes of hepatitis virus are hepatitis A, hepatitis B, and hepatitis C.
- Tuberculosis is a chronic pulmonary disease. It is acquired by inhaling a tubercle bacilli. The infection is passed mainly by infected persons coughing or sneezing the bacteria into the air or from contact with sputum that contains virulent TB bacilli. The infection is characterized by stages of early infection (frequently asymptomatic), latency, and a potential for recurrent postprimary disease.
- Meningococcal meningitis refers to inflammation of the membranes that surround the spinal cord and brain. It can be caused by bacteria, viruses, and other microorganisms.
- Pneumonia is an acute inflammatory process of the respiratory bronchioles and alveoli. Agents responsible for this disease may be bacterial, viral, or fungal.
- Tetanus is a serious, sometimes fatal, disease of the CNS. It is caused by infection of a wound with spores of the bacterium *Clostridium tetani*. The most common symptom is trismus. This symptom makes it difficult to open the mouth.
- Rabies is an acute viral infection of the CNS. Humans are highly susceptible to the rabies virus after being exposed to saliva from a bite or scratch of an infected animal.
- Hantaviruses are carried by rodents. They are transmitted by inhaling material contaminated with rodent urine and feces. Many forms of this disease occur in specific geographical areas.
- Rubella is a mild, febrile, and highly communicable viral disease. It is characterized by a diffuse punctate macular rash. The CDC recommends that all health care providers receive immunization if they are not immune from previous rubella infection.
- Rubeola is an acute, highly communicable viral disease. (It is caused by the measles virus.) It is characterized by fever, conjunctivitis, cough, bronchitis, and a blotchy red rash.
- Mumps is an acute, communicable systemic viral disease. It is characterized by localized unilateral or bilateral edema of one or more of the salivary glands. There is occasional involvement of other glands.
- Chickenpox is highly communicable. It is characterized by a sudden onset of low-grade fever, mild malaise, and a maculopapular skin eruption for a few hours and vesicular for 3 to 4 days, leaving a granular scab. The virus may reactivate during periods of stress or immunosuppression. At that time, it may produce an illness known as *shingles*.
- Pertussis is an infectious disease that leads to inflammation of the entire respiratory tract. It causes an insidious cough. The cough becomes paroxysmal in 1 to 2 weeks and lasts for 1 to 2 months.
- Influenza is mainly a respiratory infection. It is spread by influenza viruses A, B, and C.
- Severe acute respiratory syndrome (SARS) is a viral illness. It is spread by exposure to infected droplets. It was first detected in 2003. The illness begins with a fever and mild respiratory symptoms. It can progress to respiratory failure and death.
- Mononucleosis is caused either by the Epstein-Barr virus or cytomegalovirus. Both of these are members of the herpesvirus family.

- Syphilis is a systemic disease. It is characterized by a primary lesion; a secondary eruption involving skin and mucous membranes; long latency periods; and eventual seriously disabling lesions of the skin, bone, viscera, CNS, and cardiovascular system.
- Gonorrhea is caused by the sexually transmitted bacterium *Neisseria gonorrhoeae*. Gonorrhea is treatable with antibiotics. However, some strains brought into the United States from other countries do not respond to the usual antibiotic therapy.
- Chlamydia is a major cause of sexually transmitted nonspecific urethritis or genital infection. Signs and symptoms are similar to gonorrhea.
- Herpes simplex virus is transmitted by skin-to-skin contact with an infected area of the body. The primary infection produces a vesicular lesion (blister). This lesion heals spontaneously. After the primary infection, the virus travels to a sensory nerve ganglion. It remains there in a latent stage until reactivated.
- Lice are small, wingless insects that are ectoparasites of birds and mammals. During biting and feeding, secretions from the louse cause a small, red macule and pruritus.
- The human scabies mite is a parasite. It completes its life cycle in and on the epidermis of its host. Scabies bites are usually concentrated around the hands and feet, especially between the webs of the fingers and toes.
- Reporting a possible communicable disease exposure permits immediate medical follow-up. It also enables the designated officer to make changes that might prevent exposures in the future. Moreover, it helps employees to get the proper evaluation and testing.
- Part of the paramedic's professional duty related to infectious disease transmission is to know when not to go to work. Paramedics also have a duty to use the proper BSI at all times.

REVIEW QUESTIONS

Match the infectious diseases listed in Column II with their descriptions in Column I. Use each disease only once.

Column I	Column II
1. ـــــ Infection that produces influenza-like symptoms, dark-colored urine, and light-colored stools	a. Chlamydia
	b. Gonorrhea
	c. Hepatitis
2. ـــــ Macular rash that can cause severe birth defects if a susceptible mother is exposed in pregnancy	d. Herpes simplex
	e. Human immunodeficiency virus
3. ـــــ Bacterial pulmonary infection spread by airborne droplets	f. Meningitis
	g. Rubella
4. ـــــ Viral infection that impairs the ability of the body to fight other infectious disease	h. Syphilis
	i. Tuberculosis
5. ـــــ Sexually transmitted disease characterized in the early stage by a painless chancre	j. Varicella
6. ـــــ Inflammation of lining of the central nervous system that may produce headache, stiff neck, seizures, and coma	
7. ـــــ Bacterial infection that produces mucopurulent discharge but rarely causes septicemia	
8. _____ Generalized illness accompanied by vesicular lesions, fever, and malaise	

9. List the six components of the chain of elements that must be present for an infectious disease to occur.

    a.

    b.

    c.

    d.

    e.

    f.

10. Describe two situations that interfere with the external bodily barriers to infection, thereby increasing the risk of infection.

   a.

   b.

11. Name two factors that can affect the ability of the internal barriers of the body to fight infectious disease.

   a.

   b.

12. For each of the following patient care scenarios, describe the personal protective measures that you should take.

   a. A 23-year-old woman is about to deliver her fourth child. The baby's head is crowning, and you are preparing for delivery.

   _____

   b. A 50-year-old man is complaining of severe substernal chest pain. You are preparing to initiate an intravenous line to administer medications.

   _____

   c. You are preparing to administer epinephrine subcutaneously to a 25-year-old patient with dyspnea because of anaphylaxis.

   _____

   d. A 17-year-old girl ingested a large amount of alcohol and barbiturates, vomited, and rapidly lost consciousness. You elect to intubate her trachea.

   _____

   e. A 55-year-old man attempted suicide by holding a shotgun under his chin and firing. He is combative and thrashes about as you try to control the large amount of bleeding and secure his airway.

   _____

   f. A butcher sustained a laceration to her hand at work. The wound is oozing a small amount of blood.

   _____

Questions 13 to 16 refer to the following case study:

   While caring for a 40-year-old man who has nausea, vomiting, right upper quadrant abdominal pain, and jaundice, you puncture your finger with a needle contaminated with the patient's blood. The hospital notifies you the next day that he tested positive for hepatitis.

13. What type or types of hepatitis can produce the symptoms experienced by this patient?

   _____

14. What are the most effective measures you can take to prevent yourself from becoming infected with hepatitis at work?

   _____

15. Describe the modes of transmission for hepatitis B.

   _____

16. Can you do anything now that you are exposed so that you will not get hepatitis?

_____

17. What signs and symptoms may be evident on the prehospital examination of a patient in each of the following stages of infection from the human immunodeficiency virus?

   a. Acute retroviral infection:

_____

   b. Asymptomatic infection:

_____

   c. Early symptomatic infection:

_____

   d. Late symptomatic infection:

_____

18. You are transporting a patient with human immunodeficiency virus to the hospital after he sustained a sprained ankle at a volleyball game. No other injuries are evident.

   a. What personal protective measures should you take while caring for this patient?

_____

   b. How should the ambulance be cleaned before transport of the next patient?

_____

19. What is the best way for emergency care workers to monitor whether they have been exposed to a patient with tuberculosis?

_____

20. A 23-year-old man has a severe headache and a temperature of 102° F (38.9° C) and complained earlier of a stiff neck. Now he is limp and arouses only to a loud voice. You suspect meningitis.

   a. What personal protective measures should you use on this call? (You plan to initiate an intravenous line and apply oxygen by mask.)

_____

   b. If the emergency department contacts you later to inform you that the patient has bacterial meningitis, should you report an exposure?

_____

   c. What is the likelihood that you will be given prophylaxis if you have used appropriate body substance isolation from the beginning of this call?

_____

21. List three chronic signs or symptoms that may develop if syphilis is untreated for a number of years.

    a.

    b.

    c.

22. What personal protective measures should be taken when examining the mouth of a child with an outbreak of herpes simplex on the lips?

23. For each of the following ailments, list the signs and symptoms and site of infestation:

    a. Pubic lice:

_____

    b. Head lice:

_____

    c. Scabies:

_____

Questions 24 to 26 refer to the following case study:

You transport a child who has a temperature of 101° F (38.3° C) and a generalized skin rash that began the previous day. Some lesions are flat and red, some are raised blisters, and others have scabbed. On arrival to the emergency department, the pediatrician confirms that the child has chickenpox.

24. Is this disease communicable at this stage?

_____

25. If you have never had chickenpox, how long would you expect to wait before symptoms appear?

_____

26. Are you contagious during this entire time?

_____

Questions 27 to 35 refer to the following case study:

During your care of a patient at the scene of a motor-vehicle crash, you had blood splash into your eyes while your partner was intubating the patient and you were holding in-line immobilization of the cervical spine. You had gloves on at the time.

27. Has a significant exposure to blood or body fluids occurred?

_____

28. When should you report this exposure?

_____

29. Besides evaluation for postexposure prophylaxis, what other emergency care will you need in this situation?

_____

The patient refuses to give permission to test for human immunodeficiency virus.

30. Can the emergency department ignore the patient's refusal and run a test for human immunodeficiency virus in this situation? Why?

_____

31. What other questions should you ask the patient?

_____

32. What are your options for postexposure prophylaxis if the patient refuses testing?

_____

_____

33. After counseling and examination by the emergency department staff, you are offered a course of medicine for postexposure prophylaxis. How will you decide whether to take the medicine?

_____

34. Why do you think some paramedics might need psychological counseling after this incident?

_____

35. How could this exposure have been prevented?

_____

STUDENT SELF-ASSESSMENT

36. Which agency is responsible for establishing the guidelines for body substance isolation and universal (standard) precautions?
   a. Centers for Disease Control
   b. Department of Health
   c. Department of Transportation
   d. Occupational Safety and Health Administration

37. Which of the following could be used to interrupt the portal of entry in the chain of elements of an infectious disease?
   a. Administering antibiotics to kill a bacterium
   b. Cleaning a blood spill with an appropriate agent
   c. Receiving immunizations at appropriate intervals
   d. Using gloves as defined in the body substance isolation guidelines

38. Which of the following is an internal barrier to infection?
   a. Flora
   b. Leukocytes
   c. Nasal hairs
   d. Prostatic fluid

39. The internal defense that provides antibodies to destroy invading organisms is produced by which of the following?
   a. Cell-mediated immunity
   b. Complement
   c. Humoral immunity
   d. Killer cells

40. The infectious disease phase that begins when the agent invades the body and ends when the disease process begins is which period?
   a. Communicability
   b. Disease
   c. Incubation
   d. Latent

41. Death caused by hepatitis is most likely to occur from which strain of the virus?
   a. Hepatitis A
   b. Hepatitis B
   c. Hepatitis C
   d. Non-A, non-B hepatitis

42. What type of organism causes hepatitis?
    a. Bacteria
    b. Fungus
    c. Parasite
    d. Virus
43. Which sign or symptom can help to distinguish pneumonia from other respiratory illness?
    a. Fatigue and loss of appetite
    b. Headache and muscle aches
    c. Shaking chills and chest pain
    d. Yellow mucus from productive cough
44. Which of the following is a classic sign or symptom of tetanus?
    a. Flaccid paralysis
    b. Seizures
    c. Trismus
    d. Urticaria
45. What is the reaction causing muscle spasms that prevents a patient with rabies from drinking called?
    a. Hydropenia
    b. Hydrophobia
    c. Polydipsia
    d. Polyuria
46. What is the primary mode of transmission for rubella, mumps, and varicella?
    a. Blood-to-blood contact
    b. Fecal contamination
    c. Lesion contact
    d. Respiratory droplets
47. Complications of varicella may include all of the following *except* which disease?
    a. Bacterial infection
    b. Croup
    c. Meningitis
    d. Reye's syndrome
48. Which treatment measure usually is given to patients with chickenpox, influenza, or herpes simplex?
    a. Antibiotic therapy
    b. Aspirin for pain and fever
    c. Comfort measures
    d. Intravenous therapy
49. Which childhood disease is characterized by a violent cough that can persist for 1 to 2 months?
    a. Influenza
    b. Mumps
    c. Pertussis
    d. Pneumonia
50. What secondary complication of influenza often is associated with severe illness or death?
    a. Aspiration
    b. Dehydration
    c. Meningitis
    d. Pneumonia
51. Which sign or symptom associated with mononucleosis could produce a life-threatening condition if the patient is not maintained at rest?
    a. Fever
    b. Lymphadenopathy
    c. Oral rash
    d. Splenomegaly
52. A patient has a headache, malaise, fever, lymphadenopathy, and a symmetrical rash that involves the palms and soles. He states that an ulcerated sore on his penis healed spontaneously 3 weeks earlier. Which infectious disease do you suspect?
    a. Chlamydia
    b. Gonorrhea
    c. Herpes
    d. Syphilis
53. Which body system harbors the dormant herpesvirus?
    a. Cardiovascular system
    b. Gastrointestinal system
    c. Integumentary system
    d. Nervous system
54. Which of the following is the most effective measure that you can take to prevent the spread of severe acute respiratory syndrome?
    a. Antibiotic treatment if exposure is suspected
    b. Hand washing and respiratory protection
    c. Immunization with a pneumonia vaccine
    d. Treatment with bronchodilator drugs

WRAP IT UP

You are dispatched to a store for "difficulty breathing." The patient is a thin 40-year-old who bystanders say lives in the adjacent park. The man is coughing vigorously, and you note a strong smell of whiskey as you approach him. His vital signs are BP 142/88 mm Hg, P 104, R28, SaO_2 92%, so you apply a nasal cannula. He is cooperative but has slurred speech and tells you that he just cannot seem to catch his breath, so you listen and hear diffuse, coarse crackles in his lungs. You note some purple skin lesions around his bare feet, which he says are numb, and his mouth is coated with white plaque. His arms and feet are scarred with old track marks. Although initially reluctant to tell you much about his history, when you move him to the ambulance, he discloses that he has AIDS. He says he has not been compliant with his medications and has not been to see a doctor for about 6 months. When you ask about this cough and dyspnea, the patient says that it has been going on for about 3 months and that he has lost weight, has night sweats, and now is coughing up blood. You and your partner don N-95 HEPA masks, replace the patient's nasal cannula with an oxygen face mask, and open the window in the back of the ambulance. As you move the patient to the ER stretcher, he has a coughing spasm and expectorates a large amount of bloody sputum, which sprays into your face and eyes. You immediately wash with soap and water and have the ED staff irrigate your eyes. After contacting your supervisor, the appropriate exposure reporting papers are completed, and after the patient's HIV and tuberculosis risk factors and health status is determined, the ED physician sits down to explain your options. You are told the benefits and risks of tuberculosis and HIV transmission by this exposure, and the side effects associated with the prophylactic drugs. You decide to take the prophylactic drugs, and subsequently miss the next 2 days of work sick from them. Your pregnant wife is upset and fearful that she may become HIV positive. In 6 months and finally a year, the HIV screening tests come back negative, and at last you stop waking in the night, fearful that you will contract this life-threatening illness.

1. What additional personal protective measure(s) could have decreased your risk for this exposure?

2. Identify (a) each of the elements in the chain of transmission of infectious disease that are present on this call and (b) actions that were taken to reduce the risk of transmission at some links in the chain.

Link	How is it present on this call?	Actions taken to reduce the risk of transmission?
Pathogenic agent(s)		
Reservoir		
Portal of exit		
Transmission		
Host susceptibility		

3. Place a check mark beside the complications of human immunodeficiency virus or acquired immunodeficiency syndrome that are seen in this patient.
   a. _____ *Candida*
   b. _____ Dementia
   c. _____ Kaposi sarcoma
   d. _____ Pulmonary tuberculosis
   e. _____ *Pneumocystis carinii* pneumonia
   f. _____ Sensory neuropathy
   g. _____ Wasting syndrome

4. What risk factors does this patient have for tuberculosis?

5. Which is true regarding follow-up after infectious disease exposure?
   a. If proper immunizations have been obtained, medical follow-up is not needed.
   b. Prophylaxis should not be taken without information regarding risks and benefits.
   c. Reporting should be deferred until the end of the paramedic's shift.
   d. The final decision regarding prophylaxis is the choice of the treating physician.

REVIEW QUESTIONS

1. c
   (Objective 5)

2. g
   (Objective 7)

3. i
   (Objective 5)

4. e
   (Objective 5)

5. h
   (Objective 9)

6. f
   (Objective 5)

7. b
   (Objective 9)

8. j
   (Objective 9)

9. A pathological agent, a reservoir, a portal of exit from the reservoir, an environment conducive to transmission of the pathogenic agent, portal of entry, and susceptibility of the new host to the infectious disease
   (Objective 2)

10. Burns, lacerations, abrasions, intravenous therapy, and urinary catheter
    (Objective 3)

11. Human immunodeficiency virus, chemotherapy, and prolonged steroid therapy
    (Objective 3)

12. a. Gloves, gown, mask, and eyewear
    b. Gloves
    c. Nothing is necessary according to the Centers for Disease Control and Prevention; however, if bleeding is likely and because the prehospital setting is high risk, gloves are indicated.
    d. Gloves, mask, and eyewear
    e. Gloves, gown, mask, and eyewear
    f. Gloves
    (Objective 1)

13. Hepatitis A, B, or C
    (Objective 5)

14. Take hepatitis B virus vaccination, and use strict universal (body substance isolation) precautions as warranted by each situation.
    (Objectives 1 and 5)

15. Direct introduction of infected blood by needle or transfusion, introduction of serum or plasma through skin cuts, absorption of infected serum or plasma through mucosal surfaces, absorption of saliva or semen through mucosal surfaces, and transfer of infective serum or plasma via inanimate surfaces
(Objective 5)

16. Yes. If the patient is found to have hepatitis A, you may be given an immune globulin injection. If he has hepatitis B and if you are not immune to the hepatitis B virus, a hepatitis B virus vaccine will be given to protect against future exposures, and hepatitis B immune globulin will be given to provide temporary passive immunity to the hepatitis B virus. No immunization or immune globulin exists that is effective to prevent hepatitis C.
(Objective 5)

17. a. Fever, swollen lymph nodes, and sore throat; b. enlarged lymph nodes; c. bacterial pneumonia, oral lesions, shingles, and pulmonary tuberculosis; d. diarrhea, tumors, dementia, neurological symptoms, and opportunistic infections
(Objective 5)

18. a. You should take the same precautions you would take with any patient with this type of injury. If no open wounds are present, no body substance isolation is indicated.
b. Clean the ambulance as you would after any patient.
(Objectives 1 and 5)

19. Periodic skin test with purified protein derivative (of tuberculin) and chest x-ray study if purified protein derivative (of tuberculin) test is positive or other history exists indicating the need
(Objective 5)

20. a. Gloves and mask (respiratory spread); wear eye shield if risk of splash or spray exists (for example, if the patient vomits or needs to be intubated)
b. An exposure should be reported if you did not have appropriate personal protective equipment on or if you had contact with blood or body fluids.
c. The need for prophylaxis will be determined by your occupational health provider but is not likely indicated if all body substance isolation precautions were used for the entire call.
(Objective 5)

21. Paresis, wide gait, ataxia, psychosis, and signs of myocardial insufficiency
(Objective 9)

22. Gloves (mask and protective eyewear if any risk of splash or spray of body fluids exists)
(Objective 1)

23. a. Pubic lice look like crabs or gray-blue spots, and nits appear on abdomen, thighs, eyelashes, eyebrows, and axillary hair.
b. Head lice have an elongated body with narrow head and three pair of legs, and nits look like dandruff that cannot be brushed off.
c. Scabies produces bites concentrated around webs of hands and feet, a child's face and scalp, a female's nipples, and a male's penis, and vesicles and papules that become easily infected because of scratching.
(Objective 10)

24. Yes. Chickenpox is contagious for 1 to 2 days before the onset of the rash until all of the lesions are crusted and dry.
(Objective 7)

25. 13 to 17 days
(Objective 7)

26. Varicella can be transmitted 1 to 2 days before eruption of the rash until the lesions have all scabbed over. (Objective 5)

27. Yes. Blood that came in contact with your mucous membranes is a significant exposure. (Objective 5)

28. Immediately report the exposure as soon as you arrive at the hospital with the patient. If you did not transport the patient to the hospital, you should go there immediately (or follow your local protocol). (Objective 5)

29. You should irrigate your eyes immediately after the eye splash exposure. (Objective 5)

30. No. The emergency department cannot ignore the patient's request. The patient has the legal right to refuse a test for human immunodeficiency virus. (Objective 5)

31. Ask if the patient has human immunodeficiency virus and assess for risk factors that would indicate the potential for such infection (intravenous drug use, unsafe sex practices). (Objective 5)

32. The emergency department or occupational medicine staff still may offer you prophylactic drug treatment based on the nature of the exposure and the patient's risk factors (antiviral and possibly protease inhibitor drugs). (Objective 5)

33. The benefits to you (risk of human immunodeficiency virus infection) versus complications of the prophylaxis therapy based on your personal health status will need to be weighed before you decide whether to take the medicine. (Objective 5)

34. For a year, you will undergo periodic evaluation to determine whether you have converted to HIV-positive status. Until that time, you should alter your sexual practices and discontinue breast-feeding if you are lactating. This can be a difficult time for paramedics and their significant others, wondering if the next test will be positive. Counseling may provide an opportunity to verbalize those feelings in a healthful manner. (Objective 5)

35. Use of eye shield and face mask likely would have prevented this exposure. (Objectives 5 and 12)

36. a. The Centers for Disease Control and Prevention establishes guidelines that often are adopted by the Occupational Safety and Health Administration and are incorporated by agencies such as the Department of Health and Department of Transportation into other documents (for example, National Standard Paramedic Curriculum). (Objective 1)

37. d. All of the answers reflect something that could break a link in the chain of transmission. Antibiotics can kill the pathogenic agent; cleaning agents with appropriate disinfectants destroy the environment conducive to transmission; immunizations decrease host susceptibility. (Objective 2)

38. b. All other answers are external barriers to infection. (Objective 3)

39. c. Antibodies can fix complement. Killer cells are part of cell-mediated immunity.
(Objective 3)

40. c. The communicability period begins when the latent period ends and continues as long as the agent is present and can spread to others. The latent period begins with invasion of the body and ends when the agent can be shed or communicated. The disease period follows the incubation period and has variable lengths.
(Objective 4)

41. b. Short- and long-term mortality is higher from hepatitis B.
(Objective 2)

42. d
(Objective 2)

43. c. The patient with pneumonia also may have all of the other signs and symptoms.
(Objective 5)

44. c. Trismus (lockjaw) often occurs and makes opening the mouth difficult. The patient often has muscle tetany and spasms but not urticaria or seizures.
(Objective 6)

45. b. Hydropenia is a lack of water in tissues; polydipsia is increased thirst; and polyuria is increased urination.
(Objective 6)

46. d
(Objective 7)

47. b
(Objective 7)

48. c. Antibiotic therapy would be indicated only if a secondary bacterial infection develops. Aspirin is contraindicated for children and patients with chickenpox. Intravenous therapy would be needed only if an acute complication of these viral illnesses develops.
(Objectives 7, 8, and 9)

49. c. Influenza and pneumonia can produce cough; however, they do not persist as long as pertussis.
(Objective 7)

50. d. Pneumonia is an especially dangerous secondary complication for patients who are elderly or have preexisting lung or heart disease.
(Objective 8)

51. d. The enlarged spleen increases the chance of injury if the patient sustains a blow to the abdomen.
(Objective 8)

52. d. Syphilis is associated with systemic and chronic signs and symptoms.
(Objective 9)

53. d. The virus migrates along the sensory nerve pathways and remains in a latent stage on the ganglion.
(Objective 9)

54. b. There is no vaccine to prevent severe acute respiratory syndrome, nor is the disease treatable with antibiotics. Bronchodilators may be used to manage signs and symptoms of severe acute respiratory syndrome but do not prevent its spread.
(Objective 8)

WRAP IT UP

1. Protective eyewear could have prevented this exposure.
   (Objective 5)

2.

Link	How is it present on this call?	Actions taken to reduce the risk of transmission?
Pathogenic agent(s)	Human immunodeficiency virus, tuberculosis (bacteria)	Face washed with soap and water; eyes irrigated
Reservoir	Patient in poor heath	Mask on patient
Portal of exit	Cough with bloody sputum	Mask on patient
Transmission	Cough with bloody sputum	Mask on patient, N-95 mask, gloves, on paramedics, window open in ambulance
Host susceptibility		Human immunodeficiency virus, tuberculosis prophylaxis drugs

(Objective 2)

3. a (white, coated tongue), b (slurred speech, confusion), c (skin discoloration on feet), d (cough, hemoptysis, night sweats), f (numbness in feet), g (thin, wasted appearance)
   (Objective 5)

4. Alcohol use, intravenous drug user (or former user), positive for human immunodeficiency virus, homeless
   (Objective 5)

5. b. Follow-up should be initiated as soon as possible after the exposure for maximum effectiveness. The paramedic should make the decision after being given adequate information about risks/benefits of treatment.
   (Objective 11)

40

Behavioral and Psychiatric Disorders

READING ASSIGNMENT

Chapter 40, pages 1042-1061, in *Mosby's Paramedic Textbook,* ed. 3

OBJECTIVES

Upon completion of this chapter, the paramedic student will be able to:

1. Define what constitutes a behavioral emergency.
2. Identify potential causes for behavioral and psychiatric illnesses.
3. List three critical principles that should be considered in the prehospital care of any patient with a behavioral emergency.
4. Outline key elements in the prehospital patient examination during a behavioral emergency.
5. Describe effective techniques for interviewing a patient during a behavioral emergency.
6. Distinguish between key symptoms and management techniques for selected behavioral and psychiatric disorders.
7. Identify factors that must be considered when assessing suicide risk.
8. Formulate appropriate interview questions to determine suicidal intent.
9. Explain prehospital management techniques for the patient who has attempted suicide.
10. Describe assessment of the potentially violent patient.
11. Outline measures that may be used in an attempt to safely diffuse a potentially violent patient situation.
12. List situations when patient restraints can be used.
13. Discuss key principles in patient restraint.
14. Describe safety measures taken when patient violence is anticipated.
15. Explain variations in approach to behavioral emergencies in children.

SUMMARY

- A behavioral emergency is a change in mood or behavior. This change cannot be tolerated by the involved person or others. It calls for immediate attention.
- Physical or biochemical disturbances can result in significant changes in behavior. Psychosocial mental illness is often the result of childhood trauma, parental deprivation, or a dysfunctional family structure.
- Changes in behavior caused by interpersonal or situational stress are often linked to specific incidents, such as environmental violence, death of a loved one, economic or employment problems, or prejudice and discrimination.

- When dealing with behavioral emergencies, the paramedic should contain the crisis. He or she should provide the proper emergency care as well. Also, the paramedic should transport the patient to an appropriate health care facility.
- During the patient assessment, an attempt should be made to determine the patient's mental state, name and age, significant past medical history, medications (and compliance), and past psychiatric problems, as well as the precipitating situation or problem.
- Effective interviewing techniques include active listening, being supportive and empathetic, limiting interruptions, and respecting the patient's personal space.
- All cognitive disorders result in a disturbance in thinking that may manifest as delirium or dementia.
- Schizophrenia is characterized by recurrent episodes of psychotic behavior. This behavior may include abnormalities of thought process, thought content, perception, and judgment.
- Anxiety disorders may cause a panic attack. Anxiety disorders include phobias, obsessive-compulsive disorders, and posttraumatic syndrome.
- Depression is an impairment of normal functioning. A person with depression may have feelings of hopelessness, loss of appetite, decreased libido, and feelings of worthlessness and guilt.
- Bipolar disorder is a manic-depressive illness. In this illness, depressive and manic episodes alternate with one another.
- Somatoform disorders are conditions in which there are physical symptoms for which no physical cause can be found. The cause is thought to be psychological. These include somatization disorder and conversion disorder.
- Factitious disorders are disorders in which symptoms mimic a true illness. However, the symptoms have been invented. They are under the control of the patient.
- Dissociative disorders are a group of psychological illnesses. In these disorders, a particular mental function is separated from the mind as a whole.
- The most common eating disorders considered to be forms of psychiatric illness are anorexia nervosa and bulimia nervosa.
- Impulse control disorders are characterized by the inability to resist an impulse or temptation to do some act that is unlawful, socially unacceptable, or self-harmful.
- Personality disorders are conditions characterized by failing to learn from experience or adapt appropriately to changes. This results in personal distress and impairment of social functioning.
- A threat of suicide is an indication that a patient has a serious crisis. This crisis requires immediate intervention.
- Questions that determine the patient's ideation, plan, intent, and means to commit suicide should be asked.
- After ensuring scene safety, the first priority in patient management after a suicide attempt is medical care. If the patient is conscious, developing rapport as soon as possible is crucial.
- Assessment of a potentially violent patient should include past history of violence, posture, vocal activity, and physical activity.
- When trying to defuse a situation involving a potentially violent patient, the paramedic should ensure a safe environment, gather the patient's history, try to gain the patient's cooperation, avoid threats, and explain the paramedic's role in providing care.
- Severely disturbed patients who pose a threat to themselves or others may need to be restrained.
- Reasonable force to restrain a patient should be used as humanely as possible. An adequate number of personnel is needed. This will ensure patient and rescuer safety during restraint. The risk of personal injury and legal liability is always present.
- Personal safety measures while responding to a behavioral emergency should include not allowing the patient to block the exit, keeping large furniture between you and the patient, working as a team, avoiding threatening statements, and using soft objects to absorb the impact of thrown objects.
- When caring for children with behavioral emergencies, the paramedic should attempt to gain their trust, tell them they won't be hurt, keep questions brief, be honest, involve parents (if appropriate), and take threats of violence seriously.

REVIEW QUESTIONS

Match the psychiatric conditions in Column II with their descriptions in Column I. Use each condition only once.

Column I

1. _____ Feelings of worthlessness and guilt
2. _____ Unfounded fear of situation or object
3. _____ Loss of touch with reality in this major mental disorder
4. _____ Loss of sensory or motor function without organic cause
5. _____ Excessive elation, irritability, talkativeness, and delusions
6. _____ Logical, highly developed delusions

Column II

a. Conversion hysteria
b. Depression
c. Mania
d. Neurosis
e. Panic attack
f. Paranoia
g. Phobia
h. Psychosis

7. You arrive at the home of a 60-year-old man whose behavior is erratic. He alternates between hysterical bursts of laughter, irritability, sitting quietly, and crying. You find metformin HCL (Glucophage), hydralazine, and thyroxine in the medicine chest and note an ecchymotic area on his left temple. His skin is hot and moist. Based on this patient's history, what are some likely organic causes of his behavior that must be ruled out before assuming that this is a behavioral emergency?

_____

_____

_____

8. a. List three psychosocial causes of mental illness.

_____

b. List three sociocultural causes of mental illness.

_____

Questions 9 to 11 refer to the following patient case study:

You are called to a private residence to care for a behavioral emergency. Police report that the patient is "OBS." On arrival, you find a 34-year-old woman sitting quietly in a living room chair. She is complaining of depression.

9. What four general management principles should you consider on this and all behavioral calls?

a.

b.

c.

d.

10. What should your scene survey include?

_____

_____

11. What minimum patient data should be obtained if possible?

_____

_____

12. Should a detailed secondary survey be performed on a patient with a behavioral emergency?

13. Complete the missing information in the following table.

Illness	Classification	Clinical Presentation	Treatment (Medical or EMS)
Dementia			
Schizophrenia			
Posttraumatic syndrome			
Bipolar disorder			
Somatization disorder			
Bulimia nervosa			

14. A patient with a phobia of heights must be rescued by ladder from a high bridge. What measures can you take to prevent a panic attack?

15. A manic patient is being transported to the hospital for psychiatric evaluation. Describe effective patient management techniques in this situation.

16. Family members call you to the home of a 25-year-old man who has become increasingly out of touch with reality. He feels that aliens are trying to kidnap him so that they can remove his brain. He tells you that they are trying to control his thoughts. He states, "They're here. Can't you hear them laughing?"

a. What behavioral illness does this presentation suggest?

b. What approach will enable therapeutic communication with this patient?

17. You are on the scene with a 25-year-old woman who cut her wrist with a razor blade. She is crying, "Let me go. Why didn't you let me do it?" She has a small laceration with controlled bleeding, minimal blood loss, and stable vital signs.

a. How can you best assess the patient's suicidal risk?

b. What are your goals in caring for this patient during transport?

Questions 18 to 22 refer to the following case study:

A distraught family calls you to take their son to the hospital for a court-ordered, involuntary psychiatric evaluation. They state that he has been breaking furniture for the past few hours and refuses to take his antipsychotic drugs.

18. What four factors should you assess rapidly to determine the potential for violence in this patient?

a.

b.

c.

d.

Your patient is pacing, is verbally abusive, and is threatening injury to those who approach. He is not armed.

19. You elect to restrain him. What help should you request?

_____

20. When approaching the patient to prepare for restraint, what should you note about the physical environment?

_____

21. Assuming that the patient meets the standard for involuntary detention in your state, how should he be restrained (including position and ways to secure extremities and torso)?

_____

_____

22. After restraints are applied, what should you monitor en route to the hospital?

_____

STUDENT SELF-ASSESSMENT

23. What is a change in mood or behavior that cannot be tolerated by the involved person or others and needs immediate attention called?
  a. Behavioral emergency
  b. Delusion
  c. Neurosis
  d. Psychosis

24. What is the characteristic of abnormal (maladaptive) behavior?
  a. Deviates from the person's normal behavior
  b. Does not conform to your idea of normal behavior
  c. Interferes with a person's ability to function
  d. Violates a societal law

25. Which of the following questions would be most appropriate to begin a conversation with a mentally ill patient?
  a. Did you start feeling this way today?
  b. Are you feeling bad now?
  c. How did this all begin?
  d. Are you okay?

26. Which response by the paramedic is most likely to lead to an effective interview in the prehospital setting?
  a. Everything will be fine.
  b. I know exactly how you feel.
  c. Yes, I see those scary bugs too.
  d. You look very sad.

27. Which condition is a state of acute mental confusion commonly brought on by a physical illness?
  a. Delirium
  b. Delusions
  c. Dementia
  d. Depression

28. A middle-aged woman suddenly loses the ability to speak after catching her husband in an extramarital affair. What behavioral illness may have caused her problem?
  a. Conversion hysteria
  b. Depression
  c. Panic attack
  d. Phobia

29. Which of the following feelings commonly characterizes depression?
    a. Hopelessness
    b. Hunger
    c. Increased libido
    d. Restlessness

30. You are transporting a man who believes he is Elvis Presley. His wife states that he quit his job, keeps calling her Priscilla, and is preparing to move to Graceland. You suspect that he is suffering from which of the following?
    a. Delusions
    b. Neurosis
    c. Paranoia
    d. Phobia

31. A panic attack typically occurs with any of the following *except* which symptom?
    a. Chest pain and vertigo
    b. Hyperventilation
    c. Suicidal intent
    d. Trembling and sweating

32. What is the highest priority on a suicide call?
    a. Ensuring safety of crew members
    b. Managing life threats
    c. Talking the person out of it
    d. Listening empathetically

33. Which of the following statements regarding suicide is true?
    a. Those who talk about killing themselves rarely do it.
    b. Men commit suicide more often than women.
    c. Suicide is an inherited tendency.
    d. When depression lifts, suicide risk disappears.

34. When should a violent patient be released from physical restraints?
    a. Immediately after administration of haloperidol intramuscularly
    b. As soon as the patient assures cooperation
    c. When the police have adequate personnel to control the patient
    d. When a physician at the hospital determines the patient is no longer dangerous

35. You are caring for a violent psychiatric patient. Which of the following drugs would *not* be appropriate for chemical restraint?
    a. Diazepam
    b. Diphenhydramine
    c. Haloperidol
    d. Lorazepam

36. Which strategy should be used to maintain emergency medical services crew safety when on a behavioral emergency call?
    a. Be firm and tell the patient to behave or you will have to use restraints.
    b. Interview the patient privately while your partner waits outside of the room.
    c. Kneel and put your arm on the patient's shoulder to show you care.
    d. Stay closer to the exit than the patient, with furniture between you and the patient.

37. Which strategy will be helpful when caring for a child who is experiencing a behavioral emergency?
    a. Avoid having the parents present during care.
    b. Do not be concerned about the possibility of violence.
    c. Keep the interview questions brief.
    d. Lie if you need to gain cooperation.

WRAP IT UP

You immediately recognize your patient when you arrive at the call. "Herb" is a 30-year-old homeless man with a history of schizophrenia. He is in and out of treatment facilities, and he is difficult to predict. When he is taking his medications, he is usually reasonable, but when he runs out of his medications or chooses not to take them, he can be dangerous. The police are with him and have called because he was threatening to kill himself. You introduce yourself, call him by name, and ask how he is feeling. He says, "The voices are telling me to end it all." "What do you mean by end it all?" you ask. "Kill myself you silly, x#@$er," he replies, "What did you think I meant?" His voice tone gets louder as he speaks, and he begins to lean forward menacingly toward you. "I'm here to help you, Herb," you tell him. "Have you thought about how you would do it?" you ask. "Hanging, it's what the voices say I should do," he replies, "that's why I'm headed to the park, lots of good trees for it over there." "Herb, we'd like to take you to the hospital to get you some medicine so you don't hurt yourself," you explain. With that, he suddenly lunges toward you, screaming, "You'll never get me to go back to that place." With police assistance, you subdue him and restrain him supine on your cot, where he continues to struggle forcefully. Then, with the approval of online medical direction, you administer haloperidol intramuscularly. You manage to get a pulse oximeter reading every few minutes and monitor his respirations carefully. Just as you arrive at the hospital, 30 minutes later, you note marked relaxation, and his voice calms. You give report to the ED staff and assist them to secure him to their stretcher after the physician briefly examines him. As you return to the station, you express your frustration about this patient to your partner: it just doesn't seem right that they can't find a treatment to make him well for more than a month or so at a time.

1. What clues led you to believe that the patient's behavior might become violent?

_____

2. Which of the following is true regarding schizophrenia?
   a. It is more common in men than women.

_____

   b. It typically resolves when the patient is in his or her 40s.

_____

   c. Delusions and auditory hallucinations are common.

_____

   d. Suicide rarely is associated with this disease.

_____

3. Explain why asking a patient directly about suicidal intent would or would not be a helpful strategy.

_____

4. Explain your rationale for administering haloperidol.

_____

CHAPTER 40 ANSWERS

REVIEW QUESTIONS

1. b
2. g
3. h
4. a
5. c
6. f
   (Questions 1 to 6, Objective 5)

7. Metformin (Glucophage) indicates that he is diabetic; assess for hypoglycemia or hyperglycemia. Thyroxine is prescribed for thyroid disorders, which can cause behavioral alterations. Treatment with hydralazine suggests he has a history of hypertension or heart disease, so he may have had a transient ischemic attack, stroke, or cardiac dysrhythmia. The ecchymotic area on his head could indicate cerebral injury from trauma, causing his behavior. His warm, moist skin could indicate many problems. If he has a fever, an infectious process will have to be ruled out as a cause for his mental status change.
   (Objective 2)

8. a. Childhood trauma, parental deprivation, or a dysfunctional family structure
   b. War, riots, rape, assault, death of a loved one, economic and employment problems, or prejudice and discrimination
   (Objective 2)

9. a. Ensure scene safety.
   b. Contain the crisis.
   c. Render appropriate emergency care.
   d. Transport to the appropriate medical facility.
   (Objective 3)

10. Look for evidence of violence, substance abuse, a suicide attempt, and any weapons that may be accessible to the patient.
    (Objective 4)

11. The patient's mental status, name, age, significant medical history, medications, allergies, and the precipitating event for this crisis should be ascertained from the patient, family, or other bystanders.
    (Objective 4)

12. The need to perform a physical assessment should be guided by your initial patient interview. If no possibility to exacerbate a violent situation arises and no life threat exists, the survey can be deferred until you arrive at the hospital. Bulky clothing and bags should be examined for the presence of weapons by law enforcement before transport.
    (Objective 4)

13.

Illness	Classification	Clinical Presentation	Treatment (Medical or EMS)
Dementia	Cognitive disorder	General decline in mental functioning; inability for self-care	Medical interventions
Schizophrenia	Schizophrenia	Recurrent psychotic behavior; abnormal thought processes, delusions, hallucinations, poor judgment	Drug therapy; paramedic should be friendly but neutral; do not respond to anger or speak to family in hushed tones; be firm, maintain personal safety.

Illness	Classification	Clinical Presentation	Treatment (Medical or EMS)
Posttraumatic syndrome	Anxiety disorder	Reaction to severe psychosocial event producing depression, sleep disturbances, nightmares, survivor guilt	Psychotherapy; medication
Bipolar disorder	Mood disorder	Alternating depressive and manic behaviors	Medications; paramedic should be calm and provide firm emotional support; minimize stimulation (no lights or sirens)
Somatization disorder	Somatoform disorder	Chronic physical complaints without any physical problems identified; associated with anxiety, depression	Psychotherapy
Bulimia nervosa	Eating disorder	Binge eating followed by purging (vomiting or laxatives), depression, self-deprivation	Medication, psychotherapy, hospitalization

(Objective 5)

14. Talk through the steps (rehearse) of the rescue slowly and calmly with the patient.
(Objective 5)

15. Provide calm, firm, emotional support, and minimize sensory stimuli.
(Objective 6)

16. a. Schizophrenia or paranoia is suggested by this presentation.
b. Be friendly but neutral; modulate your voice so that it does not get louder if the patient does. Do not talk to the family in whispers. Use firmness and tact to guide the patient to the ambulance. Consider asking for police assistance if you suspect a risk of violence.
(Objective 5)

17. a. Ask, "Why did you do that? Were you trying to kill yourself?" Determine whether she had a plan (did she leave a note or call significant others to say good-bye?).
b. Ensure safety (protect the patient from escape or injury), listen in a nonjudgmental way, observe the dressing to ensure bleeding is controlled.
(Objectives 7 to 9)

18. a. Does the patient have a history of violent, aggressive, or hostile behavior?
b. What is the patient's posture? Is he sitting or standing? Does he appear tense or rigid?
c. What does his voice sound like? Is his speech loud, obscene, or erratic?
d. Is he pacing or agitated or displaying aggressive behaviors?

19. Ask for police assistance.
(Objective 14)

20. Look for any objects that the patient could use as a weapon.
(Objective 14)

21. A minimum of two rescuers should move swiftly toward the patient and position themselves close to and slightly behind the patient. Each rescuer then should position an inside leg in front of the patient's leg to force the patient into a prone position if needed. The least restrictive restraints needed for a given situation should be used.
(Objective 13)

22. Monitor the patient's level of consciousness, airway, breathing, circulation, vital signs, oxygen saturation (if available), and peripheral pulses while the patient remains in restraints.
(Objective 13)

23. a. Delusional behavior, neurosis, or psychosis may be present during a behavioral emergency.
(Objective 1)

24. c. Many persons break laws without demonstrating abnormal behavior. One person (the paramedic) does not establish norms for society. A person may deviate from usual, normal behavior and not meet the standard for abnormal behavior.
(Objective 1)

25. c. All of the other questions elicit a yes or no answer and yield limited information.
(Objective 5)

26. d. You may acknowledge and label a patient's feelings, but do not patronize or give false reassurances. Correct cognitive misconceptions or distortions in a nonconfrontational manner.
(Objective 4)

27. a. Common signs and symptoms include inattention, memory impairment, disorientation, clouding of consciousness, and vivid visual hallucinations.
(Objective 5)

28. a. In conversion hysteria, painful emotions are converted unconsciously into physical symptoms.
(Objective 5)

29. a. The depressed patient has low self-worth, a loss of appetite, and decreased libido and is tense and irritable.
(Objective 5)

30. a. Neurosis is a faulty or inefficient way of coping. Paranoia is an abnormal way of thinking, characterized by delusions of persecution or grandeur usually centered on a theme. A phobia occurs when a person transfers feelings of anxiety onto a situation or object in the form of an irrational, intense fear.
(Objective 5)

31. c
(Objective 5)

32. a. A small percentage of suicidal patients also will be homicidal. All of the other options are important, but crew safety is your primary responsibility.
(Objective 9)

33. b. Women attempt suicide more often, but men succeed at a higher rate. All talk or threats of suicide should be taken seriously. When depression lifts, the person finally may have the energy to follow through on a suicide plan.
(Objective 7)

34. d. Releasing a patient from restraints en route can place the crew in great danger.
(Objective 13)

35. b. Diphenhydramine is an antihistamine and would not be effective in this situation.
(Objective 13)

36. d. Be sure you can exit quickly if the situation deteriorates. Do not threaten the patient. Do not allow the patient to be alone or to be alone with an emergency medical services crew member on the scene. Remain a safe distance from the patient until your assessment reveals no danger.
(Objective 14)

37. c. Usually the parents can be helpful in the interview and help to relieve anxiety in children (if the situation worsens when they are present, immediately remove them). Children can become violent and injure themselves or others. Do not lie to children.
(Objective 15)

WRAP IT UP

1. His voice was getting louder, his posture became more threatening, and he started to use profane language.
(Objective 10)

2. c. The disease occurs as often in woman as in men. Schizophrenia is a chronic, lifelong disease that is associated with about a 10% risk of suicide.
(Objective 6)

3. It is important to determine suicide risk by asking patients direct questions about their intent, method, and timing of when they intend to commit suicide. This often is not associated with an escalation of the patient's violent behavior.
(Objectives 5, 7, and 8)

4. Haloperidol is an antipsychotic drug that can help control violent, aggressive behavior.
(Objective 11)

CHAPTER

41

Gynecology

READING ASSIGNMENT

Chapter 41, pages 1062-1071, in *Mosby's Paramedic Textbook,* ed. 3

OBJECTIVES

Upon completion of this chapter, the paramedic student will be able to:
1. Describe the physiological processes of menstruation and ovulation.
2. Describe the pathophysiology of the following nontraumatic causes of abdominal pain in females: pelvic inflammatory disease, ruptured ovarian cyst, cystitis, dysmenorrhea, mittelschmerz, endometriosis, ectopic pregnancy, vaginal bleeding.
3. Describe the pathophysiology of traumatic causes of abdominal pain in females, including vaginal bleeding and sexual assault.
4. Outline the prehospital assessment and management of the female with abdominal pain.
5. Outline specific assessment and management for the patient who has been sexually assaulted.
6. Describe specific prehospital measures to preserve evidence in sexual assault cases.

SUMMARY

- Menstruation is the normal, periodic discharge of blood, mucus, and cellular debris from the uterine mucosa. Ovulation is the release of a secondary oocyte from the ovary.
- Pelvic inflammatory disease (PID) results from infection of the cervix, uterus, fallopian tubes, and ovaries and their supporting structures.
- Ruptured ovarian cyst occurs when a thin-walled, fluid-filled sac located on the ovary ruptures. This can cause internal hemorrhage.
- Cystitis is inflammation of the inner lining of the bladder. It usually is caused by a bacterial infection.
- Dysmenorrhea is characterized by painful menses. It may be associated with headache, faintness, dizziness, nausea, diarrhea, backache, and leg pain.
- Mittelschmerz is German for "middle pain." This pain may occur from the rupture of the graafian follicle and bleeding from the ovary during the menstrual cycle.
- Endometritis is inflammation of the uterine lining. Endometriosis is characterized by endometrial tissue growing outside of the uterus.
- An ectopic pregnancy is one that develops outside the uterus.
- Vaginal bleeding is the loss of blood from the uterus, cervix, or vagina.
- Traumatic causes of vaginal bleeding include straddle injuries, blows to the perineum, blunt forces to the lower abdomen, foreign bodies in the vagina, injury during intercourse, abortion attempts, and soft tissue injuries from sexual assault.
- The goal of prehospital care of lower abdominal pain in the female is to obtain a history (including a gynecological history); provide airway, ventilatory, and circulatory support as needed; and provide transport for physician evaluation.

- Sexual assault is a crime of violence. It can have serious physical and psychological effects.
- Paramedics should be aware of the need to preserve evidence from a sexual assault crime scene.

REVIEW QUESTIONS

Match the gynecological problems in Column II with their description in Column I. Use each term only once.

Column I	Column II
1. _____ Abdominal pain at ovulation	a. Dysmenorrhea
2. _____ Beginning of menses	b. Endometriosis
3. _____ Intraabdominal growth of the uterine lining	c. Endometritis
4. _____ Infection of the female pelvic organs	d. Menarche
5. _____ Menstrual cramps	e. Mittelschmerz
6. _____ Fluid sac that ruptures	f. Pelvic inflammatory disease
	g. Ruptured ovarian cyst

7. The normal menstrual cycle is about **(a)** _____ days. The average menstrual flow is

(b) _____ to _____ mL and usually lasts from **(c)** _____

to _____ days. During the menstrual cycle, some of the primary follicles become

(d) _____. These enlarge and form a lump on the surface of the ovary and when mature are

known as the **(e)** _____ or _____ The release of the oocyte from the follicle

is called **(f)** _____ After ovulation, the follicle turns into a glandular structure called the

(g)_____ the cells of which secrete large amounts of **(h)** _____ and some

(i) _____ If pregnancy occurs, the fertilized oocyte **(j)** (_____) begins

releasing a hormonelike substance called **(k)** _____ that keeps the corpus from degenerating.

8. Other than pain, list three signs or symptoms that a woman may experience during menses.

   a.

   b.

   c.

Questions 9 to 12 refer to the following case study:

> You are called to a private residence to evaluate a 19-year-old woman who is complaining of severe pelvic pain. Her pain began yesterday, and she says it is unbearable now. She has no allergies, takes no medicines, and has no significant medical history.

9. What specific questions related to her obstetrical history should you ask her?

   a. _____

   b. _____

   c. _____

   d. _____

e. _____

f. _____

g. _____

h. _____

i. _____

j. _____

She tells you that she has never been pregnant, that she presently has her menstrual period, and that it is of normal color and amount. She denies vaginal discharge or the possibility of pregnancy because she uses birth control pills. She states that she has not had intercourse in 4 months. She denies other symptoms of pregnancy and any history of gynecological problems.

10. What should you specifically assess on the physical examination?

_____

_____

Her lower abdomen is diffusely tender. Vital signs are within normal limits, and her skin is warm and dry.

11. What are some potential causes of her pain?

_____

_____

12. What prehospital interventions will you provide for this patient?

_____

_____

13. What measures can be taken in the prehospital environment to minimize the fear and stress experienced by a victim of sexual abuse?

_____

14. Describe five guidelines for evidence preservation on a sexual abuse call.

a.

b.

c.

d.

e.

STUDENT SELF-ASSESSMENT

15. How often does a typical woman have menstrual flow?
a. Every 14 days
b. Every 21 days
c. Every 28 days
d. Every 35 days

16. Which hormone initiates the ovarian cycle leading to ovulation?
    a. Estrogen
    c. Luteinizing hormone
    b. Follicle-stimulating hormone
    d. Progesterone
17. What is the most common cause of pelvic inflammatory disease?
    a. Gonorrhea
    b. Herpes virus
    c. Human immunodeficiency virus
    d. Syphilis
18. Which of the following factors increases the incidence of dysmenorrhea?
    a. Increased age
    c. Childbirth
    b. Frequent exercise
    d. Infection
19. A ruptured ovarian cyst may mimic all of the following *except* which disorder?
    a. Appendicitis
    c. Ectopic pregnancy
    b. Cholecystitis
    d. Salpingitis
20. Which of the following is a normal sign or symptom of cystitis?
    a. Blood in the urine
    c. Inability to urinate
    b. Flank pain
    d. Painless urination
21. Which of the following is true regarding endometriosis?
    a. It is an inflammation of the uterine lining.
    b. It is common in young women.
    c. It has no effect on fertility.
    d. Its pain may increase during menstruation.
22. Which of the following gynecological problems may cause severe internal hemorrhage?
    a. Dysmenorrhea
    c. Salpingitis
    b. Mittelschmerz
    d. Ruptured ovarian cyst
23. Which of the following is a traumatic cause of vaginal bleeding?
    a. Abortion attempts
    c. Onset of labor
    b. Disorders of the placenta
    d. Pelvic inflammatory disease
24. What is your most important role in caring for a victim of sexual abuse?
    a. Allow only a paramedic of the same gender to care for the patient.
    b. Provide a safe and secure environment for the patient.
    c. Preserve evidence exactly as outlined by protocol.
    d. Perform a complete history and thorough examination.
25. Which of the following should you do to preserve evidence on a sexual abuse call?
    a. Ask the patient to shower.
    c. Place the clothing in a paper bag.
    b. Thoroughly clean wounds.
    d. Search the scene for evidence.

WRAP IT UP

"Unit twelve, respond to one-two-five-six Weston, cross-street Thames, abdominal pain." You and your partner look hungrily at the dinner you have just set on the table, and you quickly move to the ambulance. Your patient is a 26-year-old female whose abdominal pain began 2 hours ago. She is pale and her skin is cool. She is anxious and appears to be in significant pain, especially guarding her left lower quadrant when you palpate her abdomen. Her vital signs are BP 90/50 mm Hg, P 128, R 20, and SaO_2 95%. She has been pregnant 4 times but has miscarried each within the first 8 weeks. Her last normal menstrual period was 8 weeks ago, so she is concerned that her pain may be related to the pregnancy. She started spotting yesterday but has not soaked a pad yet. You quickly apply oxygen by mask, elevate her legs, and tell your partner to start en route. During transport, you start one IV of normal saline with blood tubing and another with macrodrip tubing using lactated Ringer's. When you reassess her vital signs, her blood pressure is 74/50 mm Hg, P 134, R 28, so you open the IVs to administer a fluid challenge. You call the receiving hospital so that they can prepare to resuscitate this patient. On arrival, uncrossmatched blood is given to her, and within 20 minutes, they are rushing her to surgery to treat her ectopic pregnancy.

1. Place a check mark beside the gynecological condition that you might suspect if this patient's pregnancy status were not known.
   a. _____ Cystitis   d. _____ Mittelschmerz
   b. _____ Dysmenorrhea   e. _____ Pelvic inflammatory disease
   c. _____ Endometriosis   f. _____ Ruptured ovarian cyst

2. Which is true of ectopic pregnancy?
   a. It usually occurs in the fallopian tube.
   b. It is a fluid-filled sac on the ovaries.
   c. Uterine inflammation occurs because of placental tissue retention.
   d. There is ectopic growth and functioning of uterine tissue.
3. Why was it critical to evaluate the possibility of pregnancy in this patient?

_____

_____

4. Explain your rationale for the following interventions.
   a. Elevation of her legs

_____

_____

   b. Intravenous fluid bolus

_____

_____

   c. Oxygen therapy

CHAPTER 41 ANSWERS

GYNECOLOGY

1. e
2. d
3. b
4. f
5. a
6. g
   (Questions 1 to 6, Objective 2)

7. a. 28; b. 25, 60; c. 4, 6; d. secondary follicles; e. vesicular, graafian follicles; f. ovulation; g. corpus luteum; h. progesterone; i. estrogen; j. zygote; k. chorionic gonadotropin.
   (Objective 1)

8. Headache, faintness, dizziness, nausea, diarrhea, backache, leg pain, chills, nausea, and vomiting
   (Objective 2)

9. a. Have you ever been pregnant? If yes, how many pregnancies and how many have you carried to term?
   b. Have you ever had a cesarean delivery?
   c. When was your last menstrual period? How long did it last? Was it normal? Do you have a regular menstrual cycle? Have you had any bleeding between your periods?
   d. Could you be pregnant now? Is your period late or did you miss one? Do you have any breast tenderness, increased need to urinate, or morning sickness? Have you had any unprotected sexual activity?
   e. Do you have a history of any gynecological (female) problems such as bleeding, infections, pain during intercourse, miscarriage, abortion, or ectopic pregnancy?
   f. Are you having any bleeding now? If you are, what color is it, how many pads have you soaked, and how long have you been bleeding?
   g. Do you have any vaginal discharge? What color and how much is there? Does it smell bad?
   h. What kind of birth control do you use? Have you ever forgotten to use it?
   i. Have you had any injury to your genital area?
   j. How are you feeling now?
   (Objective 4)

10. Evaluate vital signs and check for signs of blood loss (skin signs, orthostatic vital signs). Palpate the abdomen to assess for masses, tenderness, guarding, distention, and rebound tenderness.
    (Objective 4)

11. Pelvic inflammatory disease, ruptured ovarian cyst, dysmenorrhea, endometritis, endometriosis, or appendicitis are potential causes. Ectopic pregnancy and miscarriage should not be discounted completely because sometimes patients do not give a completely accurate sexual history.
    (Objective 4)

12. Consider oxygen administration; however, because no signs of shock exist, this may not be necessary. Consider initiating intravenous therapy. Transport in a position of comfort.
    (Objective 4)

13. Move to a private, safe location; allow paramedic who is the same sex as the patient to provide care if possible; minimize questions and physical examination as appropriate; and listen and provide comfort.
    (Objective 5)

14. Handle clothes as little as possible, do not clean wounds, use paper bags for clothing and bag each item separately, ask the victim not to change clothing, and try not to disturb the crime scene.
(Objective 6)

15. c. Menstrual flow varies according to each individual.
(Objective 1)

16. c. Follicle-stimulating hormone stimulates development of the follicle. Estrogen causes a surge in the production of luteinizing hormone, which initiates the ovarian cycle.
(Objective 1)

17. a. *Chlamydia* organisms and *Chlamydia trachomatis* also often are associated with pelvic inflammatory disease.
(Objective 2)

18. d. All of the other factors often decrease the severity of this condition.
(Objective 2)

19. b. The pain of cholecystitis is usually in the right upper quadrant of the abdomen. All other conditions cause lower abdominal pain.
(Objective 2)

20. a. Urination is usually painful and frequent in cystitis. Flank pain may indicate that the infection has moved to the kidneys.
(Objective 2)

21. d. Endometriosis is an ectopic placement of uterine lining and causes inflammation of the endometrium. It is common in women in their late 30s and is associated with infertility.
(Objective 2)

22. d
(Objective 2)

23. a. All other answers are nontraumatic causes of vaginal bleeding.
(Objective 3)

24. b. Having a paramedic of the same sex as the patient perform care is desirable but may not always be possible. You should attempt to preserve evidence, but this is not always possible if a life-threatening condition exists that requires rapid intervention. Perform only the necessary history and physical examination.
(Objective 5)

25. c. Bag items separately if possible. The patient should not shower, wash, or have wounds cleansed until evidence can be gathered.
(Objective 6)

WRAP IT UP

1. f. She gave no urinary signs or symptoms, so cystitis would not be a consideration. Pelvic inflammatory disease is possible, but there is no report of vaginal discharge. The pain of dysmenorrhea and mittelschmerz is not usually so severe and are not associated with shock.

2. a. It can occur less often in the ovary, abdominal cavity, or cervix.
   (Objective 2)

3. If the pregnancy status is known, the differential diagnosis can be narrowed.
   (Objective 2)

4. a. Elevating her legs may improve her shock temporarily.
   b. An intravenous fluid bolus will increase the preload and temporarily increase the blood pressure.
   c. Because this patient is in shock, oxygenation is critical, especially because she has internal bleeding.
   (Objective 2)

CHAPTER 42

Obstetrics

READING ASSIGNMENT
Chapter 42, pages 1072-1097, in *Mosby's Paramedic Textbook,* ed. 3

OBJECTIVES
Upon completion of this chapter, the paramedic student will be able to do the following:
1. Describe the organization and function of the specialized structures of pregnancy.
2. Outline fetal development from ovulation through adaptations at birth.
3. Explain normal maternal physiological changes that occur during pregnancy and how they influence prehospital patient care and transportation.
4. Describe appropriate information to be elicited during the obstetrical patient's history.
5. Describe specific techniques for assessment of the pregnant patient.
6. Describe general prehospital care of the pregnant patient.
7. Discuss the implications of prehospital care after trauma to the fetus and mother.
8. Describe the assessment and management of patients with preeclampsia and eclampsia.
9. Explain the pathophysiology, signs and symptoms, and management of the processes that cause vaginal bleeding in pregnancy.
10. Outline the physiological changes that occur during the stages of labor.
11. Describe the role of the paramedic during normal labor and delivery.
12. Compute an Apgar score.
13. Describe assessment and management of postpartum hemorrhage.
14. Discuss the identification, implications, and prehospital management of complicated deliveries.

SUMMARY
- The placenta is a disklike organ. It is composed of interlocking fetal and maternal tissues. It is the organ of exchange between the mother and fetus. Blood flows from the fetus to the placenta through two umbilical arteries. These arteries carry deoxygenated blood. Oxygenated blood returns to the fetus through the umbilical vein. The amniotic sac is a fluid-filled bag. It completely surrounds and protects the embryo.
- The developing ovum is known as an embryo during the first 8 weeks of pregnancy. After that time and until birth it is called a fetus. Gestation (fetal development) usually averages 40 weeks from the time of fertilization to the delivery of the newborn.
- The pregnant woman undergoes many physiological changes that affect the genital tract, breasts, gastrointestinal system, cardiovascular system, respiratory system, and metabolism.
- The patient history should include obstetrical history; presence of pain; presence, quantity, and character of vaginal bleeding; presence of abnormal vaginal discharge; presence of "bloody show"; current general health and prenatal care; allergies and medicines taken; and maternal urge to bear down.

- The goal in examining an obstetrical patient is to rapidly identify acute life-threatening conditions. A part of this involves identifying imminent delivery. Then the paramedic must take the proper management steps. In addition to the routine physical examination, the paramedic should assess the abdomen, uterine size, and fetal heart sounds.
- If birth is not imminent, the paramedic should limit prehospital care for the healthy patient. It should be limited to basic treatment modalities. It should include transport for physician evaluation as well.
- Causes of fetal death from maternal trauma include death of the mother, separation of the placenta, maternal shock, uterine rupture, and fetal head injury.
- Preeclampsia occurs after 20 weeks' gestation. The criteria for diagnosis include hypertension, proteinuria, and excessive weight gain with edema. Eclampsia is characterized by the same signs and symptoms with the addition of seizures or coma.
- Vaginal bleeding during pregnancy can result from abortion (miscarriage), ectopic pregnancy, abruptio placentae, placenta previa, uterine rupture, or postpartum hemorrhage. Abortion is the termination of pregnancy from any cause before 20 weeks' gestation. Ectopic pregnancy occurs when a fertilized ovum implants anywhere other than the uterus. Abruptio placentae is partial or complete detachment of the placenta at more than 20 weeks' gestation. Placenta previa is placental implantation in the lower uterine segment partially or completely covering the cervical opening. Uterine rupture is a spontaneous or traumatic rupture of the uterine wall.
- The first stage of labor begins with the onset of regular contractions. It ends with complete dilation of the cervix. The second stage of labor is measured from full dilation of the cervix to delivery of the infant. The third stage of labor begins with delivery of the infant and ends when the placenta is expelled and the uterus has contracted.
- One of the primary responsibilities of the EMS crew is to prevent an uncontrolled delivery. The other is to protect the infant from cold and stress after birth.
- Criteria for computing the Apgar score include appearance (color), pulse (heart rate), grimace (reflex irritability), activity (muscle tone), and respiratory effort.
- More than 500 mL of blood loss after the delivery of the newborn is called a postpartum hemorrhage. It often results from ineffective or incomplete contraction of the uterus.
- Paramedics should be alert to factors that point to a possible abnormal delivery.
- Cephalopelvic disproportion produces a difficult labor because of the presence of a small pelvis, an oversized uterus, or fetal abnormalities. Most infants are born head first (cephalic or vertex presentation). However, sometimes a presentation is abnormal. In breech presentation, the largest part of the fetus (the head) is delivered last. Shoulder dystocia occurs when the fetal shoulders impact against the maternal symphysis pubis. This blocks shoulder delivery. Shoulder presentation (transverse presentation) results when the long axis of the fetus lies perpendicular to that of the mother. The fetal arm or hand may be the presenting part. Cord presentation occurs when the cord slips down into the vagina or presents externally.
- A premature infant is born before 37 weeks' gestation.
- A multiple gestation is a pregnancy with more than one fetus. It is accompanied by an increased complication rate.
- A precipitous delivery is a rapid spontaneous delivery with less than 3 hours from onset of labor to birth. The main danger to the fetus is from cerebral trauma or tearing of the umbilical cord.
- Uterine inversion is a rare complication of childbirth. It is a serious complication. With this condition, the uterus turns "inside out."
- The development of pulmonary embolism during pregnancy, labor, or the postpartum period is one of the most common causes of maternal death.
- Premature rupture of the membranes is a rupture of the amniotic sac before the onset of labor, regardless of gestational age.
- An amniotic fluid embolism may occur when amniotic fluid enters the maternal circulation during labor or delivery or immediately after delivery.

REVIEW QUESTIONS

Match the types of abortion in Column II with their description in Column I. Use each term only once.

Column I

1. _____ Abortion before 12 weeks not externally induced
2. _____ Legal termination of pregnancy to preserve the mother's health
3. _____ All the products of conception passed before 12 weeks
4. _____ Symptoms of impending abortion with a closed cervix
5. _____ Failure to pass a fetus after 4 weeks of fetal death
6. _____ Intentional termination of pregnancy

Column II

a. Complete abortion
b. Incomplete abortion
c. Induced abortion
d. Missed abortion
e. Spontaneous abortion
f. Therapeutic abortion
g. Threatened abortion

Match the problems of pregnancy in Column II with their description in Column I. Use each problem only once.

Column I

7. _____ Painless bleeding in third trimester of pregnancy
8. _____ Hypertension, proteinuria, and visual disturbance in the third trimester
9. _____ Severe abdominal pain, shock, and easily palpable fetal parts
10. _____ Painful third-trimester bleeding
11. _____ Third-trimester seizure after a new onset of hypertension
12. _____ Abdominal pain, scant vaginal bleeding, and shock in the first trimester

Column II

a. Abortion
b. Abruptio placentae
c. Eclampsia
d. Ectopic pregnancy
e. Placenta previa
f. Preeclampsia
g. Uterine rupture

13. In what lunar month do the following fetal development characteristics typically occur?

   a. Fetal movement felt by the mother:

   _____

   b. Fetal heart beat:

   _____

   c. Distinct fingers and toes:

   _____

   d. Eyebrows and fingernails:

   _____

   e. Possible viability if born:

   _____

14. What causes the arteriovenous shunts to close at birth?

   _____

   _____

15. What do the following pregnancy terms mean?

   a. A patient is gravida 6 para 5 (G6 P5).

   _____

b. She is a multipara.

_____

c. The patient has postpartum bleeding.

_____

d. You are called to care for a nullipara who is term.

_____

16. A woman in her fortieth week of pregnancy complains of heartburn, dizziness, and frequency of urination. Her heart rate is 100; respirations are 20 and deep; and blood pressure is 90/60 mm Hg. (She says her normal is 100/70 mm Hg.) She has slight edema of the ankles and tortuous varicose veins. Explain how the physiological alterations of pregnancy cause each of the signs or symptoms she is experiencing.

a. Heartburn:

_____

_____

b. Dizziness:

_____

_____

c. Frequency of urination:

_____

_____

d. Hypotension:

_____

_____

e. Pedal edema and varicose veins:

_____

_____

17. Briefly explain why each of the following historical findings would cause concern if delivery is imminent in the field:

a. No prenatal care:

_____

_____

b. Diabetic mother:

_____

_____

c. Vaginal bleeding:

_____

_____

d. Current heroin intoxication:

_____

_____

Questions 18 to 20 refer to the following case study:

A 28-year-old woman who is in her third trimester complains of abdominal pain after an automobile accident in which she was the unrestrained driver. She is pale, and her vital signs are blood pressure, 90/60 mm Hg; pulse, 134; and respirations, 28. Her abdomen is tender to palpation, and you note some vaginal bleeding.

18. What other subjective information do you need from the mother?

_____

_____

19. How can you determine whether the infant is in distress?

_____

_____

20. Describe prehospital care and transport of this patient.

_____

_____

_____

Questions 21 to 24 refer to the following case study:

A 30-year-old woman says she is 9 weeks' pregnant and complains of severe cramping pain in the lower abdomen and vaginal bleeding. She states that she has saturated six sanitary napkins and passed some "white, stringy stuff" that her husband shows you in the toilet.

21. What condition of pregnancy do you suspect?

_____

22. What actions should you take so that the physician can determine whether she has had a complete abortion?

_____

23. Estimate her blood loss if you feel the history was accurate.

_____

24. Why might this patient be exhibiting a grief reaction?

_____

_____

25. An obstetrician calls you to his office to transport a 28-year-old woman who has an ectopic pregnancy (determined by ultrasound). She complains of severe abdominal pain and has frank signs of shock.

   a. What other signs or symptoms might she experience?

   _____

   b. Describe interventions you will use on your 20-minute trip to the emergency department.

   _____

   _____

26. What general patient care measures should be taken for any patient who has third-trimester bleeding without shock?

   _____

   _____

   _____

Questions 27 to 31 refer to the following case study:

   A 40-year-old primipara in the third trimester complains of headache, dizziness, and nausea. Vital signs are blood pressure, 160/100 mm Hg; pulse, 110; and respirations, 20. Her hands and feet are considerably swollen, and you note intermittent facial twitching. She says her doctor was worried about protein in her urine.

27. What complication do you suspect?

   _____

28. In what position should you transport this patient?

   _____

29. List two drugs with appropriate doses that may be ordered by medical direction to stop seizure activity in these types of patients.

   _____

30. Besides medication, what emergency medical services actions can minimize the risk of seizures?

   _____

31. What risks to the fetus exist with this condition?

   _____

   _____

Questions 32 to 36 refer to the following case study:

   You are called to a private residence 30 minutes from the nearest hospital to care for a woman in labor.

32. What information in the patient's medical history is important to help gauge how quickly labor will progress?

   _____

   _____

33. What specific signs or symptoms during labor would lead you to believe that delivery is imminent?

_____

_____

34. As the baby's head delivers, what assessment and interventions should you perform?

_____

_____

35. Describe the procedure to clamp the umbilical cord.

_____

_____

36. When should the Apgar score be calculated?

_____

37. If necessary, when should oxytocin be administered, and what is the proper dose and route?

_____

38. Labor fails to progress after a baby in breech position is delivered to the level of the chest. Describe the steps you should take in this situation.

_____

_____

39. After the head of a baby with shoulder dystocia is delivered, what can you do to deliver the shoulders while minimizing fetal injury?

_____

_____

40. A 35-year-old woman who is G6 P5 states that she is ready to deliver her baby at home. Her membranes have ruptured, her contractions are frequent, and she wants to push. When you examine her perineum, you see the umbilical cord protruding from the vagina.

   a. What actions should you take immediately to prevent fetal hypoxia?

_____

_____

   b. Should you attempt to deliver this baby on the scene?

_____

STUDENT SELF-ASSESSMENT

41. Functions of the placenta include all except which of the following?
    a. Excretion of wastes
    b. Hormone production
    c. Metabolism of drugs
    d. Transfer of gases

42. The primary role of amniotic fluid is which of the following?
    a. Excretion
    b. Hydration
    c. Nutrition
    d. Protection

43. The fetal structure that allows blood to bypass the liver and go directly into the inferior vena cava is which of the following?
    a. Ductus arteriosus
    b. Ductus venosus
    c. Foramen ovale
    d. Umbilical vein

44. The umbilical cord carries which of the following?
    a. Deoxygenated blood by one umbilical artery and oxygenated blood by one umbilical vein
    b. Deoxygenated blood by two umbilical arteries and oxygenated blood by one umbilical vein
    c. Oxygenated blood by one umbilical artery and deoxygenated blood by one umbilical vein
    d. Oxygenated blood by two umbilical arteries and deoxygenated blood by one umbilical vein

45. Where should the uterus be palpable at week 20 of gestation?
    a. At the lower border of the umbilicus
    b. Between the symphysis pubis and umbilicus
    c. Halfway between the umbilicus and the xiphoid
    d. Just above the symphysis pubis

46. Which of the following is the normal fetal heart rate?
    a. 80 to 120 beats/min
    b. 120 to 160 beats/min
    c. 160 to 200 beats/mine
    d. 200 to 240 beats/min

47. In which of the following positions should the hypotensive pregnant patient who is more than 4 months gestation be transported?
    a. High Fowler's
    b. Left lateral recumbent
    c. Prone
    d. Supine

48. Immediately after the delivery of a healthy baby, your patient's eyes roll back and she becomes pulseless. She has no previous medical history. Which of the following may have caused her cardiac arrest?
    a. Abruptio placentae
    b. Amniotic fluid embolism
    c. Aortic dissection
    d. Congestive cardiomyopathy

49. When attempting to resuscitate a patient in cardiac arrest who is 8 months pregnant, what special care measures should you use to be most effective?
    a. Decrease ventilation volumes to minimize gastric distention.
    b. Increase the dose of epinephrine to maximize vasoconstriction.
    c. Perform chest compressions lower on the sternum.
    d. Tilt her torso laterally to prevent compression of the vena cava.

50. By which of the following signs is eclampsia distinguished from preeclampsia?
    a. Edema
    b. Glucosuria
    c. Hypertension
    d. Seizures

51. The primary complication from administration of magnesium sulfate is which of the following?
    a. Increased hypertension
    b. Precipitous delivery
    c. Respiratory depression
    d. Ventricular dysrhythmias

52. Excessive traction on the umbilical cord during placental delivery may cause which of the following?
    a. Fetal distress
    b. Placenta previa
    c. Uterine inversion
    d. Uterine rupture

53. Which of the following occurs in the second stage of labor?
    a. Cervical dilation
    b. Delivery of the infant
    c. Expulsion of the placenta
    d. Fetal descent into the birth canal

54. When delivering a baby's head, you note that the umbilical cord is wrapped around the baby's neck. Which of the following is the first action you should take?
    a. Cut the cord in two places, clamp, and proceed with delivery.
    b. Elevate the mother's hips and have her pant until you reach the hospital.
    c. Gently unloop the cord around and over the baby's head.
    d. No special action is needed; the cord will free itself as the shoulders deliver.

55. A minute after delivery, a baby has a weak cry, a pink body with blue extremities, and a pulse of 128; he actively moves about and sneezes when a catheter is introduced into his nose. The Apgar score is which of the following?

    a. 6   **c.** 8

    b. 7   **d.** 9

56. Hemorrhage control in the postpartum period may include all of the following *except* which?

    a. Elevation of the mother's hips

    b. Delivery of oxytocin intravenously

    c. Breast-feeding of the baby

    d. Vigorous uterine massage

57. For which of the following is the premature infant at risk?

    a. Gestational diabetes   **c.** Placenta previa

    b. Hypothermia   **d.** Prolapsed umbilical cord

58. Which of the following is a frequent complication of multiple gestation?

    a. Eclampsia   **c.** Premature delivery

    b. Placenta previa   **d.** Uterine rupture

59. Which of the following complications of pregnancy is most likely to require delivery by cesarean section?

    a. Breech presentation   **c.** Shoulder dystocia

    b. Cephalopelvic disproportion   **d.** Vaginal bleeding

60. A 30-year-old woman develops dyspnea and severe chest pain 24 hours after delivery of her third child. She is hypotensive and in acute distress. Based on her history, you suspect which of the following?

    a. Eclampsia   **c.** Pneumonia

    b. Myocardial infarction   **d.** Pulmonary embolism

61. Which of the following is the primary danger to an infant delivered during a precipitous delivery?

    a. Abruptio placentae   **c.** Nuchal cord

    b. Cerebral trauma   **d.** Placenta previa

62. Which of the following describes chorioamnionitis?

    a. Amniotic fluid embolism

    b. Excessive amniotic fluid

    c. Infection of fetal membranes

    d. Premature rupture of the membranes

WRAP IT UP

At 1630 your crew is sitting around the kitchen table, reviewing some QI data with your supervisor, when you are dispatched for a "maternity case." When you arrive, your 30-year-old patient is on the sofa, saying, "I've got to push!" As you prepare to check her perineum, you obtain a quick history: She is due in 8 weeks, her bag of waters ruptured with clear fluid, there is one fetus, and she denies using narcotic drugs. Her perineum is bulging, and there is evidence of mucousy bloody show, so you call for additional personnel. Your partner listens for fetal heart tones, which he finds inferior to the umbilicus at 150 beats/min. The patient has another contraction, moaning loudly, "the baby's coming." The baby's head is now visible at the perineum so you prepare for imminent delivery and open the OB kit. You continue to obtain her history and note that she has two children at home, and no miscarriages or other health problems. Your partner moves to the ambulance to open the pediatric resuscitation bag and set up for neonatal resuscitation. You don a face shield, gown, and a clean pair of gloves, and then the patient's next contraction begins—you estimate they are 2 to 3 minutes apart. You encourage her to push, and see the baby's forehead appear and then retract slightly when the contraction ends. Coaching her breathing, you arrange towels under her buttocks, elevating them slightly, and prepare some clean towels and blankets for the baby. With the next contraction, the baby's head delivers face down. While supporting the baby's head with one hand, you insert a finger in the vagina and sweep around the neck to feel for the presence of the cord; there is none. Then, taking the bulb syringe from your kit, you suction the fluids from the baby's mouth and then nose, clearing the thick clear mucus. As the next contraction begins, the baby rotates laterally, and you guide it downward to deliver the first shoulder and up to free the other; then the baby slips quickly from the birth canal. It's a girl, and she is very slippery and hard to hold on to. You hold her level with her mother's perineum, as you again suction her nose and mouth and then begin to warm and dry her, vigorously rubbing her back to stimulate the floppy baby to breathe. The cord is clamped and cut, and at 1 minute, you note the baby is still pale and blue, her heart rate is 90 beats/min, she grimaces when you put the bulb syringe in her nose, she has some flexion, but her muscle tone is generally floppy, and she has slow, irregular respirations. You apply oxygen, position her on her back with her shoulders slightly elevated, and flick her feet to stimulate her. She is becoming pinker and has brisk capillary refill, and at 5 minutes her heart rate is 140 beats/min, but even though she is breathing, there is no brisk cry or cough, she grimaces to suction, and her body is now completely pink, in fact it looks very red. You remove the wet towel and cover her (including her head) with warm blankets, apply an oxygen saturation monitor and continue the blowby oxygen, continually monitoring her respiratory effort. She is very small, around 5 lb you guess. In the meantime, your partner has been caring for the mother, who by now has delivered the placenta. She has brisk bleeding from the vagina and cramping. He has started an IV and administered oxytocin intramuscularly. Her vital signs are stable, and she is asking about her baby. Your partner massages the mother's fundus, which she finds uncomfortable. You arrive at the hospital in 8 minutes, where the neonatal resuscitation team is awaiting your arrival. They immediately take the baby, evaluate her in the ED, where her saturation and heart rate are good, allow the mother to hold her for a moment, then take her to the neonatal ICU, where they tell the mother they will intubate her because of her premature status. A week later, baby is discharged to home in good health.

1. What stage of labor is the mother in when you arrive?

_____

2. Why is this baby at risk for complications during or after delivery?

_____

3. What was the baby's Apgar score?
   a. At 1 minute:

_____

   b. At 5 minutes:

_____

4. What additional resuscitation measures would you have performed immediately if the baby's color and heart rate did not improve after oxygen administration?
   a. Begin ventilation using a bag-mask device and oxygen.
   b. Give epinephrine 0.01 mg/kg.
   c. Initiate vascular access by cannulation of the umbilicus.
   d. Intubate the trachea and ventilate at a rate of 20 per minute.
5. a. What head presentation did you note at delivery?
   b. Is this normal or abnormal?

_____

6. What action would you have taken if you palpated the cord around his neck?

_____

7. Why did you hold the baby at the level of the mother's perineum until the cord was cut?

_____

8. What should be done with the placenta?

_____

9. Where should the cord be cut?

_____

10. Explain your rationale for the following interventions:
   a. Stimulation of the baby

   _____

   b. Suctioning of fluids from the mouth and nose

   _____

   c. Elevation of the baby's shoulders

   _____

   d. Massage of the mother's abdomen

   _____

   e. Administration of oxytocin

CHAPTER 42 ANSWERS

REVIEW QUESTIONS

1. e
(Objective 9)

2. f
(Objective 9)

3. a
(Objective 9)

4. g
(Objective 9)

5. d
(Objective 9)

6. c
(Objective 9)

7. e
(Objective 9)

8. f
(Objective 8)

9. g
(Objective 9)

10. b
(Objective 9)

11. c
(Objective 8)

12. d
(Objective 9)

13. a. Fifth
b. Fourth
c. Third
d. Sixth
e. Eighth
(Objective 2)

14. The rapid increase in systemic vascular resistance, aortic pressure, and left ventricular and left atrial pressures after placental flow stops and the decrease in pulmonary vascular resistance resulting from expansion of the lungs cause atrioventricular shunts to close within a few hours after birth.
(Objective 2)

15. a. She has had six pregnancies and delivered five children.

b. She has had two or more deliveries.

c. The patient had bleeding after delivery of her baby.

d. You are called to care for a woman who has never delivered and whose pregnancy has reached 40 weeks of gestation.

(Objective 4)

16. a. Decreased tone and motility of the gastrointestinal tract, which leads to slow gastric emptying and relaxation of the pyloric sphincter

b. Decreased PCO_2 caused by increased respiratory rate and tidal volume late in pregnancy

c. Pressure that the gravid uterus places directly on the bladder when the fetal head moves down in the pelvis near term

d. Blood pressure decreases 10 to 15 mm Hg during the second semester and gradually increases to prepregnant levels near term. (The patient should be questioned about her normal blood pressure.)

e. Impaired venous return resulting from the pressure the uterus exerts

(Objective 3)

17. a. Problems such as maternal nutrition, growth of fetus, maternal diabetes, and preeclampsia would not have been managed; an increased risk of fetal and maternal problems at birth exists.

b. Increased birth weight of the baby may make field delivery difficult or impossible if cephalopelvic disproportion is present.

c. Vaginal bleeding may indicate abruptio placentae, placenta previa, or uterine rupture. All of these conditions cause an increase in fetal mortality rate and pose a risk of maternal shock and death.

d. Recent maternal narcotic intoxication causes neonatal respiratory depression and increases the risk of complications in the field.

(Objective 4)

18. When did she last feel fetal movement? What other medical problems does she have? What other medications does she take? Is she having any contractions?

(Objective 7)

19. Assess fetal heart tones. (A persistent fetal heart rate of greater than 160 or less than 120 is an early sign of fetal distress and fetal or maternal hypoxia.) Ask the mother to report fetal movement to you.

(Objective 7)

20. Administer 100% oxygen by non-rebreather mask (monitoring oxygen saturation with pulse oximeter, if available). Immobilize the patient on a backboard and roll the backboard to the left side. Consider applying pneumatic antishock garments in case the patient's condition deteriorates (controversial). Initiate intravenous lactated Ringer's solution or normal saline (two large-bore lines) en route to the nearest appropriate trauma center and frequently reassess vital signs, fetal heart tones, and the amount of vaginal bleeding en route.

(Objective 7)

21. Spontaneous abortion

(Objective 9)

22. Retrieve the tissue from the toilet and give it to the emergency department staff so that a pathologist can examine it for completeness.

(Objective 9)

23. 6 sanitary napkins × 20 to 30 mL/pad = 120 to 180 mL of blood lost.

(Objective 9)

24. Pregnant women are often attached to the fetus and grieve when they know that their baby has died. This fact is especially true if a similar event has happened to the patient in the past.

(Objective 9)

25. a. Vaginal bleeding, shoulder pain, nausea, vomiting, and syncope
   b. Administer 100% oxygen by non-rebreather mask. Consider use of pneumatic antishock garments (controversial). While en route, initiate two large-bore intravenous lines and infuse boluses of normal saline or lactated Ringer's solution. Place the patient in modified Trendelenburg's position if signs and symptoms of shock do not improve, and report her condition and diagnosis to the receiving hospital so that operative preparations can be made.
   (Objective 9)

26. Administer 100% oxygen by a non-rebreather mask. Place the patient in left lateral recumbent position. Initiate precautionary intravenous lactated Ringer's solution or normal saline en route to the hospital. Rapidly transport the patient to the closest appropriate medical center and monitor maternal vital signs and fetal heart tones.
   (Objective 6)

27. Preeclampsia
   (Objective 8)

28. Left lateral recumbent
   (Objective 8)

29. Magnesium sulfate 10% (1 to 4 g slow intravenous infusion) and diazepam (5 mg slow intravenous) over 2 minutes
   (Objective 8)

30. Minimized stimulation and gentle patient handling
   (Objective 8)

31. Abruptio placentae is a complication, and maternal apnea during a seizure may cause fetal hypoxia.
   (Objective 8)

32. How many previous deliveries has she had, and how quickly did they progress? How long has she been in labor, and how close are the contractions?
   (Objective 11)

33. Contractions lasting 45 to 60 seconds at 1- to 2-minute intervals; measurement from beginning of one contraction to the beginning of the next; patient who wants to bear down or have a bowel movement; large amount of bloody show; crowning; and mother's feeling that delivery is imminent
   (Objective 11)

34. Examine for the presence of a nuchal cord. If this cord is present, gently slip it over the infant's head or, if this is not possible, clamp it in two places and cut between the clamps to release the cord. If the cord is cut, ensure that the rest of the delivery proceeds rapidly because the baby has no source of oxygen. Suction the fluids from the baby's mouth and nose with a bulb syringe. Deliver the shoulders.
   (Objective 11)

35. Clamp 6 to 9 inches from the infant in two places. Cut between the clamps with sterile scissors or a scalpel. Examine the cord to ensure that no bleeding exists.
   (Objective 11)

36. At 1 minute and 5 minutes of age
   (Objective 12)

37. After delivery of the baby, 10 units of oxytocin in 1000 mL of lactated Ringer's solution infused at 20 to 30 gtt/min on microdrip tubing
   (Objectives 11 and 13)

38. If the head does not deliver immediately, place a gloved hand in the vagina with the palm toward the baby's face. Form a V, with the index and middle fingers on either side of the baby's nose, and push the vaginal wall from the face until delivery. If the head does not deliver within 3 minutes, maintain the airway as described and transport the patient to the receiving hospital.
(Objective 14)

39. Position the mother on her left side in the knee-chest position. Guide the baby's head downward to allow the anterior shoulder to slip under the symphysis pubis; avoid excess force. Rotate the fetal shoulder girdle into the wider oblique pelvic diameter and deliver the posterior and then the anterior shoulders.
(Objective 14)

40. a. Elevate the mother's hips, administer oxygen, and ask the mother to pant with contractions to avoid bearing down. With gloved hand, gently push the baby's presenting part back into the vagina and elevate it to relieve pressure on the cord. Maintain this position while rapidly transporting the patient to the receiving hospital.
b. No, this baby will have to be delivered by cesarean section.
(Objective 14)

41. c
(Objective 1)

42. d. Although amniotic fluid originates from fetal urine and secretions from the respiratory tract, skin, and amniotic membranes, its primary function is protection.
(Objective 1)

43. b. The ductus arteriosus connects the aorta and pulmonary artery, and the foramen ovale provides a passageway for blood directly from the right to the left atrium. The umbilical cord connects the placenta to the embryo and is its lifeline.
(Objective 2)

44. b
(Objective 1)

45. a. At week 12, the uterus is just above the symphysis pubis; at week 16, between the symphysis pubis and the umbilicus; and at week 28, halfway between the umbilicus and the xiphoid.
(Objective 5)

46. b. A persistent rate greater than 160 or below 120 is a sign of fetal distress and fetal or maternal hypoxia.
(Objective 5)

47. b. This position prevents pressure from being exerted on the inferior vena cava.
(Objective 6)

48. b. Maternal mortality from pregnancy-related causes is rare. If the patient had abruptio placentae, a healthy delivery would be unlikely. Aortic dissection and congestive cardiomyopathy may cause maternal death, but amniotic fluid embolism is more likely at the time of delivery.
(Objective 6)

49. d. Drug doses and ventilations do not need to be modified. Chest compressions should be performed higher on the sternum.
(Objective 6)

50. d. Edema and hypertension are found in both.
(Objective 8)

51. c. Magnesium also can cause clinically significant hypotension.
(Objective 8)

52. c. Uterine inversion also may happen, although less frequently, after a contraction, cough, or sneeze.
(Objective 14)

53. b. During the prodromal period, the fetus descends into the birth canal. In the first stage the cervix dilates completely, and in the third stage the placenta is delivered.
(Objective 10)

54. c. Usually the cord can be freed in this manner. If this action fails and the decision is made to cut the cord after your medical direction protocols, delivery must be expedited or the baby will suffer severe hypoxia and risk of death.
(Objectives 11 and 14)

55. c. Weak cry (1); plus pink body and blue extremities (1); plus pulse at 128 (2), plus active movement (2); plus sneeze (2) = 8
(Objective 12)

56. a. Having the baby suckle stimulates the production of oxytocin.
(Objective 13)

57. b. The premature infant has a large surface area-to-mass ratio and is susceptible to hypothermia. In addition, a potential for cardiorespiratory dysfunction exists because of immaturity.
(Objective 14)

58. c. Other complications include abruptio placentae, postpartum hemorrhage, and abnormal presentation.
(Objective 14)

59. b. In this condition the pelvic ring is too small to allow passage of the baby's head.
(Objective 14)

60. d. Pulmonary embolism or, more rarely, amniotic fluid embolism can cause these signs and symptoms.
(Objective 14)

61. b. Tearing of the umbilical cord is also a risk.
(Objective 14)

62. c. This condition often occurs after prolonged premature rupture of the membranes.
(Objective 14)

WRAP IT UP

1. Stage II (expulsion stage)
(Objective 10)

2. Baby is premature based on mother's history
(Objective 14)

3. a. 1-minute Apgar: 4
b. 5-minute Apgar: 7
(Objective 12)

4. a. Assisted ventilation may be all that is necessary to open the small airway and stimulate normal breathing in the infant.
(Objectives 7 and 14)

5. a. Vertex (cephalic); this is normal
(Objective 10)

6. Gently try to slip the cord over the head.
(Objective 14)

7. Elevation of the baby below the perineum could result in undertransfusion of blood from the cord; lowering the baby below the perineum could result in overtransfusion of cord blood.
(Objective 11)

8. The placenta surface should be inspected to see whether it is intact (retained fragments can cause postpartum hemorrhage); and then it should be placed in a plastic bag and transported with the mother to the hospital.
(Objective 11)

9. Clamp the cord in two places 4 to 6 inches from the baby and then cut between the clamps.
(Objective 11)

10. a. Stimulation of the baby is designed to promote effective respiratory effort.
b. Suctioning of fluids from the mouth and nose clears the upper airway of mucus and other secretions to promote normal unobstructed breathing
c. Elevation of the baby's shoulders positions the airway in the most effective manner to promote effective ventilation.
d. Massage of the mother's abdomen stimulates uterine contractions that help to slow vaginal bleeding.
e. Administration of oxytocin causes uterine contraction and slows vaginal bleeding.
(Objective 11)

PART NINE

CHAPTER 43

Neonatology

READING ASSIGNMENT

Chapter 43, pages 1100-1115, in *Mosby's Paramedic Textbook,* ed. 3

OBJECTIVES

Upon completion of this chapter, the paramedic student will be able to:
1. Identify risk factors associated with the need for neonatal resuscitation.
2. Describe physiological adaptations at birth.
3. Outline the prehospital assessment and management of the neonate.
4. Describe resuscitation of the distressed neonate.
5. Discuss postresuscitative management and transport.
6. Describe signs and symptoms and prehospital management of specific neonatal resuscitation situations.
7. Identify injuries associated with birth.
8. Describe appropriate interventions to manage the emotional needs of the neonate's family.

SUMMARY

- When oxygenation and continued ventilations do not improve the infant's condition or they begin to deteriorate further, ET intubation and administration of drugs may be required. The drugs most often used during neonatal resuscitation are epinephrine, volume expanders, and naloxone.
- Some of the more common congenital anomalies include choanal atresia, cleft lip, diaphragmatic hernia, and Pierre Robin syndrome.
- At birth, newborns make three major physiological adaptations necessary for survival: (1) emptying fluids from their lungs and beginning ventilation, (2) changing their circulatory pattern, and (3) maintaining body temperature.
- The initial steps of neonatal resuscitation (except for those born through meconium) are to prevent heat loss, clear the airway by positioning and suctioning, provide tactile stimulation and initiate breathing if necessary, and further evaluate the infant.
- The three most common complications during the postresuscitation period are endotracheal position change (including dislodgment), tube occlusion by mucus or meconium, and pneumothorax. During transport of the neonate, it is important to maintain body temperature, oxygen administration, and ventilatory support.
- Specific situations that may require advanced life support for the neonate include meconium staining, apnea, diaphragmatic hernia, bradycardia, premature infants, respiratory distress and cyanosis, hypovolemia, seizures, fever, hypothermia, hypoglycemia, and vomiting and diarrhea.
- Premature infants have an increased risk of respiratory suppression, hypothermia, and head and brain injury. In addition to low birth weight, various antepartum and intrapartum risk factors may affect the need for resuscitation.
- About 2% to 7% of every 1000 live births result in avoidable and unavoidable mechanical and anoxic trauma during labor and delivery.

- The paramedic should be aware of the normal feelings and reactions of parents, siblings, other family members, and caregivers while providing emergency care to an ill or injured child.

REVIEW QUESTIONS

Match the structures described in Column I with the correct term in Column II.

Column I	Column II
1. _____ A vertical split in the lip	**a.** Choanal atresia
2. _____ Abnormalities that include a small mandible and defects of the eyes and ears	**b.** Cleft lip
3. _____ Occlusion that blocks the passage between the nose and pharynx	**c.** Diaphragmatic hernia
	d. Gastroesophageal reflux
4. _____ Protrusion of stomach through the diaphragm	**e.** Pierre Robin syndrome

5. List two risk factors that may indicate the need for neonatal resuscitation in each of the following categories:

    a. Antepartum risk factors

_____

    b. Intrapartum risk factors

_____

6. What three major adaptations are necessary for the survival of the neonate at birth?

    a.

    b.

    c.

7. List three actions that help maintain body warmth of the neonate.

    a.

    b.

    c.

8. Arrange the following steps in neonatal resuscitation (assuming you have a blue infant with slightly decreased respirations and a heart rate of 70 that does not improve at each step) in the correct order in the following table.

Incorrect Order	Correct Order
Administer epinephrine.	
Obtain vascular access.	
Administer oxygen at 5 L/min.	
Ventilate with bag-mask device.	
Perform chest compressions.	
Warm, dry, suction, and stimulate.	

Questions 9 to 14 pertain to the following case study:

A 3-kg baby is delivered, his airway has been suctioned, and he has been positioned properly. Tactile stimulation has been provided; however, he is still not breathing.

9. At what rate should you ventilate the neonate?

_____

After ventilations are initiated, you detect a pulse of 70 per minute.

10. Where should you palpate the pulse on a neonate?

_____

11. What steps should you take now?

_____

After you initiate chest compressions, there is no improvement. Your partner has intubated the baby.

12. What size of endotracheal tube would be appropriate for this infant?

_____

13. What are your options to obtain vascular access?

_____

14. What drug/dose should you administer when vascular access has been established?

_____

15. List an intervention for each of the following neonatal postresuscitation complications:

   a. Endotracheal tube dislodgment

   _____

   b. Endotracheal tube occlusion by mucus

   _____

   c. Pneumothorax

   _____

STUDENT SELF-ASSESSMENT

16. In which of the following situations will you anticipate the need for neonatal resuscitation?
    a. Contractions have been occurring for 6 hours.
    b. Physician states the baby weighs 3600 g (7½ lb).
    c. Rupture of the membranes occurred 12 hours ago.
    d. The baby is at 36 weeks' gestation.
17. What initiates respiration in the newborn?
    a. Chemical and temperature changes
    b. Chest compression
    c. Closure of the patent ductus
    d. Cutting the umbilical cord
18. What is a proper position to maximize the airway of a neonate?
    a. Prone with neck slightly extended
    b. Supine with neck slightly flexed
    c. Supine with towel under the shoulders
    d. Supine with towel under the head
19. Which neonatal suctioning technique is appropriate after delivery if no meconium has been observed?
    a. Cut the umbilical cord before suctioning.
    b. Suction secretions from the mouth first and then the nose.
    c. Suction secretions from the nose first and then the mouth.
    d. Suctioning is unnecessary if meconium is not observed.

20. Priorities of care for neonatal resuscitation are as follows:
    a. Prevent heat loss, administer intravenous fluids, and allow the infant to feed at the breast.
    b. Position the neonate, suction to clear the airway, minimize external stimulation, and initiate intravenous fluids.
    c. Prevent heat loss, position the neonate, suction to clear the airway, and provide stimulation.
    d. Position the infant, suction to clear the airway, administer intravenous fluids, and provide stimulation.
21. Deep suctioning of the posterior pharynx of the neonate may cause which of the following?
    a. Bradycardia
    b. Central nervous system depression
    c. Hypocarbia
    d. Tachypnea
22. After delivery the infant is warmed, dried, and stimulated. Respirations are 30 per minute and heart rate is 110, but the baby's lips and ears are still blue. What should you do?
    a. Administer oxygen at 5 L/min by holding the tubing ½ inch from the nose.
    b. Begin bag-mask ventilation with 100% oxygen until the color improves.
    c. Initiate bag-mask ventilation and chest compressions.
    d. No intervention is needed; this is a normal finding in the newborn.
23. Which of the following is an acceptable method of neonatal stimulation?
    a. Shouting loudly close to the baby's ear
    b. Holding the baby by the ankles and slapping the buttocks
    c. Slapping or flicking the soles of the feet or rubbing the back
    d. Vigorously shaking the baby by firmly grasping the shoulders
24. When should the paramedic consider intubation of the neonate?
    a. If the heart rate increases after bag-mask ventilation is performed
    b. If prolonged ventilation is likely to be needed
    c. Immediately after absent respirations are noted
    d. When the gestational age is less than 39 weeks
25. What is the normal heart rate of an infant?
    a. 60 beats/min
    b. 80 beats/min
    c. 120 beats/min
    d. 160 beats/min
26. Which finding may indicate a postresuscitation complication related to intubation in the neonate?
    a. Decreased resistance to ventilation
    b. Diminished breath sounds
    c. Increase in chest expansion
    d. Return of tachycardia
27. Apnea in infants may be related to which of the following?
    a. Central nervous system disorders
    b. Excessive stimulation
    c. Meconium aspiration
    d. Use of stimulants
28. The most common factor for respiratory distress and cyanosis in a neonate is prematurity. Which of the following factors also can be responsible for this condition?
    a. Cleft lip congenital anomaly
    b. Mucus obstruction of the nasal passages
    c. Premature rupture of membranes
    d. Postterm delivery
29. What is the correct first drug and dose used for the treatment of neonatal bradycardia in the presence of adequate ventilation and oxygenation?
    a. Atropine 0.01 mg/kg IV
    b. Atropine 0.02 mg/kg IV
    c. Epinephrine 0.01 mg/kg (1:1000) IV
    d. Epinephrine 0.01 mg/kg (1:10,000) IV
30. Which of the following is a risk factor associated with cardiac arrest in the newborn?
    a. Amniotic fluid aspiration
    b. Gestational diabetes
    c. Intrauterine asphyxia
    d. Premature cutting of the cord after birth

31. Which is true regarding vomiting in the neonate?
    a. An intravenous line should be established if this is observed.
    b. It is unusual and is associated with serious illness.
    c. It is a frequent occurrence and should be of no concern.
    d. Persistent bile-stained vomit may indicate a bowel obstruction.
32. What sign or symptom can be found following phototherapy for hyperbilirubinemia?
    a. Bradycardia   c. Seizures
    b. Diarrhea   d. Vomiting
33. You are called to evaluate a 4-day-old breast-fed infant whose mother states the child has diarrhea. When asked, she says the child is having five or six "loose" yellow stools per day. What is your assessment of this situation?
    a. This number of stools is normal for a breast-fed baby.
    b. This indicates a serious situation that requires immediate intravenous therapy.
    c. This indicates bowel obstruction from a congenital defect.
    d. The yellow stools could indicate hepatitis, and the mother should be assessed for risk.
34. A mother states that she has observed repetitive eye deviation and blinking and sucking and swimming movements of the 2-day-old infant's arms. This may indicate which of the following?
    a. Focal clonic seizures   c. Subtle seizures
    b. Multifocal seizures   d. Tonic seizures
35. What should be assessed in the prehospital setting when evaluating an infant with apparent seizures?
    a. Blood glucose level   c. Child's ability to feed normally
    b. Blood pressure   d. Glasgow Coma Scale
36. Which is true of a temperature of 100.4° F (38.0° C) in a neonate?
    a. It is a normal result of immature temperature control and does not require treatment.
    b. It may indicate a life-threatening infection and requires immediate transport.
    c. It often results in the development of febrile seizures that are difficult to control.
    d. Prehospital care should involve ice packs in the groin area to lower temperature.
37. A 3-kg infant delivered at home yesterday is limp and has irregular respirations. You assess the child, maintain warmth, assist ventilations, and initiate vascular access. The blood glucose drawn when the intravenous line was started is 40 mg/dL. What should you administer?
    a. 3 g of a $D_{10}W$ solution   c. 6 g of a $D_{10}W$ solution
    b. 3 g of a D50W solution   d. 6 g of a D50W solution
38. Which of the following injuries may occur during childbirth?
    a. Clavicle or extremity fracture   c. Spine or spinal cord injury
    b. Liver or spleen injury   d. All of the above
39. Which of the following statements by the paramedic would be helpful when speaking to the parents of an infant who is being resuscitated in the prehospital setting:
    a. Everything's going to be okay.
    b. Everything possible is being done for your baby.
    c. I can't tell you anything at all about your baby.
    d. I think your baby's going to make it; this is a great crew.

WRAP IT UP

You hear the dispatcher say, "Respond to a call for maternity ... ," and you figure this will just be another person who thinks she is in labor. However, when you arrive, the father meets you at the door yelling, "The baby, the baby." You find an 18-year-old woman squatting by the bed, pants around her ankles, screaming, and can see thick, chunky, green liquid running down her legs and a baby's head crowning at her perineum. You quickly pull out the OB kit, while your partner calls for a pumper assist and hurries to get the pediatric resuscitation bag from your ambulance. As the head delivers, you suction secretions from the mouth and then nose with the bulb syringe, pulling out thick meconium with each aspiration. The chest delivers, and there is no immediate spontaneous respiration, so you insert an endotracheal tube, quickly applying suction to the end. As you pull it out some residual green meconium is aspirated, and you repeat it twice until there is no aspirate. Your partner holds an oxygen mask close to the baby's face and checks his heart rate after you position him on his side, dry him, and stimulate him; it is 50 per minute, and he is floppy and does not grimace to suction, so your partner begins ventilation with a bag mask. After 30 seconds, there is no improvement in heart rate, so you have a firefighter perform chest compressions while you intubate his trachea and verify placement. You explain quickly to the mother that the baby has not responded to initial treatment, so you are helping his blood circulate with chest compressions and are going to give him some medicines to help stimulate his heart. There is still no improvement, so you initiate an umbilical line and administer epinephrine. Reassessment shows a heart rate of 150 beats/min, which quickly slows when you stop ventilation for a moment. You continue ventilation with frequent reevaluation of tube placement and cover him to keep him warm until you arrive at the ED 10 minutes later. After a month in NICU, he is released home and his mother brings him to visit 2 months later.

1. What scene finding made you prepare for neonatal resuscitation?
   a. Age of the mother
   b. Baby crowning on arrival
   c. Presence of meconium on the mother's legs
   d. Resuscitation is needed on most field deliveries
2. What physiological change at birth explains the
   a. Presence of secretions in the baby's nose and mouth that need suctioning.

   _____

   b. Need to dry and warm the infant. _____

   c. Circulatory changes after the cord is cut. _____
3. Place a check mark beside the steps in the neonatal resuscitation pyramid that you performed on this baby.
   a. _____ Position, suction, stimulate   d. _____ Chest compression
   b. _____ Oxygen   e. _____ Intubation
   c. _____ Bag-mask ventilation   f. _____ Medication
4. Why was the baby intubated and secretions suctioned before any other resuscitation measures?
   a. All babies with meconium in the amniotic fluid need intubation.
   b. If the paramedic is skilled at intubation, it should be done first.
   c. It takes longer to insert an umbilical catheter, so it is left until later.
   d. The baby was depressed, and the meconium was thick.
5. Why is it important to give the family some preliminary information about the baby's condition?

   _____

CHAPTER 43 ANSWERS

Review Questions

1. b
(Objective 1)

2. e
(Objective 1)

3. a
(Objective 1)

4. c
(Objective 1)

5. a. Multiple gestation, inadequate prenatal care, mother's age, history of perinatal morbidity or mortality, postterm gestation, drugs/medication, toxemia, hypertension, and diabetes
b. Premature labor, meconium-stained amniotic fluid, rupture of membranes more than 24 hours before delivery, use of narcotics within 4 hours of delivery, abnormal presentation, prolonged labor or precipitous delivery, prolapsed cord, bleeding
(Objective 1)

6. a. Emptying fluid from the lungs and beginning ventilation
b. Changing the circulatory pattern
c. Maintaining body temperature
(Objective 2)

7. a. Dry the infant's head and body thoroughly; remove any wet coverings; cover the head and body of the baby with warm blankets; turn the heat up high in the ambulance; use chemical warm packs (with blankets between the pack and the infant).
(Objective 3)

8.

Incorrect Order	Correct Order
Administer epinephrine.	Warm, dry, suction, and stimulate.
Obtain vascular access.	Administer oxygen at 5 L/min.
Administer oxygen at 5 L/min.	Ventilate with bag-mask device.
Ventilate with bag-mask device.	Perform chest compressions.
Perform chest compressions.	Obtain vascular access.
Warm, dry, suction, and stimulate.	Administer epinephrine.
(Objective 4)	

9. Initiate positive pressure breathing with 100% oxygen by bag mask at 40 to 60 breaths/min.
(Objectives 3 and 4)

10. At the brachial artery, at the umbilical cord, or by auscultation
(Objective 3)

11. Continue positive pressure ventilations for 30 seconds; if heart rate does not begin to improve, start chest compressions ½ to ¾ inch at 120 per minute.
(Objective 4)

12. 2.5 or 3.0
(Objective 4)

13. Initiate a peripheral intravenous line, an intraosseous line, or an umbilical vein cannulation.
(Objective 4)

14. Epinephrine 0.01 mg/kg (1:10,000)
(Objective 4)

15. a. If breath sounds are audible only on the right, pull back slightly and reevaluate; if tube is in the correct location, secure. If breath sounds are absent, remove the tube and reintubate.
(Objective 5)

b. Suction the tube with a suction catheter and reevaluate.
(Objective 5)

c. Assess for presence of tension pneumothorax, and treat if present. If at hospital, prepare to assist with chest tube placement.
(Objective 5)

16. d. A premature infant refers to a baby born before 37 weeks' gestation (weight usually 0.6 to 2.2 kg [1½ to 5 lb]). The incidence of complications increases as gestational age (and weight) decreases. A normal birth weight is 7½ lb; 6 hours is not a lengthy labor. Rupture of membranes more than 24 hours before birth would be a concern.
(Objective 1)

17. a. As the chest recoils during delivery, chemical and temperature changes initiate the first breath. Cutting the umbilical cord initiates changes in fetal circulation.
(Objective 2)

18. c. The torso should be elevated ¾ to 1 inch so that the neck is slighted extended.
(Objective 3)

19. b. The mouth should be suctioned before the nose, and then the cord can be cut.
(Objective 3)

20. c. Intravenous fluids are rarely necessary in the normal infant if appropriate resuscitation is done.
(Objective 3)

21. a
(Objective 3)

22. a. Continue the oxygen administration until the color improves (keep the baby warm).
(Objective 3)

23. c. The goal is to stimulate the neonate without risk of injury.
(Objective 3)

24. b. Often the infant will initiate adequate spontaneous respirations after a brief period of bagging and will not require intubation. Increasing heart rate is a positive indicator.
(Objective 4)

25. c. A heart rate greater than 100 beats/min is desirable. Chest compressions should be initiated for a persistent heart rate less than 80 beats/min that does not respond to ventilation.
(Objective 3)

26. b. Decreased chest wall movement, return of bradycardia, unilateral decrease in chest expansion, altered intensity to pitch or breath sounds, and increased resistance to hand ventilation are signs that may point to tube migration, occlusion, or pneumothorax.
(Objective 5)

27. a. Other causes include narcotic/central nervous system depressant use, airway or respiratory muscle weakness, oxyhemoglobin dissociation curve shift, septicemia, and metabolic disorders.
(Objective 6)

28. b. Infants are obligate nose breathers; suctioning of mucus from the nasal passages will correct this problem.

29. d. Inadequate ventilations and oxygenation are the most common causes of bradycardia and should be reassessed continually.
(Objective 6)

30. c. Other causes are drugs taken by the mother, congenital diseases or malformations, and intrapartum hypoxemia.
(Objective 6)

31. d. Some vomiting is normal; however, if it is persistent or bile-stained or contains dark blood, a serious underlying illness may exist. Vascular access would not be indicated unless needed to treat dehydration or bradycardia because of the vagal stimulation this can produce.
(Objective 6)

32. b. Other causes of diarrhea in the neonate are gastroenteritis, lactose intolerance, neonatal abstinence syndrome, thyrotoxicosis, and cystic fibrosis
(Objective 6)

33. a. The baby should be assessed for clinical signs of dehydration or other signs of illness (e.g., fever, lethargy, and feeding habits), but typically this stool pattern is normal in this situation.
(Objective 5)

34. c. All types of seizures in this age group are considered pathological.

35. a. Hypoglycemia may produce seizure activity. Determining the presence of this condition and correcting it are urgent matters.
(Objective 6)

36. b. Even small temperature elevations in this age group can signal impending sepsis. Febrile seizures are unusual in this age group and would not be expected (especially at this temperature). Ice packs should never be applied to a neonate.
(Objective 6)

37. a
(Objective 6)

38. d. Brain and hypoxic injuries may occur as well.
(Objective 7)

39. b. Honest, frequent updates about the baby's condition should be given during the resuscitation so that family members can prepare themselves for the outcome.
(Objective 7)

WRAP IT UP

1. c. Meconium points to a high-risk delivery, especially if it is thick and dark. Other indicators of birth complications are early delivery, maternal use of drugs, and multiple births.
(Objective 1)

2. a. Fluid is squeezed from the chest into the nose and mouth during delivery and should be suctioned.
b. Infants have a large body surface area, immature temperature regulation mechanisms, and are born into a cool, wet environment. Maintaining warmth is a critical aspect of neonatal resuscitation.
c. Cutting the cord shuts down placental circulation, closing some of the circulatory pathways established in utero.
(Objective 2)

3. a, b, c, d, e, f. On most deliveries, progression past (a) or (b) is never needed.
(Objectives 3 and 4)

4. d. This is the only situation when intubation would be near the first step.
(Objectives 4 and 6)

5. Family should be given brief, accurate information often to give them a realistic idea of the condition of their baby.
(Objective 8)

CHAPTER
44

Pediatrics

READING ASSIGNMENT
Chapter 44, pages 1116-1159, in *Mosby's Paramedic Textbook,* ed. 3

OBJECTIVES
Upon completion of this chapter, the paramedic student will be able to:
1. Identify the role of the Emergency Medical Services for Children program.
2. Identify modifications in patient assessment techniques that assist in the examination of patients at different developmental levels.
3. Identify age-related illnesses and injuries in pediatric patients.
4. Outline the general principles of assessment and management of the pediatric patient.
5. Describe the pathophysiology, signs and symptoms, and management of selected pediatric respiratory emergencies.
6. Describe the pathophysiology, signs and symptoms, and management of shock in the pediatric patient.
7. Describe the pathophysiology, signs and symptoms, and management of selected pediatric dysrhythmias.
8. Describe the pathophysiology, signs and symptoms, and management of pediatric seizures.
9. Describe the pathophysiology, signs and symptoms, and management of hypoglycemia and hyperglycemia in the pediatric patient.
10. Describe the pathophysiology, signs and symptoms, and management of infectious pediatric emergencies.
11. Identify common causes of poisoning and toxic exposure in the pediatric patient.
12. Describe special considerations for assessment and management of specific injuries in children.
13. Outline the pathophysiology and management of sudden infant death syndrome.
14. Describe the risk factors, key signs and symptoms, and management of injuries or illness resulting from child abuse and neglect.
15. Identify prehospital considerations for the care of infants and children with special needs.

SUMMARY
- The Emergency Medical Services for Children program was designed to enhance and expand emergency medical services for acutely ill and injured children. The program has defined 12 basic components of an effective Emergency Medical Services for Children system.
- Children have unique anatomical, physiological, and psychological characteristics, which change during their development.
- Some childhood diseases and disabilities can be predicted by age group.
- Many elements of the initial evaluation can be done by observing the child. The child's parent or guardian also should be involved in the initial evaluation. The three components of the pediatric assessment triangle are appearance, work of breathing, and circulation.

- Obstruction of the upper or lower airway by a foreign body usually occurs in toddlers or preschoolers. Obstruction may be partial or complete.
- Croup is a common inflammatory respiratory illness. It usually is seen in children between the ages of 6 months and 4 years. Symptoms are caused by inflammation in the subglottic region.
- Bacterial tracheitis is an infection of the upper airway and subglottic trachea often seen in infants and toddlers; it often occurs with or after croup.
- Epiglottitis is a rapidly progressive, life-threatening bacterial infection. It causes edema and swelling of the epiglottis and supraglottic structures. It often affects children between 3 and 7 years of age.
- Asthma is common in children over 2 years of age. Asthma is characterized by bronchoconstriction that results from autonomic dysfunction or sensitizing agents.
- Bronchiolitis is a viral disease frequently caused by respiratory syncytial virus infection of the lower airway; it usually affects children age 6 to 18 months of age.
- Pneumonia is an acute infection of the lower airways and lungs involving the alveolar walls and the alveoli.
- Several special differences must be remembered when caring for a child in shock. These include circulating blood volume, body surface area and hypothermia, cardiac reserve, and vital signs and assessment. A child in shock may appear normal and stable until all compensatory mechanisms fail. At that point, pediatric shock progresses rapidly, with serious deterioration.
- When dysrhythmias occur in children, they usually result from hypoxia or structural heart disease.
- The most common causes of seizure in adult and pediatric patients are noncompliance with a drug regimen for the treatment of epilepsy, in addition to head trauma, intracranial infection, metabolic disturbance, or poisoning. The most common cause of new onset of seizure in children is fever.
- Hypoglycemia and hyperglycemia should be suspected whenever a child has an altered level of consciousness with no explainable cause.
- Children with infection may have a variety of signs and symptoms. These depend on the source and extent of infection and the length of time since the patient was exposed.
- Most poisoning events in the United States involve children. Signs and symptoms of accidental poisoning vary, depending on the toxic substance and the length of time since the child was exposed.
- Blunt and penetrating trauma is a chief cause of injury and death in children. Head injury is the most common cause of death in pediatric trauma patients. Early recognition and aggressive management can reduce morbidity and mortality caused by traumatic brain injury in children.
- Because of the pliability of the chest wall, severe intrathoracic injury can be present without signs of external injury. The liver, kidneys, and spleen are the most frequently injured abdominal organs. Extremity injuries are more common in children than adults.
- Sudden infant death syndrome is the leading cause of death in American infants under 1 year of age. The syndrome is defined as the sudden death of a seemingly healthy infant. The death cannot be explained by history and an autopsy.
- Child abuse and neglect is the maltreatment of children by their parents, guardians, or other caregivers. Forms of maltreatment include infliction of physical injury, sexual exploitation, and infliction of emotional pain and neglect.
- Some infants and children are born with or develop conditions that pose special needs. These children may require special medical equipment to sustain life. Often these children are cared for at home. Many are dependent on specialized medical equipment such as tracheostomy tubes, home artificial ventilators, central venous lines, gastrostomy tubes, and shunts.

REVIEW QUESTIONS

Match the drugs in column II with their appropriate initial *pediatric* dose in column I. Use each drug only once.

Column I	Column II
1. _____ 0.1 mL/kg	**a.** Adenosine
2. _____ 2 to 20 μg/kg/min	**b.** Amiodarone
3. _____ 1 mEq/kg per dose	**c.** Atropine sulfate
4. _____ 0.1 to 0.2 mg/kg	**d.** Diazepam
5. _____ 1 mg/kg	**e.** Dopamine hydrochloride
6. _____ 0.02 mg/kg	**f.** Epinephrine (1:10,000)
7. _____ 5 mg/kg	**g.** Lidocaine
	h. Sodium bicarbonate

8. In what pediatric age group(s) are you most likely to see the following illness or injuries?

a. Sepsis:

_____

b. Febrile seizures:

_____

c. Jaundice:

_____

d. Ingestions:

_____

e. Falls:

_____

f. Child abuse:

_____

g. Drowning or near drowning:

_____

h. Suicidal gestures:

_____

Questions 9 to 12 pertain to the following case study:

A 7-year-old boy is in acute respiratory distress after visiting a friend's home. He gives a history of asthma and allergy to dogs (his friend has three). His home medicines include an Atrovent inhaler, montelukast sodium (Singulair) tabs, which he takes daily, and albuterol by nebulizer as necessary, which he has not used for a week. He has circumoral cyanosis, is working very hard to breathe, and has faint inspiratory and expiratory wheezes.

9. What interventions are appropriate for this child? Include two possible beta-agonist drugs you could administer (with appropriate doses and routes).

_____

10. What side effects do you anticipate from the administration of these drugs?

_____

11. In 15 minutes, you see no clinical improvement and your estimated arrival time is still 20 minutes. What do you do?

_____

12. What aspects of the physical examination will change when the patient improves?

_____

_____

13. List three characteristic signs or symptoms of epiglottitis.

    a.

    b.

    c.

14. A 20-month-old with croup is in mild respiratory distress on a cool October evening.

    a. What intervention should you try before entering the ambulance that may cause rapid improvement in the patient's signs and symptoms?

_____

    b. When in the ambulance, how will you care for this child?

_____

_____

Questions 15 to 19 pertain to the following case study:

A limp, 11-month-old boy is carried into the ambulance base by his mother. She states that he has had a fever with vomiting and diarrhea for 3 days. His eyes are sunken, his tongue is furrowed, and his lips are cracked. Physical examination reveals rapid respirations; cold, mottled extremities; and the electrocardiogram shown in Fig. 44-1.

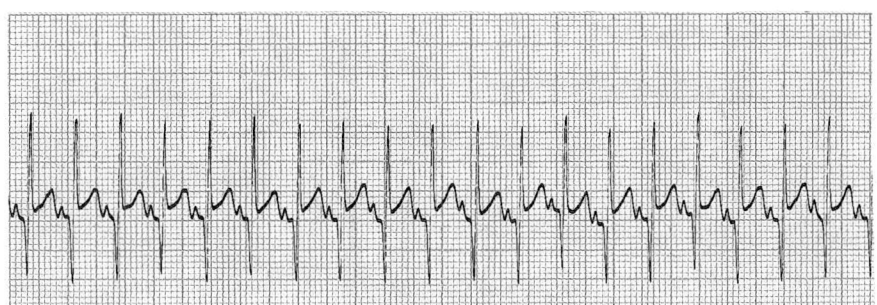

Figure 44-1

15. What condition does this child have?

_____

16. Interpret the electrocardiogram.

_____

17. Describe management of this child, assuming a 45-minute transport time.

_____

_____

18. What are the appropriate vital signs for this child?

_____

19. What clinical signs of improvement will you watch for in addition to improvement in vital signs?

_____

Questions 20 to 23 refer to the following case study:

A 3-year-old, 33 pound (15 kg)-child is found unconscious after suffocation with a plastic bag. On arrival, you find a dusky, pale child who is unresponsive and apneic. Occasionally you can palpate a faint pulse at the carotid artery, but you obtain no blood pressure reading. The electrocardiogram is shown in Fig. 44-2.

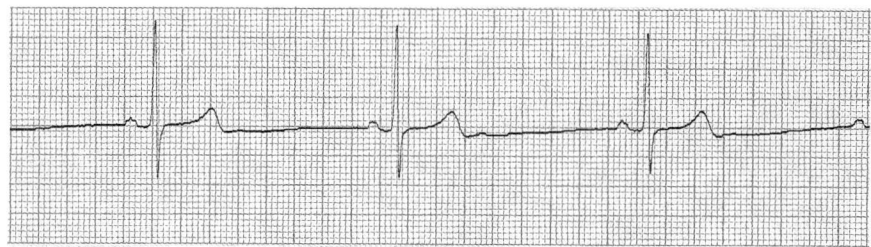

Figure 44-2

20. Interpret the electrocardiogram tracing.

_____

21. What actions will you take immediately, up to and including the first drug (with appropriate dose and route).

_____

_____

22. If an intravenous line cannot be immediately established, what two actions can be taken?

    a.

    b.

23. After your initial interventions result in no patient improvement, what is the next drug (and dose and route) indicated?

_____

24. A 3-week-old, 5 kg infant with a history of congenital heart defects suddenly loses consciousness and stops breathing. On arrival, you find him pulseless and apneic. Cardiopulmonary resuscitation is initiated, the child's trachea is intubated, and lactated Ringer solution is given intravenously. The electrocardiogram tracing in Fig. 44-3 is noted.

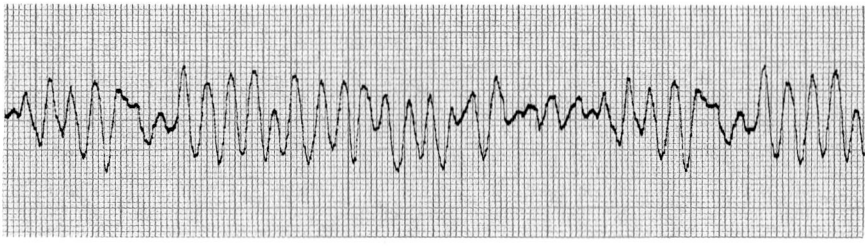

Figure 44-3

a. Outline your continued care of this patient, up to and including the first two drugs (including doses and routes).

_____

_____

_____

b. If a repeat dose of epinephrine is necessary, what is the correct dose and concentration?

_____

Questions 25 to 27 refer to the following case study:

A frightened mother tells you that when she put her 4-year-old, 14-kg child to bed, he complained of a slight earache and had a low-grade temperature. She heard a noise several hours later and found her child having a grand mal seizure, which stopped after approximately 1 minute. The child's temperature is 105.5° F (40.8° C). He appears to be postictal at this time.

25. After you have ensured that the child is stable, what history should you obtain from the mother?

_____

_____

26. What care should be provided en route to the hospital?

_____

_____

27. If the child has a seizure during transport, list two anticonvulsant drugs that may be given, including the appropriate doses and routes.

a.

b.

28. You are called to an elementary school to care for a 6-year-old who is "acting funny." She is responsive only to pain. The nurse says the child has a history of diabetes. You check a finger-stick glucose level and determine that this child's blood sugar is 35 mg/dL.

a. What drug should you administer (including dose and route)?

_____

b. What other signs or symptoms may this child have had before becoming this ill?

_____

_____

29. Your 3-year-old patient weighs 17 kg. He was involved in a head-on motor vehicle collision and was restrained only by a lap belt. He says his "tummy hurts." The physical examination reveals an anxious, pale child with a rigid, tender abdomen. Discuss the significance of the following physiological differences in children and specific ways they will influence your care of this child.

a. Children have a greater percentage of circulating blood volume than adults.

_____

_____

b. Children have a large body surface area in proportion to body weight.

_____

_____

c. Children's hearts function at near-maximal performance in a normal, healthy state.

_____

_____

d. Volume replacement in children is weight related.

_____

_____

_____

e. Intravenous access is difficult to establish in children.

_____

_____

30. How do you determine whether an intraosseous needle has been properly placed?

_____

Questions 31 to 33 pertain to the following case study:

At 1 AM on a cool February morning, you are dispatched for a "baby choking." On arrival you find a well-nourished 4-month-old baby boy apneic and pulseless in his crib. There is frothy sputum in the nose and mouth, and his diaper is wet and full of stool. The child is cold, and dependent lividity is present. The hysterical mother states that he and his older sister have both had a slight cold but that otherwise he was healthy.

31. What characteristics of sudden infant death syndrome are consistent with this call?

_____

32. What other findings should you document in this situation?

_____

You spend some time at the scene comforting the family and making the appropriate notifications and then ride back quietly to the firehouse with your normally talkative partner. You ask if he is OK, and he says, "Of course, I'm fine." Then he immediately rushes to the phone, where you hear him awaken his wife and ask her to check on their 6-month-old daughter.

33. Should you ignore your partner's unusual behavior, since he told you he is OK? If not, what action(s) can you take?

_____

_____

Questions 34 to 36 pertain to the following case study:

A mother tells you that her 8-month-old son fell off his tricycle early in the day but seemed to be feeling fine. Later, she could not wake him from his nap. On physical examination you find a dirty child who has agonal respirations, a slow pulse, and extension posturing. No visible signs of trauma are present on the head, although small bruises are noted on the shoulders.

34. What should your immediate interventions be for this child?

_____

_____

35. What findings might lead you to suspect child abuse?

_____

_____

36. After you deliver the child to the appropriate medical center, what are your responsibilities?

_____

_____

37. What history and physical examination should be performed on a child who is a victim of sexual abuse?

_____

_____

STUDENT SELF-ASSESSMENT

38. Which of the following is a component of an effective EMSC system?
    a. Access to care   **c.** Legislative committees
    b. Immunization programs **d.** Medical direction

39. Which examination strategy can help reduce anxiety in school-age children?
    a. Allow them to take part in decisions about their care.
    b. Reassure them that they are not being punished.
    c. Let them play with equipment.
    d. Use deep breathing and relaxation techniques.

40. Which age group fears bodily injury and mutilation and interprets words literally?
    a. Adolescents   **c.** School-age children
    b. Preschoolers   **d.** Toddlers

41. You are called to care for a 6-month-old child who has respiratory distress. Which of the following would be the most likely cause of this complaint in this age group?
    a. Asthma
    b. Bronchiolitis
    c. Epiglottitis
    d. Foreign body airway obstruction

42. A great deal of the child's physical examination can be done by which step?
- **a.** Assessing the skin temperature and moisture.
- **b.** Auscultating the breath sounds.
- **c.** Observing the child's behavior.
- **d.** Palpating the central and distal pulses.

43. Which of the following is a sign of respiratory distress in a child?
- **a.** Crying
- **b.** Elevated temperature
- **c.** Flushed skin
- **d.** Head bobbing

44. Which of the following is a bacterial infection of the upper airway and subglottic trachea that occurs during or after croup?
- **a.** Bronchiolitis
- **b.** Epiglottitis
- **c.** Pneumonia
- **d.** Tracheitis

45. Which of the following may be indicated for the management of severe respiratory distress associated with bronchiolitis?
- **a.** Albuterol, 0.15 mg/kg by inhalation
- **b.** Atropine, 0.01 mg/kg by inhalation
- **c.** Epinephrine, 0.1 mg/kg subcutaneously
- **d.** Terbutaline, 0.2 mg/kg subcutaneously

46 Which of the following is an appropriate intervention for a child in whom epiglottitis is suspected?
- **a.** Lay the child supine on the mother's lap.
- **b.** See if the epiglottis is swollen.
- **c.** Infuse intravenous normal saline fluids at 20 mL/kg.
- **d.** Give humidified oxygen by mask.

47. Which drug may be administered to relieve respiratory distress in a child with bronchiolitis?
- **a.** Albuterol
- **b.** Alupent
- **c.** Epinephrine
- **d.** Diphenhydramine

48. Which of the following findings would be your first indication that an infant is developing dehydration and needs a fluid bolus?
- **a.** Decreasing blood pressure and poor skin turgor
- **b.** Flat fontanelle and warm skin
- **c.** Loss of appetite and nausea
- **d.** Very dry mucous membranes and tachycardia

49. A 20-kg child is lethargic and tachycardic and has dry mucous membranes after a 3-day history of "flu." Medical direction asks for a fluid bolus of normal saline. How much will you administer initially?
- **a.** 20 mL
- **b.** 100 mL
- **c.** 200 mL
- **d.** 400 mL

50. You are caring for a child who has fatigue, difficulty breathing, and peripheral edema. Crackles are audible in the bases of both lungs. Which illness do you suspect?
- **a.** Anaphylaxis
- **b.** Asthma
- **c.** Cardiomyopathy
- **d.** Pneumonia

51. A 5-year-old, 44-lb child is in ventricular fibrillation. Which is the correct *initial* energy level for defibrillation?
- **a.** 20 joules
- **b.** 40 joules
- **c.** 80 joules
- **d.** 88 joules

52. What is the maximum single dose of atropine that should be given to a 6-year-old child?
- **a.** 0.05 mg
- **b.** 0.01 mg
- **c.** 0.1 mg
- **d.** 0.5 mg

53. What is the correct sequence of interventions for a bradycardic, hypotensive child after the airway has been secured, an intravenous line has been established, and cardiopulmonary resuscitation has been initiated?
- **a.** Atropine and epinephrine
- **b.** Epinephrine and atropine
- **c.** Atropine only
- **d.** Epinephrine only

54. An infant who "wasn't acting right" has a heart rate of 230/min. He is awake but somewhat lethargic, and his skin is pale with delayed capillary refill. You determine that he has SVT, and your partner has established vascular access. What is the initial treatment of choice for this child?
- **a.** Adenosine
- **b.** Digoxin
- **c.** Synchronized cardioversion
- **d.** Verapamil

55. Which of the following is *not* likely to cause seizures?
- **a.** CNS infection
- **b.** Metabolic abnormalities
- **c.** Prolonged dehydration
- **d.** Serious head trauma

56. After intravenous administration of diazepam, you should monitor closely for which of the following?
- **a.** Decreased pulse
- **b.** Increased blood pressure
- **c.** Respiratory depression
- **d.** Vomiting or nausea

57. Your 7-year-old patient is lethargic and has a blood pressure of 70/50 mm Hg and a pulse of 138/min. Respirations are 40/min and smell fruity. His mother says he has been losing weight and has had increased urination and thirst for several weeks. What condition should you consider?
- **a.** Head injury
- **b.** Hydrocarbon ingestion
- **c.** Hyperglycemia
- **d.** Hyperthermia

58. What life-threatening condition may be found in a child after ingestion of alcohol?
- **a.** Hypoglycemia
- **b.** Hypothermia
- **c.** Hypokalemia
- **d.** Hypocalcemia

59. What clinical finding may be present in a child who has ingested a large amount of aspirin?
- **a.** Bradycardia
- **b.** Hiccoughs
- **c.** Hypothermia
- **d.** Tachypnea

60. You are caring for a teenager who was "huffing" toluene. What effects could this produce?
- **a.** Pulmonary edema
- **b.** Renal failure
- **c.** Uncontrolled bleeding
- **d.** Visual disturbances

61. A 14-year-old is experiencing anxiety, tremors, and chest pain after smoking crack cocaine. His vital signs are BP, 180/100 mm Hg; P, 130/min; and R, 20/min. Which of the following drugs would *not* be indicated in the initial care of this child?
- **a.** Aspirin
- **b.** Epinephrine
- **c.** Lorazepam
- **d.** Nitroglycerin

62. A 4-year-old has taken 10 tricyclic antidepressant tablets. Her BP is 60 mm Hg by palpation; P is 130/min; and she is drowsy. Which intervention would be indicated to improve her cardiac output?
- **a.** Lidocaine (1 mg/kg)
- **b.** Normal saline (30 mL/kg bolus)
- **c.** Oxygen (2 L/min)
- **d.** Sodium bicarbonate (1 mEq/kg)

63. Glucagon may be helpful as an antidote to an overdose of
- **a.** Beta blockers
- **b.** Calcium channel blockers
- **c.** Cocaine
- **d.** Tricyclic antidepressants

64. Which mechanism of injury accounts for the largest number of trauma deaths in children?
- **a.** Drowning
- **b.** Falls
- **c.** Fire
- **d.** Motor vehicle crashes

65. Which is a sign of increasing intracranial pressure unique to an infant?
- **a.** Bulging fontanelle
- **b.** Cheyne-Stokes respirations
- **c.** Hypotension
- **d.** Tachycardia

66. Why is the child more vulnerable to liver and splenic injuries?
- **a.** Those organs are larger in children under the age of 8 years.
- **b.** Mechanisms of injury in children are more likely to affect these areas.
- **c.** The abdominal musculature is minimal and does not protect these organs.
- **d.** These organs are more fragile in a child and injure more easily.

67. Which is a risk factor associated with a higher incidence of SIDS?
- **a.** High maternal or paternal age
- **b.** Rank of first in the birth order
- **c.** Premature birth and low birth weight
- **d.** Higher socioeconomic groups

68. Which of the following injuries should be considered the result of possible abuse?
- **a.** Any fractures in a child less than 5 years of age.
- **b.** Injuries localized to one area of the body.
- **c.** Bruises or burns in unusual patterns.
- **d.** Lacerations on the forehead of a toddler.

69. You are called to care for a 10-month-old child who "didn't wake up from his nap." He is unconscious and has vomited. What other physical findings may indicate abuse?

a. Dirty diaper
b. Increased respiratory rate
c. Other children in the room
d. Retinal hemorrhage

70. Respiratory distress is reported in a child who has a tracheostomy. The tube appears to be partly obstructed. Which of the following should be your first intervention?

a. Intubate the child orally.
b. Insert a tracheal dilator to enlarge the hole.
c. Remove and replace the tracheostomy.
d. Suction the tracheostomy.

71. A child is experiencing signs and symptoms of hypoxia while on a home ventilator. On arrival you should immediately perform which of the following?

a. Begin ventilation with a bag-valve device.
b. Check the connections on the machine and oxygen.
c. Contact medical direction to help trouble-shoot.
d. Request that the home health agency repair the ventilator.

72. A frantic mother calls you to check her son's central venous catheter because it is leaking. On arrival you note that the catheter is cracked and leaking. The child's condition is stable. What action should you take?

a. Clamp the line
b. Flush the line
c. Remove the line
d. Tape around the crack

73. A child with a gastric feeding tube develops respiratory distress. For what complication should you assess?

a. Allergic reaction
b. Aspiration
c. Hypoglycemia
d. Pulmonary embolism

WRAP IT UP

You are dispatched to a home for an "unresponsive child." As you pull up to the house, a woman runs toward your ambulance with a limp, 3-week-old infant in her arms. "He's had a runny nose and been listless today," she explains, "then he started shaking all over, and now I can't wake him." "Febrile seizure," you hear your partner mutter under his breath. In the ambulance, oxygen is administered as you begin to assess the baby. He is floppy and limp, but he grimaces, whines weakly, and opens his eyes when you rub his sternum, and his arms flex. You note rapid breathing, with retractions of the ribs. The skin is pale and cool and shows sluggish capillary refill (about 3 seconds). Vital signs are BP, 70/50 mm Hg; P, 168/min; and R, 40/min. Oxygen saturation is intermittently showing about 95%, and the infant's lungs are clear. A temperature shows 99° F (37° C) axilla, and the diaper is wet when you remove it. Pupils are 3 mm and react to light; skin turgor seems normal; ECG shows a rapid, narrow complex tachycardia; and blood glucose is 98 mg/dL. No other significant findings are noted on the detailed exam. The baby's mother says he was term with no birth complications and no illnesses or injuries that she is aware of. You are able to start a 22 g IV in the AC space TKO and continue to monitor the baby's condition, which is unchanged en route. In the ED a determination of sepsis is made, and the infant is admitted to the ICU.

1. Put a ✓ beside some possible causes of this baby's condition, based on your initial impression.

a. _____ Abuse
b. _____ Croup
c. _____ Dehydration
d. _____ Febrile seizure
e. _____ Jaundice
f. _____ Meningitis
g. _____ Sepsis

2. Which aspects of the physical examination indicated that the baby was in distress?

_____

_____

3. What treatment should have been given to treat the heart rate/rhythm?

a. Adenosine
b. Diltiazem
c. Vagal maneuvers
d. None of the above

4. What was the baby's score on the Glasgow Coma Scale?

_____

5. What should you monitor most closely as you continue transport?

_____

_____

6. a. List at least three possible causes of seizure in a baby this age.

_____

_____

    b. What interventions would you consider if the child has another seizure?

_____

_____

7. Why should you assess the blood glucose level in this child even though you know that the onset of type 1 diabetes does not usually occur until later in childhood?

_____

_____

CHAPTER 44 ANSWERS

REVIEW QUESTIONS

   1. f
   2. e
   3. h
   4. a
   5. g
   6. c
   7. b
(Questions 1-7: Objective 7)

   8. a. Neonate
       b. Infant, toddler, and preschooler
       c. Neonate
       d. Infant and toddler
       e. Infant, toddler, and school-age child
       f. Young infant, infant, toddler, school-age child, and adolescent (sexual abuse)
       g. Preschooler and school-age child
       h. Adolescent
       (Objective 3)

   9. Humidified oxygen by nonrebreather mask, position of comfort (to maximize respiratory efficiency), albuterol 0.01 to 0.03 mL (0.05 to 0.15 mg)/kg/dose to maximum of 0.5 mL/dose diluted in 2 mL of 0.9% NS, or epineph-rine 0.01 mL/kg subcutaneous (1:1000), maximum 0.3 mL
       (Objective 5)

  10. Tachycardia and anxiousness
       (Objective 5)

  11. Repeat drugs, initiate IV, and continue to reassess.
       (Objective 5)

  12. Patient will state improvement, respiratory rate will decrease, oxygen saturation will improve, use of accessory muscles will decrease, wheezing will diminish (inspiratory wheeze and then expiratory wheeze should dissi-pate), and heart rate may decrease (although possibly not because of the effects of beta agonists).
       (Objective 5)

  13. Drooling, stridor, sudden onset of high fever, and dysphagia
       (Objective 5)

  14. a. Take the patient into the cool night air or into a steam-filled bathroom. b. Allow the child to assume a posi-tion of comfort and administer high-flow oxygen (humidified) by whatever means is least threatening to the child.
       (Objective 5)

  15. Moderate to severe dehydration
       (Objective 6)

  16. Sinus tachycardia
       (Objective 6)

17. Open airway, ventilate with 100% oxygen; initiate lactated Ringer solution or normal saline intravenously (intraosseously if intravenous line cannot be established), and infuse initial fluid bolus of 20 mL/kg; reassess and repeat until perfusion improves.
(Objective 6)

18. BP, 82/44 mm Hg; P, 80 to 140/min; R, 30 to 40/min
(Objective 4)

19. Improved level of consciousness, skin color, and temperature
(Objective 6)

20. Sinus bradycardia, rate 30/min
(Objective 7)

21. Assess ABCs, secure airway, administer 100% oxygen using bag-mask device, perform chest compressions, start an intravenous or intraosseous line, assess vital signs, and if bradycardia continues, administer epinephrine 0.1 mL/kg (1:10,000) intravenously or intraosseously.
(Objective 7)

22. Infuse the medication intraosseously or administer epinephrine 0.1 mL/kg (1:1000) endotracheally diluted to 3 to 5 mL. NOTE: Endotracheal dose is 10 times greater than the intravenous dose.
(Objective 7)

23. Atropine 0.02 mg/kg intravenously to a maximum single dose of 0.5 mg (child) and 1 mg (adolescent); minimum dose: 0.1 mg
(Objective 7)

24. a. Defibrillate at 2 joules/kg and then at 2 to 4 joules/kg and 4 joules/kg; continue cardiopulmonary resuscitation, administer epinephrine 0.1 mL/kg (1:10,000), defibrillate at 4 joules/kg, and administer amiodarone 5 mg/kg intravenously or intraosseously or lidocaine 1 mg/kg intravenously or intraosseously or magnesium 25 to 50 mg/kg intravenously or intraosseously for torsades de pointes or hypomagnesemia (maximum: 2 g)
b. Epinephrine 0.1 mL/kg (1:1000) intravenously or intraosseously, repeated every 3 to 5 minutes
(Objective 7)

25. Description of seizure activity, vomiting during seizure, history of epilepsy or another major medical illness, other current medicines, potential for toxic ingestion, recent head injury, and complaints of headache or stiff neck
(Objective 8)

26. Maintain airway and breathing; monitor vital signs; cool child with tepid water and fanning; monitor electrocardiogram and oxygen saturation (if available); depending on patient's vital signs and level of consciousness, initiate lactated Ringer solution intravenously to keep vein open and obtain blood sample; assess blood sugar and treat if it is below 60 mg/dL.
(Objective 8)

27. a. Diazepam 1 mg every 2 to 5 minutes by slow IV; if intravenous or intraosseous infusion is not possible, administer medication rectally at higher dose (0.5 mg/kg).
b. Lorazepam 0.05 to 0.15 mg/kg/dose intramuscularly, intravenously, or intraosseously to maximum dose 4 mg (rectal dose: 0.1 to 0.2 mg/kg)
(Objective 8)

28. a. 50% dextrose 1 to 2 mL/kg/dose or 25% dextrose 2 to 4 mL/kg/dose intravenously
(Objective 9)

b. Presenting symptoms of mild hypoglycemia may be hunger, weakness, tachypnea, and tachycardia. Presenting symptoms of moderate hypoglycemia may be sweating, tremors, irritability, vomiting, mood swings, blurred vision, stomachache, headache, and dizziness.
(Objective 9)

29. a. Because a relatively small loss of blood can be devastating, fluid resuscitation should be anticipated for blood volume losses that would seem small in an adult.
b. This makes children susceptible to hypothermia. Measures should be used on the scene to maintain body warmth.
c. This leaves them little reserve for a stressed situation such as shock. Energy and oxygen requirements should be reduced to a minimum by assisting ventilations and using measures to decrease anxiety and promote body warmth.
d. Volume replacement with lactated Ringer solution or normal saline should be initiated at 20 mL/kg given rapidly and repeated if no response is seen. If good response is obtained, the fluids should be continued at a weight-related maintenance rate obtained from medical direction.
e. Intravenous access should first be attempted in a peripheral vein in the arms, hands, or feet. If access cannot be easily established and the patient's condition deteriorates, intraosseous infusion should be used.
(Objectives 6, 12)

30. Aspiration of marrow may rarely be obtained. The intravenous fluid will run freely with no evidence of infiltration.
(Objectives 4, 6)

31. Occurrence between midnight and 6 AM, male child under 6 months, occurrence between October and March, frothy sputum, wet diaper with stool, second child, and recent mild viral illness.
(Objective 13)

32. Document death as required by protocol and observe carefully for any obvious external signs of trauma.
(Objective 13)

33. Encourage your partner to verbalize, perhaps stating, "It's frightening to go on a call like this when you have a baby at home." Listen if he wants to talk; if he does not, check on him again in the morning. Initiate the CISD team, following local protocol (if available).
(Objective 13)

34. Protect the cervical spine while opening the airway; hyperventilate with 100% oxygen and consider intubation; verify perfusion with slow pulse; if it is inadequate, initiate cardiopulmonary resuscitation; en route to the hospital initiate an intravenous or intraosseous line and administer medicines if indicated.
(Objective 12)

35. The story does not match the physical findings or the child's developmental stage. An 8-month-old child is too young to ride a tricycle. A fall from a tricycle is unlikely to produce intracerebral bleeding. The child had no external signs of head trauma but had bruises at the shoulders that may suggest shaking. The child was dirty (this could be normal).
(Objective 14)

36. Report the suspected abuse to the receiving facility and to other authorities as indicated by local protocol. Carefully document all physical findings and statements made by the mother, using exact quotes if possible. This document is likely to be questioned in court if abuse is suspected.
(Objective 14)

37. Only enough data to address the immediate threats to the health of the sexually abused child should be elicited. The child should be made to feel safe and secure, and the detailed history and physical examination should be performed by child sexual abuse specialists if they are available in your area.
(Objective 14)

STUDENT SELF-ASSESSMENT

38. a. The other 11 components are system approach, education, data collection, quality improvement, injury prevention, prehospital care, emergency care, definitive care, rehabilitation, finance, and ongoing health care from birth to young adulthood.
(Objective 1)

39. b. Have them repeat things back to you in their words to be sure they understand. Give them choices when possible. Anticipate questions about the long-term effect of care, injuries, and so on.
(Objective 2)

40. b. Toddlers fear separation and loss of direction; school-age children fear bodily injury and mutilation but are less likely to interpret words literally.
(Objective 2)

41. b. Asthma is usually not diagnosed until a child is 3 to 5 years of age. Epiglottitis is more common in children 3 to 5 years of age. Foreign body airway obstruction would be unlikely in this age group because children usually do not eat solid food at this age.
(Objective 3)

42. c. Each component is important, but information about level of consciousness, color, respiratory effort, and muscle tone often can be assessed by observing children before touching them.
(Objective 4)

43. d. Other signs are use of accessory muscles, nasal flaring, tachypnea, bradypnea, irregular breathing pattern, grunting, and absent or abnormal breath sounds.
(Objective 4)

44. d. It may produce stridor and complete airway obstruction.
(Objective 5)

45. a. The correct dose of epinephrine is 0.01 mL/kg subcutaneously (1:1000), and the correct dose of terbutaline is 0.01 mg/kg of a 1 mg/mL solution subcutaneously.
(Objective 5)

46. d. The child should be permitted to assume a position of comfort, which typically is sitting up with the chin jutted forward to maximize airflow. Examination of the airway can produce obstruction and is contraindicated. Initiation of an intravenous infusion will not improve the child's condition and may cause the child to become agitated and cry, increasing the respiratory distress.
(Objective 5)

47. a. Albuterol can provide temporary symptomatic relief with limited side effects.
(Objective 5)

48. d. Fluid resuscitation should not be delayed until the blood pressure drops, or resuscitating the child may be difficult. The fontanelle likely would be flat and the skin cool.
(Objective 6)

49. d. The recommended fluid bolus is 20 mL/kg.
20 mL/kg × 20 kg = 400 mL
(Objective 6)

50. c. Crackles and edema are characteristics of congestive heart failure associated with cardiomyopathy.
(Objective 6)

51. b. 44 lb = 20 kg; initial defibrillation is 2 joules/kg; 2 joules × 20 kg = 40 joules
(Objective 7)

52. d. Atropine 0.02 mg/kg to a maximum dose of 0.5 mg in a child
(Objective 7)

53. b. Epinephrine is the drug of choice in patients with bradycardia with hemodynamic compromise, followed by atropine if no improvement results.
(Objective 7)

54. a. If his condition deteriorates, synchronized cardioversion may be considered.
(Objective 7)

55. c. Unless the dehydration produces severe electrolyte imbalance, it is much more likely to produce shock and death than seizures.
(Objective 8)

56. c. Ventilatory equipment should be available, and the respiratory rate and depth should be closely monitored. Pulse oximetry should be used if available.
(Objective 8)

57. c. Undiagnosed type 1 diabetes can manifest in this manner with severe hyperglycemia and ketoacidosis. This child is critical and needs urgent transport with airway management, oxygenation, and fluid resuscitation.
(Objective 9)

58. a. Hypoglycemia can lead to death if left uncorrected.
(Objective 11)

59. d. Tachypnea, GI irritation, hypoglycemia, cardiac dysrhythmias (ventricular), seizure, coma, coagulation defects, and death can occur from salicylate poisoning.
(Objective 11)

60. d. Changes in color perception, hallucinations, and blindness can occur, as well as other CNS and GI effects.
(Objective 11)

61. b. Epinephrine would be indicated only if cardiac arrest ensues. Aspirin may be given to counteract the platelet aggregation property of cocaine; lorazepam is administered to treat anxiety and/or seizures; and nitroglycerin is used as a vasodilator to treat chest pain.
(Objective 11)

62. d. Sodium bicarbonate may be given to improve myocardial contractility and cardiac output. Lidocaine would be given to treat ventricular dysrhythmias (if present). Normal saline 10 mL/kg bolus may be given to improve cardiac output. Oxygen should be given at high flow based on the patient's physical findings.
(Objective 11)

63. a. Other prehospital interventions may include oxygen administration, ventilatory support (if indicated), ECG monitoring, treatment for shock, epinephrine infusion, sodium bicarbonate, and calcium chloride (controversial).
(Objective 11)

64. d. Motor vehicle crashes are the leading cause of death and serious injury in children.
(Objective 12)

65. a. Other findings include hypertension, bradycardia, and Cheyne-Stokes respirations.
(Objective 12)

66. c
(Objective 12)

67. c. Low maternal/paternal age, low socioeconomic group, and rank of second or third in the birth order are associated with an increased incidence.
(Objective 13)

68. c. Fractures in a child less than 2 years of age should be cause for suspicion.
(Objective 14)

69. d. Retinal hemorrhage is a sign of a shaken baby.
(Objective 14)

70. d. If suctioning does not improve the situation, removing and replacing the tracheostomy may be necessary. If this is not possible or proves unsuccessful, oral intubation or intubation through the stoma may be necessary.
(Objective 15)

71. a. Correcting the hypoxia is the priority. The machine can be checked and fixed after the hypoxia has been corrected.
(Objective 15)

72. a. If the child develops signs of air embolism, position him on the left side with his head lowered and administer high-flow oxygen.
(Objective 15)

73. b. If the tube becomes dislodged, the feeding could be delivered to the lung, causing aspiration.
(Objective 15)

WRAP IT UP

1. a, c, f, g. The baby is too young for croup and for febrile seizures (and the temperature is not high). No evidence of yellow skin or eyes was noted, which would be apparent in jaundice. Dehydration is less likely because skin turgor is normal and the diaper is wet.
(Objective 3)

2. Decreased muscle tone and level of consciousness; labored, rapid breathing; rapid heart rate; skin color.
(Objective 4)

3. d. Based on the information available, this baby's rapid heart rate probably is sinus tachycardia. If the rhythm were SVT, the heart rate could be expected to be about 220/min. Treatment should focus on the underlying cause of the tachycardia.
(Objective 7)

4. Opens eyes to pain (2) + flexion to pain (4) + whines (3) = 9
(Objective 4)

5. Respiratory status should be monitored closely by observing rate, effort, Sao_2, skin color, heart rate, and, if available, end-tidal CO_2.
(Objective 4)

6. a. Head trauma, intracranial infection, metabolic disturbance, poisoning, epilepsy
b. Secure the airway, manage breathing, and consider administration of lorazepam or diazepam.
(Objective 8)

7. Blood glucose can be altered by other illnesses and should be assessed in any child with altered level of consciousness.
(Objective 4)

45

Geriatrics

READING ASSIGNMENT
Chapter 45, pages 1160-1183, in *Mosby's Paramedic Textbook*, ed. 3

OBJECTIVES
Upon completion of this chapter, the paramedic student will be able to:
1. Explain the physiology of the aging process as it relates to major body systems and homeostasis.
2. Describe general principles of assessment specific to older adults.
3. Describe the pathophysiology, assessment, and management of specific illnesses that affect selected body systems in the geriatric patient.
4. Identify specific problems with sensations experienced by some geriatric patients.
5. Discuss effects of drug toxicity and alcoholism in the older adult.
6. Identify factors that contribute to environmental emergencies in the geriatric patient.
7. Discuss prehospital assessment and management of depression and suicide in the older adult.
8. Describe epidemiology, assessment, and management of trauma in the geriatric patient.
9. Identify characteristics of elder abuse.

SUMMARY
- The aging process proceeds at different rates in different persons. Respiratory function in the older adult generally is compromised. This is a result of changes in pulmonary physiology that go along with the aging process. Cardiac function also declines with age. This is a result of normal physiological changes and the high incidence of coronary artery disease. Renal blood flow falls an average of 50% between 30 and 80 years of age. A gradual decrease in neurons, decreased cerebral blood flow, and changes in the location and amounts of specific neurotransmitters probably contribute to changes in the CNS. As the body ages, muscles shrink, muscles and ligaments calcify, and the intervertebral disks become thin. Other physiological changes that occur with aging include changes in body mass and total body water, a decreased ability to maintain internal homeostasis, a decrease in the function of immunological mechanisms, nutritional disorders, and decreases in hearing and visual acuity.
- Normal changes with aging and existing illnesses may make evaluation of an ill or injured geriatric patient a challenge.
- Pneumonia is a leading cause of death in the geriatric age group. It often is fatal in frail adults. Chronic obstructive pulmonary disease (COPD) is a common finding in the geriatric patient who has a history of smoking. The disease usually is associated with various other diseases that result in reduced expiratory airflow. Pulmonary embolism is a life-threatening cause of dyspnea. Pulmonary embolism is associated with venous stasis, heart failure, COPD, malignancy, and immobilization. All of these are common in older adults.
- A lack of the typical chest pain can cause MI to go unrecognized in the geriatric patient. Heart failure is more frequent in geriatric patients and has a larger incidence of noncardiac causes. The most common cause of

dysrhythmias in the geriatric patient is hypertensive heart disease. Abdominal aortic aneurysm affects 2% to 4% of the U.S. population over 50 years of age. This aneurysm is most prevalent between 60 and 70 years of age. The incidence of hypertension in the geriatric patient increases when atherosclerosis is present.

- Risk factors for cerebral vascular disease in the older adult include smoking, hypertension, diabetes, atherosclerosis, hyperlipidemia, polycythemia, and heart disease.
- Delirium is an abrupt disorientation of time and place. Delirium is commonly a result of physical illness.
- Dementia is a slow, progressive loss of awareness of time and place. It usually involves an inability to learn new things or remember recent events. This condition often is a result of brain disease. Alzheimer's disease is the most common cause of dementia. Alzheimer's disease is a condition in which nerve cells in the cerebral cortex die and the brain substance shrinks.
- Parkinson's disease is a brain disorder. It causes muscle tremor, stiffness, and weakness.
- About 20% of older adults have diabetes. Almost 40% have some impaired glucose tolerance. Hyperglycemic hyperosmolar nonketotic coma is a serious complication of elderly type 2 diabetic patients. It has a mortality rate of 20% to 50%. Thyroid disease is more common in geriatric patients. It may not present in the classic manner.
- Gastrointestinal bleeding most often affects patients between 60 and 90 years of age. It has a mortality rate of about 10%. Bowel obstruction generally occurs in patients with prior abdominal surgeries or hernias. It also occurs in those with colonic cancer. Some geriatric patients may have problems with continence or with elimination as well.
- Aging results in a gradual decrease in epidermal cellular turnover. It also results in loss of deep and dermal vessels. Capillary circulation leads to changes in thermal regulation and skin-related complications.
- Osteoarthritis is a common form of arthritis in geriatric patients. It results from cartilage loss and wear and tear on the joints. The loss in bone density from osteoporosis causes bones to become brittle. These bones may fracture easily.
- As persons age, they may experience problems with vision, hearing, and speech.
- Geriatric patients are at an increased risk for adverse drug reactions. This is due to age-related changes in body makeup and drug distribution. It also is the result of metabolism and excretion. Moreover, the risk for adverse drug reactions often stems from multiple prescribed drugs. Alcohol abuse is a common problem in geriatric patients.
- The geriatric patient may develop hypothermia while indoors. This may be the result of cold surroundings and/or an illness that alters heat production or conservation. Hyperthermia most likely results from exposure to high temperatures that continue for several days.
- Depression is common in geriatric patients. It can result from physiological and psychological causes. The rate of completed suicides for geriatric patients is higher than that of the general population.
- One third of traumatic deaths in persons 65 to 74 years of age result from vehicular trauma. Twenty-five percent result from falls. In those older than 80 years of age, falls account for 50% of injury-related deaths. The risk of fatality from multiple trauma is estimated to be 3 times greater at 70 years of age than at 20 years of age.
- Elder abuse is classified as physical abuse, psychological abuse, financial or material abuse, and neglect.

REVIEW QUESTIONS

1. An 85-year-old woman falls down an escalator at a department store. Explain how age-related changes in each of the following areas increase her risk of suffering a traumatic injury or influence her body's response to a major injury.

   a. Respiratory system:

   _____

   _____

   b. Cardiovascular system:

   _____

   _____

c. Renal system:

_____

_____

d. Musculoskeletal system:

_____

_____

e. Thermoregulation:

_____

_____

2. A woman calls you to the home of her 70-year-old father, who has fallen. He says he is just fine. On your arrival, she states that he has a history of diabetes, a heart attack, heart failure, and lung disease. His home medications include Lanoxin, insulin, Dyazide, Slow-K, Theo-Dur, and a number of vitamins and laxatives. He is on oxygen at 2 L/min by nasal cannula.

a. What factors will make it difficult to assess and determine the nature of his acute problem?

_____

_____

_____

_____

b. List eight possible causes of his fall.

a.	**e.**
b.	**f.**
c.	**g.**
d.	**h.**

Questions 3 to 5 pertain to the following case study:

A 70-year-old man calls you to his home complaining of dyspnea and weakness. He has no underlying pulmonary problems. His ECG is shown in Fig. 45-1.

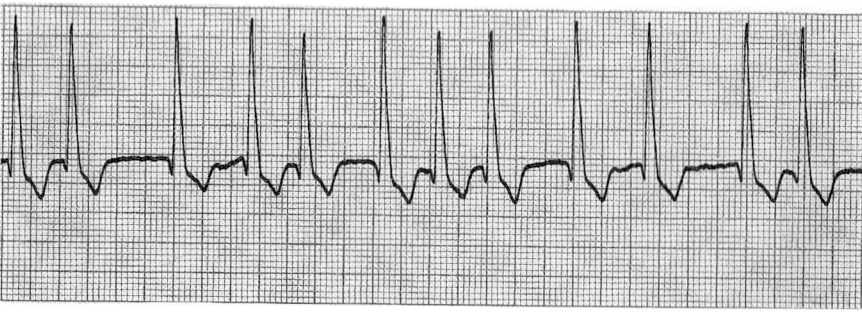

Figure 45-1

3. Why should you assess the appropriate history and physical examination for myocardial infarction and pulmonary embolism on this patient?

_____

4. What is your interpretation of the ECG rhythm?

_____

5. List two complications associated with this dysrhythmia.
   a.

   b.

6. A 76-year-old woman complains of diffuse abdominal pain. Identify four conditions that can cause this symptom.
   a.

   b.

   c.

   d.

7. Briefly describe the following characteristics of delirium:

   a. Onset:

   _____

   b. Duration:

   _____

   c. Metabolic causes:

   _____

8. List four reversible causes of dementia.
   a.   c.
   b.   d.

Questions 9 to 11 pertain to the following case study:

An 80-year-old man experiences a syncopal episode in church. He is conscious but pale and diaphoretic. His blood pressure is 80/50 mm Hg. His ECG is shown in Fig. 45-2.

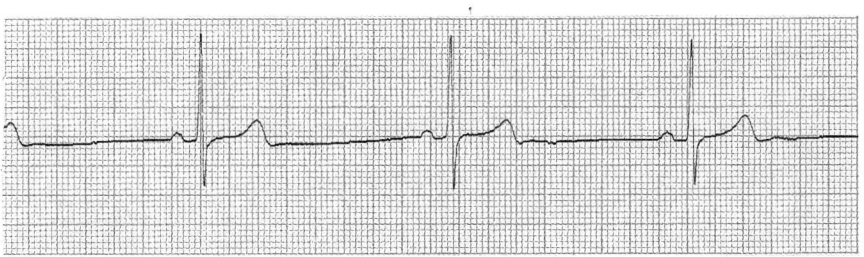

Figure 45-2

9. What is your interpretation of the rhythm?

_____

10. a. State the dose and route of administration of the drug used to treat this rhythm.

_____

    b. What other intervention should be considered if drug therapy is unsuccessful?

_____

11. List two possible causes of the signs and symptoms this patient is experiencing.
    a.
    b.

Questions 12 to 15 pertain to the following case study:

On arrival at a call for "difficulty breathing," you find a 69-year-old woman complaining of dyspnea and chills. She states that she has been ill with a mild cough and weakness for approximately 1 week. Her skin is cold and clammy. Vital signs are BP, 108/70 mm Hg; P, 135/min; and R, 30/min. Breath sounds in the right base are diminished with scattered crackles. Her ECG is shown in Fig. 45-3.

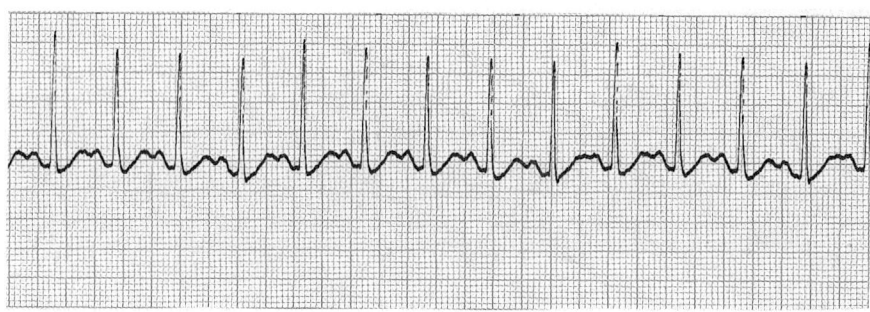

Figure 45-3

12. Identify the rhythm.

_____

13. What illness do you suspect?

_____

14. Should you use synchronized cardioversion or adenosine to treat the rhythm?

_____

15. What other interventions would be indicated for this patient?

_____

_____

16. An older man with a history of chronic lung disease is being transferred to another hospital. He has applied a Venturi mask that supplies oxygen at 24%. His vital signs are within normal limits. His ECG tracing is shown in Fig. 45-4.

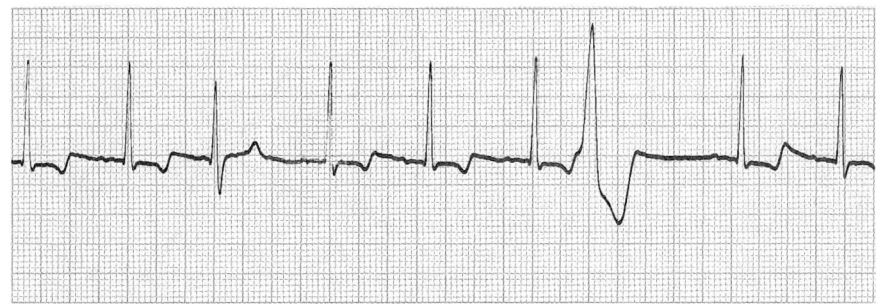

Figure 45-4

a. Identify the rhythm strip.

_____

b. What interventions are indicated with this rhythm?

_____

c. For what signs and symptoms of acute decompensation of COPD will you observe?

_____

17. An older patient who had a syncopal episode is now awake and has the following vital signs: BP, 108/70 mm Hg; P, 50/min; and R, 18/min and unlabored. The lungs are clear. The ECG is shown in Fig. 45-5.

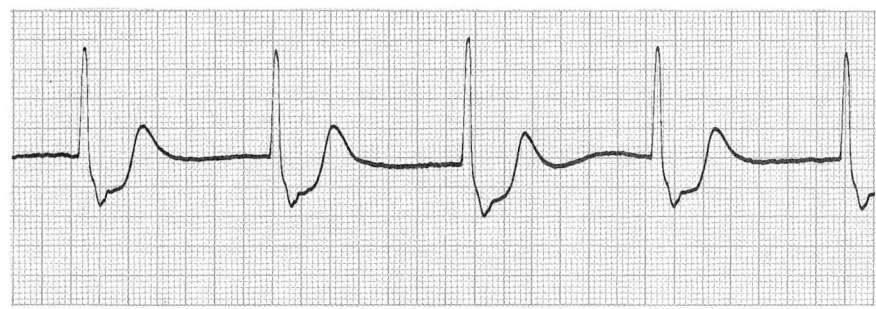

Figure 45-5

a. Identify the rhythm strip.

_____

b. After oxygen has been administered and intravenous therapy started, what interventions should be performed en route to the medical center?

_____

c. What age-related changes predispose this patient to developing this rhythm?

_____

Questions 18 to 21 refer to the following case study:

The family of a 72-year-old man states that he suddenly became confused and disoriented to time and place over the past few hours. His vital signs are BP, 168/110 mm Hg; P, 100/min; and R, 20/min. His ECG is shown in Fig. 45-6.

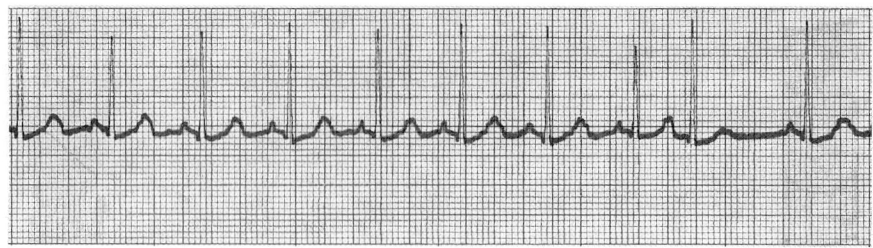

Figure 45-6

18. Is he likely experiencing dementia or delirium?

_____

19. Identify the rhythm strip.

_____

20. Are his symptoms related to his ECG tracing?

_____

21. List two factors that could cause this change in behavior.

  a.

  b.

Questions 22 and 23 refer to the following case study:

An 80-year-old woman complains of dizziness and shortness of breath. Her vital signs are BP, 82/50 mm Hg; P, 50/min; and R, 24/min. Her ECG tracing is shown in Fig. 45-7.

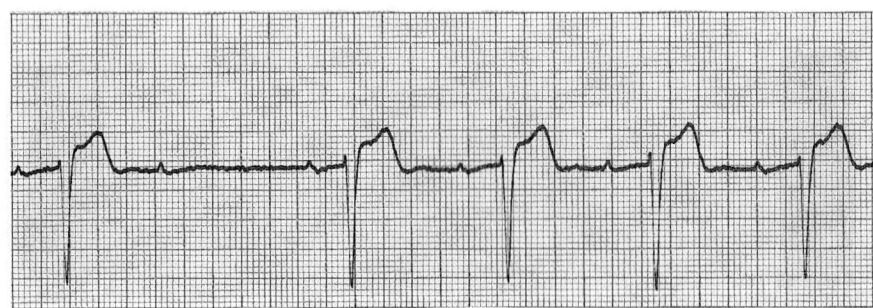

Figure 45-7

22. Identify the rhythm strip.

_____

23. a. What illness may be causing her signs and symptoms?

_____

b. List prehospital interventions that you will consider for this patient.

_____

24. A 94-year-old woman who was found in her apartment is confused and difficult to arouse. You note that it feels very cold inside, and her temperature is 95° F (35° C). List at least nine reasons (physiological, social, or medical) that she is at risk for hypothermia.

_____

_____

_____

25. Adverse drug reactions are common in older adults. For each of the following drugs or drug groups, list two signs or symptoms associated with overdose or adverse effects.

a. Anticoagulants:

_____

_____

b. Diuretics:

_____

_____

c. Digitalis:

_____

_____

d. Tricyclic antidepressants:

_____

_____

e. Sedative-hypnotic drugs:

_____

_____

f. Propranolol:

_____

_____

g. Theophylline:

_____

_____

h. Quinidine:

_____

_____

Questions 26 to 29 refer to the following case study:

You are on the scene of a single-car accident in which a compact car struck a bridge abutment at high speed. The driver, an anxious 75-year-old man, complains of mild abdominal discomfort. Vital signs are BP, 90/70 mm Hg; P, 70/min; and R, 24/min and somewhat labored. His skin is pale and clammy, and his nail beds are dusky.

26. What vital sign assessment does *not* fit with this man's clinical picture?

_____

27. What aspect of his history may explain this discrepancy?

_____

28. Because he has just mild abdominal pain, should you be concerned?

_____

29. What prehospital treatment should be given after the cervical spine has been appropriately immobilized?

_____

_____

30. You are at the home of an older patient who appears dehydrated and very dirty. You note large ecchymotic areas on the back and hips. The daughter, who lives with the patient, says these were caused by a fall.

a. If you suspect elder abuse, what should you do?

_____

_____

b. Does the caregiver have any characteristics of an elder abuser?

_____

STUDENT SELF-ASSESSMENT

31. Alterations in lung and chest wall compliance in the older adult result in a decrease in which of the following?
- **a.** Alveolar diameter
- **b.** Residual volume
- **c.** Total lung capacity
- **d.** Vital capacity

32. Humpback posture that develops as a result of osteoporosis is known by which of the following terms?
- **a.** Kyphosis
- **b.** Lordosis
- **c.** Osteoarthritis
- **d.** Scoliosis

33. An elderly patient presents with a sudden onset of dyspnea. The patient has crackles and wheezes. He had an MI 3 years ago and has no other history. Vital signs are BP, 170/94 mm Hg; P, 124/min; R, 28/min; and SaO_2, 90% on room air. You administer oxygen. What drug is indicated next?
- **a.** Albuterol
- **b.** Aspirin
- **c.** Epinephrine
- **d.** Furosemide

34. An elderly patient, whose only past medical history is metastatic breast cancer, has been on bed rest. She suddenly develops dyspnea and tachycardia. Which of the following would be the *least* likely cause of her symptoms?
    a. Chronic obstructive pulmonary disease
    b. Myocardial infarction
    c. Pneumonia
    d. Pulmonary embolus

35. Which of the following are possible causes of dementia?
    a. Alzheimer disease   c. Hyperglycemia
    b. Epilepsy   d. Pneumonia

36. Which illness causes trembling, a rigid posture, slow movement, and a shuffling, unbalanced walk?
    a. Alzheimer disease   c. Dementia
    b. Delirium   d. Parkinson disease

37. Administration of which of the following would be a critical prehospital intervention for an unconscious diabetic patient suffering from hyperglycemic hyperosmolar nonketotic coma?
    a. Dextrose   c. IV fluids
    b. Glucagon   d. Sodium bicarbonate

38. Which of the following is a consequence of thyroid dysfunction that might lead to a call for EMS?
    a. Altered mental status   c. Diarrhea
    b. Bradycardia   d. Weight gain

39. Your elderly male patient complains that he is unable to urinate. What condition should you inquire about specifically when obtaining his history?
    a. Constipation   c. Kidney stones
    b. Epididymitis   d. Prostate enlargement

40. Pressure ulcers are caused by which of the following?
    a. Burns   c. Infection
    b. Hypoxia   d. Tears of the tissue

41. Which eye condition causes damage to the optic nerve and can result in blindness if untreated?
    a. Cataracts   c. Corneal abrasion
    b. Conjunctivitis   d. Glaucoma

42. A patient is being treated for Parkinson disease. What sign, if present, might you attribute to drug toxicity?
    a. Altered vision   c. Paresthesias
    b. Hypokalemia   d. Tardive dyskinesia

43. Which of the following medications may increase the elderly patient's risk of hyperthermia?
    a. Amitriptyline (Elavil)   c. Cimetidine (Tagamet)
    b. Aspirin   d. Coumadin

44. Which of the following may be a physiological cause of depression in an elderly patient?
    a. Hyperglycemia   c. Hyponatremia
    b. Hypertension   d. Hypothermia

45. What is the most common psychiatric disorder in older adults?
    a. Bipolar disorder   c. Hysteria
    b. Depression   d. Schizophrenia

46. Why might the symptoms of increased intracranial pressure be delayed in an older patient?
    a. Altered blood-brain barrier   c. Decreased cerebral blood flow
    b. Cerebral atrophy   d. Fragile bridging veins

47. Which of the following is most often fractured in falls by older adults?
    a. Ankle   c. Hip
    b. Clavicle   d. Wrist

48. Which of the following home medications increases the older person's risk of falling?
    a. Alprazolam   c. Hydrochlorothiazide
    b. Digoxin   d. Dipyridamole

WRAP IT UP

Your partner groans as your dispatcher sends you to a familiar address for a "person down with possible forcible entry." The 80-year-old patient is well known because of her frequent 9-1-1 calls to "assist the invalid" when she misses her walker and slides to the floor. Since her stroke 3 months ago, she has been calling 9-1-1 several times a week despite attempts to identify appropriate social services. Her home is locked up tight, and you can see that she is sitting on the floor, but she oddly won't acknowledge the knocking on the window. The fire captain quickly breaks out a pane of glass on a rear door and unlocks it, permitting you to enter her steamy home. "Mabel, what's going on today?" you call out. As you approach her, you recognize that something is wrong; instead of her typical crooked smile, she is staring blankly ahead, showing no sign she recognizes you. Her skin color isn't right either; she looks pale and sweaty, and her usually neatly coifed hair is disheveled and dirty. As you grasp her wrist, you feel her rapid, irregular pulse and note that her breathing seems labored and fast. The oxygen saturation monitor is registering only 89%, much lower than her normal reading, and you can hear some basilar crackles when you listen to her lungs. A quick scan of her body reveals no obvious injuries. "Mabel, what's wrong? Are you in pain? Did you fall?" you ask. She looks blankly at you, and the usually polite and articulate woman mumbles some obscenities and pushes you away. You administer oxygen and assess her vital signs, which are BP, 102/60 mm Hg; P, 124/min; and R, 24/min. Her pupils are 3 mm, equal, and reactive to light. By then your partner has the cot at her side, and you guide her onto it and secure the straps. In the ambulance her ECG shows atrial fibrillation, and a blood sugar reading of 78 mg/dL is obtained as you start her IV. As you look through her sack of familiar medicines (furosemide, Persantine, aspirin, Glucophage, Lipitor, Lanoxin, Paxil), you realize that some of them are empty and, based on the date they were pre-scribed, they should not be. Her Sao_2 is improving on oxygen, and her vital signs are unchanged, but she is still mut-tering obscenities. You look more carefully head to toe to see if you've missed something on your initial exam, but you find nothing additional. As you sit writing your report at the hospital, you recall your last visit, 3 days ago, and try to think of anything unusual that may have occurred, but nothing seemed out of place.

1. Based on the information given, list five chronic problems this patient is likely to have.
   a.

   b.

   c.

   d.

   e.

2. Place a ✓ beside some possible causes for this patient's altered level of consciousness.

   a. _____ Delirium   f. _____ Hypoxia

   b. _____ Dementia   g. _____ Hypoglycemia

   c. _____ Head injury   h. _____ Overdose

   d. _____ Hyperthermia   i. _____ Sepsis

   e. _____ Depression   j. _____ Stroke

3. a. Would this patient be a candidate for fibrinolytic therapy if an acute stroke were diagnosed? Yes/No

   b. Explain your answer: _____

   _____

   _____

4. Which of the patient's social or medical conditions would *not* put her at high risk for complications related to her diabetes?
   a. Aspirin use
   b. Decreased ability to care for herself
   c. Living alone
   d. Other illnesses

5. If you think she has taken an overdose, what problems should you anticipate during transport based on your knowledge of her prescription drugs.

626

CHAPTER 45 ANSWERS

REVIEW QUESTIONS

1. a. Because the baseline Pao_2 is lower, the body is less able to compensate if chest trauma is sustained or if the patient is hypoxic because of trauma (e.g., inhalation injury). The chest wall is less elastic and more susceptible to injury.

b. Myocardial contusion can cause pump failure stemming from poor cardiac reserve. Decreased ability to increase the heart rate can result in a decreased ability to compensate for shock, and dysrhythmias can cause syncope and precipitate a fall.

c. Renal blood flow is decreased, therefore a sudden traumatic event that causes shock and hypoperfusion to the kidneys can precipitate the onset of renal failure; decreased renal function can make an older adult more susceptible to toxic drug effects, leading to CNS depression, disturbances in balance, hypotension, and dysrhythmias, all of which can increase the risk of falls.

d. Kyphosis may alter balance and predispose a person to falls, and osteoporosis increases the incidence of fractures after falls.

e. Advancing age can result in decreased peripheral vasoconstriction, a lowered metabolic rate, and poor peripheral circulation and can impair the body's ability to regulate temperature effectively, especially during stressful events such as traumatic injury. Hypothermia may occur rapidly.
(Objective 1)

2. a. His multiple illnesses and drugs make it difficult to assess for new onset of signs or symptoms. Diabetes: Impairs pain perception and retards healing. Heart attack and heart failure: Cardiac output may be impaired from chronic conditions, and dysrhythmias may be chronic. Lung disease: Patient's baseline must be determined. Cyanosis, increased respiratory rate, and abnormal lung sounds may be chronic. Lanoxin: Therapeutic effects slow heart rate; patient may not become tachycardic in response to trauma, and toxic effects may cause dysrhythmias. Insulin: Excessive amounts may cause hypoglycemia and produce CNS impairment. Dyazide: Diuretics may cause an electrolyte imbalance that can affect muscle strength and may precipitate dysrhythmias that can cause syncope and falls.
(Objective 2)

b. Dysrhythmias, visual impairment, neurological disabilities, arthritis, changes in gait, postural hypotension, syncope, cerebrovascular accident or transient ischemic attack, medications, slippery surfaces, loose rugs, objects on floors, poor lighting, pets, low beds or toilet seats, defective walking equipment, and lack of handrails on stairs.
(Objective 8)

3. In an older adult, dyspnea and weakness may be the only presenting history for myocardial infarction. Carefully obtain a patient history; perform a physical examination, including a 12-lead ECG; and treat with a high index of suspicion for myocardial infarction (these signs and symptoms also accompany pulmonary embolus).
(Objective 3)

4. Atrial fibrillation
(Objective 3)

5. Cerebrovascular accident and pulmonary embolism
(Objective 3)

6. Cholecystitis, colonic diverticular disease, appendicitis, aortic abdominal aneurysm, mesenteric artery occlusion, and mesenteric vein thrombosis
(Objective 2)

7. a. Rapid
b. Variable: It is usually self-limited and can be corrected quickly when the cause is identified.
c. Electrolyte imbalance, hypoglycemia, hyperglycemia, acid-base imbalance, hypoxia, vital organ failure, and Wernicke encephalopathy
(Objective 3)

8. Hypothyroidism, Cushing syndrome, vitamin deficiencies, and hydrocephalus
(Objective 3)

9. Sinus bradycardia, rate 30/min
(Objective 3)

10. a. Atropine 0.5 to 1 mg IV
(Objective 3)

b. Transcutaneous pacing
(Objective 3)

11. Acute myocardial infarction, drug toxicity, or vagal response
(Objective 3)

12. Sinus tachycardia
(Objective 3)

13. Bacterial pneumonia or pulmonary embolus
(Objective 3)

14. No to both; you must treat the patient and her underlying problem.
(Objective 3)

15. Administer high-flow oxygen via nonrebreather mask, initiate intravenous therapy, and monitor the patient's response and vital signs closely en route.
(Objective 3)

16. a. Normal sinus rhythm with a premature atrial contraction and a premature ventricular contraction
b. Continue to monitor the patient and the electrocardiographic rhythm.
c. Assess for limited airflow, increased work of breathing, dyspnea, hypoxemia, or hemodynamic compromise. Measure $EtCO_2$ if available.
(Objective 3)

17. a. Junctional rhythm
b. Observe the patient for any signs of hemodynamic compromise related to the slow rhythm (monitor vital signs and electrocardiogram). Consider drug administration or pacing if unstable.
c. Functional cells are lost in the SA and AV nodes during aging, which contributes to dysrhythmias.
(Objectives 2, 3)

18. Delirium (sudden onset)
(Objective 3)

19. Normal sinus rhythm with a premature atrial contraction
(Objective 3)

20. There is no reason for this ECG to cause these symptoms.
(Objective 3)

21. Intoxication or poisoning, withdrawal from drugs, metabolic disturbances, infectious processes, CNS trauma, and stroke.
(Objective 3)

22. Second-degree heart block Mobitz type II
(Objective 3)

23. a. Myocardial infarction is the most likely cause.
(Objective 3)

b. Administer high-concentration oxygen. Continue assessment to include breath sounds and observe for signs of congestive heart failure; perform head to toe survey. Initiate IV therapy at a TKO rate. Prepare to apply transcutaneous pacing. Consult with medical direction regarding administration of sedation (with caution because of dyspnea and hypotension). Provide rapid transport for definitive cardiac care. Perform a 12-lead ECG if available.
(Objective 3)

24. Decreased ability to sense changes in ambient temperature, less total body water to store heat, reduced likelihood of becoming tachycardic to compensate for cold stress, decreased ability to shiver, inability to pay utilities for heat, insufficient insulation, malnutrition, arthritis, drug overdose, hepatic failure, hypoglycemia, infection, Parkinson disease, stroke, thyroid disease, and uremia.
(Objective 6)

25. a. Bleeding problems, increased hemorrhage from trauma, multiple contusions, and allergic reactions.
b. Electrolyte abnormalities (sodium and potassium) and dehydration.
c. Influenza-like symptoms, multiple dysrhythmias, and bradycardia.
d. Dry mouth, tachycardia, ventricular dysrhythmias, seizures, and impaired level of consciousness.
e. Impaired perception (increased risk of falls) and decreased level of consciousness with respiratory depression.
f. Decreased heart rate (excessive), bronchoconstriction, and mood alteration.
g. Tachycardia, dysrhythmias, and CNS stimulation.
h. Dysrhythmias and clotting abnormalities.
(Objective 5)

26. His heart rate is slow relative to the rest of his clinical picture (everything else indicates impending shock or hypoxia).
(Objective 8)

27. He may have a pacemaker or may be taking medications (e.g., digitalis or beta blockers) that prevent his heart rate from becoming tachycardic in response to a decrease in cardiac output.
(Objective 8)

28. Yes, abdominal injuries are frequently lethal in older adults. His perception of pain may be impaired, and this situation could deteriorate quickly, especially with signs of shock.
(Objective 8)

29. Ensure a patent airway; deliver high-flow oxygen by nonrebreather mask; apply pneumatic antishock garments (if indicated by local protocol); en route to a trauma center, start two large-bore intravenous lines and administer small fluid challenges in consultation with medical direction; frequently monitor vital signs and lung sounds (for increased rales [crackles]) to make sure the patient is not developing a volume overload.
(Objective 8)

30. a. Follow local protocols and report to appropriate authority (e.g., local law enforcement, abuse hotline, medical direction) as indicated; report findings to receiving hospital and document findings thoroughly on prehospital run report.
b. Yes, daughter lives with parent.
(Objective 9)

STUDENT SELF-ASSESSMENT

31. d. Total lung capacity remains unchanged because the loss of chest wall compliance balances the weakened respiratory muscles. The residual volume increases as a result of variable increases in alveolar diameter and the tendency for distal airways to collapse on expiration.
(Objective 1)

32. a. *Lordosis* is the normal S curve of the spine. *Osteolysis* is degeneration of bone. *Scoliosis* is lateral curvature of the spine, usually found in childhood.
(Objective 3)

33. d. The patient has no history of COPD. His history and clinical presentation point to left-sided heart failure. Furosemide would be the drug of choice.
(Objective 3)

34. a. The risk of myocardial infarction increases in postmenopausal women. Myocardial infarction may manifest without pain in elderly patients. Pneumonia is a complication seen in immunocompromised patients or those who have other chronic illnesses, and it may have an atypical presentation in older adults. Pulmonary embolus is a higher risk in patients with cancer and in bedridden patients.
(Objective 3)

35. a. The other conditions may cause delirium.
(Objective 3)

36. d. These signs can be reduced or eliminated with drug therapy.
(Objective 3)

37. c. This condition results from excessive glucose in the blood and causes serious dehydration; IV fluids are indicated in the prehospital setting to treat the severe dehydration. Sodium bicarbonate may be indicated after arterial blood gas analysis or if the patient experiences cardiac arrest.
(Objective 3)

38. a. Thyroid dysfunction may also cause tachydysrhythmias, constipation, weight loss, anemia, or musculoskeletal complaints.
(Objective 3)

39. d. Prostate enlargement is a cause of dysuria commonly found in this age group.
(Objective 3)

40. b. The ulcers often become infected because of the poor blood supply to the area.
(Objective 3)

41. d. *Cataracts* are a loss in transparency of the lens of the eye. *Conjunctivitis* is an inflammation of the conjunctiva of the eye. *Corneal abrasion* is a scraping-off of the outer layer of the cornea.
(Objective 4)

42. d. Some of the older drugs prescribed for patients with Parkinson disease may produce this reaction.
(Objective 5)

43. a. Cyclic antidepressants, antidysrhythmics, and beta blockers may increase the risk of hyperthermia.
(Objective 6)

44. c. This may result from diuretic or other drug therapy and can have a very slow onset.
(Objective 7)

45. b. It may be caused by physiological or psychological factors.
(Objective 7)

46. b. The venous blood of a subdural hematoma takes longer to fill the larger space between the skull and the brain.
(Objective 8)

47. c
(Objective 8)

48. a. Sedative-hypnotic drugs put older patients at greater risk for falls.
(Objective 8)

WRAP IT UP

1. Stroke (in history and Coumadin); congestive heart failure (Lanoxin, furosemide); atrial fibrillation (Lanoxin); type 2 diabetes (Glucophage); high cholesterol (Lipitor); depression or anxiety (Paxil).
(Objectives 2, 3)

2. a (sudden onset of confusion); c (altered level of consciousness); d (house is hot); e (age and Paxil); f (Sao_2 and crackles); h (missing pills); i (elders are at high risk; crackles in lungs); j (prior stroke, atrial fibrillation)
(Objective 3)

3. a. No
b. Unknown time of onset of symptoms (must be less than 3 hours)
(Objective 2)

4. a
(Objective 3)

5. Possibility for bleeding (Coumadin, aspirin); acidosis (aspirin); hypoglycemia (Glucophage); bradycardia or dysrhythmias (Lanoxin); depressed respirations (Paxil).
(Objective 2)

CHAPTER 46

Abuse and Neglect

READING ASSIGNMENT

Chapter 46, pages 1184-1195, in *Mosby's Paramedic Textbook*, ed. 3

OBJECTIVES

Upon completion of this chapter, the paramedic student will be able to do the following:
1. Define battering.
2. Describe the characteristics of abusive relationships.
3. Outline findings that indicate a battered patient.
4. Describe prehospital considerations when responding to and caring for battered patients.
5. Identify types of elder abuse.
6. Discuss legal considerations related to elder abuse.
7. Describe characteristics of abused children and their abusers.
8. Outline the physical examination of the abused child.
9. Describe the characteristics of sexual assault.
10. Outline prehospital patient care considerations for the patient who has been sexually assaulted.

SUMMARY

- Battering is the establishment of control and fear in a relationship through violence and other forms of abuse.
- Domestic violence follows a cycle of three phases. Phase one involves arguing and verbal abuse. Phase two progresses to physical and sexual abuse. Phase three consists of denial and apologies. Certain personality traits may predispose a person to abusive relationships.
- The paramedic may have a hard time identifying the battered patient. Injuries from domestic violence often involve contusions and lacerations of the face, neck, head, breast, and abdomen.
- The paramedic must ensure scene and personal safety in domestic violence events. The paramedic should manage physical injuries according to standard protocols. The paramedic should direct special attention toward the emotional needs of the victim as well.
- Elder abuse is classified into four categories: physical abuse, psychological abuse, financial or material abuse, and neglect.
- All 50 states have elder abuse statutes. Reporting of suspected elder abuse also is mandatory under law in most states.
- Most child abusers are the child's parents (77%). Eleven percent are other relatives of the victim. Abused children often exhibit behavior that provides key clues about abuse and neglect. The paramedic should observe carefully the child under 6 years of age who is passive or the child over 6 years of age who is aggressive.
- If the child volunteers the history of the event without hesitation and matches the history that the parent provides (and the history is suitable for the injury), child abuse is unlikely.

- Injuries may include soft tissue injuries, fractures, head injuries, and abdominal injuries.
- *Sexual assault* generally refers to any genital, anal, oral, or manual penetration of the victim's body by way of force and without the victim's consent. The highest incidence of sexual assault occurs in women who live alone in isolated areas.
- After managing all threats to life, the paramedic should provide emotional support to the victim. The paramedic should deliver care in a way that preserves evidence.

REVIEW QUESTIONS

Questions 1 to 5 pertain to the following case study:

> You are called to a private residence by a woman who says her husband "beat her up." On arrival, you hear loud shouting coming from the house.

1. What measures should be taken before entering the home?

_____

_____

2. When you begin your examination, what measures should you take to enhance safety and allow for a better history and examination?

_____

_____

   The patient's vital signs are stable. She has several bruises around her face, but she is alert and oriented and does not want further care. You contact medical direction, and despite both your and their recommendations, the patient refuses transport.

3. What reasons might someone have for staying with an abusive partner?

_____

_____

4. If you tell her to move out immediately, would that be the safest course of action without planning on her part? Why or why not?

_____

_____

5. What advice and resources can you offer her before you leave the scene?

_____

_____

Questions 6 to 8 refer to the following case study:

> You are dispatched to a residence in a middle-class neighborhood for an "accidental injury." On arrival, you find an 80-year-old widow with a tender, swollen, ecchymotic left upper arm. She is awake and alert but very withdrawn. You note multiple other bruises on both arms and her back that are yellow, brown, and green. Her 60-year-old daughter lives with her and says that her mother tripped and fell. When you ask the patient to confirm this, she nods slowly; when you ask about the old bruises, she just shrugs. She has a history of heart disease, emphysema, and adult-onset diabetes. Her vital signs are normal.

6. What characteristics typical of an "average" victim of elder abuse does this woman have?

_____

7. What physical findings suggest possible abuse?

_____

8. What action should you take if you suspect abuse on this call?

_____

_____

Questions 9 to 12 refer to the following case study:

You are dispatched to an address in your district that is well-known to you and your partner. Both the woman that lives at this address and her boyfriend are heavy drinkers, and you have responded to multiple calls at their home. When you arrive, you find a 2-year-old girl with bilateral circumferential second-degree burns to her feet, lower legs, and buttocks. The mother says that when she was filling the tub to bathe the child after she dirtied her pants, the child stepped into the tub and got burned. You take the child to the ambulance to provide care and notice that she does not cry for her mother to be with her. She shudders when you touch her to begin your assessment and jumps every time someone approaches or opens a door.

9. What characteristics of an abusive family situation are present in this situation?

_____

_____

10. What specific characteristics of the injuries increase your suspicion of possible abuse?

_____

_____

11. How does the child's behavior suggest the possibility of an abusive family situation?

_____

_____

12. What are your legal responsibilities with regard to this situation?

_____

_____

13. List five measures to help preserve evidence on a sexual assault call.
   a.

   b.

   c.

   d.

   e.

14. List at least four injuries that may accompany sexual assault.

   a.

   b.

   c.

   d.

STUDENT SELF-ASSESSMENT

15. The establishment of control and fear in a relationship through violence and other forms of abuse is known by which of the following terms?
   a. Assault
   b. Battering
   c. Intimidation
   d. Terrorism

16. What typically occurs in the third phase of the domestic violence cycle?
   a. An argument occurs, and the situation escalates.
   b. Threats of violence and harm are made to the victim.
   c. Physical or sexual abuse occurs.
   d. The abuser apologizes for what has happened.

17. What does the victim of domestic violence often fear most?
   a. That her children will be harmed or taken away.
   b. That she will be humiliated in front of their friends.
   c. That she will not be able to achieve financial independence.
   d. That the abuser will hurt himself if the victim leaves.

18. Which of the following characteristics may an abuser or victim of domestic violence have?
   a. Alcohol or drug dependence
   b. Dislike of discipline
   c. Fear of love and affection
   d. Rigid personal boundaries

19. Which of the following injury patterns is more suggestive of domestic abuse?
   a. Contusions of the breast
   b. Fracture of the ankle
   c. Laceration of the finger
   d. Scald burn of the hand

20. What is an effective way to treat a patient whom you suspect has been injured in a domestic violence situation?
   a. Ask the police to speak to her partner so that you can examine her privately.
   b. Don't pry if she doesn't volunteer any information about abuse.
   c. If she won't talk, ask her, "You've been abused, haven't you?"
   d. Force her to go to the hospital even if she doesn't want to.

21. Which is an example of psychological abuse of an elder?
   a. Sexual molestation
   b. Theft of property
   c. Verbal threats
   d. Withholding food

22. What action should the paramedic take if elder abuse is suspected?
   a. Confront the suspected abuser about the abusive behavior and threaten to report it.
   b. Report your suspicions to medical direction and the appropriate state agency.
   c. Discuss the patient's rights and ways to follow up with authorities.
   d. Wait to see whether it happens again before you take action so that you can be sure.

23. Which of the following descriptions is most characteristic of a child abuser?
   a. 20-year-old mother
   b. 45-year-old female neighbor
   c. 50-year-old father
   d. 70-year-old uncle

24. What is helpful in most cases in assessing whether a child's injury is accidental or inflicted by an adult?
   a. Assessing the family for the characteristics of abusers
   b. Checking with the police to see whether a record of abuse exists
   c. Matching the description of the event to the injury
   d. Performing a careful, detailed physical examination

25. Which of the following statements about sexual assault is true?
   a. All victims of sexual assault are women.
   b. Rape is motivated by sexual desire.
   c. Threats of harm or use of weapons during the attack are rare.
   d. Victims often know their attackers.

26. What statement by the paramedic may be most helpful to a child who has been sexually assaulted?

    a. "Don't worry about anything; you are OK."

    b. "They'll probably get the person who did this."

    c. "You didn't do anything wrong; this wasn't your fault."

    d. "You're really lucky; it could have been a lot worse."

WRAP IT UP

You are dispatched to a large, elegant home for a "maternity case." En route, the dispatcher notes that the caller requests no lights and sirens and that the crew use a rear entrance. The patient's husband meets you; you recognize him, from his frequent television commercials, as a prominent injury claims attorney. He tells you that his wife has gone into labor. The patient is crying and telling you, "It's too early." She has two other children, has miscarried several times, and is at 30 weeks' gestation. She tells you her contractions began about an hour ago, are very painful, and are coming every 3 minutes. You note her pale skin and assess her vital signs, which are BP, 80/50 mm Hg; P, 132/min; and R, 28/min. The Sao$_2$ does not register. When you drape the patient and examine her perineum during a contraction to determine if she is crowning, you are alarmed to see that her undergarments are soaked with dark red blood, much different from the mucousy bloody show you've seen in the past. Your partner looks alarmed when she is unable to dopple fetal heart tones. The patient grimaces in pain when the Doppler is pressed against her abdomen, where you note an ecchymotic area lateral to her umbilicus. When you ask the patient if she has any risk factors for abruption, toxemia, high blood pressure, or trauma, she glances nervously at her husband but denies all. He quickly interrupts and says, "Well, she did fall down a couple of steps this morning." As you administer oxygen, she whispers to you that her husband punched her in the abdomen during an argument earlier today. As you quickly secure the patient to your cot and raise her legs, you explain to her that her pain and blood pressure concern you, therefore you will be staring an IV and transporting her to the closest hospital with high-risk OB services. The husband is crying and telling her that he loves her as you wheel her out the door. The patient appears embarrassed and tells you, "I should have left him years ago, but I know he'll take the other kids. He's really a good person, but he just has a bad temper. It's all my fault." You start an IV line en route and deliver her to the labor and delivery unit, where a team is waiting with four units of blood to rush her for an emergency C-section based on your report. Subsequently you learn that the patient survived but her baby did not. Her husband plea bargained, so you are thankful you did not have to testify at trial.

    1. Which is true about battered women?

        a. City dwellers are at higher risk of abuse.

        b. Domestic abuse calls pose little threat to rescuers.

        c. Fifteen percent to 25% of pregnant women are battered.

        d. Wife batterers do not usually abuse their children.

    2. What clues to abuse did you note before the patient told you she had been assaulted?

_____

_____

    3. Which action or actions could have increased the potential for violence directed at the EMS crew?

_____

_____

_____

    4. Put a ✔ beside interventions related to this patient's abuse that would have been appropriate for you to provide during transport.

        a. _____ Listen with a nonjudgmental attitude

        b. _____ Encourage the patient to get control of her life

        c. _____ Provide access to community resources

        d. _____ Provide a written list of community resources for the patient

        e. _____ Confirm that she is not at fault

        f. _____ Treat her in a sensitive manner

CHAPTER 46 ANSWERS

REVIEW QUESTIONS

1. Request and await police to help assess and maintain scene safety. Domestic violence calls are very dangerous. (Objective 4)

2. Move the patient to the ambulance as soon as possible. Do not ask about the violence until you have the patient alone. Have police remain with the alleged abuser while you perform your examination. (Objective 4)

3. The patient may fear for her own safety or the safety of her children if she leaves. A victim often believes that the offender's behavior will change. She may not have money or emotional support to help her leave. She may believe that she is the cause of the behavior or that abuse is a normal part of marriage. (Objective 2)

4. Often the perpetrator is released from jail within several hours. A woman who leaves is 75% more likely to be killed by her partner. A woman who leaves should be directed to community support agencies that can maximize her safety. Sometimes it is more prudent for her to stay and carefully plan a safe departure than to leave suddenly. (Objective 4)

5. Accept her decision and support her by confirming that she is not at fault and doesn't deserve to be abused. Give her written information (preferably on something small enough to hide) about community agencies that can provide financial, emotional, safety-related, and legal resources to assist her. Help her prepare a quick way out. Identify safety precautions for her. (Objective 4)

6. The victim is a widow who is over 75 years of age. She has multiple chronic health problems and lives with a child. (Objective 7)

7. The patient seems hesitant to confirm the source of the injury and has aging bruises. (Objective 5)

8. If you suspect abuse, you should report your suspicions to medical direction and call the agency mandated by law to report suspected elder abuse. (Objective 6)

9. This child is with a parent, and alcohol abuse is evident, which greatly increases the risk of physical abuse. You also have received many calls to this home. (Objective 7)

10. The burns involve both extremities and the buttocks and are circumferential, indicating that the child was probably forcibly held in the hot water. (Objective 8)

11. The child does not mind separation from the parents, appears fearful, and does not like to be touched. (Objective 7)

12. This case should be reported to the appropriate state agency for child abuse on arrival at the hospital (refer to local reporting protocols). (Objective 7)

13. a. Take steps to preserve evidence.
 b. Do not allow the patient to urinate, defecate, douche, or bathe.
 c. Do not remove evidence from areas of sexual contact.
 d. Notify law enforcement immediately.
 e. Maintain a chain of evidence with clothing and other items.
 (Objective 10)

14. a. Abrasions or bruises on the upper limb, head, and neck
 b. Forcible signs of restraint
 c. Petechiae of the face and conjunctiva
 d. Broken teeth, swollen jaw or cheekbone, or eye injuries
 e. Muscle soreness or stiffness of the shoulder, neck, knee, hip, or back
 (Objective 9)

STUDENT SELF-ASSESSMENT

15. b. Battering may include physical abuse (assault) or psychological abuse such as intimidation, isolation, or threats to control another person.
 (Objective 1)

16. d. This is known as the *honeymoon phase*.
 (Objective 2)

17. a. Usually all these fears exist, but children most often are the most compelling reason for the victim to stay.
 (Objective 2)

18. a. Abusers may feel that abuse is a form of discipline. Abusers or victims often have an intense need for love and affection and are unable to set personal boundaries.
 (Objective 2)

19. a. Abusive injuries are more commonly found on the face, head, neck, breasts, and abdomen.
 (Objective 3)

20. a. The partner may be reluctant to leave the victim alone and may need to be distracted for you to be able to conduct an effective history. If the victim does not volunteer information, you could say something nonthreatening, such as, "I'm concerned for you because I've seen these types of injuries in people who have been hit by others." Do not intimidate or accuse the victim. You cannot insist on transport if the adult patient is competent.
 (Objective 4)

21. c. Sexual molestation is physical abuse, theft is financial or material abuse, and withholding food is neglect.
 (Objective 5)

22. b. Report it to the authorities so that they will have complete information if a pattern of abuse exists.
 (Objective 6)

23. a. Most perpetrators are a parent, female, and under 40.
 (Objective 7)

24. c. If the child volunteers the same story as the parents without prompting and the story is consistent with the injuries you see, abuse is not likely. You probably will not have time in the field to assess the family or check police records.
 (Objective 8)

25. d. About 49,000 men report sexual assault each year. Rape is a crime of violence, not a sexual act. Threats of harm or the use of weapons for intimidation are common.
(Objective 9)

26. c. Abused children should understand that the assault was not their fault and that they won't be punished. False reassurances serve no purpose.
(Objective 10)

WRAP IT UP

1. c. Abuse is also common in rural and suburban areas. Domestic violence calls pose a high risk of violence toward police and EMS. More than half of wife batterers also abuse their children.
(Objective 2)

2. The request to respond on the quiet; the obvious trauma to the abdomen (characteristic of abuse); a pregnant patient with possible abruption (trauma is a possible cause); the changing story (no mention of trauma initially); and the high incidence of abuse during pregnancy.
(Objective 3)

3. Confronting or questioning the husband about the abuse.
(Objective 4)

4. a, e, f. The patient is experiencing a life-threatening injury, and the other interventions would not be appropriate at this time. A detailed report to hospital staff members, who can refer her to the appropriate social services after her recovery, would also be indicated.
(Objective 4)

Patients with Special Challenges

READING ASSIGNMENT
Chapter 47, pages 1196-1209, in *Mosby's Paramedic Textbook*, ed. 3

OBJECTIVES
Upon completion of this chapter, the paramedic student will be able to do the following:
1. Identify considerations in prehospital management related to physical challenges such as hearing, visual, and speech impairments; obesity; and patients with paraplegia or quadriplegia.
2. Identify considerations in prehospital management of patients who have mental illness, are developmentally disabled, or are emotionally or mentally impaired.
3. Describe special considerations for prehospital management of patients with selected pathological challenges.
4. Outline considerations in management of culturally diverse patients.
5. Describe special considerations in the prehospital management of terminally ill patients.
6. Identify special considerations in management of patients with communicable diseases.
7. Describe special considerations in the prehospital management of patients with financial challenges.

SUMMARY
- Certain accommodations may be needed for a hearing-impaired patient. These include helping with a patient's hearing aid, providing paper and pen to aid in communication, speaking softly into the patient's ear, and speaking in clear view of the patient.
- When caring for the visually impaired patient, the paramedic should help the patient use his or her glasses or other visual aids. The paramedic also should describe all procedures before performing them.
- Allow extra time for the history of a patient with a speech impairment. If appropriate, provide aids such as a pen and paper to assist in communication.
- When caring for an obese patient, use the proper sized diagnostic devices. Also, secure extra personnel if needed to move the patient for transport.
- When transporting patients with paraplegia or quadriplegia, extra personnel may be needed to move special equipment.
- Once rapport and trust have been established with a patient who has mental illness, the paramedic should proceed with care in the standard manner.
- When caring for a patient with developmental delays, the paramedic should allow enough time to obtain a history, perform an assessment, deliver care, and prepare for transport.
- The challenge in assessing patients with emotional impairments is distinguishing between symptoms produced by stress and those caused by serious medical illness.

- Pathological conditions may call for special assessment and management skills. The paramedic should ask about current medications and the patient's normal level of functioning.
- Diversity refers to differences of any kind. These include race, class, religion, gender, sexual preference, personal habitat, and physical ability. Good health care depends on sensitivity toward these differences.
- Often, calls involving the care of a terminally ill patient will be emotionally charged. They require a great deal of empathy and compassion for the patient and his or her loved ones.
- Some infectious diseases will take a toll on the emotional well-being of affected patients, their families, and loved ones. Paramedics should be sensitive to the psychological needs of the patient and his or her family.
- Financial challenges can deprive a patient of basic health care services. These patients may be reluctant to seek care for illness or injury.

REVIEW QUESTIONS

Match the pathological condition in column II with the appropriate description in column I. Use each condition just once.

Column I	Column II
1. _____ Nonprogressive disorders of movement and posture	**a.** Arthritis
2. _____ Inherited disorder that causes slow muscle deterioration	**b.** Cerebral palsy
3. _____ Congenital defect that exposes part of the spinal cord	**c.** Cystic fibrosis
4. _____ Autoimmune disorder that weakens the muscles of the head and extremities	**d.** Multiple sclerosis
	e. Muscular dystrophy
5. _____ Inflammation of the joints	**f.** Myasthenia gravis
6. _____ Inherited disease of the lungs and digestive tract	**g.** Poliomyelitis
7. _____ Autoimmune disease that affects the CNS	**h.** Spina bifida

For the patient situations in questions 8 to 20, identify which of the following prehospital considerations may be necessary to accommodate the patient's special needs. More than one answer may be required.

    a. Provide communication aids
    b. Allow additional time for history and management
    c. Obtain detailed information about the preexisting condition
    d. Determine baseline level of functioning
    e. Obtain additional resources and manpower to prepare for transport

8. _____ The patient had a stroke 6 months ago, has weakness on the right side, and speaks slowly and with a stutter. He called you today complaining of inability to urinate.

9. _____ Your patient complains of crushing chest pain. He weighs approximately 375 lb (170 kg).

10. _____ You are providing an interfacility transfer for a quadriplegic patient who is in halo traction.

11. _____ A man with a history of schizophrenia is having difficulty breathing because of his asthma.

12. _____ A 12-year-old girl with Down syndrome is having extreme weakness after chemotherapy for her leukemia.

13. _____ A moderately retarded man lacerated his finger at his job in the cafeteria.

14. _____ A severely arthritic patient was involved in a motor vehicle crash.

15. _____ A 14-year-old patient with quadriplegic spastic paralysis and mental retardation caused by cerebral palsy is febrile and congested.

16. _____ A child with cystic fibrosis has vomiting and diarrhea.

17. _____ A 43-year-old woman with multiple sclerosis complains of severe vertigo.

18. _____ An 8-year-old boy with Duchenne muscular dystrophy says he can't breathe.

19. _____ A 45-year-old patient who suffered a head injury 5 years ago is confused and pale.

20. _____ A 65-year-old man tells you he is being treated for tuberculosis.

21. Which of the following accommodations might be helpful to many patients with hearing impairment?
    a. No accommodation is necessary.
    b. Speaking very loudly into the patient's ear
    c. Speaking very slowly with very exaggerated lip movements
    d. Writing key questions or instructions on a piece of paper

22. Which of the following fits the definition of obesity?
    a. A person who is impaired as a result of excessive weight
    b. A person who weighs 20% or more than the maximum desirable weight relative to height
    c. A person who weighs 50 lb (23 kg) more than the average weight for someone of that age
    d. A person who weighs more than 250 lb (114 kg)

23. During the initial examination of a patient with a mental illness, what is your priority?
    a. To determine whether the patient is aware of the mental illness
    b. To determine whether the patient is dangerous
    c. To determine the patient's specific form of mental illness
    d. To determine the type of medications the patient is taking

24. What challenge is posed by caring for a patient who is emotionally impaired?
    a. Determining whether symptoms are produced by stress or medical illness
    b. Determining whether the patient is lying or telling the truth
    c. Obtaining an accurate medical history from caregivers
    d. Winning the patient's trust so that you can perform the examination

25. A patient with severe arthritis of the spine falls down some steps. What is likely to be the most significant challenge in caring for this patient?
    a. Communicating so that you can understand the patient
    b. Determining whether the patient has any serious injuries
    c. Obtaining a reliable patient history and medication list
    d. Securing the patient to a spine board to minimize pain

26. Which of the following terms describes the involuntary writhing movements found in some patients with cerebral palsy?
    a. Ataxia   c. Diplegia
    b. Athetosis   d. Mucoviscidosis

27. During transport of a patient with severe cystic fibrosis, you should anticipate the need for which of the following?
    a. Antidysrhythmic treatment c. Nitrous oxide inhalation
    b. Blood glucose monitoring   d. Suctioning

28. Which of the following is true about cultural diversity in prehospital patient care?
    a. All generations in a culture share the same beliefs.
    b. Personal prejudices and belief systems should not interfere with patient care.
    c. People must accept your explanation of the cause of their illness.
    d. You should agree with every aspect of a patient's cultural beliefs.

29. What is a primary consideration during transport of a terminally ill patient?
    a. The family should be encouraged to deal with the imminent death.
    b. Talking to the family may interfere with their grieving process.
    c. Pain management is usually the priority of care.
    d. Rapid transport is essential for definitive care.

30. How can you show respect for the dignity of a patient with AIDS during transport?
    a. Don't discuss their disease process.
    b. To keep the patient from feeling ashamed, don't use BSI.
    c. Encourage the patient to express feelings related to the disease.
    d. Respecting the patient's dignity should not be a primary concern during prehospital care.

31. What statement may be helpful when transporting a patient who has serious financial concerns?
    a. "Don't worry; the ambulance bill won't come for a couple of months."
    b. "I don't see why you're worried. You're sick now—worry about the money later."
    c. "I'll ask the nurse to contact social services to see whether there is a program to help you."
    d. "We have people who never pay a dime for our service, and they abuse us all the time."

WRAP IT UP

You could have predicted it; a light, drizzly rain always precipitates multiple "fender benders" at this very busy corner. As you approach the scene, you can see that a van has struck the rear of a large dump truck. There is almost no visible damage to the truck, but the van has considerable front-end damage. The van's driver, a woman in her thirties, is crying and calling out to her rear-seat passenger, a 13-year-old boy who was thrown out of his wheelchair, which had been secured in the specialized van. He is crying, making a high-pitched, moaning sound. As you approach him, the driver, his mother, tells you that his name is Michael, he has cerebral palsy with diplegic spasticity, and he is blind and has mental retardation. She tries to calm him, but his persistent cries pierce the environment, making it difficult to concentrate and impossible to hear anything on your assessment. You find him recumbent with his arms and legs drawn toward his chest in a fetal-like position. "Michael," you say loudly as you grasp one wrist and place the other hand on his shoulder, "I'm here to help you." His pulse is rapid, breathing is normal, and his skin is warm and dry. He has a laceration on the left temporal area of his head but no other visible soft tissue injury or any evidence of deformity or crepitus distally. Vital signs are BP, 96 mm Hg by palpation; P, 120/min; R, 20/min; and Sao_2, 97%. His pupils are 3 mm, equal, round, and react to light. By now your partner has evaluated the mother; her vital signs are stable, she denies any injury, and she refuses any care. You ask her to help you to calm her son. She moves close to him and rubs his back while singing a familiar song into his ear, and the moaning begins to slow. After realizing that standard spinal immobilization would be impossible because of the rigid spasticity of the boy's limbs, you and your partner determine that applying a cervical collar and a half spine board device will provide stabilization of the spine. Medical direction concurs. In simple language you explain each step of the process, which his mother relays to him. Although his agitation increases, it is manageable. After the immobilization has been applied, you position him on the stretcher in a semisitting position with blankets and pillows supporting his legs. You allow his mother to sit seat belted in the CPR seat beside him, where she continually soothes him on the way in and tells you that she thinks his behavior is appropriate for the situation. He is treated in the ED and released several hours later.

1. What difficulties were posed by the assessment of this patient?

_____

2. Why is it appropriate to have the parent remain with the child in this situation?

_____

3. What does *diplegic spasticity* mean?
   a. It affects both arms and legs.
   b. It is intermittent.
   c. It affects both limbs on one side of the body.
   d. It causes involuntary writhing movements.

_____

4. Explain why it would be appropriate to deviate from standard spinal immobilization protocol in this situation.

_____

_____

CHAPTER 47 ANSWERS

REVIEW QUESTIONS

1. b
2. e
3. h
4. f
5. a
6. c
7. d
   (Questions 1-7: Objective 3)

8. a, b, c, d
   (Objective 1)

9. c, e
   (Objective 1)

10. b, c, d, e
    (Objective 1)

11. c, d
    (Objective 2)

12. b, c, d
    (Objective 2)

13. b, d
    (Objective 2)

14. b, c, e (possibly)
    (Objective 3)

15. c, d, e
    (Objective 3)

16. c, d
    (Objective 3)

17. c, d
    (Objective 3)

18. c, d
    (Objective 3)

19. c, d
(Objective 3)

20. c
(Objective 6)

STUDENT SELF-ASSESSMENT

21. d. Speak in low tones into the patient's ear if residual hearing exists. Otherwise, if the patient reads lips, speak at a regular speed in view of the patient.
(Objective 1)

22. b
(Objective 1)

23. b. The safety of the patient, crew, and bystanders should always be prioritized.
(Objective 2)

24. a. Anxiety can produce a host of symptoms that mimic serious medical illness.
(Objective 2)

25. d. The arthritic pain and deformity can make spinal immobilization challenging.
(Objective 3)

26. b. Ataxia is a loss of coordination and balance. Diplegic cerebral palsy affects all four limbs, the legs more severely than the arms. Mucoviscidosis is cystic fibrosis.
(Objective 3)

27. d. These patients often have excessive secretions, and the paramedic should anticipate the need for suctioning.
(Objective 3)

28. b. Individual beliefs exist even within specific cultures. People may choose to have their own beliefs about the cause of their illness despite your explanations. You need not agree with all aspects of a patient's cultural beliefs, but do not let your opinion interfere with patient care or interaction.
(Objective 4)

29. c. Some families will not be fully prepared for the death regardless of the length of illness. The paramedic should support the patient and family with honest and empathetic care. Talking to the patient and family should be encouraged if the patient's condition permits.
(Objective 5)

30. c. There is no reason not to mention the disease to the patient, but the condition should remain confidential with regard to others. Use BSI as you would for any other patient care situation. The dignity of each patient is an important part of prehospital patient care delivery.
(Objective 6)

31. c. The patient may worry about receiving poor credit ratings, adding to a mounting debt, and being a deadbeat. Offer constructive suggestions related to their financial concerns rather than empty statements.
(Objective 7)

WRAP IT UP

1. He is unable to communicate effectively, he is blind and so is probably terrified because he has no idea what happened to him, and he is mentally retarded.
(Objective 2)

2. The mother knows how to communicate with her child, can calm him, and can tell medical providers what behaviors are normal or abnormal for her son.
(Objective 1)

3. a. All four limbs are affected, the legs more than the arms. *Athetosis* describes writhing movements.
(Objective 3)

4. Positioning this patient supine on a long spine board would be impossible. Adaptations in care should take into consideration the physical needs of the patient and the potential for injury. Consultation with medical direction can be helpful.
(Objective 3)

CHAPTER

48

Acute Interventions for the Home Health Care Patient

READING ASSIGNMENT

Chapter 48, pages 1210-1229, in *Mosby's Paramedic Textbook*, ed. 3

OBJECTIVES

Upon completion of this chapter, the paramedic student will be able to:
1. Discuss general issues related to the home health care patient.
2. Outline general principles of assessment and management of the home health care patient.
3. Describe medical equipment, assessment, and management of the home health care patient with inadequate respiratory support.
4. Identify assessment findings and acute interventions for problems related to vascular access devices in the home health care setting.
5. Describe medical equipment, assessment, and management of the patient with a gastrointestinal or genitourinary crisis in the home health care setting.
6. Identify key assessments and principles of wound care management in the home health care patient.
7. Outline maternal/child problems that may be encountered early in the postpartum period in the home health care setting.
8. Describe medical therapy associated with hospice and comfort care in the home health care setting.

SUMMARY

- About 25% of home health care patients have heart and circulatory diseases as their primary diagnosis. Other common diagnoses of home health care patients include cancer, diabetes, and hypertension. Typical EMS calls to a home health care setting may include respiratory failure, cardiac decompensation, septic complications, equipment malfunction, and other medical problems.
- After arrival at the scene of a home health care patient, the scene size-up should include standard precautions, elements of scene safety, and environmental setting. The initial assessment should focus on illness or injury that poses a threat to life. The paramedic should take appropriate measures as indicated.

- Patients with diseases of the respiratory system being cared for at home are at increased risk for airway infections. In addition, the progression of their illnesses may lead to difficulty breathing, making current support equipment inadequate.
- Assessment findings that may require acute interventions in patients with VADs include infection, hemorrhage, hemodynamic compromise from circulatory overload or embolus, obstruction of the vascular device, and catheter damage with leakage of medication.
- Patients with diseases of the digestive or genitourinary system may have medical devices such as urinary catheters or urostomies, indwelling nutritional support devices (e.g., percutaneous endoscopic gastrostomy tube or gastrostomy tube), colostomies, and nasogastric tubes. Acute interventions required for these patients can result from UTI, urosepsis, urinary retention, and problems with gastric emptying or feeding.
- Home health care patients with acute infections have an increased death rate from sepsis and severe peripheral infections. Many also have a decreased ability to perceive pain or perform self-care.
- Maternal/child conditions that one may encounter in the home health care setting during the postpartum period include postpartum hemorrhage, infection, pulmonary embolism, postpartum depression, septicemia in the newborn, infantile apnea, and failure to thrive.
- Hospice services include supportive social, emotional, and spiritual services for the terminally ill. They also provide support for a patient's family. Palliative care is directed mainly at providing relief to a terminally ill person. They do this through symptom and pain management.

REVIEW QUESTIONS

Questions 1 to 4 refer to the following case study:

You are called to care for a patient who has difficulty breathing. When you arrive at his home, you find a man who has a tracheostomy and is on a ventilator. The low pressure alarm is sounding.

1. What signs and symptoms might the patient have if he were hypoxic?

_____

_____

2. What should your first action be?

_____

_____

3. What will you check on the ventilator to assess the problem?

_____

_____

4. How can you calm the patient before reconnecting him to the ventilator?

_____

_____

_____

Questions 5 to 7 refer to the following case study:

An elderly patient has a home IV infusion. You are called to treat her for difficulty breathing. She has a history of multiple myeloma. Her husband thinks the pump hasn't been working correctly and too much has run in.

5. What specifically would you assess to check for fluid overload?

_____

The patient has crackles bilaterally in the bases of her lungs, and her neck veins are slightly distended. Her vital signs are 160/84 mm Hg; P, 100/min; and R, 24/min. Her Sao$_2$ is 93% on room air.

6. What interventions should you perform in cooperation with medical direction?

_____

_____

7. Should you transport the patient for evaluation by a physician?

_____

Questions 8 to 13 pertain to the following case study:

You are called to a home for an "assist invalid" call. An elderly woman greets you, and after you help her husband to bed (he couldn't get off the commode), she asks you to check his arm. She says that he burned it 4 days ago. When you remove the dressing, you note a green wound bed surrounded by black tissue. The drainage is green and foul smelling.

8. What does the appearance of this wound suggest?

_____

9. How would it look if it were healing normally?

_____

10. What should you look for in the surrounding skin?

_____

The skin around the wound is reddened and warm to the touch.

11. What does this assessment suggest?

_____

_____

12. What systemic assessment should you perform on this patient?

_____

The patient's vital signs are BP, 150/80 mm Hg; P, 110/min; and R, 16/min. His skin feels hot to the touch. The rest of the exam is normal.

13. What action should you take?

_____

_____

Questions 14 to 17 refer to the following case study:

You respond to a call for "baby not breathing." On arrival you find a woman sobbing while holding her 4-day-old infant in her arms. The baby is awake, lying quietly in her mother's arms. The parents state that they had just put her down for a nap, when they noticed that she wasn't breathing and her color looked bad. They state that the episode lasted about 15 to 20 seconds.

14. What assessments should you perform?

_____

_____

_____

The baby's examination looks normal. While you are on the phone with medical direction, your partner shouts at you. She states that the baby stopped breathing for approximately 15 seconds and was very pale, and the heart rate dropped to 80/min on the monitor. Now she is breathing normally.

15. What are some possible causes of infantile apnea?

_____

_____

16. What interventions should you perform?

_____

_____

17. What equipment should you prepare and keep easily accessible during transport?

_____

_____

STUDENT SELF-ASSESSMENT

18. What was the historical focus of home health care?
   a. To benefit the rich
   b. To care for rural patients
   c. To provide wider physician care
   d. To provide preventative care

19. Home health care services in the United States include which of the following?
   a. Diagnostic radiology
   b. Minor surgical procedures
   c. IV antibiotic therapy
   d. Physician visits for acute illness

20. The Haddon matrix states that any injury or disease can be broken down into three components. Which of the following shows the correct three?
   a. Agent, host, environment
   b. Agent, host, mechanical force
   c. Patient, host, environment
   d. Agent, disease, environment

21. What type of infection control standards should be practiced in the home health setting?
    a. No precautions are needed.
    b. Use precautions only for HIV patients.
    c. Wear reusable rubber gloves.
    d. Observe universal precautions.
22. Assessment of the milieu in home care includes evaluation to ensure which of the following?
    a. Infectious waste is disposed of properly.
    b. Dogs and other pets are contained.
    c. No hazards are present in the home.
    d. The home has heat, water, and electricity.
23. On arrival at a call in which home care is provided, your priority (after making sure the scene is safe) is to assess for which of the following?
    a. Abusive caregivers
    b. Equipment failure
    c. Life-threatening illness or injury
    d. Medical device malfunction
24. Which of the following systems will not work during a power failure?
    a. Demand valve
    b. Liquid oxygen
    c. Oxygen concentrators
    d. Oxygen cylinders
25. You are called because the high pressure alarm keeps sounding on a home care ventilator. What might this indicate?
    a. Cuff leak
    b. Disconnected tubing
    c. Insufficient oxygen
    d. Water in tubing
26. Which of the following is a peripheral vascular access device?
    a. Groshon
    b. Hickman
    c. Intracath
    d. Mediport
27. Which of the following complications of vascular access devices does not pose an immediate life threat?
    a. Circulatory overload
    b. Embolus
    c. Hemorrhage
    d. Site infection
28. Which of the following is a sign of air embolus that may occur if air enters a vascular access device?
    a. Distended neck veins
    b. Fever
    c. Hypotension
    d. Pulmonary congestion
29. How much heparin should be used when flushing a peripheral vascular device?
    a. 2.5 to 3 mL (10 U/mL)
    b. 2.5 to 3 mL (100 U/mL)
    c. 3 to 5 mL (10 U/mL)
    d. 3 to 5 mL (100 U/mL)
30. What complication can result from an untreated urinary tract infection in a patient with a urinary catheter?
    a. Kidney stones
    b. Prostatic hypertrophy
    c. Sepsis
    d. Urinary retention
31. Which complication of tube feedings can cause serious skin breakdown and fluid and electrolyte imbalances?
    a. Bowel obstruction
    b. Choking
    c. Diarrhea
    d. Irritable bowel syndrome
32. What is a critical step in the insertion of a urinary catheter?
    a. Do not retract the foreskin, if present.
    b. Inflate the balloon with 10 to 15 mL of sterile saline after insertion.
    c. Use aseptic technique until the catheter is inserted and the balloon inflated.
    d. Use significant force to overcome resistance during catheter insertion.
33. Which of the following enhances wound repair?
    a. Environmental contamination
    b. Eschar
    c. Moisture
    d. Necrotic tissue
34. Your patient delivered a baby 3 days ago. She is complaining of severe abdominal pain, weakness, and shaking chills. What postpartum complication should be anticipated?
    a. Appendicitis
    b. Endometritis
    c. Hemorrhage
    d. Pulmonary embolism
35. You are called to the home of a woman who appears to have signs and symptoms of postpartum depression. Your priority should be to assess for which of the following?
    a. Depressive psychosis
    b. Forgetfulness or memory loss
    c. Severe sleep disturbances
    d. The well-being of the baby

36. A mother calls you to evaluate her 11-day-old infant. She says she has been nursing him, but he doesn't "seem right." He is difficult to awaken and pale, and he has dry mucous membranes and a sunken fontanelle. She thinks he hasn't wet a diaper in about 18 hours. What do you suspect?
    a. Apnea
    b. Dehydration
    c. Jaundice
    d. Sepsis

37. Which of the following terms describes abnormal retardation of growth and development in an infant caused by maternal deprivation or malnutrition?
    a. Cerebral palsy
    b. Cystic fibrosis
    c. Failure to thrive
    d. Muscular dystrophy

38. What is the primary goal of palliative care?
    a. To make sure that optimal nutritional requirements are met
    b. To help families accept the reality of impending death
    c. To improve the quality of a person's life as death approaches
    d. To provide complete relief of any pain or discomfort

WRAP IT UP

When you walk into the neat, single-story home, you are surprised to see your patient, a 35-year-old man, sitting upright in a wheelchair using a ventilator. With great difficulty he tells you that he is a high-level quadriplegic, and he directs you to some papers that describe his medical history. He has a ventilator, a G tube, a urinary catheter, and several splints on his extremities. You note that he has an oral antibiotic that was prescribed today. He says he is "sick; just doesn't feel well," and his doctor would like him transported to the ED for evaluation. His skin is hot, and his pulse is rapid. His vital signs are T, 102.6° F (38.8 °C) axilla; BP, 90/68 mm Hg; and P, 128/min. His ventilator is set at a rate of 12 with a tidal volume of 500 mL on room air; his Sao_2 is 90%. You can hear some wheezes in his lungs, so you connect some oxygen to the ventilator. You note that the urine in his catheter bag is a milky color. The rest of his exam is unremarkable. It takes a few moments for you and your partner to plan how to effectively move him to the cot without disturbing the ventilator. You make sure the G tube is clamped securely and move the urinary catheter so that you won't pull on it. The patient says he can breathe spontaneously for several minutes on his own, so you momentarily disconnect him as you perform the lift. In the ambulance, you administer bronchodilator updraft treatment while your partner starts an IV and delivers a 200 mL fluid bolus. Reassessment in a few minutes shows that his vital signs are now BP, 100/70 mm Hg; P, 120/min; and Sao_2, 97%.

1. Why is it important to review the medical papers of the home care patient if they are available?

_____

2. Put a ✔ beside the type(s) of home care services this patient is likely to need on an ongoing basis.
    a. _____ Cardiopulmonary care
    b. _____ Dermatological or wound care
    c. _____ Catheter management
    d. _____ Gastroenterological care
    e. _____ Hospice care
    f. _____ Orthopedic care
    g. _____ Pain management
    h. _____ Rehabilitative care

3. What complications requiring emergency care could occur based on this patient's use of a
    a. Ventilator
    b. G tube
    c. Foley catheter

4. If you could not transport the patient with his ventilator, what should you do?

_____

_____

CHAPTER 48 ANSWERS

REVIEW QUESTIONS

1. A hypoxic patient may be restless, confused, tachycardic, hypertensive, dyspneic, or cyanotic or may have a headache. When you monitor the patient, you may find a low Sao_2 or cardiac dysrhythmias.
   (Objective 3)

2. If he appears to be in distress, immediately begin ventilation with a bag-valve device and 100% O_2. Then you can evaluate the equipment problem. Determine the need for suctioning.
   (Objective 3)

3. Check the ventilator for disconnected tubing or power cords; check the settings; make sure the tracheostomy tube is in the proper place and the balloon is adequately inflated.
   (Objective 3)

4. Reassure the patient that the problem has been fixed, perhaps showing him how you fixed it. Tell him you will remain with him for several minutes after you reconnect him to the ventilator to make sure that everything continues to work properly.
   (Objective 3)

5. Assess the patient's level of consciousness and level of distress; respiratory rate and lung sounds; neck for signs of JVD; skin color, temperature, and moisture; and vital signs.
   (Objective 4)

6. Slow the infusion to a keep-open rate; provide high-concentration oxygen; elevate the patient's head; maintain body warmth; monitor vital signs; reassess. If her condition does not improve, consider the need for a diuretic.
   (Objective 4)

7. The need to transport depends on the patient's response to your interventions, other anticipated complications based on the contents of the infusion, and the patient's wishes with regard to transport. The decision should be made in consultation with medical direction.
   (Objective 4)

8. The wound has many signs of infection and necrosis.
   (Objective 6)

9. A properly healing wound has a pink or red wound bed, clear or serosanguineous drainage, and no odor.
   (Objective 6)

10. The surrounding skin should be assessed for color, warmth, and swelling.
    (Objective 6)

11. The redness and warmth of the surrounding skin suggest infection.
    (Objective 6)

12. A full assessment is necessary. Specifically, vital signs, including temperature and lung sounds, should be evaluated.
    (Objective 6)

13. His physical examination suggests systemic infection. You should administer high-concentration oxygen, start IV fluids, assess his temperature, and transport.
    (Objective 6)

14. A full assessment is indicated, including initial assessment, vital signs, blood glucose, and ECG and oxygen saturation monitoring.
(Objective 7)

15. Infantile apnea may be caused by hypoglycemia, hypocalcemia, hypothermia, sepsis, pneumonia, meningitis, CNS hemorrhage, hypoxic injury, seizures, respiratory distress, hyaline membrane disease, and obstruction.
(Objective 7)

16. Keep the baby warm; administer dextrose if the glucose level is low; administer high-concentration oxygen by mask or blow-by; start an IV line (in consultation with medical direction); continually monitor breathing, color, oxygen saturation, and ECG; transport.
(Objective 7)

17. Make sure that resuscitation equipment is within easy reach. Open the appropriate size bag-mask for the child and connect it so that it is easily accessible should another apneic episode occur.
(Objective 7)

STUDENT SELF-ASSESSMENT

18. d. The growing population of immigrants in large cities stimulated the growth of nurse-provided home care for the poor.
(Objective 1)

19. c. The home health field may continue to expand, perhaps offering these services in the future.
(Objective 1)

20. a. These factors occur in three phases: preinjury, injury, and postinjury.
(Objective 1)

21. d. The same precautions should be used as in the hospital setting.
(Objective 1)

22. d. Environmental assessments include infectious waste, pets, and hazards.
(Objective 2)

23. c. Life threats should be identified before further assessment is done.
(Objective 2)

24. c. The patient should keep an oxygen cylinder on hand in case this happens.
(Objective 3)

25. d. Cuff leakage and disconnected tubing trigger a low pressure alarm. The oxygen alarm sounds if the oxygen supply is inadequate.
(Objective 3)

26. c. The rest are central venous access devices.
(Objective 4)

27. d. Although a site infection is not an immediate life threat, it can cause sepsis and possibly death if it spreads and becomes systemic.
(Objective 4)

28. c. Fever is a sign of infection. Distended neck veins and pulmonary congestion are signs of fluid overload. Other signs and symptoms of embolus include cyanosis; weak, rapid pulse; and loss of consciousness.
(Objective 4)

29. b
(Objective 4)

30. c. Urosepsis is managed with antibiotic therapy.
(Objective 5)

31. c. Excessive diarrhea can cause skin to break down rapidly, as well as dehydration and electrolyte imbalances. A change in the volume or type of tube feeding may remedy the problem.
(Objective 5)

32. c. The foreskin should be retracted to visualize the urethra. The balloon should be inflated with 3 to 5 mL of sterile water. Excessive force should not be necessary and may injure the urethra.
(Objective 5)

33. c. An adequate blood supply and sufficient oxygen and nutrition are also essential.
(Objective 6)

34. c. Fever and abdominal pain are the most common signs and symptoms of postpartum hemorrhage.
(Objective 7)

35. d. Some women who suffer from this condition fantasize about harming their babies. All the other symptoms should be assessed after the physical well-being of the mother and baby have been ensured.
(Objective 7)

36. b. Further evaluation is necessary, but the patient's clinical presentation suggests severe dehydration, which requires immediate fluid resuscitation and rapid transport.
(Objective 7)

37. c. This condition can also be caused by chromosomal abnormalities and major organ system defects.
(Objective 7)

38. c. Palliative care customizes treatment for patients and their families, providing pain and symptom management if needed and mental and spiritual guidance with the goal of improving quality of life.
(Objective 8)

WRAP IT UP

1. To determine his normal state of functioning, other medical conditions, home medications, any special instructions regarding care, legal papers, including advanced directives, normal vital signs, and private physician and hospital of choice.
(Objective 2)

2. a, b, c, d, h
(Objective 1)

3. a. The ventilator could fail as a result of power loss, kinks or water in the tubing, and excessive secretions. Patients can develop pneumothorax or experience anxiety attacks if they feel as if they are not being ventilated. Oxygen supply (if present) can fail.

b. G tube: Aspiration and severe diarrhea can occur.

c. A urinary catheter can become infected, resulting in sepsis. It can cause urethral trauma if pulled out forcefully with the balloon inflated, and the patient can develop serious signs and symptoms if the catheter is removed and urinary retention occurs.

(Objectives 3, 5)

4. Ventilate the patient with a bag-mask device or place on an automatic transport ventilator adjusted closely to the settings the patient was on at home.

(Objective 3)

PART TEN

CHAPTER
49

Ambulance Operations

READING ASSIGNMENT

Chapter 49, pages 1230-1239, in *Mosby's Paramedic Textbook,* ed. 3

OBJECTIVES

Upon completion of this chapter, the paramedic student will be able to do the following:

1. List standards that govern ambulance performance and specifications.
2. Discuss the tracking of equipment, supplies, and maintenance on an ambulance.
3. Outline the considerations for appropriate stationing of ambulances.
4. Describe measures that can influence safe operation of an ambulance.
5. Identify aeromedical crew members and training.
6. Describe the appropriate use of aeromedical services in the prehospital setting.

SUMMARY

- The federal KKK A-1822 standards provide the foundation of uniformity for the design of ambulance vehicles.
- Completing an equipment and supply checklist at the start of every work shift is important. It is essential for safety, patient care, and risk management. It also helps to ensure proper handling and safekeeping of scheduled medications.
- The methods for estimating ambulance service needs and placement in a community have changed. Compliance in providing EMS services within time frames that meet national standards is the method that now is commonly used.
- Factors that influence safe ambulance operation include proper use of escorts, environmental conditions, proper use of warning devices, proceeding safely through intersections, parking at the emergency scene, and operating with due regard for the safety of all others.
- The staffing of air ambulances includes a pilot and various health care professionals. These individuals undergo specialized training in flight physiology and the use of special medical equipment and procedures.
- When paramedics request aeromedical service, the flight crew should be advised of the type of emergency response, the number of patients, and the location of the landing zone and any prominent landmarks and hazards. Paramedics should always follow strict safety measures during helicopter landings. This helps to prevent injury to air medical crews, ground crews, the patient, and bystanders.

REVIEW QUESTIONS

1. Cite the standard that defines ambulance design or performance.

   _____

2. List three types of prehospital care supplies that should be routinely checked on an ambulance.

   a. _____

   b. _____

   c. _____

3. What would be a consequence of the following supply/equipment problems?

   a. The batteries aren't charged on the portable suction unit, and your patient is trapped in a car with a mouth full of blood and vomit.

   _____

   b. The defibrillator doesn't work, and the patient is in ventricular fibrillation.

   _____

   c. You run out of strips to check blood glucose levels on a call with an elderly man who has an altered level of consciousness and no available history.

   _____

   d. Someone forgot to replace the OB (delivery) kit after the last delivery.

   _____

   e. You run out of oxygen while on a call for pulmonary edema.

   _____

4. EMS and community planners must consider a number of factors when determining ambulance placement to provide acceptable availability and response times. List four of these factors.

   a.

   b.

   c.

   d.

5. Explain how you can reduce the risk of vehicle accidents in each of the following situations:

   a. You are being followed by a police escort.

   _____

   b. It's 0500, and driving conditions include a light rain and heavy fog.

   _____

   c. The lights and sirens are on, and you are preparing to proceed through a red light at an intersection.

   _____

Questions 6 to 10 refer to the following case study:

> You respond to a rollover MVC with a patient ejected at 0800. On arrival you find a 4-year-old girl who was thrown 20 feet from the vehicle. She is unconscious, has rapid, shallow respirations, and shows signs of shock. The nearest hospital is 40 minutes away; a pediatric trauma center is 45 minutes away by ground, 20 minutes by air. Air medical ETA to your location would be 10 minutes.

6. Give two reasons why this is an appropriate situation for use of air medical transport.

    a.

    b.

7. What information should you give the dispatcher when you call to activate the air medical transport?

_____

_____

_____

8. Describe landing zone selection and preparation for this air medical response.

_____

_____

> The crash occurred across from a baseball diamond that is easily accessible, and the LZ is set up there.

9. What patient management procedures should be performed before the helicopter arrives?

_____

_____

10. List three safety measures that should be taken as you approach the helicopter to load the patient when it lands.

    a.

    b.

    c.

STUDENT SELF-ASSESSMENT

11. Which of the following is true of the KKK A-1822 standards?
    a. They contradict the AMD 001-009 performance standards.
    b. They designate design standards for types I, II, and III ambulances.
    c. They define performance specifications for air ambulances.
    d. They outline ambulance driving standards and qualifications.

12. Why are routine ambulance equipment checks essential?
    a. So that accurate patient billing and reimbursement can occur in a timely manner
    b. So that disciplinary action will not be necessary if an equipment failure occurs
    c. So that essential equipment is available and in working order during patient care
    d. So that state laws and regulations can be met and licensure can be maintained

13. Emergency vehicle placement in a community should be determined by which of the following?
    a. Average response times that meet national standards
    b. The number of receiving hospitals in the region
    c. The projected revenue flow from reimbursement
    d. Where the citizens would like to have ambulances

14. Which of the following help promote safety when driving an ambulance?
    a. Drive no faster than 20 miles per hour over the speed limit on routine calls.
    b. Make sure that only the driver and the patient are always restrained.
    c. Use extreme caution at intersections, especially when using lights and sirens.
    d. Use lights and sirens often so that other drivers will yield the right of way.
15. How can the paramedic promote safety when responding to a vehicle crash on the highway?
    a. Park 100 feet past the crash.
    b. Park downhill from hazardous materials.
    c. Park on the opposite side of the road.
    d. Turn off emergency lights.
16. All air medical crew members should receive specialized training in which of the following areas?
    a. Airway management techniques
    b. Flight physiology
    c. Medication administration
    d. Vascular access techniques
17. Which of the following situations would justify the use of air medical transport by an advanced life support unit with an ETA of 40 minutes?
    a. Possible fractured tibia with good pulses
    b. Possible aneurysm with absent pedal pulses
    c. Home delivery with both patients stable
    d. Asthma patient with P, 100/min; R, 20/min
18. Which of the following safety measures should be used when approaching the helicopter to load patients?
    a. Approach the aircraft as soon as it lands.
    b. At least six people should help load the aircraft.
    c. Long objects should be carried vertically to maintain control.
    d. The aircraft should be approached from the front.

WRAP IT UP

"C-crew," your partner mutters as you begin your morning ambulance check. It's frustrating, because things just don't seem as neat and clean as you like them, and there's always some little thing missing or out of place. You complete the equipment checklist and then go to the office to fill out a maintenance request for the broken latch on the medication drawer. Because it's the first day of the month, the sealed pediatric bag is opened and checked to make sure that none of the drugs have expired. Just as break time begins, you are dispatched to a call for an electrocution. The pumper is responding with you, so you and your partner follow it at a distance, taking care to change the siren as you pass motorists that have pulled to the right. At each light you change your siren and sound the air horn, stop, and make sure all traffic has stopped before you proceed. En route, you ask dispatch to place the air medical team on standby because the burn center is an hour away. You are thankful that your new engine house is so close to the scene; it will probably save you a couple of minutes on this response.

When you arrive on the scene, you find that the patient touched some high-voltage wires with a tree trimmer and is critically burned, so you immediately ask that the aircraft be launched. Your captain sends two of his crew members to set up the landing zone in an adjacent parking lot while the rest of the team works to assess and treat the patient. When the flight crew lands, you give a report, explaining that intubation is impossible because the man's jaw is clenched. After assessing the patient, the air crew performs rapid sequence induction and intubates the patient, ensuring a secure airway in flight. You help them with loading, being careful to stay to the front of the aircraft, away from the tail rotor. Back at the station, you restock and document the call and then get your well-deserved cup of coffee.

1. Put a ✔ beside the consequences of failing to check the ambulance equipment or to maintain it properly.
   a. _____ Batteries dead in saturation monitor
   b. _____ Inability to defibrillate
   c. _____ Break down en route to hospital
   d. _____ Drugs expired
   e. _____ Traction splint unavailable
   f. _____ No oxygen available
   g. _____ Appropriate drug not on ambulance
   h. _____ Ambulance tire blowout

2. What advantage of constructing a new station is described here?

3. List two additional safe driving considerations that were not mentioned in this case study.

_____

_____

4. List two advantages of aeromedical transport that were described in this situation.

_____

_____

CHAPTER 49 ANSWERS

REVIEW QUESTIONS

1. KKK A-1822D
   (Objective 1)

2. a. Supplies (airway, vascular access, dressings)
   b. Medications (number and expiration dates, oxygen supply)
   c. Equipment (including routine maintenance, battery loads, supplementary supplies)
   (Objective 2)

3. a. The patient may aspirate and die.
   b. You will be unable to defibrillate until another unit arrives, and the patient may deteriorate into asystole and die.
   c. You will be unable to determine whether the altered consciousness is due to hypoglycemia. If you administer glucose and the patient's altered level of consciousness is related to a stroke, this action may worsen his condition.
   d. You will have to search for other appropriate supplies, wasting time to care for the patient and baby. What will you use to cut the cord and then clamp it?
   e. The patient's hypoxia may worsen, resulting in death.
   (Objective 2)

4. a. National response time standards
   b. Geographical area
   c. Population and patient demand
   d. Traffic conditions
   Others include time of day and appropriate placement of vehicles.
   (Objective 3)

5. a. Make sure that the police follow at a safe distance. Use a siren tone different from that used by the police.
   b. Slow the ambulance to a safe speed and use the low beam lights.
   c. Remember that not all drivers will hear your sirens or see your lights. Stop and look to make sure that all traffic is stopping (make eye contact if possible). Use the yelp mode of the siren and remain vigilant as you proceed.
   (Objective 4)

6. Your patient is critical and requires specialized resources, and you are far from a hospital.
   (Objective 6)

7. Advise the flight crew that you are at an MVC with a critically ill child. Let them know the location of the landing zone and any prominent landmarks or hazards.
   (Objective 6)

8. The landing zone should be 100 × 100 feet. It should have few vertical structures and should be relatively flat and free of high grass, crops, debris, or rough terrain (check local standards for specific variations).
   (Objective 6)

9. As many patient care procedures as possible should be done, depending on the ETA of the helicopter. The airway should be secured, and the patient ventilated appropriately. The patient should be secured to a long spine board with straps and cervical immobilization. Vascular access should be obtained, and other patient assessment and care continued (e.g., maintain warmth) until the helicopter arrives.
   (Objective 6)

10. Do not approach the aircraft unless directed to do so by the crew. Approach from the front of the aircraft and stay clear of the tail rotor. Allow a minimal number of people to help load. Secure loose objects. Walk in a crouched position. Carry objects at waist height. Depart from the front in view of the pilot. Wear eye protection.
    (Objective 6)

STUDENT SELF-ASSESSMENT

11. b. The AMD 001-009 performance standards have been incorporated into the latest KKK standards. (Objective 1)

12. c. Lack or failure of essential patient equipment could mean the difference between life and death. (Objective 2)

13. a. A number of factors will affect those times, and they can vary by time of day and other variables. This should be monitored on a continuing basis. (Objective 3)

14. c. Paramedics driving an ambulance should remain at or below the speed limit except in extreme circumstances. For maximal safety, the paramedic attendant should also be restrained except when patient care requires movement. Lights and sirens should be used only on emergency responses (as dictated by policy) and when a patient in critical condition is being transported. (Objective 4)

15. a. Ideally, the ambulance should be on the same side of the road as the crash. Emergency lights should be left on. Ambulances should be parked uphill and upwind from hazardous materials incidents. (Objective 4)

16. b. Some air medical services require training in specialized airway and vascular access techniques, as well as expanded medication administration knowledge. This varies by agency. (Objective 5)

17. b. Unless inclement weather or impassable roads prohibit transport, all the other patients could be appropriately transported by ground ALS service. (Objective 6)

18. d. No one should approach the aircraft until a crew member signals that it is OK. A minimal number of people should approach the aircraft. No objects should be held up. (Objective 6)

WRAP IT UP

1. a (are replacements available on the ambulance, are the batteries fully charged on the defibrillator, and are there defibrillator pads on truck); c (is preventive maintenance being done); d (what effect would giving an expired drug have); e (how will that affect the patient's pain and further damage/bleeding); f (what if your patient is critical; would you have to call another ambulance); g (how would you explain that in court); h (what might the consequence be; are you checking the tires each day and reporting wear) (Objective 2)

2. Reduction in response time (Objective 3)

3. Wearing seatbelts; driving the speed limit, except as allowed by law; parking safely at the scene. (Objective 4)

4. The crew is trained and authorized to perform advanced techniques; a specialized resource center can be reached more quickly. (Objectives 5, 6)

CHAPTER

50

Medical Incident Command

READING ASSIGNMENT

Chapter 50, pages 1240-1256, in *Mosby's Paramedic Textbook*, ed. 3

OBJECTIVES

Upon completion of this chapter, the paramedic student will be able to:
 1. Identify the components of an effective incident command system.
 2. Outline the activities of the preplanning, scene management, and postdisaster follow-up phases of an incident.
 3. Identify the five major functions of the incident command system.
 4. List command responsibilities during a major incident response.
 5. Describe the section responsibilities in the incident command system.
 6. Identify situations that may be classified as major incidents.
 7. Describe the steps necessary to establish and operate the incident command system.
 8. Given a major incident, describe the groups and/or divisions that would need to be established and the responsibilities of each.
 9. List common problems related to the incident command system and to mass casualty incidents.
 10. Outline the principles and technology of triage.
 11. Identify resources for the management of critical incident stress.

SUMMARY

- The ICS organizational structure should be adaptable to any agency or to any incident requiring emergency management. The ICS also must be expandable. It must be able to expand from dealing with a nonmajor incident to a major one in a logical way.
- All participating response agencies must agree to the preplan (phase 1 of the ICS). The preplan must address common goals and the specific duties of each group. Phase 2 requires the development of a strategy to manage the emergency scene. Phase 3 includes a postdisaster review of lessons learned from the incident and the determination of ways to improve.
- The five major functions of the ICS organization are command, planning, operations, logistics, and finance/administration.
- The responsibility of command should belong to one person. This should be a person who can effectively manage the emergency scene. In multiagency and/or multijurisdictional incidents, unified command may be used.
- The planning section should provide past, present, and future information about the incident and the status of resources. The operations section directs and coordinates all operations. It also ensures the safety of all personnel.

The logistics section is responsible for providing supplies and equipment (including personnel to operate the equipment), facilities, services, food, and communications support. The finance/administration section tracks incident and reimbursement costs.

- The need to expand the ICS at a medical incident is based on the number of casualties and the nature of the event.
- The first EMS unit to arrive at the scene should make a quick and rapid assessment of the situation. Command must immediately establish radio contact with the communications center or emergency operations center. Additional units should be requested as soon as the need has been identified.
- Common divisions or groups that may need to be established include extrication/rescue, treatment, and transportation. A staging area and support branch may also be needed. The rescue/extrication group is responsible for managing trapped patients at the scene. The treatment group provides advanced care and stabilization until the patients are transported to a medical facility. The transportation group communicates with the receiving hospital, ambulances, and aeromedical services for patient transport. The staging area is used in large incidents to prevent vehicle congestion and delays in response. The rehabilitation area allows rescue personnel to receive physical and psychological rest. The support branch coordinates the gathering and distribution of equipment and supplies for all divisions and groups.
- Problems of mass casualty incidents and incident command systems stem from numerous issues related to communication, resource allocation, and delegation.
- Triage is a method used to categorize patients for priorities of treatment. START triage uses a 60-second assessment. It focuses on the patient's ability to walk, respiratory effort, pulses/perfusion, and neurological status. The METTAG system is one of a number of tape, tag, and label systems used to categorize patients during triage.
- Critical incident stress debriefing is part of a critical incident stress management program. Such debriefing should be part of postdisaster standard operating procedures.

REVIEW QUESTIONS

Match the terms in column II with their definitions in column I. Use each term only once.

Column I	Column II
1. _____ Contracts agreeing to interagency exchange of resources when necessary	a. Apparatus
2. _____ Pumpers, ladder trucks, rescue trucks	b. Command
3. _____ Rendezvous location for all arriving EMS, fire, and rescue equipment	c. Command post
4. _____ Responsible for coordination of major incident situation	d. Communication center
	e. Mutual aid
	f. Sector
	g. Staging area

Questions 5 to 13 refer to the following case study:

Dispatch radios your crew to respond to a local sports stadium for a bleacher collapse at a college football game. During your initial size-up, you determine that 50 to 100 people are injured, with a substantial number of victims still trapped under the fallen concrete seats. It is rush hour, and traffic conditions will be heavy for at least 2 more hours.

5. List three actions that should be taken by the first unit arriving at the scene.

_____

_____

6. a. How will command be determined?

_____

_____

b. Will single or unified command be used?

_____

_____

7. List nine command responsibilities during this incident.

   a.

   b.

   c.

   d.

   e.

   f.

   g.

   h.

   i.

8. Fill in Fig. 50-1 with the appropriate positions needed in this incident command situation.

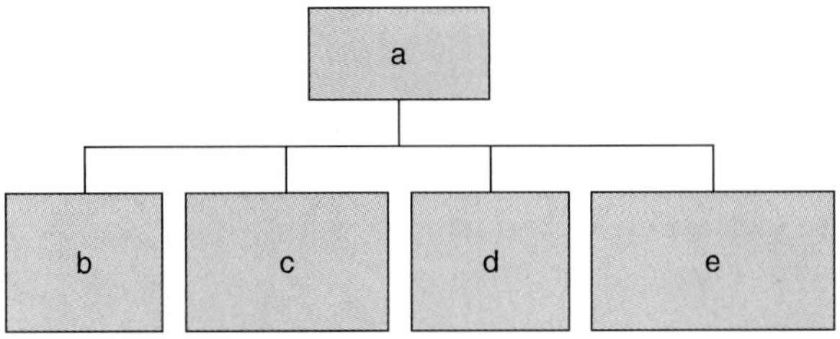

Figure 50-1

9. Briefly describe the responsibilities of each of the following sectors that command has established for this incident.

   a. Support branch:

_____

_____

   b. Staging area:

_____

_____

   c. Extrication group:

_____

_____

   d. Treatment group:

_____

_____

e. Transportation:

_____

_____

10. Explain how communications can be initiated in an effective manner in this situation.

_____

_____

_____

11. a. What special resources will be needed during this incident?

_____

_____

b. How will command know where to obtain those resources?

_____

_____

12. Triage each of the following patients injured at this scene using START triage and METTAG categories.

a. A man walks over to you complaining of chest pain.

_____

b. A woman has a respiratory rate of 20/min and no radial pulse, but a carotid pulse is present.

_____

c. A man is lying under a bleacher. His respiratory rate is 24/min; a radial pulse is present; he can't touch his nose with his index finger; he knows his name but not the date or year.

_____

d. A woman is leaning against a bleacher, unable to walk. Her respiratory rate is 16/min; a radial pulse is present; she can stick out her tongue and touch her nose with her index finger; she knows her name, the date, and the year.

_____

e. A man has a respiratory rate of 8/min. He has no radial pulse, but a carotid pulse is present.

_____

f. A woman is trapped under a post. She is not breathing and has no pulse.

_____

13. During triage, what care should be provided to the patients in question 12?

_____

STUDENT SELF-ASSESSMENT

14. An ideal incident command system would have which of the following characteristics?
    a. It would be able to expand to a larger incident in a logical manner.
    b. It would be used only for large or complex mass casualty situations.
    c. It would provide for just single jurisdiction involvement.
    d. It would respond to one specific incident or situation.

15. Which phase of major incident planning involves establishing an inventory of community resources needed for selected disasters?
    a. Logistics operations
    b. Postdisaster follow-up
    c. Scene management
    d. The preplan

16. What are the five major components of FEMA's ICS organization?
    a. Communications, logistics, operations, staging, support
    b. Communications, finance, staging, support, treatment
    c. Command, finance, logistics, operations, planning
    d. Command, operations, planning, transportation, treatment

17. Which of the following should have the highest priority when the incident commander is considering whether to expand the ICS organization during an incident?
    a. Cost
    b. Incident stability
    c. Life safety
    d. Property conservation

18. What is the primary responsibility of the section chiefs in an MCI situation?
    a. To assume overall accountability for the MCI situation
    b. To make sure that section members are working toward a common goal
    c. To operate rescue equipment and supervise staff in the area
    d. To provide patient care and stabilization within a defined area

19. Which section has overall responsibility for the areas that provide care to medical staff?
    a. Finance
    b. Logistics
    c. Operations
    d. Planning

20. Which of the following situations would be *least* likely to be declared a major incident?
    a. Rural EMS service, motor vehicle collision requiring four EMS units
    b. City EMS service, train derailment, possible hazardous materials leak
    c. Rural EMS service, two-patient incident with high-angle rescue
    d. City EMS service, two-person motor vehicle collision, no patient trapped

21. Except in unusual circumstances, patient care and stabilization should be provided by which group?
    a. Extrication
    b. Support
    c. Treatment
    d. Triage

22. What is an appropriate role for a physician brought to the scene from a local hospital?
    a. Incident commander
    b. Extrication group resource
    c. Staging area resource
    d. Transport group resource

23. The most appropriate *radio* communication during a mass casualty incident would be between which of the following crew members?
    a. Command and sector officers
    b. Individuals within each unit
    c. Treatment group and hospital
    d. Public information officer and press

24. Which of the following may create a problem at an MCI?
    a. Organizing patients rapidly at a treatment area
    b. Transporting patients prematurely
    c. Performing rapid "initial" stabilization of patients
    d. Wearing identification vests

25. Patient classification during mass casualty incidents should be based on which of the following?
    a. Physiological signs, mechanism of injury, and anatomical injury
    b. Mechanism of injury, anatomical injury, and patient age
    c. Chief complaint, physiological signs, and anatomical injury
    d. Physiological signs, anatomical injury, and concurrent disease

26. Your patient has a gunshot wound to the chest, is conscious, and has a respiratory rate of 36/min. Which of the following would be the appropriate triage category, using the triage systems discussed in the text?
    a. Urgent, yellow   **c.** Dead/dying, black
    b. Critical, red   **d.** Delayed, green
27. Mental status examination during START triage should include which of the following?
    a. Asking the patient to touch his nose
    b. AVPU
    c. Glasgow coma scale
    d. Observing for arm drift
28. What information should be included on the patient tracking log?
    a. Patient's age   **c.** Patient's next of kin
    b. Patient's injuries   **d.** Patient's priority
29. Which of the following is *not* typically provided in a critical incident stress management program?
    a. Advice to command during large-scale incidents
    b. Defusing services immediately after a large-scale incident
    c. Long-term psychiatric counseling
    d. On-scene support for distressed personnel

WRAP IT UP

At 0828 on this foggy morning, a large passenger aircraft runs off runway M2R, striking the perimeter fence around the airport. Your ambulance is the first to arrive on the scene. The local fire chief is the incident commander, and he immediately delegates your supervisor to assume EMS command. She, in turn, asks that you lead the rescue/extrication group. You send your partner to do a quick size-up of the patients who are out of the aircraft. The initial assessment reveals that the pilot was found not breathing and pulseless; three crew members and three passengers are noted to have inhalation injury and severe respiratory distress; the other 19 patients appear on initial exam to be walking, complaining of minor injuries. The next several hours are frantic and chaotic at times as the patients are sorted, treated, and finally transported.

During an incident debriefing 3 days later, you review the whole situation. The incident commander shows how he laid out the groups: rescue/extrication (triage, treatment, transport), staging, and transportation. A PIO officer was definitely an asset for dealing with the huge media presence, and a liaison officer helped to communicate with the unified command. Problems identified in the situation included difficulty with communication, a delay in getting ambulances to the scene, a traffic jam at the scene, difficulty identifying branch leaders, and failure to update the hospitals about incoming patients. Some suggestions are offered for remedying these problems, and another planning meeting is scheduled for 2 weeks later.

1. What additional support staff person should have been appointed by command, in addition to the public relations and liaison officers?

2. What are some possible causes of the difficulties identified in this situation, and which sectors or branches are responsible for identifying solutions?

Problem	Possible Causes	Sector or Branch Responsible for Solution
a. Difficulty with communication		
b. Delay in ambulance arrival		
c. Traffic jam on scene		
d. Difficulty identifying command		
e. Failure to update hospitals		

3. Based on the limited information you have, how many patients would you triage as
   a. Dead or dying
   b. Critical
   c. Urgent
   d. Delayed

CHAPTER 50 ANSWERS

REVIEW QUESTIONS

1. e
2. a
3. g
4. b
(Questions 1-4: Objective 1)

5. A rapid scene assessment should be performed. Communication should be established with the communications center or emergency operations center (as dictated by local policy). Additional units should be requested as soon as the need has been identified.
(Objective 7)

6. a. Command is determined by the preplanned system of arriving emergency units. The person assuming command must be familiar with ICS structure and the operating procedures of responding units.
(Objective 7)

b. It will likely be a unified command involving EMS, fire/rescue, and police. Some communities have public safety departments that incorporate all three functions. In that case, a single command will likely be used.
(Objective 4)

7. Assuming an effective command position that has a good vantage point and is away from any danger of the bleachers, some responsibilities would be: transmitting initial radio reports to the communications center; evaluating the scene rapidly (visually and with reports of other first responders); developing a strategy to safely extricate, triage, treat, transport, and provide security on scene; requesting additional equipment and personnel resources and assigning command roles; assigning sectors and identifying objectives in cooperation with section chiefs; evaluating information to determine the progress of the event; sending units no longer needed back into service; terminating command at an appropriate time; and evaluating the effectiveness of operations (may be done retrospectively).
(Objective 4)

8. Incident command organizational chart completed. a. Command b. Finance c. Logistic d. Operation e. Planning
(Objective 3)

9. a. Procuring and distributing supplies (medicine, food, water, protective gear) and resources (heavy equipment, special tools).
b. Designating and staffing a safe helicopter landing zone and designating and staffing a staging area where all arriving apparatus will report and be assigned to areas where needed.
c. Triaging victims and moving them to a designated treatment area; securing necessary experts to determine the safest extrication procedures for this structure; coordinating physical rescue operations (including direction of heavy equipment); and ensuring scene safety.
d. Selecting a site close to but at a safe distance from the collapse site; categorizing patients on arrival and sending them to the appropriate segment of the treatment area or immediate or delayed zones; providing patient care and stabilization until transport can be provided; and communicating frequently with the transportation sector so that appropriate patient transfers can be facilitated.
e. Coordinating patient transport with the staging area manager and treatment groups; communicating with receiving hospitals so that appropriate resources can be selected; and assigning patients to ambulances or helicopters and directing them to the appropriate facilities.
(Objective 8)

10. Effective communications can be enhanced by using a common frequency (command frequency) for interdisciplinary communication when necessary; using the radio frequencies designated in the plan; using different frequencies for fire, EMS, and other support agencies; making sure that common terminology is used; ensuring clear, concise radio traffic; preparing messages before transmitting; limiting use of radios; and identifying the speaker only by sector.
    (Objective 7)

11. a. Air medical transport, because of heavy traffic and heavy equipment needed to extricate victims from under the bleachers.
    (Objective 8)

    b. The preplan should identify the availability and location of specialized resources that may be needed during an MCI situation.
    (Objective 2)

12. a. Delayed, yellow (may be upgraded after retriage in treatment sector)
    b. Critical, red
    c. Critical, yellow
    d. Delayed, green
    e. Critical, red
    f. Dead/dying, black
    (Objective 10)

13. The airway may be opened if necessary and hemorrhage controlled.
    (Objective 10)

STUDENT SELF-ASSESSMENT

14. a. The ICS should be adaptable to small or large situations involving one or more jurisdictions as the need arises.
    (Objective 1)

15. d. Preidentification of resources ensures rapid deployment by logistics during a disaster.
    (Objective 2)

16. c. Command, finance, logistics, operations, and planning (C-FLOP) are the foundations on which the ICS is built.
    (Objective 3)

17. c. The priority is always the safety of the emergency responders and the public.
    (Objective 4)

18. b. The incident commander has overall responsibility. The section chiefs should be directing staff in their sectors, not performing physical tasks or providing patient care.
    (Objective 3)

19. b. The rehab branch falls under the command of the logistics section.
    (Objective 3)

20. d. In most city EMS systems, this type of patient situation should not overwhelm the system, requiring a mass casualty plan.
    (Objective 6)

21. c. In triage, patients are sorted, airways are opened, and hemorrhage is controlled.
(Objective 8)

22. b. Physicians are probably not appropriately trained for command. Their services may be more useful in assisting with triage and providing emergency surgery to facilitate extrication (all extrication sector responsibilities). A physician may also be assigned to the treatment sector.
(Objective 3)

23. a. As much verbal communication as possible should take place during the mass casualty incident to permit essential communication on the airwaves.
(Objective 7)

24. b
(Objective 9)

25. d. Abnormal vital signs, obvious anatomical injury, and other obvious preexisting illnesses and injuries should be considered when triaging patients.
(Objective 10)

26. b. A respiratory rate over 30/min indicates critical status in the START triage method. This patient obviously has a serious anatomical injury and abnormal physiological signs, indicating that urgent care is necessary.
(Objective 10)

27. a. The patient should also be asked to state his name and the current date, including the year.
(Objective 10)

28. d. Patient identification, transporting unit, and hospital destination should also be noted.
(Objective 10)

29. c. The services provided depend on the local CISM team.
(Objective 11)

WRAP IT UP

1. There should always be a safety officer.
   (Objective 1)

2.

Problem	Possible Causes	Sector or Branch Responsible for Solution
a. Difficulty with communication	Failure to designate specific channels in preplan and/or early in incident Excessive talking on the radio; failure to use face-to-face communication	Incident command Sector officers
b. Delay in ambulance arrival	Possible failure to request resources early Possible failure to adequately control the perimeter and access roads	Incident command
c. Traffic jam on scene	Failure to designate staging area early; failure to designate areas spread apart (e.g., transportation, staging, command)	Law enforcement Incident command
d. Difficulty identifying command	Possible failure to declare who is in command on the radio Failure to wear identification vests or to mark the command area adequately	Incident command
e. Failure to update hospitals	Failure to give hospitals a brief report when wounded are leaving	Transportation group leader

(Objective 9)

3. a. 1
   b. 3
   c. 0
   d. 19

(Objective 10)

CHAPTER

51

Rescue Awareness and Operations

READING ASSIGNMENT

Chapter 51, pages 1256-1275 in *Mosby's Paramedic Textbook*, ed. 3

OBJECTIVES

Upon completion of this chapter, the paramedic student will be able to do the following:

1. Describe factors that must be considered to ensure appropriate timing of medical and mechanical skills during a rescue.
2. Outline each phase of a rescue operation.
3. Identify the appropriate personal protective equipment (PPE) for rescue operations.
4. Describe important considerations for emergency medical services (EMS) crews in a surface water rescue.
5. Discuss important considerations for EMS crews in rescues associated with hazardous atmospheres, including confined spaces and trench or cave-in situations.
6. Describe hazards that may be present during an EMS rescue operation on a highway.
7. Describe important considerations for EMS crews in a rescue involving hazardous terrain.
8. Outline special considerations for prehospital assessment and management during a rescue operation.

SUMMARY

- Rescue is a patient-driven event. It calls for specialized medical and mechanical skills. The right amount of each must be applied at the right time. The main role of the paramedic in rescues is to have the proper training and the appropriate PPE. These allow safe access to the patient and the provision of treatment at the site and throughout the incident.
- The seven phases of a rescue operation are arrival and scene size-up, hazard control, gaining access to the patient, medical treatment, disentanglement, patient packaging, and transportation.
- The standards for protective clothing and personal protection equipment established by the National Fire Protection Association and OSHA have been adopted by many fire and EMS agencies. The appropriate PPE depends on the level of rescuer involvement and the nature of the incident.
- Water rescue should never be attempted by a single rescuer or by one who is untrained.
- Water hazards include obstructions to flow and foot or extremity pins that can trap victims and drag them under water. Some factors that contribute to flat water drowning are alcohol or other drug use. Also, cool water temperatures contribute to such drownings.

- Hazardous atmospheres are environments with low oxygen. These environments can occur in confined spaces. The six major hazards associated with confined spaces are oxygen-deficient atmospheres, chemical/toxic exposure and explosion, engulfment, machinery entrapment, electricity, and structural concerns.
- Traffic flow is the biggest hazard in EMS highway operations. Other scene hazards associated with highway operations include fuel or fire hazards, electrical power, unstable vehicles, airbags and supplemental restraint systems, and hazardous cargoes.
- Hazardous terrain can create major difficulties during rescue events. Three common classifications of hazardous terrain are low-angle, high-angle, and flat terrain with obstructions.

REVIEW QUESTIONS

Questions 1 and 2 refer to the following case study:

A woman who is kayaking on a winter day is swept under the ice. You can see her about 3 feet (1 meter) from the edge of the ice where the water is rolling up over a large rock. Her team is frantically screaming at you to do something.

1. What hazards do you face if you enter the water to attempt a rescue?

_____

Additional equipment is requested, and a cut is made in the ice to retrieve the woman. However, she does not survive the 90-minute submersion.

2. What services of the local CISM team might your crew need after this incident?

_____

Questions 3 to 8 refer to the following case study:

A party-goer falls into an open sewer standpipe. You estimate that he is approximately 30 feet down the 48-inch pipe. Bystanders report that he was talking to them when they arrived, but you hear him moaning only occasionally at this time.

3. What additional assistance will you request?

_____

4. What potential injuries should you worry about in this patient?

_____

5. Why must the rescue team test the air quality at several levels in the pipe?

_____

6. Why might the rescuer who enters the pipe wear an SABA instead of an SCBA during this rescue?

_____

7. What can cause problems when using an SABA?

_____

8. Aside from a confined-space rescue, what other hazardous rescue situation exists here?

_____

_____

Questions 9 to 18 refer to the following case study:

You are called to the scene of a motor vehicle collision at a busy urban shopping center. On arrival, you find that a large sedan has hit the side of a compact car, wedging it between the sedan and a storefront. A large crowd of spectators has gathered and is impeding your access to the patient. You note a trickle of gasoline coming from one of the vehicles. No other equipment or law enforcement personnel have been dispatched.

9. What should you be looking for as you do your scene size-up?

_____

10. What information/assistance did you receive on your response?

_____

_____

11. What steps should you take to gain control of the crowd?

_____

_____

_____

One patient was pulled from the sedan by bystanders before your arrival. He is pale and complains of abdominal pain. Your partner begins care. A second patient in the compact car is unconscious. He is trapped and inaccessible.

12. List the additional equipment and other resources you should request at this time.

_____

13. What hazards have you identified that should be reported to incoming crews?

_____

14. What actions can be taken to reduce the risks associated with the hazards you identified?

_____

_____

A rescue truck arrives, and the crew breaks a window in the compact car, providing limited access to the patient while rescue operations proceed.

15. What can you do for your patient at this time?

_____

16. How can you ensure patient safety during the rescue?

_____

_____

A brief primary survey reveals an unconscious patient with gurgling respirations and a strong radial pulse of 70/min. You observe a large ecchymotic area on the temporal region of the patient's head.

17. You have limited time and access to the patient. What are your priorities of care?

_____

_____

18. Describe the disentanglement, packaging, and removal segments of the rescue operation and your responsibilities to the patient during these phases.

_____

_____

_____

_____

_____

19. At the scene of an accident in which an energized wire is in contact with an involved automobile, what safety measures should be taken for

   a. Rescuers:

_____

_____

   b. People trapped in the involved automobile:

_____

_____

20. Give two examples of equipment that may be used to disentangle a person who is trapped inside a vehicle.

   a.

   b.

STUDENT SELF-ASSESSMENT

21. Aside from ensuring safety, the rescue operations should be guided by which of the following?
   a. Performance of techniques in the standardized manner
   b. The desire of the rescue team to complete the task
   c. The medical and physical needs of the patient
   d. The number of bystanders observing the scene

22. What is the responsibility of the paramedic in any rescue situation?
    a. To coordinate overall scene safety
    b. To direct scene and tactical operations
    c. To know when it is safe to attempt rescue
    d. To operate all rescue and extrication equipment
23. The safety of which of the following should be the *first* priority at the scene of any rescue?
    a. Bystanders   c. Injured
    b. Crew   d. Trapped
24. When does scene size-up begin on a call for rescue?
    a. On arrival to the scene   c. When the call is received
    b. When specialized teams arrive   d. When the patient is visible
25. Which is true regarding medical treatment during a rescue situation for a safely accessible patient?
    a. All standardized procedures should be followed.
    b. Medical treatment should be directed by the rescue commander.
    c. No treatment should be attempted until the patient has been freed.
    d. Rapid assessment and basic stabilization should be attempted.
26. What routine safety measures should be used to protect the patient during a vehicle rescue that does not involve fire or hazardous materials?
    a. Blanket   c. Surgical mask
    b. Air bags   d. An SCBA
27. According to NFPA and OSHA standards, EMS rescue personnel should have access to all the following personal protective equipment *except*
    a. Ear plugs   c. Rubber boots
    b. Protective helmet   d. Waterproof gloves
28. Which is true when responding to a rescue in swift water?
    a. A foot trapped in water should be freed the opposite way it went in.
    b. Do not walk through fast-moving water that is over knee deep.
    c. Flat water does not create any serious hazard.
    d. High dams create more dangerous situations than low dams.
29. What factors contribute to drowning?
    a. Cool water temperature   c. PFDs worn properly
    b. Advanced patient age   d. Swimming after eating
30. What factor would be an acceptable reason *not* to resuscitate a person who has drowned?
    a. More than 5 minutes of submersion was documented by witnesses.
    b. Evidence of activation of the mammalian diving reflex exists.
    c. Patient is cold, and temperature can't be detected on a regular thermometer.
    d. Rigor mortis or dependent lividity is present.
31. What is the first measure that should be used to attempt rescue for a person in the water?
    a. Go   c. Row
    b. Reach   d. Throw
32. Which of the following oxygen levels is considered hazardous?
    a. Over 19.5%   c. Over 21%
    b. Over 22%   d. Under 21%
33. Which is a clue to help identify an oxygen-limiting silo?
    a. An audible tone will sound.
    b. The color is usually blue.
    c. The placard states this information.
    d. The smell will be sweet.
34. You arrive at the scene of a trench collapse. When do you enter the trench to rescue the patient without specialized rescue equipment?
    a. The patient is unconscious.
    b. The patient is completely covered.
    c. The trench is less than waist deep.
    d. The trench is more than 3 feet wide.

35. Which of the following techniques may be used to increase safety at the scene of a vehicle accident with a gasoline leak at night?
    a. Put flares adjacent to the involved vehicles to alert motorists.
    b. Stage all apparatus on the highway and not on side roads.
    c. Use all warning lights and headlights to increase visibility.
    d. Wear high-visibility clothing, such as orange highway vests.
36. To reduce the risk of fire at the scene of a motor vehicle collision in which gasoline is leaking, a paramedic should *always* do which of the following?
    a. Disconnect the battery cable
    b. Douse the vehicle with foam
    c. Place a tarp over the spilled fuel
    d. Turn off the automobile ignition
37. Which type of extinguisher can be used to suppress a combustible metal fire?
    a. Class A
    b. Class B
    c. Class C
    d. Class D
38. What type of equipment is helpful for vehicle stabilization during rescue?
    a. Chain saws
    b. Cribbing
    c. Hurst tools
    d. Pry bars
39. You respond to a vehicle crash involving an undeployed air bag. What measure may create a hazard for rescuers?
    a. Using tools that generate sparks
    b. Cutting the steering column to disable the system
    c. Disconnecting or cutting both battery cables
    d. Cutting into the air bag module
40. What is the primary risk associated with hazardous terrain rescue?
    a. Avalanche of debris
    b. Dropping the patient
    c. Injury from falls
    d. Injury from projectiles
41. Which term describes rescue on steep terrain that can be walked on without use of the hands?
    a. Graded terrain rescue
    b. High-angle rescue
    c. Low-angle rescue
    d. Rescue on flat terrain with obstructions
42. Which of the following factors that can interfere with a paramedic's ability to adequately assess and treat a patient is unique to a rescue situation?
    a. Cumbersome personal protective equipment
    b. Lack of cooperation among your team members
    c. Hostile, uncommunicative patient
    d. Unstable vital signs and neurological status
43. Which is a complication of crush syndrome?
    a. Hypertension
    b. Metabolic alkalosis
    c. Myoglobinemia
    d. Sepsis
44. You are trying to free a driver involved in a head-on crash who is seriously injured. The car shows major front-end damage; also, the passenger air bag has deployed, but the driver-side air bag has not. How will this affect your approach to the rescue?
    a. When the ignition is off, the bag will not open unless there is a fire.
    b. It will not affect your approach to this patient.
    c. You will put a board between the patient and the unopened bag.
    d. You will keep at least 10 inches or more away from the path of the bag.

WRAP IT UP

You can sense the panic as you pull up to the scene of a mine explosion. Six men were down in the narrow shaft when a rumbling noise was heard, and then a plume of dark smoke slowly wound out of the mine. The incident commander and mine supervisor are reviewing the situation, trying to determine the best approach. An alternate shaft is available, but there is a fear of secondary danger. One garbled radio transmission from below indicates that there are survivors, but several are trapped under the rubble. It is determined that you and your partner will go in first because of your advanced rescue training. The two of you don an SABA and rappelling harness and are lowered slowly down the secondary shaft. At the bottom, water is slowly creeping up the walls of the enclosure. Your lamps provide a glimpse of some movement through the haze, and you carefully move along the side of the wall, taking care not to catch your air hoses on the protruding rocks. When you reach the miners, two are dead, three are in good condition, and one is entangled in some twisted rebar. Over the next 4 hours, first the three men in good condition are lifted up the narrow shaft in a rescue harness; then the rebar is cut, the fourth miner is removed from the wreckage, his wounds are treated, and he is pulled to the top wrapped securely in a Stokes basket. Finally, the agonizing job of respectfully packaging and lifting the bodies is undertaken.

1. Put a ✓ beside potential hazards faced by the rescuers in this situation.
   a. _____ Collapse/engulfment   d. _____ Hypothermia
   b. _____ Electrical   e. _____ Oxygen deficiency
   c. _____ Explosion   f. _____ Toxic gases

2. Identify steps that should be taken to minimize the risks you indicated for the trapped miners and for the rescuers.

   _____

   _____

   _____

3. What personal protective equipment should the rescuers be using in this situation?

   _____

4. Which phase of the rescue operation was it when the rescuers cut the rebar and freed the miner?
   a. Disentanglement
   b. Gaining access to the patient
   c. Hazard control
   d. Patient packaging

5. Which elements of low- or high-angle rescue did the rescuers need to consider during this situation?

   _____

   _____

CHAPTER 51 ANSWERS

REVIEW QUESTIONS

1. Drowning, foot/extremity entrapment, hypothermia, recirculating current
   (Objective 4)

2. Defusing immediately after the incident if the emotional impact is high; critical incident stress debriefing 24 to 72 hours after the incident; follow-up to ensure that specific crew members are recovering; specialty debriefing for the people with the patient (if your team provides that service)

3. Rescue truck, possibly specialized hazardous materials team, high-angle rescue specialists
   (Objective 2)

4. Asphyxiation, toxic inhalation, trauma, drowning, and exposure (depending on time of year)
   (Objective 5)

5. Toxic gas may exist, or oxygen levels may be low, and these conditions may vary at different levels in the pipe.
   (Objective 5)

6. It may be difficult to maneuver in the pipe with a standard air tank, and the time required for the rescue may exceed the tank capacity.
   (Objective 5)

7. The line may kink or tangle, or the equipment may fail.
   (Objective 5)

8. High-angle rescue probably will be necessary to retrieve the patient.
   (Objective 7)

9. During arrival and scene size-up, you should look for environmental risks, the number of patients, and the need for medical care and/or rescue and then request additional resources.
   (Objectives 2, 6)

10. Information was limited to location and the fact that a crash had occurred. No additional equipment was dispatched (or has arrived).
    (Objective 2)

11. Immediately delegate several crowd members to move the crowd to a safe distance to allow for patient care and the arrival of additional equipment. Call for law enforcement officers to take charge of crowd control.
    (Objective 2)

12. Advanced life support ambulance, rescue truck, pumper, and law enforcement officers
    (Objective 2)

13. Hazards identified are a crowd and the gasoline spill.
    (Objective 2)

14. Make sure no one is smoking near the crash. Also, disconnect the vehicle battery cables.
    (Objective 2)

15. Begin initial patient assessment and airway management (if indicated).
    (Objective 8)

16. Protect the patient with blankets, shields, or flame-retardant coverings.
(Objective 8)

17. Securing an open airway, protecting the cervical spine, and assisting ventilations with high-concentration oxygen if possible.
(Objective 8)

18. Disentanglement involves removing the wreckage from the patient. Rescuers must protect the patient and maintain the airway, cervical spine immobilization, and breathing to the best of their ability. Packaging involves immobilization and removal of the patient from the scene to the emergency response vehicle. Rescuers must protect the patient's spine, splint or bandage injuries if appropriate (based on the acuteness of the patient's condition), and make sure that the patient is adequately secured before removal begins. The paramedic should oversee safe transport of the patient by the rescue team to the ambulance.
(Objective 2)

19. a. Contact utility workers to move downed wires or shut off power, keep bystanders away, and secure energized wires with a dry fire hose or other appropriate means.
b. Advise occupants to stay in the car.
(Objective 6)

20. Ropes, air bags, pry bars, jacks, wedges, cutters, spreaders, and winches
(Objective 6)

STUDENT SELF-ASSESSMENT

21. c. Other than safety, the patient is the primary focus of the rescue.
(Objective 1)

22. c. Unless responding as part of a specialized fire/rescue team, the paramedic is not responsible for coordinating the rescue, serving as the safety officer, or operating equipment. Although everyone on the scene should be alert for overall safety considerations, the paramedic's responsibilities are to recognize when a rescue is safe before arrival of specialized teams and to provide patient care and monitoring during a rescue situation.
(Objective 1)

23. b. Initial efforts should ensure that the crew is uninjured so that their EMS functions can be maintained.
(Objective 1)

24. c. The dispatch call can provide the first information paramedics need to size up a rescue situation and respond to it with the appropriate safety measures.
(Objective 2)

25. d. Moving all standardized equipment into the rescue area is not practical. Basic assessment and stabilization should be attempted until the patient is in the ambulance. In certain situations, when the surroundings are unsafe or the patient is inaccessible, delivery of care may not be possible.
(Objective 2)

26. a. Ear and eye protection may also be necessary. A face mask with supplemental air or oxygen would be needed only in situations in which the oxygen supply is inadequate or toxic fumes are present.
(Objective 2)

27. a. Although ear plugs are helpful during the response, they may impair communication on a rescue.
(Objective 3)

28. b. Walking in swift water could result in a foot becoming trapped, and the paramedic could be dragged under the surface.
(Objective 4)

29. a. Alcohol and drug use also contribute to drowning. Properly worn PFDs reduce the risk of drowning.
(Objective 4)

30. d. Survival after cold water drowning is difficult to predict; rigor mortis, dependent lividity, or putrefaction indicates death.
(Objective 4)

31. b. If the person is close enough, the rescuer should reach out with a long device. The next measure would be to throw a device to the person. Then, if this is unsuccessful, a boat should be taken to rescue the person. Finally, if no other option exists, a trained rescuer with appropriate PPE should enter the water in an attempt to rescue the individual.
(Objective 4)

32. b. High oxygen concentrations create a risk of rapid combustion to fuel fire or explosion. Concentrations below 19.5% are considered an atmospheric hazard.
(Objective 5)

33. b. Personnel on the scene may be helpful and may also provide that information.
(Objective 5)

34. c. Rescuer safety should be the primary concern.
(Objective 5)

35. d. Flares would be dangerous in the presence of a gasoline leak. Apparatus should be staged off the highway if possible. Placing one large apparatus in front of the scene so that safe loading can occur may be helpful. Use warning lights cautiously and make sure that headlights are not pointed at oncoming traffic.
(Objective 6)

36. d. In some cases the battery may be left connected. The other measures would be unnecessary in the absence of flames.
(Objective 6)

37. d. Class A is used to extinguish ordinary combustibles; class B, flammable liquids; and class C, energized electrical equipment.
(Objective 6)

38. b. The other tools are used for disentanglement.
(Objective 6)

39. c. The steering column should not be cut.
(Objective 6)

40. c. Both the rescuers and patient are at risk for falls during rescue from hazardous terrain.
(Objective 7)

41. c. *High angle* refers to cliffs or the sides of buildings or other structures; rope or aerial apparatus is needed for such rescues. Flat terrain with obstacles may include large rocks, loose soil, and waterbeds or creeks.
(Objective 7)

42. a. Ideally, team cooperation is a standard on all scenes. Hostile or unstable patients are not unique to rescue situations.
(Objective 8)

43. c. When the muscles are crushed, they release their pigment (myoglobin), which can cause renal failure. Hypotension and metabolic acidosis may also occur.
(Objective 8)

44. d. If possible, avoid that side of the car for your safety.
(Objective 8)

WRAP IT UP

1. a, b, c, d, e, f
(Objective 5)

2. Collapse: The incident commander should confer with the site engineer to determine the risk of further collapse.
Electrical: The incident commander and site engineer should make sure that power is disabled if the risk of electrical injury exists.
Explosion: The cause of the initial explosion should be identified, if possible, and the risk of secondary explosion determined. Measurements should be taken in the shaft to determine if explosive gas levels are present.
Hypothermia: The depth of the cold water and the potential for the water to rise to a dangerous level, posing the risk of hypothermia and/or drowning, should be determined.
Oxygen deficiency and toxic gases: Gas levels should be monitored.
(Objective 5)

3. Helmet, light, face shield or goggles, gloves, boots with steel toe shank, Nomex jumpsuit, PFD if risk of water rising exists
(Objective 3)

4. a. Gaining access to the patient was accomplished if the patient were accessible at first contact. Hazard control should have started before the rescuers entered the shaft and continued until conclusion of the rescue. Packaging covered the activities involved in securing the patient in the Stokes basket.
(Objective 2)

5. Low-angle rescue considerations would develop as the rescuers moved through the obstructions and hazards in the shaft. High-angle rescue principles would have been applied when the rescuers were lowered into the shaft and the miners were removed.
(Objective 7)

CHAPTER

52

Crime Scene Awareness

READING ASSIGNMENT

Chapter 52, pages 1276-1285, in *Mosby's Paramedic Textbook*, ed. 3

OBJECTIVES

Upon completion of this chapter, the paramedic student will be able to:

1. Describe general techniques for determining whether a scene is violent and choosing the appropriate response to a violent scene.
2. Outline techniques for recognizing and responding to potentially dangerous residential calls.
3. Outline techniques for recognizing and responding to potentially dangerous calls on the highway.
4. Describe signs of danger and emergency medical services (EMS) response to violent street incidents.
5. Identify characteristics of and EMS response to situations involving gangs, clandestine drug labs, and domestic violence situations.
6. Outline general safety tactics that EMS personnel can use if they find themselves in a dangerous situation.
7. Describe special EMS considerations when providing tactical patient care.
8. Discuss EMS documentation and preservation of evidence at a crime scene.

SUMMARY

- A key point in ensuring scene safety is to identify and respond to dangers before they threaten. If the scene is known to be violent, the EMS crew should remain at a safe and out-of-sight distance from the area. They should remain at this distance until the scene has been secured.
- The paramedic should look for warning signs of violence during response to a residence. He or she should retreat from the scene if danger becomes evident.
- A response to a highway incident may present the dangers associated with traffic and extrication. However, it may present danger from violence as well. Occupants may be armed, wanted or fleeing felons, intoxicated or drugged, or violent/abusive from an altered mental state.
- The paramedic should monitor for warning signs of danger in violent street incidents. He or she should retreat from the scene if necessary.
- A gang is any group of people who take part in socially disruptive or criminal behavior. Some gangs are involved in violent criminal activities. EMS personnel often look like law enforcement officers. Thus, they should be very cautious about personal safety when working in gang areas.

- Clandestine lab activities can produce explosive and toxic gases. Other risks include booby traps that can maim or kill an intruder, and armed or violent occupants.
- EMS personnel who respond to a scene of domestic violence should be aware that acts of violence may be directed toward them by the perpetrator; they should take all safety precautions.
- Tactics for safety include avoidance, tactical retreat, cover and concealment, and distraction and evasive maneuvers.
- Tactical patient care refers to care activities that occur inside the scene perimeter. This is known as the "hot zone." Providing care in this area calls for special training and authorization, body armor and a tactical uniform, compact and functional equipment, and in some operations, personal defensive weapons.
- The paramedic's observations at a crime scene are important. They should be carefully documented. Evidence should be protected while caring for the patient. This can be done by not unnecessarily disturbing the scene or destroying evidence.

REVIEW QUESTIONS

Questions 1 and 2 apply to the following case study:

> You are responding to a routine call in a residential neighborhood.

1. When should your scene size-up begin?

_____

2. List six warning signs of danger that you should look for on this call.

   a.

   b.

   c.

   d.

   e.

   f.

3. List strategies to increase safety as you approach each of the following:
   a. A darkened residence:

_____

_____

   b. A vehicle stopped on the side of the highway:

_____

_____

4. For each of the situations below, indicate which of the following tactics would best increase your safety and describe how you would use it.

Avoidance	Cover and concealment
Tactical retreat	Distraction and evasive maneuvers

   a. You respond to a school shooting. En route, you determine that several shots fired in a school classroom have been reported; however, there is no confirmation that the perpetrator has been apprehended.

_____

_____

b. You are providing care to an injured fan at a large soccer match when irate fans begin to hurl bottles at you and your partner.

_____

_____

c. You are on bike patrol at a community picnic. You respond to a call for a "person injured." You find a teenager dressed in known gang attire who was punched in the face. As you begin your care, you hear the sound of gunfire nearby.

_____

_____

d. During assessment of a patient with an altered level of consciousness in the living room of a small home, his behavior escalates suddenly and he starts yelling and threatening to hurt you as he lunges toward you.

_____

_____

5. List six types of physical evidence that may be found at a crime scene.

a.

b.

c.

d.

e.

f.

STUDENT SELF-ASSESSMENT

6. When should assessment of the potential for violence at the scene begin?
  a. If the patient threatens the crew
  b. On arrival at the scene
  c. When the patient is encountered
  d. En route to the call

7. Which of the following may indicate that the residence you are about to enter is potentially dangerous?
  a. Darkened residence   **c.** No car in the driveway
  b. History of multiple calls   **d.** Person waving you in

8. Which represents the safest approach to a single vehicle stopped on the highway?
  a. Approach from the passenger side of the vehicle
  b. Simultaneous approach by both crew members
  c. Ambulance lights turned off to eliminate glare
  d. Walking between the ambulance and the other vehicle

9. Which of the following is most likely to protect the paramedic from danger during a violent street scene?
  a. Allow police to control the scene and proceed as usual.
  b. Attempt to disperse the crowd while providing care.
  c. Retreat immediately from the scene with the patient.
  d. There is no danger; crowds will not attack paramedics.

10. How can you learn about gang-related activity in your EMS response area?
  a. Police   **c.** Social service agencies
  b. School officials   **d.** All of the above

11. Which of the following drugs are commonly produced or altered in drug labs?
    a. Codeine
    b. Marijuana
    c. Methamphetamine
    d. Morphine
12. Which of the following may signal a situation that includes domestic violence?
    a. Darkened rooms
    b. Excessive nervous talking
    c. Inaccurate medical history
    d. Inconsistent injuries
13. Which of the following is a common EMS safety strategy in a dangerous situation?
    a. Avoidance
    b. Contact
    c. Negotiation
    d. Use of weapons
14. Which is an appropriate location for cover during gunfire?
    a. Bushes
    b. Car door
    c. Large tree
    d. Wooden sign
15. Which of the following provides a clue that a patient may become violent?
    a. Crossed legs
    b. Hands on hips
    c. Quiet dialogue
    d. Verbal abuse
16. Body armor is least effective against which of the following weapons?
    a. Air guns
    b. Handguns
    c. Ice picks
    d. Knives
17. Which of the following does tactical paramedic training usually include?
    a. HAZMAT decontamination
    b. Minor surgical techniques
    c. Radiographic interpretation
    d. Suturing and advanced wound care
18. Which of the following is an appropriate way to approach a crime scene?
    a. Document any suspicions you may have.
    b. Follow the same path to and from the victim.
    c. Move visible evidence so that police can find it.
    d. Save patient items in a plastic bag.

WRAP IT UP

As you respond to a call for a suicidal patient, dispatch notifies you that this address is flagged because the occupant is heavily armed and has shown violent behavior in the past. The dispatcher notifies you that the police are en route. The 9-1-1 call was placed by the patient's girlfriend, who said that he was threatening to "blow his brains out." You stage a block away from the home, out of sight of the scene, until dispatch notifies you, "The scene is safe; you may proceed in." You enter the darkened house and find your patient, a very tall, muscular man in his sixties. He is a retired police officer and has many weapons, which are evident to you. You hear loud barking from behind a closed bedroom door. Police tell you that a German shepherd that had been trained as an attack dog was secured in that room. As you begin to question the patient, he somehow escapes the grip of the police and grabs a gun. You and your partner quickly flee the house and run behind the ambulance, where you seek cover. A prolonged standoff with the police ensues, until finally the tactical police squad throws a stun grenade into the home, subduing the patient, and the incident is over.

1. What is the rationale for staging a block away from this scene?

2. Aside from known information about previous violent episodes, what are some other situational clues that this may be a violent scene?

3. Put a ✔ beside the safety tactics that were used at this scene.
    a. _____ Avoidance
    b. _____ Cover and concealment
    c. _____ Distraction and evasive maneuvers
    d. _____ Tactical retreat

4. If you were to hide behind the ambulance box, which of the following would be true?
    a. It would provide cover.
    b. It would protect you from gunfire.
    c. It would provide protection from any potential danger.
    d. It would provide temporary concealment.

5. a. Is this a crime scene? Yes/No
   b. If you answered yes, what additional responsibilities do you have on the call?

CHAPTER 52 ANSWERS

REVIEW QUESTIONS

1. Scene size-up for danger should begin during response and be based on dispatch information, knowledge of the area, and physical assessment of the scene during the approach.
   (Objective 1)

2. a. Past history of problems or violence
   b. Known drug or gang area
   c. Loud noises indicating violent activity
   d. Presence of alcohol or drug use
   e. Presence of dangerous pets
   f. Unusual silence or darkened residence
   (Objective 2)

3. a. Avoid use of lights and sirens as you get close; use unconventional pathways to approach the house; avoid positioning yourself between the ambulance lights and the residence; listen for signs of danger before entry; and stand on the doorknob side of the entry door.
   (Objective 2)

   b. One crew member should approach the car while the other remains in the ambulance; ambulance lights should be used to light the vehicle; the approach should be made from the passenger side; and the paramedic should not walk between the ambulance and the other vehicle. Observe for unusual activity in the rear seat and do not move forward from post C if a threat is suspected. If any warning signs of danger are noted, retreat until law enforcement secures the scene.
   (Objective 3)

4. a. Avoidance should be used. The EMS crew should stage their ambulance at a safe distance until law enforcement officers indicate that the scene is safe enough to proceed.
   b. Tactical retreat should be used and cover should be sought. The paramedics should immediately retreat to a safe area of cover for protection against the projectiles and the possibility of further crowd violence.
   c. Cover and concealment should immediately be sought. Seek cover behind a solid object that will not allow penetration of a bullet and conceal yourself from the perpetrator until the scene is safe or retreat can be done safely.
   d. Distraction and evasive maneuvers may be attempted during retreat. Try to move something between you and the patient to slow an attack as you quickly retreat.
   (Objective 6)

5. a. Fingerprints
   b. Footprints
   c. Blood or other body fluids
   d. Hair
   e. Carpet fibers
   f. Clothing fibers
   (Objective 8)

STUDENT SELF-ASSESSMENT

6. d. Locations of unsafe scenes may be known, as may the presence of crowds, intoxicated people on the scene, violence on the scene, or weapons.
   (Objective 1)

7. a. Other indications of a potentially dangerous residence are a history of violence, known drug or gang area, loud noises, witnessing acts of violence, alcohol or drug use, or dangerous pets.
    (Objective 2)

8. a. Lights should be left on, and only one crew member should approach, leaving the second crew member to call for help if needed.
    (Objective 3)

9. c. Police may lose control of the scene, which would put you, your partner, and the patient in danger. Leave the scene as quickly as possible. Angry people may direct violence at uniformed paramedics.
    (Objective 4)

10. d. Gang-related activity varies by region. All these agencies may provide you with information that can alert you to danger related to gang activities.
    (Objective 5)

11. c. This process can produce hazardous gases, explosive forces, or fires.
    (Objective 5)

12. d. Injuries that aren't consistent with the history or mechanism of injury should be viewed with suspicion. An inaccurate medical history may reflect poor patient knowledge. Excessive nervous talking may be related to many factors.
    (Objective 5)

13. a. Avoidance requires alertness to detect and avoid dangerous situations.
    (Objective 6)

14. c. The other choices provide concealment but can easily be penetrated by a bullet and therefore should not be used for cover.
    (Objective 6)

15. d. The boxer stance and clenched fists are also signs of increasing aggression.
    (Objective 6)

16. c. High-velocity rifle bullets or thin- or dual-edged weapons, such as ice picks, may penetrate body armor.
    (Objective 7)

17. a. Other areas of training include hostage survival, care under fire, weapons and ballistics, medical threat assessment, forensic medicine, assessment under special situations, safe searches, dental injury management, medical issues related to drug lab raids, and rescue and extraction.
    (Objective 7)

18. b. Document only objective findings; try not to disturb any evidence; save patient items in a paper bag.
    (Objective 8)

WRAP IT UP

1. If the patient is violent, he may come after the EMS crew, injuring or killing crew members or taking a hostage.
    (Objectives 1, 2)

2. The house is dark, the patient has numerous visible weapons, and a dangerous pet is on the premises.
    (Objective 2)

3. a (staging); b (behind ambulance); d (running from house)
(Objective 6)

4. d. It would temporarily hide you from the perpetrator, but it does not afford complete protection from gunfire.
(Objective 6)

5. Yes. Objective observations should be carefully worded. Any significant statements from the patient should be recorded in quotes.
(Objective 8)

CHAPTER

53

Hazardous Materials Incidents

READING ASSIGNMENT

Chapter 53, pages 1286-1305, in *Mosby's Paramedic Textbook,* ed. 3

OBJECTIVES

Upon completion of this chapter, the paramedic student will be able to:
1. Define hazardous materials terminology.
2. Identify legislation about hazardous materials that influences emergency health care workers.
3. Describe resources to assist in identification and management of hazardous materials incidents.
4. Identify the protective clothing and equipment needed to respond to selected hazardous materials incidents.
5. Describe the pathophysiology, signs, and symptoms of internal damage caused by exposure to selected hazardous materials.
6. Identify the pathophysiology, signs and symptoms, and prehospital management of selected hazardous materials that produce external damage.
7. Outline the prehospital response to a hazardous materials emergency.
8. Describe medical monitoring and rehabilitation of rescue workers who respond to a hazardous materials emergency.
9. Describe emergency decontamination and management of patients who have been contaminated by hazardous materials.
10. Outline the eight steps to decontaminate rescue personnel and equipment at a hazardous materials incident.

SUMMARY

- A hazardous material is any substance or material that is capable of posing an unreasonable risk to health, safety, and property.
- The Superfund Amendments and Reauthorization Act of 1986 established requirements for federal, state, and local governments and industry regarding emergency planning and the reporting of hazardous materials-related incidents. In 1989 OSHA and the EPA published rules to govern training requirements, emergency plans, medical checkups, and other safety precautions for workers at uncontrolled hazardous waste sites and those responding to hazardous chemical spills. In addition, the NFPA has published standards that address competencies for EMS workers at hazmat scenes.
- There are two methods used to identify hazardous materials. One is informal product identification. (This includes visual, olfactory, and verbal clues.) The other is formal product identification. (This includes, for

694

example, placards and shipping papers.) Resources for hazardous materials reference include the North American Emergency Response Guidebook, regional poison control centers, CHEMTREC, CHEMTEL, and CAMEO.

- It is crucial that anyone dealing with hazardous materials use proper protection. This includes using the proper respiratory devices. It also includes wearing protective clothing. This clothing is made of a variety of materials. The clothing is designed for certain chemical exposures. Thus, the manufacturer's guidelines must be followed.
- Hazardous materials may enter the body through inhalation, ingestion, injection, and absorption. Internal damage to the human body from hazardous materials exposure may involve the respiratory tract, CNS, or other internal organs. Chemicals producing internal damage include irritants, asphyxiants, nerve poisons, anesthetics, narcotics, hepatotoxins, cardiotoxins, nephrotoxins, neurotoxins, and carcinogens.
- Exposure to hazardous materials may result in burns. It also may result in severe tissue damage.
- The first agency to arrive at the scene of a hazardous materials incident must detect and identify the materials involved, assess the risk of exposure to rescue personnel and others, consider the potential risk of fire or explosion, gather information from on-site personnel or other sources, and confine and control the incident.
- A hazmat medical monitoring program may include medical examination for members of hazmat response teams, providing medical care, record-keeping, and periodic evaluation of the surveillance program.
- The primary goals of decontamination are to reduce the patient's dosage of material, decrease the threat of secondary contamination, and reduce the risk of rescuer injury.
- Rescuers should follow strict protocols for proper decontamination of themselves, their clothing, and any contaminated equipment.

REVIEW QUESTIONS

Match the HAZMAT terms in column II with the appropriate definition in column I. Use each term *only* once.

Column I

1. _____ Weight of pure vapor compared with the weight of an equal volume of dry air
2. _____ Dose of chemical that will kill 50% of animals
3. _____ Exposure limit of 15 minutes
4. _____ Gas or vapor concentration that will burn or explode with ignition source
5. _____ Safe exposure for a 40-hour work week
6. _____ Minimum temperature to ignite gas without spark or flame
7. _____ Atmosphere that causes immediate harm
8. _____ Vapor's ability to mix with water
9. _____ Maximum concentration not to be exceeded even for a moment
10. _____ Temperature at which liquid produces enough vapor to ignite and flash over but not continue to burn without more heat

Column II

a. Flammable/exposure limits
b. Flash point
c. IDLH
d. Ignition temperature
e. LD50
f. PEL
g. TLV-C
h. TLV-STEL
i. Vapor density
j. Vapor pressure
k. Vapor solubility

Match each of the hazardous chemicals in column I with *all* the terms in column II that describe the chemical's associated health hazards. Answers may be used *more* than once.

Column I

11. _____ Arsenic
12. _____ Halogenated hydrocarbons
13. _____ Hydrochloric acid
14. _____ Hydrogen cyanide
15. _____ Lead
16. _____ Malathion
17. _____ Mercury

Column II

a. Asphyxiant
b. Anesthetic
c. Carcinogen
d. Cardiotoxin
e. Hemotoxin
f. Hepatotoxin
g. Irritant
h. Nephrotoxin
i. Nerve poison
j. Neurotoxin

18. Briefly describe each of the five categories of emergency response personnel who may respond to a hazardous materials situation:

   a. First responder–awareness:

   _____

   _____

   b. First responder–operations:

   _____

   _____

   c. Hazardous materials technician:

   _____

   _____

   d. Hazardous materials specialist:

   _____

   _____

   e. On-scene incident commander:

   _____

   _____

19. You arrive on the scene of a motor vehicle collision involving an overturned tanker truck. You note a cloud of white vapor escaping from a relief valve on top of the truck. Describe the formal and informal means of identifying hazardous materials that may be involved in this situation.

   a. Formal:

   _____

   _____

b. Informal:

_____

20. After a hazardous material has been identified, what other resources can help the emergency response crew to determine the dangers and management of the scene?

_____

_____

21. Describe the protective clothing needed in the following hazardous materials response situations:

   a. The hazardous materials crew provides emergency care to a seriously injured worker who is lying in an area contaminated with a liquid acidic chemical. No contaminated gas is present from the spill.

_____

_____

   b. Your fire rescue team must enter a burning building to extricate trapped victims. No known hazardous materials are reported on the scene.

_____

_____

   c. An equipment malfunction inside a chemical manufacturing plant has resulted in the release of toxic gases. Hazardous materials specialists must enter to attempt to locate a victim known to be just inside the hot zone.

_____

_____

22. Describe the health problems that can be encountered when an individual is exposed to the following agents:

   a. Irritants:

_____

   b. Asphyxiants:

_____

   c. Nerve poisons, anesthetics, and narcotics:

_____

   d. Hepatotoxins:

_____

   e. Cardiotoxins:

_____

   f. Neurotoxins:

_____

g. Hemotoxins:

_____

h. Carcinogens:

_____

23. You respond to the scene of a fire in which hazardous materials of unknown origin are involved. Describe signs and symptoms shown by scene workers that may cause you to suspect exposure to hazardous materials.

_____

24. Your crew arrives at an industrial chemical manufacturing plant where a worker has sustained a splash exposure of a corrosive chemical to the eyes. Describe patient management in this situation.

_____

25. Label Fig. 53-1 and briefly describe each of the three safety zones for a hazardous materials situation that have been established by hazardous materials specialists.

A. _____

B. _____

C. _____

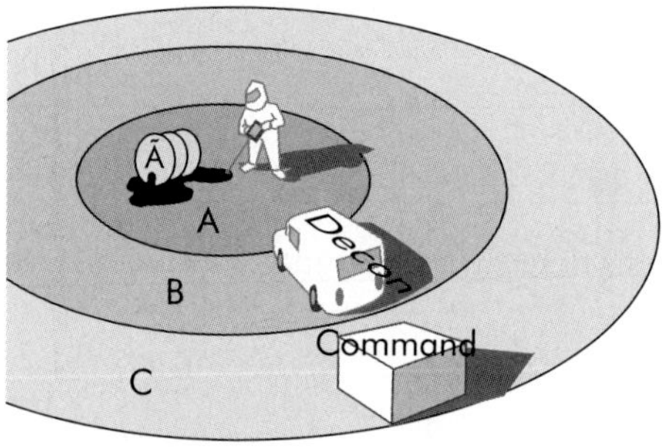

Figure 53-1

Questions 26 to 28 refer to the following case study:

You are the first team dispatched to the scene of a train derailment where three victims remain trapped. The bystanders who called in the incident report that several of the involved train cars have placards indicating the presence of hazardous materials.

26. Describe any actions you should take during your initial response to this situation.

_____

_____

_____

_____

_____

_____

27. Describe special considerations in the prehospital management of contaminated patients.

_____

_____

_____

_____

_____

28. The incident commander at this scene delegates your EMS crew to establish a medical monitoring station. Describe the responsibilities of this role.

_____

_____

_____

29. What measures should rescuers follow as they leave the hot zone of a HAZMAT scene?

_____

_____

STUDENT SELF-ASSESSMENT

30. What term is used for substances and materials that can pose an unreasonable risk to health, safety, and property?
   a. External hazards
   b. Hazardous materials
   c. Immediately dangerous to life and health
   d. Internal hazards

31. What term describes the legislation, enacted in 1986, that established requirements for federal, state, and local governments and industry regarding emergency planning and the reporting of hazardous materials?
   a. Hazardous Materials Control Act
   b. Occupational Health and Safety Law
   c. Ryan White Law
   d. Superfund Amendments and Reauthorization Act

32. According to the HAZWOPER rules, the five categories of individuals who may respond to an emergency involving hazardous materials include all of the following _except_
   a. First responder-operations
   c. Hazardous material specialist
   b. Hazardous material technician
   d. Rescue operation technician

33. Which of the following is a formal means of identifying hazardous products?
   a. Container characteristics
   c. Patient signs and symptoms
   b. Incident location
   d. United Nations labeling system

34. Which agency requires Material Safety Data Sheets when chemicals are stored, handled, or used in the workplace?
   a. International Air Transport Association
   b. National Fire Protection Association
   c. Occupational Safety and Health Administration
   d. U.S. Department of Transportation

35. General signs or symptoms of inhalation exposure to a hazardous material may include which of the following?
   a. Hemiplegia
   b. Hematemesis
   c. Seizure
   d. Urticaria

36. External exposure to corrosive chemicals generally causes which of the following?
   a. Acidosis
   b. Burns
   c. Coughing
   d. Systemic effects

37. Which of the following signs or symptoms should prompt a rescuer to seek immediate medical attention at the site of a hazardous materials incident?
   a. Confusion and lightheadedness
   b. Shortness of breath and coughing
   c. Tingling of the extremities
   d. Nausea and vomiting
   e. Any of the above

38. When responding to the scene of a hazardous materials incident, the EMS crew should approach from which direction?
   a. Downhill and downwind
   b. Downhill and upwind
   c. Uphill and downwind
   d. Uphill and upwind

39. The "pre-suit" medical monitoring of an individual who will be entering a hazardous materials situation should include all of the following *except* which one?
   a. Heart rate
   b. Reflexes
   c. Temperature
   d. Weight

40. General recommendations for emergency management of contaminated patients include all of the following *except* which one?
   a. Emergency patient care overrides all safety considerations.
   b. All patients in the hot zone are considered contaminated.
   c. Intravenous therapy should be initiated only with a physician's order.
   d. The patient's clothing should be completely cut off.

41. Which of the following is an appropriate step in the decontamination of a rescuer leaving a HAZMAT site?
   a. Shave all body hair.
   b. Shake clothing vigorously before reapplying.
   c. Take HAZMAT suit to the ambulance to be used later.
   d. Shower and wash with soap.

WRAP IT UP

The crash isn't too impressive; a car struck the rear of a delivery truck, causing it to topple over onto its side. All the occupants of both vehicles are out and moving around, but as approach, you note tears streaming down their faces, and a man is standing next to the truck coughing vigorously. "Stop," you tell your driver, "let's park upwind aways." You pick up the microphone for the loud speaker. "Move away from the truck," you command, instructing the group to follow your ambulance to a higher location, several hundred feet away from the truck. You contact dispatch to ask for fire department and HAZMAT team response. You notice a faint ammonia smell that is becoming weaker as you move away from the scene, and you pull out your binoculars to get a better look at the scene. No placards are visible, nor do you see any liquid pools around either vehicle.

When the truck driver and the two occupants of the car get to the ambulance, they report a very strong smell of ammonia and severe burning of their eyes, noses, and throats, as well as difficulty breathing. They say that they didn't see anything spilled, or any gas cloud. You immediately administer oxygen, and when you listen to their lungs, you hear diffuse wheezes. The patients are tachycardic and tachypneic but have normal blood pressure. Fire department crews douse the three with water to grossly decontaminate any affected skin and remove the patients' clothing. In the ambulance you begin treatment with a bronchodilator and place a nasal cannula over their eyes to begin continuous irrigation with normal saline. You ask the truck driver about his cargo and request his shipping papers, but he is evasive; he gets up and tries to run from the scene, but the police tackle and subdue him, confiscating a handgun from his pocket. HAZMAT teams arrive, establish zones around the contaminated area, and find a variety of hazardous chemicals in the back of the truck, which turns out to be a mobile methamphetamine lab. Apparently an ammonia tank ruptured in the collision, releasing the irritant gas and exposing your patients.

1. What methods of identification of the hazardous materials did the first rescuers attempt to use in this situation?
    a. Informal:

    _____

    _____

    b. Formal:

    _____

    _____

2. What additional resources were contacted immediately to assist with the incident?

3. Put a ✓ beside the signs or symptoms of hazardous materials exposure that were observed in these patients.
    a. _____ Confusion, dizziness   g. _____ Numbness
    b. _____ Chest tightness   h. _____ Loss of coordination
    c. _____ Double vision   i. _____ Nausea, vomiting
    d. _____ Changes in skin color   j. _____ Drooling, rhinorrhea
    e. _____ Coughing   k. _____ Tearing
    f. _____ Difficulty breathing   l. _____ Unconsciousness

4. Why was gross water decontamination done even though the situation involved a gas exposure?

    _____

    _____

5. Could the ambulance crew be charged with abandonment for pulling past the scene of an emergency? Explain your answer.

    _____

    _____

6. Describe the zones that the HAZMAT team established around the scene.

    _____

    _____

CHAPTER 53 ANSWERS

REVIEW QUESTIONS

1. i
2. e
3. h
4. a
5. f
6. d
7. c
8. k
9. g
10. b
(Questions 1-10: Objective 1)

11. j, e
12. f, d
13. g
14. a
15. j, e
16. i
17. h, j, e
(Questions 11-17: Objective 5)

18.

Category	Description
a. First responder–awareness	May witness or discover hazardous materials release but job does not include emergency response duties pertaining to hazardous materials
b. First responder–operations	Responds to hazardous materials release to protect nearby people, property, or the environment without trying to stop the release
c. Hazardous material technician	Responds to hazardous materials situations to stop the release
d. Hazardous materials specialist	Has direct or specific knowledge of various hazardous substances and provides support to hazardous materials technicians
e. On-scene incident commander	Trained to assume control of a hazardous materials event

(Objective 2)

19. a. Placards on trucks, shipping papers, and material safety data sheets
b. Visual indicators (vapor), container characteristics, company name on truck, and smell
(Objective 3)

20. Hazardous materials texts, poison control centers, CHEMTREC, federal agencies, commercial agencies, subject experts, site coordinators, and regional, state, and local agencies
(Objective 3)

21. a. Chemical splash protective clothing to protect the skin and eyes from direct chemical contact.
b. Structural firefighting clothing, including helmet, positive-pressure self-contained breathing apparatus, turnout coat and pants, gloves and boots, and a protective hood of fire-resistant material.
c. Vapor-protective clothing (suit with a self-contained breathing apparatus worn inside or outside the suit or a supplied-air breathing apparatus with emergency escape capabilities).
(Objective 4)

22. a. Irritants damage the upper and lower respiratory tracts and irritate the eyes.

b. Asphyxiants deprive the body tissues of oxygen.

c. Nerve gases, anesthetics, and narcotics act on the nervous system, causing disruption of cardiorespiratory function.

d. Hepatotoxins destroy the liver's ability to function in a normal capacity.

e. Cardiotoxins may induce myocardial ischemia and cardiac dysrhythmias.

f. Neurotoxins may cause cerebral hypoxia or neurological or behavioral disruption.

g. Hemotoxins cause destruction of red blood cells, resulting in hemolytic anemia.

h. Carcinogens are cancer-causing agents.

(Objective 5)

23. Confusion, anxiety, dizziness, visual disturbances, changes in skin color, shortness of breath or burning of the upper airway, tingling or numbness of extremities, loss of coordination, seizures, nausea and vomiting, abdominal cramps, diarrhea, unconsciousness.

(Objective 5)

24. Don protective gear, remove contact lenses, and flush with copious amounts of water, normal saline, or lactated Ringer solution.

(Objective 6)

25. A. The *hot zone* is the area that includes the hazardous material and any associated wastes. Only specially trained and clothed personnel may enter this area.

B. The *warm zone* is the area that can become contaminated if the hot zone is unstable. Decontamination and patient care activities take place here.

C. The *cold zone* is the area around the warm zone. Minimal protective clothing is required. The command post and other support agencies are located here.

(Objective 7)

26. En route to the emergency scene, the EMS crew should attempt to identify the hazardous material and obtain preliminary information about the potential hazards and recommended safety equipment, initial first aid, and a safe distance factor for response to the area. Medical control should be notified so that appropriate measures can be taken at the hospital for potential victims. If the involved substance is identified, the dispatching agency should contact the appropriate authorities and other experts (e.g., CHEMTREC) to get additional information and support. The scene should be approached from uphill and upwind, and the EMS crew should call for additional help as needed. The arriving crew should be alert to any fire hazards and leakage of gas or liquid from the involved cars and remain clear of all vapors and spills.

(Objective 7)

27. Nonambulatory patients should be removed from the hot zone by trained personnel who have adequate protective clothing. All patients in the hot zone should be considered contaminated. Patient care in the hot zone should consist only of airway and breathing management, spinal immobilization, and control of hemorrhage. Intravenous lines should be avoided unless absolutely necessary to prevent internal introduction of contaminants. Decontamination should be attempted only with adequate protection of the rescue workers; often, removal of the victim's clothing removes most of the contaminant, with the remainder being washed with copious amounts of water and mild detergent soap. All contaminated clothing from the patient and rescuers should be left in the decontamination area. Further patient care should be provided in the support area before transport. The patient should be wrapped tightly in blankets.

(Objective 9)

28. Pre-suit examination: Assess baseline vital signs and instruct rescuers about possible symptoms to anticipate if contamination or exposure occurs. Postentry examination: Assess vital signs and monitor rescuer for signs or symptoms of exposure or heat-related illness.

(Objective 8)

29. Outer gloves and boots should be removed and placed in a receptacle. Remove contaminated breathing apparatus. Remove protective clothing and assess the need to remove outer clothing (based on type of chemical). Shower and wash twice. Put on clean clothing. Obtain medical evaluation.
(Objective 8)

STUDENT SELF-ASSESSMENT

30. b. The term *external hazards* refers to materials that produce external damage, whereas *internal hazards* cause internal damage. Not all HAZMAT substances are IDLH.
(Objective 1)

31. d. The Ryan White law pertains to exposure to infectious diseases.
(Objective 2)

32. d. The categories are first responder–awareness, first responder–operations, hazardous materials technician, hazardous materials specialist, and on-scene incident commander.
(Objective 2)

33. d. All other responses are informal means of recognizing and identifying hazardous materials.
(Objective 3)

34. d. The U.S. Department of Transportation regulates hazardous materials in transit.
(Objective 3)

35. c. The others would not usually be associated with this type of exposure.
(Objective 5)

36. b. The other signs described are systemic effects, which are not the most common findings in external exposure to corrosive chemicals.
(Objective 6)

37. e. A high index of suspicion for rescuer exposure should always be maintained.
(Objective 5)

38. d. This ensures that hazardous gases and liquids are moving away from the ambulance.
(Objective 7)

39. b
(Objective 8)

40. a. Safety overrides all considerations.

41. d. Shaving may permit internal entry of chemicals. Clothing should be left at the exit point and appropriately cleaned or discarded.
(Objective 9)

WRAP IT UP

1. a. Observation of the patient's signs and symptoms; smell
   b. Checking for placards, shipping papers
   (Objective 3)

2. Fire department, HAZMAT team
   (Objective 7)

3. e, f, k
   (Objectives 5, 6)

4. To remove any chemical irritant present on the skin or clothes and to prevent subsequent off-gassing of chemicals.
   (Objective 9)

5. The first priority in an incident, especially a HAZMAT incident, is scene safety. Pulling onto the scene would have been dangerous, therefore no abandonment claim could be made.
   (Objective 7)

6. Hot (contamination) zone: Area where actual contaminant is located; only personnel in appropriate PPE are allowed entry.
   Warm (control) zone: Surrounds hot zone and is location of decontamination
   Cold (safe) zone: Normal operations
   (Objective 7)

Bioterrorism and Weapons of Mass Destruction

READING ASSIGNMENT
Chapter 54, pages 1306-1319, in *Mosby's Paramedic Textbook*, ed. 3

OBJECTIVES
Upon completion of this chapter, the paramedic student will be able to do the following:
1. List five types of weapons of mass destruction.
2. Identify actions, signs and symptoms, methods of distribution, and management of biological weapons of mass destruction.
3. Identify actions, signs and symptoms, methods of distribution, and management of chemical weapons of mass destruction.
4. Identify actions, signs and symptoms, methods of distribution, and management of nuclear weapons of mass destruction.
5. Describe security threat levels as defined by the Department of Homeland Security.
6. Identify measures to be taken by paramedics who respond to incidents with suspected weapons of mass destruction involvement.

SUMMARY
- There are five categories of weapons of mass destruction. These include biological, nuclear, incendiary, chemical, and explosive.
- Biological agents include anthrax, botulism, plague, ricin, tularemia, and smallpox.
- Person-to-person spread is possible in patients who are infected with plague or smallpox.
- Nerve agents include Sarin, Soman, Tabun, and VX. Exposure causes a cholinergic overdrive. The antidote for nerve agent exposure is atropine and pralidoxime chloride.
- Poisonous gases such as chlorine and phosgene cause severe respiratory problems. They also can cause skin and eye injury. Move exposed patients to safety, remove their clothing, and treat their symptoms.
- Dirty bombs could cause heat damage and radiation sickness, severe burns, and cancer.
- The Department of Homeland Security has identified five terrorist threat levels. Each level has specific community-wide emergency preparedness activities to be taken.

- Emergency responders at a WMD incident should recognize hazmat incidents, know protocols to detect WMD, use PPE, know crime-scene procedures, know how to activate more resources, and implement incident operations.

REVIEW QUESTIONS

Match the terms in column II with the description in column I. A term may be used more than once.

Column I

1. _____ Illness caused by bacteria found in rodents
2. _____ Nerve agent that has a camphorlike odor
3. _____ Thick, odorless liquid used as a nerve agent
4. _____ Gray, poisonous gas that smells like mown hay
5. _____ Odorless nerve agent
6. _____ Bacterial disease spread by rodent fleas
7. _____ Poisonous cytotoxin from a plant
8. _____ Nerve agent that has a fruity odor

Column II

a. Anthrax
b. Chlorine
c. Phosgene
d. Plague
e. Ricin
f. Sarin
g. Soman
h. Tabun
i. Tularemia
j. VX

9. Supply the words that form the following acronym for weapons of mass destruction.

B—

N—

I—

C—

E—

Match the categories in column II with the characteristics of biological agents in column I. Each category may be used *more* than once.

Column I

10. _____ Emerging pathogen
11. _____ Q fever
12. _____ Second highest priority agents
13. _____ Nipah virus
14. _____ National security risk
15. _____ Anthrax

Column II

a. Category A
b. Category B
c. Category C

16. Provide the missing information for each of the following biological weapons of mass destruction.

Agent	Signs/Symptoms	Outcomes	Treatment
a. Anthrax			
b.	Fever, fainting, shortness of breath, cough, bloody sputum, GI symptoms		
c.		35% mortality from septicemia	
d. Botulism			
e.			Antibiotics, supportive treatment; vaccine under study
f. Ricin			
g.		DIC, respiratory failure, death (5%)	

17. You are called to investigate multiple reports of difficulty breathing at the airport. When you arrive, approximately 30 people rush toward the ambulance with tears streaming down their faces. They report a sudden onset of difficulty breathing, blurred vision, headache, and weakness. Most were in the baggage pickup area when their symptoms began. You note that they are sweating profusely, some are faint, and they have fasciculations.

   a. List four agents that can cause this clinical presentation.

   b. What precautions should you take prior to transport of these patients?

   c. List three drugs that may be indicated in the management of these patients.

18. Your patients were working at an immigration center when they smelled an odor they described as "like fresh cut hay." They then developed severe dyspnea, a burning sensation in the chest, and a nonproductive cough.

   a. What WMD agent do you suspect?

b. What interventions would you perform?

_____

_____

_____

19. List three factors that would affect the degree of contamination from a dirty bomb.

a.

b.

c.

20. Describe three special considerations for a paramedic responding to a WMD incident.

a.

b.

c.

STUDENT SELF-ASSESSMENT

21. People in your community are becoming very ill with a rash and severe respiratory symptoms. Many have died, and new cases are spreading among people who appear to have had contact with the first group. What WMD infectious agent may be involved?
   a. Anthrax   **c.** Smallpox
   b. Plague   **d.** Tularemia

22. According to the CDC categorization of biological agents, which category includes agents that cause moderate morbidity and low mortality and includes Q fever?
   a. Category A   **c.** Category C
   b. Category B   **d.** Category D

23. Which WMD exposure route has the potential for the greatest number of casualties?
   a. Aerosol   **c.** Liquid ingestion
   b. Direct contact   **d.** Solid ingestion

24. Which of the following is _true_ about anthrax infection?
   a. All those who come in contact with the infected patient should be quarantined.
   b. It can cause severe respiratory distress and sepsis in later stages.
   c. Treatment with antibiotics is not indicated and is ineffective.
   d. Vaccination is routinely recommended for health care workers.

25. A large number of patients who ate at the salad bar of a local restaurant are complaining of nausea, blurred vision, and dry mouth. Several have difficulty swallowing and complain that they are having trouble breathing. Which of the following may be associated with this presentation?
   a. Botulism   **c.** Soman
   b. Ricin   **d.** Tularemia

26. Which of the following WMD agents can be spread from person to person?
   a. Botulism   **c.** Ricin
   b. Plague   **d.** Tularemia

27. You are caring for a patient who has just been exposed to a WMD agent. You know that you must remove the patient's clothing to protect yourself from illness or injury caused by which of the following?
   a. Chlorine
   b. Smallpox
   c. VX
   d. All of the above

28. You are called to a government building where a large number of patients have excessive tearing, salivation, severe dyspnea with wheezing, weakness, drooling, and hypotension. After HAZMAT teams have decontaminated the patients and while oxygen is administered, which treatments should you give next to improve their condition?
    a. Albuterol, fluid bolus
    b. Albuterol, atropine
    d. Atropine, fluid bolus
    d. Atropine, pralidoxime chloride

29. A tanker transporting chlorine has collided with a van carrying six occupants. A slow gas leak is streaming from the side of the truck. All those involved in the accident are ambulatory but complaining of severe burning of the eyes, coughing, and difficulty breathing. You have staged away from the incident. After calling for appropriate additional resources, what should your immediate priorities be for these patients?
    a. Administer oxygen and an antidote.
    b. Have them remain in place until the HAZMAT team arrives.
    c. Instruct them to move upwind to higher ground.
    d. Take oxygen and albuterol to the patients to begin care.

30. When a yellow Homeland Security threat level is activated, what special measures should be taken?
    a. Consider canceling or alternative venues for special events.
    b. Implement appropriate contingency and emergency response plans.
    c. Monitor, redirect, or constrain transportation systems.
    d. Refine and exercise preplanned protective measures.

31. According to the Office for Domestic Preparedness, what are the responsibilities of EMS providers in preparing for and responding to incidents of terrorism involving WMD agents?
    a. Contain hazardous materials.
    b. Detect and identify agents used as a WMD.
    c. Implement incident operations.
    d. Protect the crime scene perimeter.

WRAP IT UP

As you pull up on the scene, you see more than 100 people streaming from a church where your dispatcher tells you there have been multiple calls for difficulty breathing. People report noticing a faint "fruity" odor when the minister lit the incense oil pots, and watering eyes, drooling, sweating, and coughing quickly developed. You call for an MCI response and a HAZMAT team. Several people have fallen to the ground, and you note a child having a grand mal seizure on the grass. Other people are running from the scene to their cars. The incident commander and HAZMAT team arrive, and a decision is quickly made that a vaporized nerve agent has been used. Therefore the patients' clothing should be removed and gross decontamination should be performed before treatment and transport to eliminate any possibility of off-gassing. You and your partner are in charge of the triage sector and direct next-arriving crews to initiate START triage. The supply sector is in charge of locating and procuring MARK-I kits deployed in the city and having them sent to the treatment sector and appropriate receiving hospitals. After disrobing and undergoing gross decontamination, patients are moved to the treatment sector, where antidote administration and supportive care begin until appropriate transport can be arranged. It is 2 hours before the ninety-seventh patient is transported to the hospital, leaving only seven who were tagged unsalvageable to be transported to the county medical examiner's office and the police and HAZMAT teams to finish up their work.

1. Which nerve agent has the characteristics described in this scenario?

2. Put a ✔ beside the signs or symptoms that a patient exposed to a nerve agent may experience (even if not described in the above scenario).

a. _____ Blurred vision

b. _____ Bradycardia

c. _____ Cardiac arrest

d. _____ Drooling

e. _____ Dry skin

f. _____ Headache

g. _____ Hypertension

h. _____ Hypotension

i. _____ Renal failure

j. _____ Seizures

k. _____ Sweating

l. _____ Watery eyes

m. _____ Wheezing

n. _____ Loss of consciousness

3. What drugs does the MARK-I kit contain?

4. What additional interventions are needed for patients poisoned by a nerve agent?

CHAPTER 54 ANSWERS

REVIEW QUESTIONS

1. d, i
   (Objective 2)

2. b
   (Objective 3)

3. j
   (Objective 3)

4. c
   (Objective 3)

5. f
   (Objective 3)

6. d
   (Objective 2)

7. e
   (Objective 2)

8. h
   (Objective 3)

9. B—biological; N—nuclear; I—incendiary; C—chemical; E—explosives
   (Objective 1)

10. c
11. b
12. b
13. c
14. a
15. a
    (Questions 10-15: Objective 2)

16.

Agent	Signs/Symptoms	Outcomes	Treatment
a. Anthrax	Itching, papular lesion that becomes vesicular, black eschar; signs and symptoms resembling those of a cold, followed by respiratory distress, sepsis	High mortality if untreated	Antibiotics, vaccines (controversial)
b. Plague (*Yersinia pestis*)	Fever, fainting, short of breath, cough, bloody sputum, GI symptoms	Septic shock; high mortality	Antibiotics, post-exposure drug therapy, isolation
c. Smallpox (variola virus)	High fever, fatigue, headache and backache; within 2 to 3 days, rash and skin lesions that crust and scar; joint deformities; blindness	35% mortality from septicemia	Vaccine, antivirals (experimental), supportive care, isolation
d. Botulism	Nausea, dry mouth, blurred vision, dysphagia, fatigue, dyspnea	Recovery may occur with weeks of supportive care	Antitoxin, mechanical ventilation
e. Tularemia	Fever, HA, chills, malaise, GI illness, DIC, ARF; death possible	Severe incapacitation; low death rate	Antibiotics, supportive treatment; vaccine under study
f. Ricin	Severe respiratory symptoms within 8 hours; respiratory failure in 36 to 72 hours; severe GI symptoms; vascular collapse; seizures	Respiratory failure, shock, death	No antidote; only supportive care possible; avoid exposure, eliminate toxin, and decontaminate
g. Tularemia	Fever, chills, general malaise, GI illness	DIC, respiratory failure, death (5%)	Antibiotics, supportive care; vaccine under review

(Objective 2)

17. a. Sarin, soman, tabun, VX
b. Secondary exposure is possible from off-gassing of clothes; clothing should be removed before transport.
c. Atropine, pralidoxime chloride, and diazepam or lorazepam are indicated for the management of nerve agent poisoning.
(Objective 3)

18. a. Phosgene gas; b. decontamination if needed, supportive care with oxygen and management of symptoms.
(Objective 3)

19. The size of the explosive, the amount and type of radioactive material used, and the weather (Objective 4)

20. Danger to EMS crews from secondary devices or armed resistance; crowd control and public panic situations; the need to preserve the crime scene.
(Objective 6)

STUDENT SELF-ASSESSMENT

21. c. Smallpox is spread easily from person to person, causes a progressive rash, and has a high mortality rate in unvaccinated individuals.
(Objective 2)

22. b. Category A agents (which include anthrax) have a high morbidity and mortality; category C agents (which include Nipah virus) are emerging pathogens. There is no category D.
(Objective 2)

23. a. Aerosolized agents can be distributed easily over a wide area, exposing large numbers of victims in a short time.
(Objective 2)

24. b. Person-to-person contact does not transmit the infection. Antibiotics should be given as soon as possible to minimize the risk of death. Vaccination is recommended only for military personnel and for researchers who work with anthrax.
(Objective 2)

25. a. Ricin produces pulmonary symptoms; soman is a nerve agent; and tularemia does not typically cause blurred vision or dysphagia.
(Objective 2)

26. b. Botulism and tularemia are not known to spread from person to person. Ricin is not an infectious agent.
(Objective 2)

27. d. Direct skin contamination or secondary contamination from off-gassing is possible with many WMD agents. As a precaution, if full decontamination is not indicated, clothing should be removed before transport to prevent secondary exposure.
(Objective 3)

28. d. Atropine and pralidoxime chloride (PAM) are direct antidotes to nerve agents and should be given immediately to reverse the effect of the nerve poisons.
(Objective 3)

29. c. Any attempt to move to the contaminated area without appropriate PPE would be dangerous. Supportive care can begin after patients are in a safe area and their clothing has been removed.
(Objective 3)

30. b. In an orange level activation, public event modifications would be considered. In a red condition situation, transportation modifications may need to be made. Preplanning should be done at the green level and modified as needed at each level of activation.
(Objective 4)

31. c. HAZMAT teams are typically responsible for containing the hazardous material and identifying specific agents using special monitoring devices. Police should control the perimeter of the crime scene.
(Objective 5)

WRAP IT UP

1. Tabun; it has a fruity odor, vaporizes when heated, causes symptoms within seconds of exposure to the vapor, and produces the signs and symptoms described.
(Objective 3)

2. a, b, c, d, f, h, i, j, k, l, m
(Objective 3)

3. Atropine and pralidoxime chloride
(Objective 3)

4. IV fluids, oxygen, and diazepam or lorazepam for seizures
(Objective 3)

Emergency Drug Index

1. List the actions, indications, and side effects of steroids.

   _____

   _____

2. For each of the following two drugs, list the time of onset, duration, and dose:
   a. Methylprednisolone:

   _____

   b. Dexamethasone:

   _____

   For each of the scenarios in questions 3 to 28, complete the corresponding flashcard (after the electrocardiogram flashcards at the end of this workbook) with the appropriate drug information, including trade name, class, description, indications, contraindications, adverse reactions, onset, duration, dose (adult and pediatric, if appropriate), and special considerations. Verify your drug choice before completing the flashcard by looking at the generic drug name on the back.

3. Your patient is experiencing urticaria and severe itching resulting from an allergic reaction. His vital signs are

   stable, and no wheezes are audible on auscultation of his lungs. You administer _____.
   (Complete Flashcard 23.)

4. After delivering three shocks to your patient who is in ventricular fibrillation cardiac arrest, you wish to give a

   potent vasoconstrictor with a long duration of action. What do you administer? _____.
   (Complete Flashcard 24.)

5. Your crew is unable to initiate an intravenous line on an unconscious diabetic patient who is known to be hypoglycemic. Transport time is 45 minutes. The drug of choice to increase the blood glucose level is

   _____. (Complete Flashcard 25.)

6. Your patient is in ventricular fibrillation cardiac arrest. After you defibrillate three times and administer epinephrine, medical direction asks you to administer an antidysrhythmic drug. List two specific antidysrhythmic

   drugs other than lidocaine that you may administer. _____. (Complete Flashcards 26 and 27.)

7. A 65-year-old woman calls you and complains of shortness of breath and chest pain radiating down her left arm.

   Her blood pressure is 110/70 mm Hg. The initial drug of choice to relieve her pain is _____.
   (Complete Flashcard 28.)

8. You place a 22-year-old patient with a pounding sensation in her chest on a monitor and discover ventricular tachycardia. The patient's blood pressure is normal, she has no chest pain, and the rest of the history and physical examination is unremarkable. The appropriate drug to use to suppress ventricular dysrhythmia in this situation is _____. (Complete Flashcard 29.)

9. Your 30-year-old patient fell while in-line skating and has obvious deformity of the right wrist with significant pain.

   What nonnarcotic analgesic can you give him intramuscularly or intravenously? _____
   (Complete Flashcard 30.)

10. You are called to an outpatient surgery center to evaluate a nurse who is unconscious. Co-workers confide that they have suspected drug abuse for some time, and an empty meperidine (Demerol) tubex is found in her pocket. All other available medical history is negative. Pupils are pinpoint, and respirations are 12 and shallow.

    What drug do you administer first if an overdose is suspected? _____ (Complete Flashcard 31.)

11. You are performing transcutaneous pacing on a conscious patient who is complaining of severe discomfort related to the procedure. What short-acting intravenous medicine can you administer to reduce anxiety, relax skeletal muscles, and provide amnesia? _____ (Complete Flashcard 32.)

12. You are called to a nursing home to care for an 88-year-old woman who has fainted. The patient is extremely bradycardic (pulse 40) and has a blood pressure of 80 mm Hg systolic by palpation. Her only history is hypertension. What emergency care drug is indicated initially to correct her sinus bradycardia?

    _____ (Complete Flashcard 33.)

13. Initial electrical countershocks do not successfully convert your cardiac arrest patient from ventricular fibrillation. An adrenergic drug that should be repeated every 3 to 5 minutes is _____.
    (Complete Flashcard 34.)

14. A 32-year-old patient fell while playing softball and has an apparent dislocation of the left shoulder, which is very painful. Medical direction wishes to administer a short-acting analgesic so that accurate emergency department evaluation will be possible. What is an appropriate, self-administered analgesic in this situation?

    _____ (Complete Flashcard 35.)

15. You have been trying without success to resuscitate a 73-year-old woman who is in cardiac arrest. Tricyclic antidepressant overdose is suspected. What drug may be considered at this point? _____
    (Complete Flashcard 36.)

16. The police call you to evaluate an unconscious person. The patient is a known alcoholic, and friends say that he has not eaten for several days. He has a blood glucose level of 40 mg/dL (normal range 80 to 120 mg/dL). No drug use is suspected. The two drugs indicated for this patient are _____ and _____. (Complete Flashcards 37 and 38.)

17. A frantic husband calls you to evaluate his wife, who has been having seizures for 10 minutes. You find that she is experiencing repetitive grand mal seizures. The husband tells you that she is a known epileptic who has not taken any phenytoin (Dilantin) for 2 days. What is your drug of choice under these circumstances?

    _____ (Complete Flashcard 39.)

18. Your 24-year-old patient is a known asthmatic who is experiencing an acute attack. Inspiratory and expiratory wheezes are audible throughout the chest, and the patient is tachypneic. What drug would you initially administer by inhalation? _____ (Complete Flashcard 40.)

19. A 56-year-old woman has severe crushing substernal chest pain and diaphoresis. You administer vasodilators and a narcotic analgesic to relieve pain. What antiplatelet drug should you administer en route?

    _____ (Complete Flashcard 41.)

20. You are called to treat a 32-year-old woman with a sudden onset of palpitations. The electrocardiogram reveals a rapid supraventricular tachycardia. The patient states that she has Wolff-Parkinson-White syndrome. What is the safest drug to use to convert this rhythm to sinus rhythm? _____ (Complete Flashcard 42.)

21. Airport authorities call you to care for a mechanic whose arm is trapped in the landing gear of a small aircraft. Extrication time is lengthy, and the patient is in extreme distress because of pain. Vital signs are stable, and no other injuries are noted. List two narcotic analgesics that may be administered to this patient. _____ and _____ (Complete Flashcards 43 ands 44.)

22. Your 67-year-old patient is experiencing a severe headache and blurred vision resulting from his blood pressure, which is now 230/160 mm Hg. He is awake and cooperative. Which alpha- and beta-adrenegic blocker drug may improve this potentially disastrous situation by lowering the blood pressure? _____ (Complete Flashcard 45.)

23. A 21-year-old took an overdose of an antidepressant 10 minutes ago and is awake and alert. What drug may be used to prevent absorption of the antidepressant in the gastrointestinal tract? _____ (Complete Flashcard 46.)

24. Your patient is 8 months pregnant and has been diagnosed with preeclampsia. Co-workers found her experiencing a grand mal seizure in the restroom. The patient appears to be in a postictal state. Blood pressure is 160/116 mm Hg. What drug may be given if she has a recurrence of seizure activity? _____ (Complete Flashcard 47.)

25. You have a 30-minute estimated time of arrival to the hospital with an 86-year-old patient from a nursing home whose vital signs are blood pressure, 80/50 mm Hg; pulse, 124; and respirations, 24. The urine in her Foley catheter bag is milky green and foul smelling. Cardiac history is negative, and no reason exists to suspect blood or fluid volume loss. What is the drug of choice to treat her hypotension quickly after fluid resuscitation in this situation? _____ (Complete Flashcard 48.)

26. The 65-year-old patient you are called to evaluate has the following vital signs: blood pressure, 130/90 mm Hg; pulse, 160; and respirations, 24. The electrocardiogram monitor shows atrial fibrillation with a rapid ventricular response. She has mild signs of congestive heart failure, but all other physical findings are negative. What Class IV antidysrhythmic drug is indicated for this patient? _____ (Complete Flashcard 49.)

27. Your 72-year-old patient is experiencing severe dyspnea that began suddenly during the night. She is in obvious distress, with cyanosis of the nail beds and lips. Lung sounds reveal rales and wheezes throughout, and she has a cough that produces frothy, pink sputum. History reveals two previous myocardial infarctions. Vital signs are blood pressure, 170/108 mm Hg; pulse, 132; and respirations, 32. Identify the diuretic to administer in an attempt to improve this patient's condition. _____ (Complete Flashcard 50.)

28. You have just delivered a healthy baby boy, followed minutes later by a complete placenta. Despite vigorous massage, the patient's uterus is very soft, and she is experiencing profuse vaginal bleeding. What pharmacological agent can you administer to help control this bleeding? _____ (Complete Flashcard 51.)

Complete the remaining flashcards with drugs not included in the previous questions that are administered within your emergency medical services system.

STUDENT SELF-ASSESSMENT

29. When is the use of dopamine most clearly indicated?
    a. Cardiac arrest
    b. Cardiogenic shock
    c. Head injury
    d. Internal bleeding
30. Which of the following is the appropriate drug to administer to a patient who was in a motor vehicle collision and is complaining of severe abdominal pain?
    a. Meperidine
    b. Morphine
    c. Nitrous oxide
    d. None of the above

31. Which of the following is an indication for administration of epinephrine 1:1000 subcutaneously?
    a. Anaphylaxis
    c. Electromechanical dissociation
    b. Asystole
    d. Ventricular fibrillation
32. Which drug is recommended to control atrial fibrillation with a rate of 170 beats/min when the patient has Wolff-Parkinson-White syndrome?
    a. Adenosine
    c. Atenolol
    b. Amiodarone
    d. Diltiazem
33. Which of the following is *not* true regarding use of atropine?
    a. It is indicated for management of bradycardia.
    b. The initial dose in bradycardia is 0.5 mg intravenously.
    c. It should be given in asystole.
    d. It is an antidote for verapamil.
34. Dopamine, when administered at low doses (1.0 to 2.0 mcg/kg/min), has which of the following effects?
    a. Renal and mesenteric vessel dilation
    b. Profound arteriolar constriction
    c. Decreased cerebral edema
    d. Ventricular dysrhythmias
35. Your patient has severe chest pain and is nauseated and diaphoretic. His 12-lead electrocardiogram shows ST segment elevation in leads II, III, and aV_F. His breath sounds are clear and his blood pressure is 86/50 mm Hg, pulse is 64 per minute, and respirations are 20 per minute. Which of the following drugs would be indicated during your 10-minute transport to the emergency department?
    a. Aspirin
    c. Nitroglycerin
    b. Morphine
    d. Verapamil
36. Your patient is in ventricular fibrillation and has been shocked 3 times. An intravenous infusion has been started. Your first choice for drug therapy is which of the following?
    a. Epinephrine
    c. Morphine
    b. Hydralazine
    d. Nifedipine
37. Which of the following drugs does *not* cause bronchodilation?
    a. Albuterol
    c. Diphenhydramine
    b. Epinephrine
    d. Isoproterenol
38. Verapamil is contraindicated if the patient can be described as which of the following?
    a. Complaining of palpitations
    c. Tachycardic
    b. Hypotensive
    d. Under age 45
39. Which of the following drugs is self-administered by mask for relief of pain?
    a. Albuterol
    c. Nitroglycerin
    b. Morphine sulfate
    d. Nitrous oxide:oxygen
40. Which of the following is a drug indicated for the management of hypertension?
    a. Dobutamine
    c. Phenytoin
    b. Hydralazine
    d. Procainamide
41. Which of the following drugs affects blood clotting by inhibition of platelets?
    a. Aspirin
    c. Streptokinase
    b. Reteplase
    d. Tissue plasminogen activator
42. Pharmacological management of the patient suffering from coma of unknown origin includes which of the following?
    a. Naloxone, glucagon, and D50W
    b. Butorphanol (Stadol), glucagon, and thiamine
    c. Naloxone, thiamine, and D50W
    d. Dexamethasone, glucagon, and D50W
43. In which of the following situations is mannitol indicated?
    a. Myocardial infarction
    c. Digoxin toxicity
    b. Acute cerebral edema
    d. Shock
44. Which of the following pharmacological agents is useful in status epilepticus, as an antianxiety agent, and as a skeletal muscle relaxant?
    a. Diazepam
    c. Naloxone
    b. Morphine
    d. Phenytoin

45. Which of the following drugs is indicated for management of postpartum bleeding?
    a. Dopamine   **c.** Magnesium sulfate
    b. Insulin   **d.** Oxytocin

46. Diphenhydramine is contraindicated in which of the following situations?
    a. Anaphylactic shock   **c.** Allergic reactions
    b. An acute asthma attack   **d.** Patients over 35 years of age

47. Syrup of ipecac may be given to which of the following patients within 30 minutes of the ingestion?
    a. Those without a gag reflex
    b. Those who have ingested prochlorperazine (Compazine)
    c. Those who have ingested phenytoin (Dilantin)
    d. Those who have ingested gasoline

48. Naloxone is an antagonist to all of the following, except which?
    a. Propoxyphene   **c.** Meperidine
    b. Heroin   **d.** Phenobarbital

49. Which of the following medications may cause respiratory depression?
    a. Atropine   **c.** Magnesium sulfate
    b. Dexamethasone   **d.** Thiamine

50. A patient has monomorphic ventricular tachycardia at 160 beats/min (normal Q-T interval). Her blood pressure is 100 mm Hg, and the patient has crackles in both lung bases. Which drug is indicated initially to manage this rhythm?
    a. Lidocaine   **c.** Metoprolol
    b. Magnesium sulfate   **d.** Procainamide

51. Which of the following side effects may occur after nitroglycerin ingestion?
    a. Headache   **c.** Burning under the tongue
    b. Hypotension   **d.** All of the above

52. Which of the following drugs exerts a positive chronotropic effect?
    a. Adenosine   **c.** Haloperidol
    b. Epinephrine   **d.** Propranolol

53. Furosemide is indicated in the management of which of the following?
    a. Angina   **c.** Hypotension
    b. Dysrhythmias   **d.** Pulmonary edema

54. Which of the following is a calcium channel blocker that slows conduction and is useful to slow the heart rate in atrial flutter?
    a. Adenosine   **c.** Dobutamine
    b. Albuterol   **d.** Diltiazem

55. All of the following drugs are indicated to manage pulmonary edema that develops from left ventricular failure, except which?
    a. Atropine   **c.** Morphine
    b. Furosemide   **d.** Nitroglycerin

56. When meperidine is given alone, which of the following side effects should be anticipated?
    a. Increased heart rate   **c.** Vasoconstriction
    b. Nausea and vomiting   **d.** Hyperactivity

57. Your patient is a 35-year-old man who is psychotic and violent. Which of the following is the drug of choice for his care?
    a. Haloperidol   **c.** Meperidine
    b. Hydroxyzine   **d.** Nifedipine

58. Dexamethasone and methylprednisolone belong to which of the following classes of drugs?
    a. Analgesics   **c.** Sympathomimetics
    b. Inotropics   **d.** Steroids

EMERGENCY DRUG INDEX ANSWERS

1. Actions: suppress acute or chronic inflammation and potentiate relaxation of vascular smooth muscle by beta-adrenergic agonist. Indications: anaphylaxis, asthma, shock, and spinal cord injury. Adverse reactions: hypertension, sodium and water retention, hypokalemia, hypocalcemia, alkalosis, and headache

2. a. Onset: 1 to 2 hours. Duration: 8 to 24 hours. Dose: 40 to 125 mg intravenously (in spinal cord injury, initial dose of 30 mg/kg, followed by intravenous infusion of 5.4 mg/kg/hr)
   b. Onset: 4 to 8 hours. Duration: 24 to 72 hours. Dose: 4 to 24 mg intravenously

3. Diphenhydramine (Benadryl). *Class:* antihistamine. *Description:* drug that prevents histamine from reaching H_1 and H_2 receptor sites. *Indications:* allergic reactions, anaphylaxis, and acute extrapyramidal reactions. *Contraindications:* asthma attacks, patients taking monoamine oxidase inhibitors, hypersensitivity, narrow-angle glaucoma, newborns, and nursing mothers. *Adverse reactions:* drowsiness, sedation, disturbed coordination, hypotension, palpitations, tachycardia or bradycardia, thickening of bronchial secretions, and dry mouth and throat. *Onset:* maximal effects in 1 to 3 hours. *Duration:* 6 to 12 hours. *Dose:* adult—25 to 50 mg deep intramuscular or intravenous injection; pediatric—5 mg/kg/day in divided doses intravenously or intramuscularly. *Special considerations:* pregnancy category C.

4. Vasopressin (Pitressin). *Class:* naturally occurring antidiuretic hormone. *Description:* direct stimulation of smooth muscles; when given in high doses acts as a nonadrenergic peripheral vasoconstrictor. *Indications:* adult shock—refractory ventricular fibrillation; vasodilatory shock. *Contraindications:* responsive patients with coronary artery disease. *Adverse reactions:* ischemic chest pain, abdominal distress, sweating, nausea, vomiting, tremors. *Onset:* immediate. *Duration:* variable. *Dose:* adult cardiac arrest—40 U intravenous push 1 time; pediatric—not recommended. *Special considerations:* Drug may cause cardiac ischemia and angina. Drug may be given intraosseously.

5. Glucagon. *Class:* pancreatic hormone and insulin antagonist. *Description:* drug used to elevate blood glucose level if sufficient stores of glycogen are available; also has a positive inotropic effect on the heart. *Indications:* altered level of consciousness resulting from hypoglycemia if glucose administration not possible; calcium channel blocker or beta-blocker toxicity. *Contraindications:* hypersensitivity to proteins. *Adverse reactions:* tachycardia, hypotension, nausea, vomiting, and urticaria; may potentiate the effects of oral anticoagulants. *Onset:* within 1 minute. *Duration:* 60 to 90 minutes. *Dose:* adult—0.5 to 1.0 mg intramuscularly; pediatric—0.025 to 1.0 mg intramuscularly (may repeat in 7 to 10 minutes). Calcium channel blocker or beta-blocker toxicity, adult 1 to 5 mg over 2 to 5 minutes. *Special considerations:* not first-line choice for hypoglycemia.

6. a. Procainamide (Pronestyl). *Class:* antidysrhythmic (Class Ia). *Description:* drug that reduces automaticity of ectopic pacemakers and suppresses reentry dysrhythmias by slowing intraventricular conduction. *Indications:* suppression of premature ventricular contractions refractory to lidocaine, suppression of ventricular tachycardia (with a pulse) refractory to lidocaine, suppression of ventricular fibrillation refractory to lidocaine, and paroxysmal supraventricular tachycardia with wide-complex tachycardia of unknown origin (especially if Wolff-Parkinson-White syndrome is present). *Contraindications:* second- and third-degree atrioventricular block, complete heart block, tricyclic antidepressant toxicity, digitalis toxicity, and torsades de pointes. *Adverse reactions:* hypotension, bradycardia, reflex tachycardia, atrioventricular block, widened QRS complex, prolonged P-R or Q-T interval, premature ventricular contractions, ventricular tachycardia, ventricular fibrillation, asystole, central nervous system depression, confusion, and seizure. *Onset:* 10 to 30 minutes. *Duration:* 3 to 6 hours. *Dose:* adult—20 mg/min slow intravenous (IV) infusion (100 mg IV push in refractory ventricular fibrillation) to maximum dose 17 mg/kg, maintenance infusion after resuscitation or after initial bolus; 1 g mixed in 250 mL of solution infuse at (1 to 4 mg/min). *Special considerations:* Administration should be discontinued if dysrhythmia is suppressed, hypotension develops, the QRS complex widens by 50% of its original width, or a total of 17 mg/kg has been given; use caution with patients with asthma, digitalis-induced dysrhythmias, acute myocardial infarction, or cardiac, renal, or hepatic insufficiency. Do not use in combination with other drugs that prolong the Q-T interval.
   b. Amiodarone (Cordarone). *Class:* Class III antidysrhythmic. *Description:* multiple mechanisms of action; prolongs action potential and refractory period; alpha adrenoreceptor and calcium channel blocker. *Indications:* treatment and prophylaxis of frequently recurring ventricular fibrillation and unstable ventricular tachycardia. *Contraindications:* pulmonary congestion, cardiogenic shock, hypotension, sensitivity to amiodarone. *Adverse reactions:* hypotension, bradycardia, headache, dizziness, atrioventricular conduction abnormalities, flushing, abnormal salivation. *Onset:* within minutes. *Duration:* variable. *Dose:* adult cardiac arrest—300 mg IV push; supplemental bolus for cardiac arrest—150 mg IV push in 3 to 5 minutes; loading infusion after reestablishment of spontaneous circulation—360 mg (diluted) over 6 hours.

7. Nitroglycerin (Nitrostat). *Class:* vasodilator. *Description:* drug that dilates peripheral venous and arteriolar blood vessels and reduces cardiac workload and oxygen demand. *Indications:* ischemic chest pain, pulmonary hypertension, hypertensive emergencies, and congestive heart failure. *Contraindications:* hypersensitivity, hypotension, head injury, and cerebral hemorrhage. *Adverse reactions:* headache, postural syncope, reflex tachycardia, hypotension, nausea, vomiting, and diaphoresis. *Onset:* 1 to 3 minutes. *Duration:* 30 to 60 minutes. *Dose:* tablet—0.3 to 0.4 mg sublingually that may be repeated in 5 minutes, twice; metered spray—0.4 mg/spray, one sublingual spray that may be repeated in 5 minutes, twice; infusion—200 to 400 mcg/mL at a rate of 10 to 20 mcg/min, increased by 5 to 10 mcg/min every 5 to 10 minutes to desired effect. *Special considerations:* The drug must be kept in an airtight container protected from light; older adults have an increased risk of hypotension.

8. Lidocaine (Xylocaine). *Class:* antidysrhythmic, local anesthetic (Class Ib). *Description:* drug that suppresses premature ventricular contractions and raises ventricular fibrillation threshold. *Indications:* ventricular fibrillation, ventricular tachycardia, significant ventricular ectopy in the presence of myocardial ischemia or infarction; wide-complex tachycardia of unknown origin. *Contraindications:* hypersensitivity, Stokes-Adams syndrome, and second- or third-degree heart block in the absence of an artificial pacemaker. *Adverse reactions:* light-headedness, confusion, blurred vision, hypotension, cardiovascular collapse, bradycardia, and central nervous system depression (including seizures) with high doses. *Onset:* 30 to 90 seconds. *Duration:* 10 to 20 minutes. *Dose:* adult—administration intravenously or via endotracheal bolus (at 2 to 2{1/2} times intravenous dose) followed by a continuous infusion; for ventricular fibrillation, 1.0 to 1.5 mg/kg intravenously repeated in 3 to 5 minutes to a total loading dose of 3 mg/kg; for ventricular ectopy or stable ventricular tachycardia, 1 to 1.5 mg/kg intravenously repeated in 5 to 10 minutes at 0.5 to 0.75 mg/kg to a total dose of 3 mg/kg; given via infusion—dilution of 1 g of lidocaine in 250 mL of D_5W and infusion at 2 to 4 mg/min; pediatric—1 mg/kg/dose intravenous or intraosseously; infusion—20 to 50 mcg/kg/min. *Special considerations:* The drug has a short half-life; if bradycardia is present with premature ventricular contractions, the bradycardia is treated first with atropine; high doses can result in coma or death; decrease dose in elderly. Avoid lidocaine in reperfusion dysrhythmias after thrombolytic therapy; use extreme caution in patients with hepatic disease, heart failure, marked hypoxia, severe respiratory depression, hypovolemia, or shock.

9. Ketorolac tromethamine (Toradol). *Class:* nonsteroidal antiinflammatory. *Description:* an antiinflammatory drug that also exhibits peripherally acting nonnarcotic analgesic activity by inhibiting prostaglandin synthesis. *Indications:* Short-term management of moderate to severe pain. *Contraindications:* hypersensitivity, allergies to aspirin or other nonsteroidal antiinflammatory drugs, bleeding disorders, renal failure, active peptic ulcer disease. *Adverse reactions:* anaphylaxis from hypersensitivity, edema, sedation, bleeding disorders, rash, nausea, and headache. *Onset:* within 10 minutes. *Duration:* 6 to 8 hours. *Dose:* adult— 30 to 60 mg intramuscularly, followed by 15 to 30 mg q6h prn up to 5 days; or 30 mg intravenously over 1 minute (patients ***65 years); one half dose (15 mg) for patients more than 65 years old and those with renal impairment. *Special considerations:* pregnancy category B safety; clear, slightly yellow solution; use with caution and reduce dose in elderly.

10. Naloxone (Narcan). *Class:* synthetic opioid antagonist. *Description:* a competitive narcotic antagonist used to manage and reverse overdoses caused by narcotics and synthetic narcotic agents. *Indications:* complete or partial reversal of narcotic depression and ventilatory depression resulting from opioids, including narcotic agonists (heroin, morphine sulfate, hydromorphone [Dilaudid], methadone, meperidine [Demerol], paregoric, fentanyl [Sublimaze], oxycodone [Percodan], and codeine), narcotic agonist/antagonists (butorphanol tartrate [Stadol], pentazocine [Talwin], propoxyphene [Darvon], and nalbuphine [Nubain]); decreased level of consciousness, coma of unknown origin, and circulatory support in refractory shock (investigational), phencyclidine, and ethanol ingestion (investigational). *Contraindications:* hypersensitivity and caution with narcotic-dependent patients, who may experience withdrawal syndrome. *Adverse reactions:* tachycardia, hypertension, dysrhythmias, nausea, vomiting, blurred vision, withdrawal, and diaphoresis. *Onset:* within 2 minutes. *Duration:* 30 to 60 minutes. *Dose:* adult— 0.4 to 0.8 mg intravenously or intramuscularly; 0.8 mg subcutaneously may be repeated in 5-minute intervals to a maximum of 10 mg; infusion—mix 8 mg in 1000 mL of D_5W and infuse at two thirds of the reversal dose titrated to desired effect; children less than 5 years old or less than 20 kg—0.1 mg/kg/dose intravenously, intramuscularly, or subcutaneously or via endotracheal administration (diluted). *Special considerations:* Seizures have been reported; drug may not reverse hypotension and may cause withdrawal syndrome; use caution if patient is a suspected narcotic addict. Naloxone has shorter duration than some narcotics; monitor patient carefully after administration.

11. Midazolam hydrochloride (Versed). *Class:* short-acting benzodiazepine. *Description:* benzodiazepine that may be administered for conscious sedation to relieve apprehension or impair memory before tracheal intubation or cardioversion. *Indications:* premedication for trachea intubation or cardioversion. *Contraindications:* hypersensitivity to midazolam; glaucoma; shock; coma; alcohol intoxication (relative); depressed vital signs; concomitant use of barbiturates, alcohol, narcotics, or other central nervous system depressants. *Adverse reactions:* respiratory depression, hiccups, cough, oversedation, pain at injection site, nausea and vomiting, headache, blurred vision, fluctuations in

vital signs, hypotension, and respiratory arrest. *Onset:* 1 to 3 minutes. *Duration:* 2 to 6 hours, dose dependent. *Dose:* adult—1 to 2.5 mg slow intravenously (over 2 to 3 minutes); repeat as needed in small increments (total maximum dose not to exceed 0.1 mg/kg); elderly—0.5 mg slow intravenously (maximum of 1.5 mg in a 2-minute period); pediatric—loading dose 0.05 to 0.2 mg/kg, followed by continued infusion at 1 to 2 mcg/kg/min. *Special considerations:* pregnancy category D; continuously monitor respiratory and cardiac function; have resuscitation equipment and medication readily at hand; never administer medication as an intravenous bolus.

12. **Atropine sulfate (atropine and others).** *Class:* anticholinergic agent. *Description:* drug that inhibits the action of acetylcholine at postganglionic parasympathetic receptor sites; blocks vagus nerve and causes increased heart rate and enhanced atrioventricular conduction. *Indications:* hemodynamically significant bradycardia, asystole, pulseless electrical activity, organophosphate or nerve-gas poisoning, and exercise-induced pulmonary disorders. *Contraindications:* tachycardia, hypersensitivity, unstable cardiovascular status in acute hemorrhage and myocardial ischemia, and narrow-angle glaucoma, obstructive disease of the gastrointestinal tract, obstructive uropathy, and thyrotoxicosis. *Adverse reactions:* tachycardia; paradoxical bradycardia when pushed slowly or when used at doses less than 0.5 mg; palpitations; dysrhythmias; headache; dizziness; anticholinergic effects (dry mouth, nose, skin, photophobia, blurred vision, urine retention); nausea; vomiting; flushed, hot, dry skin; and allergic reactions. *Onset:* rapid. *Duration:* 2 to 6 hours. *Dose:* Bradydysrhythmias: adult—0.5 to 1.0 mg intravenously every 3 to 5 minutes as needed (maximum total dose 0.03 to 0.04 mg/kg); pediatric—0.02 mg/kg/dose intravenously or intraosseous (minimum total dose dose 0.1 mg; maximum single dose 0.5 mg for a child and 1.0 mg for an adolescent; may repeat in 5 minutes for maximum total dose of 1.0 mg child and 2.0 mg adolescent). Asystole: adult—1.0 mg intravenously or endotracheally; repeat to total dose 0.03 to 0.04 mg/kg; pediatric—same dose as bradycardia. Pulseless electrical activity: if absolute or relative bradycardia, same dose as asystole. Anticholinesterase poisoning: adult—2 mg intravenously every 5 to 15 minutes to dry secretions, repeated as needed; pediatric—0.05 mg/kg/dose (usual dose 1 to 5 mg) intravenously, repeated as needed every 20 minutes until atropine effect is observed. *Special considerations:* potential adverse effects when given with digitalis, cholinergics, and neostigmine; effects of atropine may be enhanced by antihistamines, procainamide, quinidine, antipsychotics, antidepressants, and benzodiazepines.

13. **Epinephrine (Adrenalin).** *Class:* sympathomimetic. *Description:* drug that stimulates alpha- and beta-receptors; causes bronchodilation and, when administered via rapid intravenous injection, causes rapid increases in systolic pressure, ventricular contractility, and heart rate; causes vasoconstriction of the arterioles of the skin, mucosa, and splanchnic areas; and antagonizes the effects of histamine. *Indications:* bronchial asthma, acute allergic reactions, asystole, pulseless electrical activity, ventricular fibrillation, and pulseless ventricular tachycardia. *Contraindications:* hypersensitivity, hypovolemic shock, coronary insufficiency (should be used with caution). *Adverse reactions:* headache, restlessness, weakness, dysrhythmias, hypertension, and precipitation of angina pectoris and tachycardia. *Onset:* 5 to 10 minutes (subcutaneously), 1 to 2 minutes (intravenously). *Duration:* 5 to 10 minutes. *Dose:* Asystole, pulseless electrical activity, pulseless ventricular tachycardia, or ventricular fibrillation: adult—1 mg intravenous push repeated every 3 to 5 minutes; pediatric—first dose: standard (0.1 ml/kg 1:10,000) intravenously or intraosseously, high (0.1 mL/kg 1:1000) via endotracheal administration (diluted to 3 to 5 mL); second and subsequent doses: high (0.1 mL/kg 1:1000) intravenously or intraosseously, high (0.1 mL/kg 1:1000) via endotracheal administration. Bradycardia refractory to other interventions: adult—2 to 10 mcg/min (1 mg 1:1000 in 500 mL of normal saline or D_5W); pediatric—dilute 0.6 mg/kg to create 100 mL solution; begin infusion at 1 mL/hr (0.1 mcg/kg/min) and adjust every 5 minutes for desired effect (0.1 to 1.0 mcg/kg/min). Anaphylactic reaction or bronchoconstriction: adult—mild to moderate: 0.3 to 0.5 mL (1:1000) subcutaneously; severe: 1 to 2 mL (1:10,000) slow intravenous injection; pediatric—0.01 mL/kg subcutaneously (1:1000), maximum of 0.3 mL. *Special considerations:* Syncope has been reported after administration in children; it may increase myocardial oxygen demand.

14. **Nitrous oxide:oxygen (50:50; Nitronox).** *Class:* gaseous analgesic and anesthetic. *Description:* drug that depresses the central nervous system and causes anesthesia. *Indications:* moderate to severe pain. *Contraindications:* impaired level of consciousness, head injury, chest trauma, inability to comply with instructions, decompression sickness, undiagnosed abdominal pain, bowel obstruction, hypotension, shock, and chronic obstructive pulmonary disease. *Adverse reactions:* dizziness, apnea, cyanosis, nausea, vomiting, and malignant hyperthermia. *Onset:* 2 to 5 minutes. *Duration:* 2 to 5 minutes. *Dose:* adult—invert cylinder several times before use and instruct the patient to inhale deeply through the mask or mouthpiece, which the patient must hold; pediatric—same. *Special considerations:* The drug increases the incidence of spontaneous abortion; it diffuses into gas-filled pockets trapped in the patient (for example, pneumothorax, intestinal obstruction) and may cause rupture; nitrous oxide is a nonexplosive gas.

15. **Sodium bicarbonate.** *Class:* buffer, alkalinizing agent, electrolyte supplement. *Description:* drug that reacts with hydrogen ions to form water and carbon dioxide to buffer metabolic acidosis. *Indications:* known preexisting

metabolic acidosis, tricyclic antidepressant overdose, and alkalinization for treatment of specific intoxications. *Contraindications:* patients with chloride loss from vomiting or gastrointestinal suction, metabolic and respiratory alkalosis, hypernatremia, hypokalemia, hypocalcemia, and abdominal pain of unknown origin. *Adverse reactions:* metabolic alkalosis, hypoxia, rise in intracellular PCO_2 and increased tissue acidosis, hypernatremia, seizures, and tissue sloughing at injection site. *Onset:* 2 to 10 minutes. *Duration:* 30 to 60 minutes. *Dose:* urgent forms of metabolic acidosis: adult—1 mEq/kg intravenously repeated in 5 minutes with 0.5 mEq/kg every 10 minutes; pediatric—same. *Special considerations:* If possible, arterial blood gas analysis should guide administration of this drug; it may increase edematous or sodium-retaining states; it initially may worsen cellular acidosis; it may worsen congestive heart failure.

16. a. Thiamine (Betaxin). *Class:* vitamin (B_1). *Description:* vitamin necessary for carbohydrate metabolism. *Indications:* coma of unknown origin (with administration of dextrose 50% or naloxone), delirium tremens, beriberi, and Wernicke's encephalopathy. *Contraindications:* none significant. *Adverse reactions:* hypotension (from rapid injection or a large dose), anxiety, diaphoresis, nausea, vomiting, and allergic reaction (rare). *Onset:* rapid. *Duration:* depends on degree of deficiency. *Dose:* adult—100 mg slow intravenous or intramuscular injection. *Special considerations:* Anaphylactic reactions have been reported.

    b. Dextrose 50%. *Class:* carbohydrate and hypertonic solution. *Description:* the principal carbohydrate used in the body. *Indications:* hypoglycemia, altered level of consciousness, coma of unknown cause, seizure of unknown cause. *Contraindications:* intracranial hemorrhage, increased intracranial pressure, or suspected cerebral vascular accident in the absence of hypoglycemia. *Adverse reactions:* warmth, pain, burning from medication infusion, thrombophlebitis. *Onset:* less than 1 minute. *Duration:* depends on degree of hypoglycemia. *Dose:* adult—12.5 to 25 g slow intravenous injection (may repeat once); pediatric—0.5 to 1 g/kg/dose intravenously or intraosseously; 1 to 2 mL/kg 50%; 2 to 4 mL/kg 25%; 5 to 10 mL/kg 10%. *Special considerations:* Blood glucose analysis should be performed before administration, if possible; extravasation may cause tissue necrosis; it may sometimes precipitate severe neurological symptoms (Wernicke's encephalopathy) in patients with thiamine depletion, such as alcoholics; high-risk groups should receive thiamine before dextrose 50%.

17. Diazepam (Valium and others). *Class:* benzodiazepine. *Description:* drug that raises the seizure threshold in the cerebral cortex and acts on the limbic, thalamic, and hypothalamic regions of the brain to potentiate the effects of inhibitory neurotransmitters. *Indications:* acute anxiety states, acute alcohol withdrawal, muscle relaxation, seizure activity, and premedication to countershock or transcutaneous pacing. *Contraindications:* hypersensitivity, substance abuse, coma, shock, central nervous system depression following head injury, respiratory depression. *Adverse reactions:* hypotension, reflex tachycardia, respiratory depression, ataxia, psychomotor impairment, confusion, and nausea. *Onset:* 1 to 5 minutes (intravenously); 15 to 30 minutes (intramuscularly). *Duration:* 15 minutes to 1 hour (intravenously), 15 minutes to 1 hour (intramuscularly). *Dose:* Seizure activity: adult—5 mg intravenously over 2 minutes (may give up to 10 mg for most adults); pediatric—infants more than 30 days to 5 years: 0.2 to 0.5 mg slow intravenously or intraosseously every 2 to 5 minutes as necessary (maximum total dose 5 mg); children greater than 5 years: 1 mg every 2 to 5 minutes to maximum 10 mg slow intravenously. Premedication for cardioversion: adult—5 to 15 mg intravenously 5 to 10 minutes before procedure. *Special considerations:* Diazepam may cause local venous irritation; dose should be reduced by 50% in older adults; resuscitation equipment should be readily available; anticonvulsant effect has a short duration.

18. Albuterol (Proventil, Ventolin). *Class:* sympathomimetic bronchodilator. *Description:* a beta$_2$-specific sympathomimetic stimulant that relaxes bronchiolar smooth muscle and peripheral vasculature. *Indications:* relief of bronchospasm in patients with reversible obstructive airway disease and prevention of exercise-induced bronchospasm. *Contraindications:* hypersensitivity, cardiac dysrhythmias associated with tachycardia. *Adverse reactions:* restlessness, apprehension, dizziness, palpitations, increased blood pressure, and dysrhythmias. *Onset:* 5 to 15 minutes via inhalation. *Duration:* 3 to 4 hours via inhalation. *Dose:* bronchial asthma: adults—via metered dose inhaler, 1 to 2 inhalations (90 to 180 mcg) every 4 to 6 hours (5 minutes between inhalations); via inhalation, 2.5 mg (0.5 mL of 0.5% solution) diluted to 3 mL with 0.9% NaCl administered over 5 to 15 minutes; pediatric—via solution, 0.01 to 0.03 mL (0.05 to 0.15 mg) per kilogram per dose to a maximum of 0.5 mL/dose diluted in 2 mL of 0.9% normal saline (may be repeated every 20 minutes, 3 times). *Special considerations:* Sympathomimetics may exacerbate adverse cardiac effects; drug may potentiate hypokalemia; it may precipitate angina pectoris and dysrhythmias; it should be used with caution with patients with diabetes mellitus, hyperthyroidism, prostatic hypertrophy, cardiovascular disorder or seizure disorder; it should be administered only by inhalation in prehospital care.

19. Aspirin (ASA, Bayer, Ecotrin, St. Joseph, others). *Class:* analgesic, antiinflammatory, antiplatelet, antipyretic. *Description:* drug that blocks pain impulses in the central nervous system, dilates peripheral vessels, and decreases platelet aggregation. *Indications:* mild to moderate pain or fever; prevention of platelet aggregation in

ischemia and thromboembolism; unstable angina; prevention of myocardial infarction or reinfarction. *Contraindications:* hypersensitivity to salicylates; gastrointestinal bleeding; active ulcer disease; hemorrhagic stroke; bleeding disorders; children. *Adverse reactions:* stomach irritation, heartburn or indigestion, nausea or vomiting, allergic reaction. *Onset:* 15 to 30 minutes. *Duration:* 4 to 6 hours. *Dose:* adult—mild pain or fever: 325 to 650 mg PO q4h; myocardial infarction—160 to 325 mg PO (chew).

20. Adenosine (Adenocard). *Class:* endogenous nucleotide, miscellaneous antidysrhythmic agent. *Description:* drug that slows tachycardia associated with the atrioventricular node via modulation of the autonomic nervous system without causing negative inotropic effects and acts directly on sinus pacemaker cells and vagal nerve terminals to decrease chronotropic and dromotropic activity. *Indications:* treatment of supraventricular tachycardia. *Contraindications:* second- or third-degree atrioventricular block, sick sinus syndrome, and hypersensitivity to adenosine; adenosine will not convert atrial flutter, atrial fibrillation, and ventricular tachycardia. *Adverse reactions:* light-headedness, paresthesia, headache, diaphoresis, palpitations, chest pain, hypotension, dyspnea, nausea, and metallic taste. Transient sinus bradycardia, sinus pause, bradyasystole ventricular ectopy. *Onset:* immediate. *Duration:* 10 seconds. *Dose:* adult—initial, 6 mg over 1 to 3 seconds, if no response in 1 to 2 minutes, administration of 12 mg over 1 to 3 seconds, 12-mg dose repeated once as necessary; pediatric—0.1 mg/kg rapid intravenous injection; may be doubled once (maximum single dose 12 mg). *Special considerations:* Methylxanthines antagonize the action of adenosine; dipyridamole potentiates the effect of adenosine; carbamazepine may potentiate the atrioventricular-nodal blocking effect of adenosine; adenosine may produce bronchoconstriction in patients with asthma or bronchopulmonary disease; asystole (up to 15 seconds) followed by normal sinus rhythm is common after administration.

21. a. Morphine sulfate (Astramorph/PF and others). *Class:* opioid analgesic. *Description:* drug that increases peripheral venous capacitance and decreases venous return; promotes analgesia, euphoria, and respiratory and physical depression; decreases myocardial oxygen demand; a Schedule II drug. *Indications:* chest pain associated with myocardial infarction, moderate to severe acute or chronic pain, and pulmonary edema with or without pain. *Contraindications:* hypersensitivity to narcotics, hypovolemia, hypotension, head injury or undiagnosed abdominal pain, and patients who have taken monoamine oxidase inhibitors within 14 days; increased intracranial pressure; and severe respiratory depression. *Adverse reactions:* hypotension, tachycardia, bradycardia, palpitations, syncope, facial flushing, respiratory depression, euphoria, bronchospasm, dry mouth, and allergic reaction. *Onset:* 1 to 2 minutes. *Duration:* 2 to 7 hours. *Dose:* adult—2 to 4 mg intravenously every 5 to 30 minutes titrated to relief of pain; pediatric—0.1 to 0.2 mg/kg/dose intravenously (maximum 15-mg total dose). *Special considerations:* Narcotics rapidly cross the placenta; drug should be used with caution with older adults, patients with asthma, and patients susceptible to central nervous system depression; naloxone should be readily available; drug may worsen bradycardia or heart block in inferior myocardial infarction (vagotonic effect).

   b. Meperidine (Demerol). *Class:* opioid analgesic. *Description:* an opioid agonist that produces analgesia, euphoria, and respiratory and central nervous system depression. *Indications:* moderate to severe pain, preoperative medication, obstetrical analgesia. *Contraindications:* hypersensitivity to narcotics, concurrent use of monoamine oxidase inhibitors or selective serotonin reuptake inhibitors, labor or delivery of a premature infant, and head injury. *Adverse reactions:* respiratory depression, euphoria, delirium, agitation, hallucination, seizures, headache, visual disturbances, coma, facial flushing, hypotension, circulatory collapse, dysrhythmias, allergic reaction, nausea, and vomiting. *Onset:* 10 to 45 minutes (intramuscularly), within 5 minutes (intravenously). *Duration:* 2 to 4 hours. *Dose:* adult—50 to 100 mg every 3 to 4 hours (intramuscularly), 15 to 35 mg (intravenously); pediatric—1 to 2 mg/kg/dose (intramuscularly) every 3 to 4 hours. *Special considerations:* Drug should be used with caution in patients with asthma and chronic obstructive pulmonary disease and may aggravate seizures in patients with convulsive disorders; nalaxone should be readily available.

22. Labetalol (Normodyne, Trandate). *Class:* alpha- and beta-adrenergic blocker. *Description:* competitive alpha$_1$-receptor blocker and a nonselective beta-receptor blocker used to lower blood pressure in hypertensive crisis. *Indications:* hypertensive emergencies. *Contraindications:* bronchial asthma (relative), uncompensated congestive heart failure, second- and third-degree heart block, bradycardia, cardiogenic shock, pulmonary edema. *Adverse reactions:* dose-related orthostatic hypotension, headache, dizziness, edema, fatigue, vertigo, ventricular dysrhythmias, dyspnea, allergic reaction, facial flushing, diaphoresis. *Onset:* within 5 minutes. *Duration:* 3 to 6 hours. *Dose:* adult—10 mg slow intravenous bolus over 2 minutes; additional injections at 10-minute intervals as needed (maximum 150 mg); infusion—mix 200 mg in 250 mL D$_5$W (0.8 mg/mL) and infuse at a rate of 2 to 8 mg/min, titrated to supine blood pressure (maximum 300 mg). *Special considerations:* pregnancy safety category C; monitor blood pressure, pulse, electrocardiogram continuously; observe for signs of congestive heart failure, bradycardia, bronchospasm; administer with patient in supine position.

23. Activated charcoal (Actidose-Aqua, Liqui-Char). *Class:* adsorbent, antidote. *Description:* drug that binds and adsorbs ingested toxins. *Indications:* many oral poisonings and medication overdoses. *Contraindications:* corrosives, gastrointestinal bleeding, caustics, and petroleum distillates. *Adverse reactions:* nausea (indirectly), vomiting, and constipation. *Onset:* immediate. *Duration:* continual in gastrointestinal tract. *Dose:* prepared in a slurry and administered by mouth or slowly by gastric tube; adult—30 to 100 g; pediatric—15 to 30 g; infant less than 1 year—1 g/kg. *Special considerations:* Drug does not adsorb all drugs and toxic substances (for example, phenobarbital, aspirin, cyanide, lithium, iron, lead, and arsenic).

24. Magnesium sulfate. *Class:* electrolyte, anticonvulsant. *Description:* drug that reduces striated muscle contractions and blocks peripheral neuromuscular transmission by reducing acetylcholine release at the myoneural junction. *Indications:* seizures resulting from eclampsia, torsades de pointes, refractory ventricular fibrillation, or suspected hypomagnesemia. *Contraindications:* heart block or myocardial damage. *Adverse reactions:* diaphoresis, facial flushing, hypotension, depressed reflexes, hypothermia, reduced heart rate, circulatory collapse, diarrhea, and respiratory depression. *Onset:* (intravenously) immediate. *Duration:* 30 minutes. *Dose:* seizures associated with pregnancy: 1 to 4 g (8 to 32 mEq) intravenously; maximum dose of 1.5 mL/min. Pulseless arrest (torsades de pointes, or hypomagnesemic state): adult—1 to 2 g in 10 mL of D_5W intravenously over 1 to 2 minutes; pediatric—25 to 50 mg/kg over 10 to 20 minutes. *Special considerations:* Other central nervous system depressants may enhance central nervous system depressant effects; drug should not be administered in the 2 hours before delivery; calcium gluconate or calcium chloride should be available as antagonist; drug may be needed for up to 48 hours after delivery; use with caution in patients with renal failure.

25. Dopamine (Intropin). *Class:* sympathomimetic. *Description:* drug that acts on alpha$_1$- and beta-adrenergic receptors, increasing systemic vascular resistance and exerting a positive inotropic effect on the heart, and dilates renal and splanchnic vasculature at low doses (dopaminergic effect), maintaining blood flow. *Indications:* hemodynamically significant hypotension in the absence of hypovolemia. *Contraindications:* tachydysrhythmias, ventricular fibrillation, and patients with pheochromocytoma. *Adverse reactions:* dose-related tachycardias, hypertension, and increased myocardial oxygen demand. *Onset:* 2 to 4 minutes. *Duration:* 10 to 15 minutes. *Dose:* adult—begin infusion at 2 to 5 mcg/kg/min; intravenously (titrated to patient response); final dosage range of 5 to 20 mcg/kg/min recommended; low dose—1 to 5 mcg/kg/min; cardiac dose—5 to 20 mcg/kg/min; vasopressor—10 to 20 mcg/kg/min; pediatric—2 to 20 mcg/kg/min; intravenously or intraosseously titrated to patient response (not to exceed 20 mcg/kg/min). *Special considerations:* Drug should be infused through a large, stable vein to avoid extravasation injury; patient should be monitored for signs of compromised circulation; infusion pump is recommended.

26. Verapamil (Isoptin). *Class:* calcium channel blocker (Class IV antidysrhythmic). *Description:* antidysrhythmic, antianginal, antihypertensive; inhibits the movement of calcium ions across cell membranes, decreases atrial automaticity, reduces atrioventricular conduction velocity, prolongs the atrioventricular nodal refractory period, decreases myocardial contractility, reduces vascular smooth muscle tone, and dilates coronary arteries and arterioles. *Indications:* paroxysmal supraventricular tachycardia (unresponsive to adenosine), atrial flutter with rapid ventricular response, and atrial fibrillation with a rapid ventricular response; vasospastic and unstable angina; chronic stable angina. *Contraindications:* hypersensitivity, sick sinus syndrome (unless the patient has a pacemaker), second- or third-degree heart block, hypotension, cardiogenic shock, severe congestive heart failure, Wolff-Parkinson-White syndrome with atrial fibrillation or flutter, patients receiving intravenously administered beta-blockers, wide-complex tachycardias. *Adverse reactions:* dizziness, headache, nausea, vomiting, hypotension, bradycardia, complete atrioventricular block, and peripheral edema. *Onset:* 2 to 5 minutes. *Duration:* 30 to 60 minutes. *Dose:* adult—2.5 to 5.0 mg intravenous bolus over 2 minutes; repeat with 5 to 10 mg in 15 to 30 minutes, as necessary (maximum of 30 mg). *Special considerations:* Vital signs should be monitored closely; be prepared to resuscitate the patient; atrioventricular block or asystole may occur because of slowed atrioventricular conduction; decrease dose when administering to elderly or borderline hypotensive patients.

27. Furosemide (Lasix). *Class:* loop diuretic. *Description:* drug that inhibits reabsorption of sodium and chloride in the proximal tubule and loop of Henle; intravenous doses can increase venous capacitance and decrease preload. *Indications:* pulmonary edema associated with congestive heart failure, and hepatic or renal disease. *Contraindications:* anuria, hypersensitivity; states of severe electrolyte depletion; dehydration; known allergy to sulfonamides. *Adverse reactions:* hypotension, electrocardiogram changes, dry mouth, hypercalcemia, hypochloremia, hypokalemia, hyponatremia, and hyperglycemia; may cause hearing loss if infusion of large doses is too rapid. *Onset:* vascular effects within 5 minutes intravenously; diuresis, 15 to 20 minutes. *Duration:* 2 hours. *Dose:* adult—0.5 to 1.0 mg/kg slow intravenous injection (not to exceed 20 mg/min); if no response, double dose to 2 mg/kg slow over 2 minutes; pediatric—1 mg/kg/dose. *Special considerations:* Drug has been known to cause fetal abnormalities; it should be protected from light.

28. Oxytocin (Pitocin). *Class:* pituitary hormone. *Description:* drug that indirectly stimulates uterine smooth muscle contractions, which transiently reduce uterine blood flow, and stimulates the mammary gland to increase lactation. *Indications:* postpartum hemorrhage after infant and placental delivery; induces labor at term (not a prehospital indication). *Contraindications:* presence of a second fetus; hypertonic or hyperactive uterus. *Adverse reactions:* tachycardia, hypertension, dysrhythmias, angina pectoris, anxiety, seizure, nausea, vomiting, allergic reaction, and uterine rupture (excessive dose). *Onset:* intravenous—immediate; intramuscular—3 to 5 minutes. *Duration:* intravenous—20 minutes; intramuscular—30 to 60 minutes. *Dose:* intramuscular—3 to 10 units after delivery of the placenta; intravenous—mix 10 units in 1000 mL normal saline or lactated Ringer's solution and infuse at 20 to 30 drops/min, titrated to the severity of bleeding and uterine response. *Special considerations:* Vasopressors may potentiate hypertension; vital signs and uterine tone should be monitored closely.

29. b. Dopamine is used to increase stroke volume.

30. d. Narcotic analgesics and nitrous oxide are contraindicated in undiagnosed abdominal pain because they may mask symptoms.

31. a. Epinephrine 1:10,000 intravenously is indicated for all other conditions listed.

32. b. Adenosine, beta-blockers (atenolol), and calcium blockers (diltiazem) are Class III recommendations to control rate in atrial fibrillation/flutter in the presence of Wolff-Parkinson-White syndrome.

33. d. Calcium and pacemaker are used to treat calcium channel blocker overdose.

34. a. It causes vasoconstriction at high doses.

35. a. Aspirin and oxygen should be administered. The patient's legs should be elevated, and a fluid bolus should be administered in an attempt to increase the blood pressure. His electrocardiogram and clinical presentation suggest the probability of right ventricular infarction, so nitroglycerin would not be given. Morphine would not be given until the blood pressure increases. Verapamil is not indicated in this setting.

36. a. Hydralazine is an antihistamine used to treat nausea. Morphine is a narcotic analgesic. Nifedipine is a calcium channel blocker used to treat hypertension.

37. c. All others are beta-agonists.

38. b. Verapamil vasodilates and further decreases blood pressure.

39. d

40. b. It dilates blood vessels and decreases peripheral vascular resistance and blood pressure.

41. a. The other drugs listed increase the plasmin in the blood, which causes degradation of fibrin threads and fibrinogen.

42. c. Naloxone is administered to reverse potential narcotic intoxication. Thiamine promotes uptake of glucose in the brain and prevents the development of Wernicke's encephalopathy when glucose is administered. Dextrose 50% in water corrects underlying hypoglycemia.

43. b. It is an osmotic diuretic and pulls excess fluid from the brain, temporarily decreasing intracranial pressure.

44. a

45. d. Oxytocin should be administered only after delivery of all the babies.

46. b. Benadryl causes thickening of the bronchial secretions and exacerbates an asthma attack.

47. c. Syrup of ipecac is contraindicated in patients without gag reflexes because aspiration may occur. Prochlorperazine (Compazine) is an antiemetic and decreases the effect of the ipecac. Hydrocarbons such as gasoline pose a large risk of aspiration, so ipecac is not indicated.

48. d. It is not effective against barbiturates.

49. c. It also may cause hypotension.

50. a. Magnesium would be given if the Q-T interval were prolonged. Beta-blockers would be an option for polymorphic ventricular tachycardia. Procainamide would be indicated in the absence of signs of congestive heart failure.

51. d

52. b

53. d. Furosemide decreases intravascular volume and causes vasodilation, which causes decreased preload and therefore less fluid to back up in the lungs.

54. d. Adenosine is not a calcium channel blocker and is not used to treat atrial flutter.

55. a. Atropine would increase the heart rate and the work of the heart and make the patient's condition worse.

56. b. Vistaril or phenergen often is ordered concurrently to prevent this side effect.

57. a. Haloperidol (Haldol) is a major tranquilizer.

58. d

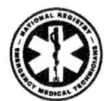

Candidate: _____ Examiner: _____

Date: _____ Signature: _____

Scenario # _____

Time Start: _____   NOTE: Areas denoted by "**" may be integrated within sequence of Initial Assessment

	Possible Points	Points Awarded
Takes or verbalizes body substance isolation precautions	1	
SCENE SIZE-UP		
Determines the scene/situation is safe	1	
Determines the mechanism of injury/nature of illness	1	
Determines the number of patients	1	
Requests additional help if necessary	1	
Considers stabilization of spine	1	
INITIAL ASSESSMENT/RESUSCITATION		
Verbalizes general impression of the patient	1	
Determines responsiveness/level of consciousness	1	
Determines chief complaint/apparent life-threats	1	
Airway -Opens and assesses airway (1 point) -Inserts adjunct as indicated (1 point)	2	
Breathing -Assess breathing (1 point) -Assures adequate ventilation (1 point) -Initiates appropriate oxygen therapy (1 point) -Manages any injury which may compromise breathing/ventilation (1 point)	4	
Circulation -Checks pulse (1point) -Assess skin [either skin color, temperature, or condition] (1 point) -Assesses for and controls major bleeding if present (1 point) -Initiates shock management (1 point)	4	
Identifies priority patients/makes transport decision	1	
FOCUSED HISTORY AND PHYSICAL EXAMINATION/RAPID TRAUMA ASSESSMENT		
Selects appropriate assessment	1	
Obtains, or directs assistant to obtain, baseline vital signs	1	
Obtains SAMPLE history	1	
DETAILED PHYSICAL EXAMINATION		
Head -Inspects mouth**, nose**, and assesses facial area (1 point) -Inspects and palpates scalp and ears (1 point) -Assesses eyes for PERRL** (1 point)	3	
Neck** -Checks position of trachea (1 point) -Checks jugular veins (1 point) -Palpates cervical spine (1 point)	3	
Chest** -Inspects chest (1 point) -Palpates chest (1 point) -Auscultates chest (1 point)	3	
Abdomen/pelvis** -Inspects and palpates abdomen (1 point) -Assesses pelvis (1 point) -Verbalizes assessment of genitalia/perineum as needed (1 point)	3	
Lower extremities** -Inspects, palpates, and assesses motor, sensory, and distal circulatory functions (1 point/leg)	2	
Upper extremities -Inspects, palpates, and assesses motor, sensory, and distal circulatory functions (1 point/arm)	2	
Posterior thorax, lumbar, and buttocks** -Inspects and palpates posterior thorax (1 point) -Inspects and palpates lumbar and buttocks area (1 point)	2	
Manages secondary injuries and wounds appropriately	1	
Performs ongoing assessment	1	
TOTAL	43	

Time End: _____

CRITICAL CRITERIA

____ Failure to initiate or call for transport of the patient within 10 minute time limit
____ Failure to take or verbalize body substance isolation precautions
____ Failure to determine scene safety
____ Failure to assess for and provide spinal protection when indicated
____ Failure to voice and ultimately provide high concentration of oxygen
____ Failure to assess/provide adequate ventilation
____ Failure to find or appropriately manage problems associated with airway, breathing, hemorrhage or shock [hypoperfusion]
____ Failure to differentiate patient's need for immediate transportation versus continued assessment/treatment at the scene
____ Does other detailed/focused history or physical exam before assessing/treating threats to airway, breathing, and circulation
____ Orders a dangerous or inappropriate intervention

You must factually document your rationale for checking any of the above critical items on the reverse side of this form.

p301/8-003k

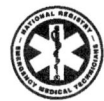

PATIENT ASSESSMENT - MEDICAL

Candidate: _____ Examiner: _____

Date: _____ Signature: _____

Scenario: _____

Time Start: _____

	Possible Points	Points Awarded
Takes or verbalizes body substance isolation precautions	1	
SCENE SIZE-UP		
Determines the scene/situation is safe	1	
Determines the mechanism of injury/nature of illness	1	
Determines the number of patients	1	
Requests additional help if necessary	1	
Considers stabilization of spine	1	
INITIAL ASSESSMENT		
Verbalizes general impression of the patient	1	
Determines responsiveness/level of consciousness	1	
Determines chief complaint/apparent life-threats	1	

Assesses airway and breathing
    -Assessment (1 point)
    -Assures adequate ventilation (1 point)
    -Initiates appropriate oxygen therapy (1 point)
	3	

Assesses circulation
    -Assesses/controls major bleeding (1 point)   -Assesses skin [either skin color, temperature, or condition] (1 point)
    -Assesses pulse (1 point)
	3	

Identifies priority patients/makes transport decision	1	
FOCUSED HISTORY AND PHYSICAL EXAMINATION/RAPID ASSESSMENT		

History of present illness
    -Onset (1 point)   -Severity (1 point)
    -Provocation (1 point)   -Time (1 point)
    -Quality (1 point)   -Clarifying questions of associated signs and symptoms as related to OPQRST (2 points)
    -Radiation (1 point)
	8	

Past medical history
    -Allergies (1 point)   -Past pertinent history (1 point)   -Events leading to present illness (1 point)
    -Medications (1 point)   -Last oral intake (1 point)
	5	

Performs focused physical examination [assess affected body part/system or, if indicated, completes rapid assessment]
    -Cardiovascular   -Neurological   -Integumentary   -Reproductive
    -Pulmonary   -Musculoskeletal   -GI/GU   -Psychological/Social
	5	

Vital signs
    -Pulse (1 point)   -Respiratory rate and quality (1 point each)
    -Blood pressure (1 point)   -AVPU (1 point)
	5	

Diagnostics [must include application of ECG monitor for dyspnea and chest pain]	2	
States field impression of patient	1	
Verbalizes treatment plan for patient and calls for appropriate intervention(s)	1	
Transport decision re-evaluated	1	
ON-GOING ASSESSMENT		
Repeats initial assessment	1	
Repeats vital signs	1	
Evaluates response to treatments	1	
Repeats focused assessment regarding patient complaint or injuries	1	

Time End: _____

CRITICAL CRITERIA   **TOTAL**   **48**

_____ Failure to initiate or call for transport of the patient within 15 minute time limit

_____ Failure to take or verbalize body substance isolation precautions

_____ Failure to determine scene safety before approaching patient

_____ Failure to voice and ultimately provide appropriate oxygen therapy

_____ Failure to assess/provide adequate ventilation

_____ Failure to find or appropriately manage problems associated with airway, breathing, hemorrhage or shock [hypoperfusion]

_____ Failure to differentiate patient's need for immediate transportation versus continued assessment and treatment at the scene

_____ Does other detailed or focused history or physical examination before assessing and treating threats to airway, breathing, and circulation

_____ Failure to determine the patient's primary problem

_____ Orders a dangerous or inappropriate intervention

_____ Failure to provide for spinal protection when indicated

You must factually document your rationale for checking any of the above critical items on the reverse side of this form.

p302/8-003k

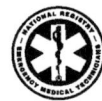

VENTILATORY MANAGEMENT - ADULT

Candidate:_____ Examiner:_____

Date: _____Signature: _____

NOTE: If candidate elects to ventilate initially with BVM attached to reservoir and oxygen, full credit must be awarded for steps denoted by "**" so long as first ventilation is delivered within 30 seconds.

	Possible Points	Points Awarded
Takes or verbalizes body substance isolation precautions	1	
Opens the airway manually	1	
Elevates tongue, inserts simple adjunct [oropharyngeal or nasopharyngeal airway]	1	
NOTE: Examiner now informs candidate no gag reflex is present and patient accepts adjunct		
**Ventilates patient immediately with bag-valve-mask device unattached to oxygen	1	
**Hyperventilates patient with room air	1	
NOTE: Examiner now informs candidate that ventilation is being performed without difficulty and that pulse oximetry indicates the patient's blood oxygen saturation is 85%		
Attaches oxygen reservoir to bag-valve-mask device and connects to high flow oxygen regulator [12-15 L/minute]	1	
Ventilates patient at a rate of 10-20/minute with appropriate volumes	1	
NOTE: After 30 seconds, examiner auscultates and reports breath sounds are present, equal bilaterally and medical direction has ordered intubation. The examiner must now take over ventilation.		
Directs assistant to pre-oxygenate patient	1	
Identifies/selects proper equipment for intubation	1	
Checks equipment for: -Cuff leaks (1 point) -Laryngoscope operational with bulb tight (1 point)	2	
NOTE: Examiner to remove OPA and move out of the way when candidate is prepared to intubate		
Positions head properly	1	
Inserts blade while displacing tongue	1	
Elevates mandible with laryngoscope	1	
Introduces ET tube and advances to proper depth	1	
Inflates cuff to proper pressure and disconnects syringe	1	
Directs ventilation of patient	1	
Confirms proper placement by auscultation bilaterally over each lung and over epigastrium	1	
NOTE: Examiner to ask, "If you had proper placement, what should you expect to hear?"		
Secures ET tube [may be verbalized]	1	
NOTE: Examiner now asks candidate, "Please demonstrate one additional method of verifying proper tube placement in this patient."		
Identifies/selects proper equipment	1	
Verbalizes findings and interpretations [compares indicator color to the colorimetric scale and states reading to examiner]	1	
NOTE: Examiner now states, "You see secretions in the tube and hear gurgling sounds with the patient's exhalation."		
Identifies/selects a flexible suction catheter	1	
Pre-oxygenates patient	1	
Marks maximum insertion length with thumb and forefinger	1	
Inserts catheter into the ET tube leaving catheter port open	1	
At proper insertion depth, covers catheter port and applies suction while withdrawing catheter	1	
Ventilates/directs ventilation of patient as catheter is flushed with sterile water	1	
TOTAL	**27**	

CRITICAL CRITERIA

_____ Failure to initiate ventilations within 30 seconds after applying gloves or interrupts ventilations for greater than 30 seconds at any time
_____ Failure to take or verbalize body substance isolation precautions
_____ Failure to voice and ultimately provide high oxygen concentrations [at least 85%]
_____ Failure to ventilate patient at a rate of at least 10/minute
_____ Failure to provide adequate volumes per breath [maximum 2 errors/minute permissible]
_____ Failure to pre-oxygenate patient prior to intubation and suctioning
_____ Failure to successfully intubate within 3 attempts
_____ Failure to disconnect syringe **immediately** after inflating cuff of ET tube
_____ Uses teeth as a fulcrum
_____ Failure to assure proper tube placement by auscultation bilaterally **and** over the epigastrium
_____ If used, stylette extends beyond end of ET tube
_____ Inserts any adjunct in a manner dangerous to the patient
_____ Suctions the patient for more than 15 seconds
_____ Does not suction the patient

You must factually document your rationale for checking any of the above critical items on the reverse side of this form.

p303/8-003k

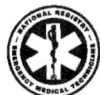

National Registry of Emergency Medical Technicians
Advanced Level Practical Examination

DUAL LUMEN AIRWAY DEVICE (COMBITUBE® OR PTL®)

Candidate: _____ Examiner: _____

Date: _____ Signature: _____

NOTE: If candidate elects to initially ventilate with BVM attached to reservoir and oxygen, full credit must be awarded for steps denoted by "**" so long as first ventilation is delivered within 30 seconds.

	Possible Points	Points Awarded
Takes or verbalizes body substance isolation precautions	1	
Opens the airway manually	1	
Elevates tongue, inserts simple adjunct [oropharyngeal or nasopharyngeal airway]	1	
NOTE: Examiner now informs candidate no gag reflex is present and patient accepts adjunct		
**Ventilates patient immediately with bag-valve-mask device unattached to oxygen	1	
**Hyperventilates patient with room air	1	
NOTE: Examiner now informs candidate that ventilation is being performed without difficulty		
Attaches oxygen reservoir to bag-valve-mask device and connects to high flow oxygen regulator [12-15 L/minute]	1	
Ventilates patient at a rate of 10-20/minute with appropriate volumes	1	
NOTE: After 30 seconds, examiner auscultates and reports breath sounds are present and equal bilaterally and medical control has ordered insertion of a dual lumen airway. The examiner must now take over ventilation.		
Directs assistant to pre-oxygenate patient	1	
Checks/prepares airway device	1	
Lubricates distal tip of the device [may be verbalized]	1	
NOTE: Examiner to remove OPA and move out of the way when candidate is prepared to insert device		
Positions head properly	1	
Performs a tongue-jaw lift	1	

☐ **USES COMBITUBE®**	☐ **USES PTL®**		
Inserts device in mid-line and to depth so printed ring is at level of teeth	Inserts device in mid-line until bite block flange is at level of teeth	1	
Inflates pharyngeal cuff with proper volume and removes syringe	Secures strap	1	
Inflates distal cuff with proper volume and removes syringe	Blows into tube #1 to adequately inflate both cuffs	1	
Attaches/directs attachment of BVM to the first [esophageal placement] lumen and ventilates		1	
Confirms placement and ventilation through correct lumen by observing chest rise, auscultation over the epigastrium, and bilaterally over each lung		1	
NOTE: The examiner states, "You do not see rise and fall of the chest and you only hear sounds over the epigastrium."			
Attaches/directs attachment of BVM to the second [endotracheal placement] lumen and ventilates		1	
Confirms placement and ventilation through correct lumen by observing chest rise, auscultation over the epigastrium, and bilaterally over each lung		1	
NOTE: The examiner confirms adequate chest rise, absent sounds over the epigastrium, and equal bilateral breath sounds.			
Secures device or confirms that the device remains properly secured		1	
	TOTAL	**20**	

CRITICAL CRITERIA

_____ Failure to initiate ventilations within 30 seconds after taking body substance isolation precautions or interrupts ventilations for greater than 30 seconds at any time
_____ Failure to take or verbalize body substance isolation precautions
_____ Failure to voice and ultimately provide high oxygen concentrations [at least 85%]
_____ Failure to ventilate patient at a rate of at least 10/minute
_____ Failure to provide adequate volumes per breath [maximum 2 errors/minute permissible]
_____ Failure to pre-oxygenate patient prior to insertion of the dual lumen airway device
_____ Failure to insert the dual lumen airway device at a proper depth or at either proper place within 3 attempts
_____ Failure to inflate both cuffs properly
_____ **Combitube** - failure to remove the syringe immediately after inflation of each cuff
      PTL - failure to secure the strap prior to cuff inflation
_____ Failure to confirm that the proper lumen of the device is being ventilated by observing chest rise, auscultation over the epigastrium, and bilaterally over each lung
_____ Inserts any adjunct in a manner dangerous to patient

You must factually document your rationale for checking any of the above critical items on the reverse side of this form.

p304/8-003k

PEDIATRIC (<2 yrs.) VENTILATORY MANAGEMENT

Candidate: _____ Examiner _____

Date: _____ Signature: _____

NOTE: If candidate elects to ventilate initially with BVM attached to reservoir and oxygen, full credit must be awarded for steps denoted by "**" so long as first ventilation is delivered within 30 seconds.

	Possible Points	Points Awarded
Takes or verbalizes body substance isolation precautions	1	
Opens the airway manually	1	
Elevates tongue, inserts simple adjunct [oropharyngeal or nasopharyngeal airway]	1	
NOTE: Examiner now informs candidate no gag reflex is present and patient accepts adjunct		
**Ventilates patient immediately with bag-valve-mask device unattached to oxygen	1	
**Hyperventilates patient with room air	1	
NOTE: Examiner now informs candidate that ventilation is being performed without difficulty and that pulse oximetry indicates the patient's blood oxygen saturation is 85%		
Attaches oxygen reservoir to bag-valve-mask device and connects to high flow oxygen regulator [12-15 L/minute]	1	
Ventilates patient at a rate of 20-30/minute and assures adequate chest expansion	1	
NOTE: After 30 seconds, examiner auscultates and reports breath sounds are present, equal bilaterally and medical direction has ordered intubation. The examiner must now take over ventilation.		
Directs assistant to pre-oxygenate patient	1	
Identifies/selects proper equipment for intubation	1	
Checks laryngoscope to assure operational with bulb tight	1	
NOTE: Examiner to remove OPA and move out of the way when candidate is prepared to intubate		
Places patient in neutral or sniffing position	1	
Inserts blade while displacing tongue	1	
Elevates mandible with laryngoscope	1	
Introduces ET tube and advances to proper depth	1	
Directs ventilation of patient	1	
Confirms proper placement by auscultation bilaterally over each lung and over epigastrium	1	
NOTE: Examiner to ask, "If you had proper placement, what should you expect to hear?"		
Secures ET tube [may be verbalized]	1	
TOTAL	17	

CRITICAL CRITERIA

_____ Failure to initiate ventilations within 30 seconds after applying gloves or interrupts ventilations for greater than 30 seconds at any time
_____ Failure to take or verbalize body substance isolation precautions
_____ Failure to pad under the torso to allow neutral head position or sniffing position
_____ Failure to voice and ultimately provide high oxygen concentrations [at least 85%]
_____ Failure to ventilate patient at a rate of at least 20/minute
_____ Failure to provide adequate volumes per breath [maximum 2 errors/minute permissible]
_____ Failure to pre-oxygenate patient prior to intubation
_____ Failure to successfully intubate within 3 attempts
_____ Uses gums as a fulcrum
_____ Failure to assure proper tube placement by auscultation bilaterally **and** over the epigastrium
_____ Inserts any adjunct in a manner dangerous to the patient
_____ Attempts to use any equipment not appropriate for the pediatric patient

You must factually document your rationale for checking any of the above critical items on the reverse side of this form.

p305/8-003k

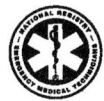

National Registry of Emergency Medical Technicians
Advanced Level Practical Examination

DYNAMIC CARDIOLOGY

Candidate: _____ Examiner: _____

Date: _____ Signature: _____

SET #_____

Level of Testing: □ NREMT-Intermediate/99   □ NREMT-Paramedic

Time Start:_____

	Possible Points	Points Awarded
Takes or verbalizes infection control precautions	1	
Checks level of responsiveness	1	
Checks ABCs	1	
Initiates CPR if appropriate [verbally]	1	
Attaches ECG monitor in a timely fashion or applies paddles for "Quick Look"	1	
Correctly interprets initial rhythm	1	
Appropriately manages initial rhythm	2	
Notes change in rhythm	1	
Checks patient condition to include pulse and, if appropriate, BP	1	
Correctly interprets second rhythm	1	
Appropriately manages second rhythm	2	
Notes change in rhythm	1	
Checks patient condition to include pulse and, if appropriate, BP	1	
Correctly interprets third rhythm	1	
Appropriately manages third rhythm	2	
Notes change in rhythm	1	
Checks patient condition to include pulse and, if appropriate, BP	1	
Correctly interprets fourth rhythm	1	
Appropriately manages fourth rhythm	2	
Orders high percentages of supplemental oxygen at proper times	1	

Time End: _____   TOTAL   24

CRITICAL CRITERIA

_____ Failure to deliver first shock in a timely manner due to operator delay in machine use or providing treatments other than CPR with simple adjuncts

_____ Failure to deliver second or third shocks without delay other than the time required to reassess rhythm and recharge paddles

_____ Failure to verify rhythm before delivering each shock

_____ Failure to ensure the safety of self and others [verbalizes "All clear" and observes]

_____ Inability to deliver DC shock [does not use machine properly]

_____ Failure to demonstrate acceptable shock sequence

_____ Failure to order initiation or resumption of CPR when appropriate

_____ Failure to order correct management of airway [ET when appropriate]

_____ Failure to order administration of appropriate oxygen at proper time

_____ Failure to diagnose or treat 2 or more rhythms correctly

_____ Orders administration of an inappropriate drug or lethal dosage

_____ Failure to correctly diagnose or adequately treat v-fib, v-tach, or asystole

You must factually document your rationale for checking any of the above critical items on the reverse side of this form.

p306/8-003k

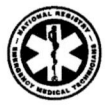

National Registry of Emergency Medical Technicians
Advanced Level Practical Examination

STATIC CARDIOLOGY

Candidate: _____ Examiner: _____

Date: _____ Signature: _____

SET # _____

Level of Testing: □ NREMT-Intermediate/99   □ NREMT-Paramedic

Note: No points for treatment may be awarded if the diagnosis is incorrect.
Only document incorrect responses in spaces provided.

Time Start: _____

	Possible Points	Points Awarded
STRIP #1 Diagnosis:	1	
Treatment:	2	
STRIP #2 Diagnosis:	1	
Treatment:	2	
STRIP #3 Diagnosis:	1	
Treatment:	2	
STRIP #4 Diagnosis:	1	
Treatment:	2	
TOTAL	12	

Time End: _____

p307/8-003k

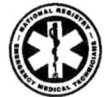

INTRAVENOUS THERAPY

Candidate: _____ Examiner: _____

Date: _____ Signature: _____

Level of Testing: ☐ NREMT-Intermediate/85   ☐ NREMT-Intermediate/99   ☐ NREMT-Paramedic

Time Start: _____

	Possible Points	Points Awarded
Checks selected IV fluid for: -Proper fluid (1 point) -Clarity (1 point)	2	
Selects appropriate catheter	1	
Selects proper administration set	1	
Connects IV tubing to the IV bag	1	
Prepares administration set [fills drip chamber and flushes tubing]	1	
Cuts or tears tape [at any time before venipuncture]	1	
Takes/verbalizes body substance isolation precautions [prior to venipuncture]	1	
Applies tourniquet	1	
Palpates suitable vein	1	
Cleanses site appropriately	1	
Performs venipuncture -Inserts stylette (1 point) -Notes or verbalizes flashback (1 point) -Occludes vein proximal to catheter (1 point) -Removes stylette (1 point) -Connects IV tubing to catheter (1 point)	5	
Disposes/verbalizes disposal of needle in proper container	1	
Releases tourniquet	1	
Runs IV for a brief period to assure patent line	1	
Secures catheter [tapes securely or verbalizes]	1	
Adjusts flow rate as appropriate	1	
TOTAL	21	

Time End: _____

CRITICAL CRITERIA

____ Failure to establish a patent and properly adjusted IV within 6 minute time limit
____ Failure to take or verbalize body substance isolation precautions prior to performing venipuncture
____ Contaminates equipment or site without appropriately correcting situation
____ Performs any improper technique resulting in the potential for uncontrolled hemorrhage, catheter shear, or air embolism
____ Failure to successfully establish IV within 3 attempts during 6 minute time limit
____ Failure to dispose/verbalize disposal of needle in proper container

NOTE: Check here (_____) if candidate did not establish a patent IV and do not evaluate IV Bolus Medications.

INTRAVENOUS BOLUS MEDICATIONS

Time Start: _____

Asks patient for known allergies	1	
Selects correct medication	1	
Assures correct concentration of drug	1	
Assembles prefilled syringe correctly and dispels air	1	
Continues body substance isolation precautions	1	
Cleanses injection site [Y-port or hub]	1	
Reaffirms medication	1	
Stops IV flow [pinches tubing or shuts off]	1	
Administers correct dose at proper push rate	1	
Disposes/verbalizes proper disposal of syringe and needle in proper container	1	
Flushes tubing [runs wide open for a brief period]	1	
Adjusts drip rate to TKO/KVO	1	
Verbalizes need to observe patient for desired effect/adverse side effects	1	
TOTAL	13	

Time End: _____

CRITICAL CRITERIA

____ Failure to begin administration of medication within 3 minute time limit
____ Contaminates equipment or site without appropriately correcting situation
____ Failure to adequately dispel air resulting in potential for air embolism
____ Injects improper drug or dosage [wrong drug, incorrect amount, or pushes at inappropriate rate]
____ Failure to flush IV tubing after injecting medication
____ Recaps needle or failure to dispose/verbalize disposal of syringe and needle in proper container

You must factually document your rationale for checking any of the above critical items on the reverse side of this form.

p309/8-003k

National Registry of Emergency Medical Technicians
Advanced Level Practical Examination

PEDIATRIC INTRAOSSEOUS INFUSION

Candidate: _____ Examiner: _____

Date: _____ Signature: _____

Time Start:_____	Possible Points	Points Awarded

Checks selected IV fluid for:
   -Proper fluid (1 point)
   -Clarity (1 point)
	2	

Selects appropriate equipment to include:
   -IO needle (1 point)
   -Syringe (1 point)
   -Saline (1 point)
   -Extension set (1 point)
	4	

Selects proper administration set	1	
Connects administration set to bag	1	
Prepares administration set [fills drip chamber and flushes tubing]	1	
Prepares syringe and extension tubing	1	
Cuts or tears tape [at any time before IO puncture]	1	
Takes or verbalizes body substance isolation precautions [prior to IO puncture]	1	
Identifies proper anatomical site for IO puncture	1	
Cleanses site appropriately	1	

Performs IO puncture:
   -Stabilizes tibia (1 point)
   -Inserts needle at proper angle (1 point)
   -Advances needle with twisting motion until "pop" is felt (1 point)
   -Unscrews cap and removes stylette from needle (1 point)
	4	

Disposes of needle in proper container	1	
Attaches syringe and extension set to IO needle and aspirates	1	
Slowly injects saline to assure proper placement of needle	1	
Connects administration set and adjusts flow rate as appropriate	1	
Secures needle with tape and supports with bulky dressing	1	
Time End: _____ **TOTAL**	23	

CRITICAL CRITERIA

_____ Failure to establish a patent and properly adjusted IO line within the 6 minute time limit
_____ Failure to take or verbalize body substance isolation precautions prior to performing IO puncture
_____ Contaminates equipment or site without appropriately correcting situation
_____ Performs any improper technique resulting in the potential for air embolism
_____ Failure to assure correct needle placement before attaching administration set
_____ Failure to successfully establish IO infusion within 2 attempts during 6 minute time limit
_____ Performing IO puncture in an unacceptable manner [improper site, incorrect needle angle, etc.]
_____ Failure to dispose of needle in proper container
_____ Orders or performs any dangerous or potentially harmful procedure

You must factually document your rationale for checking any of the above critical items on the reverse side of this form.

SPINAL IMMOBILIZATION (SEATED PATIENT)

Candidate:_____Examiner:_____

Date: _____Signature:_____

Time Start: _____	Possible Points	Points Awarded
Takes or verbalizes body substance isolation precautions	1	
Directs assistant to place/maintain head in the neutral, in-line position	1	
Directs assistant to maintain manual immobilization of the head	1	
Reassesses motor, sensory, and circulatory function in each extremity	1	
Applies appropriately sized extrication collar	1	
Positions the immobilization device behind the patient	1	
Secures the device to the patient's torso	1	
Evaluates torso fixation and adjusts as necessary	1	
Evaluates and pads behind the patient's head as necessary	1	
Secures the patient's head to the device	1	
Verbalizes moving the patient to a long backboard	1	
Reassesses motor, sensory, and circulatory function in each extremity	1	
TOTAL	12	

Time End: _____

CRITICAL CRITERIA

_____ Did not immediately direct or take manual immobilization of the head

_____ Did not properly apply appropriately sized cervical collar before ordering release of manual immobilization

_____ Released or ordered release of manual immobilization before it was maintained mechanically

_____ Manipulated or moved patient excessively causing potential spinal compromise

_____ Head immobilized to the device **before** device sufficiently secured to torso

_____ Device moves excessively up, down, left, or right on the patient's torso

_____ Head immobilization allows for excessive movement

_____ Torso fixation inhibits chest rise, resulting in respiratory compromise

_____ Upon completion of immobilization, head is not in a neutral, in-line position

_____ Did not reassess motor, sensory, and circulatory functions in each extremity after voicing immobilization to the long backboard

You must factually document your rationale for checking any of the above critical items on the reverse side of this form.

SPINAL IMMOBILIZATION (SUPINE PATIENT)

Candidate:_____Examiner:_____

Date: _____Signature:_____

Time Start: _____	Possible Points	Points Awarded
Takes or verbalizes body substance isolation precautions	1	
Directs assistant to place/maintain head in the neutral, in-line position	1	
Directs assistant to maintain manual immobilization of the head	1	
Reassesses motor, sensory, and circulatory function in each extremity	1	
Applies appropriately sized extrication collar	1	
Positions the immobilization device appropriately	1	
Directs movement of the patient onto the device without compromising the integrity of the spine	1	
Applies padding to voids between the torso and the device as necessary	1	
Immobilizes the patient's torso to the device	1	
Evaluates and pads behind the patient's head as necessary	1	
Immobilizes the patient's head to the device	1	
Secures the patient's legs to the device	1	
Secures the patient's arms to the device	1	
Reassesses motor, sensory, and circulatory function in each extremity	1	
Time End: _____ **TOTAL**	14	

CRITICAL CRITERIA
_____ Did not immediately direct or take manual immobilization of the head
_____ Did not properly apply appropriately sized cervical collar before ordering release of manual immobilization
_____ Released or ordered release of manual immobilization before it was maintained mechanically
_____ Manipulated or moved patient excessively causing potential spinal compromise
_____ Head immobilized to the device **before** device sufficiently secured to torso
_____ Patient moves excessively up, down, left, or right on the device
_____ Head immobilization allows for excessive movement
_____ Upon completion of immobilization, head is not in a neutral, in-line position
_____ Did not reassess motor, sensory, and circulatory functions in each extremity after voicing immobilization to the device

You must factually document your rationale for checking any of the above critical items on the reverse side of this form.

BLEEDING CONTROL/SHOCK MANAGEMENT

Candidate: _____ Examiner: _____

Date: _____ Signature: _____

Time Start:_____	Possible Points	Points Awarded
Takes or verbalizes body substance isolation precautions	1	
Applies direct pressure to the wound	1	
Elevates the extremity	1	
NOTE: The examiner must now inform the candidate that the wound continues to bleed.		
Applies an additional dressing to the wound	1	
NOTE: The examiner must now inform the candidate that the wound still continues to bleed. The second dressing does not control the bleeding.		
Locates and applies pressure to appropriate arterial pressure point	1	
NOTE: The examiner must now inform the candidate that the bleeding is controlled.		
Bandages the wound	1	
NOTE: The examiner must now inform the candidate that the patient is exhibiting signs and symptoms of hypoperfusion.		
Properly positions the patient	1	
Administers high concentration oxygen	1	
Initiates steps to prevent heat loss from the patient	1	
Indicates the need for immediate transportation	1	

Time End: _____   **TOTAL**   10

CRITICAL CRITERIA

_____ Did not take or verbalize body substance isolation precautions
_____ Did not apply high concentration of oxygen
_____ Applied a tourniquet before attempting other methods of bleeding control
_____ Did not control hemorrhage in a timely manner
_____ Did not indicate the need for immediate transportation

You must factually document your rationale for checking any of the above critical items on the reverse side of this form.

ILLUSTRATION CREDITS AND ACKNOWLEDGMENTS

Fig. 6-1 Thibodeau GA: *Structure & function of the body,* ed 9, St Louis, 1992, Mosby.

Figs. 6-4, 6-5, 6-13, 6-14 Thibodeau GA: *Structure & function of the body,* ed 9, St Louis, 1992, Mosby (Illustrator E.W. Beck).

Figs. 6-6, 6-8 Seeley R, Stephens T, Tate P: *Anatomy & physiology,* ed 2, St Louis, 1992, Mosby (Illustrator David J. Mascaro & Associates).

Fig. 6-18 Thibodeau GA: *Structure & function of the body,* ed 9, St Louis, 1992, Mosby (Illustrator Branislav Vidic).

Figs. 6-10, 6-11 Thibodeau GA: *Structure & function of the body,* ed 9, St Louis, 1992, Mosby (Illustrator Christine Oleksyk).

Fig. 6-15 Seeley R: *Anatomy & physiology,* ed 2, St Louis, 1992, Mosby (Sims/Illustrator Jody L. Fulks).

Fig. 6-16 Thibodeau GA: *Structure & function of the body,* ed 9, St Louis, 1992, Mosby (Illustrator Barbara Cousins).

Fig. 6-17 Thibodeau GA: *Structure & function of the body,* ed. 9, St Louis, 1992, Mosby (Illustrator William Ober).

Figs. 29-1, 29-3 Cotton S: *Mosby's paramedic study guide,* St Louis, 1989, Mosby.

Figs. 29-4, 29-12 Huszar R: *Basic dysrhythmias,* ed 2, St Louis, 1994, Mosby.

The following ECG strips and drug flashcards are included to make the task of studying easier. The cards should be completed in accordance with the questions on pages 381-389. However, they are not designed to be used in just those areas.

Challenge yourself and use the drug cards:
- With a fellow student as flashcards to study
- To review drugs in subsequent chapters
- In the cardiovascular section to enhance your instructor's lecture
- While on clinical sites as an easy reference
- Before final examinations as a quick, portable review

The ECG cards may be helpful:
- During ECG study, group them according to their similarities, and later, as you master them, mix them up and identify each one
- To make up scenarios in study groups
- When practicing for cardiac algorithm practicals
- To bring along during hospital and field clinicals as an easy reference

Be creative and invent your own uses for these flashcards. They are here so you can improve your knowledge and enhance success in study.

● **FLASHCARD 1**

Fig. 29-8

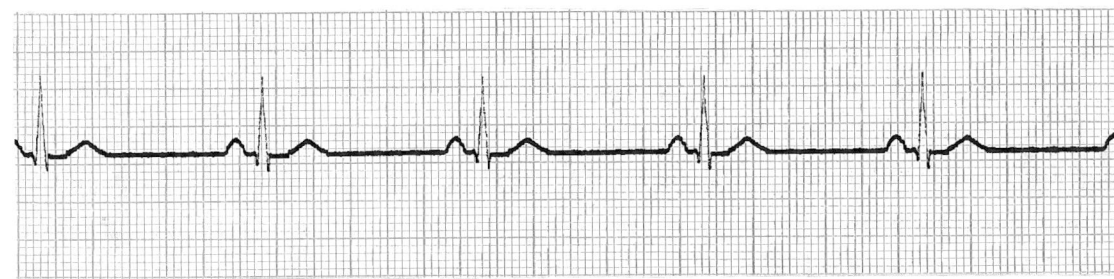

43.

QRS:_____ P wave: _____

Rate: _____ Rhythm:_____ PRI: _____

Interpretation:___**Sinus bradycardia**_____

Distinguishing features: _____

Treatment: _____

_____

● FLASHCARD 2

Fig. 29-9

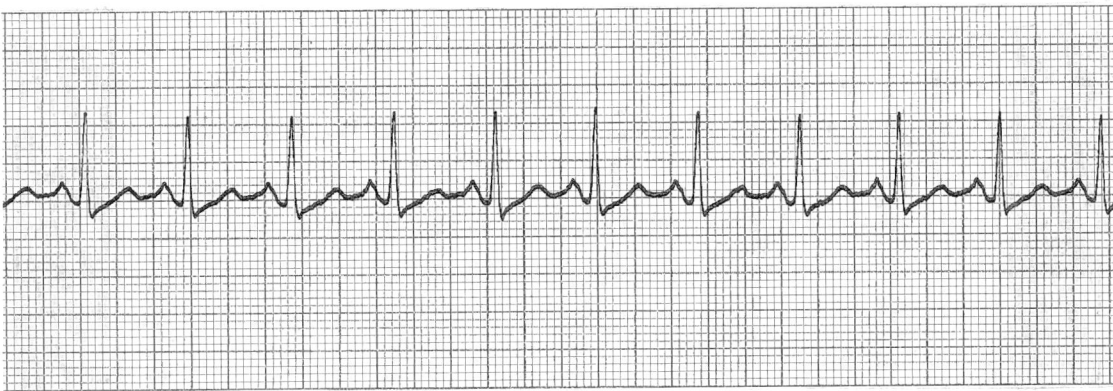

● FLASHCARD 3

Fig. 29-10

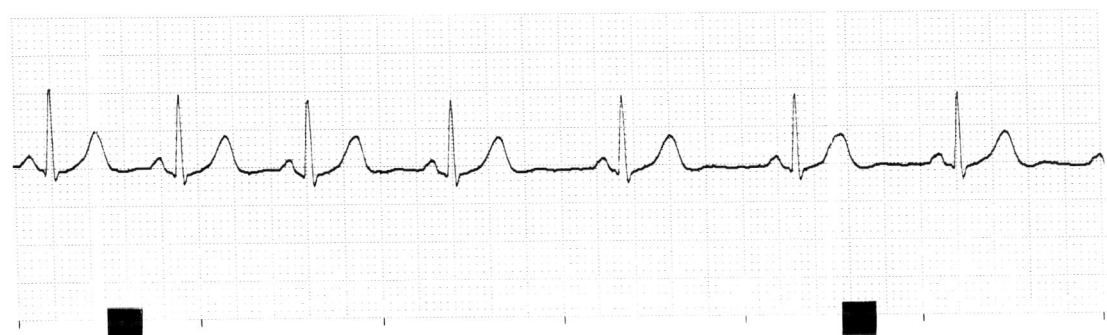

● FLASHCARD 4

Fig. 29-11

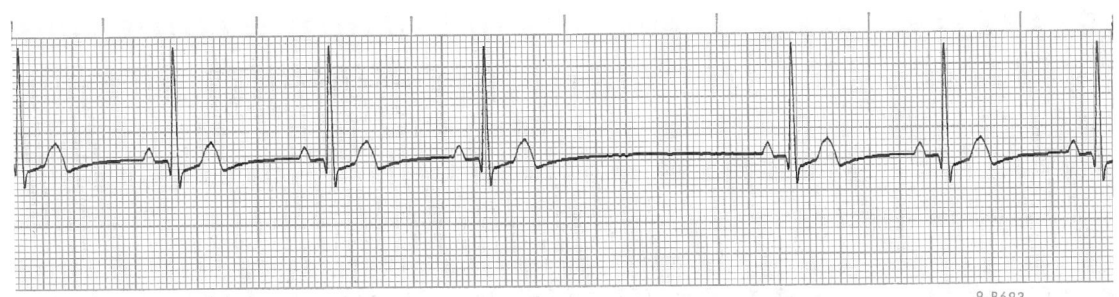

9-B693

44.

QRS:_____ P wave: _____

Rate: _____ Rhythm:_____ PRI: _____

Interpretation:___**Sinus tachycardia**_____

Distinguishing features: _____

Treatment: _____

_____

- -

45.

QRS:_____ P wave: _____

Rate: _____ Rhythm:_____ PRI: _____

Interpretation:___**Sinus dysrhythmia**_____

Distinguishing features: _____

Treatment:_____

_____

- -

46.

QRS:_____ P wave: _____

Rate: _____ Rhythm:_____ PRI: _____

Interpretation: ___**Sinus arrest**_____

Distinguishing features: _____

Treatment: _____

_____

● FLASHCARD 5

Fig. 29-12

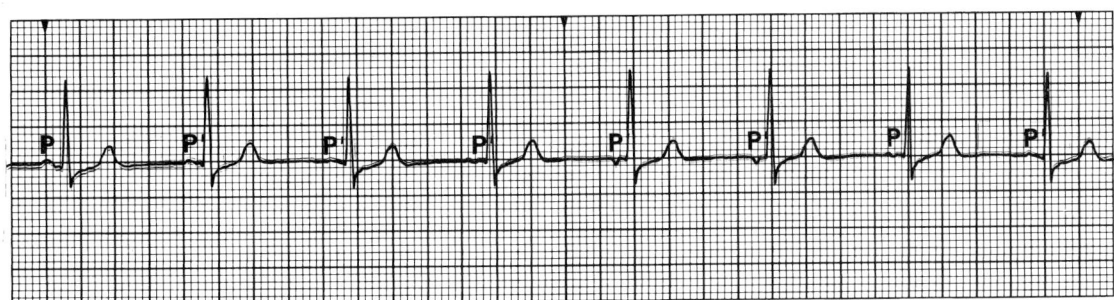

● FLASHCARD 6

Fig. 29-13

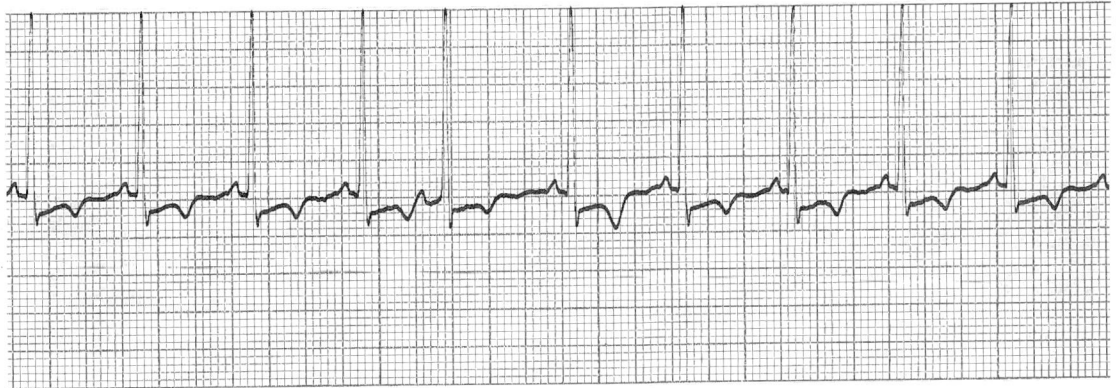

● FLASHCARD 7

Fig. 29-14

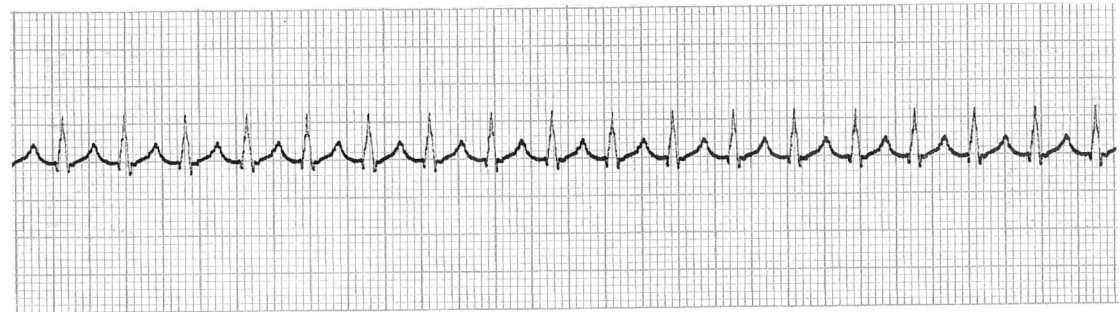

50.

QRS:_____ P wave: _____

Rate: _____ Rhythm:_____ PRI: _____

Interpretation:___**Wandering atrial pacemaker**_____

Distinguishing features: _____

Treatment: _____

_____

51.

QRS:_____ P wave: _____

Rate: _____ Rhythm:_____ PRI: _____

Interpretation:___**Premature atrial contraction**_____

Distinguishing features: _____

Treatment: _____

_____

52.

QRS:_____ P wave: _____

Rate: _____ Rhythm:_____ PRI: _____

Interpretation:___**Supraventricular tachycardia**_____

Distinguishing features: _____

Treatment: _____

_____

● FLASHCARD 8
Fig. 29-15

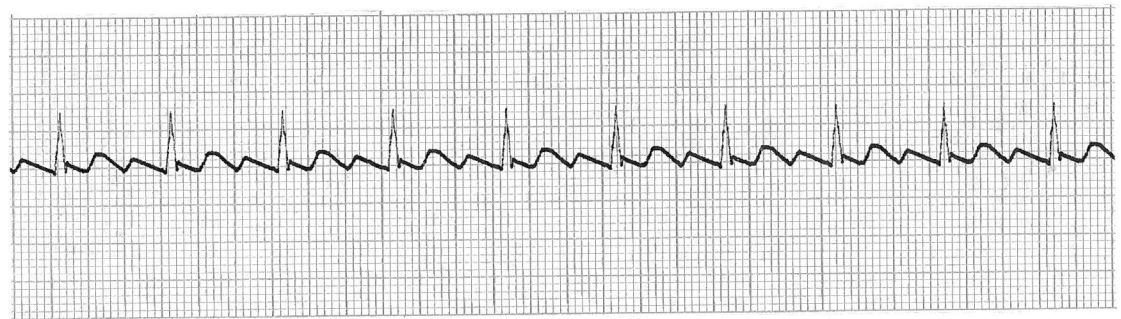

● FLASHCARD 9
Fig. 29-16

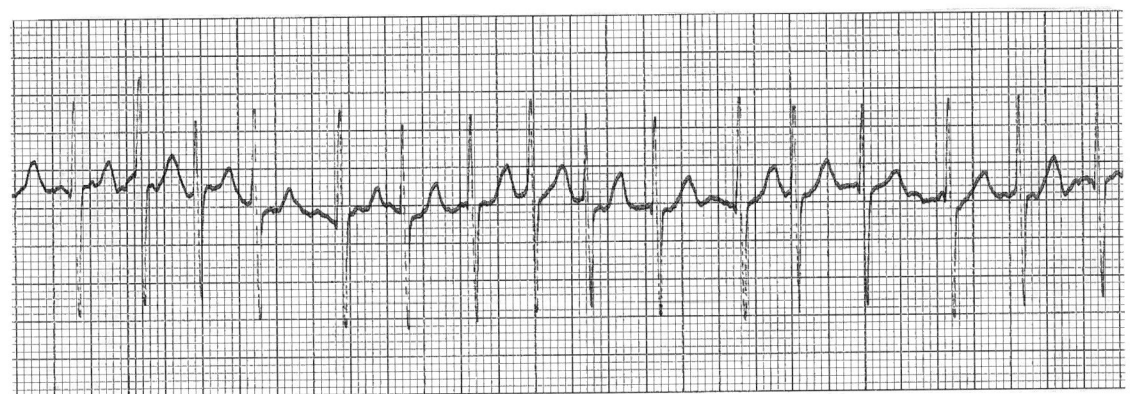

● FLASHCARD 10
Fig. 29-17

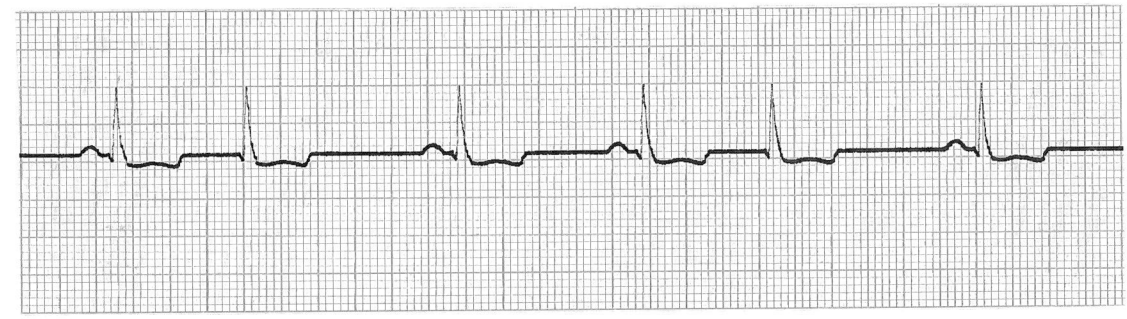

53.

QRS:_____ P wave: _____

Rate: _____ Rhythm: _____ PRI: _____

Interpretation:___**Atrial flutter with 3:1 conduction**_____

Distinguishing features: _____

Treatment: _____

_____

- -

54.

QRS:_____ P wave: _____

Rate: _____ Rhythm: _____ PRI: _____

Interpretation:___**Atrial fibrillation**_____

Distinguishing features: _____

Treatment: _____

_____

- -

57.

QRS:_____ P wave: _____

Rate: _____ Rhythm: _____ PRI: _____

Interpretation:___**Sinus rhythm (borderline bradycardia) with two premature junctional contractions**___

Distinguishing features: _____

Treatment: _____

_____

● **FLASHCARD 11**

Fig. 29-18

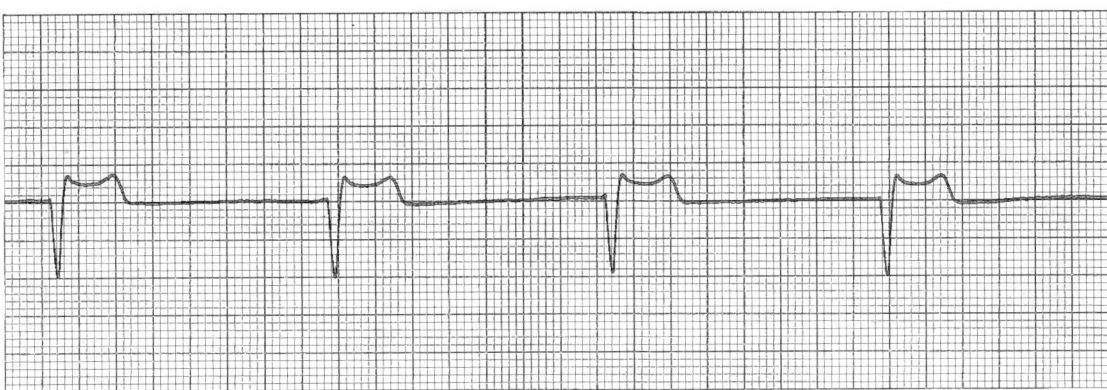

✂

● **FLASHCARD 12**

Fig. 29-19

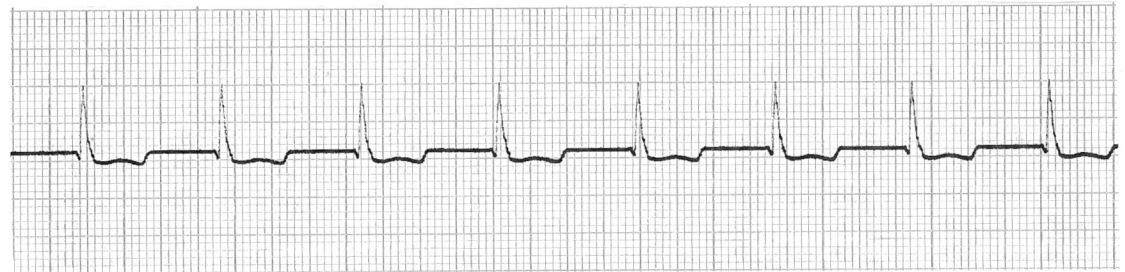

 ✂

● **FLASHCARD 13**

Fig. 29-20

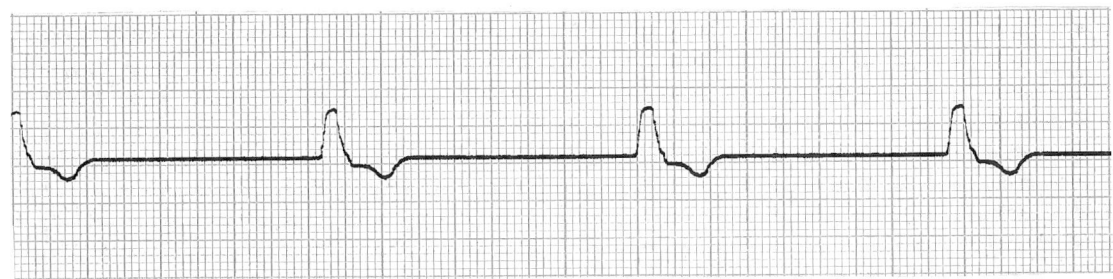

58.

QRS:_____ P wave: _____

Rate: _____ Rhythm:_____ PRI: _____

Interpretation:___**Junctional escape rhythm**_____

Distinguishing features: _____

Treatment: _____

_____

- -

59.

QRS:_____ P wave: _____

Rate: _____ Rhythm:_____ PRI: _____

Interpretation:___**Accelerated junctional rhythm**_____

Distinguishing features: _____

Treatment: _____

_____

- -

63.

QRS:_____ P wave: _____

Rate: _____ Rhythm:_____ PRI: _____

Interpretation:___**Ventricular escape rhythm**_____

Distinguishing features: _____

Treatment: _____

_____

● FLASHCARD 14
Fig. 29-21

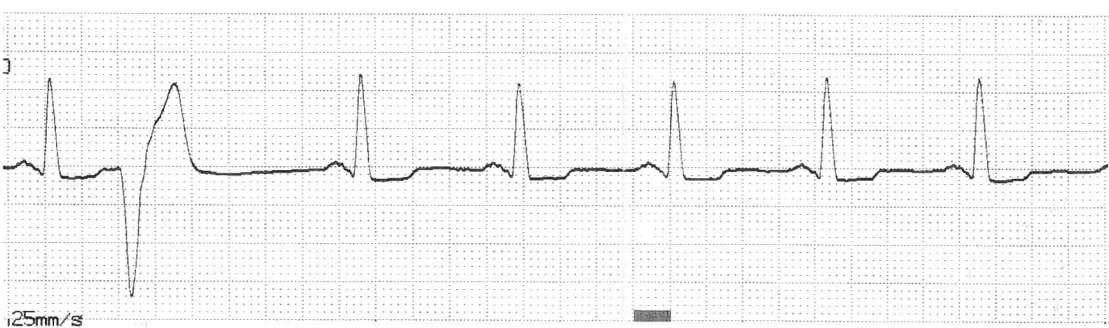

● FLASHCARD 15
Fig. 29-22

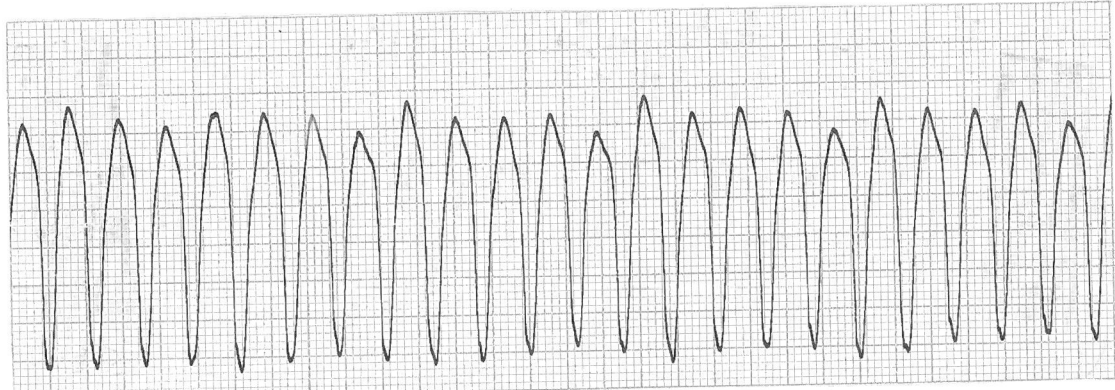

● FLASHCARD 16
Fig. 29-23

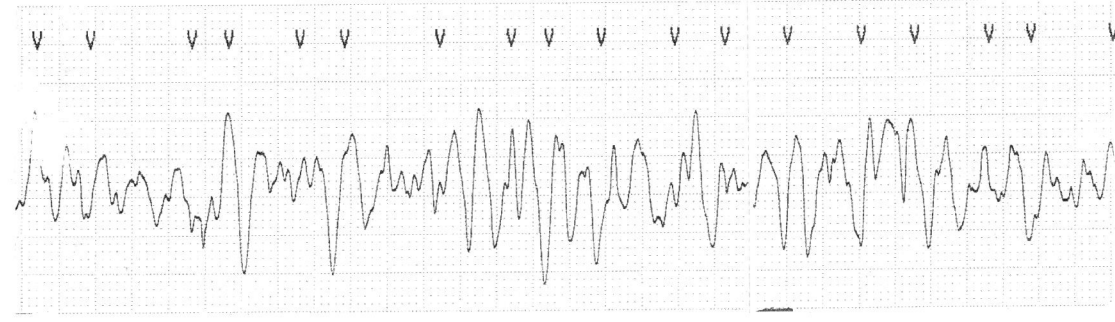

64.

QRS:_____ P wave: _____

Rate: _____ Rhythm:_____ PRI: _____

Interpretation:___**Normal sinus rhythm with one premature ventricular contraction**_____

Distinguishing features: _____

Treatment: _____

_____

- -

65.

QRS:_____ P wave: _____

Rate: _____ Rhythm:_____ PRI: _____

Interpretation:___**Monomorphic ventricular tachycardia**_____

Distinguishing features: _____

Treatment: _____

_____

- -

66.

QRS:_____ P wave: _____

Rate: _____ Rhythm:_____ PRI: _____

Interpretation:___**Ventricular fibrillation**_____

Distinguishing features: _____

Treatment: _____

_____

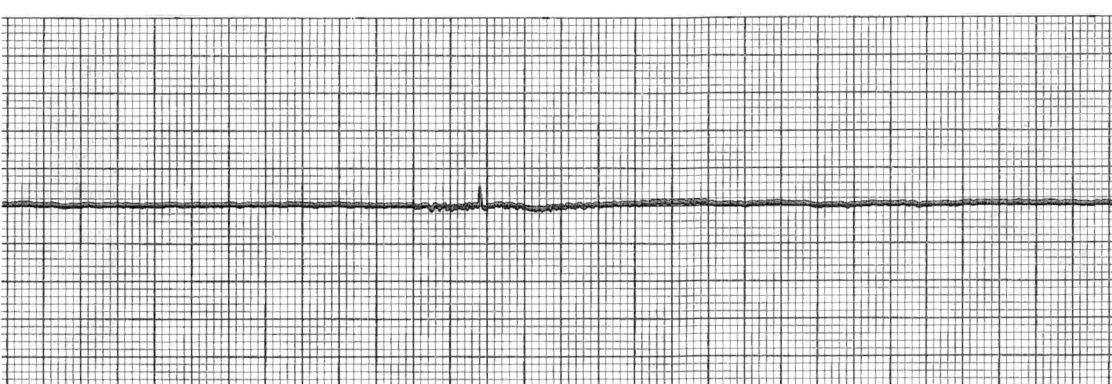
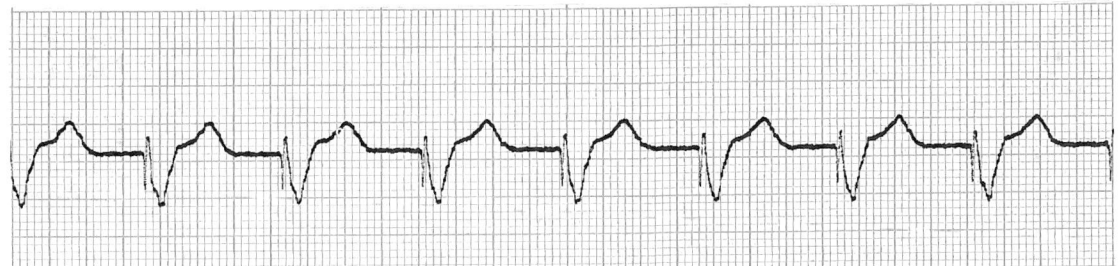

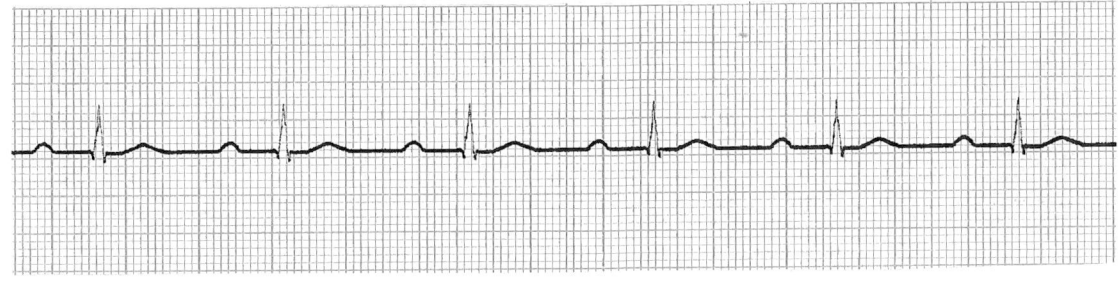

67.

QRS:_____ P wave: _____

Rate: _____ Rhythm:_____ PRI: _____

Interpretation:___**Asystole**_____

Distinguishing features: _____

Treatment: _____

_____

- -

68.

QRS:_____ P wave: _____

Rate: _____ Rhythm:_____ PRI: _____

Interpretation:___**Ventricular paced rhythm**_____

Distinguishing features: _____

Treatment: _____

_____

- -

71.

QRS:_____ P wave: _____

Rate: _____ Rhythm:_____ PRI: _____

Interpretation:___**Sinus rhythm with first-degree atrioventricular block**____

Distinguishing features: _____

Treatment: _____

_____

● **FLASHCARD 20**

Fig. 29-27

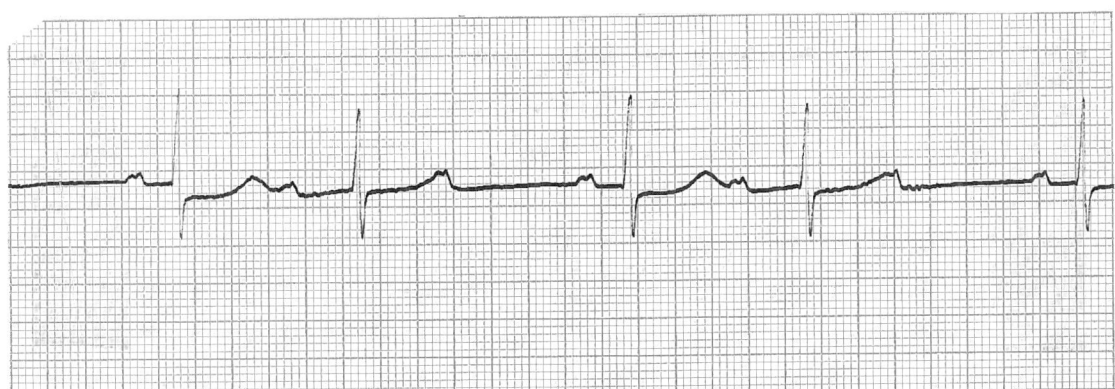

✂

● **FLASHCARD 21**

Fig. 29-28

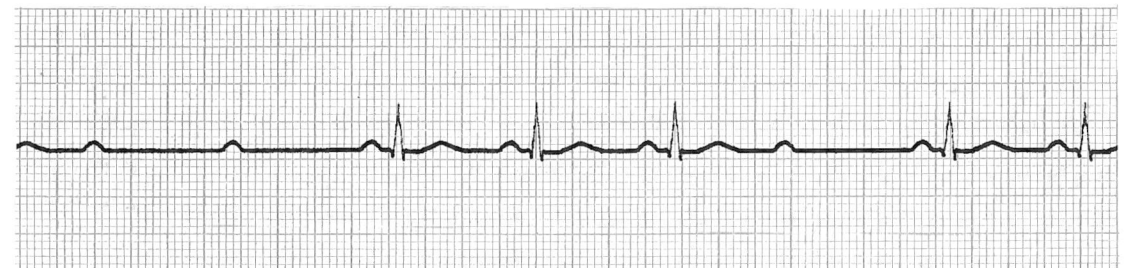

✂

● **FLASHCARD 22**

Fig. 29-29

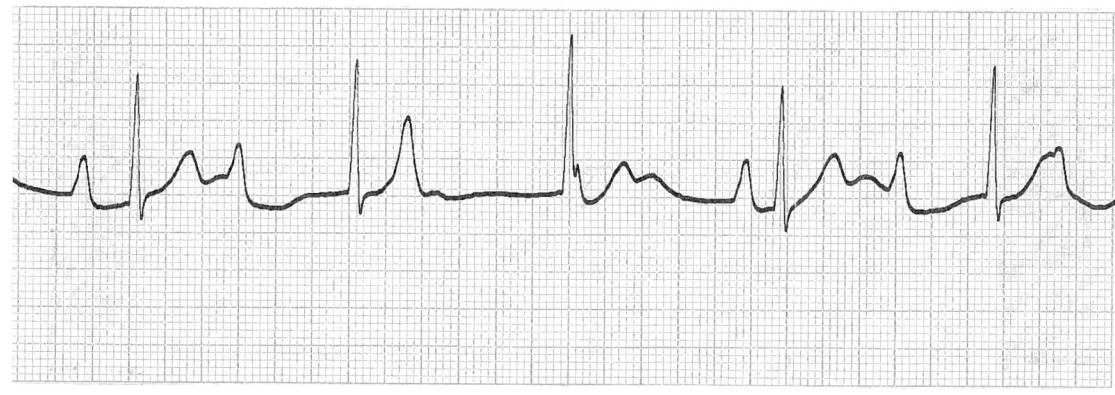

72.

QRS:_____ P wave: _____

Rate: _____ Rhythm:_____ PRI: _____

Interpretation:___**Second-degree atrioventricular block (Mobitz type I or Wenckebach)**_____

Distinguishing features: _____

Treatment: _____

_____

- -

73.

QRS:_____ P wave: _____

Rate: _____ Rhythm:_____ PRI: _____

Interpretation:___**Second-degree atrioventricular block (Mobitz type II)**_____

Distinguishing features: _____

Treatment: _____

_____

- -

74.

QRS:_____ P wave: _____

Rate: _____ Rhythm:_____ PRI: _____

Interpretation:___**Third-degree (complete) atrioventricular block**_____

Distinguishing features: _____

Treatment: _____

_____

● FLASHCARD 24

Question 4

Trade Name: _____

Class: _____

Descriptions: _____

_____

Indications: _____

_____

Contraindications: _____

_____

Adverse Reactions: _____

_____

Onset: _____

Duration _____

Dosage: _____

_____

_____

_____

Special Considerations: _____

_____

_____

● FLASHCARD 23

Question 3

Trade Name: _____

Class: _____

Descriptions: _____

_____

Indications: _____

_____

Contraindications: _____

_____

Adverse Reactions: _____

_____

Onset: _____

Duration _____

Dosage: _____

_____

_____

_____

Special Considerations: _____

_____

_____

● FLASHCARD 26

Question 6a

Trade Name: _____N/A_____

Class: _____

Descriptions: _____

_____

Indications: _____

_____

Contraindications: _____

_____

Adverse Reactions: _____

_____

Onset: _____

Duration _____

Dosage: _____

_____

_____

_____

Special Considerations: _____

_____

● FLASHCARD 25

Question 5

Trade Name: _____

Class: _____

Descriptions: _____

_____

Indications: _____

_____

Contraindications: _____

_____

Adverse Reactions: _____

_____

Onset: _____

Duration _____

Dosage: _____

_____

_____

_____

Special Considerations: _____

_____

diphenhydramine

vasopressin

glucagon

procainamide

● FLASHCARD 28

Question 7

Trade Name: _____

Class: _____

Descriptions: _____

_____

Indications: _____

_____

Contraindications: _____

_____

Adverse Reactions:_____

_____

Onset: _____

Duration _____

Dosage:_____

_____

_____

Special Considerations: _____

_____

_____

● FLASHCARD 27

Question 6b

Trade Name: _____

Class: _____

Descriptions: _____

_____

Indications: _____

_____

Contraindications: _____

_____

Adverse Reactions:_____

_____

Onset: _____

Duration _____

Dosage:_____

_____

_____

Special Considerations: _____

_____

_____

● FLASHCARD 30

Question 9

Trade Name: _____

Class: _____

Descriptions: _____

_____

Indications: _____

_____

Contraindications: _____

_____

Adverse Reactions:_____

_____

Onset: _____

Duration _____

Dosage:_____

_____

_____

Special Considerations: _____

_____

● FLASHCARD 29

Question 8

Trade Name: _____

Class: _____

Descriptions: _____

_____

Indications: _____

_____

Contraindications: _____

_____

Adverse Reactions:_____

_____

Onset: _____

Duration _____

Dosage:_____

_____

_____

Special Considerations: _____

_____

amiodarone

nitroglycerin

lidocaine

ketorolac
tromethamine

● **FLASHCARD 32**

Question 11

Trade Name: _____

Class: _____

Descriptions: _____

_____

Indications: _____

_____

Contraindications: _____

_____

Adverse Reactions:_____

_____

Onset: _____

Duration _____

Dosage:_____

_____

_____

_____

Special Considerations: _____

_____

_____

● **FLASHCARD 31**

Question 10

Trade Name: _____

Class: _____

Descriptions: _____

_____

Indications: _____

_____

Contraindications: _____

_____

Adverse Reactions:_____

_____

Onset: _____

Duration _____

Dosage:_____

_____

_____

Special Considerations: _____

_____

_____

● **FLASHCARD 34**

Question 13

Trade Name: _____

Class: _____

Descriptions: _____

_____

Indications: _____

_____

Contraindications: _____

_____

Adverse Reactions:_____

_____

Onset: _____

Duration _____

Dosage:_____

_____

_____

Special Considerations: _____

_____

● **FLASHCARD 33**

Question 12

Trade Name: _____

Class: _____

Descriptions: _____

_____

Indications: _____

_____

Contraindications: _____

_____

Adverse Reactions:_____

_____

Onset: _____

Duration _____

Dosage:_____

_____

_____

Special Considerations: _____

_____

naloxone

midazolam
hydrochloride

atropine sulfate

epinephrine

● **FLASHCARD 36**

Question 15

Trade Name: _____ N/A _____

Class: _____

Descriptions: _____

_____

Indications: _____

_____

Contraindications: _____

_____

Adverse Reactions: _____

_____

Onset: _____

Duration _____

Dosage: _____

_____

_____

_____

Special Considerations: _____

_____

_____

● **FLASHCARD 35**

Question 14

Trade Name: _____

Class: _____

Descriptions: _____

_____

Indications: _____

_____

Contraindications: _____

_____

Adverse Reactions: _____

_____

Onset: _____

Duration _____

Dosage: _____

_____

_____

_____

Special Considerations: _____

_____

_____

● **FLASHCARD 38**

Question 16b

Trade Name: _____ N/A _____

Class: _____

Descriptions: _____

_____

Indications: _____

_____

Contraindications: _____

_____

Adverse Reactions: _____

_____

Onset: _____

Duration _____

Dosage: _____

_____

_____

_____

Special Considerations: _____

_____

● **FLASHCARD 37**

Question 16a

Trade Name: _____

Class: _____

Descriptions: _____

_____

Indications: _____

_____

Contraindications: _____

_____

Adverse Reactions: _____

_____

Onset: _____

Duration _____

Dosage: _____

_____

_____

_____

Special Considerations: _____

_____

nitrous oxide

sodium bicarbonate

thiamine

dextrose 50%

● FLASHCARD 40

Question 18

Trade Name: _____

Class: _____

Descriptions: _____

_____

Indications: _____

_____

Contraindications: _____

_____

Adverse Reactions:_____

_____

Onset: _____

Duration _____

Dosage:_____

_____

_____

_____

Special Considerations: _____

_____

_____

● FLASHCARD 39

Question 17

Trade Name: _____

Class: _____

Descriptions: _____

_____

Indications: _____

_____

Contraindications: _____

_____

Adverse Reactions:_____

_____

Onset: _____

Duration _____

Dosage:_____

_____

_____

_____

Special Considerations: _____

_____

_____

● FLASHCARD 42

Question 20

Trade Name: _____

Class: _____

Descriptions: _____

_____

Indications: _____

_____

Contraindications: _____

_____

Adverse Reactions:_____

_____

Onset: _____

Duration _____

Dosage:_____

_____

_____

_____

Special Considerations: _____

_____

● FLASHCARD 41

Question 19

Trade Name: _____

Class: _____

Descriptions: _____

_____

Indications: _____

_____

Contraindications: _____

_____

Adverse Reactions:_____

_____

Onset: _____

Duration _____

Dosage:_____

_____

_____

_____

Special Considerations: _____

_____

diazepam

albuterol

aspirin

adenosine

● FLASHCARD 44

Question 21b

Trade Name: _____

Class: _____

Descriptions: _____

_____

Indications: _____

_____

Contraindications: _____

_____

Adverse Reactions: _____

_____

Onset: _____

Duration _____

Dosage: _____

_____

_____

_____

Special Considerations: _____

_____

_____

● FLASHCARD 43

Question 21a

Trade Name: _____

Class: _____

Descriptions: _____

_____

Indications: _____

_____

Contraindications: _____

_____

Adverse Reactions: _____

_____

Onset: _____

Duration _____

Dosage: _____

_____

_____

Special Considerations: _____

_____

_____

● FLASHCARD 46

Question 23

Trade Name: _____

Class: _____

Descriptions: _____

_____

Indications: _____

_____

Contraindications: _____

_____

Adverse Reactions: _____

_____

Onset: _____

Duration _____

Dosage: _____

_____

_____

_____

Special Considerations: _____

_____

_____

● FLASHCARD 45

Question 22

Trade Name: _____

Class: _____

Descriptions: _____

_____

Indications: _____

_____

Contraindications: _____

_____

Adverse Reactions: _____

_____

Onset: _____

Duration _____

Dosage: _____

_____

_____

_____

Special Considerations: _____

_____

_____

morphine sulfate

meperidine

labetalol

activated charcoal

● FLASHCARD 49

Question 26

Trade Name: _____

Class: _____

Descriptions: _____

Indications: _____

Contraindications: _____

Adverse Reactions: _____

Onset: _____

Duration _____

Dosage: _____

Special Considerations: _____

✂

● FLASHCARD 50

Question 27

Trade Name: _____

Class: _____

Descriptions: _____

Indications: _____

Contraindications: _____

Adverse Reactions: _____

Onset: _____

Duration _____

Dosage: _____

Special Considerations: _____

● FLASHCARD 47

Question 24

Trade Name: N/A _____

Class: _____

Descriptions: _____

Indications: _____

Contraindications: _____

Adverse Reactions: _____

Onset: _____

Duration _____

Dosage: _____

Special Considerations: _____

✂

● FLASHCARD 48

Question 25

Trade Name: _____

Class: _____

Descriptions: _____

Indications: _____

Contraindications: _____

Adverse Reactions: _____

Onset: _____

Duration _____

Dosage: _____

Special Considerations: _____

verapamil

furosemide

magnesium sulfate

dopamine

● **FLASHCARD 51**

Question 28

Trade Name: _____
Class: _____
Descriptions: _____
Indications: _____
Contraindications: _____
Adverse Reactions: _____
Onset: _____
Duration _____
Dosage: _____
Special Considerations: _____

● **FLASHCARD 52**

Trade Name: _____
Class: _____
Descriptions: _____
Indications: _____
Contraindications: _____
Adverse Reactions: _____
Onset: _____
Duration _____
Dosage: _____
Special Considerations: _____

● **FLASHCARD 53**

Trade Name: _____
Class: _____
Descriptions: _____
Indications: _____
Contraindications: _____
Adverse Reactions: _____
Onset: _____
Duration _____
Dosage: _____
Special Considerations: _____

● **FLASHCARD 54**

Trade Name: _____
Class: _____
Descriptions: _____
Indications: _____
Contraindications: _____
Adverse Reactions: _____
Onset: _____
Duration _____
Dosage: _____
Special Considerations: _____

Generic Name

Generic Name

Generic Name

oxytocin

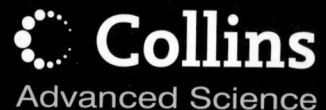
Collins
Advanced Science

Physics

Ken Dobson, David Grace & David Lovett

The complete guide to Physics

William Collins's dream of knowledge for all began with the publication of his first book in 1819. A self-educated mill worker, he not only enriched millions of lives, but also founded a flourishing publishing house. Today, staying true to this spirit, Collins books are packed with inspiration, innovation and practical expertise. They place you at the centre of a world of possibility and give you exactly what you need to explore it.

Collins. Freedom to teach.

Published by Collins
An imprint of HarperCollins Publishers
77-85 Fulham Palace Road
Hammersmith
London
W6 8JB

Browse the complete Collins catalogue at
www.collinseducation.com

© HarperCollins Publishers Limited 2008

10 9 8 7 6 5 4 3 2 1

ISBN-13 978-0-00-726749-1

International edition:

ISBN-13 978-0-00-726750-7

Ken Dobson, David Grace and David Lovett assert their moral rights to be identified as the authors of this work.

British Library Cataloguing in Publication Data. A Catalogue record for this publication is available from the British Library.

Commissioned by Penny Fowler
Project management by Laura Deacon
Edited by Mary Sanders
Proof read by Geoff Amor
Indexing by Michael Forder
Design by Newgen Imaging
Cover design by Angela English
Production by Arjen Jansen
Printed and bound in Hong Kong by Printing Express

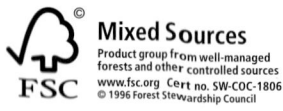

Mixed Sources
Product group from well-managed forests and other controlled sources
www.fsc.org Cert no. SW-COC-1806
© 1996 Forest Stewardship Council

FSC is a non-profit international organisation established to promote the responsible management of the world's forests. Products carrying the FSC label are independently certified to assure consumers that they come from forests that are managed to meet the social, economic and ecological needs of present and future generations.

Find out more about HarperCollins and the environment at
www.harpercollins.co.uk/green

Contents

1

Moving in space and time

1 MOVING IN SPACE AND TIME

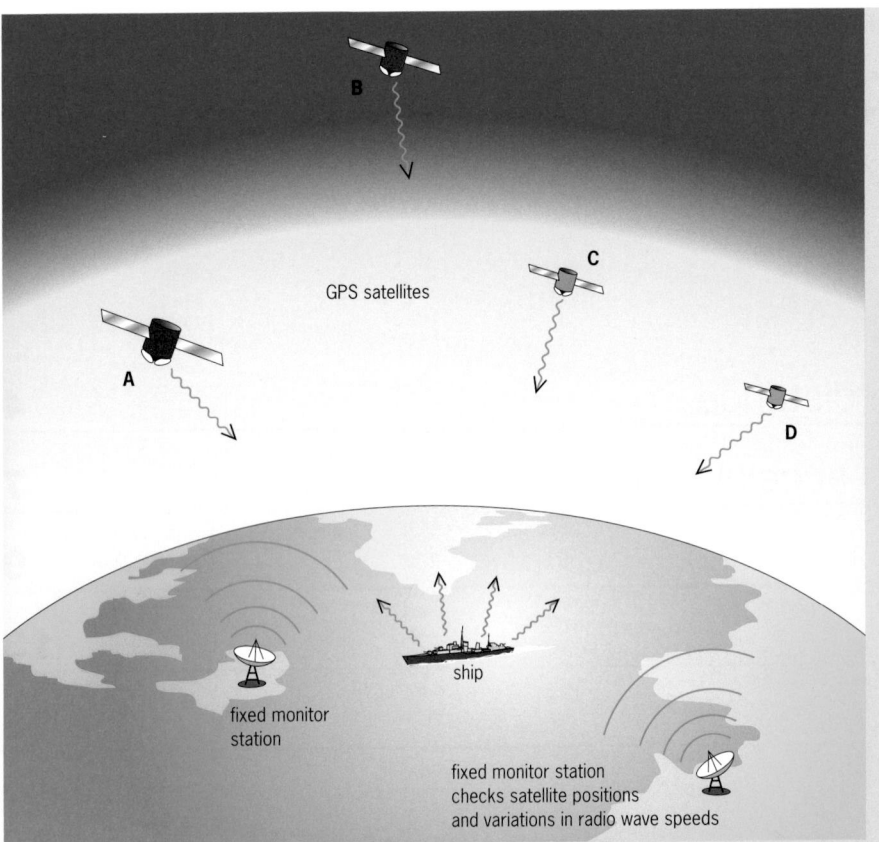

GPS satellites

ship

fixed monitor station

fixed monitor station checks satellite positions and variations in radio wave speeds

The ship's precise position is worked out using data from four satellites

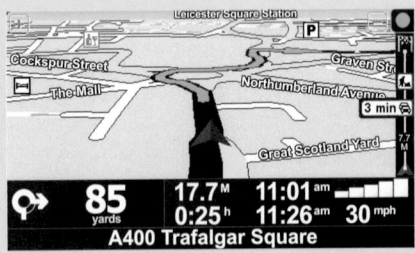

The image produced on an in-car SATNAV

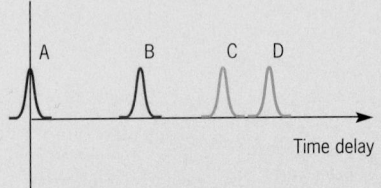

Time delay

The first satellite signal, A, arrives at a receiver, and signals B, C and D follow at different time intervals because they travel different distances. This provides enough information for a computer to fix the ship's position to a few metres

Keeping track

Satellites can pinpoint a position on the Earth to within a matter of centimetres. Travellers by land, sea or air can get a 'fix' of their positions at the press of a button on a small receiver. To get such an accurate ground position, the receiver needs to communicate with at least four satellites. Three produce a position 'fix', and the fourth provides an extra check.

Finding out where exactly you are on Earth depends on a combination of astronomy and clocks. The time intervals between the signals from the positioning satellites have to be measured to a very high degree of accuracy. For example, a hand-held receiver can tell when you move a few metres, by measuring the time that radio waves take to move that extra distance. The first important step in making accurate clocks to help in navigation was made by the watchmaker John Harrison in the eighteenth century. He won (eventually!) the prize awarded by the British Government for making a clock that was accurate enough – after a sea voyage of many weeks – to help a navigator work out his position from astronomical observations to an accuracy of less than 2 km.

The positions in space of the 24 satellites of the Global Positioning System (GPS) need to be accurately known, so they are constantly monitored from fixed ground stations. The satellites emit positioning signals using ultra-high-frequency radio waves. From the time delay at each ground station the precise position of each satellite is calculated. The position monitoring has to be continuous. Ionised layers that arise and disappear in the atmosphere slightly alter the radio wave speed. The satellites also vary slightly in position with time.

GPS receivers are now common in cars. The data received allows the vehicle's position to be calculated to about 2 metres. This position is linked to a map stored in the receiver memory which is displayed and the receiver gives visual and spoken directions to a destination fed in by the driver. Various correction factors are used to cope with such things as signal delays, unwanted reflections or absorption of the signal. The key item that allows this is a highly accurate measurement of time: each satellite contains the most accurate clock of all, an atomic clock. Clocks measure the passage of time using a regular repeated change of some kind, such a pendulum or a vibrating quartz crystal. An atomic clock makes use of the constant frequency of the radiation emitted by a particular isotope of caesium.

The ideas in this chapter

Movement is one of the most fundamental topics in the study of physics, with applications essential to our everyday lives. For example, in transport, drivers and pilots need to know how fast cars, trains and aircraft are moving, so that they can control them – while planners need to know this so that they can make timetables.

At an atomic level, knowing about the movement of particles has led to explanations of the behaviour of solids, liquids and gases.

But motion is very complicated. On a typical car journey the driver may make thousands of changes in speed and direction. Similarly, particles of gas are invisible, so how can we even think of following their movements?

Historically, the accurate study of motion began with trying to predict the movements of the Sun, the Moon, the planets and the stars. At the time, people believed that the Earth was at the centre of the Universe and everything else moved round the Earth in some way. People also believed that the stars and the planets had an effect on their lives and behaviour, and so needed accurate data to help them make *astrological* predictions. For almost 2000 years the important ideas about motion were due to the Greek scientist and philosopher Aristotle (*c.*348–322 BC). He didn't see the need to explain *why* things moved – smoke rose and apples fell from trees because it was natural for them to do so. This led him to make mistakes about falling objects and the motion of an arrow, say. Also, speed was not the important feature of everyday life that it is today. People moved slowly – on foot, on horseback or on sailing ships. Clocks were rare, and measured time no more accurately than to the nearest minute.

In the seventeenth century, many of these aspects of life began to change. First, there was a great increase in trade worldwide. As a result, there was a need to improve the skills of navigation. It was far more difficult to navigate a ship across an ocean than it had been simply to sail along the coast. The positions and movement of the Sun, the planets and the stars now needed to play a far more important role – as an aid to navigation, rather than for fortune-telling.

At the same time, the use of gunpowder was making the technology of war more sophisticated, with the development of cannons. The Italian physicist Galileo Galilei (1564–1642) studied the behaviour of moving objects and so helped to explain the movement of cannon balls. This further explained how cannons could be fired more accurately.

The result of these studies of motion in the seventeenth century was that scientists had very clear ideas of how to measure the quantities involved in motion: distance, time, speed, velocity and acceleration. See page 33 for more about Aristotle, Galileo and Newton.

The study of motion on its own is called **kinematics**. When forces are taken into account, the study becomes known as **dynamics**. Some of the world's most well-known physicists – Galileo, Newton and Einstein in particular – did their greatest work on the motion of objects.

The study of motion led to the development of accurate measuring instruments (Figs 1.1 and 1.2). Examples are telescopes, chronometers, atomic clocks and satellites for ocean navigation, radar, and lasers for surveying. Studying motion has also made physicists think deeply about the nature of space and time, and has led to theories about gravity, special and general relativity, and the origin and expansion of the Universe. Some of these more advanced ideas are dealt with in later chapters.

In this chapter, before we look closely at the movement of objects, we first see how the necessary measurements are made, and how the units of measurement have been established. In particular, we shall review the use of light as the basis of many measuring techniques today, and measurements of distances ranging from the small scale to the scale of the Universe.

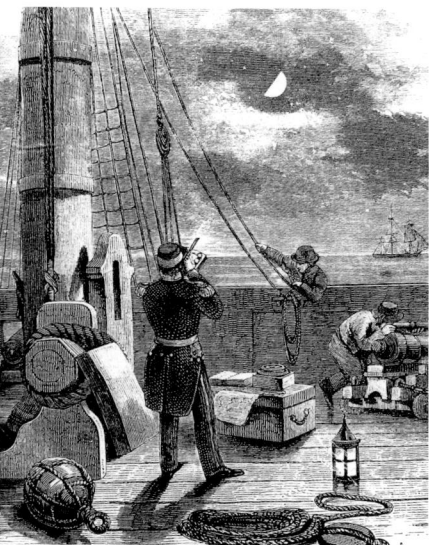

Fig 1.1 A nineteenth-century navigator uses a sextant to measure the angle of altitude of the Moon. From this he could work out the latitude of his ship. To find his longitude he needed an accurate *chronometer* (navigational clock)

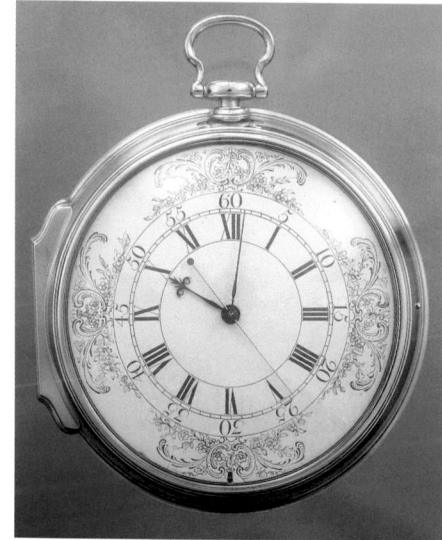

Fig 1.2 John Harrison's small watch taken to the West Indies (1761–1762) was one of the first accurate chronometers. It lost just 5 seconds during the 3 month voyage

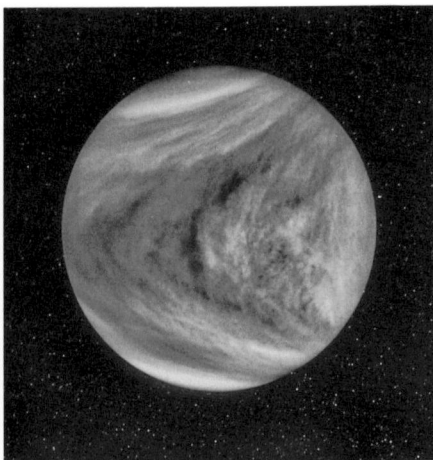

Fig 1.3 The distance of Venus from the Earth has been measured accurately using radar. This measurement is the first step in all astronomical distance measuring

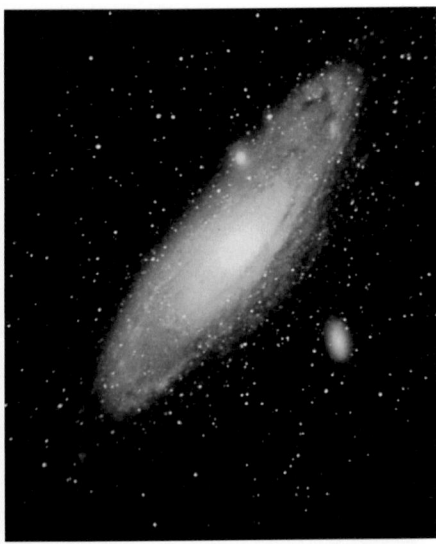

Fig 1.4 The Andromeda galaxy, a spiral galaxy and the nearest to our own Milky Way galaxy. Both are composed of countless stars, cooler objects, dust and gas. Its name is from the constellation in which it can be seen with the naked eye

1 TIME USED TO MEASURE DISTANCE

In moving, an object changes its position in space – so we need to be able to measure *distance*. Moving takes time – so *time* also has to be measured. In practice, we are often more concerned with time than distance, as these common statements show:

House for sale. Five minutes from the station.

Paris is just 40 minutes from London, by regular air shuttle.

The signposts of footpaths occasionally tell you the time it will take you to walk somewhere, rather than the distance. An assumption is being made about the speed of travel.

MEASURING DISTANCES WITH ELECTROMAGNETIC WAVES – BUT STILL USING *TIME*

Using **time units** to measure distance may seem strange, even 'unscientific'. Yet time is in fact the basis of most modern ways of measuring distance. Air traffic controllers use the time it takes radar pulses to travel to and from an aircraft to chart its position in a crowded flight pattern (see Fig 1.5). Surveyors use the time-of-flight of a pulse of laser light to measure distances accurately (see Fig 1.7, page 6). Cartographers making accurate maps now use radar or laser beams.

On the scale of distances in the Universe (Fig 1.3), astronomers also use radar to establish the precise positions of planets. As in Table 1.1, they measure far vaster distances in the **time units** based on the **speed of light** – light seconds and light years.

Table 1.1 Some distances in units of length and in time units

Object	Average distance from Earth/metres	Time units
Geostationary satellite	4.2×10^7	0.1401s
Moon	3.844×10^8	1.282s
Sun	1.496×10^{11}	499.0s
Sirius	8.2×10^{16}	8.7y
Andromeda galaxy	2.1×10^{22}	2.2×10^6y

$$\text{time unit (in seconds)} = \frac{\text{distance of an object (in metres)}}{\text{speed of light (in metres per second)}}$$

All these techniques depend on the measuring signal, light or a radio wave, having a constant speed. Many of the applications rely on the fact that electromagnetic waves are easily reflected, especially by metals. Both radio waves and light waves are electromagnetic waves of constant speed (when travelling in a vacuum). Light is now recognised as such a fundamental and useful measuring tool that the SI unit of distance, the **metre**, is defined in terms of the speed of light:

a metre is the distance travelled by light in a vacuum in the

$$\text{fraction } \frac{1}{299\ 792\ 458} \text{ of a second.}$$

? QUESTION 1

1   How long ago did the light leave the Andromeda galaxy shown in Fig 1.4?

Where does the number 299 792 458 come from? To understand this, we need to be aware that the metre is one of the seven base units that have been agreed on by scientists internationally, while other units are defined in terms of these seven. (Another base unit relevant here is the second, defined in terms of the vibrations of a caesium-133 atom.)

In 1983, it was decided that the distance light travels in a vacuum in this very tiny fraction of a second would be the new definition of a metre. This means that light is *defined* as travelling at a speed of 299 792 458 metres per second, the speed also of all electromagnetic waves in a vacuum. The speed is given the symbol c, and we can say that:

$$\textbf{distance} \quad = \quad c \quad \times \quad \textbf{time of light flight}$$
$$\text{(m)} \qquad \text{(m s}^{-1}) \qquad\qquad \text{(s)}$$

This is a use of the familiar formula:

$$\textbf{distance = speed} \times \textbf{time}$$

$$x = v \times t$$

An air traffic controller plotting the movement of an aircraft several tens of kilometres away is making more direct use of the light–distance relationship. This is because the distance of the aircraft is measured by radar waves with a 'time of flight' to the aircraft and back that is accurately measured using a quartz clock.

SCIENCE
IN CONTEXT

EXAMPLE

Q An air traffic controller uses a radar rangefinder and measures a time of 0.48 ms (0.000 48 s) for a radar pulse to go to and return from an aircraft. How far away is the aircraft in metres?

A Assuming that the radar pulse takes the same time to go out as to come back, the aircraft must be at a distance of 0.24 light-milliseconds.

Distance in metres = c × time of light-flight

$$= 2.997\,924\,58 \times 10^8 \times 0.24 \times 10^{-3}$$

$$= 7.2 \times 10^4\,\text{m}$$

Note that the limit on the accuracy of this measurement allows us to give the final answer to only two significant figures. In practice, radar range-finders can do a lot better than that. But for most exercises in this book you can take the value of c to be $3.00 \times 10^8\,\text{m s}^{-1}$.

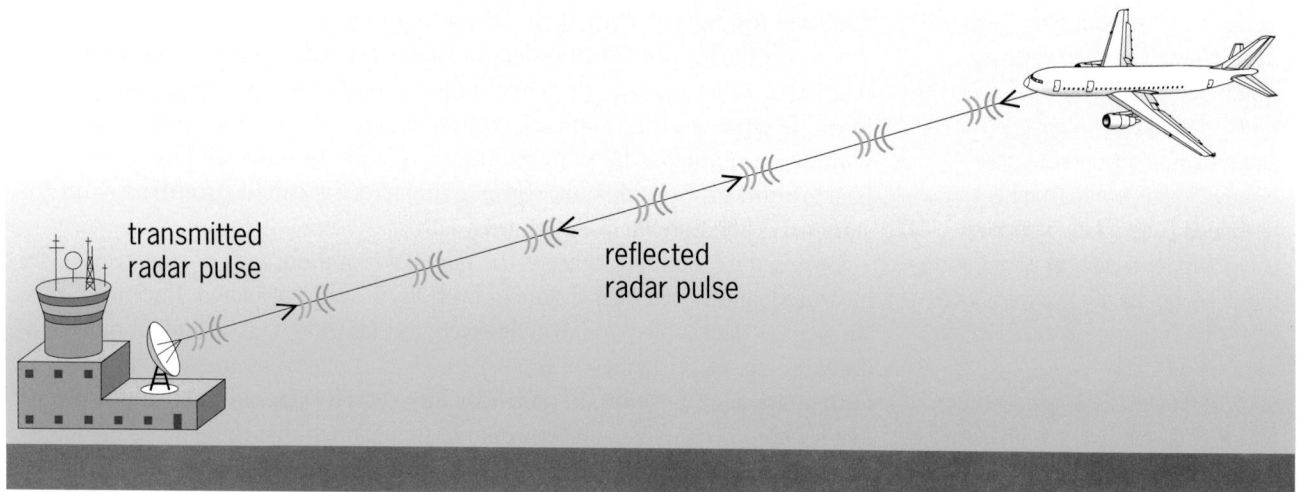

transmitted radar pulse

reflected radar pulse

Fig 1.5 Radar ranging: the time of flight of the radar pulses is measured and converted to kilometres by air traffic control

Fig 1.6 Surveying by triangulation. The angles measured from an accurately known base line will 'fix' points X and Y

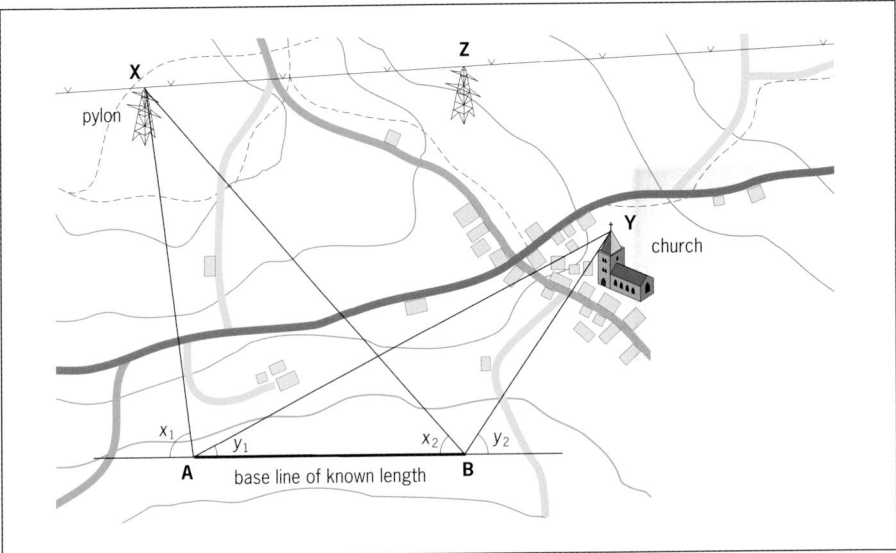

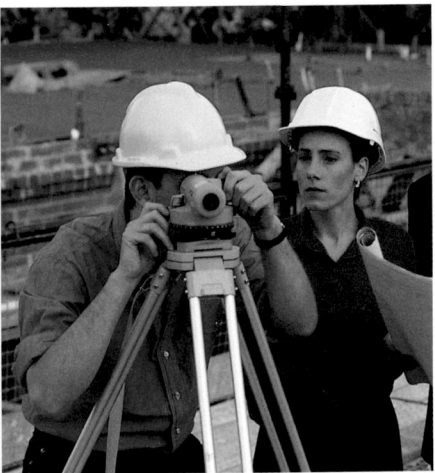

Fig 1.7 Surveyors use a laser instrument to measure distances. The instrument calculates a distance from the time a pulse travels to and from an object

 REMEMBER THIS

The letters in the word laser stand for **l**ight **a**mplification by **s**timulated **e**mission of **r**adiation, and those in radar for **ra**dio **d**irection **a**nd **r**anging.

? QUESTIONS 2–4

2   You set your watch by the radio time signal. If the broadcasting aerial is 50 km away, how 'slow' is your watch because of the finite speed of light? Should this bother you?

3   Outline some advantages and disadvantages of measuring distances such as the following using light (or radar): **a)** from Earth to the Moon, **b)** the thickness of a layer of paint on a car body, **c)** the width of a room.

4   Look at Fig 1.6. Give a reason why the objects at X and Y were used for surveying. Why was the pylon at Z not used?

MAPPING WITH LIGHT
Triangulation

Making modern maps of places on Earth involves the surveying technique called **triangulation**. This is carried out either on the ground or by using survey satellites. The technique relies on two of the properties of light:

● Light beams travel in straight lines
● Light travels at a known speed

Triangulation is a technique that was used, and probably invented, by the Ancient Egyptians. Simple triangulation needs a **base line** of carefully measured length (AB in Fig 1.6). Two distant objects (X and Y) are chosen. The angle each object makes with the base line is measured from each end of the base line. Then the distances to the objects are found using simple trigonometry. Nowadays a laser surveying instrument (Fig 1.7) measures a distance in light-seconds and converts this measurement into metres.

The accuracy of maps made using triangulation depends on very reliable clocks. Angles are also measured with great accuracy, but cannot be measured as exactly as light-times. However, a long base line increases accuracy, and accurate maps are based on lines many kilometres long.

How far away are the stars?

Stars are too far away for their distances to be measured using a base line drawn on Earth. But astronomers noticed that some stars appeared to move relative to other stars as the Earth moved round the Sun. They concluded that this effect was the same as you see when you move in front of a window: a point on the window frame appears to move against the background of more distant objects. This effect is called **parallax**, and for stars it is called stellar parallax (Fig 1.8).

During the nineteenth century, the parallaxes of thousands of stars were measured, and hence their distances from Earth were calculated. But many stars showed no detectable parallax. They were too far away for the annual motion of the Earth across a distance of 3×10^{11} metres to make any measurable difference to their apparent position. In particular there was a class of bright cloudy objects that showed no parallax, and astronomers concluded that these objects (called nebulae, the Latin for 'clouds') must be on the fringes of the Universe. Measurements on this scale, which helped reveal the expansion of the Universe, are described in Chapter 26.

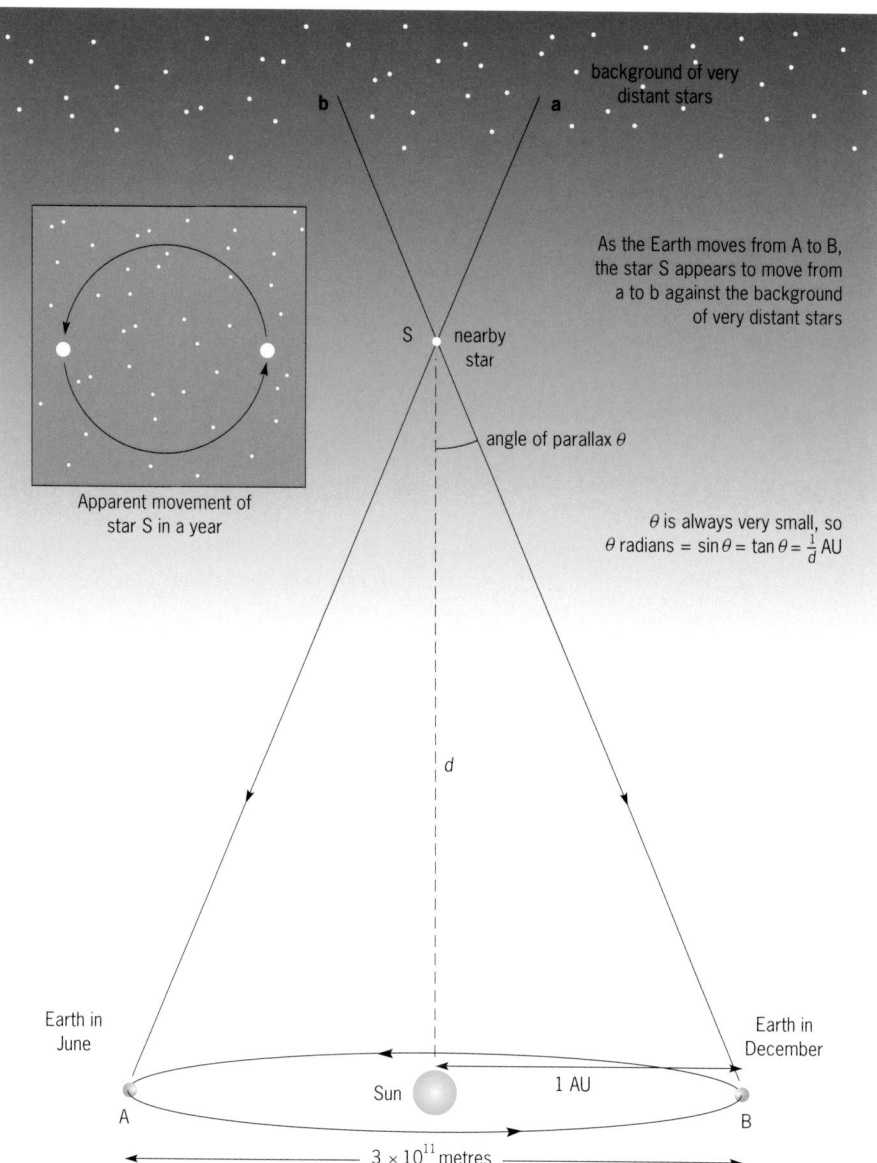

Fig 1.8 Stellar parallax, due to the motion of Earth round the Sun

As the Earth moves from A to B, the star S appears to move from a to b against the background of very distant stars

θ is always very small, so
θ radians $= \sin \theta = \tan \theta = \frac{1}{d}$ AU

2 KINEMATICS: SPEED AND ACCELERATION

Electromagnetic waves such as light and radio waves can be used to measure *speed* as well as distance. Police radar (radio) devices use the **Doppler effect** to measure the speed of a vehicle. This is the effect:

> **A signal is directed from a stationary source towards an object that is moving relative to the source. Then, the signal reflected from the moving object has a different wavelength, and hence a different frequency, from the source signal.**

For example, when an object is moving at constant speed away from the source of a signal, each wave (or pulse) has to travel a distance further than the previous wave to catch up with the moving object. A reflected wave then has a longer journey back to the source than the previous wave. This makes the reflected waves more 'spread out' – their wavelength is longer, and hence their frequency is lower, than the source frequency. The reverse happens when the reflecting object is moving towards the source.

REMEMBER THIS

The **frequency** of a wave is the number of times the wave pattern repeats itself in a second. Its **wavelength** is the distance between equivalent points from one wave pattern to the next. The **speed** of the wave is related to the frequency and wavelength:

wave speed
= frequency × wavelength

each is a wavelength

wave pattern (one wave)

Distance

Fig 1.9 The Doppler effect – the effect on radar waves directed at a vehicle **(a)** moving away from the source, **(b)** moving towards it. (Remember that the speed of all signals is *c*, the speed of light)

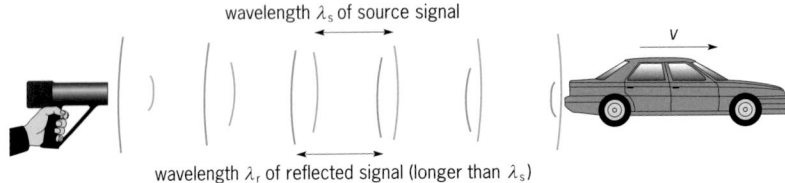

wavelength λ_s of source signal

wavelength λ_r of reflected signal (longer than λ_s)

(a) Car moving *away* from transmitter: reflected frequency is *less* than transmitted signal

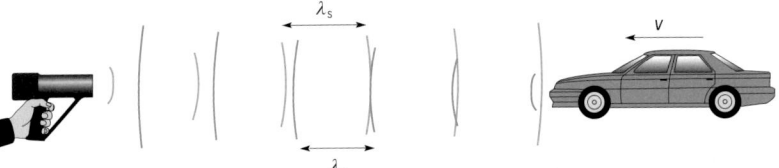

λ_s

λ_r

(b) Car moving *towards* transmitter: reflected frequency is *greater* than transmitted signal

Fig 1.10 The display on the instrument indicates whether the vehicle is speeding or not

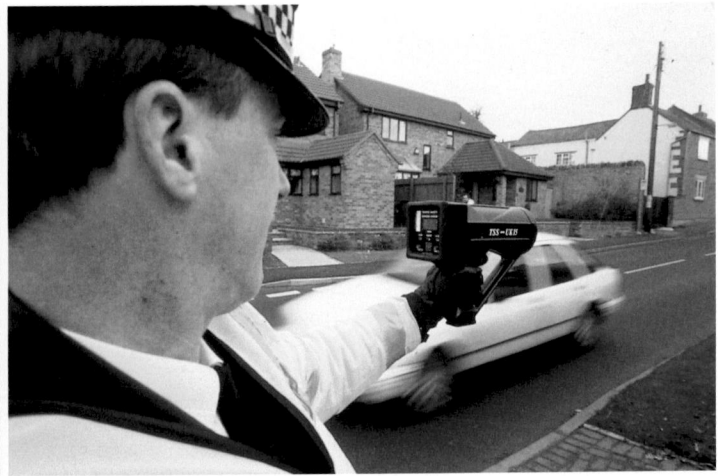

Fig 1.9 illustrates the Doppler effect for a radar signal. In (a), the wavelength of the reflected signal is longer, and the frequency lower, than that of the source signal, and in (b), with the car moving towards the source, the wavelength is shorter, and the frequency higher. The radar device used by the police measures the *difference* in frequency between the transmitted and the received signals and displays the speed of the vehicle on a screen in miles per hour (see Fig 1.10).

In the simple case when only the reflecting object is moving (such as when the speed of a vehicle is being recorded), the following formula is the basis for calculating the speed *v* of the object:

$$\Delta f = \frac{2fv}{c}$$

where Δf is the change in frequency of the radar signal and *c* the speed of light. (See Chapter 6 for a full derivation of this formula for the Doppler effect.)

SCIENCE IN CONTEXT

EXAMPLE

Q A police radar speed detector instrument uses a frequency of 10^{10} Hz. It measures a Doppler frequency change of 600 Hz when it is pointed at a moving car.

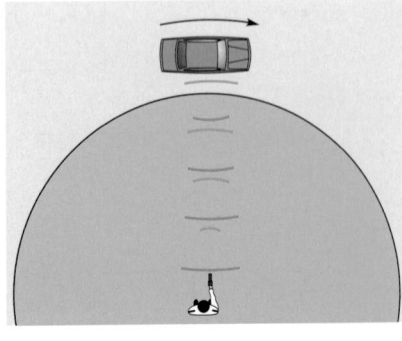

a) What speed is shown by the detector?
b) This may not be the true speed of the car. Explain why.

A

a) Using the simple Doppler formula, $\Delta f = 2fv/c$, we get:

$$600 = 10^{10} \times \frac{2v}{c}$$

So: $v = \dfrac{600 \times 3.00 \times 10^8}{2 \times 10^{10}}$

$= 9 \text{ m s}^{-1}$

Fig 1.11 Movement of a vehicle at right angles to a radar beam

b) This will be the true speed only if the direction of the radar beam is the same as the actual direction of motion of the car. At any other angle, the true speed will be greater than the measured speed. For example, if the car were moving at right angles to the beam, the speed reading would be zero, as shown in Fig 1.11 (the transmitted and reflected frequencies are the same).

SPEED FROM DISTANCE AND TIME

The simplest way to measure speed in the laboratory and in everyday life is to measure how far an object travels in a measured time:

$$\text{speed} = \frac{\text{distance moved}}{\text{time taken}}$$

in m s^{-1} or km h^{-1}, for example.

Short times can be measured, for example, using an electronic clock stopped and started by a light gate. Computers have internal clocks running at a high rate, say 1 GHz (10^9 'ticks' per second). This allows them to measure time between input signals to a high degree of accuracy – a billionth of a second. Computers coupled with some kind of sensor are very useful for the analysis of motion and any rapidly changing physical event. Speed in longer journeys may need only the accuracy of a stopwatch (to the nearest minute, second or tenth of a second). Distances are measured by metre rules, tape measures or from maps.

ACCELERATION

The police are not usually interested in measuring the **acceleration** of the car – although car manufacturers are. Acceleration of a car is a measure of how quickly its velocity changes with time:

$$\text{acceleration} = \frac{\text{change in velocity}}{\text{time for velocity to change}}$$

in *(metres per second) per second*, written as m s^{-2}.

Expressed as a formula using standard symbols:

$$a = \frac{v_1 - v_0}{t} \qquad [1]$$

where v_0 is the *initial* velocity (at the start of timing) and v_1 is the velocity t seconds later.

3 THE EQUATIONS OF MOTION

Real objects tend to move in quite complicated ways. It is better to start with the simplest possible cases and build in the complications later. We start by considering objects that move *steadily*, in a *straight line*. We deal here with the motion of objects that move at constant speeds or with constant (or *uniform*) accelerations. This is of course a very common kind of motion – for example, falling objects tend to move with a constant acceleration of 9.8 m s^{-2}.

We can describe this kind of motion by using graphs and by the *equations of motion*.

GRAPHS OF MOTION

The equations of motion (kinematic equations) can be derived most easily by analysing the graphs that illustrate the motion.

Moving at a constant speed (zero acceleration)

Graph A in Fig 1.12(a) overleaf illustrates an object moving at a steady speed. It is a **distance–time** graph. It is a straight line with a constant slope, showing that the object covers the *same* extra distance Δx in equal extra intervals of time Δt.

Speed is defined as the rate at which distance changes with respect to time. In Graph A, the object covers 5 m in any given second: its speed is 5 *metres per second* (5 m s^{-1}). In general:

$$\textbf{speed } v = \frac{\Delta x}{\Delta t}$$

Graphs of motion can be plotted using a spreadsheet. For more on this please see the How Science Works assignment for this chapter at www.collinseducation.co.uk/CAS

Fig 1.12(a) Graphs for a moving object

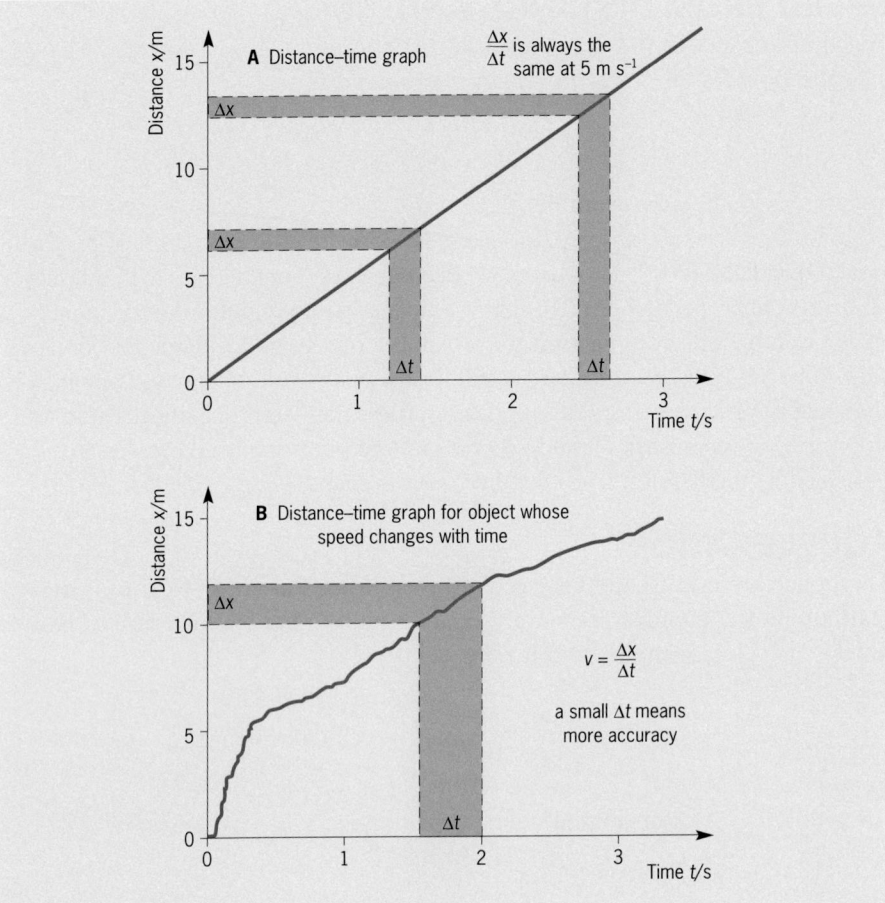

The quantity $\Delta x/\Delta t$ is the **slope** (or **tangent**) of the graph. This ratio will always give us the speed, even if the graph is not a straight line. But if the speed is changing rapidly with time as in **Graph B**, we have to make Δt very small to get an accurate result.

But in Graph A, and in Graph C of Fig 1.12(b) below, $\Delta x/\Delta t$ doesn't change with time, and so we can use the simpler equation:

$$v = \frac{x}{t} \text{ or } x = vt \qquad [2]$$

In everyday situations, such as making a long journey by car, it makes sense to consider v as an *average* speed. Drivers make an experienced guess that they can manage an average speed of, say, 80 km per hour, and so will cover 400 km in five hours' driving.

✔ REMEMBER THIS

The idea of making values like Δt very small is the basis of calculus. The equations of motion may be derived using calculus, as shown on page 19.

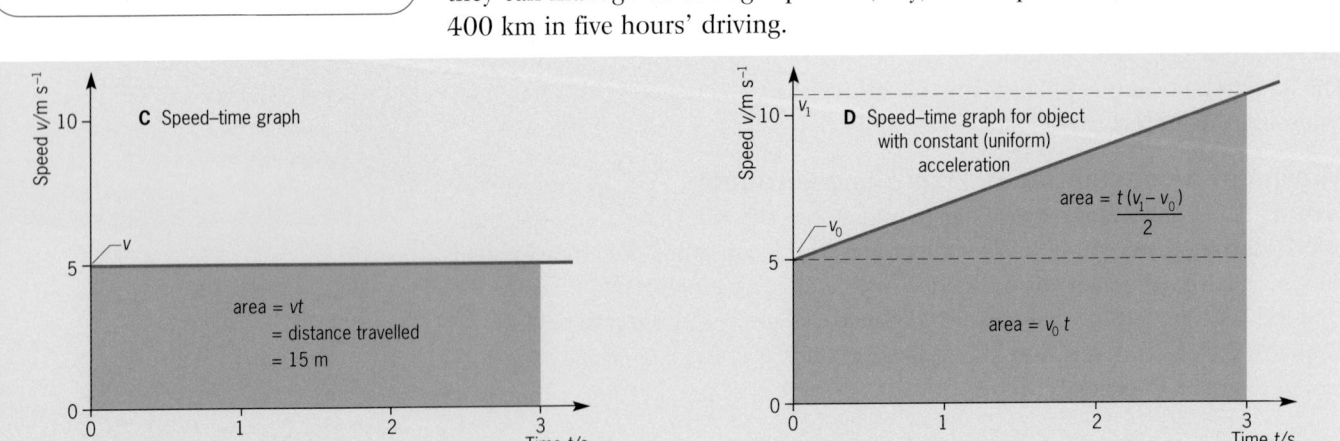

Fig 1.12(b) More graphs for a moving object

Graph C is a **speed–time** graph for movement of the object in Graph A. It shows a constant value for v. It also gives us an insight into a very useful rule:

The area between the graph line and the time axis tells us the distance travelled during any interval of time.

So the coloured area on the graph is the quantity vt (in this example, 15 metres, the distance travelled in 3 seconds at a speed of $5 \, \mathrm{m \, s^{-1}}$).

This rule works whatever the shape of the graph, however, and is useful in analysing the consequences of a changing speed, as shown in Graph B.

Moving with uniform acceleration

Graph D in Fig 1.12(b) is a **speed–time** graph for an object whose speed increases steadily with time. In other words, it is moving with a **constant (uniform) acceleration**.

The speed at the start of timing is v_0, and after t seconds it has become v_1. We often want to know what the speed v_1 of an object will be after a period of acceleration. Rearranging the defining equation 1 above for acceleration gives:

$$\text{speed after acceleration } v_1 = v_0 + at \qquad [3]$$

A graph of acceleration against time would be a straight line parallel to the time axis – showing that acceleration stays the same as time goes on.

EQUATIONS FOR CALCULATING DISTANCE TRAVELLED, x

We can use Graph D to obtain a formula for the distance travelled by an accelerating object in a time t. To do this we apply the rule that the distance travelled in time t equals the relevant area under the graph.

Graph D consists of a rectangle topped by a triangle. The area of the rectangle is $v_0 t$, where v_0 is the speed when $t = 0$ (the *initial* speed).

The area of the triangle is $\frac{1}{2}(v_1 - v_0)t$, so the equation for the total distance x travelled in time t is:

$$\text{distance} = \text{total area under graph}$$

$$x = v_0 t + \tfrac{1}{2}(v_1 - v_0)t \qquad [4]$$

This awkward bit of algebra can be rearranged to make more sense, to become:

$$x = \tfrac{1}{2}(v_0 + v_1)t \qquad [5]$$

which can be read simply as:

distance covered = average speed $\times$ time

This formula is useful if we happen to know the values of v_0 and v_1. In practice, we often know *either* v_0 *or* v_1, and the acceleration a.

? QUESTIONS 5–7

5   Estimate your average speed for your journey to school or college.

6   Think about the journey you make going to school or college. Sketch a rough distance–time graph of this journey. Label the key features and the time and place at which you are travelling at the greatest speed.

7   How long would a car take to increase its speed from $8 \, \mathrm{m \, s^{-1}}$ to $24 \, \mathrm{m \, s^{-1}}$ at a constant acceleration of $3.2 \, \mathrm{m \, s^{-2}}$?

1 Moving in space and time

8 **a)** A small boy lets go of a tyre and it rolls down a hill. It accelerates at $3\,\text{m s}^{-2}$. How far does it travel in 8 s?
b) The boy tries to run alongside it. His maximum speed is $4\,\text{m s}^{-1}$. How far does he run before the tyre runs away from him?

9 Sketch the speed–time graph you would expect for an object thrown vertically upwards. Label its main features.

When final speed v_1 is not known

We have seen that a is defined in terms of v_0, v_1 and t, as in equation 1:

$$a = \frac{v_1 - v_0}{t}$$

which can be rearranged to give:

$$v_1 - v_0 = at$$

Substituting for $(v_1 - v_0)$ in equation 4 above gives:

$$x = v_0 t + \tfrac{1}{2}at^2 \qquad [6]$$

When acceleration a is not known

Another way of looking at this situation is by using *average* speed. Where the acceleration is constant, we can assume an overall speed that is the *average* of the initial and final speeds. Then we can use equation 5:

$$\text{distance} = \text{average speed} \times \text{time}$$

or:
$$x = \tfrac{1}{2}(v_0 + v_1)t$$

When time t is not known

Finally, it would be useful to have a formula that allows us to make calculations when we have no information about the time during which speed (velocity) changes occur. This formula can be obtained by substituting for t. Rearranging equation 1 gives:

$$t = \frac{v_1 - v_0}{a}$$

Inserting this expression for t into equation 6 gives:

$$x = v_0 \left(\frac{v_1 - v_0}{a}\right) + \tfrac{1}{2}a \left(\frac{v_1 - v_0}{a}\right)^2$$

Check yourself that this simplifies to:

$$v_1^2 - v_0^2 = 2ax \qquad [7]$$

EXAMPLE

Q A hawk is hovering above a field at a height of 50 metres.
It sees a mouse directly below it and dives vertically with an acceleration of $9\,\text{m s}^{-2}$.

a) At what speed will it be travelling just before it reaches the ground?
b) How long does it take to reach the ground?

A
a) We need to calculate the final speed v_1. We know the distance, the initial velocity and the acceleration. As we don't know the time of travel, equation 7 applies here: $v_1^2 - v_0^2 = 2ax$. The initial velocity v_0 of the

hawk, relative to the ground, is zero, so:

$$v_1^2 - 0 = 2 \times 9 \times 50 = 900$$

and $v_1 = 30\,\text{m s}^{-1}$

b) Any equation that includes t (except for equation 2, zero acceleration) could be used here, but equation 3, $v_1 = v_0 + at$, is simplest:

$$30 = 0 + (9 \times t)$$

giving $t = 3.3\,\text{s}$

Note that the answer can only be approximate. The physics is likely to be a simplification of the real situation – hawks don't fly that precisely!

DECELERATION

Deceleration is a slowing down: it is a *negative* acceleration.

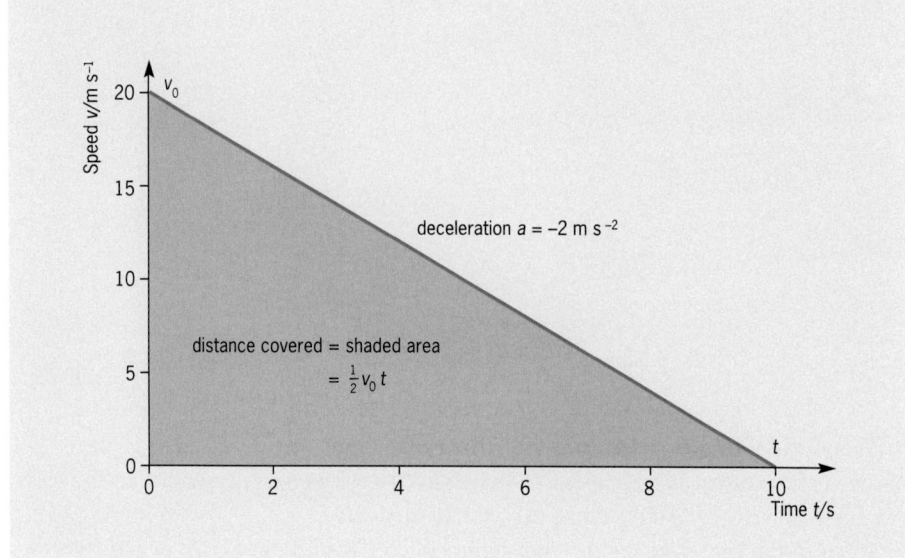

Fig 1.13 Graph of uniform deceleration. Check that the area under the graph represents a distance of 100 m

The graph in Fig 1.13 is for an object that decelerates uniformly to a stop. As before, the area of the triangle gives the distance travelled. The equations of motion still apply, but you have to be careful with the *signs*. The positive and negative signs are part of the *numbers* we put into the formulae. Suppose that the initial speed is 20 m s^{-1}, and the deceleration (negative acceleration) is -2 m s^{-2}. To calculate how far the object will travel in 10 seconds, using equation 6 we write:

$$\text{distance travelled } x = v_0 t + \tfrac{1}{2}at^2$$

$$x = (20 \times 10) + [0.5 \times (-2) \times (10)^2]$$

$$= 200 - 100$$

$$= 100 \text{ m}$$

4 FRAMES OF REFERENCE

HOW FAST ARE YOU TRAVELLING AT THE MOMENT?

The answer may seem to depend on whether you are reading this book on a train that is travelling at 140 km h^{-1}, a plane travelling at 1000 km h^{-1} or just sitting at your desk. *But in fact, as the question stands, it is meaningless.* Even if you are at your desk, both you and the desk are spinning with the Earth at a speed of just over 1000 km h^{-1} (if you are at the latitude of London). The Earth itself is moving in an orbit round the Sun at a speed of 107 000 km h^{-1}. The Sun, and its Solar System, are orbiting round the centre of the Galaxy at a speed of almost 1 000 000 km h^{-1}. You are not, of course, aware of any of these movements. The coffee in your cup is unshaken by these astronomical speeds. The question at the start of this section makes sense only when you add words such as 'relative to the room' or 'relative to the Earth' or 'relative to the Galactic centre'.

Fig 1.14 How fast would you say you are travelling?

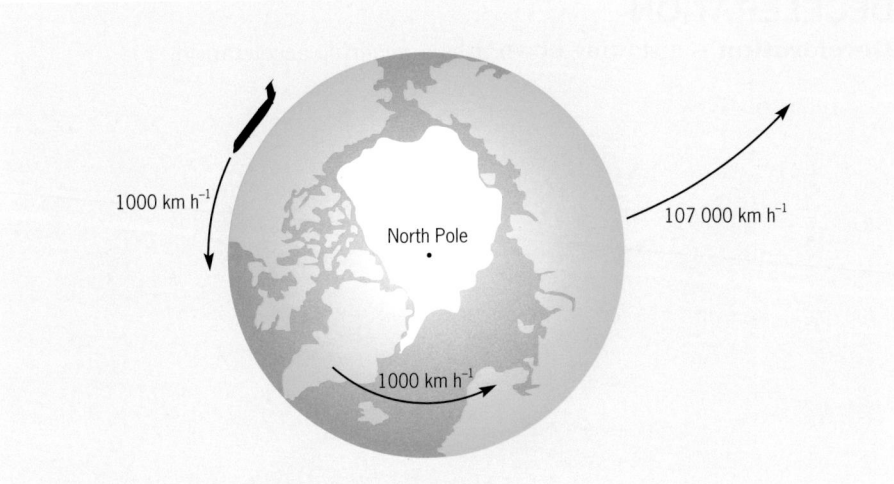

This is the **simple principle of relativity**, first stated by Galileo in the seventeenth century. His ideas of relativity were developed much further in the early twentieth century by Albert Einstein (see Chapter 23).

Much of the time we take our measurements relative to the Earth, which we assume to be still and our normal **frame of reference**. This phrase simply means that the measurements we make are with reference to our static selves and the fixed objects that surround us. So, when we measure in an experiment that a dynamics trolley is moving at 0.55 m s^{-1}, we take it for granted that this motion is relative to the walls, floor and laboratory bench. We don't keep asking ourselves, 'relative to what?' But we have some interesting problems to solve when our personal reference frame is moving relative to the Earth, as when it is a ship at sea, an aircraft in flight or a canoe on, say, a tidal river.

MOVING FRAMES OF REFERENCE

The equations of motion developed on pages 10–12 apply just as well inside an aircraft moving at speed relative to the Earth as they do for an object on the 'fixed' Earth itself.

? QUESTION 11

11 Someone says, 'The ultimate fixed point must be the centre of the Universe. Everything that moves must have a real velocity relative to that.' Do you agree with this statement? Is it likely to be of any practical use?

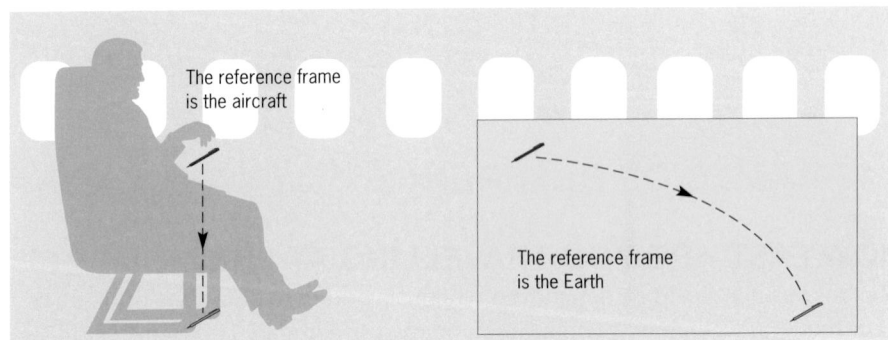

Fig 1.15 A pen dropped in an aircraft, as viewed from two frames of reference. When viewed from a different frame of reference, a straight line becomes a parabola

If you drop a pen to the floor of an aircraft (Fig 1.15) it will seem to you to move in exactly the same way as it does in your classroom on Earth. You don't need to take into account the fact that in the three-tenths of a second it takes to fall, the pen also moves forward a distance of a hundred metres or so. You too are moving forward at the same speed, so relative to you the pen falls straight downwards. You and the pen share the same reference frame – the aircraft. For both you and the pen, you could use the equation:

$$v = at$$

to calculate the speed of the pen when it hits the floor.

Galileo, who used a sailing ship as his example of a moving frame, was aware of relative motion. He needed this idea to explain why the Earth could move without our noticing its movement. But it seems to have been as hard for people in Galileo's time to understand that the Earth could possibly move without leaving behind everything on it – sea, ships, the air and flying birds – as it is for people today to grasp Einstein's theories of relativity!

? QUESTION 12

12 An airliner is travelling horizontally at 250 m s^{-1}. Someone drops a pen and it falls 0.8 m. How far from the dropping point does the pen reach the floor: **a)** relative to the airliner, **b)** relative to the Earth? Take acceleration of free fall as 10 m s^{-2}.

SCIENCE IN CONTEXT · **STRETCH AND CHALLENGE**

EXAMPLE

Q A canoe club plans a return trip on a river that flows at an average speed of 1.5 km h^{-1}. The canoeists will first paddle their canoes upstream for 6 km, then return. The leader estimates that the group can paddle at an average speed of 4.5 km h^{-1} on still water.

a) How long should the leader expect the trip to last, ignoring any stops for rest or refreshment?
b) What is the group's (expected) average speed for the journey?

A The leader must understand that the frame of reference is provided by the fixed Earth, with a map distance of 6 km each way for the trip.

a) Going upstream: The canoe speed relative to the water is 4.5 km h^{-1}, but relative to the river bank it is only 3 km h^{-1} (4.5 – 1.5).
$t = x/v = 6/3 = 2$ hours

So the group will take 2 hours of paddling time to reach their up-river destination.

Returning downstream: The distance is still 6 km, but now the speed relative to the bank is 6 km h^{-1} (4.5 + 1.5). The group should cover the distance in just 1 hour.

b) Therefore the total journey takes 3 hours. The canoeists travel 12 km at an average speed (relative to the solid Earth) of 4 km h^{-1}.

Fig 1.16 Canoeing up and down the river

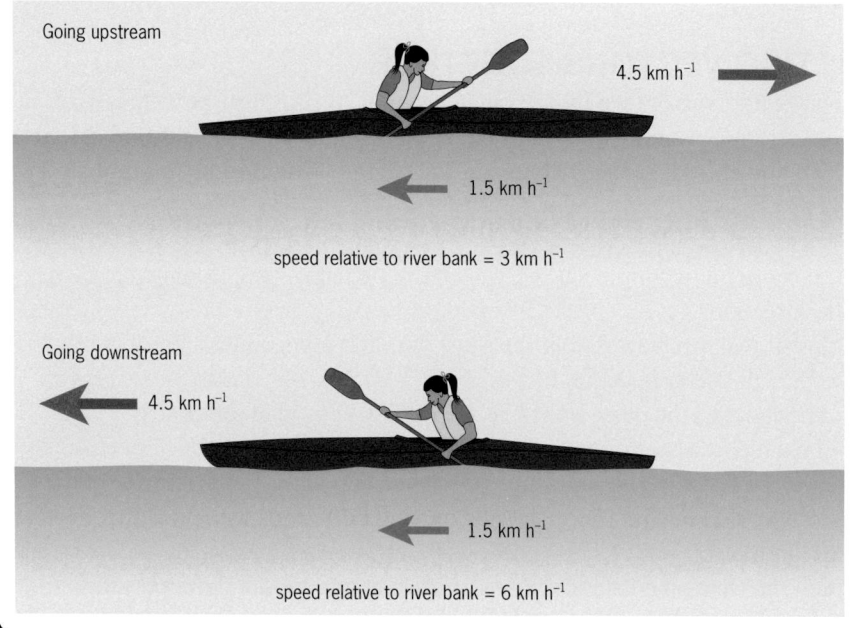

Going upstream
4.5 km h^{-1}
1.5 km h^{-1}
speed relative to river bank = 3 km h^{-1}

Going downstream
4.5 km h^{-1}
1.5 km h^{-1}
speed relative to river bank = 6 km h^{-1}

5 VECTORS

WHEN 2 + 2 DOES NOT EQUAL 4: THE IMPORTANCE OF VECTORS

As shown in Fig 1.17, if you move 2 metres to your right, and then 2 metres forwards, you have travelled 4 metres but are only 2.8 metres from where you started. This is an example of where 'how far you have travelled' is not the same as 'how far you are from where you started'.

Fig 1.17 Moving in two directions (vectors are represented by bold type)

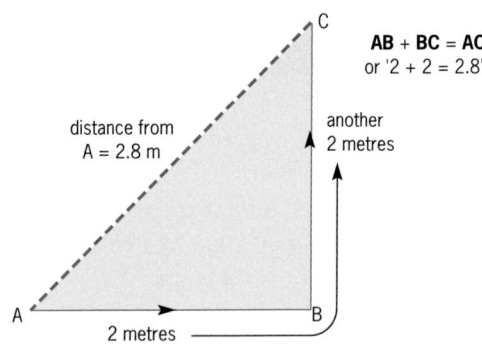

AB + **BC** = **AC**
or '2 + 2 = 2.8' !

distance from A = 2.8 m

another 2 metres

2 metres

Table 1.2 Some common vectors and scalars in physics	
Vectors	**Scalars**
displacement	frequency
velocity	speed
acceleration	mass
momentum	density
force	energy
current	charge
electric field	resistance

This is a fairly obvious example of the fact that some quantities in physics don't mean much unless you also specify a *direction* to go with them. For example, it is not very useful simply to tell friends that your house is 2 km from the station. This information isn't clear enough: as in Fig 1.18, to find your house they would have to search along the circumference of a circle 2 km in radius!

Quantities that need both a number and a direction to define them properly are called **vector quantities** (or **vectors**). Those that are useful without a direction being specified are called **scalar quantities** (or **scalars**). Table 1.2 lists some common vectors and scalars. Velocity is a vector; it refers to 'speed-in-a-given-direction'. Speed is useful, but only to describe the 'number' part of velocity. It is useful to know, for example, that the *speed* of a satellite in a circular orbit is constant, even though its *velocity* is constantly changing as the direction of travel changes. You will read more about satellite motion in Chapter 3.

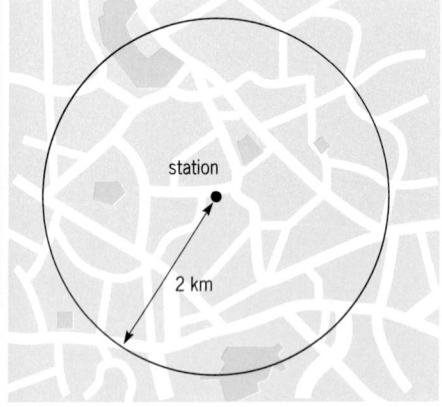

Fig 1.18 Distance alone is not enough: the circle maps the places that are 2 km from the station

station

2 km

PUTTING VECTORS TOGETHER

When we add vectors we have to take account of direction as well as size. If the directions are opposite and in the same straight line, we call one direction positive and the other negative, using the same convention as in graphs:

Going right is positive, going left is negative.

(In the canoeing example earlier, we used 'upstream' and 'downstream' to define directions.)

Think of two cars travelling in the same direction along a road, one at 30 km h^{-1}, the other at 50 km h^{-1}, as in Fig 1.19. It is obvious that the *speed* of one car relative to the other is 20 km h^{-1}. But if you were in the slow car, you would see the faster car overtake you at 20 km h^{-1}. From your (moving) frame of reference, the faster car has a relative velocity of +20 km h^{-1}. An observer in the faster car would see your car apparently moving backwards with a relative velocity of –20 km h^{-1}.

If the cars were on a collision course, travelling in opposite directions, their relative speeds would be 80 km h^{-1}.

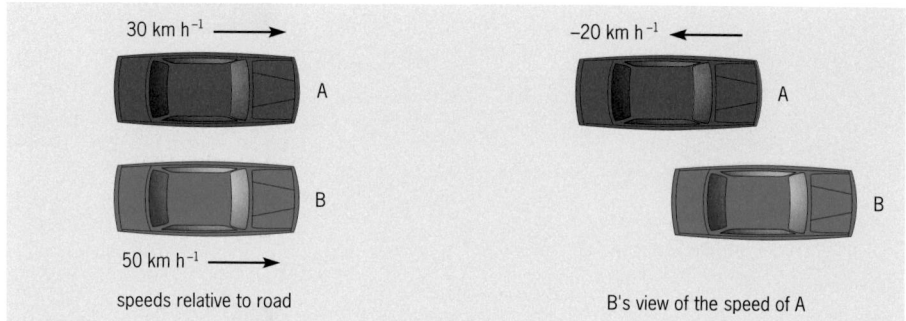

Fig 1.19 Relativity on the road

Again, think of throwing something from a moving vehicle. If it is thrown forwards with a speed of 10 km h^{-1} from a car moving with a speed of 30 km h^{-1}, it will be travelling at the even more dangerous speed of 40 km h^{-1} relative to a bystander.

THINGS MOVING AT AN ANGLE TO EACH OTHER

But how do we tackle predictions of movement when the important vectors are not in the same line? This is a problem that navigators have to deal with on water and in the air. Their vehicles may move in a medium that itself may be moving. There are usually tidal currents or winds. Suppose the canoeists in the Example on page 15 had to cross a wide estuary with a strong current of 3.0 km h^{-1}, as shown in Fig 1.20. How would this current affect their motion?

As Fig 1.20 shows, for every 4.5 units of distance they travel across the water, the current moves them downstream by 3 units. Relative to the banks of the estuary, they move along a path AC at a speed we can calculate to be 5.4 km h^{-1}, using Pythagoras' theorem. This path will *not* take them to their destination!

? **QUESTION 14**

14 A child passenger in a train rolls a ball along the floor at a speed of 5 m s^{-1}. The train is travelling at a speed of 35 m s^{-1}.
a) What other fact do you need to know to find out the speed of the ball relative to the rail track?
b) What is the range of possible values of this relative speed?

Fig 1.20 Carried along by the current

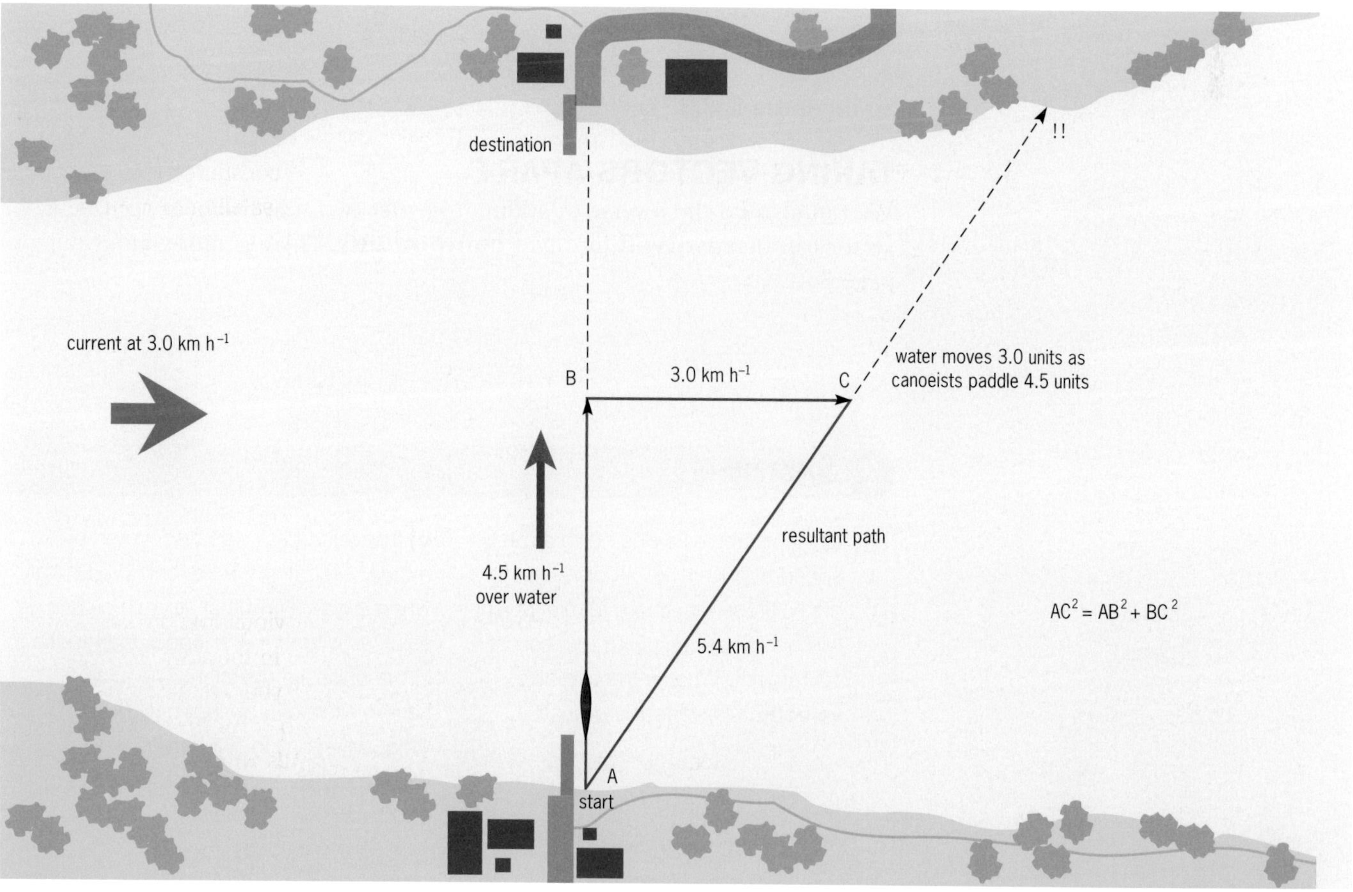

current at 3.0 km h^{-1}

destination

B 3.0 km h^{-1} C water moves 3.0 units as canoeists paddle 4.5 units

resultant path

4.5 km h^{-1} over water

5.4 km h^{-1}

$$AC^2 = AB^2 + BC^2$$

A
start

Fig 1.21 Calculating the required angle and velocity

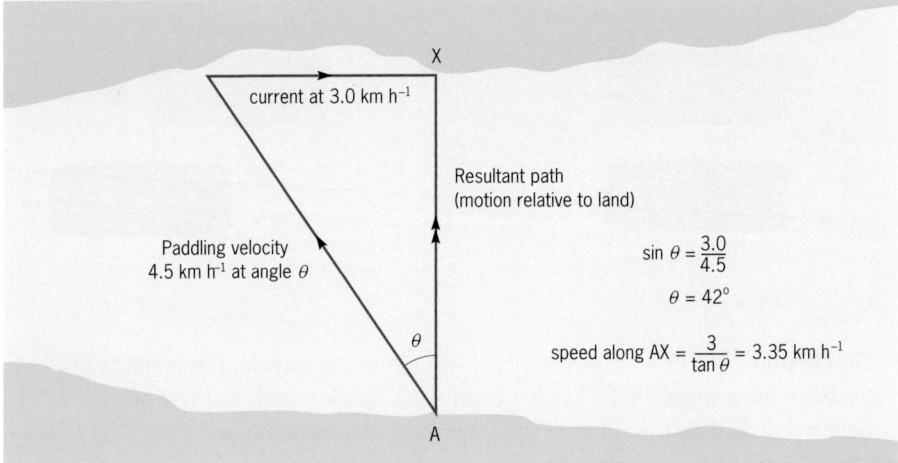

It would make more sense for the canoeists to head upstream at such an angle that the *combination* of their paddling velocity and the current velocity would lie on the path they want to move along. This combination is called the **resultant** velocity.

At what angle to the straight-across direction AX should they point the bows of the canoes? Fig 1.21 shows the situation. When the diagram is drawn to scale, it is possible to measure the angles and the value of the resultant. But it is usually quicker to use simple trigonometry to calculate the angle θ:

$$\sin \theta = \frac{3}{4.5} = 0.667$$

So:

$$\theta = 42°$$

The canoeists would travel along the line AX at a speed given by:

$$\tan \theta = \frac{3}{\text{speed}}$$

So the speed is 3.35 km h^{-1}.

TAKING VECTORS APART

We can also do the reverse of adding together two non-collinear vectors: a vector can be **resolved** into two **components**. There is more about this on page 34.

? QUESTION 15

15 **a)** An aircraft flies due north at an air speed of 500 km h^{-1}. It crosses the high altitude jet stream (of air) which is moving due east with a speed of 100 km h^{-1}. What is the aircraft's **velocity** relative to the ground?

b) The jet stream was discovered by military aircraft in the Second World War when it was found that Atlantic crossings east–west took much longer than those in the opposite direction. The aircraft has an air speed of about 400 km h^{-1}. What difference in flight times would you expect for transatlantic journeys of 6000 km?

The equations of motion using calculus

AN OBJECT MOVING AT CONSTANT SPEED

As shown in Graph A in Fig 1.22, an object is moving at a constant speed v, which is defined as the rate of change of distance with time:

$$v = \frac{dx}{dt}$$

or $$dx = v\, dt$$

In time t, it will have travelled a distance x. As the 'area under the graph' in Graph B, we can get x by integrating between the limits 0 and t:

$$\equiv dx = v \equiv dt$$

giving: $$x = vt + \text{constant} \quad [1]$$

If x was zero at the start of timing when $t = 0$, then the constant is zero and we have simply:

$$x = vt \quad [2]$$

ACCELERATED MOTION

Acceleration is the rate of change of velocity (Graph C), i.e.:

$$\frac{dv}{dt} = a$$

and so $$dv = a\, dt$$

This last equation can be integrated to relate velocity, acceleration and time:

$$\equiv dv = a \equiv dt$$
$$v = at + c \quad [3]$$

where c is a constant of integration. The physical meaning of c is that it is the velocity at time $t = 0$, so it is v_0. Also v, the velocity at time t, is v_1. So we now have the equation:

$$v_1 = v_0 + at \quad [4]$$

The equation relating distance to velocity, time and acceleration may be obtained by integrating equation 3, first putting the constant v_0 for the constant c:

$$v = at + v_0$$

i.e.: $$\frac{dx}{dt} = at + v_0$$

$$\left(\text{since } v = \frac{dx}{dt}\right)$$

So: $$\equiv dx = a \equiv t\, dt + v_0 \equiv dt$$

which comes to

$$x = a\frac{t^2}{2} + v_0 t + C$$

C is another constant of integration which represents the value of x at time $t = 0$. This is usually taken to be zero in everyday calculations, and the equation simplifies to equation 6 on page 12, namely $x = v_0 t + \frac{1}{2}at^2$.

Equation 7, $v_1^2 - v_0^2 = 2ax$, may be obtained by substitution as shown on page 12.

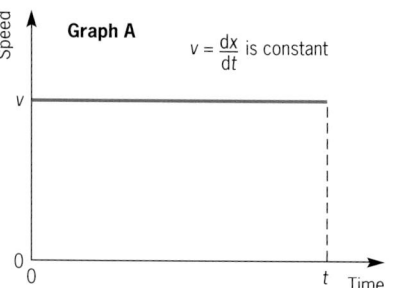

Graph A

$v = \frac{dx}{dt}$ is constant

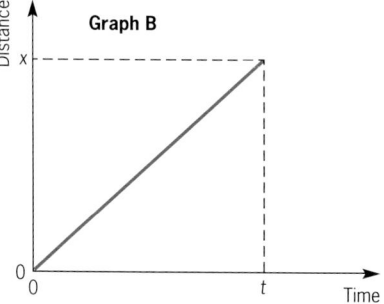

Graph B

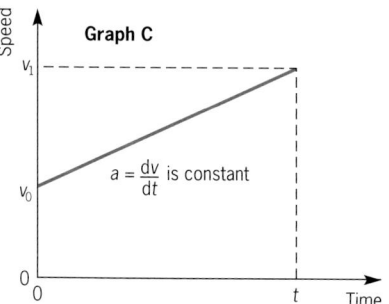

Graph C

$a = \frac{dv}{dt}$ is constant

Fig 1.22

SUMMARY

This chapter should help you to understand a number of ideas and acquire several numerical skills. Having studied it, you should:

- Understand that distance can be measured in units of time (seconds) as well as in units of distance such as metres and kilometres.
- Know that the speed of light, c, is fundamental to the measurement of distance.
- Know that measured motion is always relative to an agreed frame of reference.
- Be able to analyse distance–time and speed–time graphs.
- Be able to use the equations of motion of an object moving in a straight line with uniform acceleration.
- Know the difference between vector and scalar quantities.
- Be able to use vector diagrams and/or trigonometry to analyse vector motion.
- Understand the basic principles of triangulation.
- Know the equations of motion listed in the column on the right.
- Understand how the physics in this chapter is useful in everyday contexts, such as Satellite Navigation and Air Traffic Control.

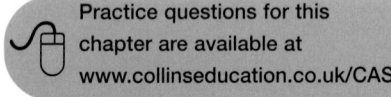

Practice questions for this chapter are available at www.collinseducation.co.uk/CAS

For motion at a constant speed (or an average speed):

distance = (average) speed × time
$$x = vt$$

For uniform (steady) acceleration:

a) acceleration = $\dfrac{\text{change in velocity}}{\text{time taken to change}}$

$$a = \frac{v_1 - v_0}{t} \quad \text{or} \quad a = \frac{\Delta v}{\Delta t}$$

which is often written as

$$v_1 = v_0 + at$$

b) distance covered = average speed × time

$$x = \frac{v_1 + v_0}{2}\, t$$

which is equivalent to:

$$x = v_0 t + \tfrac{1}{2}at^2$$

c) When t is unknown, use

$$v_1{}^2 - v_0{}^2 = 2ax$$

For non-uniform motion:
We need to deal in small changes:

$$\Delta x = v\Delta t, \quad \text{or} \quad v = \frac{dx}{dt} \text{ in calculus notation,}$$

$$\Delta v = a\Delta t, \quad \text{or} \quad a = \frac{dv}{dt} \text{ in calculus notation.}$$

2

Newton's universe

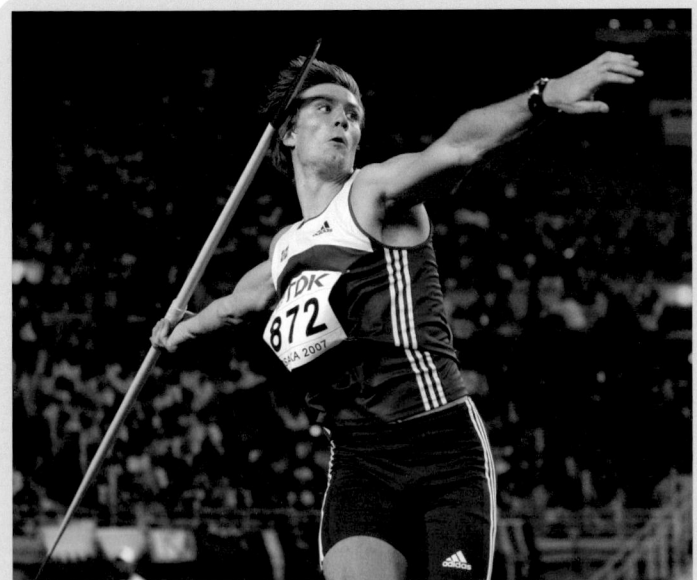

Andreas Thorkildsen, Norwegian gold medallist in the 2004 Athens Olympics, launches the javelin

A throw too far

As a weapon of war the javelin is over 5000 years old. For reasons that might puzzle a visiting Martian, the javelin is still around nowadays and has even been made more efficient. The modern javelin, used only in athletics stadiums, is a tightly controlled artefact: for the men's event it must be between 2.60 and 2.70 metres long and have a smallest mass of 800 g. It must be made so that its centre of mass is in precisely the right place. Javelins fly, not as well as aircraft, but they experience 'lift' and 'drag' for the same physical reasons. The basic physics is that of a mass hurled at an angle to the ground and then acted upon by gravity so that it moves in an (approximately) parabolic path. The bigger the lift force and the smaller the drag force the longer the javelin stays in flight and the further it goes.

In the 1908 Olympics the winning throw was just over 50 m. By 1984 (in a non-Olympic event) it had become 104.8 m – which was just about the length of a typical stadium. The athletics authorities quickly recognised the danger to spectators and brought in rules for a new design of javelin. They simply altered the position of the centre of mass of the javelin. The angle that the javelin makes as it flies is decided by a trade-off between weight (acting through the centre of mass) and lift (acting through a point decided by the shape of the javelin). In the old-style javelin, at the start of the throw, the lift force acted in front of the gravity force and the javelin tilted upwards. This increased the 'angle of attack' – and so the lift force – and made the javelin fly further.

The new design pushed the centre of mass 4 cm forward. This means that the lift acts at a point *behind* its weight. The javelin keeps its 'nose' down and there is a smaller lift force. It doesn't travel so far – and incidentally stands a better chance of sticking in the ground. As the graph shows, javelin throwing is one of the few Olympic sports in which the 'record' gets worse with time!

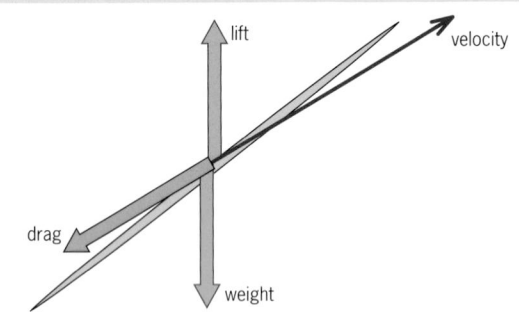

The old javelin flew in such a way that at the start of a standard throw, directed about 30° to the ground, the shaft made an angle of about 7° to its direction of movement

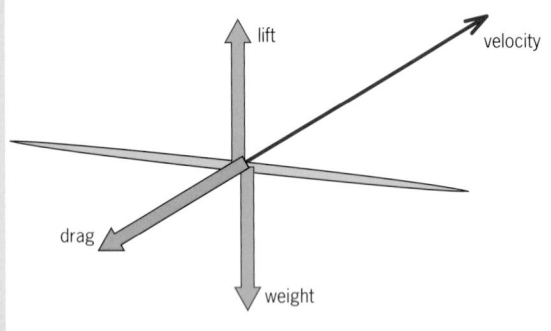

For the same upward throw, the new javelin flies nose downwards

How the Olympic javelin record has changed since 1908

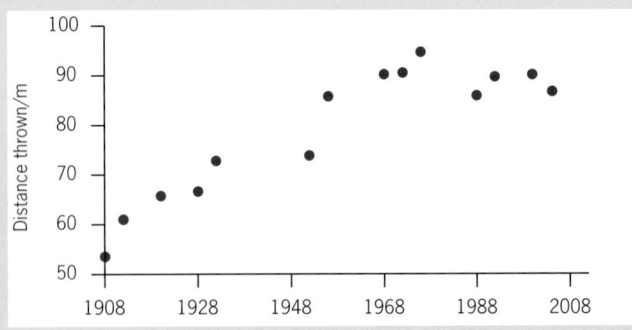

The ideas in this chapter

The ideas of **force** and **gravity** are fundamental to understanding the behaviour of objects on Earth. Objects will only start or stop moving if a force is acting on them. Gravity is a force which acts on every object. For example, if you throw a ball into the air, the force of your throw makes it move upwards. The force of gravity then causes the ball to fall back downwards.

These ideas were not fully understood by scientists until the time of Isaac Newton, over 300 years ago. In this chapter we explain Newton's theories, and then in Chapter 3 we look at some of the ways in which an understanding of forces has been used in science and engineering to transform the world we live in.

1 NEWTON'S LAWS

Suppose you roll a ball along the ground. It soon begins to slow down and eventually stops. Right from the time of Aristotle, over 300 years BC, up until Newton's time, everybody believed that this was the natural way for objects to behave. Newton showed that this belief, which had been accepted for two thousand years, was wrong. He showed that there was a force acting – the force of friction – which causes the ball to slow down. Without

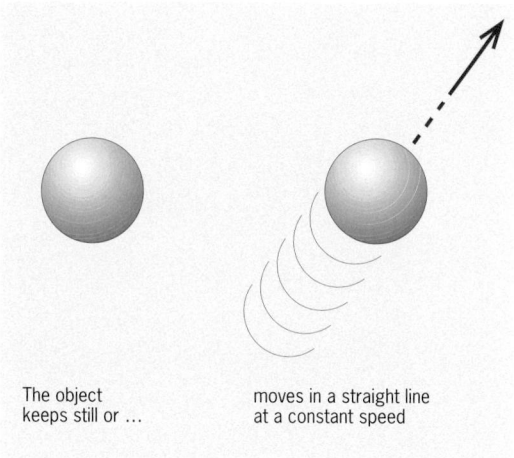

The object keeps still or …   moves in a straight line at a constant speed

Fig 2.1 Newton's imaginary, (almost) empty universe

this force, the ball would carry on, without slowing down.

Newton first of all considered an imaginary universe with just one object in it, as in Fig 2.1. This object will stay still (be 'at rest') or, if it is moving, carry on moving in a straight line at a steady speed, for ever.

It is this simple idea that led Newton to develop the fundamental laws of physics. It is a part of **Newton's first law of motion** – see the Stretch and Challenge passage on page 25. But of course our real Universe is not this simple. If it were, how could we tell if the object was moving or not? Or if it moved in a straight line? And who or where would 'we' be to ask the questions or make sense of the answers? When you do try to answer these questions you will be following closely in the footsteps of Albert Einstein – see Chapter 23.

But let us ignore these questions for now, and return to Newton. He went on to put something else in his imaginary universe: a force. If the object changes its motion in any way, by starting to move, by accelerating or slowing down, or by changing its direction of motion, then a **force must have acted on it**. This effect produced by a force defines what a force *is*, in Newton's world, and this idea completes his first law.

But where would this force come from? There must be something else in Newton's primitive universe, a 'force-causing' object or system of some kind. So far, all this seems fairly obvious – to us at least. But then Newton went on to say something really unexpected. He said that if the first object was acted

? QUESTION 1

1   You throw a ball across a field. Draw a diagram to show the ball half-way in its flight. Use labelled arrows to show any forces acting on the ball. Explain briefly the origin or cause of the force or forces you have drawn.

? QUESTIONS 2–4

2 A book lying on a table is at rest.
   a) Draw a diagram showing the sizes and directions of the forces acting on the book.
   b) One of these forces is due to gravity and, like all forces, must be one of a pair. What is the other force and on what does it act?

3 A rope is tied to a large box and pulled. You know that a force is acting on the box but observe that it doesn't move. What can you deduce from this observation?

4 What pairs of forces are involved in the following situations?
   a) A tennis ball is hit by a tennis racket.
   b) A ball is dropped but has not yet reached the ground.
   c) You start moving by taking a step forwards.

For more information on Galileo please see the How Science Works assignment for this chapter at www.collinseducation.co.uk/CAS

upon by a force, then the other 'force-causing' object must also have a force acting on it. Forces can only exist in pairs ('force' and 'antiforce'). The pair of forces must be equal in size, but act in opposite directions (Fig 2.2). This idea was expressed in the **third law of motion**.

Newton's imaginary universe was not just a science fiction story. It was based on observations made by Newton and many other scientists (see Galileo's ideas in Fig 2.3 for example). Although the basic idea might seem obvious to us, we must realise that at the time it was much more difficult to measure movement than it is now. It was a world without fuel-driven engines that move cars and trains and raise aircraft from the ground. There were no speedometers, and measurements of distance and time were, by our standards, very inaccurate.

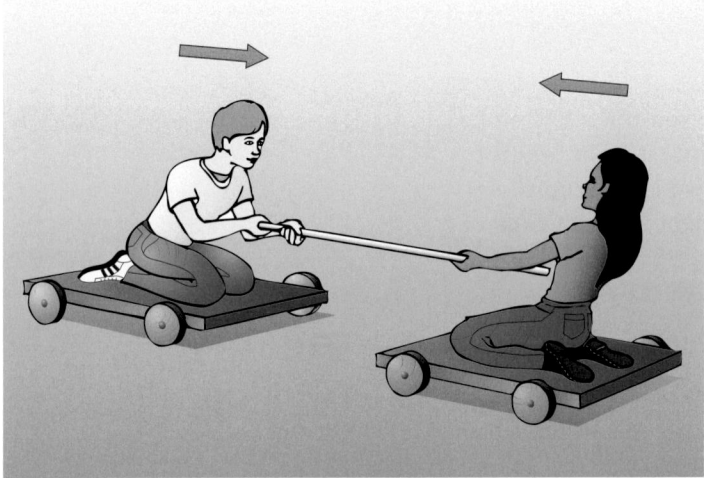

Fig 2.2 Newton's third law. If one child pulls or pushes, both move

Fig 2.3 Another scientist who studied motion was Galileo (1564–1642). These 'thought-experiments' show a ball and a slope with no frictional forces operating. In **(a)** and **(b)** the ball would roll down the slope and roll back up the other side to the same height. In **(c)** the ball would continue rolling for ever. **(d)** The Earth is round, which suggested to Galileo that 'unforced' motion is naturally circular. Newton disagreed with this idea, and showed it to be incorrect

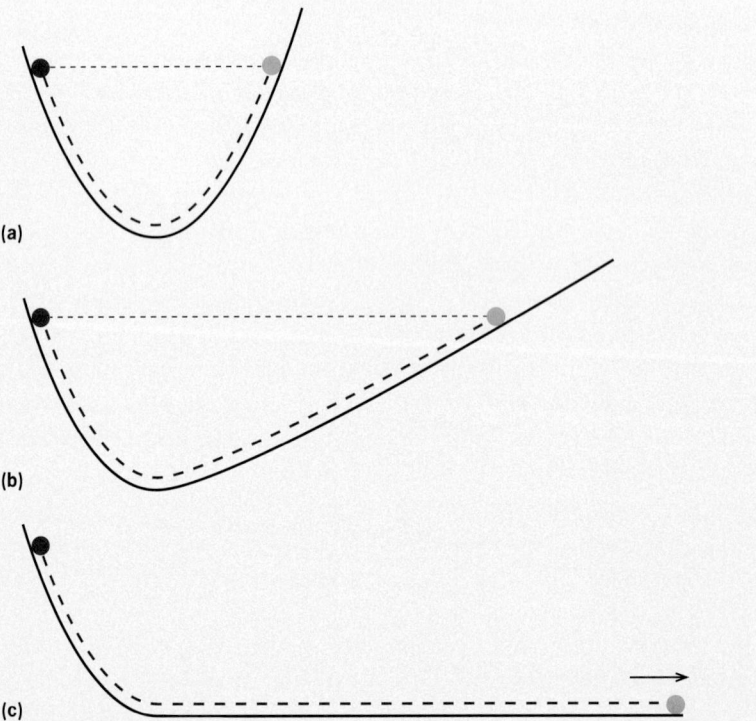
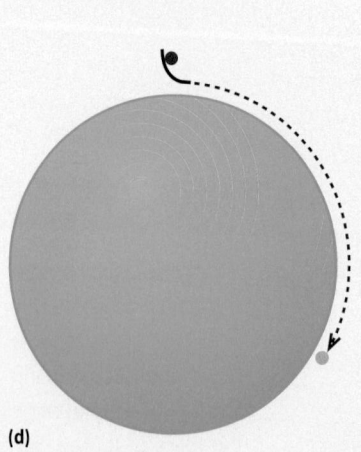

Newton's laws of motion

Newton defined three laws of motion. Law 1 defines a force. Law 2 contains a set of complex related ideas, introducing the new ideas of **momentum** (i.e. **mass** is now involved) and the rate of change of momentum with time. This law allows us to measure the size of a force. Law 3 seems very simple but is also very far-reaching, since hidden in it is probably the most fundamental law of all physics – the law of the **conservation of momentum**.

FIRST LAW

A body at rest will stay at rest, and a body moving in a straight line will continue to move in the same direction and at the same speed, unless an external (unbalanced) force acts on it.

SECOND LAW

The effect of a force is to change the speed and/or direction of motion of a body. When the force changes the momentum of the body, the rate of change of momentum is proportional to the size of the force causing the change, and is in the same direction as the force.

Law 2 leads to the equation:

$$F = ma$$

It is this law which is used to define the unit of force, the **newton** (N):

A force of 1 newton will accelerate a mass of 1 kg at 1 m s^{-2}.

It also leads to the idea of **impulse**, Ft:

$$Ft = \Delta p \text{ (see page 26)}$$

THIRD LAW

Forces occur in pairs: when a body is acted upon by a force, there must be another body which also has a force acting on it. The forces are equal in size but act in opposite directions.

USING THE PLANETS FOR MEASURING

There was, though, a class of objects whose movements had been studied with great care for thousands of years – the planets. It was vital for navigators to know about the motion and positions of the planets and stars, especially in Newton's day, which was a time when trade by sea was developing rapidly.

The planets moved in 'empty' space, with effectively no friction, and so measurements of distance and time from astronomy were the most accurate quantities that Newton could use. Indeed, all measurements of time were based on the daily and annual motion of the Earth around the Sun, and of the Moon around the Earth.

Newton is famous for solving problems posed by the motion of these astronomical objects. To achieve his results, he defined the fundamental ideas of force, mass and momentum as expressed in his three laws of motion. He put forward a law of gravity which explained the motion of the Moon and planets, and linked this to the movement of objects – like falling apples – on Earth. He also developed a new branch of mathematics, the **calculus**, which allowed him to make calculations more easily.

Newton was not the only scientist in the seventeenth century. He and his fellow 'natural philosophers', as scientists were then known, have been credited with starting the first **scientific revolution**. They proposed that theories were worthless unless matched to observation – to what really happens. In physics, this meant that theories of the motion of bodies must include mathematical formulae that could accurately describe – and predict – this motion.

Let us now look at the fundamental ideas that had to be made clear before motion could be understood, for instance the motion of such things as planets, or of more familiar objects such as ships or horses.

2 MOMENTUM

First of all, how could 'motion' be quantified, that is, be given number values? What aspects of motion could be predicted?

To answer these questions, Newton had the idea of 'quantity of motion'. This is what we now call **momentum**. Newton realised that there were two aspects to this: speed in a given direction (which is **velocity**) and **mass**.

Momentum (p) is the product of **mass** × **velocity**, or:

$$p = mv$$

A vector is a quantity with magnitude and also direction. Velocity is a vector, so momentum is also a vector. It has the same direction as the velocity.

Newton's first law of motion defines force simply and qualitatively (page 25). His second law extends the first law to give the relationship between a force and its effect on the motion of a body. A force changes the motion of a body, and is defined so that force equals the **rate of change of momentum**:

$$\textbf{force} = \frac{\textbf{change in momentum}}{\textbf{time}}$$

$$F = \frac{\Delta p}{t} \quad \text{in newtons}$$

where the symbol Δp stands for the change in momentum.

This force formula can be made more practically useful in two ways, as shown next.

IMPULSE

Rearranging the formula gives:

$$Ft = \Delta p$$

The quantity Ft, the product of force and the time for which it acts, is called the **impulse**. Thus we have:

impulse = change in momentum

This idea is particularly useful when we have situations where the force is variable, when it acts for a short time or when both force and time are hard to measure independently. This is the case in collisions, for example. There is more about the use of this way of looking at changes in motion in Chapter 3.

CHANGE IN MOMENTUM DUE TO A CONSTANT FORCE

When we are dealing with well-behaved forces that stay constant over the time interval t, we can define an initial velocity v_0 and a final velocity v_1 (see Chapter 1, page 11) such that the change in momentum is:

$$\Delta p = mv_1 - mv_0$$

Therefore

$$F = \frac{mv_1 - mv_0}{t}$$

which is tidied up to give

$$F = m\,\frac{v_1 - v_0}{t}$$

or

$$F = ma$$

This is the well-known relationship:

force = mass × acceleration

Note that this formula assumes that the mass m does not change.

? **QUESTIONS 5–6**

5   A tennis ball has a mass of 0.07 kg. It reaches a racket at a speed of 20 m s^{-1} and leaves it with a speed of 10 m s^{-1}, in exactly the opposite direction. The ball was in contact with the racket for a time of 0.15 s.
a) What was its change of momentum?
b) What was the impulse given to the ball?
c) What was the average force exerted on i) the racket, ii) the ball?

6   A force of 25 N acts for a time of 0.2 s on a body which has momentum 30 kg m s^{-1}.
a) Calculate the change in momentum produced.
b) Is it possible for the force to act in such a way that the speed of the object stays the same? Explain.

EXAMPLE

Q The engines of an airliner exert a force of 120 kN during take-off. The mass of the airliner is 40 tonnes (1 tonne = 1000 kg). Calculate

a) the acceleration produced by the engines,

b) the minimum length of runway needed if the speed required for take-off is 60 m s^{-1}.

A

a) Using the formula $F = ma$ gives:

$$a = F/m = (1.2 \times 10^5)/(4 \times 10^4)$$
$$= 3 \text{ m s}^{-2}$$

b) We use the equation of motion

$$v_1^2 = v_0^2 + 2ax$$

Rearranging this, knowing that $v_0 = 0$:

$$x = \frac{v_1^2}{2a} = \frac{3600}{6} = 600 \text{ m}$$

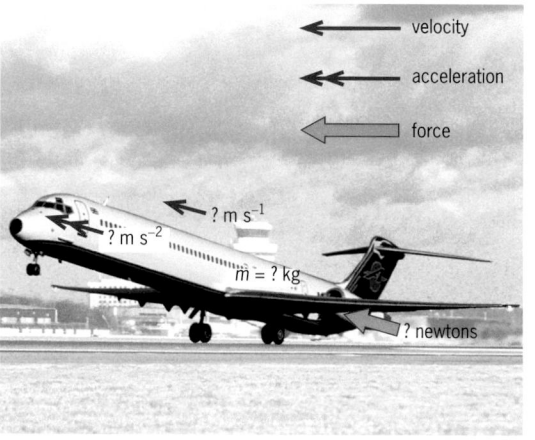

velocity
acceleration
force
? m s^{-1}
? m s^{-2}
m = ? kg
? newtons

Fig 2.4 The airliner taking off

MASS CHANGES ALSO AFFECT MOMENTUM

The simple formula $F = ma$ (or $F = m\,dv/dt$) assumes that the mass stays constant while the force is acting. But this is not true in many cases, such as rocketry, where the force is produced by expelling material from the back of the rocket. See Chapter 3 for more about this. Also, when objects are travelling at very high speeds, the mass changes with speed as a result of relativistic effects (see Chapters 23 and 24). So, using the calculus notation, a more accurate formulation of the second law relationship is:

$$F = \frac{\mathbf{d}(mv)}{\mathbf{d}t} = \frac{\mathbf{d}p}{\mathbf{d}t}$$

INERTIAL MASS AND GRAVITATIONAL MASS

It was hard for Newton to define 'mass', other than as 'quantity of matter'. It certainly was not the same as **weight** (see page 31). Finally, Newton defined mass in two ways. His first definition was equivalent to this:

> **Mass is what a body has which makes it hard to accelerate.**

This means that we can work out the mass of a body by seeing how much it accelerates when we apply a standard force to it, then apply the formula $m = F/a$. The word **inertia** means reluctance to move, so this kind of mass is called **inertial mass**.

But Newton had also produced another entirely novel theory, the **theory of gravity**. In this theory:

> **Any object with mass produces a force of attraction which acts on other masses.**

So mass can be measured by measuring the size of the force-pair exerted between two objects. This is essentially what we do when we measure the force of gravity on an object to find its 'weight', using a spring balance, say. The result we get from this kind of measurement is called **gravitational mass**.

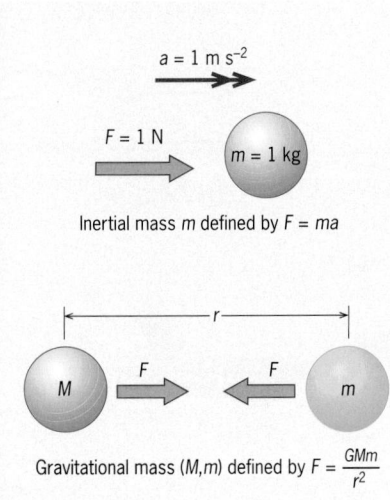

Fig 2.5 Inertial mass and gravitational mass. Are they the same?

Are these two kinds of mass equivalent?

There is no reason, in Newtonian physics, why these measurements should give the same result for a given object, but they always do. This equivalence has been tested by experiment to be exact to 1 part in 10^{12}. This might seem a rather trivial point to worry about. After all, mass is mass is mass, isn't it? But it was by thinking about this very equivalence that Einstein hit on his general theory of relativity.

CENTRE OF GRAVITY

The force of gravity acts on every 'particle' in an object. But for practical purposes we can think of this force – the weight – of an object as acting through one point in it. This point is called the **centre of gravity** or **centre of mass** of the object. This is the point about which the object will balance if it is supported there. Figure 2.6 shows the position of the centre of gravity for a number of simple objects. See also Chapter 5, page 94.

? **QUESTIONS 7–10**

7 A force of 12 N is applied to an object. Calculate its mass if it changes speed (without changing direction) from 5 m s^{-1} to 25 m s^{-1} in 4 s.

8 A net force of 15 N acts on an object and it accelerates at 5 m s^{-2}.
 a) What is the mass of the object?
 b) What force would be needed to accelerate the object by 9.8 m s^{-2}?

9 Our Universe is expanding, meaning that all the very large masses in it (such as galaxies) are moving away from each other. One theory states that this expansion may be partly due to the gravitational mass of an object being very slightly different from its inertial mass. Which mass would have to be the larger in order to produce an expanding Universe? Justify your answer.

10 Outline the principle of any experiment you can think of that would test the theory that gravitational mass and inertial mass are equivalent.

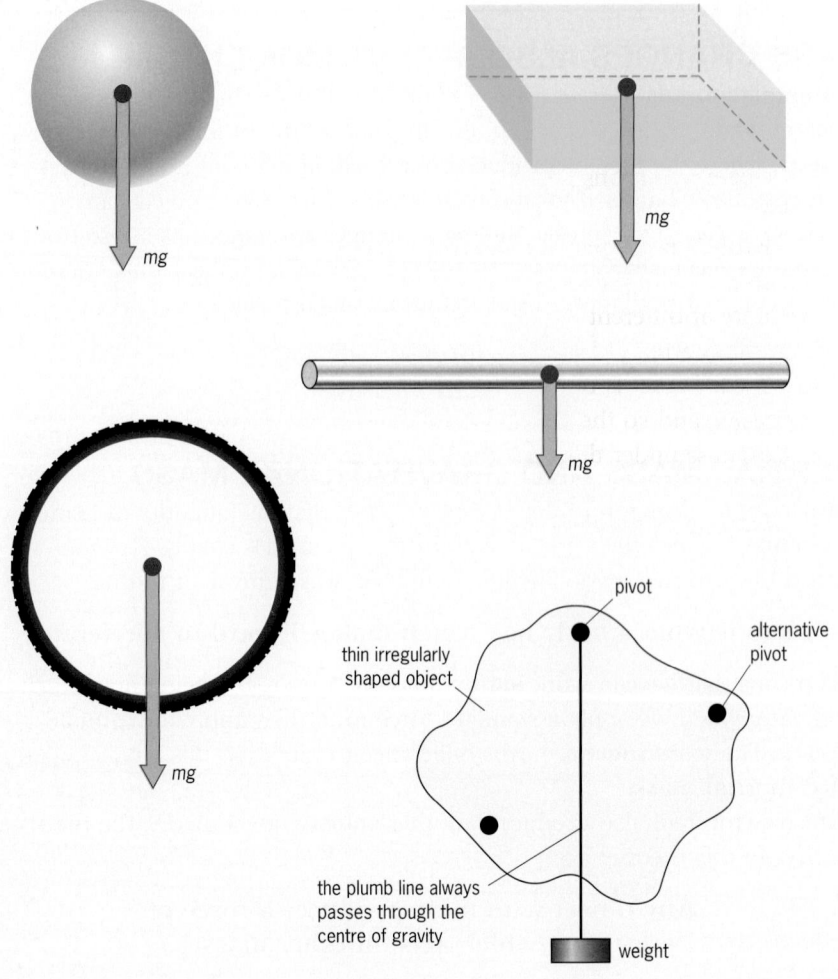

Fig 2.6 Some centres of gravity

3 THE FORCE OF GRAVITY AND THE ACCELERATION OF FREE FALL

Newton realised that objects fall because the Earth exerts a force on them – the **force of gravity**. This force causes an object to accelerate towards the ground. It was already well known that under the right conditions all objects, whatever their mass, fell with the same value of acceleration (Fig 2.7). We call this the **acceleration of free fall**. The most important condition is that the objects must be falling perfectly freely, with no friction or other opposing force to slow them down. The acceleration in air of a small lead ball is different from that of a light paper ball. This is because the objects are falling through a resistive medium, air, and the resistance is bigger in proportion to weight for the lighter object. But in a vacuum all objects accelerate at the same rate.

A simple laboratory experiment shows that the acceleration of free fall is approximately 9.8 m s^{-2}. This value is given the symbol g. More accurate experiments show that g varies over the Earth's surface. Some values are given in Table 2.1.

Table 2.1 Values of g at different places on the Earth's surface					
Location	London	Calcutta	Tokyo	Sydney	North Pole
Acceleration of free fall/m s^{-2}	9.812	9.788	9.798	9.797	9.832

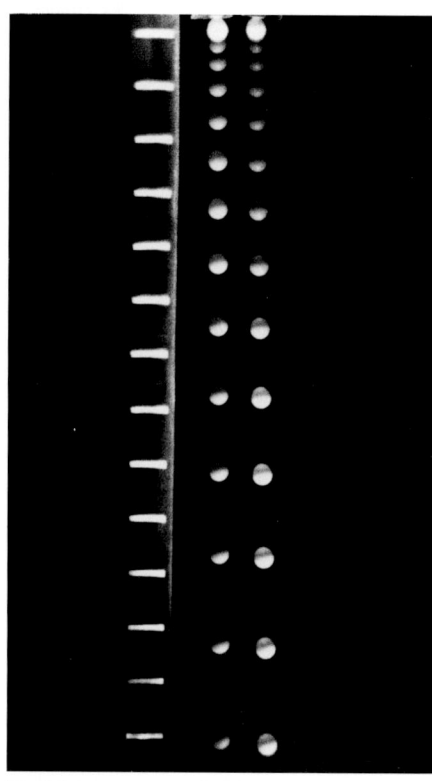

Fig 2.7 In a vacuum, all objects accelerate at the same rate
Left: golf ball; right: table-tennis ball

There are several reasons for this variation:

- The Earth is not a perfect sphere, and so different places on the Earth are at different distances from the centre.
- The Earth's crust is not uniform in density, and so there is more or less mass under different places.
- The Earth is spinning, and some places (e.g. on the Equator) are spinning with a greater speed than others.

Why these differences should change the acceleration of free fall will become clear as you work through this chapter.

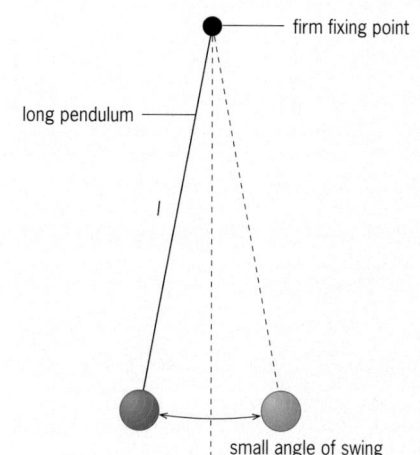

firm fixing point

long pendulum

l

small angle of swing

Fig 2.8 A simple pendulum. The period T is the time it takes for the pendulum bob to swing across and back to its starting point. At least 20 swings should be timed in order to get an accurate value

MEASURING g

Accurate measurements of g use methods based on measuring the period of a swinging pendulum, as in Fig 2.8. The period T of a simple pendulum is given by the formula:

$$T = 2\pi\sqrt{\frac{l}{g}}$$

where l is the length of the pendulum. See Chapter 6, page 121 for more about the simple pendulum. For most calculations at A-level, a value for g of 9.8 m s^{-2} is accurate enough.

? QUESTION 11

11 The simple pendulum was once the most accurate device for controlling clocks.

a) Calculate the length of a simple pendulum that would swing with a period of exactly 1 second.

b) Eighteenth-century navigators needed very accurate clocks to help locate their position at sea. Why were pendulum clocks not much use for this purpose?

WHY DO ALL OBJECTS FALL WITH THE SAME ACCELERATION?

We learn from careful experiments that the gravitational force (due to the Earth) on an object of mass m accelerates the object with the local value of g. By Newton's second law, the force F must be such that:

$$F = mg$$

Now, g is always the same at a particular place on Earth, whatever the mass of the object. This means that F must be proportional to m. If the mass doubles, for example, the force must double. (Einstein explains *why* gravity works in this way in his general theory of relativity.)

Fig 2.9 In a gravitational field, all objects at a given place have the same acceleration

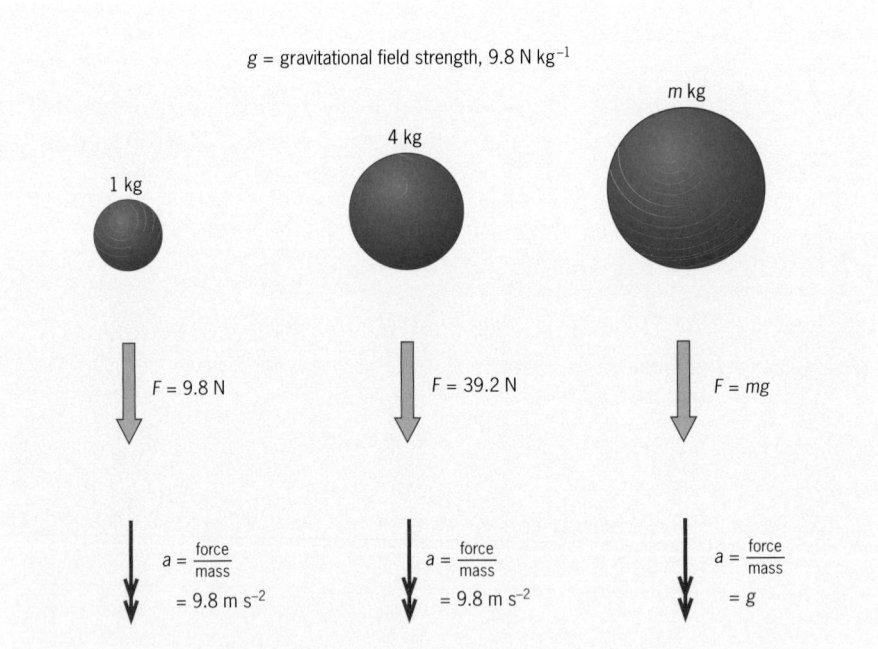

g = gravitational field strength, 9.8 N kg^{-1}

1 kg   4 kg m kg

$F = 9.8$ N $F = 39.2$ N $F = mg$

$a = \dfrac{\text{force}}{\text{mass}}$ $a = \dfrac{\text{force}}{\text{mass}}$ $a = \dfrac{\text{force}}{\text{mass}}$

$= 9.8$ m s^{-2} $= 9.8$ m s^{-2} $= g$

4 THE STRENGTH OF A GRAVITATIONAL FIELD

We use the quantity **gravitational field strength** to help define the effect of a gravity on a mass. At GCSE, you came across the idea of a magnetic or electric field to describe the pattern in space made by these types of force. We can also think of the space around any mass (such as the Earth) as having a **gravitational field**. There is more about this in Chapter 3.

The *strength* of the gravitational field is measured by the force it exerts on any object placed in the field, per unit of mass. The value of the field strength is measured to be numerically the same as the acceleration of free fall, g. So, near the surface of the Earth, the value is approximately 9.8 newtons per kilogram.

By the definition of force:

gravitational force on mass = mass × acceleration of free fall

$$F = mg$$

By our definition of gravitational field strength as force per unit mass:

$$\textbf{gravitational field strength} = \frac{\textbf{gravitational force}}{\textbf{mass}} = \frac{mg}{m} = g$$

This means that sometimes you will see g given in units of N kg^{-1}, which relates to gravitational field strength, and sometimes in units of m s^{-2}, when we are thinking about the acceleration of free fall.

MASS AND WEIGHT

Many people confuse mass and weight. This is mainly because in everyday life we use the word weight to mean what physicists call **mass**. Potatoes are sold in 2 kg packs, which have been carefully 'weighed' by the suppliers. But a kilogram is a unit of mass (and so also is a 'pound'). The **weight** is what you experience when you lift up the pack.

The simplest definition of weight is as follows:

The weight of an object is the gravitational force exerted on the object by the mass of the Earth.

This force depends on the mass of the object, as explained above. Close to the Earth's surface, a mass of 1 kg is attracted by a force of approximately 9.8 N. A mass of 2 kg feels heavier than a mass of 1 kg because the gravitational force on it is twice as great: 19.6 N.

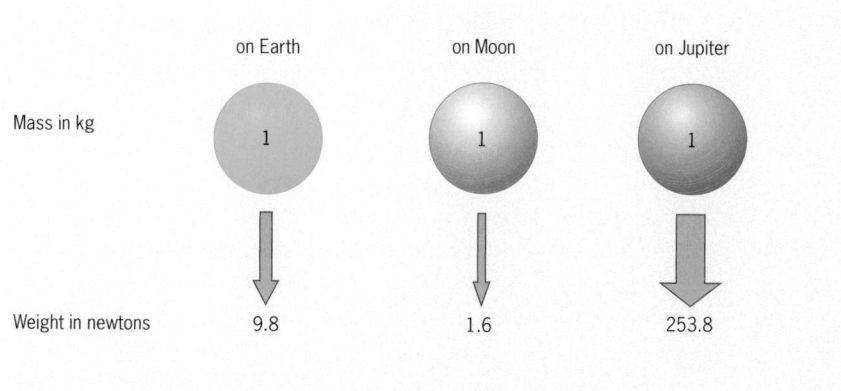

Fig 2.10 The distinction between mass and weight. Mass is the quantity of matter in a body (unit: kilogram). Weight is the force which acts on the mass in a gravitational field (unit: newton). Here, the three bodies all have the same mass, but very different weights

This force varies with distance from the centre of the Earth. But even at the height of a typical Earth satellite (say, 100 km above the surface), the force per kilogram is only slightly less at 9.5 N kg^{-1}. This is of course the force that keeps the satellite orbiting the Earth (see Chapter 3).

Weight is only one of the **pair of forces** involved. The other force is the pull of the object on the Earth, in accordance with Newton's third law (see Fig 2.11).

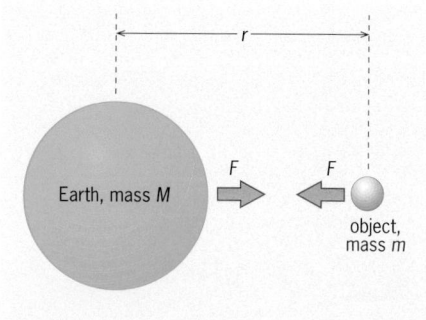

Fig 2.11 Forces always occur in pairs. Just as the object is pulled by the Earth, so the Earth is pulled by the object

? QUESTIONS 12–13

12 Explain why the quantity g is sometimes quoted as 9.8 m s^{-2} and sometimes as 9.8 N kg^{-1}.

13 The gravitational field strength at the surface of Mars is 3.8 N kg^{-1}. How long will it take a mass of 2 kg to reach a speed of 20 m s^{-1} in free fall?

? QUESTIONS 14–15

14 **a)** What was the *geocentric* model of the Universe?
b) This model was quite wrong, but using it astronomers were able to predict the movements of the planets and eclipses of the Sun and Moon. Use books and/or the internet to research and explain how they refined Aristotle's simple model to make such good predictions. [Key words: Ptolemy, epicycles]

15 **a)** Everybody knows that the Earth spins on its axis. Why do *you* believe this? Be honest!
b) Now find out any piece of evidence for the Earth's spinning that should convince a sceptical younger sibling.

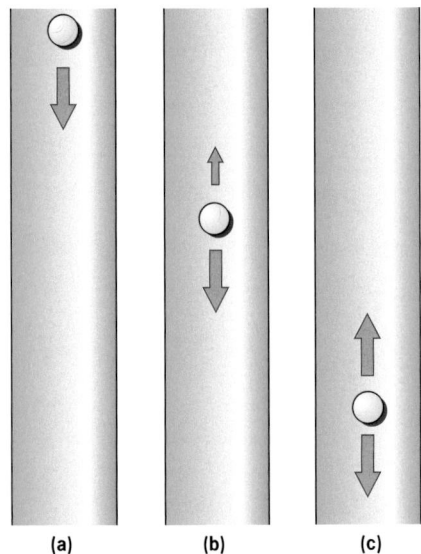

(a)   **(b)**   **(c)**

Fig 2.12 Forces on a table-tennis ball as it falls down a well.
(a) At the top the ball is stationary, so the air resistance is zero.
(b) As the ball moves down the well, air resistance increases, slowing down the rate of acceleration.
(c) The air resistance exactly balances the weight of the ball, so the ball is no longer accelerating. The speed of the ball at this time is its terminal speed

---

? QUESTIONS 16–18

16 A small steel ball is placed just above the surface of a jar of oil, about 0.5 m tall, and then let go. Describe the motion of the ball and illustrate your answer with a sketch of the speed–time graph.

17 Identify the force-pairs in the following circumstances (there might be more than one):
a) the Moon moving in its orbit;
b) a stone just after it has been dropped into a well;
c) a 'free fall' parachutist who has reached terminal speed.

18 (See Example opposite.) A boy running at 3 m s^{-1} throws a ball vertically upwards with an initial speed of 5 m s^{-1}.
a) If he carries on running at the same speed, will the ball return to him? (Ignore air resistance.)
b) How long will the ball be in the air?
c) How far has the boy run in this time?

---

5 MOVING IN A UNIFORM GRAVITATIONAL FIELD

In this section we deal with movement near the Earth's surface, so that the field strength is reasonably constant at 9.8 N kg^{-1} and the acceleration of free fall is 9.8 m s^{-2}.

EXAMPLE

Q A small coin is dropped down a well. The splash is heard 2.3 s later. How deep is the well? (Assume that sound travels quickly enough for any delaying effect to be ignored.)

A The appropriate formula, from the kinematics formulae on pages 11–12, must involve acceleration (in this case g), the initial speed (in this case zero), the distance moved x, and the time t taken to fall:

$$x = v_0 t + \tfrac{1}{2} a t^2$$

Inserting the given values:

$$x = 0 + \tfrac{1}{2} \times 9.8 \times (2.3)^2$$
$$= 26 \text{ m}$$

How fast would the coin in the example be travelling just before it hit the water? The final speed can be calculated from:

$$v_1 = v_0 + at$$
$$= 0 + 9.8 \text{ m s}^{-2} \times 2.3 \text{ s}$$
$$= 23 \text{ m s}^{-1}$$

If a table-tennis ball had been dropped into the well instead of a coin, the time taken for it to reach the water would have been a lot longer. This is because, as an object speeds up in a medium (here air), the resistive (frictional) force opposing it increases (Fig 2.12). When the opposing force is equal to the accelerating force, the *net* force on the object is zero. The object stops accelerating and carries on at a steady speed. In the case of a falling object this is called its **terminal speed** (or **terminal velocity**).

A steel ball has a terminal speed of about 80 m s^{-1}, compared with 5 m s^{-1} for a table-tennis ball. If you fell out of an aeroplane you would reach a terminal speed of about 70 m s^{-1}. A parachute increases the air resistance, producing a terminal speed of just a few metres per second, depending on its design.

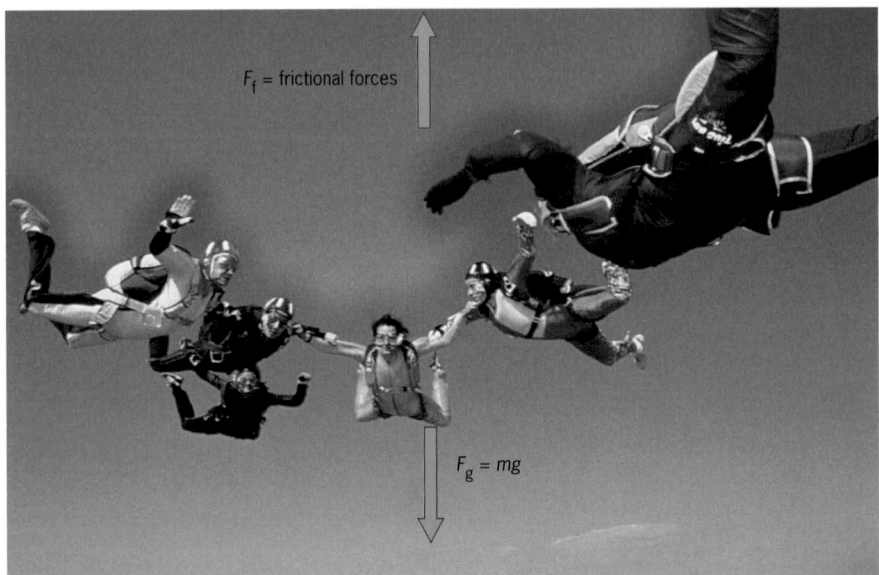

F_f = frictional forces

F_g = mg

Fig 2.13 The sky divers have reached terminal velocity: $F_f = F_g$

Aristotle to Newton, via Galileo

Aristotle was the universal genius of classical Greece. He was born in Macedonia in about 384 BC and after becoming famous in Athens became tutor to the 13-year-old Alexander (not yet the Great). He wrote about astronomy, physics, biology, psychology, medicine, philosophy, ethics, political theory, history, literature – and invented a system of formal logic still used today. His work – and reputation – lasted for two thousand years. It was the basis of medieval Christian and Islamic thought, and it took a brave spirit to criticise his ideas.

Galilei Galileo (1564–1642) was just such a spirit. In Book 3 of his Physics, Aristotle had defined some motion as 'natural' – stones fall and, smoke rises because it is in their **nature** to do so. Natural events didn't need explanation. He stated that heavy objects fell faster than light ones – this was clearly logical. Explaining how things moved sideways, like arrows and spears, was difficult. He suggested that they were pushed by the air, which moved from in front to behind the moving object. Aristotle thought heavenly objects divine: Sun, Moon, planets and stars moved in perfect circles around the Earth, the centre of the Universe.

Aristotle didn't believe in experimenting in physics – it was interfering with nature. All you need to get the right answers is to collect a few intelligent people and let them argue it out. Oddly enough, he did make very careful observations on plants, animals and human diseases.

Galileo was a mathematician with a strong interest in physics and astronomy. He did believe in experiment. He dropped cannon balls of different size from the Leaning Tower of Pisa and saw that they reached the ground at the same time. The rate of falling didn't depend on their weight. He also noted that they accelerated as they fell. He almost (but not quite) had the Newtonian idea of a force – indeed of a **gravitational** force. He also did experiments on balls rolling down inclined planes – see Fig 2.3. This led him to the (wrong) conclusion: that the natural motion for horizontal motion was circular and (correctly) that such objects would move forever in the absence of friction. He showed that missiles moved in parabolas – an idea very useful to the military technology of the time.

These ideas in physics made his reputation, but his attacks on Aristotle's physics were unpopular and he was sacked as a professor of the University of Pisa. Galileo got into even more trouble when he supported by clear arguments (and telescope observations) the idea that the Sun was at the centre of the Universe, and that the Earth moved around it. This was seen as interference with religious ideas, and he was accused of heresy. As a result, he spent the last years of his life under house arrest.

Isaac Newton was born in the year that Galileo died. He confirmed and corrected Galileo's ideas where necessary, as this section of the book shows.

EXAMPLE

Q The diagram shows a velocity–time graph for a ball thrown vertically upwards with an initial speed of 14.7 m s^{-1}. **a)** How high will it go? **b)** What is the total distance it travels? **c)** What is its time of flight? (Air resistance can be ignored.)

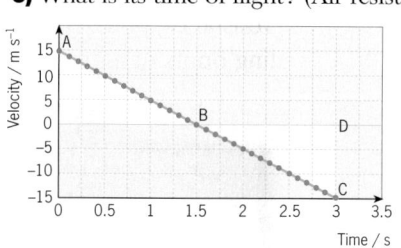

Fig 2.14 Graph of velocity against time for a ball thrown vertically upwards with an initial speed of 14.7 m s^{-1}

A

a) In this problem, direction is important, and we must be aware of the significance of the *signs* of vector quantities. We use the convention that *up* is positive and *down* is negative. The height, distance x, is given by the area under the graph for the portion A to B. The appropriate equation is:

$$v_1^2 = v_0^2 + 2ax$$

At the top of its flight, the ball has zero velocity, with $a = -9.8$ m s^{-2}.

We get:

$$0 = (14.7)^2 - (2 \times 9.8 \times x)$$

giving:

$$19.6 \times x = (14.7)^2$$

The height the ball reached:

$$x = 11.0 \text{ m}$$

b) The 'total distance travelled' can mean two things. Strictly, we could interpret it as the **displacement** of the ball from where it started. This distance is given by the sum of the two areas OAB and BCD. These areas are equal in size but opposite in sign, so add up to zero. This tells us no more than that the ball ended up in the same place as it started! How does the algebra cope with this? The final velocity is −14.7 m s^{-1}. So, using the same formula for the whole journey:

$$(-14.7)^2 = (14.7)^2 - (2 \times 9.8 \times x)$$

which also results in $x = 0$.

Taking the obvious alternative as the **non-vector** (or **scalar**) sum of the up-and-down distances, the ball has moved through a distance of 22 m.

c) What is the ball's time of flight – the time it was in the air? We can work this out using the formula $v_1 = v_0 + at$, which can be rearranged to give:

$$t = \frac{v_1 - v_0}{a} = \frac{-14.7 - 14.7}{-9.8} = 3 \text{ s}$$

Now try question 18 on the facing page.

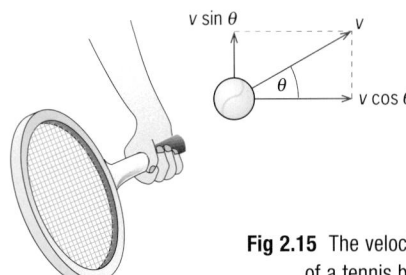

Fig 2.15 The velocity of a tennis ball

6 PROJECTILES

A projectile is an object that has been propelled by a force that acts for a short time. After you kick a football in the air or lob a tennis ball with a racket, the ball has a velocity whose direction is in between the horizontal and the vertical, as shown in Fig 2.15. It moves both upwards and sideways. The tennis ball in the diagram has a velocity v in the direction shown, when $v \sin \theta$ is the **vertical component** and $v \cos \theta$ is the **horizontal component**.

But the force of gravity acts downwards – it can only affect the up-and-down motion. Assuming air resistance is too small to worry about (though it usually isn't!), the speed in the sideways direction stays the same (Figs 2.16 and 2.17). That is, in a simple, uniform gravitational field the horizontal and vertical components of velocity are independent of each other.

You can solve problems involving the movement of projectiles as follows:
- First find the separate vertical and horizontal velocities by simple vector theory (finding components).
- Then calculate the time of flight, t, as above, using the formula $v_1 = v_0 + at$ (simplified to $v = gt$).
- Finally, use t and the horizontal component of velocity to find the horizontal distance travelled.

Fig 2.16 A ball falling in a semi-parabolic curve

? QUESTIONS 19–21

19 A tennis ball is lobbed at an angle of 50° to the ground at a speed of 16 m s⁻¹. It is hit from a point very near the ground at the baseline.
a) What is its vertical speed?
b) How long will it be in the air before reaching the ground again?
c) A tennis court has a length of 23.8 m from one base-line to the other. Will the tennis ball land in court?

20 A circus performer is fired from a cannon, hoping to land in a net 25 m away. The cannon is pointing at an angle of 45° to the horizontal. At what speed must the person leave the cannon to land in the net?

21 (Ignore air resistance here.)
A batsman hits a baseball and it moves off with a velocity of 24 m s⁻¹ at an angle of 30° to the horizontal.
a) Show that the ball should reach the ground at about 51 m away (at least).
b) A fielder is 20 m away from the expected landing point. He can run at a speed of 8 m s⁻¹. Is he likely to be in a position to catch the ball? Justify your decision, and explain what effect air resistance might have on the situation.

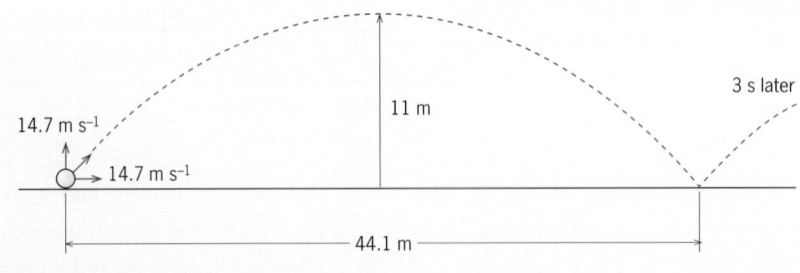

Fig 2.17 Vertical and horizontal motions are independent. The vertical movement is affected by gravity. The horizontal speed stays the same until the ball hits the ground

---

EXAMPLE

Q Suppose the ball of the last Example was kicked so that it started upwards with a speed of 14.7 m s⁻¹, and also moved sideways with the same speed. We have calculated that its time of flight would be 3 s. This is independent of whatever sideways motion it has. So, after 3 s, the ball hits the ground. How far did it move sideways before it bounced?

A It moved for 3 s at a speed of 14.7 m s⁻¹, so it must have travelled a distance of 3×14.7 m, namely 44.1 m, as shown in Fig 2.17.

7 GRAVITY ON THE WAY TO THE MOON

The most direct way of getting an object to the Moon might *seem* to be to wait until the Moon is directly overhead and then project the object vertically upwards, really fast. *How* fast we work out in the next chapter – the speed would have to be at least 11 km s^{-1}.

But it is not that simple. By the time the object reached the Moon's orbit, the Moon would have moved on. So we should have calculated when to throw the object upwards so that it reached the Moon's orbit just when the Moon happened to be there. We would also have to do some calculating to allow for the fact that the object was thrown from a spinning Earth and so would have some sideways speed as well. The path of our object moving in a gravitational field will, in general, be an ellipse. Space dynamics is not simple! (More about this in Chapter 3.)

On its way to the Moon the object would be acted on by a force due to the Earth's gravity. This acts towards Earth and would decelerate the object. Table 2.2 shows some actual data from the Apollo 11 Moon Mission of July 1969, one of a series of projects in which a space capsule was sent from Earth to the Moon.

Table 2.2 Data from Apollo 11 Moon Mission. The time interval for each pair of speed readings is 600 s			
Speed at start and end of time interval/m s^{-1}	Distance from Earth's centre at start and end of each interval/10^6 m	Acceleration in each 600 s interval/m s^{-2}	Mean distance r from Earth's centre during each time interval/10^6 m
5374	26.3	−0.45	27.65
5102	29.0		
3633	54.4	−0.12	55.4
3560	56.4		
2619	95.7	−0.04	96.45
2594	97.2		
1796	169.9	−0.01	170.4
1788	170.9		

The acceleration of the spacecraft is found by calculating the change in speed during each time interval, and dividing that by the size of the interval, 600 s. Table 2.2 shows not only that the spacecraft is slowing down on its way to the Moon, but also that the deceleration gets less as the craft gets further away from the Earth. The deceleration is due to the Earth's pull on the spacecraft, so this force must be decreasing, as shown in Fig 2.18. As explained earlier, the deceleration of the spacecraft equals the value of the Earth's gravitational field strength g at that point in space.

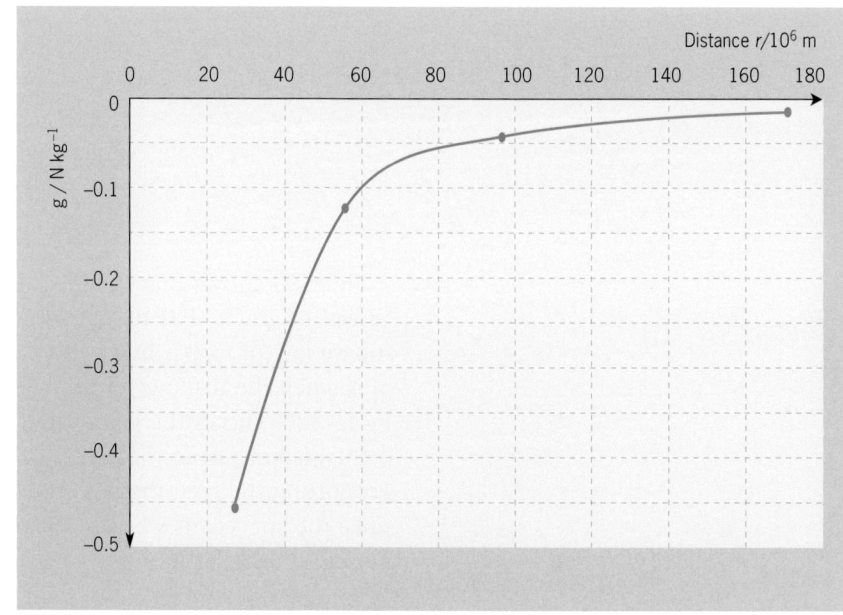

Fig 2.18 Graph of gravity strength against distance for the Apollo 11 data in Table 2.2. It shows that the value of g decreases as distance from the Earth's centre increases

THE INVERSE SQUARE LAW

The plot of the graph in Fig 2.18 shows that the measured value of g falls off rapidly with distance. It also assumes that the spacecraft kept to the straight line between Earth and the Moon. This is only roughly true, as shown in Fig 2.19.

Back in the seventeenth century, Newton proposed that the strength of the Earth's gravitational field should **vary inversely as the square of the distance from its centre**. Newton could not check this idea with spacecraft data, but he was able to confirm that the motion of the Moon in its orbit agreed with his theory to an accuracy of about 0.5 per cent, and that the motion of the planets in their orbits was also consistent with this inverse square law. Read more about this in the next chapter.

Fig 2.19 The path of Apollo 11

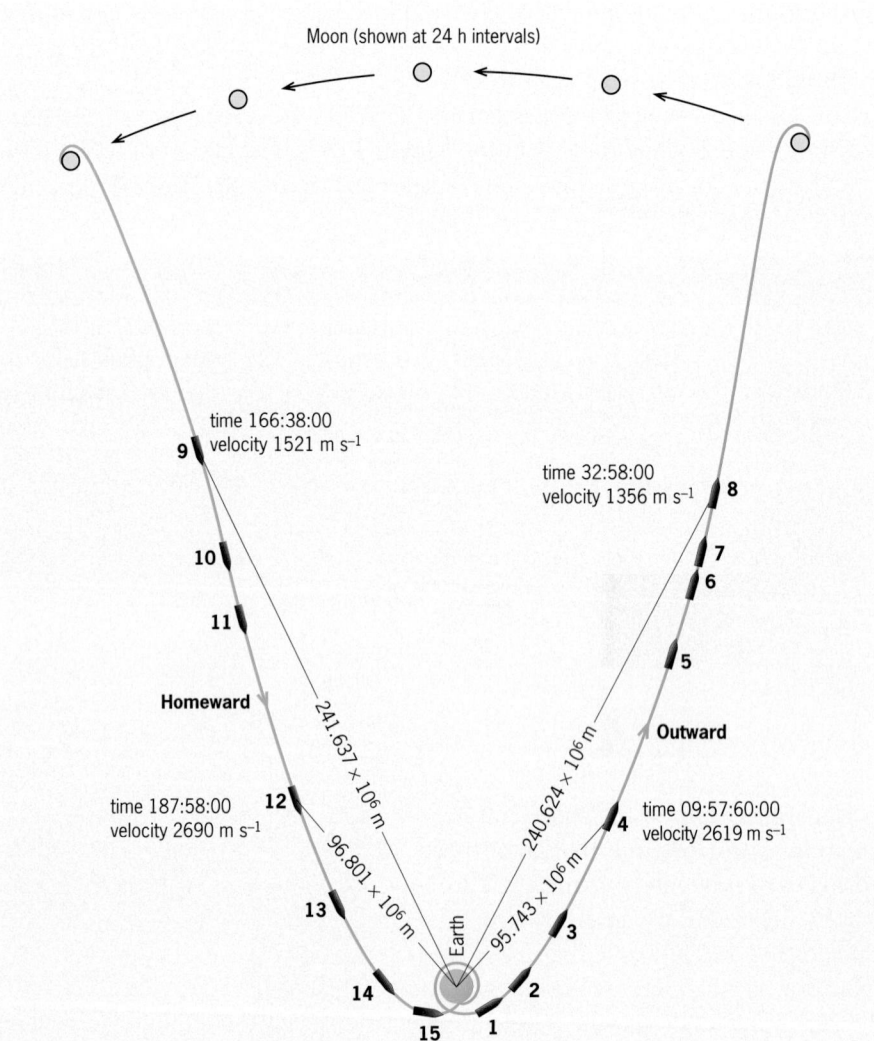

Fig 2.20 shows that the idea of an inverse square law makes sense, as the 'effect' of gravity has to spread out over larger and larger areas. In an inverse square law of force, the size of the force on any object is reduced by a factor of 4 when the distance doubles, by 9 when the distance trebles, and so on.

Fig 2.21 shows the values of g from Table 2.2 plotted against $1/r^2$, where r is the distance from the centre of the Earth. It is nearly a straight line, supporting the idea that g is proportional to $1/r^2$. The data are not ideal, since the spacecraft was not moving along a straight line joining the centres of the Earth and the Moon.

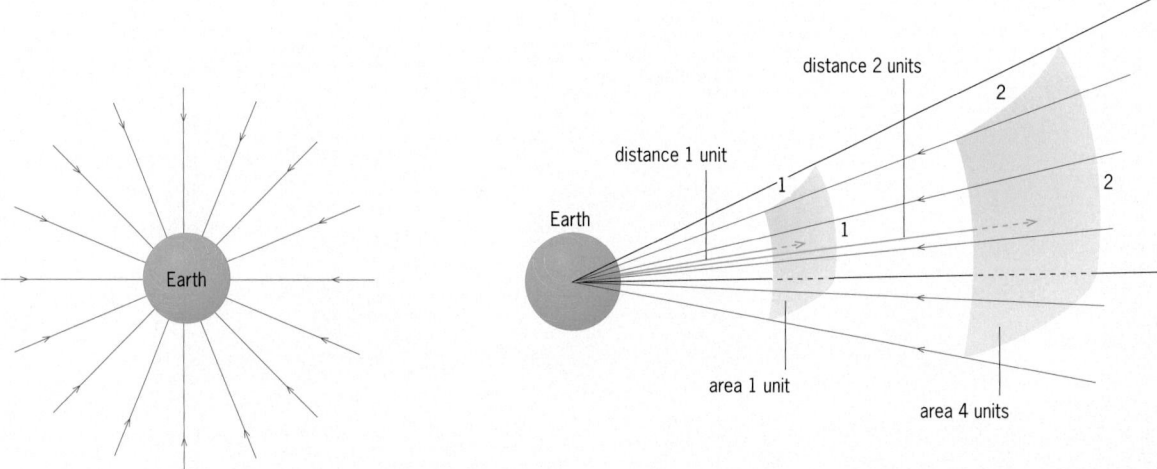

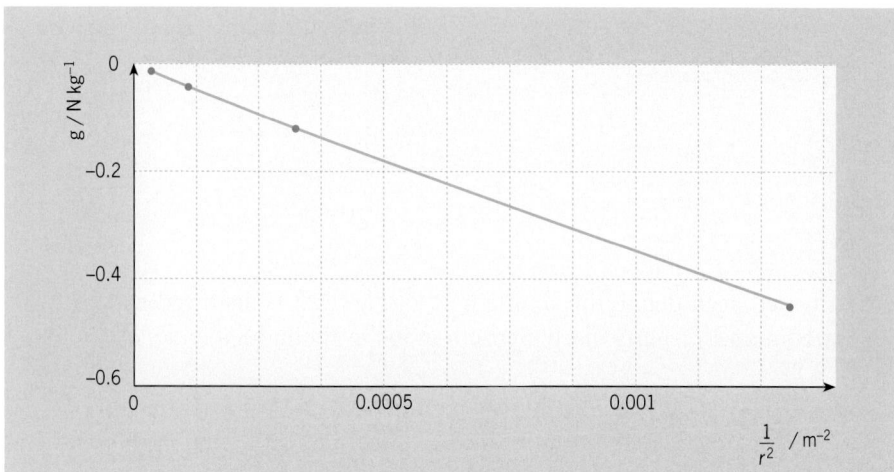

Fig 2.20 Field lines radiating from a sphere, suggesting that an inverse square law is plausible. At double the distance, a given set of force lines are spread over four times the area

Fig 2.21 Graph of g against $1/r^2$ for the data in Table 2.2. It is nearly a straight line, supporting the theory of an inverse square law

8 VISUALISING A FIELD

You can get a picture of a magnetic field by sprinkling iron filings on a sheet of paper placed on top of a magnet. Each small piece of iron acts as a kind of probe, lining itself up with the direction of the magnetic force exerted on it at that point. The field lines formed show the direction of the force field at any point (Fig 2.22). We can do similar experiments to show the shapes of electric fields (see Chapter 9).

We cannot do these experiments to show a gravitational field because the forces involved are so weak. However, we can visualise it in the same way.

All bodies with mass exert gravitational forces, and we can imagine such bodies surrounded by their gravitational fields of force. As with magnets and electrically charged bodies, the fields are defined by the directions of the forces exerted on objects situated in these fields. Gravitational fields tend to be simpler than either electrical or magnetic fields. Most masses of interest are spherical (like planets and stars), and we do not have the confusion of two kinds of charge (positive and negative) or two kinds of magnetic pole (N-seeking and S-seeking). The gravitational field lines of the Earth are shown in Fig 2.23.

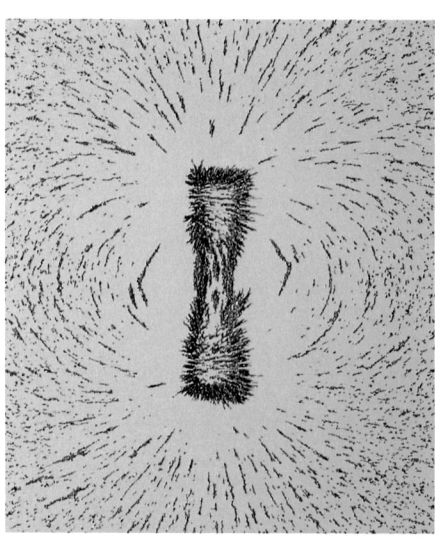

Fig 2.22 Iron filings showing the field around a magnet

Fig 2.23 The gravitational field near the Earth

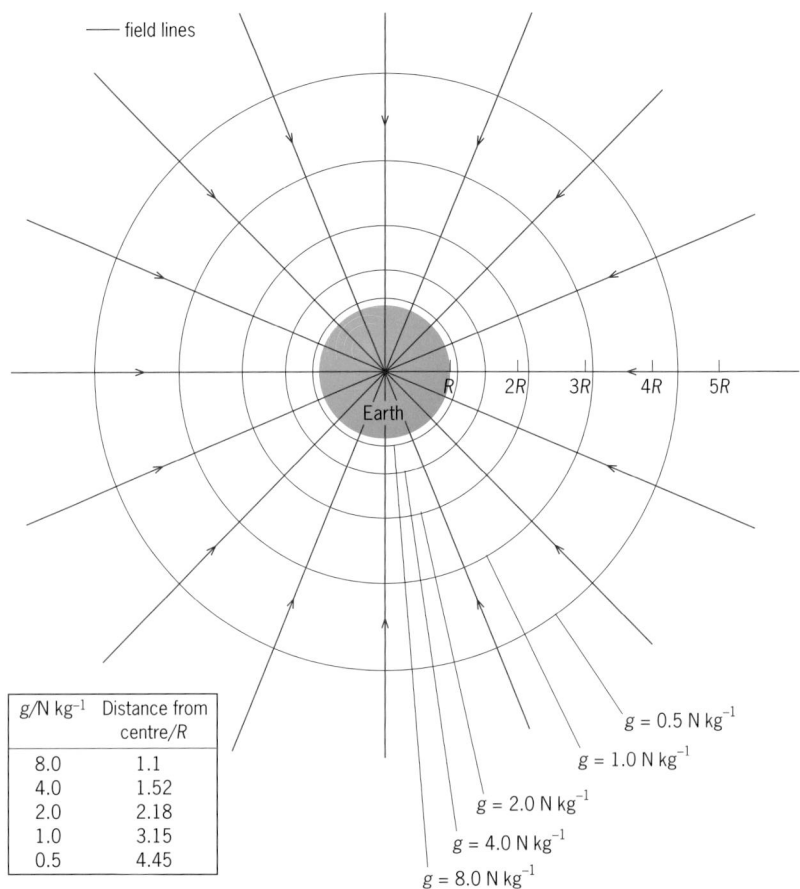

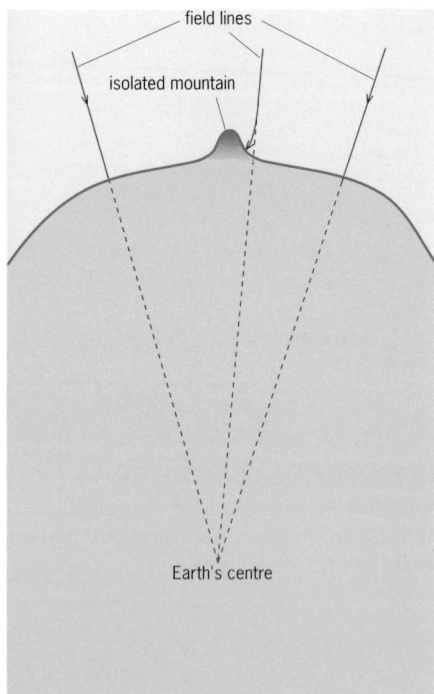

Fig 2.24 The Earth's gravitational field is distorted near the surface by large features such as mountains

g/N kg^{-1}	Distance from centre/R
8.0	1.1
4.0	1.52
2.0	2.18
1.0	3.15
0.5	4.45

$g = 0.5$ N kg^{-1}
$g = 1.0$ N kg^{-1}
$g = 2.0$ N kg^{-1}
$g = 4.0$ N kg^{-1}
$g = 8.0$ N kg^{-1}

If it is looked at in detail, the simple field of Fig 2.23 is distorted near large mountains, or particularly dense regions in the Earth's crust, as shown in Fig 2.24.

A plumb line shows the direction of the Earth's gravitational field at any point. On a perfectly still, uniform and spherical Earth the plumb line points directly towards the centre of the Earth in one direction, and towards the zenith (a point directly overhead) in the other. But, near a mountain, the plumb line veers away slightly from this line and towards the mountain.

We often picture the strength of a field by drawing lines close together for strong fields and further apart for weaker fields. So, as in Fig 2.20, drawing lines radially out from Earth represents the geometry of the inverse square law neatly and accurately. When the distance from the Earth's centre is doubled, a bundle of lines is spread over an area four times as great.

? QUESTION 22

22 The Earth's radius is 6400 km. How far apart are two places on Earth if the directions of the radial gravitational field at those places differ by 1 degree?

9 NEWTON'S LAW OF GRAVITATION

Newton proposed a law of gravitation which allows us to work out the magnitude of the force of mutual attraction between two masses. Imagine two objects of mass M and m respectively, separated by a distance r between their centres. They attract each other with a force F given by:

$$F = G \frac{Mm}{r^2}$$

G ('big G') is called the universal gravitational constant (or constant of gravitation). The currently accepted value of $G = 6.672\ 59 \times 10^{-11}$ N m^2 kg^{-2}. For most calculations we take $G = 6.67 \times 10^{-11}$ N m^2 kg^{-2}.

MEASURING *G*

It is difficult to measure *G*, the universal gravitational constant. The force between two 1 kg masses 1 m apart is very small, just 6.67×10^{-11} N. The first accurate measurement was made by the English scientist Henry Cavendish in 1798. He used a version of the apparatus that the French scientist Charles Coulomb used to measure the much larger force between two electrically charged bodies.

Fig 2.25(a) shows the type of **torsion balance** that Cavendish used in later experiments. The gravitational force between two pairs of masses is measured by the twisting (torsion) of a fine wire. Cavendish's apparatus was large, as he wanted to make the forces and movements involved as large as possible. But this produced many errors – including errors due to air currents and the effect of thermal expansion.

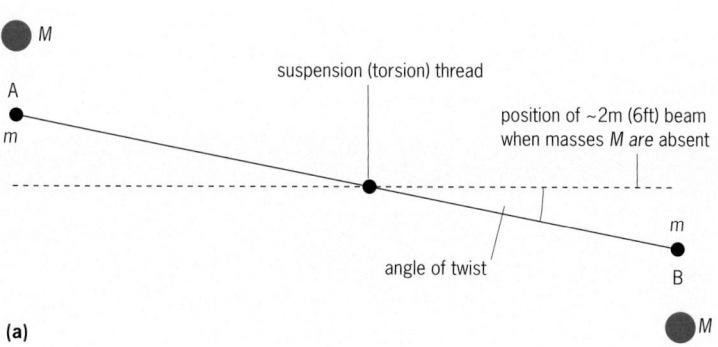

(a)

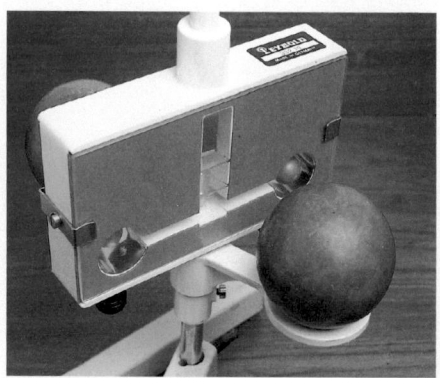

Later experimenters worked with much smaller apparatus. In 1895, C. V. Boys used a beam (AB, Fig 2.25(b)) an inch (2.54 cm) long, compared with Cavendish's 6 ft version. Boys' torsion thread was made of very thin quartz, which he made by firing melted quartz from a crossbow! He used a mirror and a beam of light to measure the twisting angle.

Once we have measured *G*, we can calculate the masses of bodies such as the Sun, the Earth, the Moon and the planets. For example, we know that the force between the Earth and a 1 kg mass on the surface of the Earth is approximately 9.81 N. Rearranging the Newtonian formula gives:

$$\text{mass of Earth, } M = \frac{Fr^2}{Gm} = \frac{9.81 \times (6.38 \times 10^6)^2}{6.67 \times 10^{-11} \times 1.00} \text{ kg}$$

$$= 5.99 \times 10^{24} \text{ kg}$$

SO WHAT EXACTLY *IS* A FORCE?

Newton was worried by his theory of gravity. It worked – in that it gave the right results – but he could not see how the force of gravity could act between objects separated by completely empty space. 'Action at a distance', with nothing to carry the action, did not seem to be scientific. What carried the pull? In the end he gave up and wrote '*Hypotheses non fingo*' – 'I don't give explanations.'

This remained the main problem with gravity for a long time – but as long as a theory gives the right results, physicists are usually happy enough to live with it!

? **QUESTION 23**

23 Use the gravitation formula to check that the units for *G* are N m² kg⁻².

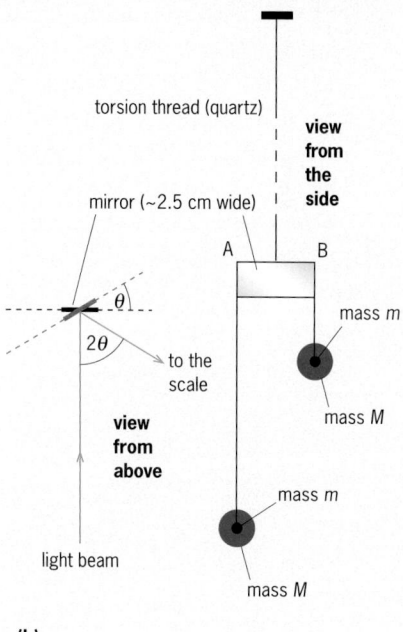

(b)

Fig 2.25 Apparatus to measure the value of the universal gravitational constant, *G*. **(a)** Principle of the Cavendish torsion balance. The masses *M* and *m* attract each other. **(b)** Boys' apparatus. The deflection of AB is measured using a beam of light, so the apparatus can be very small. The photo shows modern apparatus for measuring *G* using the principle seen in **(a)**

A hundred years after Newton, the forces of gravity, electricity and magnetism were linked by a common inverse square model (see Chapters 9 and 25). Then, early in the nineteenth century, Michael Faraday (1791–1867), discoverer of many effects in electromagnetism, proposed the idea of the **field**, as described above. With these two ideas, everything that happened to bodies could be explained and described very neatly using mathematics.

But the 'force carrier gap' still existed in these nineteenth-century field theories. Modern physics has filled the gap, using some rather strange new ideas which we deal with later. For the record, they can be briefly summarised as:

- Forces are carried through space by certain **particles** – photons, gravitons, gluons.
- Empty space isn't empty!

The point about the Newtonian model of the Universe is that it works extremely well for most everyday purposes. It is only in recent years, with the discovery of such things as radioactivity, lasers and some subatomic particles, that the model has needed to be revised. We deal with more recent models later (Chapter 26).

SUMMARY

In this chapter you have extended your knowledge about motion by considering the effect of forces: you have moved from kinematics to the beginnings of dynamics. In particular, you have learnt:

- Newton's three laws of motion.
- The significance of momentum ($p = mv$) and impulse ($Ft = \Delta p$) within these laws.
- Use of the relationships $F = ma$ and $Ft = \Delta p$.
- The distinction between inertial mass and gravitational mass.
- The acceleration of free fall, g, and its relationship to the strength of a gravitational field.

- The distinction between mass and weight.
- How to tackle problems involving motion in a uniform gravitational field (projectile motion).
- Gravitation follows the inverse square law.
- The concept of a field of force.
- How the universal gravitational constant G is measured.

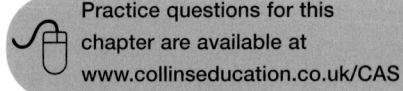

Practice questions for this chapter are available at www.collinseducation.co.uk/CAS

3

Newton's laws at work

3 NEWTON'S LAWS AT WORK

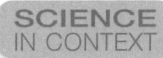
Space danger

It is very rare for an asteroid or a comet to hit the Earth. But smaller pieces of matter arrive from space all the time. Each day, 400 tonnes is added to the Earth's mass from all the pieces of metal, rock and ice travelling through 'empty' space which are trapped by the Earth's gravity and fall into its atmosphere.

Meteorites – chunks of matter in space – fall very fast, between 10 and 70 kilometres per second. Friction with the atmosphere heats them to extremely high temperatures, and that is why we can see them at night as 'shooting stars'. Even objects of 50 metres in diameter generate enough heat to melt and vaporize completely in the upper atmosphere. This is just as well, as an object of that size has the kinetic energy of a 10-megaton nuclear bomb (4.2×10^{16} J).

Massive objects have collided with the Earth about once in every 100 million years. The Earth and the other inner planets of the Solar System would have experienced many more collisions but for the giant planets Jupiter, Saturn, Uranus and Neptune, whose gravitational pull tends to divert the path of large objects. In 1994, for example, fragments of Comet Shoemaker-Levy crashed into Jupiter. It is estimated that, without the giant planets, similar collisions with the Earth could rise to once every 100 000 years. Currently groups of scientists are working on ways of detecting any large objects likely to hit the Earth – and what might be done about it if any are detected.

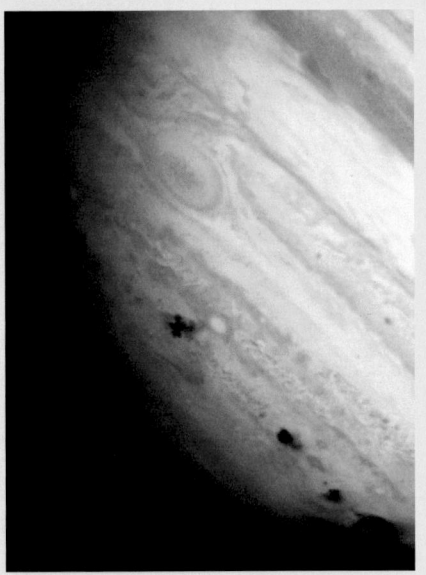

In July 1994, fragments of Comet Shoemaker-Levy hit Jupiter, a planet over 300 times the mass of the Earth. The fragments exploded on impact, and astronomers round the world recorded the fireballs which rose up through the dense atmosphere of cloud. The dark brown patches mark the sites of impact of the fragments

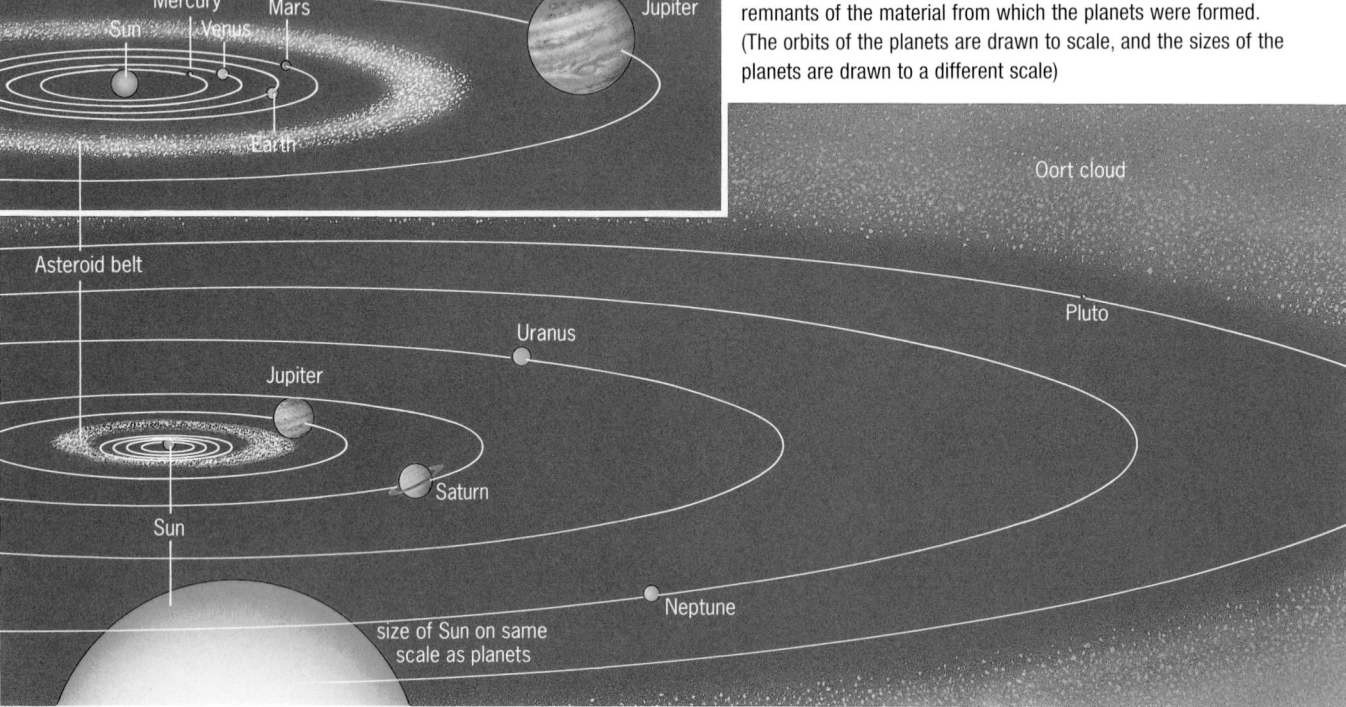

Fig 3.1 The Solar System, including the asteroid belt and Oort cloud, remnants of the material from which the planets were formed. (The orbits of the planets are drawn to scale, and the sizes of the planets are drawn to a different scale)

Energy on a massive scale

The Solar System is an arrangement of planets in orderly orbits round the Sun. But in addition, countless objects smaller than the planets take other paths, and sometimes collide with the planets. They include, for example, asteroids, and meteorites, which are smaller bodies. Near-Earth asteroids are straying members of the asteroid belt, a mass of material that lies in a wide band between the orbits of Mars and Jupiter (shown in Fig 3.1). There are at least 1800 large asteroids with a diameter greater than a kilometre that cross the Earth's orbit – and so are possible candidates for a future catastrophic collision. Fig 3.2 shows the asteroid Eros, on which the space probe NEAR (Near Earth Asteroid Rendezvous) actually landed in February 2000.

Meteorites (Fig 3.3) are smaller, mostly fragments of comets, consisting of metal and rock dust embedded in frozen water and gases, which come from the Oort cloud, on the outermost fringes of the Solar System.

An asteroid hitting the ground makes a crater far larger than itself, because of the colossal energy of its impact. An example is the 180-kilometre-wide crater at Chicxulub, Yucatan, in Mexico (Fig 3.4). The asteroid is thought to have been just over 10^{12} tonnes in mass and 10 kilometres in diameter. It collided with the Earth 65 million years ago, at the end of the geological period known as the Cretaceous, and with an estimated kinetic energy of about 4×10^{23} J. This is about a thousand times greater than the total annual global energy used by human beings today (4×10^{20} J).

The asteroid impact at Chicxulub caused a major upheaval to life on Earth. Such a massive impact sends volumes of dust into the atmosphere, which circulates round the globe for years and cuts out sunlight. Plants fail to grow, and animals that depend on them die. The decline of the dinosaurs is the best known effect thought to have been caused by the Chicxulub impact, but it is thought that about half of all marine species died out at the same time. Similarly, 160 million years earlier, 95 per cent of sea life disappeared, probably as a result of a larger impact by an asteroid whose remains have been found in the South Atlantic Ocean.

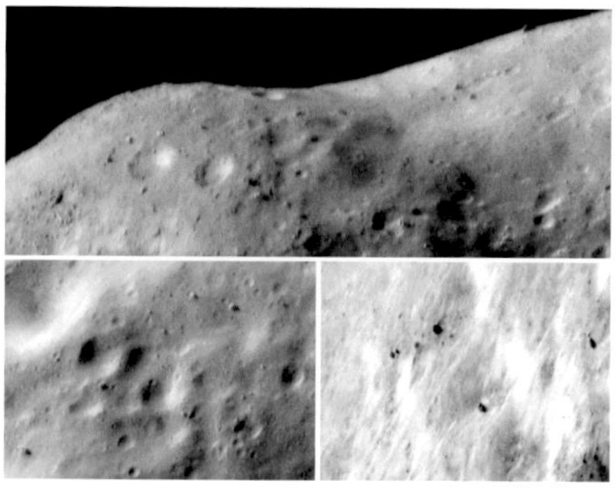

The ideas in this chapter
The physics

To work out the energy of an asteroid, you need to understand the ideas of **kinetic energy**, **gravitational potential energy** and also the **principle of the conservation of energy**. You will also be reminded about power as rate of working or transferring energy. You will develop the notion of a field of gravitational force obeying the inverse square law that you met in Chapter 2. You will learn how these forces and fields determine the **orbital motion** of asteroids, satellites and planets. You will also meet the physical principles of how rockets can put satellites into orbit, and so gain a good understanding of **momentum** and its **conservation**.

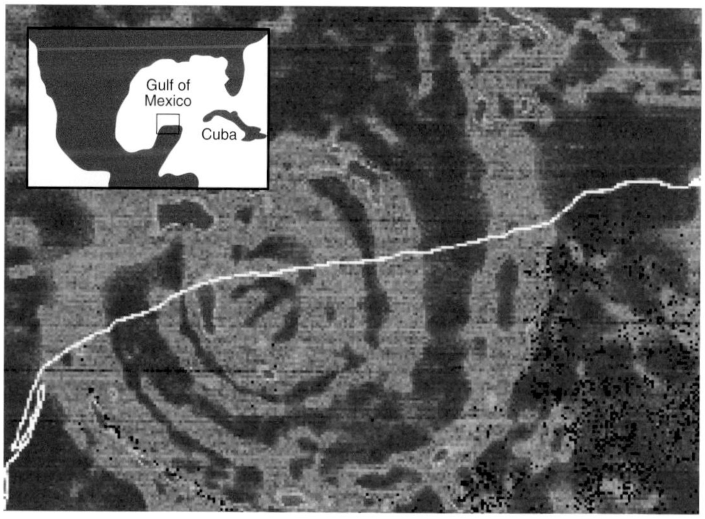

The mathematics

On the whole, simple algebra is all you need. You will be handling large numbers, interpreting graphs and learning of the importance of the area under a graph. Though not essential, integral calculus and the ability to use a spreadsheet would be helpful as well.

Fig 3.2 Eros as photographed by the NEAR spacecraft. Eros is the second largest near-Earth asteroid at about 33 km long and 13 km across. In January 1975 it came within 48 million kilometres of Earth – but its orbit is such that it is highly unlikely to hit us. The NEAR spacecraft was not designed as a lander but was set down and survived its impact velocity of 1.5 to 1.8 m s^{-1}

Fig 3.3 Travelling at great speed, a meteorite heats up and vaporizes because of friction with particles in the atmosphere. We call the streak of light we see in the sky a meteor

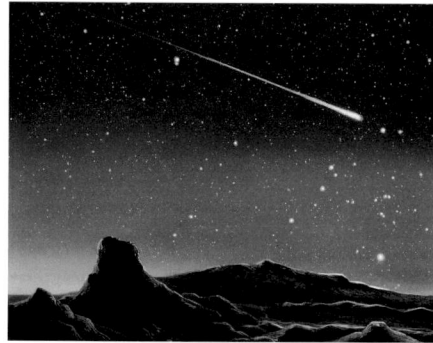

Fig 3.4 The 180-km-wide Chicxulub crater in Mexico, the largest known crater caused by an asteroid impact. The crater was gradually filled in by less dense deposits. Its size and shape are revealed by gravity measurements: the presence of less dense rock causes the gravity field to change (opposite to the effect of mountains, see page 38) and so allows us to produce an image of the crater

1 ENERGY AND WORK

We have looked at the consequences of an asteroid, an object of massive energy, hitting the Earth. Now, we turn to the concept of energy on a very much smaller, everyday level. We base our idea of energy on the concept of **work**, since the energy of a system is both defined and measured in terms of the work a system can do. The word 'work' is defined by physicists to mean something more precise than its common use, because we say that:

Work is done only when a force moves something.

For example, work is done:

- when you use muscular force to lift an object upwards against gravitational force
- when you saw through a piece of wood, again using muscular force to tear the fibres of the wood apart
- when an electrical force moves electrons through a resistor
- when water under pressure turns a turbine in a hydroelectric power station
- when the petrol–air mixture in the cylinder of a car engine explodes and pushes the piston outwards.

Forces doing no work

You are not doing any work when you stand still with a heavy rucksack on your back. You get tired because your muscles are stressed. But if the rucksack stays still, no work will be done on it. In the same way, a table wouldn't be doing any work if you took a rest and put your rucksack on it.

THE WORK FORMULA

The quantity of work done by a force is measured in joules:

work done = force × distance moved in the direction of action of the force

(in joules) (in newtons) (in metres)

$$W = Fd$$

As shown in Fig 3.5(a) and (b), the direction of the force F, and the movement of the point where the force is applied, have to be taken into account.

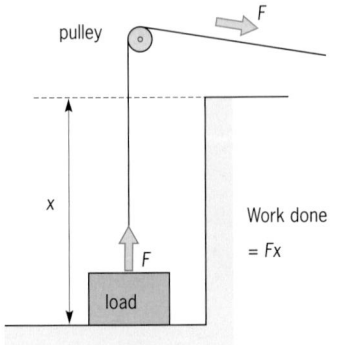

(a) Raising a load vertically, using a pulley

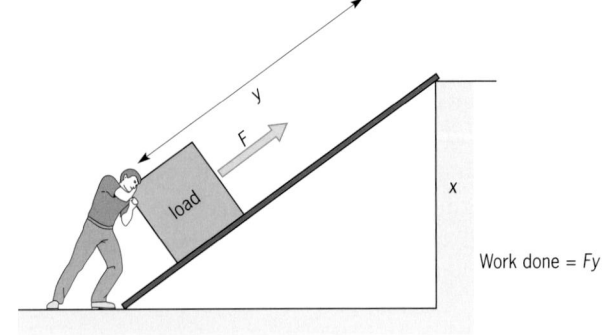

(b) Pushing a load up a ramp

Fig 3.5 Work is being done when a force is used to raise a load. The forces F in (a) and (b) depend on the load and the direction in which the force can be applied

EXAMPLE

Q A woman pushes a shopping trolley up a ramp 4 m long, as in Fig 3.6. She applies a force of 14 N along the ramp. How much work has been done?

A

$$
\begin{array}{ccc}
\text{Work done} & = & \text{force} & \times & \text{distance moved} \\
\text{(J)} & & \text{(N)} & & \text{in direction of} \\
& & & & \text{motion} \\
& & & & \text{(m)}
\end{array}
$$

$$= 14\ N \times 4\ m$$

$$= 56\ N\ m\ (56\ J)$$

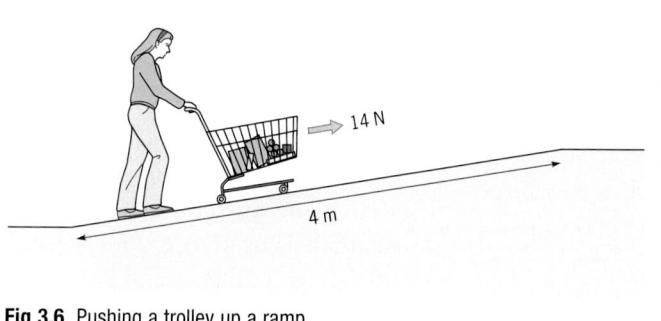

Fig 3.6 Pushing a trolley up a ramp

POWER

It has been calculated that the average citizen of Britain has at his or her disposal the **power** that only the richest Ancient Romans might have had – equivalent to several hundred slaves. Power is a measure of how quickly work is done, and so of how quickly energy can be transferred:

$$\textbf{power = rate of working} = \frac{\textbf{energy transferred}}{\textbf{time taken}}$$

$$P = \frac{E}{t}$$

Power is measured in joules per second and has its own special unit: the watt (W).

In the Example above if the woman pushing the trolley up the slope did the work in 6 seconds she would be working at the rate of 56 J/6 s or 9.3 W.

? QUESTION 3

3 Add up the power that is available to you in your kitchen. Assume that one person works steadily at a rate of 100 W. How many people would you need to replace your kitchen devices?

2 ENERGY IN A GRAVITATIONAL FIELD

Because work is usually easy to measure, we often describe the energy of a system in terms of how much work it does – or is capable of doing. Then we can define energy in this way:

A system has energy if it is capable of doing work.

We use this idea below, and in many other topics in this book.

GRAVITATIONAL POTENTIAL ENERGY

When you lift something, you are doing work. Think of taking a bag of sugar from the floor and putting it on a shelf (Fig 3.7). To do this, you have to exert a force that is just greater than the force of gravity on the sugar bag (its weight, mg), and you have to raise the bag through a height, h.

The work done on the bag = force × distance

$$W = mgh \text{ (in joules)}$$

or $$W = mg\Delta h$$

for a change in height Δh.

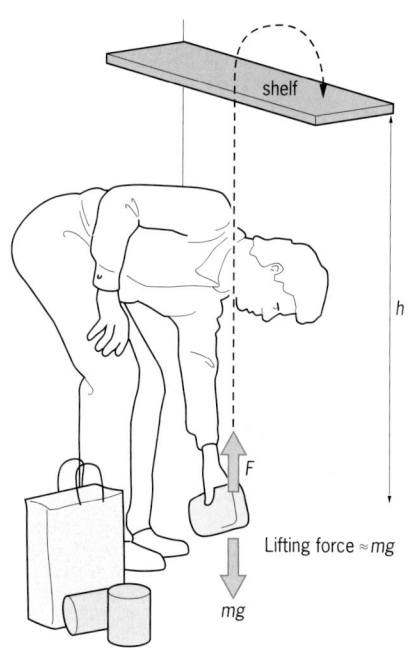

Work done on sugar bag = $Fh = mgh$

Fig 3.7 The force to lift the sugar bag just exceeds the force of gravity

? QUESTIONS 4–5

4 **a)** How much work has to be done in lifting a 5 kg mass through a vertical height of 4 m?
b) What are the energy transfers involved if this is done by someone hauling on a rope looped over a pulley?
c) Why is the energy transferred from chemicals by muscle cells less than the energy eventually transferred to the mass?

5 A force of 10.3 N is required to lift a bag of sugar from the floor to a shelf 1.8 m above the ground.
a) Use the relationship:
work done
= force x distance moved in the direction of the force
to calculate the work done on the bag of sugar.
b) Without further calculation, write down the value of the extra gravitational potential energy now stored in the Earth–bag system.
c) If the bag fell off the shelf and all the extra energy became kinetic energy, at what speed would the bag hit the floor?
(Use kinetic energy = $\frac{1}{2}mv^2$.)

? QUESTION 6

6 You pick up a stone and throw it vertically in the air. It lands back at exactly the same place from which you picked it up.
a) Did you transfer any energy in this situation?
b) What has happened to it?
c) What assumptions about energy have you had to make in giving your answers?

In a system of two objects, gravity provides a pair of forces of attraction that are equal in size but opposite in direction – the Earth pulls on the bag and the bag pulls on the Earth. If the sugar bag fell off the shelf, both bag and Earth would move towards each other (though the Earth would move only a tiny distance).

The sugar bag could do a little useful work while it is falling – for example, we could make it briefly operate a very small generator and produce an electric current to light a small bulb! On a much larger scale, the energy of waterfalls is used to produce electricity in hydroelectric power stations.

So we can think of the Earth–sugar bag system as having 'stored' energy when the bag is resting on the shelf. We call this energy **gravitational potential energy**. The word *potential* reflects the fact that the sugar bag doesn't look very energetic when it is just sitting on the shelf. But we know that it is capable of doing work when it falls. We have noted that work is done when a force moves something. If we don't use the gravitational force on the bag to do useful work (such as turning a tiny generator), then the work done simply increases the **kinetic energy** – the 'energy of movement' – of the bag: as it falls, it moves faster. The energies in their different forms are equal:

$$\text{potential energy} \rightarrow \text{kinetic energy}$$

The mass m picks up speed v so that $\frac{1}{2}mv^2 = mgh$. This is a very useful relationship. See the Stretch and Challenge passage on page 47 for the proof of the formula for kinetic energy.

3 THE PRINCIPLE OF THE CONSERVATION OF ENERGY

It is not *obvious* that the work done in lifting the sugar bag to the shelf is equal to the potential energy stored when it gets there, and that this potential energy is equal to the kinetic energy it would gain as it fell back to the floor.

In any case, you can't actually measure the potential energy directly. If you carried out a careful experiment to measure the work done and the final kinetic energy acquired, your results would probably show that the work done and the final energy were only approximately equal. It is, for example, hard to allow for work done against friction, or for experimental errors.

Nevertheless, one of the most fundamental principles of science states that:

Energy cannot be created or destroyed.

Belief in this principle grew stronger during the nineteenth century as a result of many increasingly accurate experiments, and scientists gradually came to accept it. It became known as the **principle of the conservation of energy**.

EXAMPLE

Q A rock of mass 25 kg falls from a cliff to a beach 30 metres below.
What is
a) its kinetic energy,
b) its speed just before it hits the beach?

A Relative to the beach, the gravitational potential energy of
the rock before falling can be expressed as:

$$mg\Delta h = 25 \times 9.8 \times 30 \text{ (in joules)}$$
$$= 7350 \text{ J}$$

a) Energy is conserved so, ignoring friction with the air, the kinetic
energy of the falling rock is also 7350 J.
b) Therefore: $\quad \frac{1}{2}mv^2 = \frac{1}{2} \times 25 \times v^2$

$$= 7350 \text{ J}$$
$$v^2 = 7350 \times \frac{2}{25}$$

So $\qquad v^2 = \frac{2 \times 7350}{25}$

$$v = 24 \text{ m s}^{-1}$$

Speed of rock just before it hits the beach = 24 m s^{-1}.

STRETCH
AND CHALLENGE

The kinetic energy formula

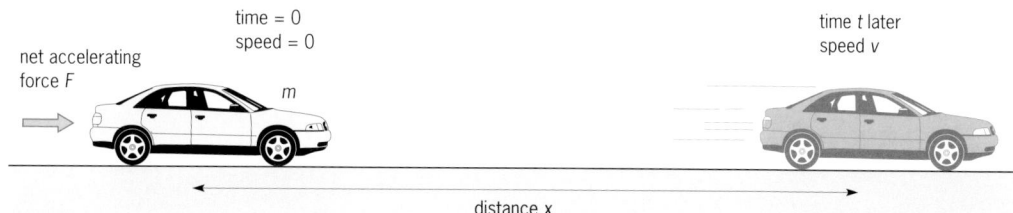

Fig 3.8 How a car gains kinetic energy

You have already used the formula for kinetic energy:

$$\text{kinetic energy} = \frac{1}{2}mv^2$$

which describes the kinetic energy of an object in terms of
its mass and speed. We can derive this formula by looking
at the kinetic energy of an object on which work is done.

Fig 3.8 shows a car having work done on it, and
gaining speed and so kinetic energy. A net accelerating
force F acts on the car, mass m, and the car moves a
distance x from rest, gaining speed, v.

According to the principle of conservation of energy, the
work done, Fx, is transferred to the kinetic energy of the
car (ignoring friction and other energy losses):

$$\text{work done} = \text{force} \times \text{distance moved}$$
$$= Fx$$
$$= max$$

(since force F = mass × acceleration)

It is this work that has given the car its kinetic energy.
We now relate ax to speed v using the kinematic
equation of motion, $v^2 = 2ax$, for an object starting at
zero speed (as in the Example on page 12).

Rearranging this equation,

$$ax = \frac{1}{2}v^2$$

So we can write:

$$\text{kinetic energy gained} = m(ax)$$
$$= m \times \frac{1}{2}v^2$$

which we normally write as:
$$E_k = \frac{1}{2}mv^2$$

Show that the kinetic energy of a moving mass may be
written as $E_k = p^2/2m$ where p is momentum mv
(see page 26).

Joule's work on heat and energy

Experience tells us that, when work is done on an object, energy can be transferred to make it hotter. Hitting metal with a hammer is an example. Conversely, we can use a substance that is hotter than its surroundings to do work, such as burning petrol in a car engine.

In the nineteenth century, the debate was over whether 'heat was a form of energy'. We now say that 'an energy input is required to make something hot, and an object hotter than its surroundings can be used to do work'.

James Prescott Joule (1818–1889) was an amateur scientist interested in heat and energy. Between 1843 and 1878, he carried out very careful experiments to establish the principle of the conservation of energy as it

applied to heating and working. He set out to show that, when frictional forces do work on a substance, it gets hotter, and that there is a direct relationship between the work done and the rise in temperature of the substance.

In his experiments, Joule measured the work done in stirring some water and the rise in temperature it produced. A paddle-wheel, which was driven by a falling weight, rotated in the water – doing work via friction on the water and heating it at the same time. Joule showed that the work done to lift the weight up to the starting position was always proportional to the 'heat energy' gained by the water as the weight fell.

At that time, 'heat' was measured not in joules but in calories, a unit still used on food packaging today. We now remember the work of Joule by the unit of energy named after him.

The principle of conservation of energy – that energy cannot be created or destroyed – is now thought of as one of the most fundamental laws of the material world. It has been extended by Albert Einstein to include the idea that mass is a form of energy. See also Chapter 13.

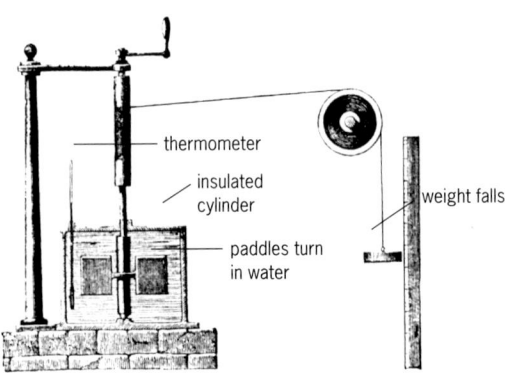

thermometer
insulated cylinder
weight falls
paddles turn in water

Fig 3.9 Using this apparatus to do work on water, Joule discovered a connection between the work done and the heating effect it produced

4 ENERGY CONSERVATION IN A UNIFORM GRAVITATIONAL FIELD

As we have seen, gravitational potential energy is measured simply as the work done to move an object directly against the force of a gravitational field, that is, upwards (refer back to Fig 3.7). So

change in gravitational potential energy = **work done when moving something against a gravitational force**

$$\Delta E = \text{gravitational force} \times \text{distance moved}$$
$$\Delta E = mg\Delta h$$

This formula for a change in gravitational potential energy is correct only if the value of g, the gravitational field strength, is constant over the whole distance Δh. The formula is accurate enough for objects moved close to the surface of the Earth, but will not be correct for distances comparable with the size of the Earth, let alone distances on the scale of the Solar System. This situation is considered more fully in the next section.

So far, you have solved some quite complicated dynamic and kinematic problems using the ideas of force, mass, acceleration and the equations of motion. These techniques are easy to use when forces on objects are uniform, and produce uniform accelerations of the objects. But in most everyday situations, things aren't so simple, and it is often more convenient to solve problems using the idea of the conservation of energy, as in the following Example.

EXAMPLE

Q A holiday park has a roller coaster shown in the diagram of Fig 3.10. The ride follows a loop path that begins and ends at D. The car is hauled from D to point A, the top of the ride, and then moves from rest, under gravity, to arrive at point D again.

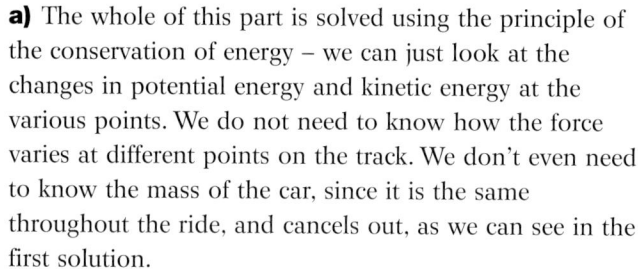

Fig 3.10 The roller coaster track

a) Ignoring frictional forces, what are the speeds of the car at: point B; point C; point D?

b) To stop at point D, the car has to be braked from a speed of 10 m s⁻¹. In practice, friction has reduced the car's speed during the ride. By point D, what proportion of the energy which the car had at point A has it lost because of friction?

A

a) The whole of this part is solved using the principle of the conservation of energy – we can just look at the changes in potential energy and kinetic energy at the various points. We do not need to know how the force varies at different points on the track. We don't even need to know the mass of the car, since it is the same throughout the ride, and cancels out, as we can see in the first solution.

Speed at point B

Gain in kinetic energy = loss in potential energy

$$\tfrac{1}{2} mv^2 = mg\Delta h \text{ (where } g = 9.8 \text{ m s}^{-2})$$
$$v^2 = 2g\Delta h \text{ (where } \Delta h = 25 - 12 = 13, \text{ in metres)}$$
$$v^2 = 2 \times 9.8 \times 13 = 254.8 \text{ m}^2 \text{ s}^{-2}$$

giving: $v = 16$ m s⁻¹

Speed at point C

The net loss in potential energy at point C is due to a drop of 5 m from point A. Check for yourself that the speed at point C is just under 10 m s⁻¹.

Speed at point D

The drop is 25 m. So, using $v^2 = 2g\Delta h$,
$$v^2 = 2 \times 9.8 \times 25 \text{ m}^2 \text{ s}^{-2}$$
$$v = 22 \text{ m s}^{-1}$$

b) Before braking, the car is travelling at 10 m s⁻¹. So, before braking, the kinetic energy $\tfrac{1}{2}v^2$ per unit mass ($m = 1$ kg) is:
$$0.5 \times 10^2 = 50 \text{ J kg}^{-1}$$

For a theoretical value for the car's kinetic energy we assume that the ride is frictionless, so the gain in kinetic energy per unit mass equals the potential energy, $mg\Delta h$, lost per unit mass:
$$9.8 \times 25 = 245 \text{ J kg}^{-1}$$

So the energy wastage due to friction per unit mass of car is:
$$245 - 50 = 195 \text{ J kg}^{-1}$$

The proportion of energy wasted during the ride
$$= 195 \sqrt{ } 245 = 0.80 \text{ or } 80\%$$

5 GRAVITATIONAL POTENTIAL ENERGY IN THE EARTH'S FIELD

As Chapter 2 explains, the gravitational field strength of an object varies with the distance from that object, and the field strength obeys the inverse square law. Earth has a **radial gravitational field** shown in Fig 3.11 overleaf. Over short distances close to the Earth's surface, the variation in gravitational field strength is too small to worry about, so here we assume that the field is uniform.

Table 3.1 summarises the relevant formulae. G is the universal gravitational constant (see Chapter 2) and M is the mass of the Earth. Some of the formulae still need to be explained.

Table 3.1 Calculating the gravitational field strength

	Uniform field	Radial field
Force	$F = mg$	$F = -GMm/r^2$
Change in gravitational potential energy	$mg\Delta h$	$GMm(1/r_1 - 1/r_2)$
Gravitational potential	(not a useful idea in a uniform field!)	$-GM/r$

REMEMBER THIS

The universal gravitational constant

$G = 6.67 \times 10^{-11}$ N m^2 kg^{-2}.

The Earth's mass

$M = 5.98 \times 10^{24}$ kg.

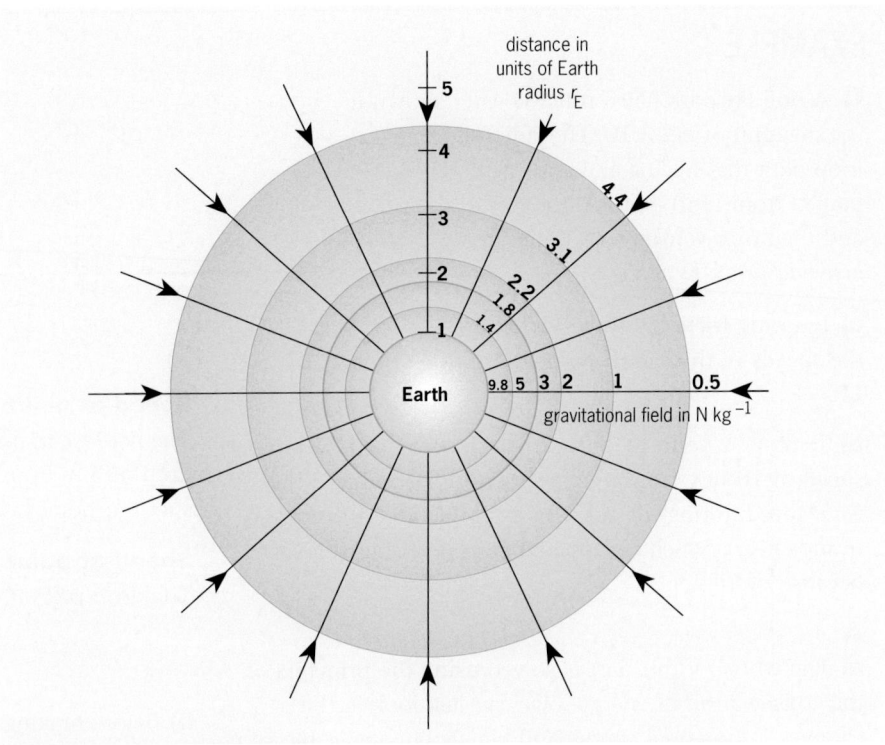

distance in units of Earth radius r_E

4.4
3.1
2.2
1.8
1.4

Earth   9.8 5 3 2   1   0.5

gravitational field in N kg^{-1}

Fig 3.11 The radial gravitational field of the Earth, showing how the value varies with distance from the Earth's surface. Radial lines are force lines, and circular lines are lines of equal gravitational field

'NEGATIVE ENERGY' – A VERY USEFUL IDEA

Before looking at the details of the radial field, we have to clear up a matter which often causes confusion – *the negative sign given to the value of gravitational potential energy.*

Imagine an object of mass m in empty space an infinite distance $r_\circ$ from any other massive body. Force in a radial field is $GMm/r_\circ{}^2$. But since $r_\circ$ is at infinity, the object will have zero force acting on it. It cannot 'fall' towards anything, so it has no potential energy and it cannot gain kinetic energy – or do any work. So it must have *zero gravitational potential energy* (Fig 3.12).

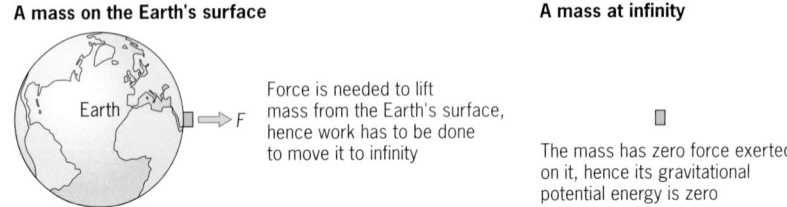

A mass on the Earth's surface

Earth ⟶ F

Force is needed to lift mass from the Earth's surface, hence work has to be done to move it to infinity

A mass at infinity

The mass has zero force exerted on it, hence its gravitational potential energy is zero

Fig 3.12 Gravitational potential energy of a mass at infinity and at the Earth's surface

Now imagine the same mass m sitting on the Earth. To move it to infinity (beyond the gravitational field of the Earth or any other body), you would have to *give* it energy – kinetic energy if you propelled it in a rocket. (Soon, we shall calculate just how much energy it needs.) But when the mass gets back to infinity again, it will of course have zero gravitational potential energy.

The only way to 'balance the books' (and so conserve energy) is to accept that when the mass rested on the Earth it had *negative* energy, and that it needed the same quantity of *positive* energy to reach infinity and stop there (with zero energy):

| some positive kinetic energy | + | same amount of negative potential energy | = | zero energy |

FINDING A VALUE FOR GRAVITATIONAL POTENTIAL ENERGY IN A RADIAL FIELD

As in Fig 3.13(a), an object of mass m is at a point r_2 from the centre of the Earth. Then it is moved to a nearby point r_1, a small extra distance Δr closer to the Earth's centre.

For a small movement, the force does not vary within distance Δr. The object is, for all practical purposes, in a **uniform field**. So the change in gravitational potential energy would simply be $mg\Delta r$, as shown in the graph of Fig 3.13(b). The change in potential energy per unit mass is $g\Delta r$, and is represented by the area ABCD under the graph.

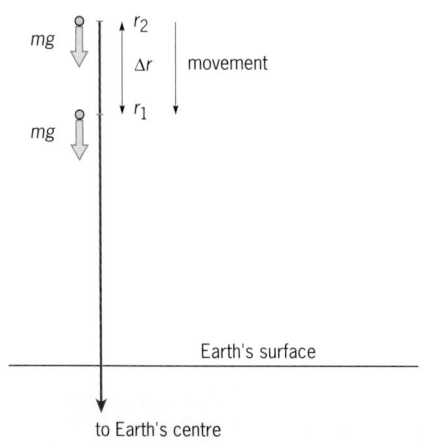

Fig 3.13(a) An object near the Earth is moved a small distance, over which the gravitational field does not significantly change

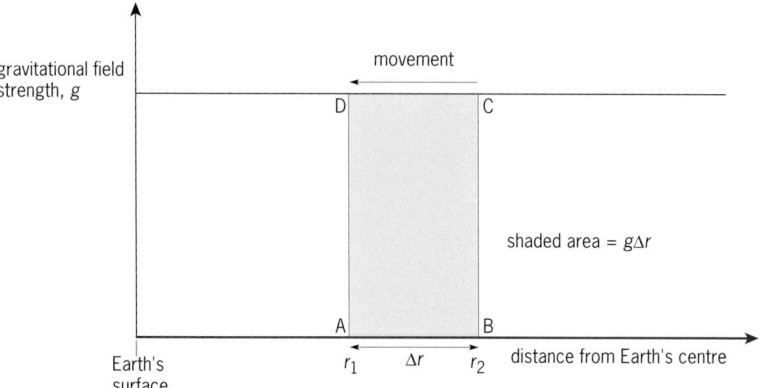

shaded area = $g\Delta r$

Fig 3.13(b) Graph of force against distance for a uniform field

Imagine a very much larger distance, on the scale of Fig 3.14(a).

Fig 3.14(a) An object is moved through a large distance from the Earth, and the gravitational field changes

? QUESTION 7

7 **a)** When objects fall towards the Earth, they lose potential energy and gain kinetic energy. Does this mean that, when an object moves in a gravitational field, the change in kinetic energy is always opposite in sign to the change in potential energy? (Look at the word equation at the bottom of page 50.)

b) A mass falls from a point A to a point B. In doing so, it gains 50 kJ of kinetic energy. If the mass had 5000 kJ of gravitational potential energy (GPE) at point B, how much GPE did it have at A?

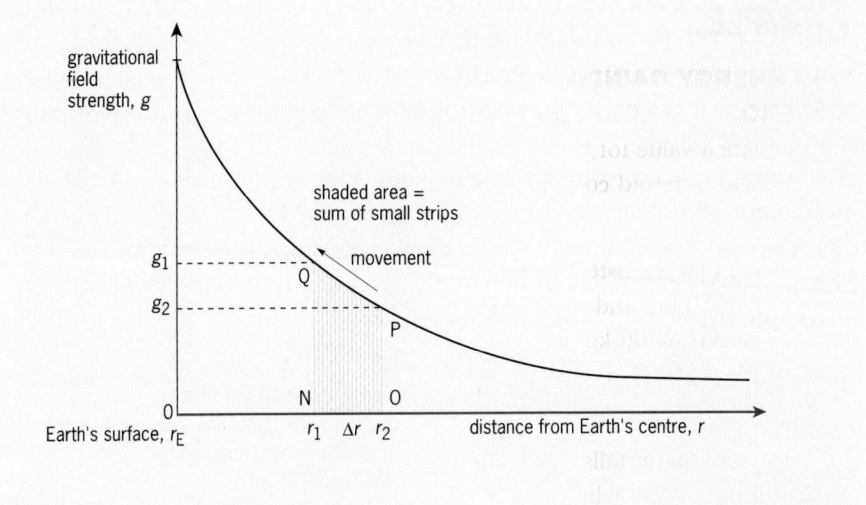

Fig 3.14(b) Graph of force against distance for a radial field such as the Earth's

The curved graph of Fig 3.14(b) represents a field of varying strength, getting less as the distance from the Earth increases. So, as the object is moved from r_2 to r_1, it experiences an increasing gravitational force. The change in potential energy per unit mass is represented by the area NOPQ under the graph. In algebraic terms this works out to be $E = GM(1/r_2 - 1/r_1)$. See the Stretch and Challenge passage below for this.

STRETCH AND CHALLENGE

Calculating the change in gravitational potential energy

GRAPHICALLY AND NUMERICALLY

We can find the value of the change in gravitational potential energy from the graph of Fig 3.14(b) by counting the squares in each small shaded strip. This is tedious! Instead, we can add them up numerically using a spreadsheet.

ALGEBRAICALLY, USING CALCULUS

We can find area NOPQ in Fig 3.14(b) more easily using a simple formula for the result. We employ calculus to get the formula, recognizing the fact that, for large distances, g depends upon r according to the inverse square law. The symbol E_p is used for gravitational potential energy.

The change in gravitational potential energy, ΔE_p, is given by using the definition of work (force × distance). The potential energy gained equals the work done in moving mass m a distance Δr between points at distances r_2 and r_1 from the centre of the Earth.

So: $\Delta E_p = -\dfrac{GMm}{r^2}\,\Delta r$

As explained on page 50, the negative sign is there to balance the books and keep potential energy negative.

The equation may be integrated to give:

$$E_p = -GMm \int_{r_2}^{r_1} \frac{1}{r^2}\,dr = GM\left[\frac{1}{r_2} - \frac{1}{r_1}\right]$$

which is usually written as:

$$E_p = \frac{GMm}{r_2} - \frac{GMm}{r_1}$$

This is the **potential energy difference formula**, where E_p is the difference in potential energy for a mass m at a point at distance r_2 from that for the same mass at distance r_1 from the centre of the Earth. If the object falls freely it equals the kinetic energy gained.

EXAMPLE

THE ENERGY GAINED BY AN ASTEROID FALLING TO EARTH

Q Estimate a value for the kinetic energy of an asteroid colliding with the Earth.

A Assume that the asteroid has a diameter of 10 km and is made of rock of density 3000 kg per cubic metre. This gives it a mass of about 1.6×10^{15} kg.

Assume, too, that it falls from infinity, that is, from a place where the gravitational potential is zero. At the Earth's surface it is at a place with a gravitational potential of $-GM/r_E$. In other words, its potential energy per kilogram has been reduced by GM/r_E.

Loss in gravitational potential (energy per unit mass):

$$-\frac{GM}{r_k} = -\frac{(6.7 \times 10^{-11})\,(6.0 \times 10^{24})}{6.4 \times 10^6}$$
$$= -6.3 \times 10^7 \text{J kg}^{-1}$$

This energy has of course been converted to kinetic energy. So the total kinetic energy of the asteroid is equal to the potential energy lost by its mass of 1.6×10^{15} kg:

gain in KE = loss in GPE
(gravitational potential × mass)

$= 6.3 \times 10^7 \text{ (J kg}^{-1}) \times 1.6 \times 10^{15} \text{ (kg)}$
$= 1.0 \times 10^{23}$ J

We can calculate its impact speed from the formula for kinetic energy:

$$E_k = \tfrac{1}{2}mv^2 = 1.0 \times 10^{23} \text{ J}$$
$$v^2 = \frac{2 \times E_k}{m}$$
$$v = \sqrt{\frac{2 \times 10^{23}}{1.6 \times 10^{15}}}$$
$$= 11.2 \times 10^3 \text{m s}^{-1}$$

So the impact speed is 11.2 km s^{-1}.

6 GRAVITATIONAL POTENTIAL

The gravitational potential (V) of an object at a point in space is a useful idea. It allows us to calculate the energy changes, or the work done, when a satellite moves to a different orbit. Gravitational potential can be compared to the concept of electrical potential, and is defined as follows:

Gravitational potential is the change in potential energy for a unit mass that moves from infinity to a point at less than infinity in a gravitational field.

If we make r_2 = infinity, $r_1 = r$ and $m = 1$ (kg), the potential energy difference formula in the Stretch and Challenge box on page 52 simplifies to:

$$V = -\frac{GM}{r}$$

For the field of the Earth, we can use this formula to calculate the potential at a point at a distance r from the centre of the Earth.

A typical meteorite enters the Earth's atmosphere at about 20 km s^{-1}, almost double the speed calculated in the Example above. This is because meteorites are already moving when they start falling towards the Earth, and the Earth is also moving. We have also ignored the gravitational effect of the Sun, which is very large.

ESCAPE SPEED

Looking the other way round at the Example above, we can see that if an object is at rest on the Earth's surface, we would have to *give* it some kinetic energy before it could escape completely from the Earth. To reach infinity, where the Earth's gravitational field doesn't affect it, we would have to give it 6.3×10^7 J of kinetic energy for every kilogram of its mass. This would convert the negative gravitational potential it had on the Earth's surface (its GPE per unit mass), of value $-GM/r_E$, to zero.

You should now use the kinetic energy formula to check what is obvious, that each kilogram of an object has to be given the right amount of energy to reach a speed of 11.2 km s^{-1} – in the right direction – for it to be able to escape from the Earth. This speed is called the **escape speed** (or escape velocity).

? QUESTION 8

8 The gravitational potential at the Earth's surface is found by inserting the following values in the formula $-GM/r$:

GM for Earth = 4.0×10^{14} N m^2 kg^{-1}

Radius of Earth, r_E = 6.38×10^6 m

Check that this calculation results in a value of -6.3×10^7 J kg^{-1}.

? QUESTION 9

9 Suggest some practical difficulties that might arise if a spacecraft is given the energy for its escape speed all at once as it leaves the ground.

? QUESTION 10

10 A neutron star has a mass of 4×10^{30} kg and a radius of 10 km. Show that the escape speed from the star is about two-thirds the speed of light.

EXAMPLE

Q The Moon has a mass of 7.3×10^{22} kg and a radius of 1.7×10^{6} m. What is the escape speed for an object on the Moon?

A The gravitational potential at the Moon's surface is:

$$- \frac{GM}{r_{\mathrm{M}}} = - \frac{(6.7 \times 10^{-11}) \times (7.3 \times 10^{22})}{1.7 \times 10^{6}}$$

$$= - 2.88 \times 10^{6} \text{ J kg}^{-1}$$

Any object has to be given an equivalent quantity of kinetic energy per unit mass to escape the Moon's gravitational pull.

So, kinetic energy per kilogram is:

$$\tfrac{1}{2}v^2 = 2.88 \times 10^6$$

$$v = \sqrt{2 \times 2.88 \times 10^6}$$

Escape speed $\quad v = 2.4 \times 10^3 \text{m s}^{-1}$

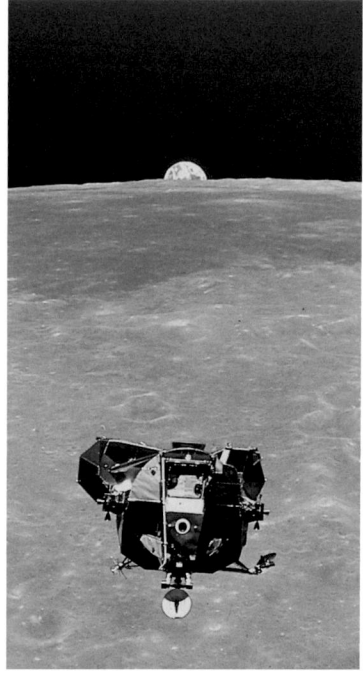

Fig 3.15 The NASA lunar module leaving the Moon to dock with the command module

7 MOVING IN AN ORBIT

The simplest orbit for an Earth satellite is circular, centred on the Earth's centre. A typical satellite used to monitor the Earth's surface has the **circumpolar orbit** shown in Fig 3.16(a). While the satellite orbits, the Earth spins underneath it. So, if a complete orbit takes 2 hours, the satellite will overfly the whole of the Earth in 12 orbits, as Fig 3.16(b) shows.

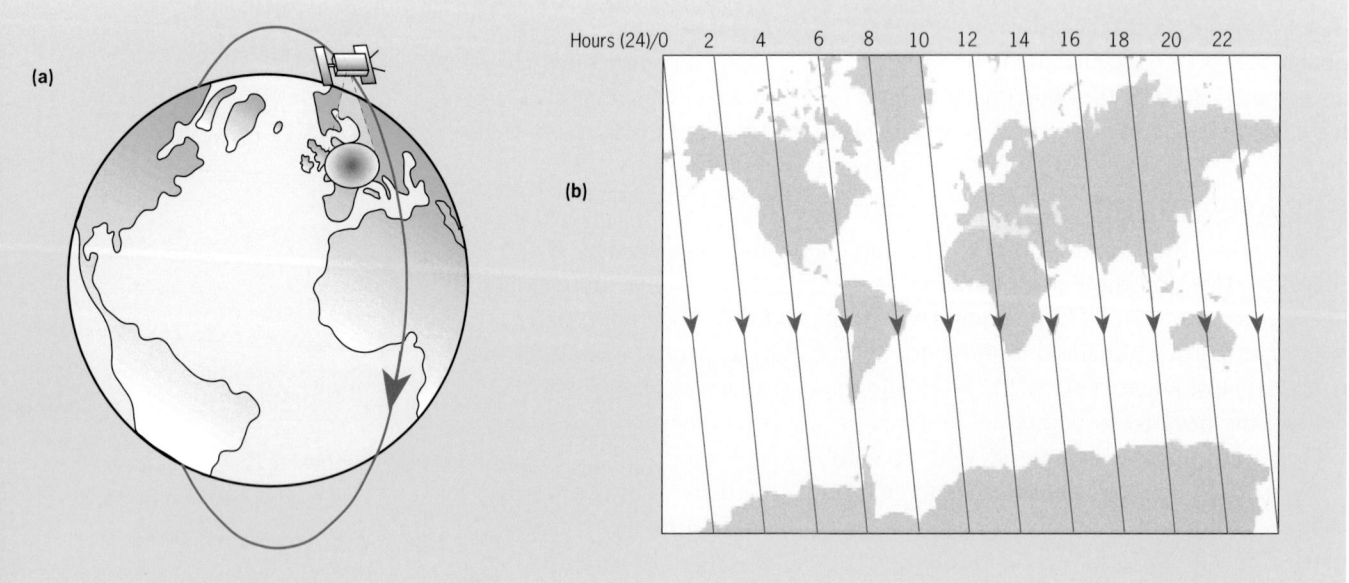

Fig 3.16 Satellites in circumpolar orbits can monitor the whole Earth as it spins beneath them

Earth satellites provide remote eyes and ears

The fact that Earth satellites can be put into orbit fairly cheaply has revolutionised everyday communications and information systems. On our television screens, we can now see events unfold in the remotest parts of the world as they happen. All a news reporter needs is a small dish aerial and a portable power supply, and access to a communications satellite. These satellites are in a high, geosynchronous orbit above the equator.

Communications satellites also carry international telephone messages that are far clearer than those transmitted by the old radio or landline systems. (Chapter 21, Communications, describes how information is sent as radio waves between satellites and ground stations, and explains the digital technology that allows a huge number of messages to be transmitted at the same time.)

Weather satellites provide the pictures of cloud systems we see on television weather reports. These satellites have polar orbits and are closer to the ground than geosynchronous satellites. The recording of land and sea temperatures, and the forecasting of climatic changes and trends in the greenhouse effect, have all become much more reliable, thanks to weather satellites. It was a British satellite collecting data over Antarctica that first provided evidence of a 'hole' developing in the ozone layer.

Links between satellite and ground computers allow us to know the positions of satellites very accurately. Similarly, satellites give us precise positions for objects on Earth. For many years, ships and aircraft have relied on navigation satellites to pinpoint their locations. On land, small receivers are now easily and cheaply available which use navigation satellite data to tell mountain walkers where they are to the nearest few metres, and drivers of vehicles their exact locations, and even the routes to take to avoid traffic jams. Bus companies use them to check where their buses are and so adjust their speeds to avoid 'bunching'.

Military satellites keep an eye on the movement of ships, troops and vehicles. They can detect when weapons are being fired, and can eavesdrop on conversations over a wide range of electronic communications systems.

The infrared satellite sensors which detect land and sea temperatures can also monitor the growth of crops – whether they are healthy or diseased, or lack water, for example. In the European Union, agricultural land is monitored to check that farmers who claim money for

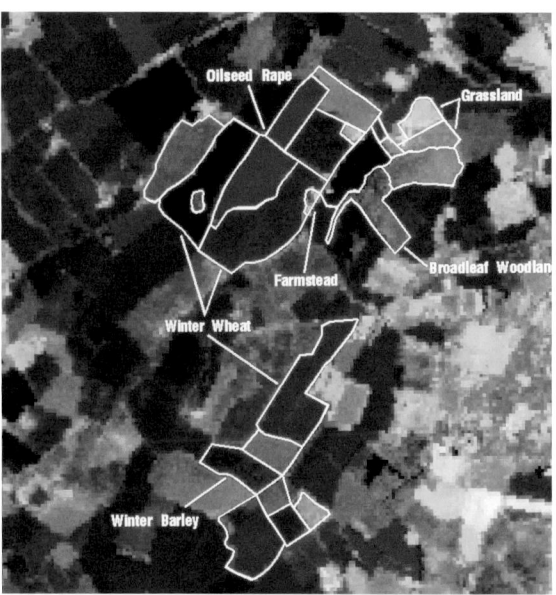

Fig 3.17(a) Infrared satellite image of a Bedfordshire farm showing that different types of crops can be identified. This picture was taken from Landsat at an altitude of 705 km

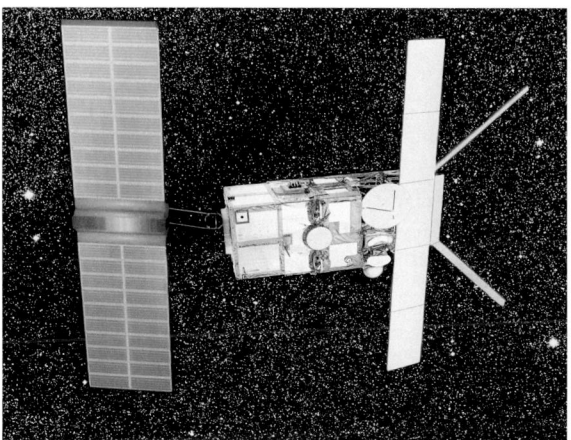

Fig 3.17(b) European Remote Sensing satellite, ERS1, surveys the structure of the Earth's surface, watches shore lines and ocean currents (it can detect oil spills), monitors crop and vegetation growth, and surveys and maps the polar ice caps

leaving land uncultivated ('set aside') are not in fact growing crops on it.

Satellites are sent into orbit either by rocket systems used once only, such as the European Ariane, or by the reusable US Space Shuttle. An increasing number of countries are putting satellites into orbit, for their own national uses such as weather monitoring, or on a commercial basis, hiring out the satellite facilities to research and communications organisations such as universities and television companies.

Newton explained how, in theory, an object shot at great speed from the Earth's surface could become an orbiting satellite. He imagined a cannon on a mountain, firing cannon balls parallel to the Earth's surface at ever-increasing speeds. Each ball lands further from the cannon than the previous one, travelling in a curved path. Newton imagined that, eventually, the curved path of a ball would match the curvature of the Earth and *then the ball would be in orbit*.

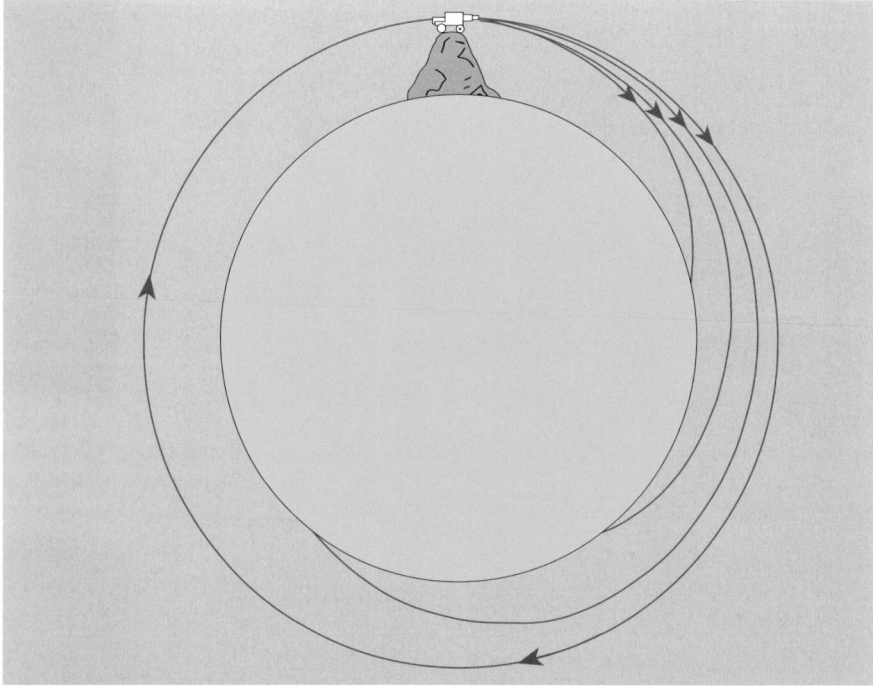

Fig 3.18 Isaac Newton's orbiting cannon ball. In his book, *System of the World*, Newton wrote: 'The greater the velocity with which [a cannon ball] is projected, the farther it goes before it falls to the Earth. We may therefore suppose the velocity to be so increased, that it would describe an arc of 1, 2, 5, 10, 100, 1000 miles before it arrived at the Earth, till at last, exceeding the limits of the Earth, it should pass into space without touching.'

? **QUESTION 11**

11 a) Suggest some practical difficulties that would arise in using Newton's cannon method for getting a satellite into orbit from the top of a high mountain. (Assume it does not then collide with anything.)
b) To what speed would the satellite have to be accelerated if fired horizontally?
(Radius of Earth = 6.4 x 10^6 m.)

✔ **REMEMBER THIS**
We say that an object is accelerating if its speed is changing, or its direction of motion is changing, or both.

It is of course the force of gravity acting on a cannon ball that makes it fall back to Earth. A ball which remains in orbit also experiences this force. Its speed may be constant, but it still obeys Newton's second law of motion because its *velocity* continuously changes – the *direction* of the ball's motion is always changing. The force of gravity is responsible, making the orbiting ball accelerate towards the centre of the Earth – in free fall.

All orbiting satellites are in free fall. Their acceleration is equal to the value of g at that distance from the Earth, and this acceleration is directed towards the centre of the Earth.

Clearly, the speed of a satellite has to be just right to stay in a circular orbit. If it is too slow, the satellite falls to Earth like the 'unsuccessful' cannon balls in Fig 3.18. Too fast, and the satellite's orbital radius may increase, or its orbit may become an ellipse. Much too fast, and the satellite leaves Earth's orbit completely.

Formula for the inward acceleration of an object moving in a circle

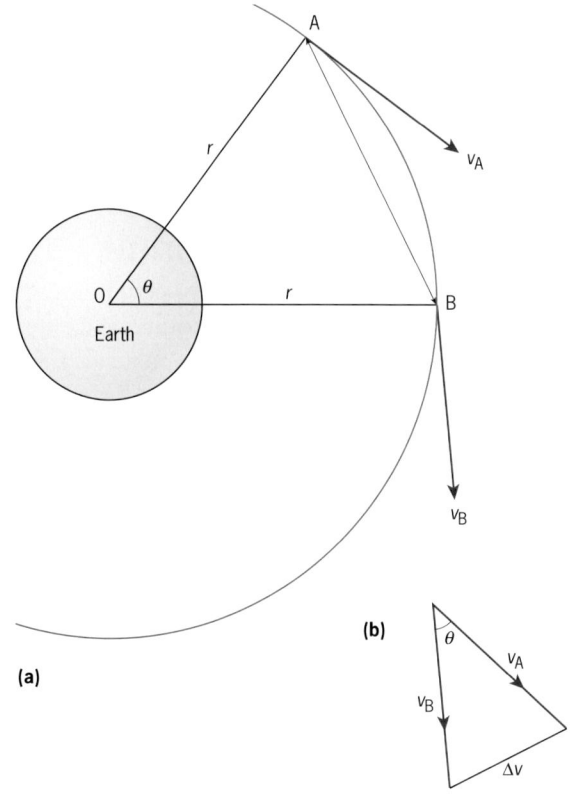

Fig 3.19(a) A satellite moving in a circle.
(b) Triangle of vectors for the satellite

The formula developed here applies to any object moving in a circle – for example, the rim of a wheel, a ball whirling on the end of a string, a car going round a bend or a satellite in orbit.

Fig 3.19(a) shows two positions, A and B, of a satellite moving in a circle round the Earth at constant speed v. The radius line, r, moves through an angle, θ, measured in radians, in a time t, and the object moves a distance $r\theta$. The gravitational force always acts along a radius, inwards towards the centre of the Earth.

Fig 3.19(b) shows how the vector representing the *velocity* of the satellite has changed in time t. Since the speed of the satellite doesn't change, vectors v_A and v_B are of equal length.

Δv shows the change in velocity using a triangle of vectors such that:

$$v_B = v_A + \Delta v$$

In these two diagrams the value of t, and therefore of θ, is large. Now see Fig 3.20, in which θ is very small, so that Δv is also very small. This also means that the *time* involved is small.

The acceleration of the body is given by

$$a = \frac{\Delta v}{t} \qquad [1]$$

Referring back to Fig 3.19(a), we can see that the object covers a distance $r\theta$ in time t at a speed v, so that

$$v = \frac{r\theta}{t} \quad \text{hence} \quad \frac{1}{t} = \frac{v}{r\theta} \qquad [2]$$

Substituting for $1/t$ in equation 1 gives

$$a = \frac{v\Delta v}{r\theta} \qquad [3]$$

v is directed along a tangent to the circle, so is always at right angles to the radius line. (Note that for small θ, sin θ = tan θ = θ radians.)

When the radius turns through an angle θ so does v. So, with the usual small-angle approximation:

$$\Delta v = v\theta \text{ (see Fig 3.20)} \qquad [4]$$

Substituting for Δv in equation 3 gives:

$$a = \frac{v^2}{r} \qquad [5]$$

As angle θ gets smaller and smaller, the direction of Δv becomes closer and closer to being at right angles to v. This means it is in the direction of the radius and acting towards the centre of the circle. This is, of course, the direction of the force causing the acceleration.

We can therefore represent the **centripetal force** F required to keep a body of mass m moving in a circle, using the relation:

$$\text{force} = \text{mass} \times \text{acceleration}$$

as: $$F = \frac{mv^2}{r}$$

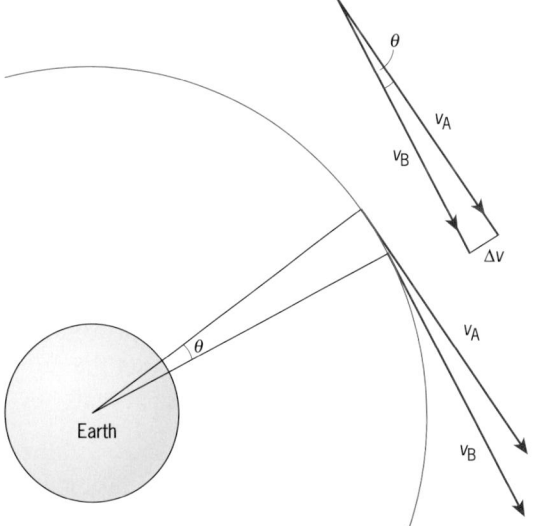

Fig 3.20 Triangle of vectors with a smaller angle

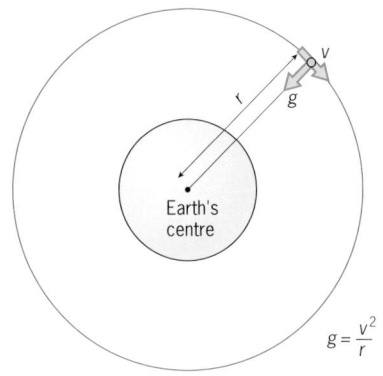

Fig 3.21 Illustrating the quantities in the formula $g = v^2/r$

SPEED AND THE RADIUS OF THE ORBIT

As shown in the Stretch and Challenge passage on page 57, a satellite that moves in a *circular* orbit has an inward gravitational acceleration g and speed v, which are linked by the equation:

$$g = \frac{v^2}{r} \qquad [6]$$

where r is the radius of the orbit (Fig 3.21).

SPEED OF A SATELLITE IN A CIRCULAR ORBIT

We saw in Fig 3.16 that a satellite in polar orbit sweeps over certain areas of the Earth which depend on the number of its orbits in 24 hours, hence on its speed. The speed is set before launch, so that the orbital time matches the purpose of the satellite – whether it is a near-Earth weather monitoring satellite, or a distant communications satellite, for example.

The satellite's speed depends both on the radius of its orbit and on the strength of the gravitational field at that height. A typical height for a satellite in near-Earth orbit is 100 km. This gives an orbital radius of 6.47×10^6 m. The inward acceleration is the value of g at that height, which is 9.53 m s^{-2}.

Thus, from equation 6 above, its speed is

$$v = \sqrt{gr}$$

Hence, $\qquad\qquad v = 7.85$ km s^{-1}

The circumference, $2\pi r$, of its orbit is 4.07×10^4 km. The satellite therefore completes an orbit in 86.3 minutes.

Now reread this section and work through the calculations for yourself.

GEOSTATIONARY SATELLITES

Communications satellites (Fig 3.22) are put into **geostationary** or **geosynchronous** orbits, meaning that the satellites stay still relative to the Earth. As a result, ground aerials which send and receive data to and from a satellite need only point in one direction, rather than having to steer to follow the satellite.

To be geostationary, an orbit has to be directly above the equator, and the satellite must complete its orbit in exactly the same time as the spot underneath rotates through *its* orbit, namely 24 hours. In theory, a geostationary satellite 'keeps up with' the point on the rotating Earth. In practice, its position shifts a little, as the satellite's speed is affected by slight changes in the Earth's gravitational field. Small adjuster rockets are fired to regain the correct position.

Using equation 6 above, we can calculate the height at which a satellite must orbit in order to remain geostationary.

Let the radius of the orbit be r_s. The satellite must have an orbital speed v such that

$$2\pi r_s = vt = v \times 86\ 400 \quad (t \text{ is } 24 \text{ hours} = 86\ 400 \text{ seconds})$$

So $\qquad\qquad\qquad\qquad v = \dfrac{2\pi r_s}{86\ 400} \qquad [7]$

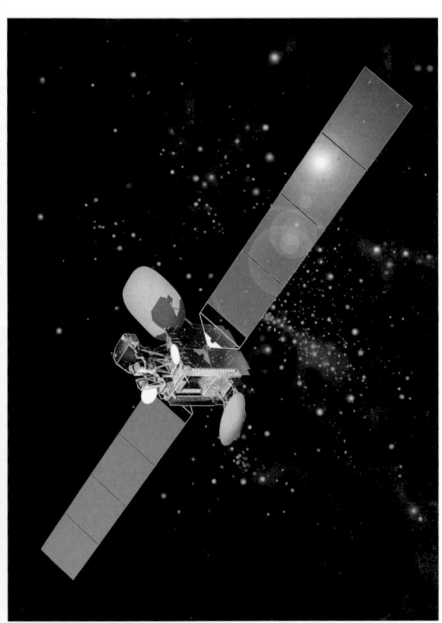

Fig 3.22 The INTELSAT IX communications satellite, used for television broadcasting and telephone communications

From equation 6,

$$v = \sqrt{gr_s} \qquad [8]$$

At distance r_s

$$g = \frac{GM}{r_s^2}$$

Putting this value for g into equation 8,

$$v = \sqrt{\frac{GM}{r_s}}$$

Equating the expressions for v in equations 7 and 8, we have

$$\frac{2\pi r_s}{86\,400} = \sqrt{\frac{GM}{r_s}}$$

Inserting the values of constants G and M, we get a value for the radius, r_s, for a geostationary orbit of 4.23×10^7 m. This is over six times the radius of the Earth and, at that distance, the value of g is 0.223 N kg^{-1}.

PUTTING SATELLITES INTO ORBIT

Fig 3.23 shows how a rocket lifts a satellite into orbit. Fuel makes up most of the mass of the main rocket with its various stages, and much of the fuel is used to get the final stage into near-Earth orbit – about 100 km above the Earth's surface. The remaining fuel propels the comparatively small payload of one or more satellites into their final orbits.

? QUESTIONS 12–13

12 An Earth satellite has a circular polar orbit at a height of 400 km above the Earth's surface.
Calculate
a) its orbital speed,
b) the time it takes to complete an orbit, and
c) how many orbits it makes in a 24-hour period.
(Use $g = 8.7$ m s^{-2} and Earth radius = 6.4×10^6 m.)

13 Work out for yourself the values calculated for the geostationary satellite.
Take $GM = 4.0 \times 10^{14}$ N m^2 kg^{-1}.

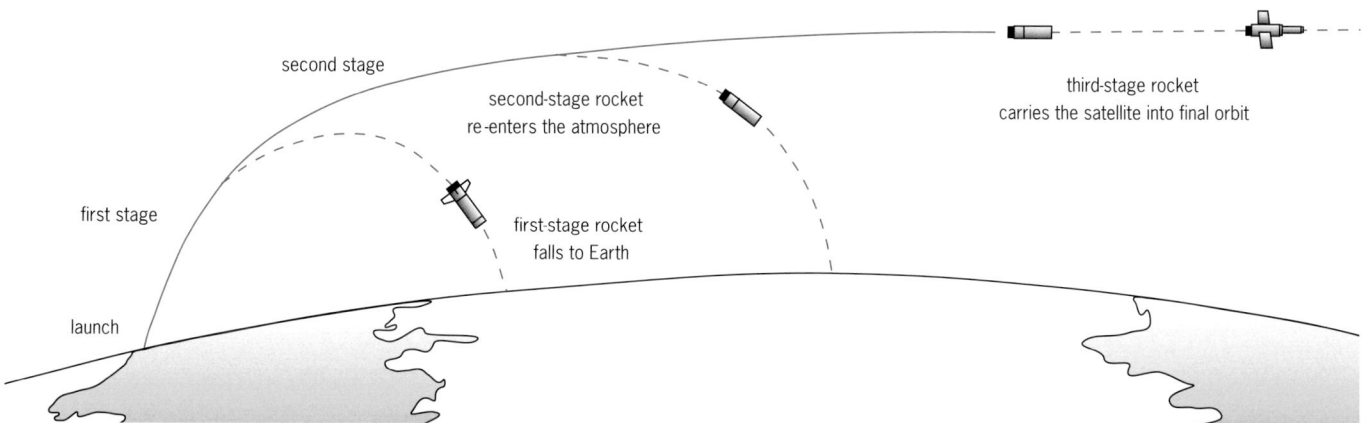

second stage

first stage

launch

second-stage rocket
re-enters the atmosphere

first-stage rocket
falls to Earth

third-stage rocket
carries the satellite into final orbit

Fig 3.23 A satellite is launched into a geostationary orbit in several stages. (More than one satellite can be put into orbit in the same launch)

WEIGHTLESSNESS

Weight is simply the force due to gravity acting on an object. We sense 'weight' when we lift something up, and we are aware of the weight of our own bodies as sensations in our muscles. Occasionally, we 'feel weightless', on a roller coaster or in a plane that suddenly loses height through air turbulence, because for a moment we are in free fall and our bodies do not need muscular support. Yet we still *have* weight, from the pull of Earth's gravity.

Astronauts in a spacecraft orbiting the Earth also experience 'weightlessness'. This is because, like the orbiting cannon ball on page 56, they are in continuous free fall towards the centre of the Earth, as explained above. Some people believe that this sensation is due to the absence of the force of gravity. This is clearly false. If there were no gravity force acting on the astronauts, they and their spacecraft would all fly off in a straight line – obeying Newton's laws of motion.

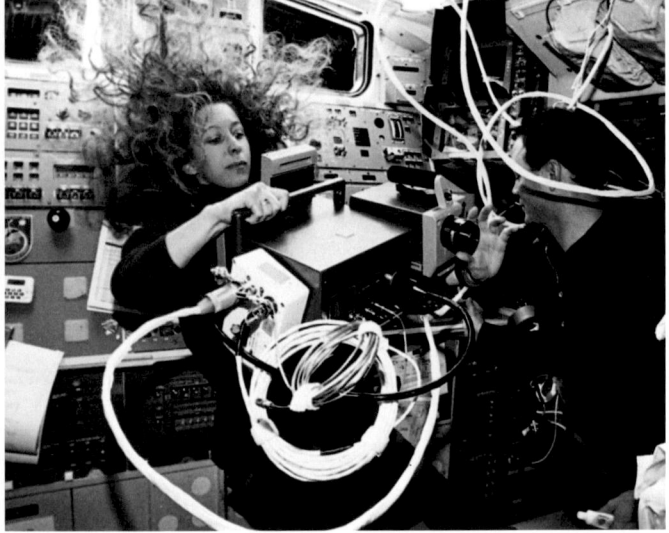 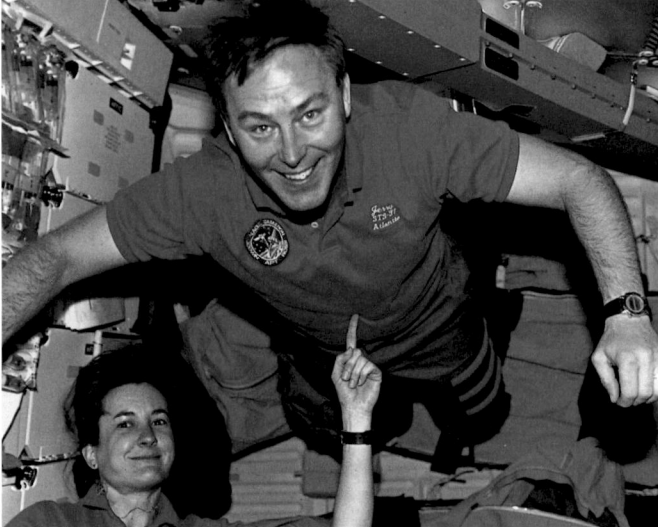

Fig 3.24 Astronauts in Earth orbit feel 'weightless' because, like their spacecraft, they are in free fall. What indicates 'weightlessness' in the left-hand picture?

? QUESTION 14

14 An astronaut is in a spacelab orbiting Earth. She has the task of moving a metal box labelled '50 kg' from one side of the lab to the other.
a) Suggest how she could check whether the box was empty or not.
b) Assuming that the box and contents did in fact have a mass of 50 kg, outline and explain a procedure which would allow the box to be moved across the lab effectively and safely.

8 MOMENTUM AND ROCKETS

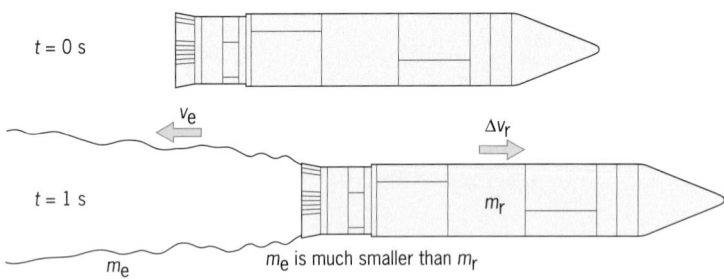

Fig 3.25 A rocket at rest, and 1 second after fuel ignition

In any interaction involving forces, *momentum is always conserved* (see also pages 26–27 in Chapter 2 on momentum). A rocket uses this principle. It gains speed by ejecting material at high speed. Fig 3.25 shows what happens. The total momentum for the whole system during flight, rocket + fuel, is constant, and in fact zero.

Initially, the rocket is at rest. Suppose that, in 1 second, the rocket ejects a mass m_e of hot gases at a velocity v_e. In this second, the ejected material carries momentum of $m_e v_e$ to the left. The rocket gains an equal quantity of momentum, moving to the right with a speed Δv_r. We assume here that the system is isolated, meaning that no other forces or bodies are involved, so there is no net change in momentum. We can write:

$$m_e v_e + m_r \Delta v_r = 0$$

and the rocket gains in speed by

$$\Delta v_r = -(m_e/m_r)v_e$$

Please see the How Science Works assignment for this chapter at www.collineducation.co.uk/CAS for a numerical, non-calculus method for investigating rocket propulsion.

STRETCH
AND CHALLENGE

EXAMPLE

Q A rocket starts firing and ejects 5.0 kg of gas per second at a speed v_e of 5.0×10^3 m s^{-1} relative to the rocket. The mass of the rocket is 4 tonnes.

a) What is the velocity of the rocket, v_r, after 1 second?

b) Will a spacecraft powered by a rocket engine move with a constant acceleration?

A

a) After 1 second, the rocket's mass has been reduced by 5 kg, but we will ignore this mass change (of about 0.1%) for the first second. Velocity is a vector, and we follow the convention that the direction of the ejected gas is *negative*:

total momentum = momentum of rocket + momentum of ejected gas = 0

$$(4 \times 10^3 \times v_r) - (5 \times 5 \times 10^3) = 0$$

So, after the first second, $v_r = 6.3$ m s^{-1}

b) No, the acceleration of a rocket-propelled spacecraft will not be constant. The rocket ejects gases at a steady rate, so that, each second, the gain in momentum of the rocket itself is constant over time. As its mass gets less, the gain in *velocity* per second has to increase in order to maintain the constant increase in momentum.

Suppose that in the short time Δt, the rocket ejects a mass of gas, Δm_e, at a velocity v_e relative to the rocket. At this time, the mass of the rocket is m_r. As a result, the rocket gains in velocity by Δv_r. We know that, in the short time Δt, by the momentum law,

change in momentum of rocket = – change in momentum of gases ejected

(mass m_r of   ×   (change in   =   (mass Δm_e of   ×   (velocity $-v_e$ of
rocket)   velocity Δv_r)   ejected fuel)   ejected fuel)

$$m_r \Delta v_r = -\Delta m_e v_e$$

Thus, the *change* in velocity of the rocket in the short time Δt is:

$$\Delta v_r = -\Delta m_e v_e / m_r$$

This equation confirms that the change in velocity – the acceleration – will get bigger as time goes on, because m_r is decreasing.

It is clear from the Example that the mass of the rocket, and consequently its acceleration, is changing constantly and uniformly.

ROCKET AND JET ENGINES

Rocket engines are designed to work in the vacuum of space. Their energy source is a fuel–oxygen mixture which is usually carried as a liquid.

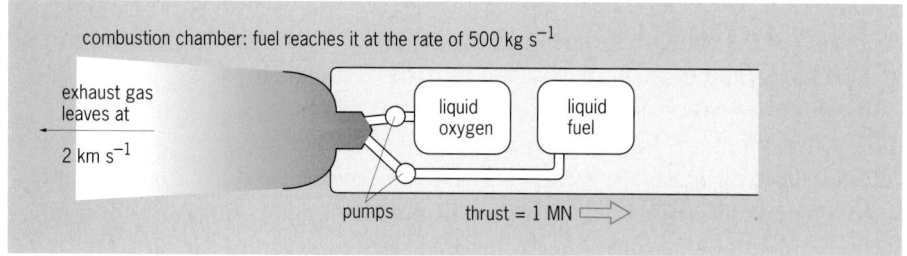

Fig 3.26 A simplified rocket engine

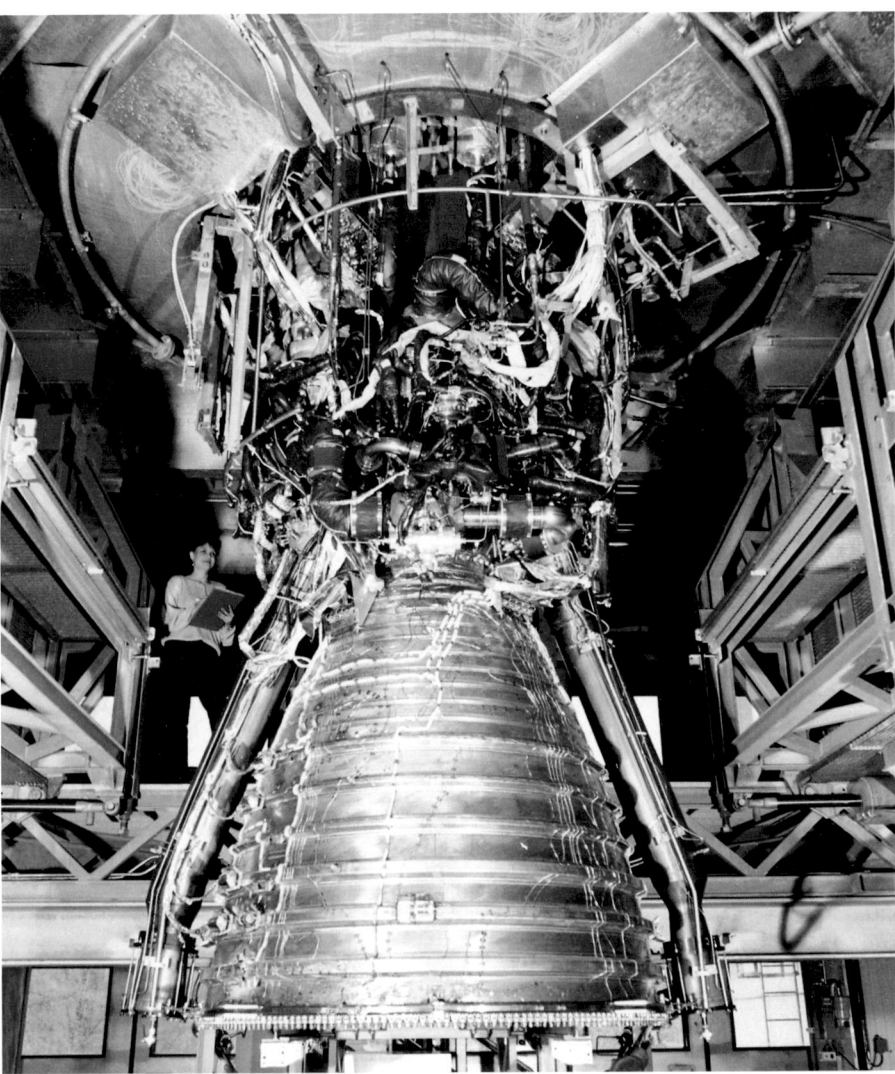

Fig 3.27 The engine of an Ariane rocket

For the US Apollo missions to the Moon (1969–1972), the Saturn rocket of the first launch stage was larger than the tower of Big Ben. It was powered by five huge engines, the most powerful ever made, and the second-stage rocket by five smaller engines. Each of the first-stage engines was 5 metres long with a mass of 8.4 tonnes, generating a thrust of 6.7 meganewtons. After the first stage was completed, and all the fuel used up, five rocket engines took over for the second stage. The kerosene–liquid oxygen fuel mixture generated a thrust of 1.14 meganewtons, and its exhaust velocity in space was 2500 metres per second.

A third stage then put the spacecraft bound for the Moon into Earth orbit. The spacecraft included its three-man astronaut team, their life support systems, the Lunar Lander and the rockets and fuel to get the craft to the Moon and back.

Thrust

A rocket engine using hydrogen and oxygen as fuel can eject hot gases at a rate of 500 kg s^{-1} and a speed of 3500 m s^{-1}. This is a change of momentum of 500×3500 kg m s^{-1} *per second*, giving a *rate of change of momentum* of 1.75×10^6 kg m s^{-2}. From Newton's second law, this is equivalent to a force of 1.75×10^6 newtons. In rocketry, this is the **thrust** produced by the engine.

A jet engine uses the same principle as a rocket engine, but can only work in the atmosphere because it uses fuel that needs oxygen in the air to burn.

SUMMARY

After studying this chapter, you should be able to do the following.

- Explain energy changes using the idea of work, $W = Fd$, and use the definition of work to make calculations involving force, $F = mg$, and distance in gravitational examples.

- Derive the formulae for a change in gravitational potential energy, $\Delta E = mg\Delta h$, and for kinetic energy, $\frac{1}{2}mv^2$, and use these ideas and formulae to explain, and make calculations for, bodies moving in uniform gravitational fields.

- Use the ideas and formulae for a change in gravitational potential energy, $GMm(1/r_1 - 1/r_2)$, and kinetic energy to explain, and make calculations for, bodies moving in radial gravitational fields.

- Have a deeper understanding of the principle of the conservation of energy as it applies to gravitational situations.

- Draw and interpret force–distance graphs for both uniform and radial gravitational fields.

- Use the idea of gravitational potential and its formula, $-GM/r$, and distinguish between gravitational potential and gravitational potential energy.

- Derive the formula for escape speed and use it to make calculations.

- Explain how gravitational force is linked to satellite motion in circular orbits and use the formula: $g = v^2/r$.

- Explain the terms circumpolar orbit, geostationary orbit, 'weightlessness' and free fall.

- Use the concept of momentum to explain the action of a rocket and a jet engine, and calculate changes of speed and of thrust for a rocket in simple situations.

- Understand how the physics in this chapter is used in real-life situations, such as amusement parks, Earth satellites and the motion of objects in gravitational fields.

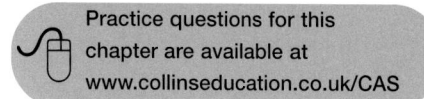 Practice questions for this chapter are available at www.collinseducation.co.uk/CAS

4

Newton on the move

4 NEWTON ON THE MOVE

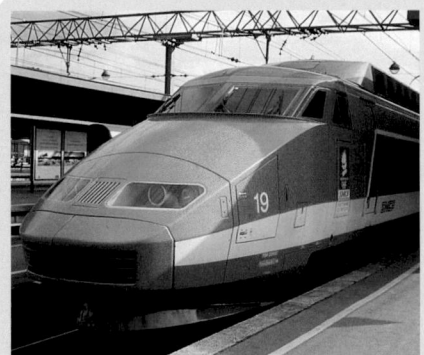

The French TGV (Train à Grande Vitesse), the world's fastest passenger train, with a front designed to reduce air friction

Going around the bend

In the design of high-speed trains (HSTs), fuel costs are minimised by reducing friction: friction with the air is kept low, while friction with the track is set at a sufficiently high level for safety. The photograph is of the front of a high-speed train. The train is shaped like this to reduce the frictional force (drag) caused by moving through a fluid (air). The resulting low 'drag coefficient' reduces the energy loss at high speed and so increases the train's maximum speed. The rear of the train, too, needs to be the right shape, to minimise air turbulence, which also wastes energy.

The mass of the train depends on the number of passengers, so the applied forces needed to accelerate and brake have to adjust to this. In emergencies, deceleration may have to be quite rapid but still safe, so great care is taken in designing the braking systems. The geography of the track is important: a longer route may save energy if it avoids inefficient changes between kinetic and potential energy, such as when a loaded train goes up and down hills.

A modern vehicle with low drag travelling at high speed experiences the same kind of force that allows aircraft to fly – aerodynamic lift. Trains and cars are unlikely to take off – but the effect is to reduce the 'supporting' force between the ground and the vehicle's wheels. There must be this supporting force to produce the frictional forces that a train needs in order to accelerate or decelerate. If friction is reduced too much, traction is lost and the driving wheels will simply skid.

When a train travels round bends at speed it needs a centripetal force to keep it moving in the arc of the circle. This is provided by the contact force of the track against the wheels. It would be better if the centripetal force acted through the centre of mass of the train, which is higher than the track contact. As it doesn't, there is a tendency for the train to topple over as a result of the turning effect of the weight and the contact force acting at a lower point. The faster the train, the worse the effect – the centripetal force varies as the *square* of the speed. It helps stability if the centre of mass is low, and this is a major feature for all HSTs. In the French TGV the centre of mass is so low that even when it is derailed the chance of the compartments turning over is very small. No modern trains have ever fallen sideways because they round a bend too quickly.

It also helps if the track is tilted (banked) at the bend so that the centripetal force acts closer to the centre of mass, reducing the turning effect. But if the track is also to be used for slower trains, passengers will tend to slide 'downhill' – and start to get worried. It is equally worrying for passengers when HSTs go around a tilted track at high speed – they are forced 'uphill' to the outside of the bend. Also, their drinks and plates slide off the table. Actually they don't – they are just stubbornly obeying Newton's first law of motion, carrying on in a straight line while the *table* slides away beneath them!

The current solution to passenger comfort is to use **tilting trains**. The carriage is made to swing as sensors detect that the track is tilting and an accelerometer measures the inward acceleration. This data is used by a computer to tilt the carriage just enough to keep passengers and coffee cups stable. It works because the contact force between cup and table (and passenger and seat) has a component towards the centre of the curve and so provides, with the help of friction, enough force to keep things stable.

Tilting trains have been in use in Italy, Spain and Scandinavia for several years. In Britain, Virgin Rail has upgraded the West Coast line between London and Glasgow to take tilting trains with a maximum speed of 225 km h^{-1} (140 mph).

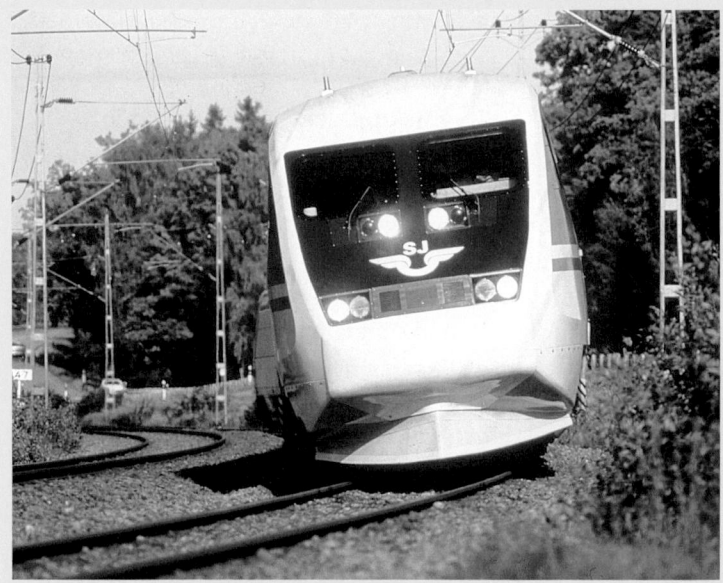

The Swedish X2000 tilting train taking a bend. It can tilt up to an angle of 8°

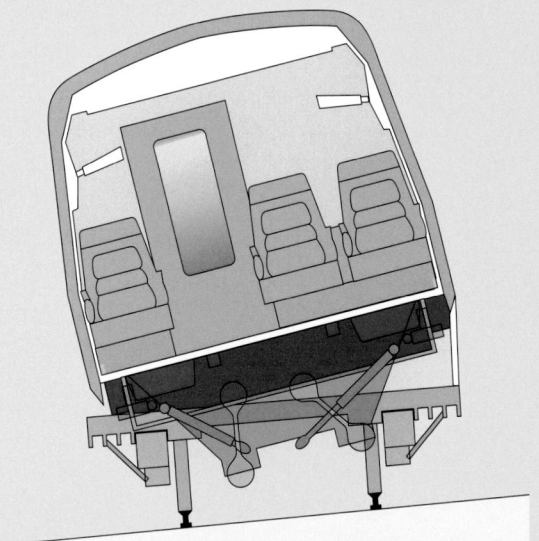

The wheels system (bogie) stays on the tilted rails as the carriage tilts even more

The ideas in this chapter

Newton's laws of motion are particularly important for an understanding of the topic of transport – and for mechanical engineering in general. The modern world relies on an ability to move materials and people quickly, efficiently and safely from place to place. We shall apply fundamental ideas about **mass**, **force**, **velocity**, **acceleration**, **momentum**, **impulse** and **energy** not only to the motion of vehicles. We shall also look at the behaviour of **fluids** (liquids and gases) to understand how ships float and aeroplanes fly. Transport systems have to take account of the fact that vehicles move through a fluid (usually air) and that the fluid is an important restraint on motion.

But a moving fluid carries kinetic energy and so can be used to do work. Moving water is used to drive turbines in hydroelectric power stations. The energy of moving air is used in wind turbines, a cheap source of energy but with an impact on the visual environment which can be controversial.

1 CONSERVATION OF MOMENTUM AND ENERGY IN TRANSPORT SYSTEMS

Chapters 2 and 3 dealt with the key ideas of momentum and energy in relation to moving objects. Both total energy and momentum are **conserved** when engines are used to move vehicles such as cars, trains and rockets – but *kinetic* energy is not conserved.

Think about a rocket: the exhaust gases and the rocket itself gain kinetic energy from burning fuel, but a significant fraction of the energy in the fuel mixture is transferred to the random motion of gas particles and does not appear as useful kinetic energy of the rocket vehicle itself. The same applies to road and rail transport vehicles, which gain their energy from burning fuels. Even electric traction engines ultimately depend on the fuels used in power stations to generate electricity.

Not all the energy transferred by a transport system appears as kinetic energy. Some energy is usually transferred to or gained from gravitational potential energy, for example when aircraft climb and land, and ground vehicles go up and down hills. But what goes up must come down and there is no net change in gravitational potential energy for a vehicle that always returns to its starting level. There are usually some friction losses: for example, energy is lost to the surroundings when vehicles brake (the brake discs get hotter).

Nevertheless, in all these changes both *total* energy and momentum are conserved – although it is more difficult to keep track of the energy transfers than the momentum changes.

TRACTION AND BRAKING

The control of a car – in accelerating, turning and braking – relies on its contact with the road surface. The key factor is **friction** between the tyres and the road surface. The area of contact is quite small, as is shown by Fig 4.1 and the Example.

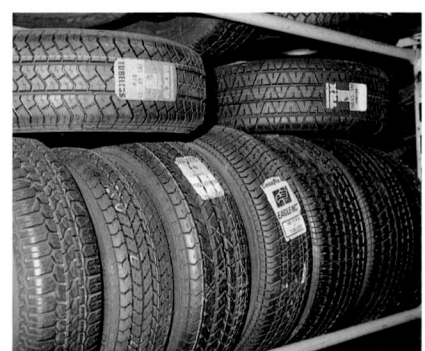

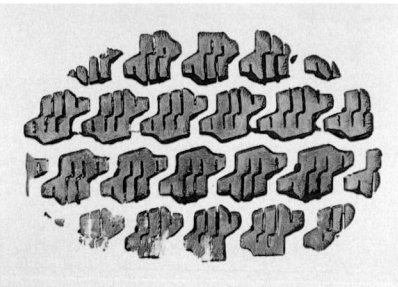

Fig 4.1 The patterned surface of tyres; and the print of a tyre showing the area in contact with the ground

EXAMPLE

Q The mass of a given car is 1000 kg. Its tyre pressure is rated as 2.4×10^5 Pa above normal atmospheric pressure: that is, about 3.4×10^5 Pa. What area of the tyre is in contact with the ground?

A Using the definition, pressure = force/area, we get:

$$\text{area of contact} = \frac{\text{weight of car}}{\text{tyre pressure}} = \frac{1000 \times 9.8 \text{ N}}{3.4 \times 10^5 \text{ N m}^{-2}}$$
$$= 0.029 \text{ m}^2$$

This is a total area of 290 cm^2. Thus the area of contact *per tyre* is 72 cm^2 – roughly the area of the palm of your hand.

As the car wheel turns, the part of the tyre in contact with the ground is instantaneously at rest with reference to the ground. If the car is accelerating or braking, the force that ultimately acts on the car as a whole must be due to the friction between the tyres and the ground. If there were zero friction the wheels would spin freely and the car would skid out of control – as tends to happen on icy roads. Fig 4.2 shows the forces acting on an accelerating car.

? QUESTION 1

1 Estimate the pressure you exert on the ground when standing barefoot on two feet.

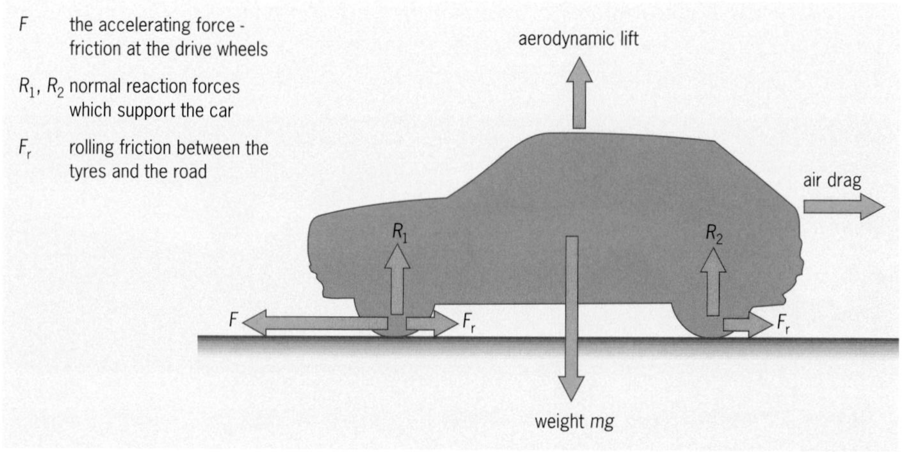

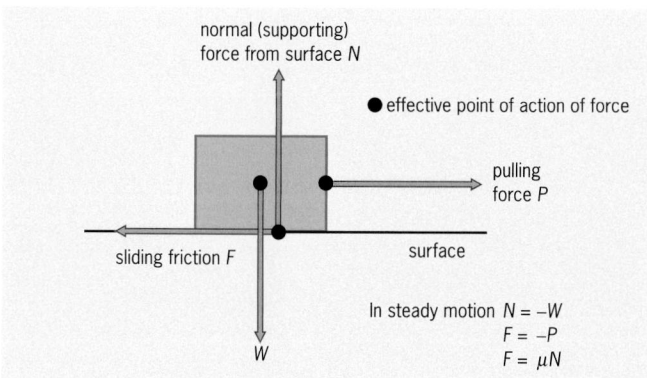

F the accelerating force - friction at the drive wheels

R_1, R_2 normal reaction forces which support the car

F_r rolling friction between the tyres and the road

The maximum value of the frictional force F is decided by the nature of the two surfaces in contact and the **normal** force N between them. Here the word 'normal' has the special mathematical meaning of 'at right angles to the surfaces at the point of contact'. This force is often called the normal *reaction*. The relationship is simple:

$$F = \mu N$$

where μ is a dimensionless number called the **coefficient of friction**. Its value depends on the nature of the surfaces, and μ is usually lower for surfaces sliding against each other than it is for the same surfaces when they are at rest relative to each other. We therefore distinguish between the coefficient of *static friction* between two particular surfaces and their coefficient of *sliding friction*. For rubber against a paved road, the static coefficient varies between 0.7 and 0.9. The coefficient for sliding friction is between 0.5 and 0.8; on a wet road this reduces to between 0.25 and 0.7. Figs 4.3 and 4.4 illustrate some simple cases involving the coefficient of friction.

normal (supporting) force from surface N

● effective point of action of force

pulling force P

sliding friction F surface

In steady motion $N = -W$
$F = -P$
$F = \mu N$

W

Fig 4.3 Friction on a flat surface

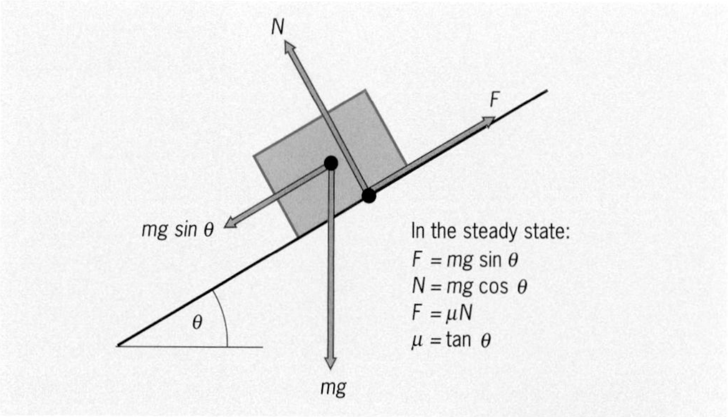

N

F

$mg \sin \theta$

In the steady state:
$F = mg \sin \theta$
$N = mg \cos \theta$
$F = \mu N$
$\mu = \tan \theta$

θ

mg

Fig 4.4 Friction on a slope

STRETCH
AND CHALLENGE

Sliding down a slope

Fig 4.4 shows the forces acting on an object that is sliding steadily down a slope. It is not accelerating, so the component of the object's weight *down* the slope must equal the frictional force acting *up* the slope. The frictional force is μN where N is the supporting force between the object and the surface of the slope. Thus:

$$mg \sin \theta = \mu N$$

But N is also due to the weight of the object. In fact, $N = mg \cos \theta$, so we can write:

$$mg \sin \theta = \mu mg \cos \theta$$

which simplifies to:

$$\mu = \frac{\sin \theta}{\cos \theta} = \tan \theta$$

This relationship can be used as a simple way of measuring the coefficient of friction between two surfaces.

Note that the frictional force F does not depend on the area of the surfaces in contact – see Figs 4.5 and 4.6. Table 4.1 gives examples of coefficients of friction for various surfaces.

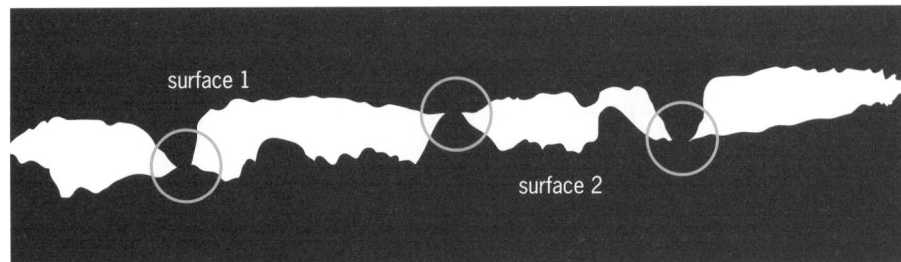

Fig 4.5 Frictional force is independent of area. No real surface is perfectly flat – it has many bumps and valleys. Just three bumps have to be in contact to support one object on another. If one of these is rubbed away by relative movement, another one takes its place. The actual area of contact is therefore very small

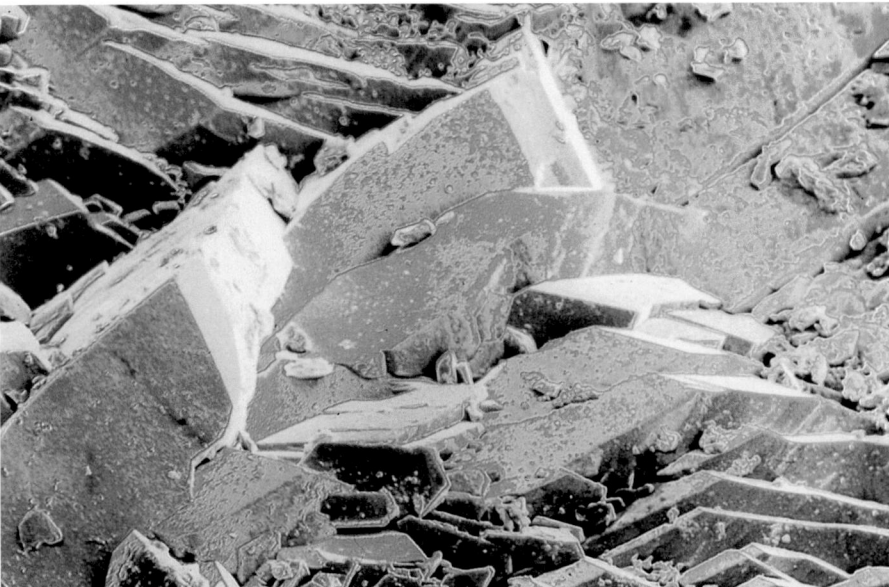

Fig 4.6 Photomicrograph showing the roughness of a coated metal surface which is smooth to the naked eye. Used in engine components, such a surface is designed to retain lubricants

Table 4.1 Coefficients of friction; these vary with temperature and humidity, so the values are approximate

Surface	Static friction	Sliding friction
Steel on steel	0.74	0.57
Rubber on concrete	0.9	0.7
Wood on wood	0.25–0.50	0.2
Ice on ice	0.1	0.03
Waxed wood on dry snow	–	0.04
Teflon on Teflon	0.04	0.04
Synovial joints in humans	0.01	0

FRICTION AND ACCELERATION

Over-keen drivers 'burn rubber' at traffic lights when they try to accelerate with forces greater than can be provided by static friction between tyres and road. The tyre moves relative to the road surface and work done against sliding friction produces local heating. Similarly you may see skid marks when vehicles brake so strongly that wheels 'lock', so that again there is relative movement between road and tyre as the tyres slide along the ground.

A car may skid if it is made to turn too sharply, that is, in too small a circle. A central force is needed to make a car move in a circle, and again this must be provided by the force of friction between car and ground, as in Fig 4.7. Look back to the start of the chapter to see why a turning vehicle might topple over.

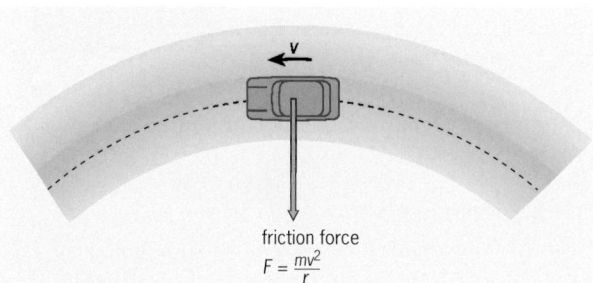

Fig 4.7 The forces acting on a car as it goes round a bend (ignoring air resistance)

friction force
$$F = \frac{mv^2}{r}$$

EXAMPLE

STRETCH AND CHALLENGE

Q A typical value for the coefficient of static friction between a particular tyre and a road is 0.8. Estimate the maximum acceleration that a car of mass 1000 kg can have.

A Maximum frictional force

$$F = \mu N = 0.8 \times 1000 \times 9.8 = 7.8 \text{ kN}$$

The acceleration produced by this force is:

$$a = \frac{F}{m} = \frac{7.8 \times 10^3}{1000} = 7.8 \text{ m s}^{-2}$$

But this is a very rough estimate – the two drive wheels share the weight of the car with the other pair of wheels, so the normal reaction N is less than the weight of the car. This means that the maximum possible acceleration is less than that calculated. Motor engineers still find the simple formula $F = \mu W$ useful, however, where W is now the load on the driving axle, which may be measured (with difficulty at speed) or calculated from theory.

? QUESTIONS 2–3

2 A bicycle has a mass of about 15 kg, and a typical adult has a mass of about 60 kg. Assuming a coefficient of friction between tyre and road of 0.8, estimate the maximum deceleration of a bicycle. Explain why both front and rear brakes should be used when stopping a bicycle as safely as possible in an emergency.

3 The estimate of F calculated in the Example is more accurate for the greatest deceleration that could be produced without the car skidding. Why is this?

2 ROTATION: WHEELS AND ROTATIONAL INERTIA

A spinning wheel has both kinetic energy and momentum due to its rotation – even when the wheel is not moving forwards. A turning force (or **torque**) is needed to get a wheel to rotate, and the force does work that appears as kinetic energy, as shown in Fig 4.8(a). Torque is measured, like the moment of a force, in newton metres (N m). Tests show that it is harder to spin a wheel of large diameter than a wheel of smaller diameter – even when both wheels have the same mass. Just as we call the resistance of a mass to being accelerated its *inertia* (m), so we can also define the resistance of a wheel to being rotated by a turning force as **rotational inertia** I (also called **moment of inertia**). The units of rotational inertia are of mass × (distance)^2, that is kg m^2.

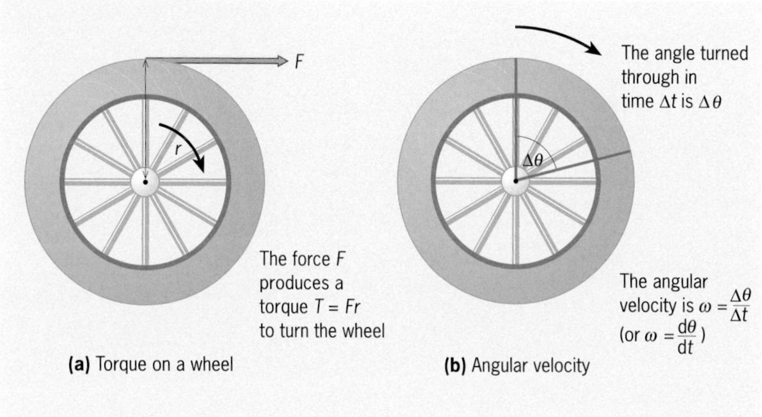

F

The force F produces a torque $T = Fr$ to turn the wheel

(a) Torque on a wheel

The angle turned through in time Δt is $\Delta \theta$

The angular velocity is $\omega = \frac{\Delta \theta}{\Delta t}$

(or $\omega = \frac{d\theta}{dt}$)

(b) Angular velocity

Fig 4.8 Torque and angular velocity

Rate of spin is measured by the angle through which a radius line turns per second, that is, its angular velocity ω, as in Fig 4.8(b). Angular velocity is measured in radians per second. Just as velocity is a vector, so is angular velocity. With a as angular acceleration, comparing linear and rotational motion:

force = mass × acceleration

$$F = ma$$

torque = rotational inertia × angular acceleration

$$T = Ia$$

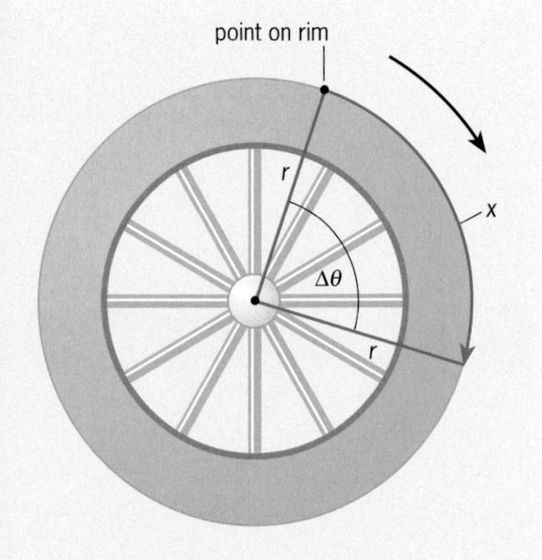

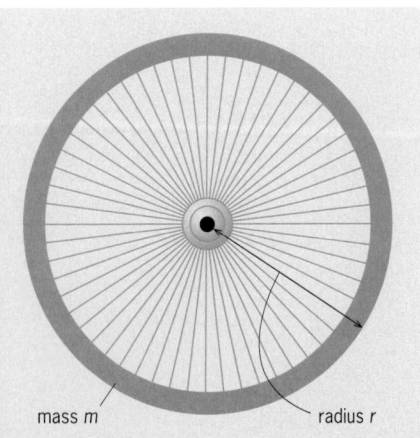

$\Delta x = r\Delta\theta$
When θ is in radians:
speed $= \dfrac{\Delta x}{\Delta t} = r\dfrac{\Delta\theta}{\Delta t} = r\omega$
where ω is angular velocity

Fig 4.9 The distance moved and the angular velocity of a point on the rim of a wheel

---

? QUESTIONS 4–5

4 A spinning ride in an activity park is 15 m in radius and at maximum speed spins once in 2 s.
   a) What is this maximum angular velocity?
   b) How fast in metres per second will a chair on the rim move?

5 A torque of 25 N m is applied to an object. After 30 s it has gained an angular velocity of 2 rad s^{-1}. What is its rotational inertia?

Fig 4.10 A simplified wheel: we assume that all the mass is in the rim

mass m radius r

EXAMPLE

Q A torque of 20 N m acts on a wheel that is initially still and has a rotational inertia of 600 kg m^2.

a) What is the angular acceleration produced?
b) At what angular velocity is the wheel spinning after 2 minutes?
c) The wheel is 30 cm in radius. How fast (in m s^{-1}) is a point on the rim moving at this time?

A

a) Angular acceleration = torque/rotational inertia:
$$a = 20/600 = 0.033 \text{ rad } s^{-2}$$

b) Angular velocity = angular acceleration × time
$$= 0.033 \times 120 = 4 \text{ rad } s^{-1}$$

c) See Fig 4.9. By the definition of a radian:

distance covered per second by a point on the rim
$$= \text{angle turned through per second} \times \text{radius}$$

So the speed of a point on the rim is $4 \times 0.30 = 1.2$ m s^{-1}.

ANGULAR MOMENTUM

Just as linear momentum is defined as mass × velocity, so we define angular momentum as:

angular momentum = rotational inertia × angular velocity = $I\omega$

As with linear motion, Newton's second law applies:

linear force = rate of change of momentum $F = \dfrac{\Delta(mv)}{\Delta t} = \dfrac{\Delta p}{\Delta t}$

rotational torque = rate of change of angular momentum
$$T = \dfrac{\Delta(I\omega)}{\Delta t}$$

ROTATIONAL INERTIA OF EVERYDAY OBJECTS

The structure of a wheel may be simplified as shown in Fig 4.10. The spokes are assumed to have negligible mass compared with the rim. All the mass (m) is then at the same distance r from the centre of rotation and the rotational inertia is simply mr^2.

In many cases, however, the mass of a spinning wheel is not evenly distributed on the rim. The rotational inertia can be calculated if the distribution is fairly simple, but may in practice have to be measured experimentally. The value of the rotational inertia of a car wheel is quite difficult to calculate mathematically, for example. As a general rule the mathematics involves adding up the contributions of all the small masses, taking into account the square of their distance from the centre of rotation:

$$I = \sum mr^2$$

Table 4.2 gives the rotational inertias of some simple shapes. Note that the value also depends on how the object is spun round an axis.

Table 4.2 Rotational inertia for simple objects

Object	Axis of rotation	Rotational inertia (m = mass of object)
Thin ring (simple wheel)	through centre, perpendicular to plane	mr^2
Thin ring	through a diameter	$\frac{1}{2}mr^2$
Disc and cylinder (solid flywheel)	through centre, perpendicular to plane	$\frac{1}{2}mr^2$
Thin rod, length d	through centre, perpendicular to rod	$\frac{1}{12}md^2$

ROTATIONAL ENERGY

The kinetic energy of a rotating body is $\frac{1}{2}I\omega^2$. This is the equivalent of the linear formula $\frac{1}{2}mv^2$.

If the wheel has mass m and is also rolling forwards with speed v it will also have *translational* kinetic energy $\frac{1}{2}mv^2$. The total kinetic energy E_k of a rolling wheel is therefore:

$$E_k = \tfrac{1}{2}I\omega^2 + \tfrac{1}{2}mv^2$$

Large vehicles (like some electric locomotives) can reduce the waste of energy in braking by storing linear kinetic energy as rotational energy in massive rotating wheels (flywheels). The track wheels are linked through a gearing system to the flywheel instead of to the usual friction brakes. As the track wheels slow down, the flywheel speeds up, and vice versa.

CONSERVATION OF ANGULAR MOMENTUM

Hold the axis of a bicycle wheel in your hands and get someone to spin it in the vertical plane. Then try to tip the wheel through a small angle away from the vertical. You will experience a mysterious force that seems to oppose the change in direction of the axis. In fact, this is a consequence of the conservation of angular momentum – and Newton's third law of motion. Changing the direction of the axis of spin means altering the angular momentum, not in size but in direction. This requires a force, and as forces occur in pairs there is an equal and opposite force exerted on you as the wheel changes direction. This 'resistance' of a spinning wheel to changing its direction of action is what makes a bicycle so stable – as long as the wheels are spinning! The importance of the conservation of angular momentum to the origin and nature of the Solar System is described in Chapter 25.

 REMEMBER THIS
Newton's third law states that, when two bodies interact, the force exerted by one body (here, the holder tipping the wheel) brings about an equal and opposite force exerted by the other body (the wheel).

3 COLLISIONS

Most traffic accidents involve **collisions** – between vehicles, between vehicles and fixed structures or between vehicles and pedestrians. We describe collisions in which the structures are permanently distorted as inelastic (see Chapter 5 for more about **elasticity**). The original kinetic energy of the colliding bodies is usually dissipated in heating the materials and the surroundings. Kinetic energy is conserved only in collisions between perfectly elastic bodies. No real objects we come across in everyday life are perfectly elastic, but rubber balls, 'superballs', steel balls and snooker balls approach elastic behaviour.

Collisions between *particles* (molecules, atoms, electrons, etc.) underpin a great deal of what happens in physics and these are often perfectly elastic, provided, that is, they collide at low enough speeds. If speeds are too high, we get chemical changes or, in specially built particle *colliders*, nuclei are smashed and other dramatic events occur. But in developing our model of the kinetic theory of gases (see Chapter 7) we assume that the collisions between the atoms or molecules of a gas are perfectly elastic.

COLLISIONS IN ONE DIMENSION
1 Inelastic collisions

The simplest example of an inelastic collision is when a moving object (such as a car) collides with a stationary object: momentarily they crunch together and then they move off together at the same time. This is a typical situation in vehicle collisions (see Fig 4.11).

The system is isolated so the total momentum is unchanged by the collision:

momentum before collision = momentum after collision

With the symbols in Fig 4.11:

$$mv_1 = (M + m)v_2$$

Suppose the car has a mass of 1000 kg and hits the lorry at a speed of 30 m s^{-1} (this is just less than the maximum motorway speed of 70 mph). The lorry has a mass of 9000 kg. Then:

$$1000 \text{ kg} \times 30 \text{ m s}^{-1} = 10\,000 \text{ kg} \times v_2$$

giving $v_2 = 3$ m s^{-1}.

The combined vehicles move off at a speed of 3 m s^{-1} but the lorry would quickly stop if it was braked. Traffic accident experts can estimate this initial speed of the combined vehicles from measurements made at the site of the accident and hence calculate the speed of the incoming vehicle to see if it was exceeding the speed limit (Fig 4.12).

Energy changes in an inelastic collision

The incoming vehicle had a kinetic energy ($\frac{1}{2}mv^2$) of 450 kJ. The combined vehicles move off with a kinetic energy of just 45 kJ. Thus only 10 per cent of the input energy remains as kinetic energy in the motion of the combined vehicles. (Check these values yourself.) The lost kinetic energy has gone to make a lot of noise, but mainly to deform (do work on) and eventually heat the material of the vehicles. Vehicles have design features that minimise both the *quantity* of this energy delivered to human bodies in the vehicles and the *rate* at which it is delivered. These features include protective shells, crumple zones, seat belts, collapsible steering wheels and rapid-inflation airbags. How these affect what happens is explained in the 'Safety first' box on pages 76–77.

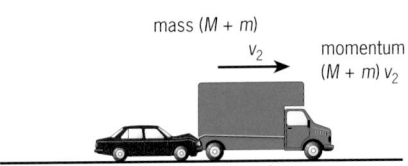

Fig 4.11 An inelastic collision: a small car colliding with a lorry

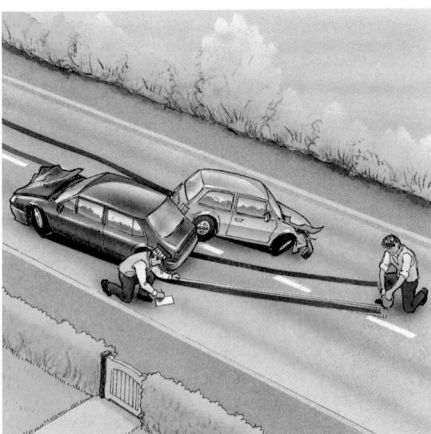

Fig 4.12 Measuring skid marks at the site of an accident enables the speed of vehicles before impact to be calculated

? QUESTION 6

6 Much expensive damage is caused in traffic accidents as inelastic materials are bent and distorted. This damage would not occur if the materials used were perfectly elastic. Would this be a good idea?

Momentum, force and energy in a traffic collision

The key relationships involved here are between:
● kinetic energy and work done in deforming structures,
● impulse and change of momentum (defining the force produced).

Imagine a car crashing into a very massive structure such as a concrete wall. Fig 4.14 on page 76 shows what happens to a car in this situation.

The forces acting on the car deform it, doing work. The work done is given by the formula $W = Fd$, where we simplify a complex situation by considering F to be the average force acting until the car is stopped, and d the distance moved by the centre of mass of the car after the front of the car hits the wall. Some of the car's kinetic energy is transferred to sound and to small pieces that fly off, but these are tiny compared with the energy transferred to produce the main structural deformation. Thus we can say:

$$\tfrac{1}{2}mv^2 = Fd$$

For a given car travelling at a given speed, kinetic energy is 'fixed'. But the force F can be reduced if d can be made larger. There is more about this in the 'Safety first' box on pages 76–77.

The significance of impulse

Somehow or other, the driver and passengers have to be brought to a stop, and safety features in a car reduce the decelerating forces to as harmless a size as possible. There is more about this on pages 76–77. We can best understand the physics of these features by using the concepts of momentum and impulse:

impulse = change of momentum

$$F\Delta t = \Delta(mv) = m\Delta v \quad \text{(remember } m \text{ is constant)}$$

Therefore: $$F = \frac{m\Delta v}{\Delta t}$$

So, if Δt is made bigger then F gets smaller. F is the force required to change the momentum. In a car collision the human body of mass m is brought to a stop from the collision speed v. The force needed to do this is applied to the body mainly by the seat belt, with some small help from the feet pressing against the floor. We consider the forces involved when a car is braked to a stop in the Example on page 78. The graphs in Fig 4.13 show a force applied to an object that stays steady (a), and one that changes with time (b). How can we calculate the effect of the varying force as an **impulse**? That is easy. The area under the steady force is simply force × time – it is the impulse produced in Newton seconds (Ns). You can *estimate* the area under the varying force graph – this will also be the impulse in Ns.

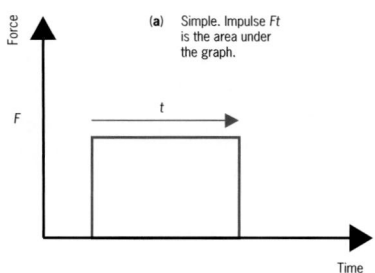

(a) Simple. Impulse Ft is the area under the graph.

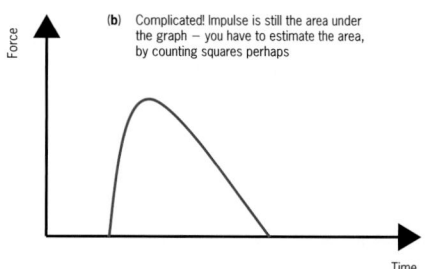

(b) Complicated! Impulse is still the area under the graph – you have to estimate the area, by counting squares perhaps

Fig 4.13 Estimating impetus when the force varies

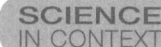

Safety first

It would seem crazy to a rational, impartial observer, from another planet, say, that ordinary human beings, after a short period of training and a simple test, are allowed to get into a metal vehicle capable of speeds of over 150 km h^{-1}. They can then drive them on narrow roads with similar vehicles approaching them at a combined relative speed of 200 km h^{-1}. And that's if they obey the speed limit. The observer would not be surprised to learn that this behaviour leads to a large number of inelastic collisions. In the European Union alone some 50 000 people die every year in road accidents, equivalent to two jumbo jets crashing a week. The World Bank and the World Health Organization estimate that in the first 20 years of the twenty-first century, 37 million people will die in such accidents. For each death there are between 4 and 12 seriously injured survivors.

Moving objects have momentum: ***mv***. To come to a stop, the object needs a force ***F*** applied for a time Δ ***t*** so that ***mv*** = $F\Delta t$ (see page 75).

Moving objects have kinetic energy $E_k = \frac{1}{2} mv^2$ (see page 47). This energy has to be dissipated when the object comes to a stop.

DESIGNING SAFETY

Car design does its best to ensure that, in an accident, the human beings in a car do not have too much force exerted on them, and that they dissipate their energy of movement in a safe way. Basic precursors to any vehicle design solutions include good road design, speed limits, good driving techniques and a simple awareness of other road users. There are three main design features of modern road vehicles that enhance safety in collisions:

1   crumple zones
2   seat belts
3   airbags

Crumple zones were invented by Mercedes engineer Bela Berenyi and were a feature of good car design by 1959. The front and rear parts of a car are designed to absorb the energy of a collision by bending and breaking in a predictable way. As the zone crumples, the time taken by a car to come to a stop also increases. For a given mv, as Δt increases, the force F gets less. The passengers are in a stronger and more rigid compartment (the safety cage) that also slows down more gently. As it does so, the metal frames that support the engine can slide under the passenger compartment (Fig 4.14).

Seat belts were invented by Nils Bohlin at Volvo at about the same time as crumple zones. The three-point seat belt holds the body across the lap and over the chest. When the passenger compartment slows or stops, the human body carries on moving (Newton's first law) until a force acts to decelerate and stop it. Without a seat belt, this force is provided by the collision with the steering wheel or fascia of the car. If these are rigid, the time of contact is small, the force large. Seat belts restrain the body to the seat and apply the stopping force. The body is still moving forward after the safety cage has stopped, so increasing the stopping, time. A perfectly unstretchable seat belt

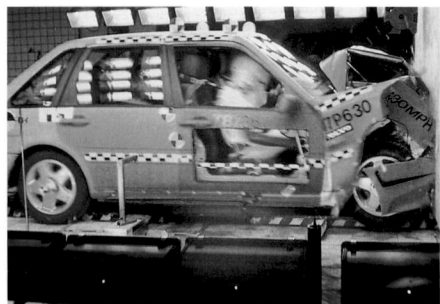

Fig 4.14 The effects of crumple zones is investigated by real collisions in a vehicle testing laboratory

would be almost as bad as not having one at all. The seat belt is designed so that the material stretches enough, without breaking.

So seat belts make good use of the key formula $mv = F\Delta t$, but even if the force F is reduced, it still acts over the small area in which it is in contact with the body. This concentration of force can cause damage to bones and tissues. Also, the head is not restrained and can move forward to make damaging contact with the steering wheel or fascia.

Airbags were an addition to and improvement on the seat belt, and protect the head and chest. They were invented in the early 1950s but only became obligatory in road vehicles in 1989. Timing is the key factor in how airbags save lives in a head-on collision. When a collision occurs, there is a sudden large deceleration of the vehicle. This triggers an explosion of gases inside a nylon or other plastic bag (Fig 4.15). The gases expand the airbag at a rate of 300 km h^{-1} (83 m s^{-1}), taking about 40 ms to inflate fully. At this stage the airbag is rock hard and a head colliding with it would be seriously injured. To avoid this, the airbag immediately starts leaking gas so that, by the time the body makes contact, the bag is comparatively soft. The benefit is twofold: the upper body is brought to a stop slowly and by a larger area, so the force exerted on the body per unit area is lowered to a safe value.

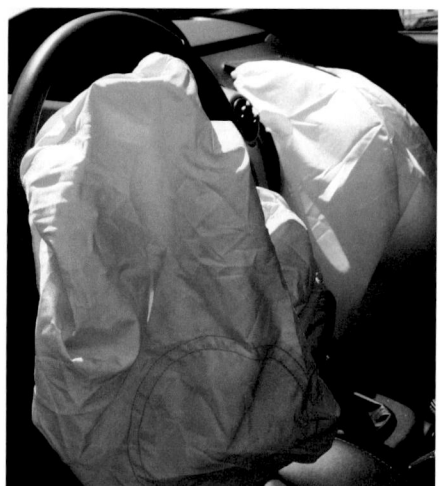

Fig 4.15 An expanded airbag

Early airbags used a simple mechanical trigger – a metal ball held inside a tube by a magnet or a spring. A large enough deceleration would let the ball move to touch a contact and complete a circuit for a heating element to trigger the explosion. Current systems are much more elaborate. The deceleration sensor is a MEMS – a Micro-Electro-Mechanical System. This is an integrated chip circuit with tiny silicon bars that move as the car decelerates. The chip monitors the movement and senses when the deceleration is large enough to have been caused by a collision, and then triggers the gas explosion.

Airbags can be dangerous. If the body hits them too soon, they can cause injury. Children and small adults tend to sit closer to the airbag and are at greater risk of injury from this effect. The most modern airbag systems include a sensor in the seat which measures the mass and deduces the size of the driver or passenger. This information can be used to limit the rate of expansion and ultimate internal pressure of the bag.

The chemical used in the bag is a solid rocket fuel: sodium azide, NaN_3. When heated to 300˚C it decomposes to produce nitrogen gas, which fills the airbag, and sodium metal. Sodium is a dangerous element, so other chemicals are used to soak up the sodium and indeed convert it into a harmless silicate.

See page 78 for an Example about collision forces.

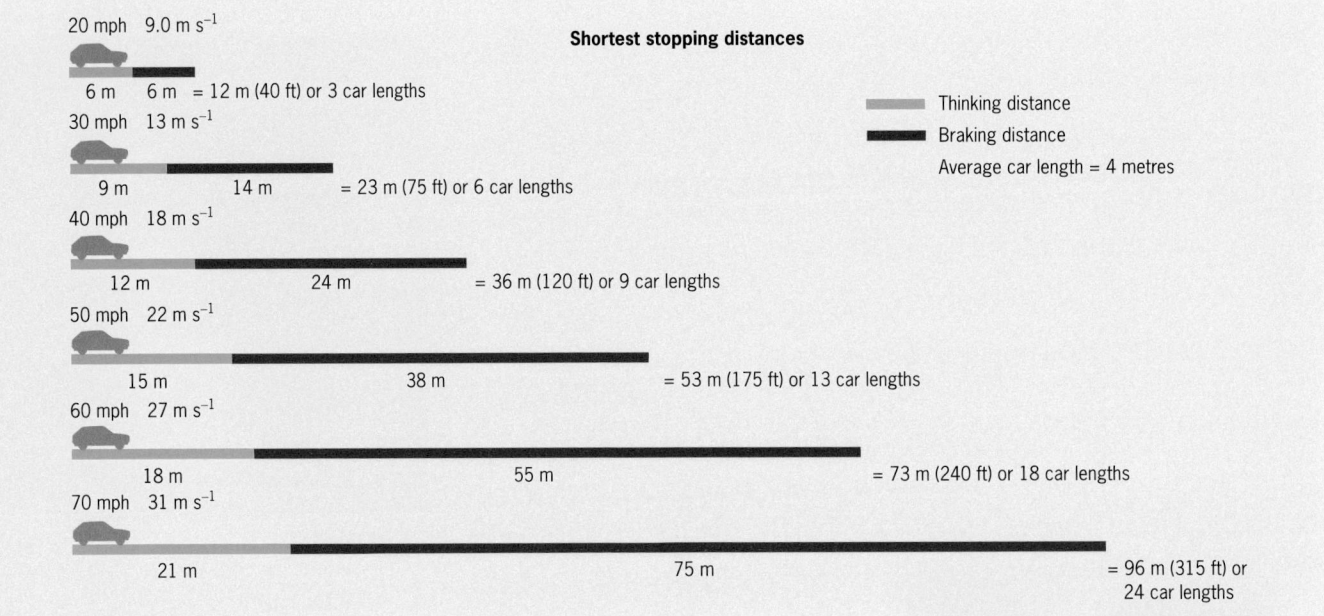

Fig 4.16 Stopping distances at various speeds (source: *Highway Code*)

SCIENCE IN CONTEXT — STRETCH AND CHALLENGE

EXAMPLE

Q Estimate the size of the force needed to stop the driver of a car when the car is braked to a stop from a speed of 13.6 m s⁻¹ (i.e. 30 mph). The *Highway Code* assumes that a car travelling at 13.6 m s⁻¹ is stopped in a distance of 14 m by normal braking, as in Fig 4.16. (A typical driver has a mass of 65 kg.)

A The time taken to stop is t, which we can estimate from the relationship:
Distance covered
= average speed × time

$$14 = \frac{13.6 + 0}{2}\,t$$

giving:

$$t = 2.06 \text{ s}$$

Using the impulse = change of momentum relation $F\Delta t = m\Delta v$, we have:

$$F \times 2.06 = 65 \times 13.6$$

or:

$$F = 429 \text{ N}$$

This force is less than the weight (say about 600 N) of the driver, which the feet are quite accustomed to coping with.

In a collision, both the car and the driver's body may be brought to a stop in 0.1 s.

The time has decreased from 2.06 s to 0.1 s, a factor of about 20, so the force is increased by the same factor to 8600 N – over 13 times the body weight.

In practice, things would be more complicated, with some of the force being applied to other parts of the body. For example, unless restrained by a seat belt, the body would pivot round the feet and would hit the steering wheel and/or the windscreen.

2 Elastic collisions

Imagine two elastic balls of equal mass colliding. Fig 4.17 shows the situation just before and just after the collision.

The system is isolated, so there is no net change in momentum. That is:

momentum before collision = momentum after collision

With quantities as in Fig 4.17:

$$mv = mv_1 + mv_2$$

This formula does not tell us which way the balls move – or their relative speeds.

Suppose $v = 10$ m s^{-1} and the masses m are both 1.0 kg. Then:

$$1.0 \text{ kg} \times 10 \text{ m s}^{-1} = 1.0 \text{ kg} \times v_1 + 1.0 \text{ kg} \times v_2$$

which simplifies to:

$$v_1 = 10 \text{ m s}^{-1} - v_2 \qquad [1]$$

We have two unknowns in the equation, and it seems that we could choose any values of the speeds so long as the left-hand side of the equation equalled the right-hand side. But there is another law that applies here – the balls are perfectly elastic, so *kinetic energy is conserved*:

$$\tfrac{1}{2}mv^2 = \tfrac{1}{2}mv_1^2 + \tfrac{1}{2}mv_2^2$$

We can solve these simultaneous equations by inserting the value of v_1 (in terms of v_2) from equation 1 and simplifying:

$$(10)^2 = (10 - v_2)^2 + v_2^2 \qquad [2]$$

This results in the quadratic equation:

$$v_2^2 - 10v_2 = 0 \qquad [3]$$

This has two solutions: the speed of the second ball v_2 is either 0 or 10 m s^{-1}. The solution $v_2 = 0$ is physically impossible: the first ball would have to move through the second at 10 m s^{-1}. But the second ball is free to move, and the second solution tells us that this ball will move off with the original speed of the first.

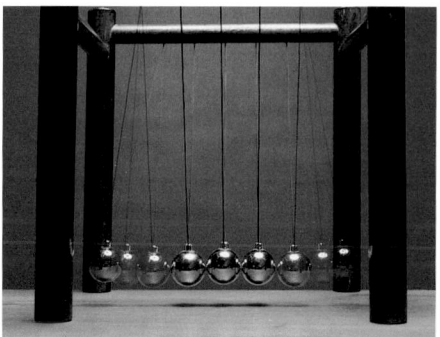

Fig 4.18 Newton's cradle. The far right ball has just hit its neighbour and the far left ball has moved out

This effect is illustrated by the toy known as Newton's cradle (Fig 4.18), but flicking one coin at another on a flat table gives you some idea of the theory. There is no momentum left for the first ball, so it will stop.

Simple experiments with steel balls or coins suggest that, when a small mass hits a larger mass at rest, the small mass is likely to bounce back and the large mass to move on. When a large mass collides with a small mass at rest, both move on with the smaller mass having the greater speed. Doing the maths – as above – tells you what exactly happens.

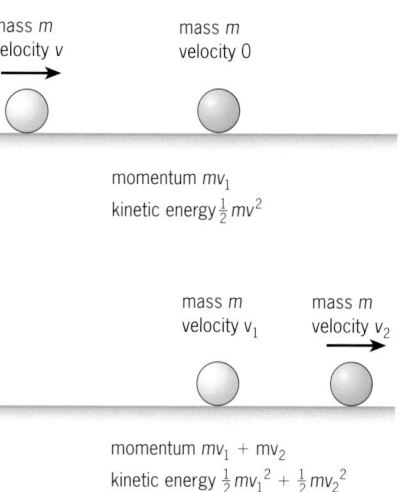

mass m
velocity v

mass m
velocity 0

momentum mv_1
kinetic energy $\tfrac{1}{2}mv^2$

mass m
velocity v_1

mass m
velocity v_2

momentum $mv_1 + mv_2$
kinetic energy $\tfrac{1}{2}mv_1^2 + \tfrac{1}{2}mv_2^2$

Fig 4.17 An elastic collision: $\mathbf{v}_1 = \mathbf{v}_2$

? QUESTION 7

7 A large steel ball and a small steel ball travelling in opposite directions collide and bounce apart elastically. Sketch graphs of force against time showing the forces acting on each ball during the collision.

4 FLUID PRESSURE: FLOATING, FLOWING AND FLYING

The movement of air over a curved surface produces unexpected forces that allow objects heavier than air to fly. These forces can be explained using Newton's laws, and can also be related to the way water flows, in pipes and rivers for example.

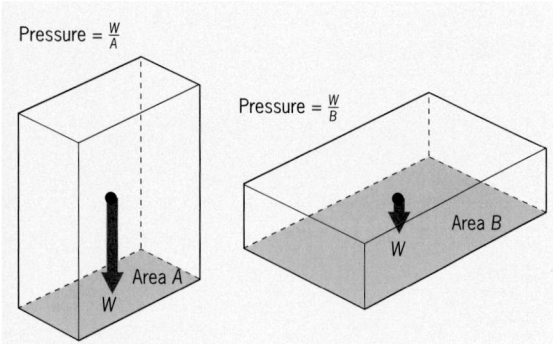

Fig 4.19 A block with weight *W* can exert different pressures on a surface

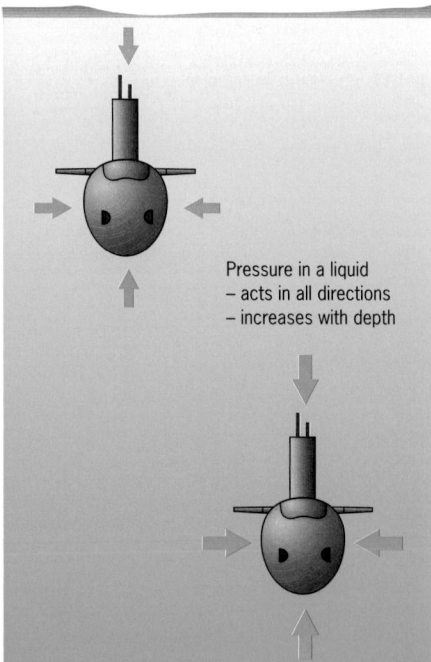

Fig 4.21 Two submarines at different depths have different pressures acting on them

Newton's laws of motion are best expressed for fluids in a statement of the Swiss mathematician Daniel Bernoulli (1700–1782) and known as **Bernoulli's principle**. Other important ideas that we use in this section of the chapter are **fluid pressure**, **thrust** and **viscosity** (the name for the *internal friction* of a fluid). We consider **hydrostatics** and **hydraulics**, which deal with the behaviour and uses of liquids under pressure. We also deal with the behaviour of fluids in response to forces. This behaviour is best explained using the **kinetic theory of matter**, which is dealt with in Chapter 7.

PRESSURE

Pressure is defined as the *force exerted on a surface per unit area* (see Fig 4.19):

$$\text{pressure = force/area}$$
$$P = F/A$$

Pressure is a scalar quantity with units of newtons per square metre. The unit of pressure has a special name, the pascal (Pa): 1 pascal = 1 N m^{-2}. This is a very tiny quantity – ordinary pressures are several thousand pascals: the pressure of the atmosphere for example is 10^5 Pa.

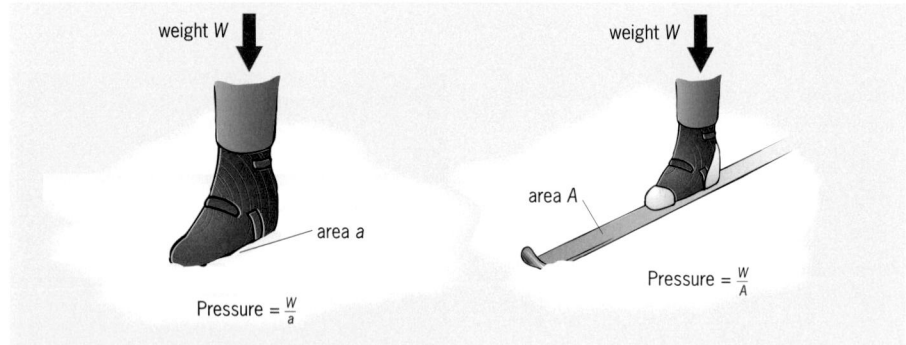

Fig 4.20 A ski reduces the pressure on snow

Fig 4.20 shows a simple example of the same force producing different pressures, due to the weight of a skier with and without skis. The large area of the ski 'spreads the load', and the weight of the body is more easily supported by the soft snow.

PRESSURE IN LIQUIDS

Pressure in a liquid has special features that are shown in Fig 4.21.

Theory and experiment show that in a liquid:
● Pressure increases with depth.
● At a given point in a liquid the pressure acts equally in all directions.
● A liquid can *transmit* a pressure exerted on it at one place so that it acts at some other place.

To say that a liquid 'finds its own level' (Fig 4.22) means that in any connected system the level of the liquid must everywhere be the same. If it isn't at any time then the difference in pressure will cause the liquid to move until the difference disappears. This is why a small clear tube outside a fuel tank can be used to show the level of the fuel inside.

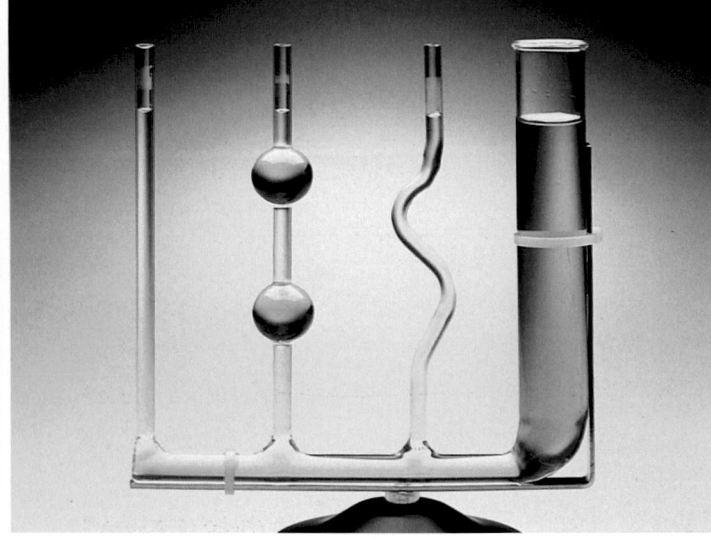

Fig 4.22 Liquid finds its own level

Hydrostatic pressure

The pressure at the bottom of a cylindrical jar of liquid is caused by the weight of the liquid and of the atmosphere above the liquid surface (Fig 4.23).

We now consider the pressure P *due to the liquid alone*.

The liquid has density ρ. The mass of water in the cylinder is thus:

$$m = \text{volume} \times \text{density} = Ah\rho$$

The weight of this mass is $mg = Ah\rho g$ and is a force acting over the area A. Thus the pressure P (force per unit area) caused by the liquid on the base of the cylinder is:

$$P = \frac{mg}{A} = h\rho g$$

Any object placed at this depth will be acted upon by this pressure. If you made a small hole in the side of the cylinder, water would be forced out sideways. It is perhaps surprising that this pressure acts *in all directions*, not just downwards as happens with, say, skis in the example on page 80.

The force due to **fluid pressure** is usually called **thrust** (see also Chapter 3, page 62):

$$\textbf{thrust} = \textbf{pressure} \times \textbf{area}$$
$$F = PA$$

Higher up we might expect that the pressure is less. For example, at a depth y the pressure should be simply

$$P = y\rho g$$

This is the basic relation in the science of **hydrostatics**, and is a simple formula that works for liquids which have a constant density. Simple experiments as shown in Fig 4.24 confirm that pressure increases with depth in a fluid and also that pressure acts in all directions. (Gases under pressure are compressed so that the density increases. This complication will be dealt with later.)

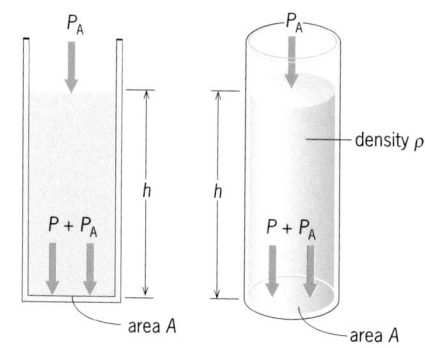

Fig 4.23 Liquid pressure in a cylinder

> **? QUESTION 8**
>
> 8 Estimate the extra pressure exerted on your body when you have dived into a swimming pool and are at a depth of 3 m. (The density of water is 1000 kg m^{-3}.)

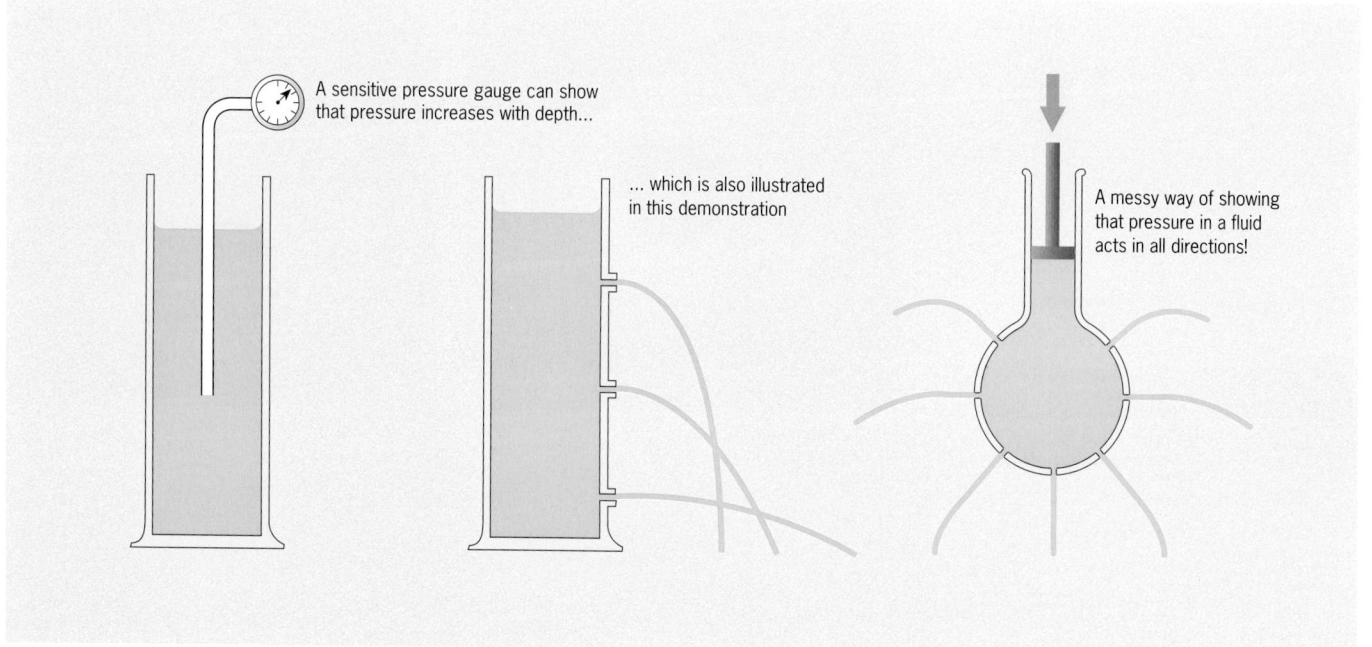

A sensitive pressure gauge can show that pressure increases with depth...

... which is also illustrated in this demonstration

A messy way of showing that pressure in a fluid acts in all directions!

Fig 4.24 Pressure increases with depth and acts in all directions

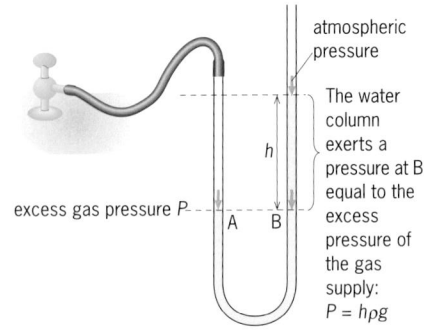

Fig 4.25 Simple U-tube manometer

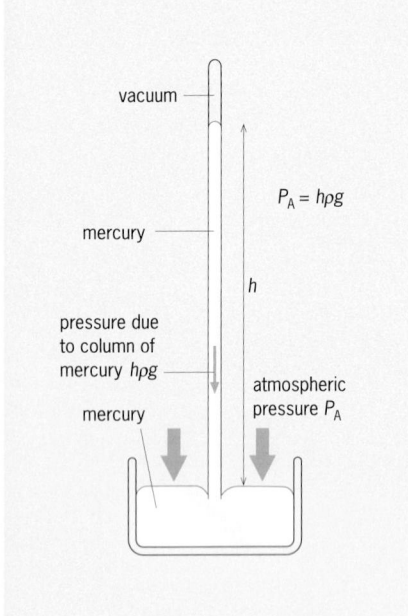

Fig 4.26 A simple mercury barometer

MEASURING PRESSURE IN FLUIDS

The simple **manometer** is being used to measure the pressure of a gas supply in Fig 4.25. The excess pressure of the gas supply compared with the pressure of the atmosphere is balancing the pressure exerted by the column of water. The pressure exerted by the liquid column, $h\rho g$, equals the excess pressure of the gas supply.

A **barometer** is used to measure atmospheric pressure. The original barometers used a column of mercury as shown in Fig 4.26. Air pressure acts on the surface of the mercury in the dish. This pressure is transmitted through the liquid and produces a thrust, acting upwards at the base of the mercury column, which exactly balances the weight of the column. The space above the column is (almost) a vacuum, created as the mercury column fell to its balancing level of about 76 cm above the surface of the mercury in the dish. The atmospheric pressure is given by $h\rho g$ where ρ is the density of mercury. (Remember that this pressure is independent of the area of the dish.)

For accurate measurements using a mercury barometer, a correction has to be made for the liquid's variation in density with temperature, and h has to be measured with great care. Barometers play an important part in weather forecasting: blocks of warm (usually damp) air and cold dry air have different densities, causing different atmospheric pressures at ground level. These pressure changes appear some distance ahead of the associated weather systems.

A cheaper instrument for measuring atmospheric pressure is an **aneroid** (liquid-free) barometer. It has a partially evacuated metal box with a corrugated shape that is kept from collapsing under the pressure of the atmosphere by a strong spring (Fig 4.27).

Changes in atmospheric pressure cause small movements in the surface of the box. These movements are amplified mechanically or electronically for display. Aneroid barometers have to be calibrated from time to time against the more direct measurements made by a mercury barometer. The aneroid principle is also used in an **altimeter** (Fig 4.28), since air pressure varies with height.

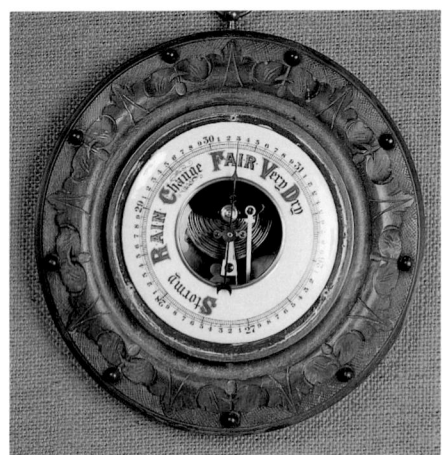

Fig 4.27 An aneroid barometer

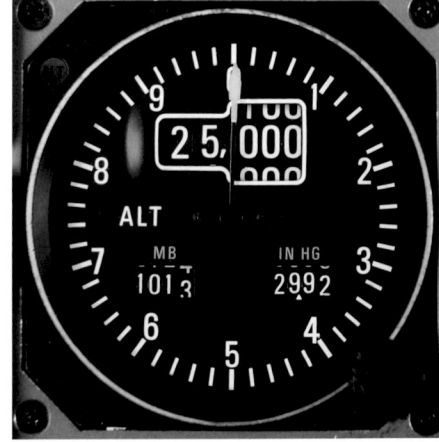

Fig 4.28 An altimeter

WHY SHIPS FLOAT: ARCHIMEDES' PRINCIPLE

Like many people, the Greek scientist and mathematician Archimedes of Syracuse (about 287 to 212 BC), had one of his best ideas in the bath – or so the fable tells us. But wherever he got the idea, Archimedes was the first scientist to realise the significance of the everyday event of the water level rising when you get into a bath. He linked this effect to a problem that he had been given to solve.

It was suspected that a royal crown was made of a silver–gold alloy, and not the pure gold supplied to the jeweller who made it. The crown's density would give Archimedes the answer. He could weigh the crown, but how could he measure its volume? Then he realised that the volume of the crown would equal the volume of water it displaced.

Archimedes also considered an object that floated either because it was hollow or because it was less dense than water. He stated that the displaced water would exert an upward force on the object. These ideas are brought together in **Archimedes' principle**, which is now stated thus:

> **When a body is wholly or partly immersed in a fluid it experiences an upward force (upthrust) equal to the weight of the fluid displaced.**

The effect is due to fluid pressure.

STRETCH AND CHALLENGE

A closer look at Archimedes' principle

Consider a block of material (assumed regular for the sake of simplicity) floating in a liquid (Fig 4.29).

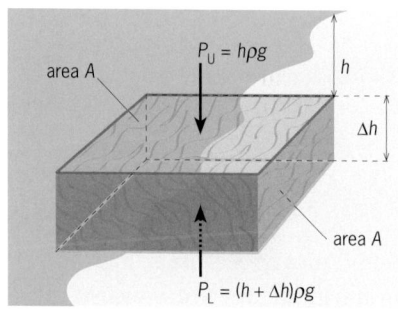

Fig 4.29 Forces acting on a floating object

The pressure on its upper surface, P_U, is $h\rho g$, where ρ is the density of the fluid. This pressure acts vertically on the surface and presses down with a force (thrust) of $Ah\rho g$.

The pressure on the lower surface is $P_L = (h + \Delta h)\rho g$ and acts upwards with a thrust $A(h + \Delta h)\rho g$. The thrusts on the vertical sides cancel out.

The net thrust on the block is thus upwards and is $A\Delta h\rho g$. But $A\Delta h$ is the volume (V) of the block and so the expression for the upthrust simplifies to $V\rho g$, which is of course the weight of the fluid displaced.

Whether the block sinks or floats depends on its own weight W. If $W > V\rho g$ it will sink. If the block is of density ρ_B, its weight is $V\rho_B g$, so the condition for sinking is simply $\rho_B > \rho$. If ρ_B is less than ρ, the block has a net upward force and will rise until it displaces just enough of the fluid for the upthrust to equal its weight.

STRETCH AND CHALLENGE

EXAMPLE

Q A block of cedar wood has a mass of 200 kg and a density of 570 kg m^{-3}. What fraction of the wood will be under the surface when the block is floating in water (density 1000 kg m^{-3})?

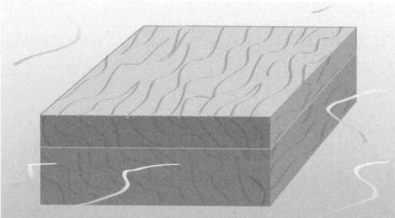

Fig 4.30 Block floating in water

A The wood will float when it displaces a weight of water equal to its own weight, which is equivalent to saying that the wood and the *displaced* water have the same mass.

Mass of water displaced = 200 kg.

Volume of water displaced = mass of water/density of water
= 200/1000 = 0.20 m^3.

The volume of the block = mass of block/density of block
= 200/570 = 0.351 m^3.

Thus the proportion of the wood under the water surface is 0.20/0.351 = 0.57.

? QUESTIONS 11–12

11 The Example on the previous page gives the proportion of wood under water as 0.57. The ratio of the densities of wood and water is also 0.57. Is this a coincidence? Explain.

12 Ships are usually made of steel, of density 7700 kg m⁻³ – much denser than water. Why do steel ships float?

FLUID FLOW: BERNOULLI'S PRINCIPLE

The principles of fluid flow were first explained over two hundred years ago by Daniel Bernoulli, although it is unlikely that he foresaw all the modern applications of his theories.

Imagine a liquid flowing through a tube shaped as in Fig 4.31. The flow is continuous – just as much liquid enters at X as leaves at Y. For this to be true, the liquid must flow *faster* in the narrow part of the pipe than it does in the wider parts.

For a liquid flowing through a tube of cross-sectional area A at a speed v, the volume passing any point each second is Av. As A varies, so will v – provided the liquid is **incompressible**. At the pressures normally found in practical situations, liquids *are* incompressible. Thus, for a liquid flowing in a pipe of varying cross-sectional area, the quantity Av stays constant. This is the **principle of continuity** for a liquid.

Gases are more easily compressed, however, and if the pressure changes as the pipe widens or narrows the gas *density* will change. What must be constant is the mass of gas that enters and the mass that leaves any section of pipe; it will help to think of this in terms of the number of molecules that enter and leave the section. At any given values of area A and speed v, the mass of gas of density ρ in the section v metres long is ρAv. In this case, we express the principle of continuity in its more general form as:

$$\rho Av = \textbf{constant}$$

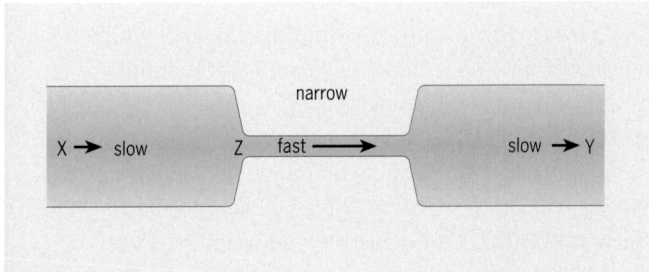

Fig 4.31 The volume of liquid flowing per second is the same in both the wide and narrow sections of the tube. This means that the liquid must flow faster in the narrow section

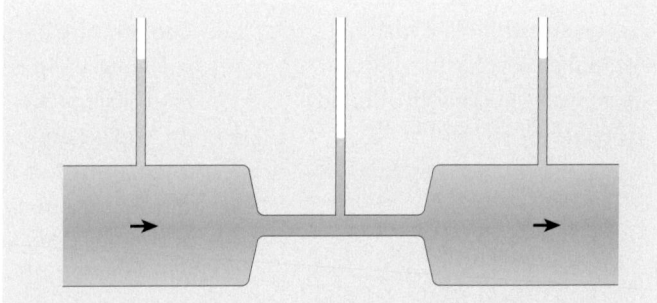

Fig 4.32 Pressure variation in a liquid flowing through a tube of varying cross-section

Returning to the case of liquid flow, the liquid moves because somewhere back along the pipe there is a pump (say) producing a pressure, which is the same everywhere within the liquid. Now think about what must be happening at Z in Fig 4.31. Here the liquid is being accelerated to increase its speed. Acceleration requires a net force acting in the direction of the acceleration. There must therefore be a greater pressure to the left of Z than there is to the right.

Fig 4.32 shows a demonstration of the pressure differences in a model of the arrangement. The vertical tubes act as manometers, with the heights of the liquid columns measuring pressure. The columns show that the pressure in the narrow tube is less than that in the wide tube in front of it, as theory predicts. The pressure increases again in the second wide tube – because the liquid is being slowed down and a force is required to decelerate it. This accounts for the differences of pressure shown in Fig 4.32, and Bernoulli's conclusion was that, in a moving fluid:

The greater the speed, the lower the pressure.

This is **Bernoulli's principle** and applies to all fluids, and is the key to understanding why 'heavier than air' aeroplanes can stay in the air – so long as they keep moving.

APPLICATIONS OF BERNOULLI'S PRINCIPLE
Fragrance spray
Fig 4.33 shows a hand-operated fragrance spray. When you press the bulb, air is forced through the tube, which has a constriction in it – that is, part of the tube is narrower than the rest. The air travels faster in the narrow part and so its pressure decreases. Liquid is drawn up the vertical tube, breaks into droplets as it meets the air jet and is carried out of the nozzle in a fine spray.

Aerofoils: the principle of flight
An **aerofoil** is the shaped wing of an aircraft (Fig 4.34). The top surface of an aerofoil is convex, which means that, while the aircraft is in flight, air travels faster over the top surface than over the bottom. This is because the air stream has to travel a greater distance over the top surface in the same time – as with a liquid, the air mass has to be continuous. The result is a smaller pressure on the upper surface than on the lower, and the aerofoil experiences a net upward thrust – called **lift**. The wing is usually angled to the direction of motion so that it has to push against the air. This produces an additional force (reaction) with an upward component to add to the lift. In general, the angle the aerofoil makes with the forward direction of motion (angle of attack) is large enough for this reaction force to be more effective in maintaining height than the aerofoil's Bernoulli effect.

STREAMLINES AND TURBULENT FLOW: FRICTION AND DRAG
The simple theory of fluid flow described above assumes that the flow is steady, so that particles of the fluid flow in smooth paths – as shown by the continuous streamlines made visible by streamers in Fig 4.35. But above a certain speed the flow becomes chaotic and we have **turbulent** flow. Energy is dissipated in sound and heating; and extra pressures are produced which can affect the straightforward motion of a vehicle.

There is often turbulent flow when two air streams that have diverged over a moving object join together again. This effect can be seen in the air behind a car being tested in a wind tunnel. The disturbed turbulent air produces a low-pressure region, which tends to pull the car backwards, contributing to the drag forces that oppose the motion of any object through a fluid. The turbulent drag force is reduced by vehicle design. The best shape is like an aerofoil, of course, but drivers would worry if, at a certain speed, the car started flying! The rear spoiler fitted to some cars, as shown in Fig 4.36, is a way of reducing the drag force by making the air flow less turbulent at the back of the vehicle. As in Fig 4.37, racing cyclists and downhill skiers wear specially shaped helmets to reduce the effect of turbulence.

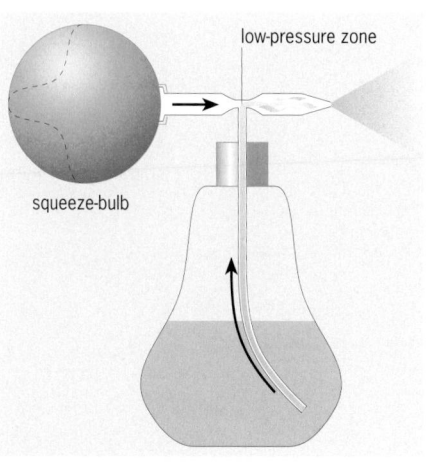

Fig 4.33 A fragrance spray

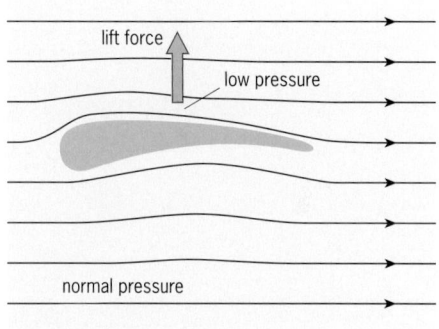

Fig 4.34 Aerofoil with lines of air flow

> **? QUESTION 13**
>
> **13** Mrs Frisbee sold her pies in dish-shaped plastic containers. Young customers discovered that a spinning pie dish (now called a Frisbee) had aerodynamic properties. Explain:
> **a)** why Frisbees fly;
> **b)** why they fly in a more controlled manner when they are spinning.

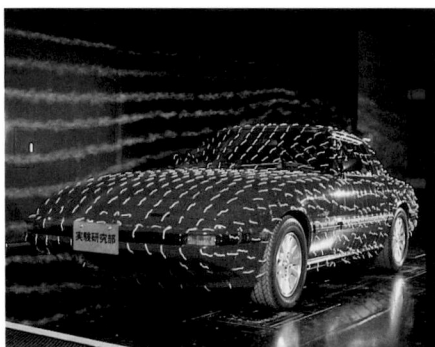

Fig 4.35 A car in a wind tunnel, with streamlines shown by streamers

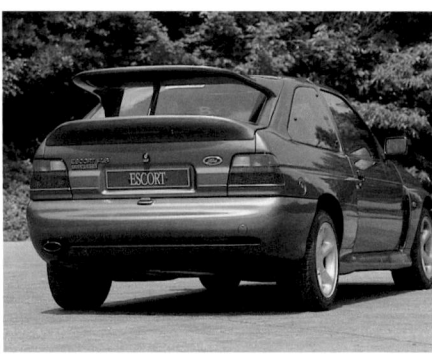

Fig 4.36 A car with a rear spoiler

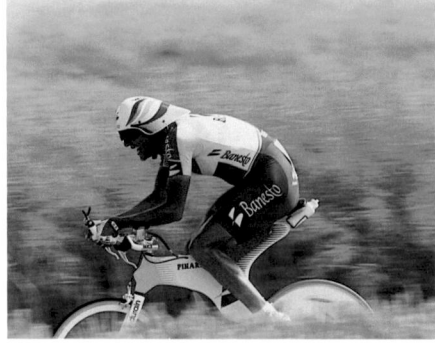

Fig 4.37 A special helmet worn by cyclists in time trials

Other drag forces act on a surface moving through a fluid. For example, air has to be pushed away as a car drives through it, and this produces a reaction force that acts on the car. Next we look at frictional forces between the vehicle's surface and the fluid.

FRICTION AND VISCOSITY

Layers of fluids move over each other very easily; for this reason a fluid cannot resist a shearing stress (see Chapter 5). But fluids do have a kind of internal friction called **viscosity**. This varies: moving a knife blade through water is much easier than moving it through honey. Similarly, viscous forces arise when adjacent layers of liquid move against each other.

In a simple model of what happens, we assume that when a fluid moves through a pipe the fluid layer next to the wall of the pipe is at rest, and that the fastest stream is at the centre of the pipe, as in Fig 4.38. There is a constant **velocity gradient** in the fluid, $\Delta v/\Delta x$, where x is the distance measured radially in the pipe. A liquid that behaves like this is called a *Newtonian liquid*. Friction between adjacent layers in the fluid determines how fast the fluid can flow – compare pouring water and treacle. A fluid has a **coefficient of viscosity** η (the Greek letter eta) which determines the size of the viscous force. The resistive viscous force is greater for a wider pipe. These factors are combined in **Newton's law of viscosity**. When F is the force due to viscosity acting on a fluid stream of cross-sectional area A, against the direction of flow, then:

$$F = \eta A \, \frac{\Delta v}{\Delta x}$$

This force is also the drag force on the sides of the container.

Viscosity has units of N s m^{-2} and values of the viscosity of some fluids are given in Table 4.3 – blood *is* thicker than water! Viscosity varies with temperature: as a general rule the coefficient decreases as temperature increases, so that liquids are more 'runny' when hot.

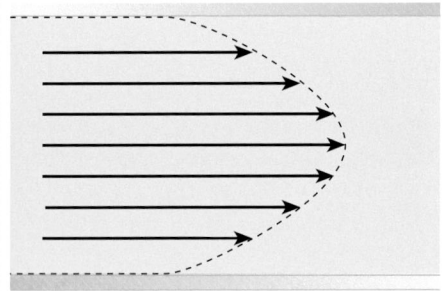

Fig 4.38 Streamline flow with viscosity. The speed at the wall is zero, and increases to a maximum at the centre of the pipe

Table 4.3 Viscosities of some common fluids	
Fluid	**Viscosity/N s m^{-2}**
Water at 20 °C	1.0×10^{-3}
Water at 100 °C	0.3×10^{-3}
Blood at 37.5 °C	2.7×10^{-3}
Typical motor oil at 20 °C	830×10^{-3}
Glycerine at 20 °C	850×10^{-3}
Air at 23 °C	0.018×10^{-3}

STOKES' LAW

Viscous forces also affect the speed of streamline motion of an object in the fluid. For a sphere in streamline motion at a speed v through a fluid, the Irish physicist George Stokes (1819–1903) proved that it would experience a drag force:

$$F = 6\pi\eta r v$$

where η is the coefficient of viscosity of the fluid and r is the radius of the sphere (Fig 4.39).

This idea may be linked to the *terminal speed* of a falling sphere (see page 32). In this case the viscous drag on the sphere equals its weight:

$$mg = 6\pi\eta r v$$

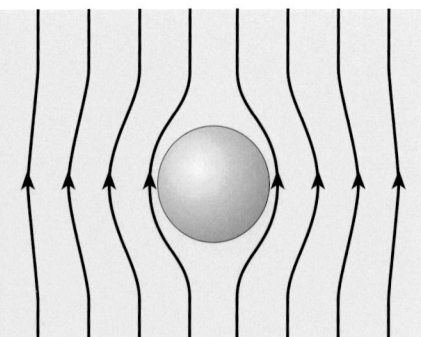

Fig 4.39 Streamline movement of a sphere through a fluid. The arrows show the velocity of the fluid relative to the sphere

EXAMPLE

Q Calculate the terminal speed of **a)** a lead sphere, **b)** a hailstone, both having a radius of 2 mm.

(The density of lead is 1.14×10^4 kg m^{-3}; the density of ice is 9.2×10^2 kg m^{-3}.)

A

a) The condition for terminal speed is that $mg = 6\pi\eta r v$, so terminal speed v is:

$$v = \frac{mg}{6\pi\eta r}$$

The mass of the lead sphere is:

$m = $ volume $\times$ density $= \frac{4}{3}\pi r^3 \times \rho$

so the equation can be simplified to:

$$v = \frac{\frac{2}{9}r^2\rho g}{\eta}$$

$$= \frac{\frac{2}{9} \times 4 \times 10^{-6} \times 1.14 \times 10^4 \times 9.8}{1.8 \times 10^{-5}}$$

giving: $v = 5.5 \times 10^3$ m s^{-1}

b) The only difference in the conditions of the problem is the density of the materials. Thus the ratio of terminal speeds is the same as the ratio of densities. Ice is less dense than lead, so it falls more slowly.

The terminal speed of the hailstone is:

$$v = \frac{5.5 \times 10^3 \times 9.2}{114} = 4.4 \times 10^2 \text{ m s}^{-1}$$

Note that in practice both spheres would fall more slowly, since turbulence would set in at much lower speeds.

? QUESTIONS 14–15

14 Calculate the terminal speed of the lead sphere in the example when it falls through water at 20 °C.

15 A parachutist has a mass of 60 kg. Assuming that Stokes' law applies in this case, what radius of circular parachute would be required to ensure a terminal speed of 4 m s^{-1}?

DRAG EFFECTS FOR A VEHICLE

Energy can be 'saved' in transportation by reducing a variety of losses. Nowadays the drag factor is taken into account in car design. This factor indicates how much energy a moving vehicle 'loses' as a result of air friction. This kind of friction loss is due to the vehicle working against a frictional **drag force** F_d. When v is the vehicle's speed, A its cross-sectional area and ρ the density of air, then:

$$F_d = \tfrac{1}{2}CA\rho v^2$$

where C is its **drag coefficient**, a constant which depends upon the shape of the vehicle.

The car is also subject to *rolling friction*, due to the contact of the tyres with the road surface. This creates a force given by μN where N is the normal reaction between car and road. The coefficient of rolling friction for a car is about 0.02. The normal reaction N gets slightly less at higher speeds as the car behaves like an aerofoil (luckily not very successfully at usual road speeds).

Rolling friction is much more important than drag for a car travelling at low speeds. However, drag increases as the square of the speed. Drag and rolling friction become equal at a speed of about 18 m s^{-1} (40 mph) for a typical car, and eventually drag is the main source of frictional loss.

The main energy losses from a car engine are not due to these effects at all. As explained in Chapter 14, heat engines are inefficient, and dissipate almost 70 per cent of the energy that comes from the burning fuel. There are other friction losses in the transmission, so that the energy available for moving the car is only about 14 per cent of the energy supplied by the fuel.

EXAMPLE

Q How much power needs to be delivered to the wheels of a car travelling at a typical motorway speed of 31 m s^{-1} (70 mph)?

(Data: At this speed, rolling friction provides a force of 210 N; the car has a cross-sectional area of 1.8 m^2; the density of air is 1.3 kg m^{-3}; the drag coefficient of the car is 0.4.)

A The drag force on the car is calculated from:

$$F_{\mathrm{d}} = \tfrac{1}{2}\, CA\rho v^2$$

$$= 0.5 \times 0.4 \times 1.8 \times 1.3 \times (31)^2 \text{ N}$$

Drag force = 450 N
Thus the total frictional force on the car is 210 N + 450 N = 660 N.

This force does work that requires energy to be supplied by the car's engine.

The work done per second
$$= \text{force} \times \text{distance moved per second (speed)}$$

that is:

power needed = work done per second
$$= \text{frictional force} \times \text{speed}$$
$$= 660 \text{ N} \times 31 \text{ m s}^{-1}$$
$$= 20.5 \text{ kW}$$

HOW FAST CAN A VEHICLE GO?

The speed of a train or a car – or a cyclist – is the result of a battle between the driving force and resistive forces. Newton's laws act as the referee. The best way to tackle many problems is from the point of view of **energy** and **power** (the rate of *transferring* energy).

The car in Fig 4.40 is travelling on a horizontal road at a steady speed of 25 m s^{-1} with its engine delivering energy at its maximum rate of 14 kW. *What is this energy being used to do?* It is in fact being used to do work against friction forces: inside the engine, the transmission, the wheels and – mostly – against the forces of drag and viscous air friction. It is also pushing air out of its way and giving it some kinetic energy. The car is not accelerating or going uphill so doesn't gain potential or kinetic energy. Suppose the total of the friction and other forces opposing motion is *F*. When the car travels 25 metres it does work of 25*F*.

>
> **REMEMBER THIS**
> Work done = energy transferred
> = force × distance travelled in direction of force

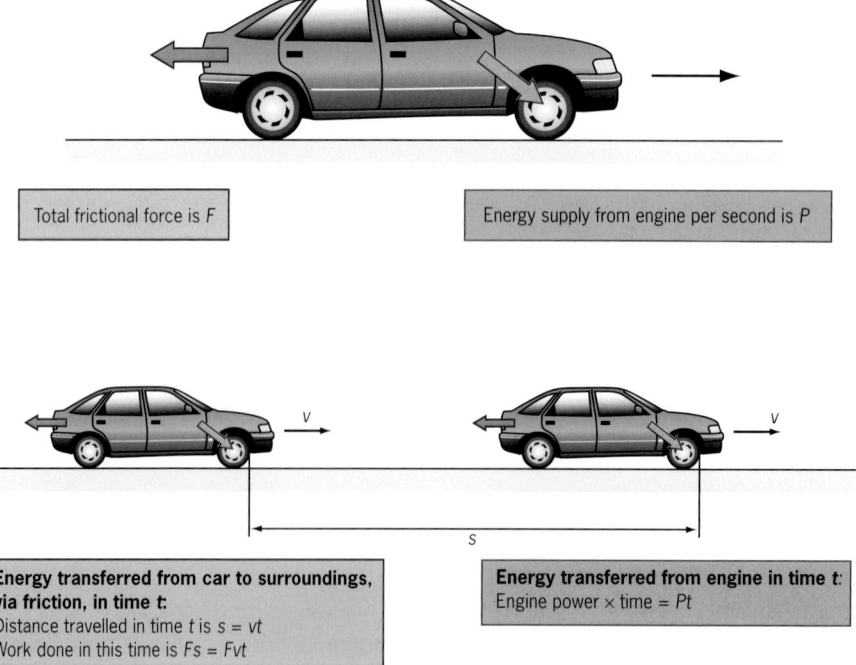

Total frictional force is *F*

Energy supply from engine per second is *P*

Energy transferred from car to surroundings, via friction, in time *t*:
Distance travelled in time *t* is *s = vt*
Work done in this time is *Fs = Fvt*

Energy transferred from engine in time *t*:
Engine power × time = *Pt*

By conservation of energy:
Pt = Fvt
and so *P = Fv*

Fig 4.40 The power relationships for a car

The car takes one second to travel 25 metres, so the work done per second is also 25F. This is the power developed by the engine of course, since all of it is being used to do work against friction.

So $25F = 14$ kW in this case. This gives the total frictional force as 560 N.

The power generated by the engine is P. What we have shown is that when the car is travelling at a steady speed on the flat

power = frictional forces × speed

$P = Fv$

Going uphill

Suppose our car is now climbing a not very steep hill that rises 1 metre for every 25 metres along the road. Some of the power from the engine has to lift the car uphill and so give it potential energy. The car can't go as fast, because the engine has an extra task:

$$P = Fv + mg\Delta h$$

Here, Δh is the increase in height of the car every second. This depends on the angle of slope and the speed of the car: $\Delta h = v \sin \theta$ (see Fig 4.41, which shows that this is simply $v/25$ in this example.

The car's speed drops:

$$Fv + mg\Delta h = P$$

$$(F + mg/25)\, v = P$$

If the car's mass is 800 kg and if (not too likely) F stays the same at 560 N, then you should be able to check that the car's speed drops to just under 16 m s^{-1}.

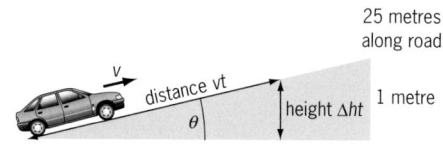

The hill rises 1 metre for every 25 metres along the road. This means that $\sin \theta = 1/25$
Also, $\sin \theta = \Delta ht/vt = \Delta h/v$

Fig 4.41 Going uphill

> Please see the How Science Works assignment for this chapter at www.collinseducation.co.uk/CAS for further practice in this topic

STRETCH AND CHALLENGE

Free-body diagrams

A good way to test your understanding of what is happening when bodies are acted upon by forces is to draw a simple diagram showing where and in which direction the forces act. To do this you need to have a good understanding of Newton's laws of motion and be able to apply them to the situation the body finds itself in. For most everyday situations the forces acting will be caused by gravity (or some other applied force), friction and any force of contact between the object and another object. This contact force is often called a *reaction* force – but this can be a confusing name because it may not be the same force as that discussed above in connection with Newton's third law.

Fig 4.42 shows some simple situations with the forces involved drawn as vectors from the points where they act.

Fig 4.42 Free-body diagrams in different situations. Note that weight W acts through the centre of mass of an object. A 'normal reaction' force acts at right angles to the supporting surface. Friction F acts at a surface of contact

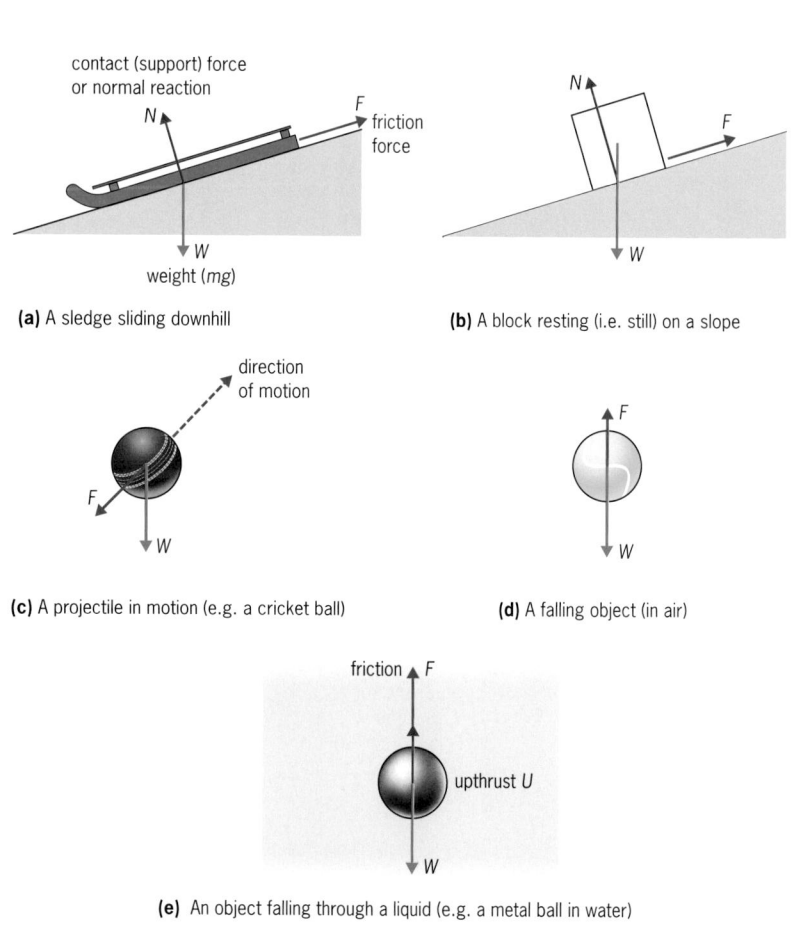

contact (support) force or normal reaction

N F friction force

W weight (mg)

(a) A sledge sliding downhill

N F

W

(b) A block resting (i.e. still) on a slope

direction of motion

F

W

(c) A projectile in motion (e.g. a cricket ball)

F

W

(d) A falling object (in air)

friction F

upthrust U

W

(e) An object falling through a liquid (e.g. a metal ball in water)

SUMMARY

After studying this chapter you should:

- Have improved your understanding of Newton's laws of motion as applied to transport and moving fluids.
- Understand the role of friction in transportation, and be able to apply the laws of static and sliding friction and coefficient of friction.
- Understand the ideas of viscosity, streamline flow and drag factor, relating these to Stokes' law and terminal speed.
- Understand the physics of rotating bodies and be able to use the ideas of angular velocity, angular acceleration, torque, rotational inertia and rotational kinetic energy.
- Be able to apply the laws of conservation of momentum and conservation of energy as appropriate to elastic and inelastic collisions.

- Be able to use the relationship: impulse = change of momentum ($F\Delta t = \Delta p$).
- Understand and be able to apply the concept of pressure in fluids and relate this to practical situations involving hydraulics and flotation.
- Understand and be able to use Archimedes' principle.
- Be able to use Bernoulli's principle to explain how fluid pressure and speed are related when a fluid moves relative to an object such as an aerofoil.
- Understand how the physics in this chapter is important in society and practical applications, such as collisions, road safety, wheels and transport in general.

Practice questions for this chapter are available at www.collinseducation.co.uk/CAS

5

Materials and forces: structures and microstructures

5 MATERIALS AND FORCES: STRUCTURES AND MICROSTRUCTURES

Building a bridge to withstand the forces of nature

The Tacoma Narrows Bridge in Washington State was opened in 1940. After only four months it collapsed (see page 129) – not as a result of an earthquake, but simply because it was badly designed. It proved not strong enough for the loads it was designed to bear when exposed to the forces of violent winds.

The need to understand how materials behave when they are subjected to forces is literally a matter of life and death.

But engineers know that they cannot just rely on theory when they are building these massive structures. They have learnt from the mistakes of the past and now test their designs on models accurate to the smallest detail before they begin to build. Then more safety tests are made at all stages during construction.

These tests can be quite spectacular. When the Japanese were building a new suspension bridge in Tokyo Bay they dropped 100-tonne hammers from a height of 60 metres on to the middle of the span. The impacts sent waves backwards and forwards along the bridge, and made it twist and turn like a corkscrew. Only because the structure survived this battering did they decide that the bridge was safe enough.

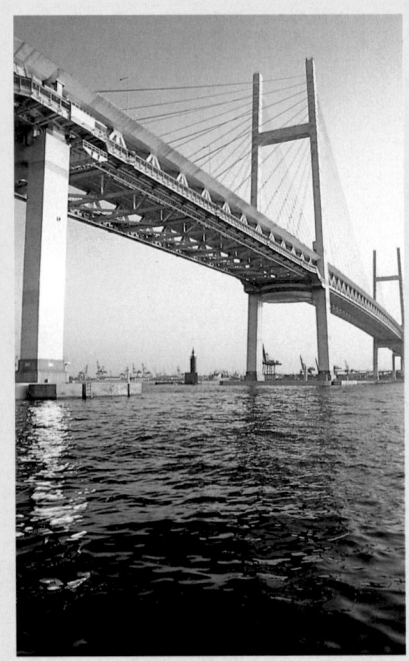

The Tokyo Bay Bridge, with a span of 570 metres

The ideas in this chapter

When we consider structures, we often think of huge engineering projects, such as the Channel Tunnel connecting Britain and France, or the Humber Bridge which for a time was the longest suspension bridge anywhere in the world, spanning 1410 metres. (The recently built Akashi Kaikyo Bridge in Japan has a span of just under 2000 metres.) Or we might think of the world's tallest buildings such as the Sears Building in Chicago (520 metres but including the TV antennas) and the Petronas Twin Towers in Kuala Lumpur (taller if the antennas are excluded). Around the world, architects and engineers are competing to build higher and the Burj, Dubai, under construction, has become the tallest. The principles behind the strength and stability of these impressive structures, and the forces affecting them, also apply on a much smaller scale to cups and saucers, fishing rods and tennis rackets, and even animal skeletons and plants.

In this chapter, we shall be looking at these forces, and at the composition and properties of the materials in the objects, noting that all materials are built up from individual atoms. We shall see that the properties of different materials arise from the ways their atoms are arranged on the molecular scale, and how the atoms and molecules pack together to form a microstructure. We shall explain the differences by creating simple models to describe the materials and then compare these models with reality.

1 STATICS – OR HOW STRUCTURES STAY UP

Large structures, such as bridges and buildings, are stationary – or move only slightly in the wind. They are subject to very large forces due to their own mass, and also due to the ground and any other point of attachment.

The forces acting on these structures must be in equilibrium – that is, their *resolved components* in any direction must balance and cancel. If the forces on an object do not balance out, then, by Newton's second law, some acceleration takes place.

The study of forces in equilibrium – of forces acting on a stationary object – is called statics.

Forces are also in equilibrium if a body is moving uniformly – that is, in a straight line without acceleration.

In order to see how forces act on an object, we must examine all the forces which are acting on it. You have seen that force is a **vector**: it has both magnitude and direction. To add two forces, we draw a parallelogram of forces as in Fig 5.1. The **resultant** force is represented by the diagonal of the parallelogram. The size and direction of the resultant force can be obtained either by scale drawing or by calculation.

CALCULATING THE RESULTANT OF FORCES ACTING AT RIGHT ANGLES

It is much easier to calculate the resultant force when the two forces act on the object at right angles. The Example shows two ways of working out the resultant force.

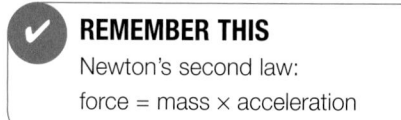

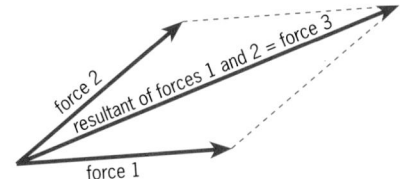

Fig 5.1 A parallelogram of two forces acting on a body. One side of the parallelogram represents the magnitude and direction of one force. An adjacent side represents the magnitude and direction of the second force. The diagonal between them is the resultant

---

EXAMPLE

1 SCALE DRAWING

In Fig 5.2, the forces acting at a point on an object are drawn to scale (1 cm ≡ 2 N).

a) The two forces are drawn acting at a single point.

b) The parallelogram (rectangle in this case) is completed.

c) The diagonal of the parallelogram is drawn starting from the point at which the forces act. This diagonal represents the resultant force.

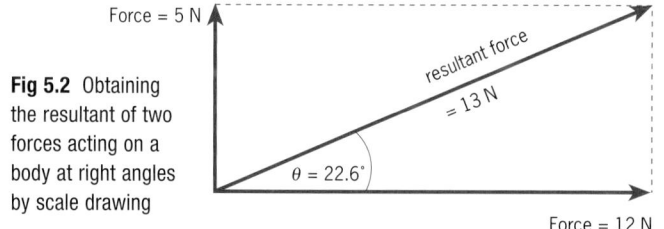

Fig 5.2 Obtaining the resultant of two forces acting on a body at right angles by scale drawing

2 CALCULATION

Alternatively, the magnitude and direction of the resultant force can be calculated by using trigonometry. Using Pythagoras' theorem:

$$(\text{resultant force})^2 = (5)^2 + (12)^2 = 169$$
$$\text{(values in newtons)}$$
$$\text{resultant force} = \sqrt{169} = 13 \text{ N}$$

The angle θ between the resultant and the 12 N force has a tangent equal to 5/12:

$$\theta = \tan^{-1}(5/12)$$
$$\text{(inverse tan on calculator)}$$
$$= 22.6°$$

COPLANAR FORCES ACTING AT A POINT

Suppose there are three forces acting at a point. We can demonstrate the effect using three newton meters (or spring balances) linked by strings to a common point and with the opposite ends of the newton meters anchored to three fixed points (Fig 5.3). The force in meter 3 must be equal and opposite to the resultant force of meters 1 and 2, as represented by the diagonal of the parallelogram. Similar parallelograms can be drawn for the pair of meters 1 and 3 and also for the pair of meters 2 and 3. These resultants in their turn will be in equilibrium with the forces on meters 2 and 1 respectively.

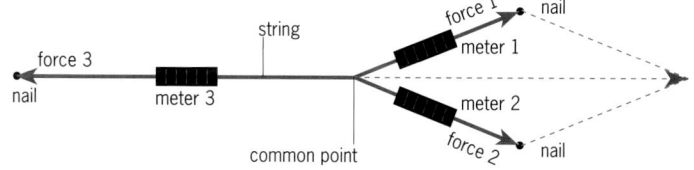

Fig 5.3 Three forces in equilibrium

? QUESTION 1

1 **a)** Sketch Fig 5.3 and draw in the parallelogram of forces for the pairs of newton meters 1 and 3, and newton meters 2 and 3. State the forces that the resultants represent.
b) Explain why we can say that the forces are in equilibrium in Fig 5.3.

✔ REMEMBER THIS

A **point object** is an object which is so small that we can consider that all the forces acting on it meet at a point. Often the forces acting on a larger body all meet at the centre of mass, so that we can consider the larger body to be equivalent to a single point.

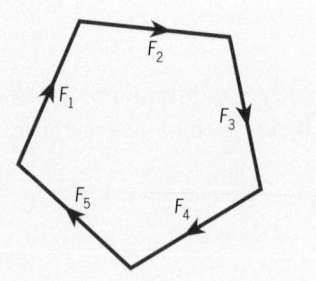

Suppose several forces all act in the same plane and we wish to find the overall resultant force. The forces are **coplanar** – they can all be represented by vectors drawn to scale on a flat sheet of paper. To find the resultant force, we can take the forces in pairs and draw parallelograms of forces for each pair. We then get a resultant for each pair. We can pair up these resultants and repeat the process until we are left with one overall resultant force. With a lot of forces to deal with, this method could be time-consuming and tedious.

We could extend to forces in three dimensions, and resolve in the x, y and z directions. But even for three-dimensional bridges and buildings, we often consider two-dimensional cross-sections. So we won't complicate our analysis here with the third dimension.

Returning to forces acting in a single x–y plane, provided these forces act through a single point in a body and the body is not being accelerated, the resultant force must be zero. We can draw the forces acting on the body as vectors and we can join up the vectors, tail-to-head, one after another. *For a body experiencing zero resultant force, the vectors will form the sides of a closed polygon (Fig 5.4).*

If the vectors do not close up, then the line F_x that closes the polygon represents both the magnitude and direction of the extra force needed for equilibrium (Fig 5.5). Without this additional vector force, the resultant force R on the body will be equal and opposite in direction, and will produce an acceleration on the body.

Fig 5.4 Left: Five forces forming a closed polygon. If these five forces act at a single point within a body, they will be in equilibrium. They will produce no acceleration of the body

Fig 5.5 Right: Five forces not in equilibrium. Resultant force **R** is in the opposite direction to the force needed to close the polygon (i.e. to achieve equilibrium)

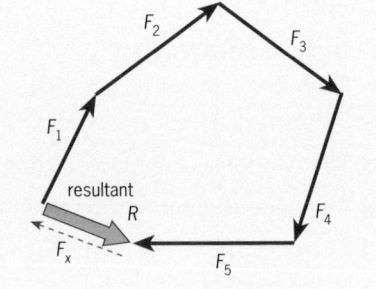

We can say that:

Any point object acted on by a number of forces will only be in equilibrium (i.e. stationary or moving with uniform velocity) if the force vectors form a closed polygon.

Centre of gravity

When we consider the gravitational force on an object of finite size we assume that this force acts through a single point within that object. We show the resultant gravitational force by a single arrow which represents the sum of the forces on all parts of the object. Thus, the **centre of gravity** is the point through which all weight appears to act.

For everyday purposes (on the Earth's surface) the centre of gravity is the **centre of mass**. This is the point through which an applied force causes no rotation of the object.

For symmetrical objects of uniform density it is easy to see where the centre of mass, and hence centre of gravity, will be. If we consider an irregular object, the centre of gravity remains the same whatever way up it is. The centre of gravity of an irregular flat object can be found by hanging it freely from two or more different points on it close to its edge. (See Fig 2.6, page 28.)

Alternative graphical method

There is another method to calculate the values of coplanar forces at a point. Take all the forces acting on a body and resolve each force into components that are at right angles. To do this graphically, set up x and y axes on graph paper and draw in the forces to scale.

- Draw to scale forces F_1, F_2 and F_3 acting in the correct directions: Fig 5.6(a).
- Draw resolved components F_{1x} and F_{1y} along the x and y axes. Similarly, draw the components for F_2 and F_3.

- Add forces as vectors along the x and y axes, taking into account plus and minus directions: Fig 5.6(b).
- Measure the lines to get the magnitude and direction of the overall force.

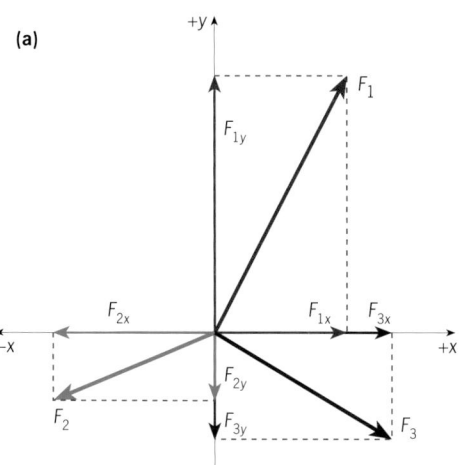

(a)

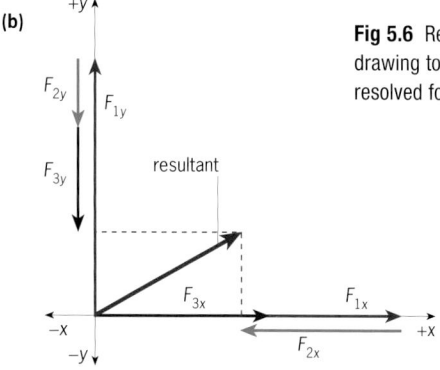

(b)

Fig 5.6 Resolving forces by drawing to scale and adding resolved forces

? QUESTION 2

2 A sailing boat with an outboard motor is subject to forces from the wind, the tide and the motor. The motor produces a force of 5 units due north, the tide creates a force of 2 units towards the north-west and the wind on the sails provides a force of 3 units towards the north-east. Obtain graphically or by calculation the magnitude and direction of the overall force.

HOW SCIENCE WORKS

Forces acting on a radio mast

Assume the mast is held in place by two cables (support wires) as shown in Fig 5.7. These give tension forces pulling down on the mast. If we split the tension force in each cable into vertical and horizontal components, we can see from the force diagram that the horizontal components of these forces will oppose each other. The vertical components are opposed by an upward force F_{ground} exerted by the ground up through the mast.

The parallelogram of forces is shown for the three forces (these are F_{cable}, F_{cable} and F_{ground}) and beneath is the closed polygon of forces (a triangle as there are three forces). In practice, a mast is held in place by two more cables acting at right angles to the plane of the paper. The force F_{ground} must oppose the vertical components of the forces exerted by all four cables.

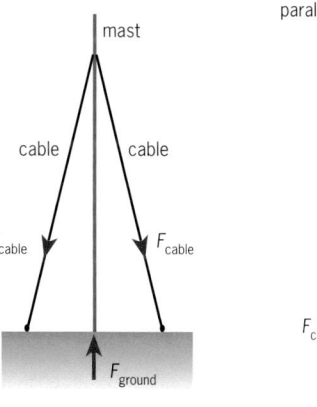
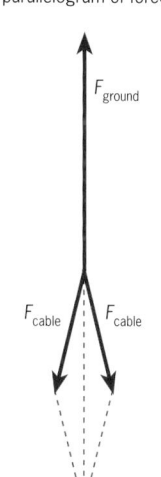
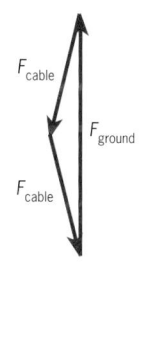

Fig 5.7 Forces acting in one plane on a radio mast, and the corresponding parallelogram and polygon of forces

REMEMBER THIS

Moments of forces

When a body is in equilibrium, the sum of anticlockwise moments about the pivot (balance point) is equal to the sum of clockwise moments. For example, where M and m are in newtons and x and y are in metres,

$$M_1 x_1 + M_2 x_2 = m_1 y_1 + m_2 y_2 \ \text{(N m)}$$

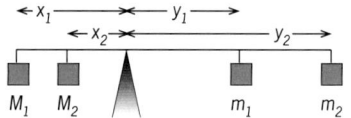

If an object is in **static equilibrium**, no resultant force acts on it and it remains at rest or moving at constant velocity.

FORCES NOT ACTING AT A POINT: INTRODUCING MOMENTS

In all the examples so far, the forces act through a single point. But for large structures it may not be possible to treat the forces as acting in this way. We may find that there are forces which are parallel to each other. To understand how static equilibrium (net force acting = zero) can exist in the case of forces not all acting at a point, we need to bring in the idea of **moments of forces** – see the reminder box in the margin. A body is in equilibrium when the net forces acting on it are zero and when the net moment of these forces is zero.

Tower crane

A good example that shows the moment of forces in action is the tower crane. Study Fig 5.8, a simplified diagram of a tower crane, and its caption carefully.

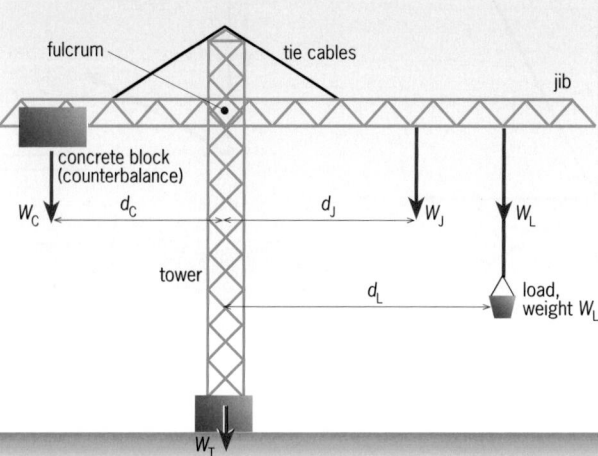

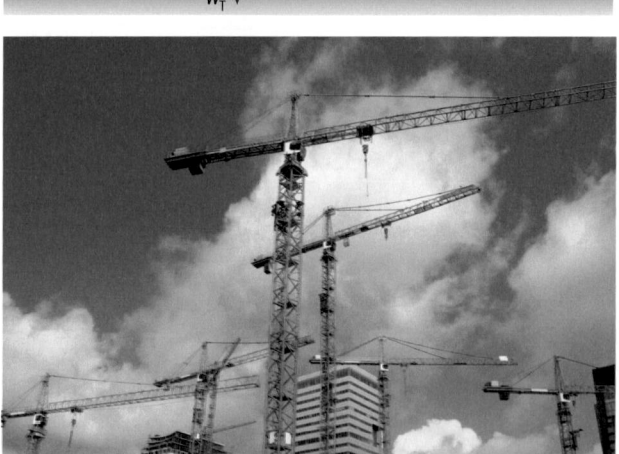

Fig 5.8 A tower crane, showing the main forces involved. The effect of gravity on the mass of the tower will produce a downward force W_T which acts directly through the tower base.

Next, the horizontal jib extends outwards from the tower on two opposite sides. But note that the jib extends further outwards on the side used for lifting the load. So the centre of gravity of the jib lies a distance d_J outwards on this side of the tower, and there is a force downwards of W_J due to the weight of the jib. Tie cables are provided to help support the jib.

A load W_L is being lifted at a distance d_L along the jib from the centre of the tower. A concrete block acting as a counterbalance is positioned at distance d_C on the opposite side, creating a downward force W_C

Remembering our use of moments, we choose a pivot point or fulcrum about which to take moments. We choose as the fulcrum the point where the jib is fixed to the tower. (Although it is important from an engineering point of view to include the tie cables to take much of the strain on the jib, we will ignore these in the calculation of moments. We can assume that they are arranged symmetrically, so that the tensions in each are equal.) From the principle of moments, we obtain:

$$W_C \times d_C = (W_J \times d_J) + (W_L \times d_L)$$
$$\text{concrete block} \qquad \text{jib} \qquad \text{load}$$

For the tower crane to remain in equilibrium and not topple, the turning moment of the block on the left of the equation must balance the sum of the turning moments of the jib and the load on the right.

Watch a tower crane in operation and you will notice that the load is moved into the required position not only by turning the crane but also by moving the load either towards or away from the fulcrum. This moves the load away from the equilibrium position we have calculated.

Now we see the need for the tie cables. As the load moves away from the equilibrium position, the tie cables take up unequal tensions so that the turning moments remain balanced. The forces in the tie cables must be balanced by forces exerted by the crane tower. The concrete block counterbalance can sometimes be moved after erection, but it cannot be precisely positioned to balance the load. In addition, there will be some distortion (extension and bending) of the crane parts to 'take up' the forces. A full calculation is complicated. In practice, a tower crane is tested for stability with appropriate loads before being put to use.

Suspension bridge

An engineer designing a suspension bridge, like the one in Fig 5.9, takes account of forces acting at points within the structure and the turning moments of the forces. The engineer considers the **forces of tension** within the steel wires supporting the roadway, and the **forces of compression** within the reinforced concrete towers, and then chooses materials that will withstand the huge forces exerted on the bridge.

Steel can withstand large tension forces, whereas concrete is suitable only for compression forces. An engineer would not suspend a bridge with concrete rods, though inserting prestressed steel into concrete does enable the resulting composite material to withstand forces of tension as well as compression. It is clear, then, that to choose the best materials for a particular application, we have to find out more about the properties of the materials.

Toppling

If a body such as a tower is vertical, the gravitational force on it acts through the centre of gravity and through the centre of its ground area. Should the tower tilt, it will remain upright, assuming that the walls remain intact, until the centre of gravity ceases to lie over the contact area of the tower with the ground. Beyond this point the tower will topple (Fig 5.10). There is now a moment of the gravitational force, operating about the contact edge of the tower as pivot point, which will cause the tower to tilt further, i.e. topple. It was because of the danger of toppling that the Leaning Tower of Pisa was brought nearer to the vertical position by civil engineers.

? QUESTION 3

3 A tower crane is used to lift a load of 1500 kg. The concrete counterbalance, a distance d_C of 12 m from the crane's fulcrum, is of mass 2000 kg. The jib of the crane creates a downward force W_J of 4000 N at a distance d_J of 3 m from the fulcrum. At what distance from the fulcrum must the load be lifted for the tower crane to be in equilibrium?

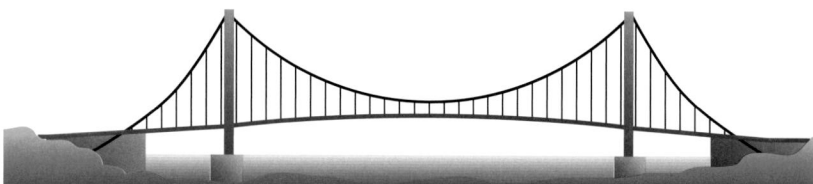

Fig 5.9 Structure of a suspension bridge

? QUESTION 4

4 Write a (non-mathematical) description of the forces acting on different parts of the bridge in Fig 5.9. Identify the parts under tension and under compression. Consider how static equilibrium is achieved. For equilibrium, forces acting at a point must balance. Turning moments about any point on the bridge must also balance. (Consider only the forces acting in the plane of the paper.)

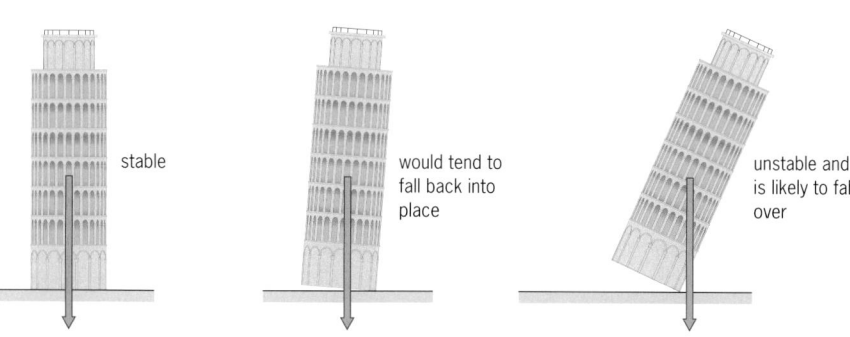

stable

would tend to fall back into place

unstable and is likely to fall over

Fig 5.10 As the tilt on a tower increases it is in danger of toppling over

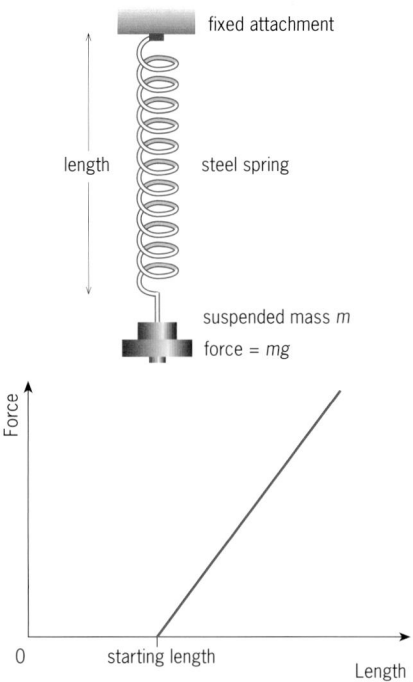

fixed attachment

length

steel spring

suspended mass m
force = mg

Fig 5.11 Force–length graph for a steel spring obeying Hooke's law

Springs are made from materials other than steel. Each material usually has a straight-line region of the graph, but its slope will be different for different materials. For example, springs made from some materials need much larger forces to produce the equivalent extension, so the gradient of the graph for these materials will be steep

? QUESTION 5

5 **a)** Suppose you obtain graphs of force against length for a number of different springs made from the same metal. The springs may have different cross-sectional areas and different starting lengths. Would you expect the gradients and intercepts to be equal for all the springs? Explain your answer.

b) Read the caption to Fig 5.11, sketch the diagram and then add a line for a spring (of the same starting length) made of a material that needs smaller forces than the steel spring to produce the equivalent extension.

2 HOOKE'S LAW AND SPRINGS

Nearly all the components of a bridge that we looked at in the last section are of rigid substances – in other words, solids. They retain their shape when forces are applied to them. To understand why a solid retains its shape, we look at the interactions of its individual atoms or molecules. A stretching force, or tension, applied to the solid tends to pull the atoms or molecules apart. Usually, the stretching is very small because of the huge forces holding atoms close together. In the same way, compressing a solid pushes the atoms closer together, but then they start to repel each other with great force.

So when we apply a force to such a solid material, we find that it distorts in some way. If the force is one of tension, the material extends. This extension is proportional to the applied force. The proportionality was first found by Robert Hooke (1635–1703) for materials shaped in the form of a spring. It was because such springs had been developed that Hooke was able to discover the law. The same effect is found when the materials are shaped as wires or rods, although the extension is much smaller.

Let's start by considering springs. When a force is applied to a spring, the coils move apart and the spring is extended. Hooke stated his law for a spring as follows:

Extension is proportional to the applied force that causes it.

Fig 5.11 shows the relationship between force and length for a typical steel spring. To apply a force to the spring, you fix the spring at one end and suspend a sequence of masses from the other. Then take measurements of the length of the spring as you change the masses, altering the applied force. Usually, we plot the quantity that we are varying along the x axis and what we measure up the y axis. But not here. In this case, the quantity we vary, the force, is plotted on the y axis, and the length we measure is on the x axis, as in Fig. 5.11.

The important result is that the graph is a straight line, *provided we keep the applied force reasonably small*. The straight line shows that the spring extends by equal amounts for equal masses added. If the applied force is too great, the spring will not return to its original shape when the force is removed. We say that the spring has gone past its **elastic limit** and Hooke's law no longer applies.

We can replot the graph in the form of force against **extension** of the spring, meaning a *change* in its length (also called **deformation**, which means change of shape). The new graph is shown in Fig 5.12. For the linear region of the graph, we have:

$$\text{gradient} = \frac{\text{force}}{\text{extension}}$$

We can relate force F and extension x by a constant k to give:

$$F = kx$$

where k is the gradient of the linear part of the graph. k is the **spring constant**, or **force constant**. It has the units of force divided by length, that is, N m^{-1}.

Springs can be compressed as well as extended. You can think of compression as a negative force causing a negative distortion, and show the *reduction* of length negatively along the x axis. The whole picture for both extension and compression of a spring is shown in Fig 5.13 and described in the caption. The slope of the Hooke's law region of the graph is the same for extension and compression.

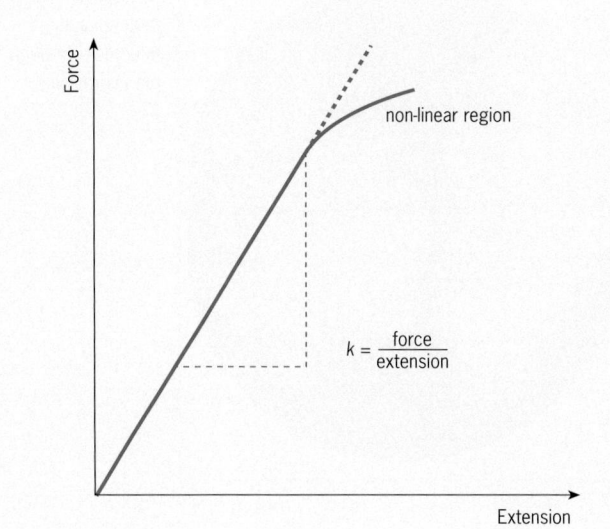

Fig 5.12 Force–extension graph for a spring

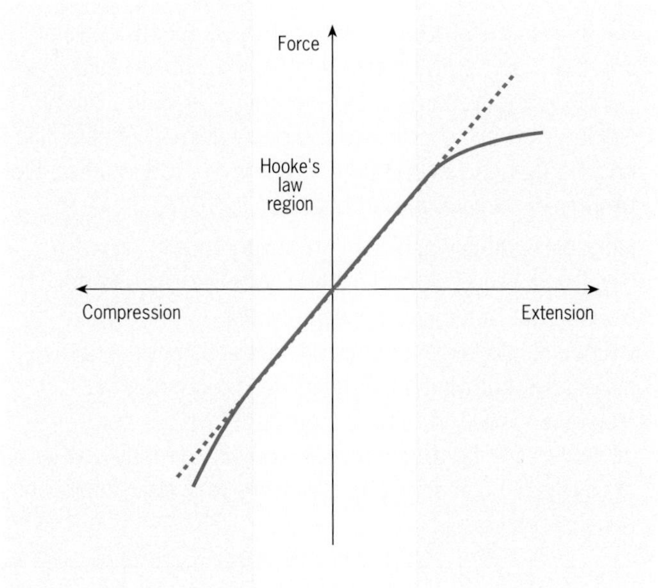

Fig 5.13 Compression and extension of a spring
The Hooke's law region is a continuous straight line, but note that the positive and negative regions are not symmetrical – the extent of the linear region is not the same, nor are the curvatures of the non-linear regions the same

HOW SCIENCE WORKS

'Non-linear' springs

Springs are usually designed to be as elastic as possible – that is, we want the relation between force and extension to be linear over as wide a range of extension and compression as possible. But some springs are designed to become harder and harder to compress by increasing forces. Such a spring can be used to stabilise vibrating machinery. In these springs, instead of compression being proportional to load (applied force) as for spring A in Fig 5.14, compression gets less with an increase in load, as shown by spring B.

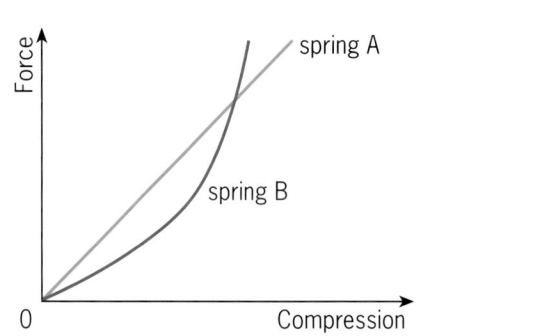

Fig 5.14 Spring A obeys Hooke's law. Spring B is non-linear – it gets harder to compress as the force increases

Coil spring

The coil spring is shown in Fig 5.15. Coil springs consist of wire wound in a helix. When a coil spring is stretched, the spring extends as each coil twists.

Hooke's law applies to the linear deformation (the change of shape in one dimension) of a spring. But it also applies, as we shall see later, to linear deformation of objects that are rods or other shapes. In addition, the law applies to other types of deformation such as twisting – **torsional deformation** – as long as the applied load is small.

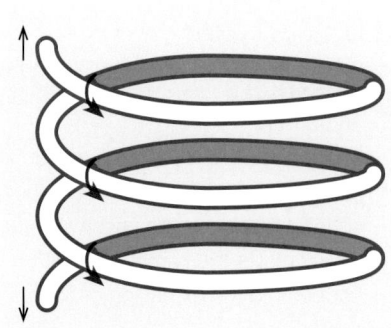

Fig 5.15 Stretching a coil spring

Robert Hooke (1635–1703)

Robert Hooke was the son of a clergyman. He went to Oxford as a chorister but soon turned to science and became the assistant to Robert Boyle, constructing an improved air pump for him. In 1660 he moved to London, and became a founder member of the Royal Society (set up to promote the development of scientific knowledge) and became its 'curator of experiments'. He proposed the law named after him in 1678.

Not only was he ingenious in his experiments, he was clever at thinking up and making scientific instruments (he devised the first spring-controlled balance wheel for a watch). Hooke's work on gravity helped Newton to arrive at his law of gravitation, and Hooke is recognised in biology for work with the microscope. In 1665, he published *Micrographia*, a book containing many beautiful drawings of microscopic observations and also details of his work on optics.

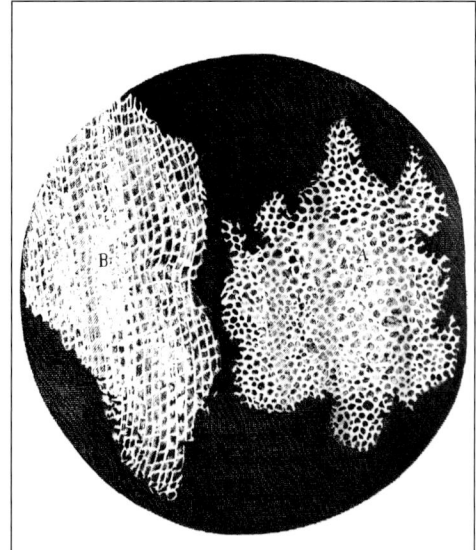

Fig 5.16 Robert Hooke's drawing in *Micrographia* of cork cells as he saw them through his microscope

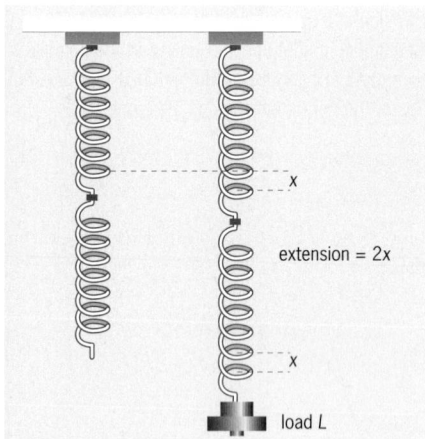

Fig 5.17 Springs in series

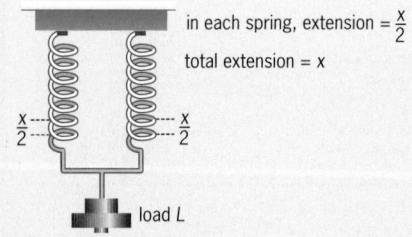

Fig 5.18 Springs in parallel

? QUESTION 6

6   A load is suspended from several identical springs in series. If another spring is added in the series and the load remains the same, what happens to the extension of each spring?

SPRINGS IN SERIES AND PARALLEL

Springs can be combined to carry a single load. The effective force constant k of the system of springs will depend on how these springs are arranged. In Fig 5.17, there are two identical springs attached end to end (in series):

● Each spring has its own force constant k, so force F equals kx.
● If a load L is suspended from the lower spring, a force F acts on both springs.
● Using $x = F/k$, we get an extension x in each spring.
● The total extension is $2x$.

So the force constant k_s of the system of **springs in series** is:

$$k_s = \frac{\text{force}}{\text{total extension}} = \frac{F}{2x} = \frac{kx}{2x} = \frac{k}{2}$$

Fig 5.18 shows the same two springs supporting the same load, but now the springs are in parallel:

● The force F exerted by the load L is shared between the springs so that each has a force of tension $F/2$.
● Extension for each spring is given by the force of tension divided by its spring constant, that is, $F/2$ divided by k. Hence the extension is $F/2k$.
● This extension $F/2k$ is the extension for the parallel system of two springs.

As we might expect, the extension is found to be half of the extension if the load was suspended from just one of the springs. The force constant k_p of the system of **springs in parallel** is:

$$k_p = \frac{\text{force}}{\text{extension}}$$

If we insert $F/2k$ for the extension that results from applying a force F, we get:

$$k_p = \frac{F}{F/2k} = 2k$$

MEASURING WITH SPRINGS

Springs are used in many force-measuring instruments such as spring balances and newton meters. An object's weight is proportional to its mass, so the scale on a spring balance can be graduated in mass units. Newton meters are graduated in force units. Only the sizes of the graduations and the labelling of the scales differ in the two instruments, even though they are designed to measure different quantities. Both instruments are calibrated using standard forces – usually the gravitational force exerted on standard masses.

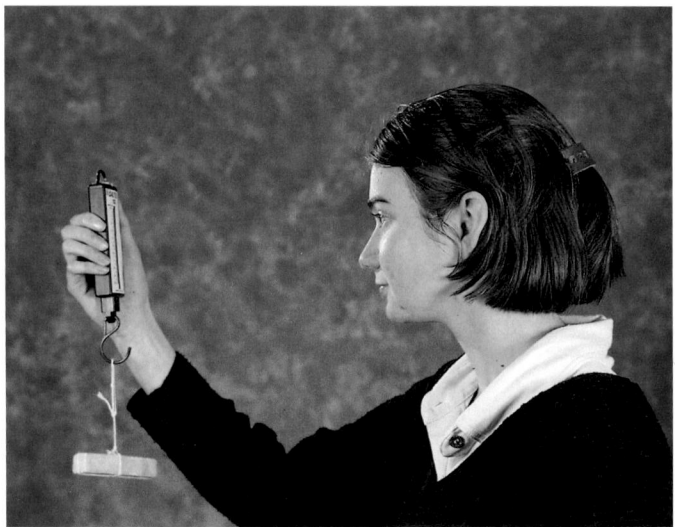 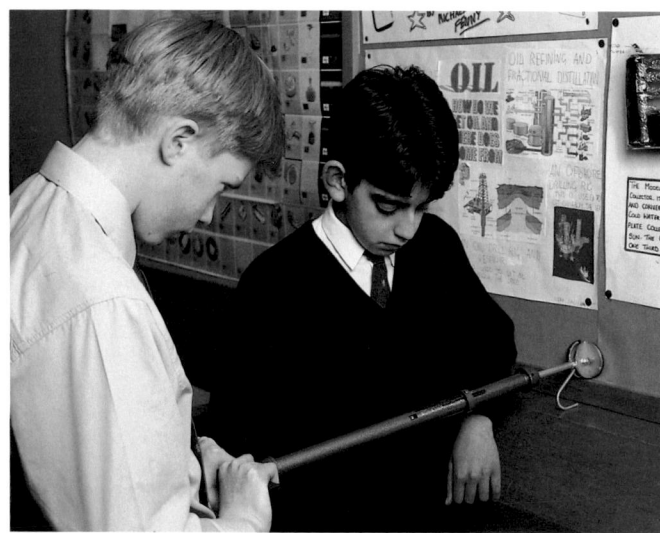

Fig 5.19 A spring balance (left) and a newton meter (right) in use

3 FORCES THAT DEFORM

As we have seen already, materials do not have to be made into springs to be deformed by forces. Most objects distort slightly when a force is applied to them. The applied forces may act in different directions and on objects of any shape. Hooke's law applies within certain limits to most everyday materials such as rubber, glass, wood and metals. But for some materials such as clay and plasticine the law does not apply at all because forces easily change their shape.

Fig 5.20 shows common effects of forces acting on a body. These effects are:

- **Tension** – forces act outwards in opposite directions and tend to lengthen the body.
- **Compression** – forces act inwards in opposite directions and tend to shorten the body.
- **Shear** – forces act in opposite directions along parallel faces, producing a tendency for parallel sections of the body to slide.
- **Torsion** – a type of shearing which twists the body lengthwise.

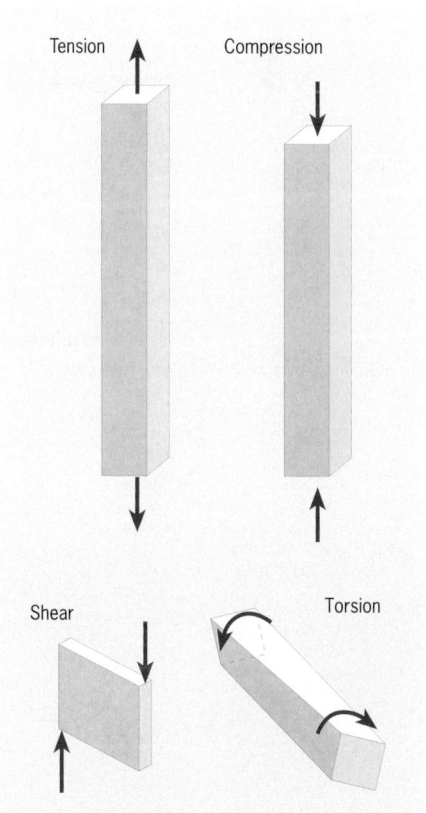

Fig 5.20 Forces acting on bodies to produce tension, compression, shear and torsion

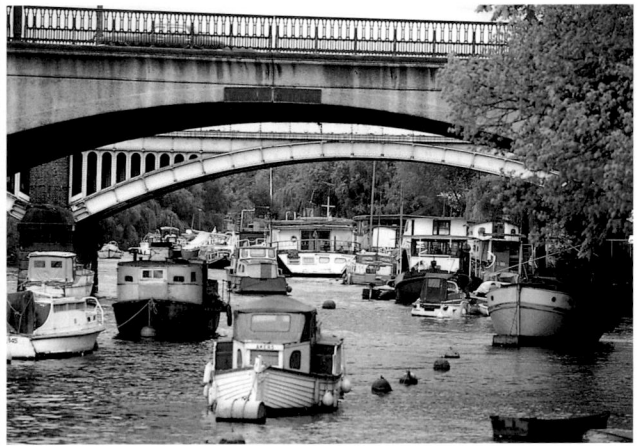

Fig 5.21 A concrete road bridge and an iron rail bridge over the Thames. Engineers take all the forces and their effects into account when designing and choosing materials for bridges

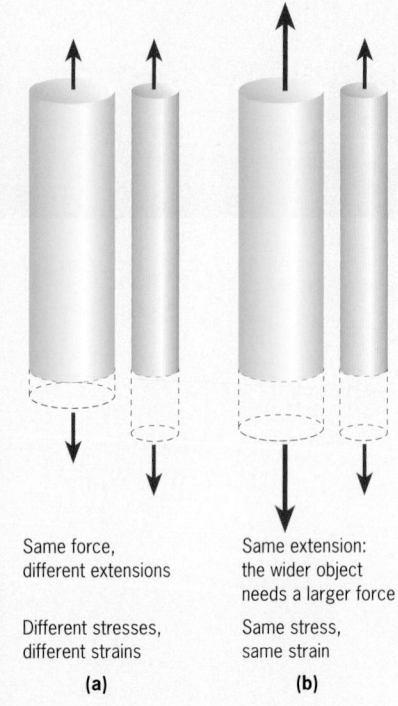

Same force, different extensions

Different stresses, different strains

(a)

Same extension: the wider object needs a larger force

Same stress, same strain

(b)

Fig 5.22 Strain: the area of cross-section affects the relationship between force and extension

In a loaded structure, there may be several effects at the same time. The response of an object to a particular force depends on its size, its shape and the material it is made from. A strong pillar may be either a thin column of a strong material or a thicker column of a weaker material. Differences in the properties of stone and iron account for the differences in design between the two bridges shown in Fig 5.21, for example.

It is not just the stiffness of the stone and iron that affects how they react to forces. Another important factor is the density of the material. Bridges have to support not only the traffic passing across them but also their own weight, and this may be many times greater than the weight of the traffic.

STRESS AND STRAIN

Which is stronger – a bridge girder or a cup? They cannot be compared directly since they are made of different materials and also have very different sizes and shapes. Before we look at the properties of objects, we should compare the properties of the materials they are made of. To do this we use measurements called **stress** and **strain**.

Stress is a relationship between the applied force and the area over which it acts:

$$\text{stress} = \text{applied force per unit area} = \frac{\text{force}}{\text{area}} = \frac{F}{A}$$

The units of stress are $N\ m^{-2}$. Notice that these are the same units as those for pressure.

In each example shown in Fig 5.22, a force is applied over a surface area. So in each case a stress is applied to the body. The shape of the body changes as a result of applying the stress. To measure this change, we compare the size or shape of the body after the forces are applied with the size or shape before. **Strain** is the measurement which does this. Precisely how we define strain depends on the type of deformation we produce in the body.

The simplest case is of forces of tension applied to opposite ends of a wire or rod. The forces produce an extension and the strain is given by:

$$\text{strain} = \frac{\text{change in length (extension)}}{\text{original length}}$$

As this is a ratio (of two lengths), strain has no units – we say it is *dimensionless*. We can express strain as a percentage change in length by multiplying the strain ratio by 100.

SCIENCE IN CONTEXT

EXAMPLE

Q The ropes of a child's swing are 3 m long. They extend by 30 mm when a child sits on the swing. What is the strain in the ropes?

A

$$\text{strain} = \frac{\text{extension}}{\text{original length}} = \frac{x}{L}$$

$$= \frac{30 \times 10^{-3}}{3} = 0.01$$

The same rules of stress and strain apply when a body has forces of compression applied to it.

Now we can see what happens if we apply the same force to two wires of different cross-sections, as in Fig 5.22(a). Although the two forces are the same, there is a smaller *stress* applied to the wire of larger cross-section, so it extends by a smaller amount. To extend this thicker wire by the same amount as the thinner wire, we must apply a larger force, as Fig 5.22(b) shows: for equal extensions, the forces need to be in the same ratio as the cross-sectional areas, and then the stress is the same for each wire.

We see from this why engineers working with structural materials find the ideas of stress and strain more useful in comparing the effects of a force on different-sized pieces of a material than merely looking at extensions using different forces.

Strain may occur through shearing or twisting an object as well as extension or compression. These different measures of strain are shown in Fig 5.23.

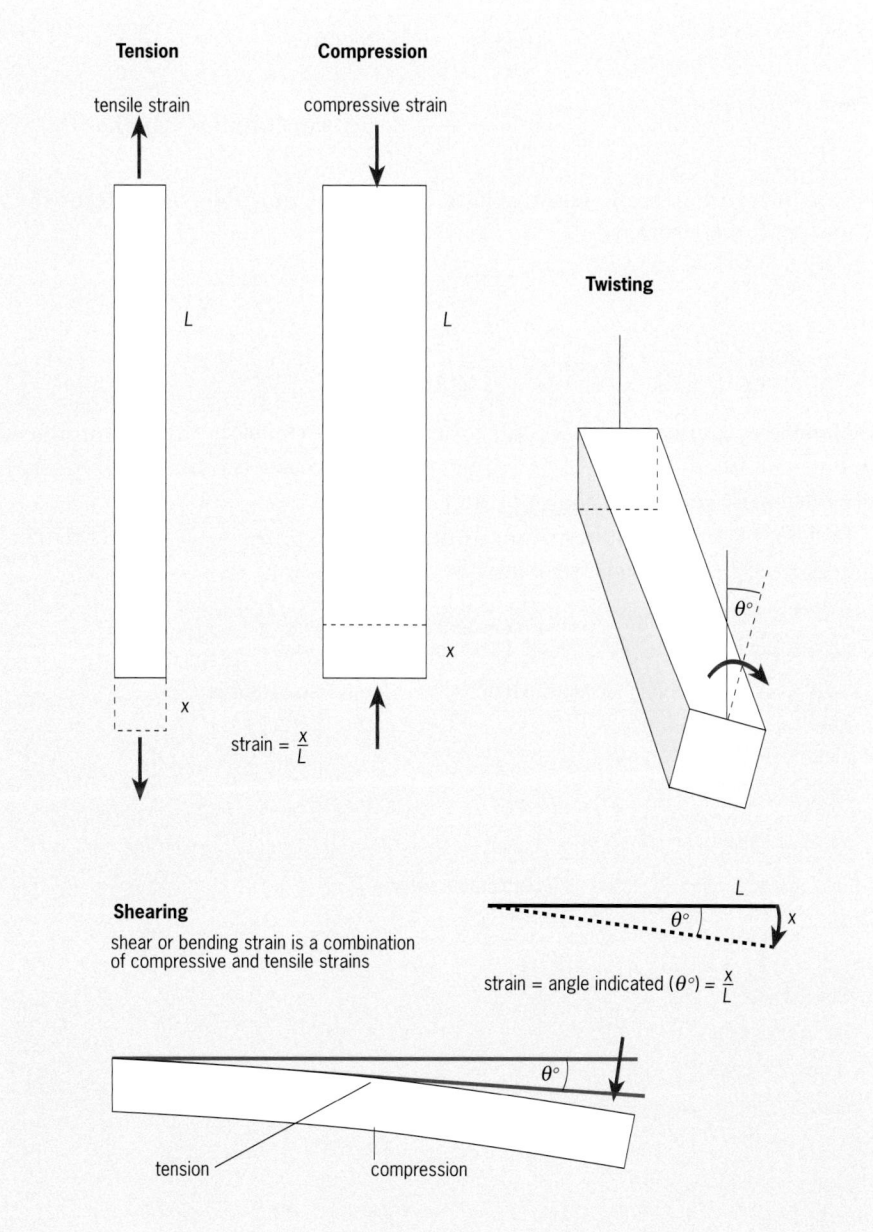

Fig 5.23 Different kinds of strain – all are dimensionless ratios

Tension

tensile strain

L

x

Compression

compressive strain

L

x

$strain = \frac{x}{L}$

Twisting

$\theta°$

L

$\theta°$

x

$strain = angle\ indicated\ (\theta°) = \frac{x}{L}$

Shearing

shear or bending strain is a combination of compressive and tensile strains

$\theta°$

tension   compression

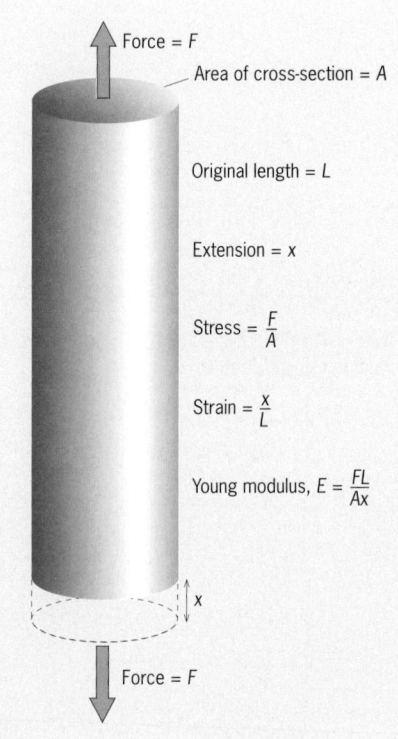

Fig 5.24 Quantities needed to measure the Young modulus

THE YOUNG MODULUS

We have seen that for springs subjected to small forces the ratio of force to extension is a constant:

$$F/x = k$$

Similarly, we can say for many materials:

The ratio of stress to strain is a constant.

This is the same as saying that many solid materials as well as springs obey Hooke's law. So, for materials that obey the law, engineers can predict the effect of applying tensile forces, whatever the size or shape of the object made from the material. Tensile forces are longitudinal forces which tend to stretch the material and pull it apart. The ratio is called the **Young modulus** of the material:

$$\text{Young modulus, } E = \frac{\text{tensile stress}}{\text{tensile strain}}$$

Strain has no units, so the Young modulus has the same units as stress, namely N m^{-2}.

We have seen that:

$$\text{stress} = \frac{F}{A} \text{ (force/area)}$$

and:

$$\text{strain} = \frac{x}{L} \text{ (extension/original length)}$$

as is shown in Fig. 5.24. Putting these expressions into the equation for the Young modulus, we have:

$$E = \frac{F}{A} \div \frac{x}{L}$$

$$= \frac{FL}{Ax} \text{ (in N m}^{-2})$$

Therefore, to measure E, we must measure the extension x that is produced by a tensile force F on an object of length L and cross-sectional area A (see the How Science Works passage opposite).

Table 5.1 gives the values of the Young modulus E for some common materials and their tensile strengths.

Table 5.1 Elasticity and strength of some materials		
Material	**Young modulus, E/N m^{-2}**	**Tensile strength/N m^{-2}**
Metals		
aluminium	7.0×10^{10}	7×10^7
copper	11×10^{10}	1.4×10^8
high tensile steel	21×10^{10}	1.5×10^9
Building and household materials (approximate values)		
rubber	7×10^6	3×10^7
brick	7×10^9	5×10^6
wood (spruce):		
along the grain	1.3×10^{10}	1×10^8
across the grain	3×10^6	
concrete	1.7×10^{10}	4×10^8
bone	2.1×10^{10}	1.4×10^8
glass (e.g. window)	7×10^{10}	$3–7 \times 10^7$
carbon fibre	7.5×10^{11}	2×10^9

? **QUESTION 7**

7   Suggest reasons why wood is stronger in one direction than another.

HOW SCIENCE WORKS

Measuring the Young modulus for a wire

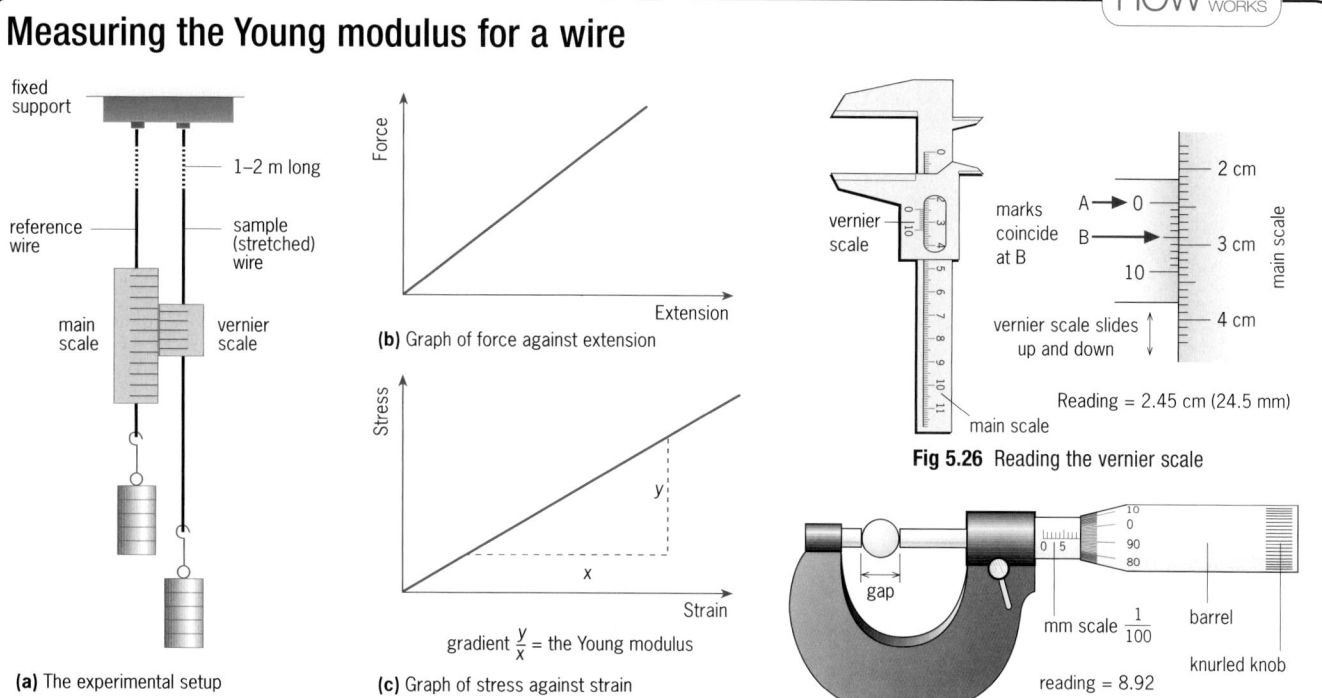

(b) Graph of force against extension

gradient $\frac{y}{x}$ = the Young modulus

(a) The experimental setup

(c) Graph of stress against strain

Reading = 2.45 cm (24.5 mm)

Fig 5.26 Reading the vernier scale

reading = 8.92

Fig 5.25 Experiment to measure the Young modulus

Fig 5.27 Reading the micrometer screw gauge

The standard way to measure the Young modulus for a wire is shown in Fig 5.25(a). The sample wire is suspended from the ceiling and is stretched by adding masses to the lower end.

Because the amount of stretch is small, the extension is usually measured with a vernier scale. A reference wire of the same material as the sample wire holds the main scale of the vernier, usually calibrated in millimetres. The vernier attachment is fixed to the sample wire.

A mass is suspended from each wire to keep them taut. The position of the vernier on the main scale is noted. Then, extra mass added to the sample wire produces an increased downward force on the wire and the vernier scale moves downwards relative to the main scale. The new position of the vernier scale is noted and the extension of the wire calculated. Further masses are added to increase the downward force, and the new values of the extension are noted.

Fig 5.25(b), of force against extension, will be linear as long as the wire remains within its elastic region. Values of strain (extension/original length) can be

calculated by measuring the length of the wire at the start of the experiment.

A micrometer screw gauge measures the diameter of the wire, so its area of cross-section is found. Fig 5.25(c), of stress against strain, can then be drawn. This graph is also linear. Its slope gives a direct value for the Young modulus for the wire.

Because the reference wire is made of the same material as the sample wire, any increase or decrease of the laboratory temperature will produce equal expansion or contraction in both wires.

USING THE VERNIER SCALE

The vernier scale, Fig 5.26, measures small distances. It has *two* scales: the zero position on the *vernier scale* gives the reading from the *main scale* to within 1 mm. The nearest lower-value millimetre reading is taken, so in Fig 5.26 it is 2.4 cm (24 mm).

The vernier scale now increases the precision of the value to ±0.1 mm. The correct value is shown by the mark *on the vernier scale* which lines up best with any mark on the main scale. In the diagram,

the fifth mark (arrowed B) lines up with a mark on the main scale. This gives a correct overall reading of 2.45 cm (24.5 mm). If no one mark quite lines up and the setting lies between two marks, you can make an estimate to ±0.05 mm.

USING THE MICROMETER SCREW GAUGE

This is used to measure thicknesses of materials accurately. The main scale gives a reading to 1 mm as with a vernier scale. The screw inside the gauge moves by 1 mm during one turn, that is, it has a pitch of 1 mm. The barrel of the screw is divided into 100 divisions, and you make a reading to 0.01 mm by noting the division which is in line with the scale line drawn on the main shaft. The reading in Fig 5.27 is 8.92 mm. Care is needed: some screw gauges have a pitch of 0.5 mm with the barrel divided into 50 divisions. In these gauges, the main scale is used first to read to 0.5 mm.

? QUESTION 8

8 A steel wire has a diameter of 0.57 mm and is 1.5 m long. What tension is required to produce an extension of 1.5 mm in the wire?

EXAMPLE

Q A lift is supported by a steel cable of diameter 2.5 cm. The maximum length of the lift cable when the lift is at the ground floor is 36 m. The Young modulus for steel is 2.1×10^{11} N m^{-2}. By how much does the cable stretch when six people of total mass 420 kg enter the lift at the ground floor?

A

First, we use the equations for the Young modulus and for stress:

$$\text{Young modulus} = \frac{\text{stress}}{\text{strain}} \qquad \text{stress} = \frac{\text{force}}{\text{area}}$$

So:

$$\text{strain} = \frac{\text{force}}{\text{area} \times E} = \frac{F}{AE}$$

Since force = mg:

$$\text{strain} = \frac{mg}{AE}$$

where m is the total mass of the six people, and A is the area of cross-section of the cable.

Now use the equation for strain:

$$\text{increase in length} = \text{original length} \times \text{strain}$$
$$= \text{original length} \times \frac{mg}{AE} \quad (A = \pi r^2)$$
$$= \frac{36 \times 420 \times 9.8}{\pi \times (1.25 \times 10^{-2})^2 \times 2.1 \times 10^{11}}$$
$$= 1.4 \times 10^{-3} \text{ m}$$

The cable extends by 1.4 mm.

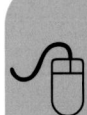

Please see the How Science Works assignment at www.collinseducation.co.uk/CAS for more practice on the Young modulus

Some useful points about the Young modulus

- Materials which are difficult to stretch have large values for the Young modulus. It takes a large stress to produce a small effect (strain).
- The values of E in Table 5.1 apply only if the *internal structure* of the object is not changed in any way (see below).
- The Young modulus for a material is only constant over the limited range of strain when the material is obeying Hooke's law – when extension (or distortion) is proportional to the applied force.

STRESS–STRAIN CURVES

Many materials obey Hooke's law only for small loads. Also, different materials have different stress–strain curves. Steels with a wide range of properties are made by varying the composition, particularly the amount of carbon which is added. Figs 5.28 and 5.29 show the stress–strain curves for two wires of very different steels. They both show a linear region AB where stress is proportional to strain. If the load is removed from either specimen anywhere along AB, the wire will return along the path BA to its original length A.

Beyond B, the force needed to extend either steel wire is no longer proportional to the extension. In this region, each specimen increases in length by a larger amount for the same increase in force compared with the linear region. What is more, if the load is removed at, say, point C, the extension (and therefore the strain) does not return to zero but stays at A′.

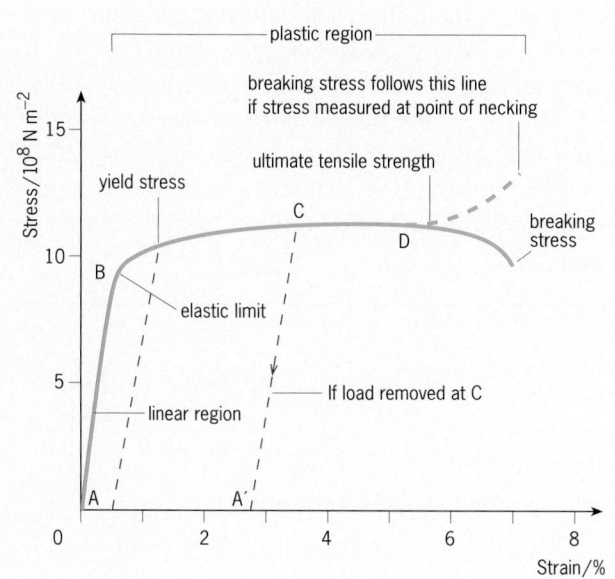

Fig 5.28 Stress–strain curve for steel wire 1

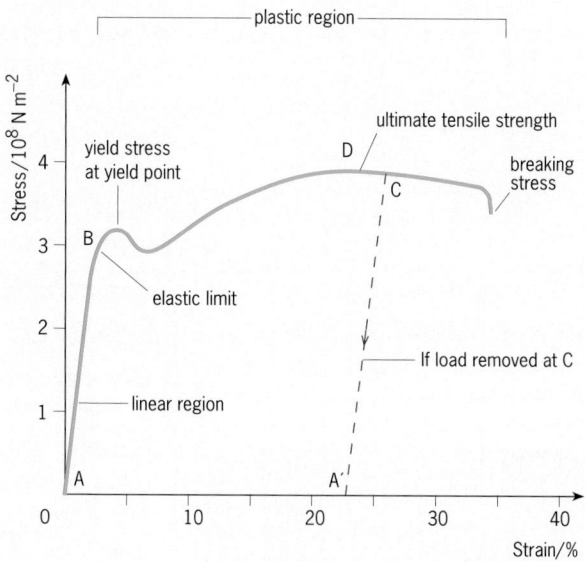

Fig 5.29 Stress–strain curve for steel wire 2

The steel wire has a permanent extension because of its inelasticity. In the curves, we can see what happens as either wire is unloaded. The stress–strain curve follows CA′. This line is parallel to the original elastic line BA. When a material behaves like this and fails to return to its original length when the load is removed, we say that **plastic strain** has occurred.

The yield point

Beyond the elastic limit, the stress–strain curves of Figs 5.28 and 5.29 for the two steel wires show different shapes. Curve 5.29 shows a peak at the point when the stress (the force required to go on extending the sample) falls very rapidly. This is the yield point and the stress at this point is called the yield stress.

Steel wire 1 also yields, but the exact yield point is not clear. In this case, we choose an arbitrary value of plastic strain: 0.5% is commonly used. This means A′ is taken to be at 0.5% along the strain axis. Follow the line parallel to AB upwards from the 0.5% point on Fig 5.28 and you meet the point of the curve marked as the yield stress point.

Tensile strength

For both specimens there is a maximum stress, different for the two samples. This maximum stress is called the **ultimate tensile strength**. The force needed to produce further extension then actually gets less. If we just leave the load on the specimen it will go on extending until it breaks. Knowledge about such possible failure is important for large-scale structures.

The tensile strength of steel is especially important because steel is used so much in construction. But notice in Table 5.1 (page 104) the value for bone – it is a factor of 10 less than steel, yet higher than the value for many materials. The skeletons of humans and other creatures are a balance between lightness and capacity to withstand the stresses of body weight and movement. Notice also that the value for carbon fibre is especially large, which is why it is used in rackets, fishing rods and high-performance bicycles (Fig 5.30).

> **? QUESTION 9**
>
> 9 A single steel wire is used to lift a cradle of mass 50 kg containing
> **a)** a woman
> **b)** an elephant.
> The type of steel used is that in Fig 5.28.
> Assume that, for safety, the stress in the steel wire should not exceed 0.1 × the ultimate tensile strength of the steel. Calculate the minimum diameter of wire required in each case. (Take the mass of the woman as 55 kg and of the elephant as 4000 kg.)

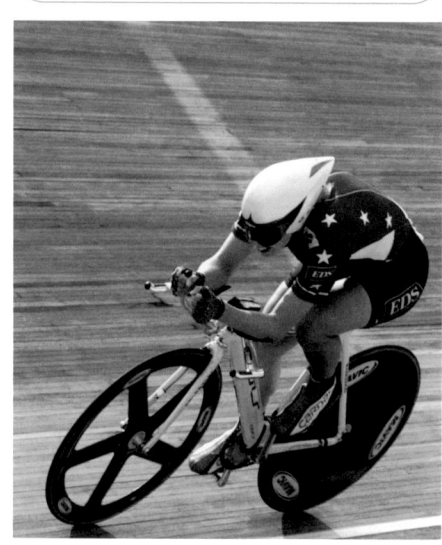

Fig 5.30 Carbon fibre bicycle frames are light but have high tensile strength

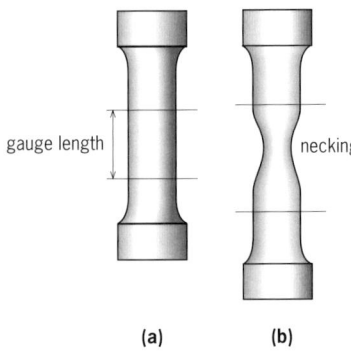

gauge length

necking

(a)   (b)

Fig 5.31 Shape of a specimen for commercial stress–strain measurements **(a)** at the start and **(b)** after necking during testing

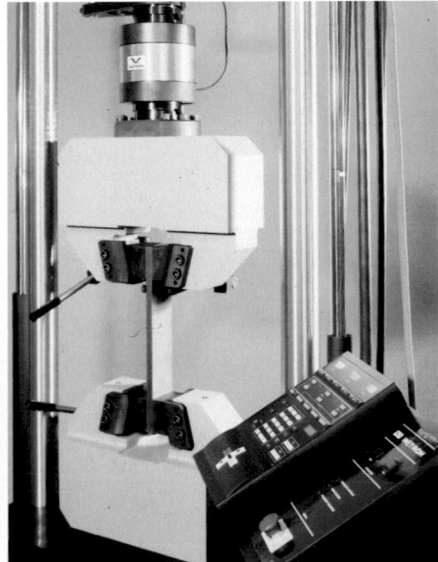

Fig 5.32 A servo-hydraulic machine stress-testing a metal sample

Commercial machines for making standard test measurements stretch samples by applying a variable load. The apparatus instantly detects any increase or decrease of force due to change in length. In this way, the equipment is able to identify the parts of the curve in Fig 5.28 where the required stress is getting less

Testing specimens

Test specimens are a particular shape to fit a standard test machine, as shown in Fig 5.31(a). As the load increases during the test, the shape eventually alters, see Fig 5.31(b), and the specimen undergoes 'necking'. If we calculate the stress at the neck, rather than for the overall sample, the stress–strain curve will go on rising and will follow the dashed line in Fig 5.28. This is because the area in the necked portion has decreased, and hence the stress (force/area) has increased. See Fig 5.32 and its caption for the operation of standard stress-testing equipment.

EXAMPLE

Q A cable is made from 100 strands of high-tensile steel wire, each of diameter 1 mm. The strain on the cable should never exceed one-fifth of the breaking strain. What is the maximum load that should be supported by the cable?

Breaking strain 0.1%.
Young modulus 2.1×10^{11} N m^{-2}.

A Total area of cable
$= 100$ times area of one strand
$= 100 \times \pi \times (0.5 \times 10^{-3})^2$ m^2

$= 7.85 \times 10^{-5}$ m^2

By definition: stress $= E \times$ strain

Breaking strain $= 10^{-3}$ (i.e. 0.1%)

Maximum allowed stress
$= E \times (0.2 \times \text{breaking strain})$
$= 2.1 \times 10^{11} \times 0.2 \times 10^{-3}$ N m^{-2}
$= 4.2 \times 10^7$ N m^{-2}

Maximum load
$= \text{stress} \times \text{area}$
$= 4.2 \times 10^7 \times 7.85 \times 10^{-5}$ N
$= 3.3 \times 10^3$ N

Creep

After a time under stress, a material may permanently retain some or all of its change in shape when the stress is removed. We say that its plastic distortion is time dependent and describe this property as **creep**. When it occurs in the plastic region, the creep is called **viscoplasticity**. Some specimens show creep even within the elastic region and return with time to their original undeformed state. This type of creep is called **viscoelasticity**.

Fig 5.33 shows stress–strain graphs for steel, copper and rubber. Although these are not to scale, they do compare relative strain. Copper can be extended more easily than steel and has passed through its plastic stage. The plastic region of steel has not been reached in the graph. Rubber stretches very easily at first, but then becomes harder to stretch. On unloading, it returns to its original length. There is no permanent strain, so rubber is also behaving elastically. Some materials do not show plastic behaviour – these are said to be brittle. Two brittle materials are glass and concrete.

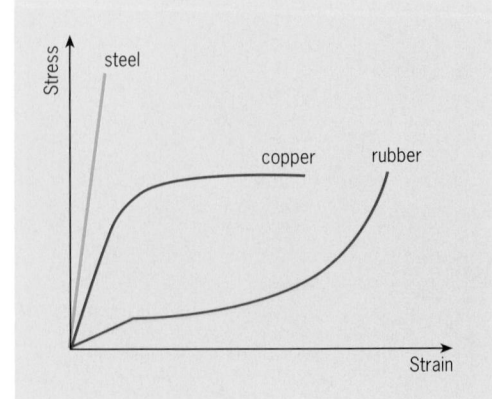

Fig 5.33 Stress–strain graphs for steel, copper and rubber (not to scale)

4 ENERGY STORED IN A STRETCHED ELASTIC MATERIAL

When an object is deformed by a force, work is done by the force. As a result, energy is transferred to the material. As long as deformation continues, we say that the energy is 'stored' in it. In the simple case of stretching a spring:

work done = force × distance moved in the direction of the force

(see page 44). That is:

W = Fd

The distance moved by the force is equal to the extension of the spring, and the force required to stretch the spring is proportional to the extension. This was shown in Fig 5.12 and is shown again in Fig 5.34. We see that there is a total extension X for a maximum force F_m. As the relationship is linear, we can take the average force applied to the spring to be $F_m/2$. The work done is the average force multiplied by the distance, since the force and the extension are in the same direction (parallel to each other):

work done = $\frac{1}{2} F_m X$

This is the energy stored in the stretched spring. It is represented by the area under the graph.

Another way of calculating the energy stored is to consider a small extension Δx of the spring – see Fig 5.34 again. By taking a very small extension, the force changes very little: we can take its average value as F. The work done in stretching the spring by this small distance Δx is $F\Delta x$. The work done is represented by the area of the dark strip. This strip is approximately a rectangle of area $F\Delta x$.

To find the work done in extending the spring, we can divide the whole of the area under the straight line graph into strips from the origin where $F = 0$ to the point on the line where $F = F_m$. The total area of these strips must equal the triangular area under the graph (area of triangle OAX). This area gives us the total work done in stretching the spring, where X is the total extension at F_m.

work done = $\frac{1}{2} F_m X$

Its value is the same as that calculated above for the work done. The work stored in the spring is sometimes called **elastic potential energy**.

Now, $F_m = kX$ where k is the force constant of the spring. By substituting this expression for F_m in the formula above, and for any given extension x (not just maximum X corresponding to force F_m), we can express the energy stored in a stretched spring in general as:

energy stored in a stretched spring = $\frac{1}{2} kx^2$

Springs may of course be compressed, and x can also refer to compression.

Similar arguments apply to solid objects that are stretched or compressed. The formulae for stretching or compressing a rod or wire are:

energy stored = $\frac{1}{2} \dfrac{EAx^2}{L}$

and:

energy stored per unit volume = $\frac{1}{2}$ stress × strain

E is the Young modulus and A and L are the area and length of the rod which has an extension or compression x.

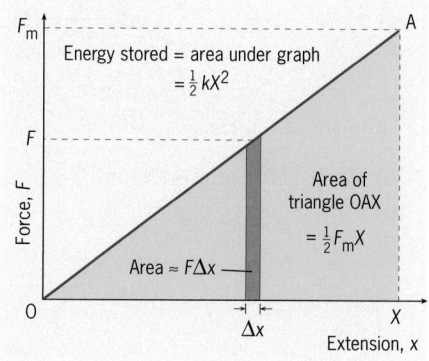

Fig 5.34 Calculating the energy stored in a stretched spring

STRETCH
AND CHALLENGE

Elastic potential energy

This section leads you through the proof that the energy stored in unit volume of a stretched material is:

$\frac{1}{2}$ stress × strain

a) Show that the energy stored in a stretched wire of length, L, area of cross-section A and Young modulus E is given by the formula:

$$\frac{1}{2} \frac{EAx^2}{L}$$

where x is the extension produced by the stretching force.

b) Which part of the formula may be replaced by strain? Complete the formula:

energy stored = $\frac{1}{2}$ strain × ?

c) Now eliminate E from the formula by putting E = stress/strain.

d) Now reinsert strain by using the definition: strain = x/L.

e) Explain how the formula obtained in part **d)** is equivalent to the statement that the energy stored in a stretched object per unit volume is $\frac{1}{2}$ stress × strain.

EXAMPLE

Q Concrete pillars are used to support the upper floor of a building. Each pillar is 200 mm in diameter and is 2.5 m tall. When the upper floor is loaded, each pillar supports a load of 8×10^4 N.

a) What is the compression of each pillar due to this load?
b) How much energy is stored in each pillar as a result of the compression?

E for high-strength concrete $= 4 \times 10^{10}$ N m^{-2}.

A
a) Strain $= x/L = $ stress$/E$

$$\text{compression } x = \frac{\text{stress} \times L}{E} = \frac{(\text{load/area}) \times L}{E}$$

$$= \frac{8.0 \times 10^4 \times 2.5}{4 \times 10^{10} \times \pi \times (0.1)^2} \text{ m}$$

$$= 1.6 \times 10^{-4} \text{ m}$$

b) Energy stored $=$ average force $\times$ compression

$$= \tfrac{1}{2} (8 \times 10^4) \times (1.6 \times 10^{-4}) \text{ J} = 6.4 \text{ J}$$

This is easier here than using:

$$\text{energy stored} = \tfrac{1}{2} EAx^2/L$$

$$= \tfrac{1}{2} \frac{4 \times 10^{10} \times \pi \times (0.1)^2 \times (1.6 \times 10^{-4})^2}{2.5} \text{ J} = 6.4 \text{ J}$$

? QUESTION 10

10 Study the graph of Fig 5.35. In terms of this graph, describe the path traced out by spot X in Fig 5.36 as the car tyre makes half a revolution.

BEHAVIOUR OF RUBBER

What are the energy implications when materials are deformed? We will consider rubber, which deforms easily. When it is stretched and compressed repeatedly and rapidly, as happens in vehicle tyres, it demonstrates what is known as **hysteresis**, when the strain, which is the effect, lags behind the stress, which is the cause. A graph of stress against strain for rubber in a car tyre is shown in Fig 5.35. The idea of finding the energy stored from the area under a graph can then be extended to the energy generated in an enclosed loop. Read the caption carefully.

The curve shows clearly that the strain in the rubber lags behind the change in the stress in the process of hysteresis. The shaded area inside the stress–strain curves represents work done on the rubber. This work generates heat within the rubber.

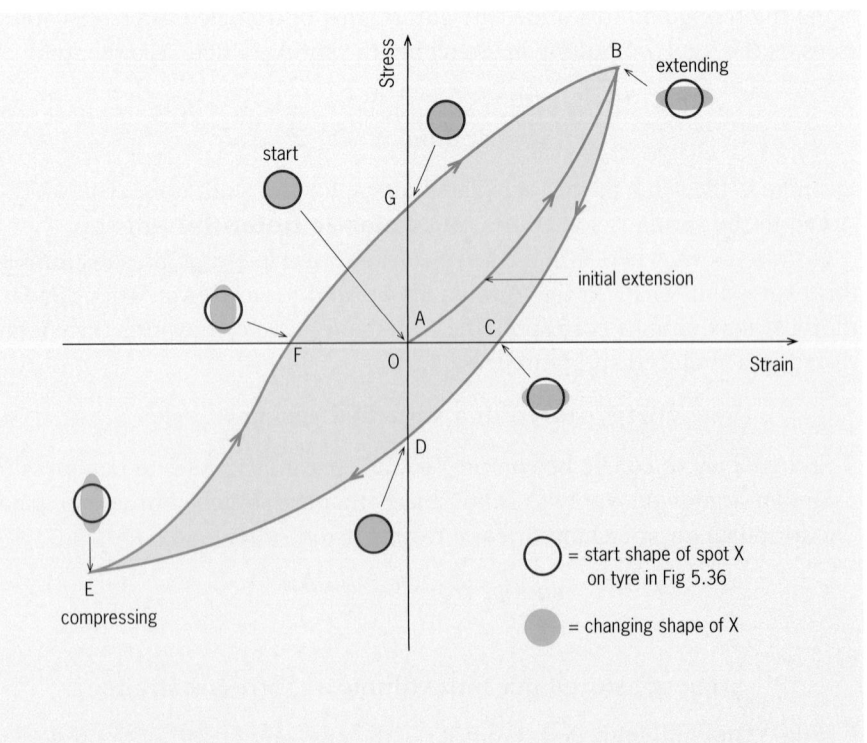

Fig 5.35 Hysteresis in a rubber car tyre

After the initial stretching along AB, stretching ceases and the rubber contracts along curve BCD. When the stress has been reduced to zero, the rubber has contracted to C, with a strain remaining that corresponds to an extension.

The rubber returns to its original size only when it experiences a compressive stress OD.

Further compression takes the stress–strain relationship to E. Compression gradually reduces, and increasing extension then takes the rubber though EFGB, and so on.

If the repetitive cycling ceases, the rubber object quickly returns to its original form

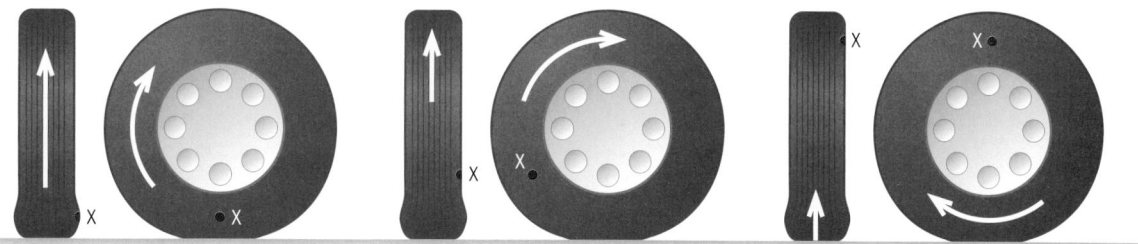

Fig 5.36 Deformation of point X on the side of a car tyre during half a revolution. Notice the change in the shape of that part of the tyre

5 MICROSTRUCTURES AND THE PROPERTIES AND BEHAVIOUR OF MATERIALS

Think of common objects around the house. In the kitchen, for example, we use copper saucepans and glass bowls. Their properties are very different, as shown if you drop them on the floor!

Everyday materials may be either simple pure chemicals or complex mixtures of chemicals. Copper is a single metallic element. Glass is several chemicals, the main one being the compound silica. *Natural* materials such as wood, leather and stone are more complex. *Artificial* materials or modified natural materials are often complex, such as brick, rubber, metal alloys, fabric mixtures such as polyester/cotton, and cardboard. *Composites* are very useful materials, combining the properties of two or more materials. Everyday examples are reinforced concrete, glass-reinforced plastic (GRP), carbon fibre and plywood.

What affects the way a given material behaves? To answer this, we have to consider many factors, including:

- the forces between atoms – chemical bonds,
- the arrangement of the atoms – whether they are in the form of molecules or form a complex extended structure,
- the nature of the molecules (if the material is molecular) – whether they are long and interlinked as in rubber and plastics, or small and weakly bonded to each other such as between atomic layers within graphite,
- its microstructure (its structure on a very small scale) – whether it is uniform or not on a small scale and whether it contains cracks and imperfections,
- its macrostructure (large-scale structure) – whether it is single-crystal, polycrystalline, fibrous, composite.

When we talk about the microscopic structure of a material we mean the structure that we can identify using an optical microscope or an electron microscope (Fig 5.37). Macroscopic structure, on the other hand, we can see with the naked eye or with a hand lens.

The forces that hold solid materials together are electrical forces. They are due to the charges on the fundamental particles of matter which make up atoms, namely **electrons** and **protons**. In a pure chemical, the atoms are either all the same – the chemical is an *element* – or different types of atoms are combined to form the molecules of one kind of *compound*.

The different types of atoms in a material, and the way these atoms link together, determine mechanical properties such as density, elasticity and strength. As a general rule, the forces (called bonds) that hold the atoms together within the molecule of a compound are stronger than the forces that hold the molecules together to form the solid material. You will learn more about the bonding of atoms in Chapter 7.

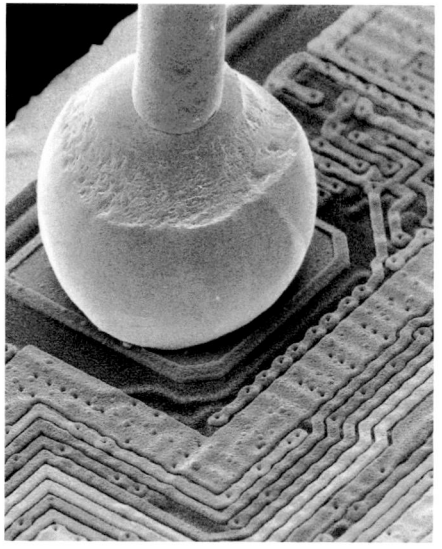

Fig 5.37 Scanning electron micrograph of a silicon chip connector in contact with microcircuitry (false colour)

STRUCTURES AND PROPERTIES OF METALS

Each atom in a metal has one or more outer electrons which can move freely between atoms. We can picture these electrons forming a 'sea' of negative charges that move amongst an ordered arrangement – a lattice – of positive metal ion spheres. It is because these electrons are so mobile that metals are good conductors of electricity.

The force of attraction between the ions and the free electrons gives rise to a 'metallic' bond. The most stable arrangement for the atoms is to occupy the minimum volume, forming a regular array of close-packed, hexagonally arranged layers. This arrangement gives a metal its regular crystalline structure.

There is no *directional* bonding between the ion 'spheres' to restrict the positions of neighbouring atoms. So, though the bonds (forces of attraction) between metal ions are strong, they can still be easily made to move to new positions. In general, then, metals are not only strong but also flexible. They can be hammered and flattened – they are **malleable** (from the Latin *malleus*, a hammer) – and can be drawn out into wires – they are **ductile**.

Usually, when a liquid metal solidifies, regions of crystal structure start to grow ('nucleate') in lots of different places. This means that many small crystals or grains (also called crystallites) form to make up the solid metal. These grains pack together with irregular **grain boundaries** in different

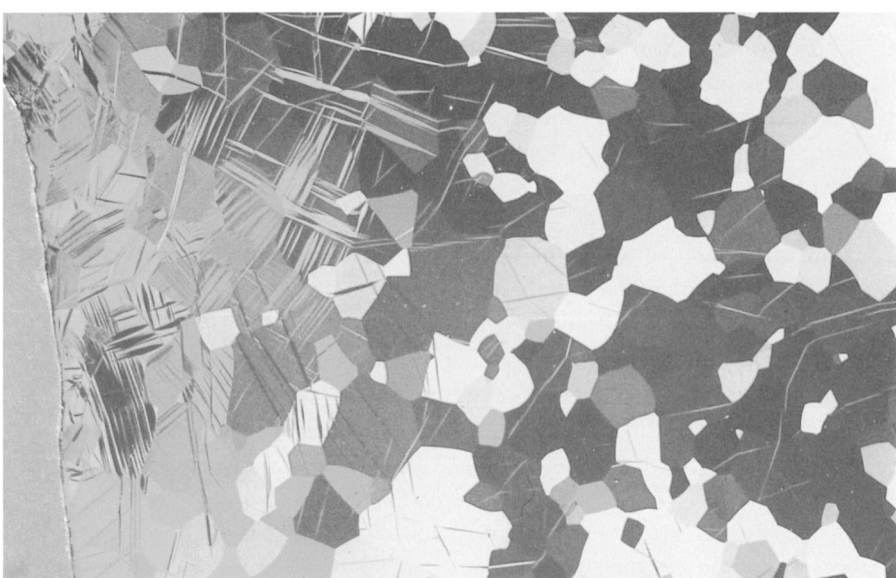

Fig 5.38 Polycrystalline titanium alloy, showing grains (crystallites) and grain boundaries. Taken with polarized light, the micrograph records different orientations of atoms

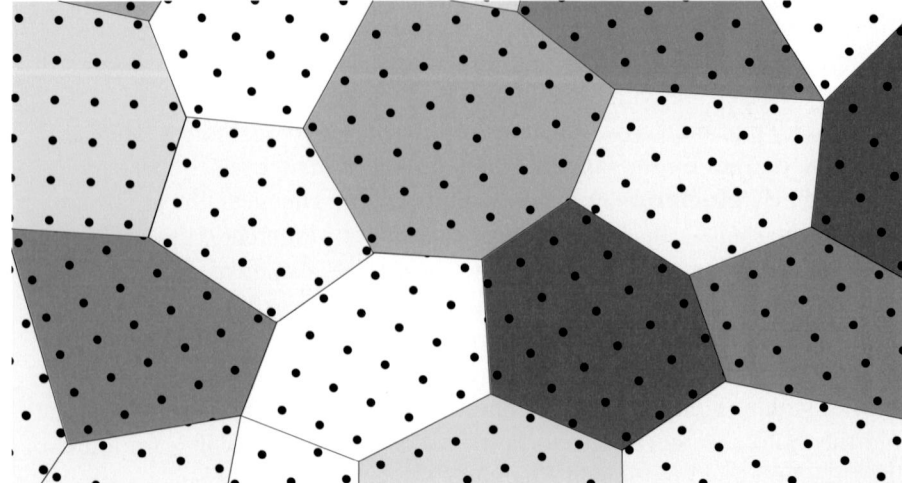

Fig 5.39 A polycrystalline metal, showing that there is the same regular lattice of atoms within the boundary of each grain, but that the lattice is differently orientated in neighbouring grains

directions. The material is said to be **polycrystalline** (Figs 5.38 and 5.39). The sizes of the grains and the presence of their boundaries affect the mechanical properties of the metal, as we shall see later.

What happens when a metal is stretched?

When a load is applied to a metal, the atoms (strictly, metal ions) move very slightly apart. Imagine the bonds between the atoms as a network of springs. The extension of the springs – the distance the atoms move apart – is proportional to the load. When the load is removed, the atoms move back to their original positions. The metal obeys Hooke's law.

Just as with a spring, once the metal is stretched to the point where the ions are separated beyond the linear region of a force–extension curve, plastic behaviour takes over. The atoms must rearrange in some way. In fact, planes of atoms move across each other (Fig 5.40) – we say they slip. The force must be large enough to break the bonds that link all the atoms in one plane to the atoms in the adjacent plane. The planes along which slip occurs most easily are called **slip planes** and the directions along which slip is easiest are called **slip directions**.

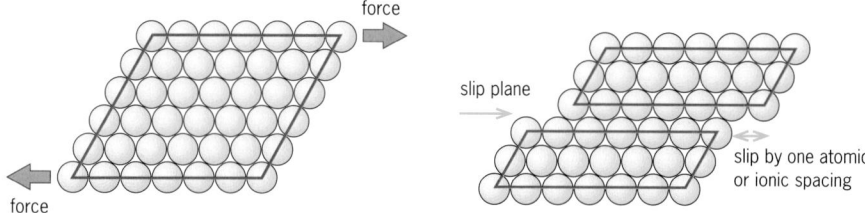

Fig 5.40 Slip occurring in a perfect crystal

Once a plane has slipped by a small amount, the bonds between neighbouring atoms can re-form. This is what happens when a specimen necks, but does not break, during a stress–strain test. We might expect that slip requires very large forces. But we shall see later that a much smaller force than we might expect can produce slip in a large metal crystal.

In a polycrystalline metal sample, the atoms in one small grain are not in the same plane as atoms in neighbouring grains: the grain boundaries interrupt these planes. This prevents slip continuing through the metal sample in any one direction. In large single metal crystals, slip occurs very much more easily because the atom planes are continuous.

Let's look at this more closely. Fig 5.40 shows whole planes of atoms sliding across each other. But, however pure a metal sample might be, it still contains imperfections. One type of imperfection is called an **edge dislocation**, a plane of atoms (or ions) missing over part of the lattice, as shown in Fig 5.41. The bonding is already weaker in the region of the missing plane. A shearing force applied to the crystal planes (Fig 5.42) will

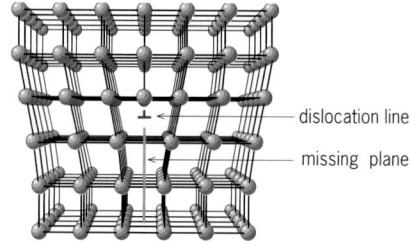

Fig 5.41 Part of a metal crystal with an edge dislocation

Fig 5.42 A shear force can move a dislocation one lattice spacing at a time. In these two-dimensional drawings, the dislocation, indicated by the conventional symbol of an inverted T, moves from one group of atoms to another

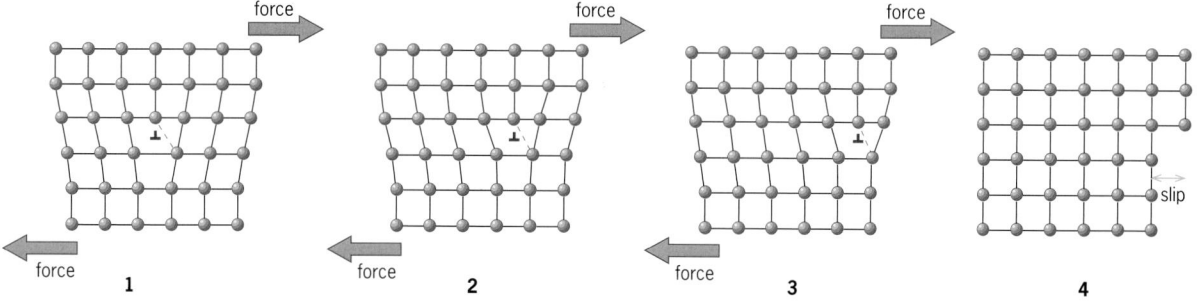

move one plane of atoms by one lattice spacing. This requires less force than it takes to move a large number of planes of atoms.

These dislocations help to give metals their properties of being ductile and malleable. We have seen that the metal atoms move and re-bond easily (we can think of the moving layers flowing over each other). This allows a metal to be drawn out into a wire – it is ductile. In general, also, a metal does not crack easily when hammered (it is not brittle), therefore it is malleable. Movement of dislocations is the major contribution to deformation or plastic strain in a metal such as steel (see Figs 5.28 and 5.29).

A material with no impurities may not be strong, particularly when it contains only a few grain boundaries. If a metal is stressed by applying forces that distort it, the number of boundaries can be increased considerably. The resulting tangle of boundaries can increase the strength.

Introducing atoms of other elements, such as atoms that are larger than those in the metal lattice, can stop dislocations from spreading and strengthen the material. The boundaries between the small grains can also hold back dislocation movement. It is therefore more difficult to deform materials consisting of small grains than materials with large crystals.

SCIENCE IN CONTEXT

Models for movement of dislocations

MOVING A RUCK IN A CARPET

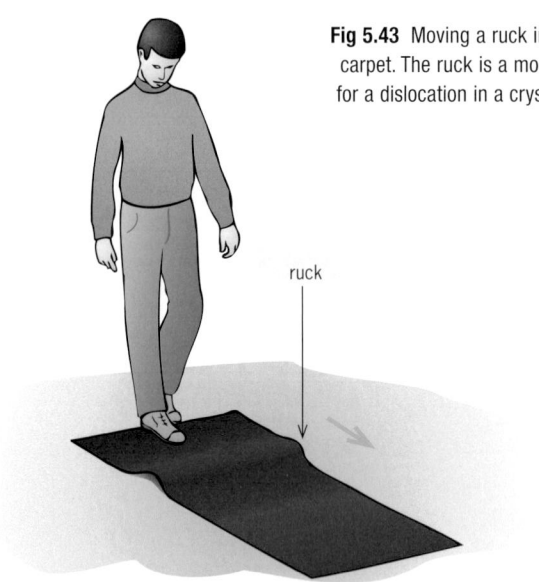

Fig 5.43 Moving a ruck in a carpet. The ruck is a model for a dislocation in a crystal

ruck

Suppose a carpet is laid flat on the floor, and we try to pull it across the floor. It is very difficult: it takes a lot of strength to overcome all the forces keeping carpet and floor together. Instead, we can create a ruck across the carpet close to one side, as in Fig 5.43 (reducing the carpet–floor forces), and then move the ruck through the carpet and across the floor. Like the steps of dislocation in a crystal in Fig 5.42, this gradual movement requires much less force.

BALL-BEARING CRYSTAL MODEL

For a simple model of a crystalline structure in two dimensions, we can place small ball bearings between parallel glass plates, as in Fig 5.44. A single layer is held in place with enough ball-bearings to pack the enclosed space almost completely to form a lattice, yet allowing movement in two dimensions.

When the model is gently tapped, dislocations and crystal boundaries appear in the lattice. There will also be small gaps. These are like the gaps, called vacancies, for missing atoms which always occur in a three-dimensional crystal lattice.

A similar model of a crystalline structure can be created using soap bubbles on a bubble raft – a small shallow tray of water onto which the bubbles are blown.

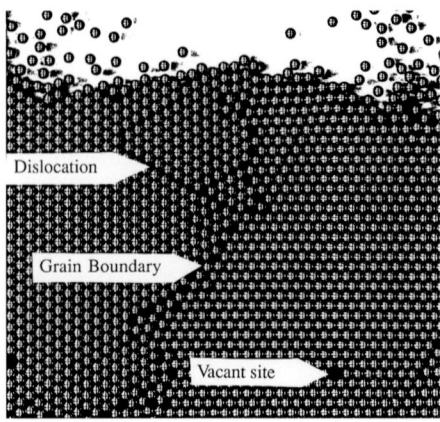

Fig 5.44 A ball-bearing model of a crystalline material showing vacancies, crystal (grain) boundaries and dislocations

Dislocation

Grain Boundary

Vacant site

FAULTS AND CRACKS IN MICROSTRUCTURES

As a rule, a material is brittle if cracks easily form and spread in it. In manufacturing, materials are often made by chemical reactions or by using heat to mould material into shapes (think of the blacksmith at his forge). During these processes, exposure to air can weaken the surface of a material. Millions of tiny imperfections on the surface can add up to form cracks. Then, these tiny cracks may **propagate** (spread) through the object when a load is applied.

This was a problem with cast iron, used extensively during the Industrial Revolution in the nineteenth century. Early railways made great use of cast iron for rails and bridges. But girders developed cracks, and many accidents occurred when bridges collapsed. It was almost as dangerous when the iron rails themselves cracked – steam engines exerting enough traction to pull loaded carriages or wagons produced a stress within the rails close to the breaking stress.

More recently, in the early days of jet passenger planes, cracks in the body of aircraft caused catastrophic accidents. Cracks develop where the strain is greatest. In the case of aircraft, cracks started at the edges of the windows. It is essential also to avoid cracks in the blades and casings of turbines such as those used in hydroelectric power stations to generate electricity. Engineers test for potential problems by using Perspex models and applying suitably scaled-down loads. In testing, the model is viewed using polarised light. The resulting interference colours (see Chapter 15) show how the strain is distributed within the model. Fig 5.45 shows an example of this for the strain in an artificial femur.

Cracks are dangerous because they are unpredictable. They are likely to occur when a material is repeatedly loaded and unloaded. For instance, in an aircraft the pressure on the outside of the body changes every time the aircraft takes off and lands. The wings are continually flexing up and down, as you may notice if you sit in a window seat in a plane. When an object fails under these conditions it is called **fatigue failure**.

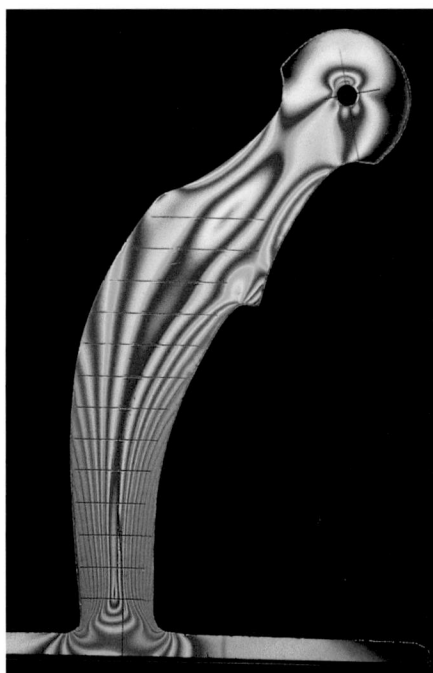

Fig 5.45 Strain patterns in the plastic model of an artificial hip bone

Hardening glass

Often, an engineer prefers to use a weaker material with larger cross-section rather than a stronger material which is more liable to crack. Wood is not as strong as glass but is less likely to break, so it has traditionally been more useful as a building material. Now, methods for treating the surface of glass make its behaviour more predictable, so it is more widely used in large buildings.

Different methods are used for making windscreens. In one method, some of the surface ions of glass are exchanged chemically with other ions of a larger diameter. These larger ions create compressive stress on the surrounding glass ions. In another method, the glass is heated until it goes soft, and cold air jets make the outer surface cooler than the interior. A compressive stress is set up in the surface, with a tensile stress in the interior.

With both methods, the surface of the glass is in compression. This makes crack propagation difficult, because whenever a crack starts, compression forces at the surface tend to close it up. But once a crack does penetrate beyond the surface, it spreads very rapidly indeed as the built-up stress is large and there is no resistance to spreading. Fig 5.46 shows what happens.

Glass is an example of an *amorphous* structure. This means that the molecules do not exist in a regular pattern. You will find out more about crystalline and amorphous materials in Chapter 7.

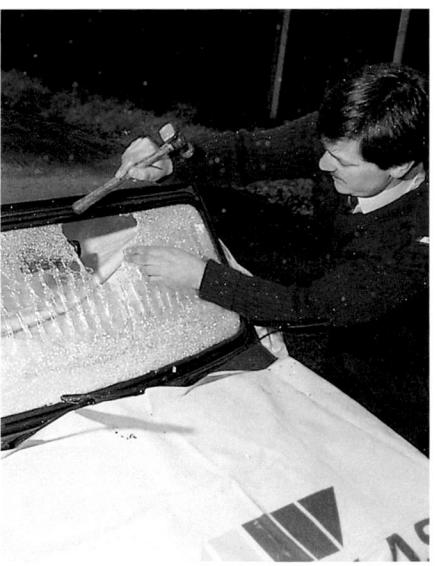

Fig 5.46 A car windscreen shatters in small pieces, so that the danger to passengers is reduced

More about rubber

Rubber is a natural polymer made of long-chain molecules. In its normal state the molecules are bent back and forth, tangled together as in Fig 5.47(a) with weak forces acting between the molecules. As in (b), when the rubber in a rubber band is pulled, the molecules straighten out and allow the rubber to become longer. Eventually, as in (c), the molecules are fully stretched and almost parallel with each other. By that time the rubber may be up to 10 times its original length. Extra force will make the rubber break. On the other hand, if the rubber is not stretched to breaking, and the force is then removed, the molecules tend to curl back again because of the attraction and cross-links between adjacent molecules. Unless there has been some reorganisation of the cross-links, the return is elastic.

Fig 5.47 The behaviour of rubber is determined by the arrangement of its molecules

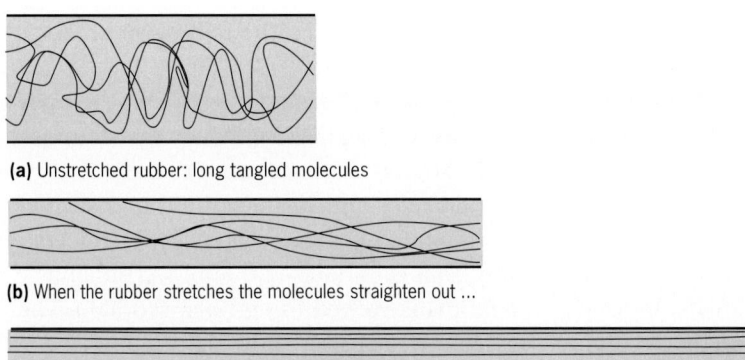

(a) Unstretched rubber: long tangled molecules

(b) When the rubber stretches the molecules straighten out ...

(c) ... until they can't get any longer without breaking

6 COMPOSITE MATERIALS

Composite materials are making an increasing contribution to modern life. They can produce combinations of properties that cannot be met by conventional metals, glass or polymers. Usually they are required to be strong, stiff, and impact- and corrosion-resistant, often for extreme applications in aerospace or underwater technology. But in our society of high-density living an alternative prime requirement for some materials is that they be good sound absorbers.

Concrete

We have seen the need to prevent cracks propagating. They may be stopped when they meet a tougher material, and it is for this reason that composites of more than one material are used. The continuous component is the **matrix**, and one or more other tougher materials are distributed in it. When a crack develops in the **matrix**, it extends until it meets the tougher component. Concrete is an example: a crack spreads in brittle cement but stops when it meets a particle of sand or gravel (Fig 5.48). (Two quite brittle materials can also be combined to make a tougher composite.)

The disadvantage of concrete is that it has low tensile strength. To get around this problem it is often strengthened with steel which has a high tensile strength. Assemblies for reinforcing steel are a common sight on building sites. They consist of a framework of steel bars which provide the tensile strength in the required directions. To take advantage of the compressive strength of concrete, prestressed concrete is used in structures involving very large forces. The concrete is set around wires which are prestressed to a high force per unit area of about 1200 MN m^{-2}.

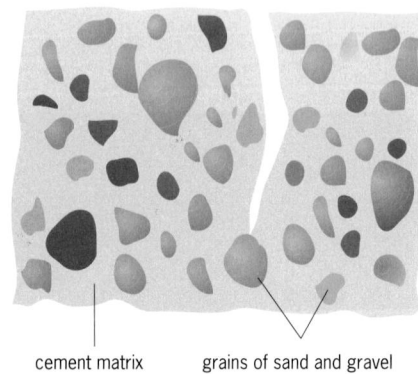

cement matrix   grains of sand and gravel

Fig 5.48 Crack-stopping in concrete

? QUESTION 11

11 Say whether either of the two steel samples shown in Figs 5.28 and 5.29 (page 107) look suitable for concrete reinforcement.

Glass-reinforced plastic (GRP)

Glass fibre is widely used to reinforce composites (see Fig 5.49). A common example is glass-reinforced plastic (GRP), used for the hulls of dinghies. A crack forming in the resin matrix spreads until it meets the glass fibre. This fibre then separates slightly from the matrix, stress around the fibre is reduced and the crack stops. A sudden blow will create thousands of tiny cracks, but they do not develop into a single catastrophic crack. In fact, the material remains almost as strong as it was before the damage.

Laminar composite and sandwich panels

Laminar products are usually made up of two-dimensional sheets or panels, each of which has a preferred high-strength direction. Wood is such an example and is commonly used in **plywood**. Laminar composites are also used for fibre-aligned plastics.

Sandwich panels consist of two strong outer sheets separated by a layer of less dense material. Often the core has a honeycomb structure. Such panels are used in aircraft fuselages and wings and in the walls of buildings. The honeycomb structures are strong. Also, because they can be made with a porous material with lots of air pockets, they can be excellent sound absorbers.

DESCRIBING THE PROPERTIES OF MATERIALS

The technical words used to describe the properties of materials have precise meanings which may not match their everyday use:

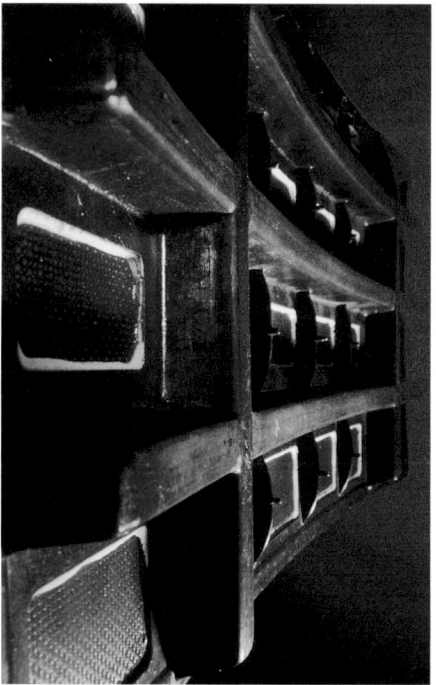

Fig 5.49 An aircraft access door made from a glass-fibre composite material; suitable for non-structural areas of an aircraft, this lightweight material gives significant fuel savings

brittle	breaks suddenly and catastrophically with rough edges; once started, cracks propagate easily; bricks and biscuits are brittle
tough	the opposite of brittle; the material resists crack propagation and so distorts rather than breaks; nylon, rope, bones, tendons and most textiles are tough
strong	the material needs a large stress to distort it; steel, titanium alloys, rubber, glass, wood (along the grain) and cotton are strong (the metals are about ten times stronger than the non-metals)
elastic	the material will return to its original length (or shape) when any load is removed; rubber, steel, glass and wood are usefully elastic – they withstand everyday forces without permanent distortion
plastic	the material distorts easily with quite small stresses but does not fracture; plasticine and wet clay are typical plastic materials; metals and ice show plastic behaviour if stresses act for a long time (metals creep, glaciers flow)
hard	hard materials are not easily cut; diamond is hard, graphite is soft (hardness is measured on a scale from 1 to 10 using the Moh scale)
soft	the opposite of hard
stiff	rigid and not easily bent
malleable	material changes shape but does not crack when subjected to sudden large forces (e.g. being hit with a hammer); many metals (e.g. copper) are malleable
ductile	material changes shape rather than cracking when subjected to a large but steadily applied force; describes the behaviour of many metals which can be drawn out into wires when forced through a small hole

? **QUESTION 12**

12 Describe as concisely and clearly as possible the mechanical properties (response to forces) of any three of the following materials: a cheese biscuit, a piece of newspaper, a piece of string, a plastic ruler, a piece of food-wrap film. Use the technical words listed, plus any others that seem relevant.

Examples

Biscuit is weak and brittle; *glass* is strong and brittle. A piece of *string* is soft, tough and fairly strong. *Rubber* is soft and elastic; *steel* is hard and elastic. *Wood* is soft, tough, fairly elastic and strong.

SUMMARY

By studying this chapter you should have learnt and understood the following about structures and materials:

- Forces act at a point, and moments of forces are in equilibrium when a body is not accelerating.
- Hooke's law states: extension x is proportional to applied force F: $F = kx$, where k is the spring constant.
- The behaviour of springs in series and in parallel.
- The key concepts of stress as force/area, F/A; and strain as extension/length, x/L.
- The Young modulus is the ratio stress/strain for an elastic material, $E = FL/Ax$.
- The types of stress that objects and structures are subject to include: tension, bending, shear.
- A metal shows elastic and plastic deformation and has an elastic limit.
- To find the energy stored in a stretched object (such as a spring), use $E = \frac{1}{2}kx^2$.

- The terms used to describe the mechanical properties and types of materials include: brittle, tough, strong, hard, elastic, plastic, malleable, ductile, crystalline, polycrystalline, amorphous, composite.
- The properties of a material can be explained by considering its microstructure at the level of forces between particles (atoms, molecules) and between larger features (crystals, grains); the significance of crystal defects.
- The importance of cracks in causing the failure of a material to withstand forces; specific methods used to stop cracks propagating.
- Ways in which materials are used in everyday structures: buildings, bridges, household objects.

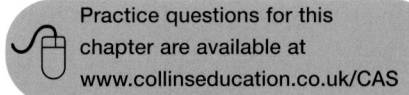

Practice questions for this chapter are available at www.collinseducation.co.uk/CAS

6

Oscillations and mechanical waves

6 OSCILLATIONS AND MECHANICAL WAVES

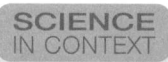
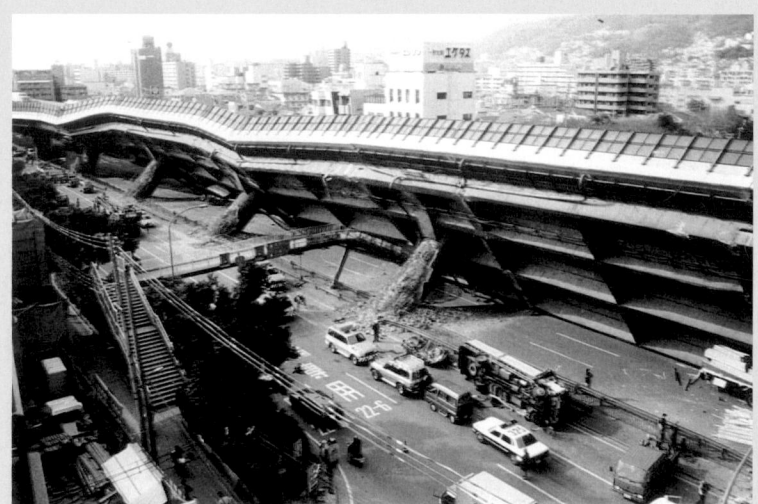

This elevated highway collapsed when a major earthquake hit the Japanese city of Kobe in 1995

Waiting for the 'big one'

The most powerful natural mechanical waves, and so potentially the most devastating, are those caused by earthquakes. They are called seismic waves from the Greek word *seismos* which means a shaking. Earthquakes can occur almost anywhere in the world, though fortunately we do not have major ones in Britain.

Severe earthquakes occur close to fault lines in the Earth's crust. Here, architects and engineers go to great lengths to protect buildings and other structures. They add strength by using more steel and more concrete than is usual elsewhere. They also introduce mechanical damping, putting rubber inserts or even metal springs into the supports.

An object, a bell for instance, can have a natural frequency at which it resonates. So can the walls of a room and even a whole building. Seismic waves at the natural frequency of a building would cause it to oscillate wildly and then collapse, so architects make sure that buildings do not have natural frequencies in a range that would make them vulnerable.

Preventing a high-rise building from toppling is difficult enough, but stopping the collapse of flyovers has proved particularly tricky, as highway engineers in Japan and California have discovered after major earthquakes which have caused chaos and death. California in particular awaits the 'big one' – a massive earthquake along the San Andreas fault line which it is predicted could occur in the next few years.

The ideas in this chapter

As the chapter opener indicates, the study of oscillations and mechanical waves is of crucial importance to our everyday safety.

In this chapter we look in some depth at the theory behind oscillations and at simple harmonic motion in particular. We also look at damping of vibrations, and the need for damping in practical applications such as car suspension systems.

Stationary, or standing, waves have special importance in music. We look at the theory behind these waves and consider their application to such instruments as guitars and organ pipes.

1 SIMPLE HARMONIC MOTION

Most of us at some time have seen a grandfather clock with a pendulum (Fig 6.1). The reason for using a pendulum is that the time taken for each swing through a small angle is constant. So, as the pendulum swings back and forth, it controls very precisely the movement of the clock's mechanism.

The pendulum is an example of an oscillator – it moves backwards and forwards in a regular (periodic) way, as in Fig 6.2(a). The period of the pendulum is the time

Fig 6.1 The time taken for the pendulum to swing is constant, provided the angle of swing is small. Galileo noticed this as he watched a lamp swing on a chain in Pisa Cathedral

it takes to go from one position in its swing through a complete oscillation back to its original position. The number of such oscillations in a unit of time is called the frequency. The distance the bob has swung away from its central equilibrium position is called its displacement, and the maximum displacement is the amplitude of swing.

Another example of an oscillator is a mass vibrating up and down on the end of a spring, see Fig 6.2(b). Here also, the mass moves up and down past a central position.

Displacement is movement in a particular direction and therefore is a vector. For the mass on the spring, displacement x (and also amplitude) is measured in metres. For the pendulum, displacement is measured as an angle, θ, usually in radians.

The period T is measured in seconds. Frequency f is the number of vibrations in a second, and so we have the inverse relationship:

$$f = \frac{1}{T}$$

We can see that the unit of frequency is second^{-1} (i.e. s^{-1}). This unit of frequency is given the special name hertz (Hz). This means that:

$$1\ \text{Hz} = 1\ \text{s}^{-1}$$

To find out more about oscillations, we can fix a pen to a pendulum and swing the pendulum over a moving strip of paper on, for example, a dynamics trolley moving at right angles to the swing of the pendulum. As shown in Fig 6.3, the pen plots a trace which represents the displacement of the pendulum with time. This is the sequence of events:

- At time $t = 0$ the pendulum is set swinging by letting it fall away from a position of maximum displacement. This displacement is the amplitude A of swing.
- The pendulum has zero displacement (it hangs vertically) at time $t = T/4$.
- At time $t = T/2$, the pendulum has maximum displacement on the side opposite its start side.
- The pendulum again has zero displacement at $t = 3T/4$ as it returns back through the vertical position.
- The pendulum takes time T to do a complete swing and return to its original position.

If you are familiar with a plot of cos θ against θ, then you will recognise this as the curve in Fig 6.3. The movement of such an oscillating system is called simple harmonic motion because many musical instruments create vibrations like this. We say that the path of the motion varies sinusoidally – that is, like a sine (or cosine) curve.

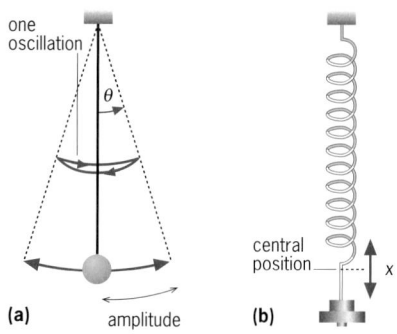

Fig 6.2 Examples of oscillating systems: (a) a pendulum; (b) a mass suspended from a spring

REMEMBER THIS
A radian is the angle subtended at the centre of a circle (in this case the pivot of the pendulum) by an arc equal in length to the radius. (Here, the radius is the length of the pendulum.)

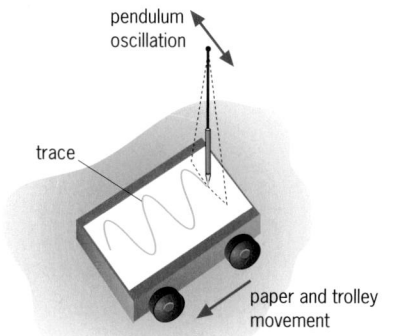

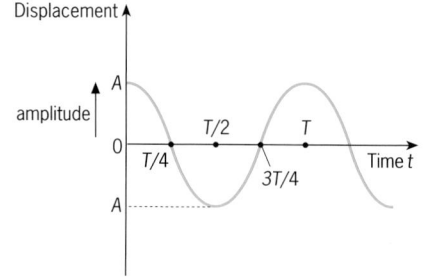

Fig 6.3 The displacement of a pendulum with time

? QUESTION 1

1 What is the frequency (in Hz) of an oscillator vibrating with a period of 1.25×10^{-3} s?

? QUESTION 2

2 **a)** Plot cos θ against θ between 0° and 360°, by hand or by graphical calculator.

b) State two ways in which the movement of the shadow in Fig 6.4 resembles the simple harmonic motion of a pendulum.

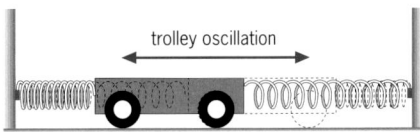

Fig 6.5 An oscillating trolley attached to two identical anchored springs undergoes simple harmonic motion

✔ REMEMBER THIS

The dynamics trolley in Fig 6.5 is demonstrating Hooke's law – see page 98.

MAPPING SIMPLE HARMONIC MOTION ONTO A CIRCLE

It helps us to understand simple harmonic motion if we link it to movement in a circle. As in Fig 6.4, we can place a sphere near the edge of a rotating turntable and project a shadow of the sphere onto a screen. As the turntable rotates, the shadow of the sphere moves across the screen with a motion similar to that of the bob of a pendulum moving back and forth.

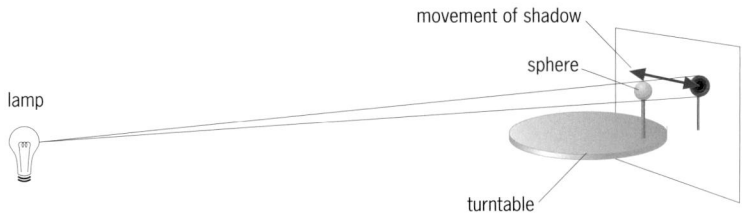

Fig 6.4 The movement of the shadow of an object rotating in a circle illustrates simple harmonic motion

For another demonstration, we can use a vibrating dynamics trolley as in Fig 6.5. The trolley is attached to two fixed posts using two identical springs. At equilibrium, the trolley sits centrally between the posts with the springs pulling equally in opposite directions. When the trolley is pulled to one side, the two springs both act, with a force proportional to the displacement x, to return the trolley to the central equilibrium position.

This restoring force F is given by:

$$F = -kx$$

where k is the spring constant for the combination of the two springs. Note that when one spring is compressed and tending to lengthen, the other is stretched and tending to shorten. When the trolley returns to its central position, it has a velocity that makes it overshoot. It goes on to achieve maximum displacement on the other side.

We can trace the change of position of the trolley with time by connecting the trolley to a ticker-tape machine as shown in Fig 6.6. We get a series of dots at equal time intervals as the trolley moves from maximum displacement on one side of the equilibrium position to maximum displacement on the other side.

We can see that the dots are not equally spaced along the strip of paper, and we can match them up with points which are equally spaced around a semicircle, as Fig 6.6 shows. It is as if a spot is moving with constant angular speed around the circle, just as the sphere in Fig 6.4 was moving uniformly around with the turntable.

The spot would make one complete revolution, covering an angle of 2ω radians, in period T. Its angular speed ω is obtained from angle turned through, divided by time. That is:

$$\text{angular speed } \omega = \frac{2\pi}{T} = 2\pi f$$

From Fig 6.6, we see that the displacement of the oscillating trolley is given by:

$$x = A \cos \theta = A \cos \omega t$$

where A is the maximum amplitude of the oscillation. This is an equation for simple harmonic motion (sometimes abbreviated to s.h.m.).

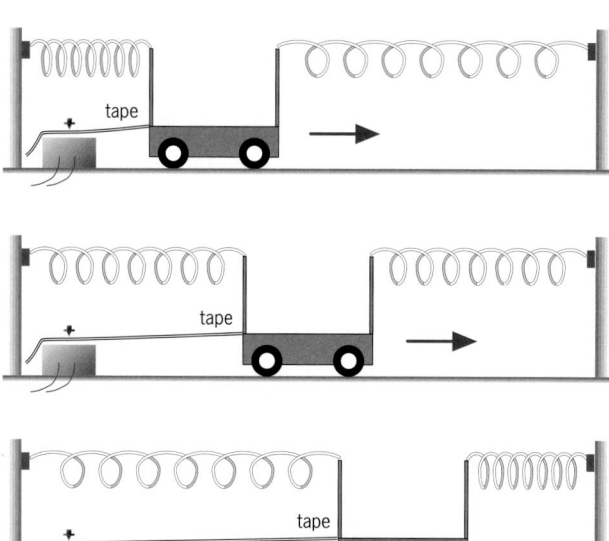

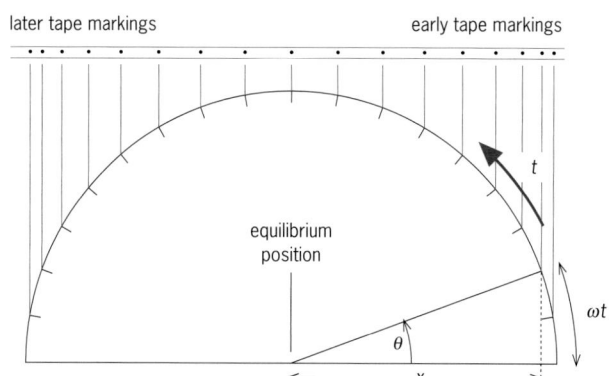

Fig 6.6 Relating movement of the trolley to uniform motion in a circle

EXAMPLE

Q A trolley oscillates with amplitude 5.0 cm and period 2.5 s. What are its displacements relative to its equilibrium position 0.4 s and 1.0 s after being set off from a position of maximum amplitude?

A We first need to find π in radians. (Your calculator needs to be in radian mode.)

We have seen that

$\omega = 2\pi f$ and $f = 1/T$

So:

$f = \dfrac{1}{2.5} = 0.4$ Hz

and

$\omega = 2\pi \times 0.40$ s^{-1}

This gives us a displacement after 0.4 s of:

$x = A \cos \omega t$
$= 5.0 \cos(2\pi \times 0.40 \times 0.4)$
$= 5.0 \cos(1.01)$
$= 2.7$ cm

That is, the trolley is 2.7 cm from the equilibrium position, on the same side as it started.

After 1.0 s:
$x = 5.0 \cos(2\pi \times 0.40 \times 1.0)$
$= 5.0 \cos(2.51)$
$= -4.0$ cm

That is, the trolley is 4.0 cm from the equilibrium position, on the opposite side from where it started.

? QUESTION 3

3 The dots along the paper in Fig 6.6 are unequally spaced. Explain this as fully as you can.

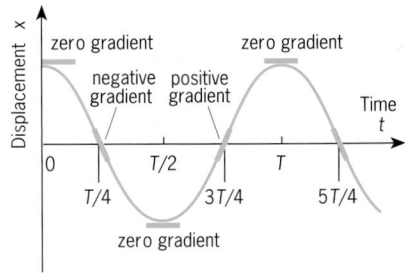

(a) Displacement–time curve

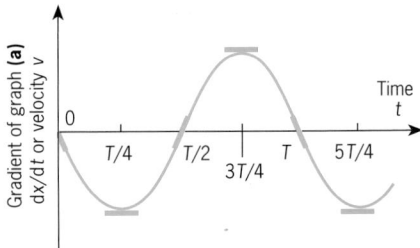

(b) Velocity–time curve

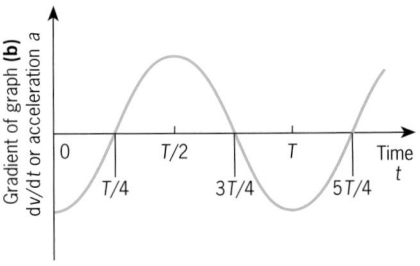

(c) Acceleration–time curve

Fig 6.7 Curves for simple harmonic motion

DISPLACEMENT, VELOCITY AND ACCELERATION

You have already encountered relationships between distance, velocity and acceleration (see Chapter 1). In simple harmonic motion, though, the displacement varies sinusoidally with time – and this is a lot more complicated than if displacement were linear with time.

Fig 6.7(a) shows the displacement for an oscillator behaving sinusoidally with time. It is plotted with maximum displacement at time $t = 0$ so that $x = A \cos \omega t = A$. The velocity of the oscillator at any time is given by the small change in displacement Δx which occurs during a small change in time Δt. That is:

$$\textbf{velocity} = \frac{\Delta x}{\Delta t}$$

This velocity is the gradient at any point on the displacement–time curve in Fig 6.7(a). We can see the following:

- At $t = 0$, the gradient is zero.
- At $t = T/4$, the gradient is negative and is the maximum possible negative value.
- At $t = T/2$, the gradient is again zero.
- At $t = 3T/4$, the gradient has the maximum possible positive value.
- At $t = T$, the oscillator has returned to its starting position and the gradient of the curve is zero.

We can plot the complete range of values of the gradient. This gives us the velocity–time curve shown in Fig 6.7(b). We see that the shape of the curve is similar to that of Fig 6.7(a) but is displaced along the time axis. The velocity is zero at time $t = 0$. It is in fact given by $\sin \omega t$; and since the velocity starts off in a negative direction, the dependence is $-\sin \omega t$. The velocity *lags* the displacement by $\pi/2$. We say that it is out of phase by $-\pi/2$; we discuss phase on page 134.

Now we take the velocity–time curve and consider the gradient $\Delta v/\Delta t$ in a similar way. This gives us the variation of acceleration with time, as shown in Fig 6.7(c). We see that acceleration is in opposite phase to the displacement – that is, they are out of phase by π, so that when one is at a maximum positive value the other is at a maximum negative value, and so on. Acceleration can be represented by $-\cos \omega t$.

STRETCH AND CHALLENGE

Proof by calculus

The relationships for velocity and acceleration can also be shown by calculus. Displacement is given by:

$$x = A \cos \omega t$$

To find the velocity, v, we differentiate:

$$v = \frac{\mathrm{d}x}{\mathrm{d}t} = \frac{\mathrm{d}}{\mathrm{d}t}(A \cos \omega t)$$
$$= -A\omega \sin \omega t$$

We differentiate again to find the acceleration, a:

$$a = \frac{\mathrm{d}v}{\mathrm{d}t} = \frac{\mathrm{d}}{\mathrm{d}t}(-A\omega \sin \omega t)$$
$$= -A\omega^2 \cos \omega t$$

But we can replace $A \cos \omega t$ by x.
So:

$$a = -\omega^2 x$$

The physics of the curves

Do the curves of Fig 6.7 make sense? We can see that the velocity is maximum at zero displacement. Think of a pendulum. It swings fastest at the centre of its swing. What about the trolley connected to the two springs? It is also moving fastest at its central position. On the other hand, in both examples, velocity is zero at maximum displacement. The pendulum and the trolley are at rest for an instant as they reverse direction of movement. But the force is a maximum here and the acceleration must be a maximum. The force is returning the pendulum or the trolley back to its central equilibrium position and so the acceleration must be negative compared with displacement. In the central position, there is no horizontal force on the pendulum. In the case of the trolley, the horizontal forces exerted by the springs exactly balance out.

So what *is* simple harmonic motion?

Simple harmonic motion (s.h.m.) is motion in which the acceleration is directly proportional to the displacement from a fixed point and is directed towards this point. We can see, both from the graphical treatment and from the calculus in the Stretch and Challenge passage opposite, that displacement varies sinusoidally with time and that acceleration is proportional to the displacement. Acceleration is oppositely directed, as shown by the negative sign.

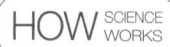

HOW SCIENCE WORKS

To show that the motion of a pendulum is simple harmonic motion

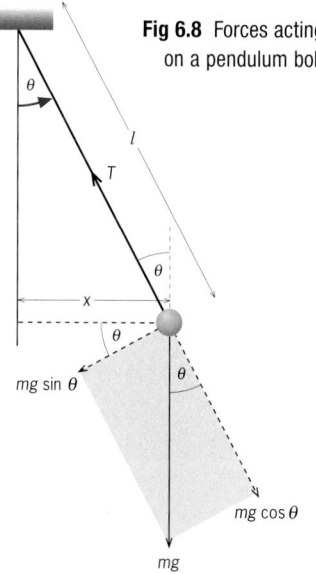

Fig 6.8 Forces acting on a pendulum bob

We need to show that the acceleration of the bob is proportional to its displacement from the centre of motion, which is taken as the vertical position. Suppose we have a bob of mass m. A gravitational force mg will act on the bob vertically downwards. There is also a tension T acting in the string. When the bob is displaced from the vertical by an angle θ, the tension acts on the bob at an angle θ to the vertical (Fig 6.8). We resolve forces along and perpendicular to the string. Along the string we have:

$$T = mg \cos \theta$$

The tension in the string must be equal and opposite to the gravitational force on the bob *as resolved in the direction of the string*.

Perpendicular to the string is an *unbalanced* force of $mg \sin \theta$. This force acting on the bob of mass m must give it an acceleration a in the direction of decreasing θ (that is, it acts in the opposite direction to the displacement). From this we can say that:

$$mg \sin \theta = -ma$$

or:

$$g \sin \theta = -a$$

If θ is very small and measured in radians, then $\sin \theta \approx \theta$ and we get:

$$g\theta = -a$$

So we see that acceleration is proportional to the angular displacement θ.

? QUESTION 4

4 Big Ben's time is finely adjusted by placing coins on the top of the vibrating pendulum bob. Why does this affect the period of vibration?

Pendulums and springs

THE PERIOD OF A SIMPLE PENDULUM

Let x be the displacement of the bob from the vertical in a horizontal direction and l be the length of the pendulum (see Fig 6.8 on the previous page). Then for small θ:

$$\theta = \frac{x}{l}$$

We know from the box on the previous page that $g\theta = -a$, so:

$$\frac{gx}{l} = -a$$

$$a = -\left(\frac{g}{l}\right)x \qquad [1]$$

The acceleration is proportional to the displacement x, in line with the definition of s.h.m. We compare equation 1 with our equation for s.h.m. on page 124:

$$a = -\omega^2 x$$

so that: $\qquad \omega^2 = \dfrac{g}{l}$

Since $\omega = 2\pi f$: $\qquad 4\pi^2 f^2 = \dfrac{g}{l}$

giving: $\quad f = \dfrac{1}{2\pi}\sqrt{\dfrac{g}{l}}$

The period of the pendulum is

$$T = \frac{1}{f}$$

so: $\qquad T = 2\pi\sqrt{\dfrac{l}{g}}$

Note that this expression is only true provided θ is small (less than approximately 10°, or less than 0.2 radians).

? QUESTION 5

5   Using the formula
$$T = 2\pi\sqrt{\frac{l}{g}}$$
calculate the period of a pendulum of length 1.20 m suspended from a fixed support. Say whether the period of the pendulum would differ (and if so, say whether the period would be larger or smaller) if the pendulum was:

a) swung on the surface of the Moon,

b) swung in a lift that is accelerating upwards.

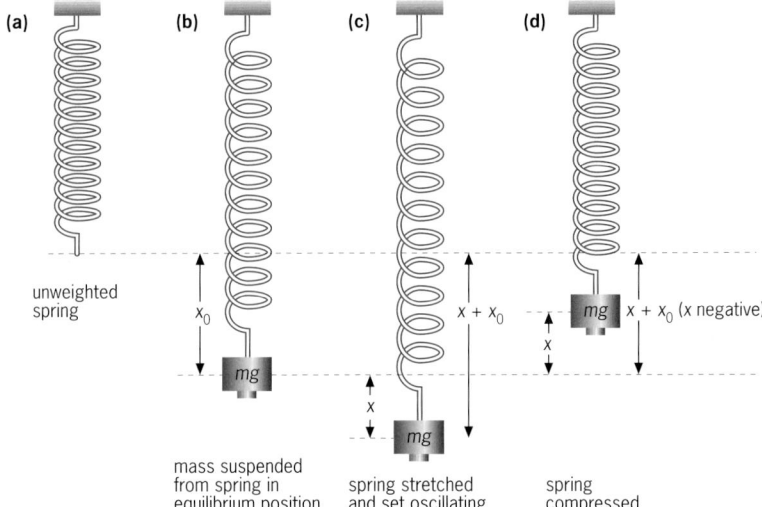

(a) unweighted spring

(b) x_0 — mass suspended from spring in equilibrium position — mg

(c) $x + x_0$ — spring stretched and set oscillating — x — mg

(d) mg — $x + x_0$ (x negative) — x — spring compressed

Fig 6.9 Obtaining an expression for the period of oscillation of a mass suspended from a spring

THE PERIOD OF OSCILLATION OF A MASS SUSPENDED FROM A SPRING

The force exerted by the spring is:

$$F = -kx$$

where x is the extension or compression of the spring from its equilibrium length, and k is the spring constant. When a mass m is suspended from the spring, it will already be stretched through an extension x_0 given by $kx_0 = mg$, see Fig 6.9(b).

After pulling the mass down a further distance x and letting go of the mass, as in (c), we have:

● a force downwards equal to mg due to the gravitational force on the mass,

● a force upwards equal to $k(x + x_0)$ due to the tension of the stretched spring.

These are not equal and so there is a net force acting on the suspended mass giving it an acceleration a. As force equals mass × acceleration, assuming that we give a downward force a plus sign and an upward force a minus sign, we have:

$$\underset{\substack{\text{force exerted}\\\text{by spring}}}{-k(x + x_0)} + \underset{\substack{\text{force due}\\\text{to gravity}}}{mg} = \underset{\substack{\text{resulting (net)}\\\text{accelerating}\\\text{force}}}{ma}$$

As the upward force $k(x + x_0)$ of the spring is greater than the downward force on the mass mg, the acceleration is upwards and hence has a negative value. The equation continues to apply as the spring contracts through its equilibrium extension.

Now, by Hooke's law we can replace mg by kx_0 in the equation to give:

So: $\qquad -k(x + x_0) + kx_0 = ma$

$$-kx = ma$$

$$a = \left(\frac{k}{m}\right)x$$

Comparing this with the equation for s.h.m.:

$$a = -\omega^2 x$$

we obtain: $\qquad \omega^2 = \dfrac{k}{m}$

This gives the period of oscillation for the suspended mass on the spring as:

$$T = \frac{2\pi}{\omega} = 2\pi\sqrt{\frac{m}{k}}$$

2 ENERGY CHANGES IN AN OSCILLATING SYSTEM

In all the examples of s.h.m. that we have considered – that is the pendulum, the mass on a spring and the vibrating dynamics trolley – the velocity v of the oscillating mass m varies in the same way. It goes from a maximum when it

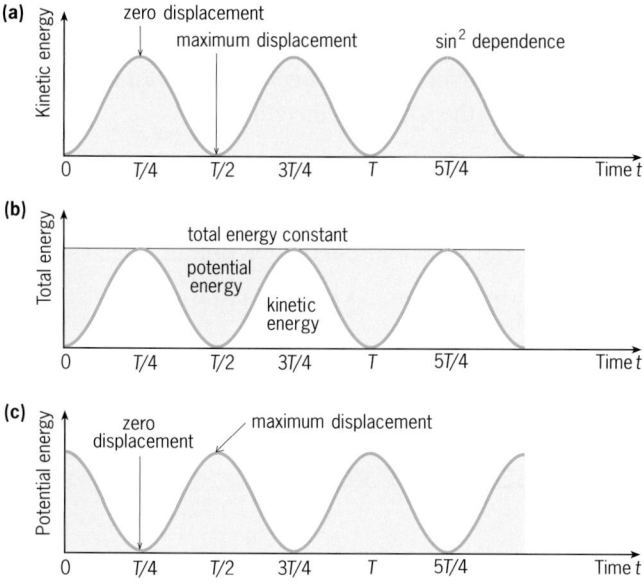

Fig 6.10 Variation of **(a)** kinetic energy, **(b)** total energy and **(c)** potential energy of an s.h.m. oscillator with time

passes through the equilibrium position to zero at maximum displacement when the direction of motion is instantaneously changing.

For each system, the kinetic energy at any time is $\frac{1}{2}mv^2$. We can now look at how this energy varies.

ENERGY–TIME CURVES

Since the velocity v changes sinusoidally with time as shown in Fig 6.7(b), the variation of kinetic energy with time can be shown by squaring the velocity, Fig 6.10(a). The total energy of the oscillating system must remain constant. So, as the kinetic energy rises and falls, it is being transferred back and forth into another form of energy. This form must be potential energy. We can see this energy as the difference (shaded areas) between the constant level of energy and the kinetic energy as in Fig 6.10(b). Alternatively, potential energy can be plotted positively in the same way as kinetic energy, as Fig 6.10(c), and is seen to be out of phase with kinetic energy by a quarter of a period.

ENERGY–DISPLACEMENT CURVES

We can also show the variation of kinetic energy and potential energy with displacement x, rather than with time t, and this gives us curves of a different shape. When working out the form of these curves, it is easiest to start with the potential energy contribution to the energy.

As before, let's consider a mass connected horizontally between two springs. (This is so that we do not need to consider gravitational potential energy.) We will take the force constant as k for the two springs acting on the mass. To move the trolley from its equilibrium position at $x = 0$ to displaced position x requires an applied force F_{applied} given by:

$$F_{\text{applied}} = kx$$

This applied force is equal and opposite to the restoring force exerted by the springs.

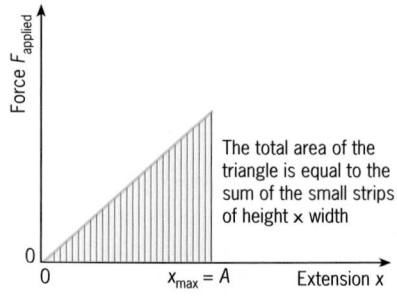

Fig 6.11 The graph shows how the applied force needs to increase in order to extend a spring system. Its maximum extension = x_{max} = A

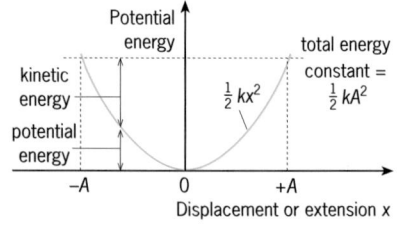

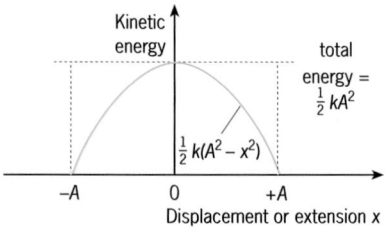

Fig 6.12 The variation of potential energy and kinetic energy with displacement x for an oscillator

The work done is force × distance and is equal to the triangular area under the applied force plot of Fig 6.11:

$$\text{work done} = \tfrac{1}{2} F_{\text{applied}}\, x_{\text{max}} = \tfrac{1}{2} k x_{\text{max}}^{2}$$

But x_{max} is the maximum displacement or amplitude of vibration. We called this A earlier. So:

$$\text{work done} = \tfrac{1}{2} k A^{2}$$

This is the potential energy now stored in the springs.

At maximum displacement, the kinetic energy is zero and this means that $\tfrac{1}{2} k A^{2}$ is the total energy of the vibrating system. The total energy of a vibrating system is therefore proportional to the square of the amplitude:

$$E_{\text{total}} \propto A^{2}$$

For a displacement $x < A$, the potential energy is $\tfrac{1}{2} k x^{2}$. Taking the difference between the total energy and the potential energy we obtain:

$$\text{kinetic energy } E_{k} = E_{\text{total}} - \tfrac{1}{2} k x^{2} = \tfrac{1}{2} k (A^{2} - x^{2})$$

Fig 6.12 shows how the potential energy and kinetic energy vary as displacement x varies.

STRETCH AND CHALLENGE

Alternative expression for velocity

$E_{k} = \tfrac{1}{2} k (A^{2} - x^{2})$

$\quad = \tfrac{1}{2} m v^{2}$

So $m v^{2} = k(A^{2} - x^{2})$, and therefore:

$$v = \pm \sqrt{\frac{k}{m} (A^{2} - x^{2})}$$

But:

$$\sqrt{\frac{k}{m}} = \omega$$

since $\omega^{2} = \dfrac{k}{m}$

(see the How Science Work box on page 126).

This gives us velocity in the form:

$$v = \pm \omega \sqrt{(A^{2} - x^{2})}$$

---

3 DAMPING

So far, we have assumed that there is no friction in our oscillating systems. However, in reality this can never happen – there will always be some friction, causing energy to be lost from the system.

The total energy of a vibrating system depends on the square of the amplitude. If energy is removed from the system, the amplitude of vibration is reduced. How rapidly this happens depends on the amount of friction, which causes what is known as damping.

? QUESTION 6

6 Suggest some practical examples of damping.

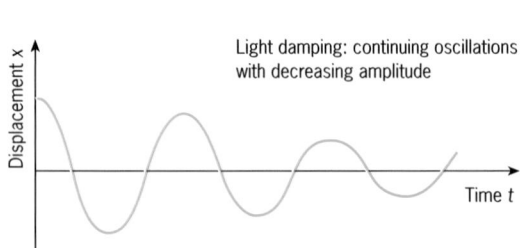

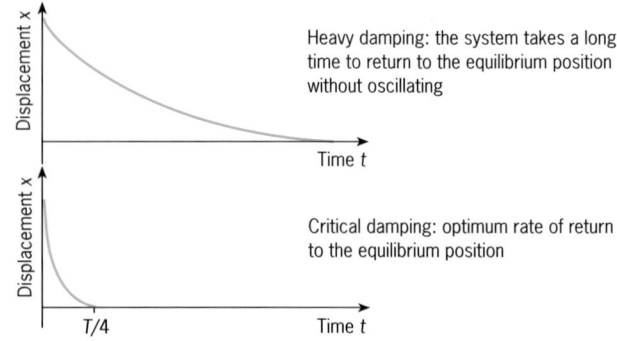

Fig 6.13 The effect of damping on an oscillating system

Smoothing out a bumpy ride

Car suspensions are fitted with springs and shock absorbers to damp out the vibrations of a moving car. The shock absorbers are pistons moving up and down in a viscous fluid (usually an oil). Without the shock absorbers, the car would bounce up and down repeatedly on the springs.

The amount of damping is set by the dimensions and materials of the spring and absorber. Car suspensions need to be slightly less than critically damped. If there is too much damping, then when the system has responded to a bump or rut in the road it does not return to its equilibrium position in time to respond to the next bump or rut. If the damping is too light, the passengers experience a lot of oscillations before the system recovers. When shock absorbers become worn, the ride of a car becomes bouncy and rather uncomfortable.

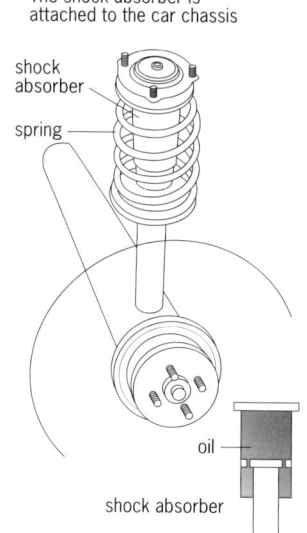

The shock absorber is attached to the car chassis

shock absorber

spring

oil

shock absorber

piston

Fig. 6.14(a) A car suspension

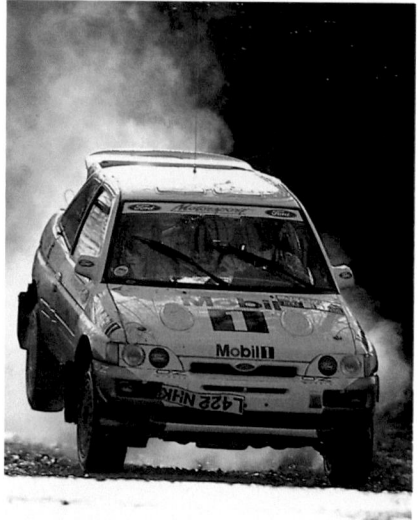

Fig 6.14(b) A rally car: the suspension allows the rough ride to be smoother than if there were no suspension in the vehicle

Damping, causing a reduction in the amplitude of vibration (Fig 6.13), is often an advantage. With light damping, the oscillations gradually reduce in amplitude but take a long time to disappear. With very heavy damping, the system does not oscillate but returns to its equilibrium position very slowly. With critical damping, the amount of friction is such that the system returns as quickly as possible to equilibrium without 'overshooting' in the opposite direction. The time for this to happen is approximately a quarter of the period for free oscillation of the system.

4 FORCED OSCILLATIONS AND RESONANCE

If the vibrating system is losing energy, it is possible to replace the energy or even increase the total energy by applying a force to the system periodically and in the correct direction. If the frequency of the applied force is the same as the natural frequency of the system, the amplitude of vibration builds up.

Think about pushing a child on a swing (Fig 6.15). You time your pushes to coincide with the natural oscillation, but have to be careful not to push too much or too often as this would cause the amplitude to get too large and the child could fall off.

It is often necessary to prevent vibrations building up in mechanical systems. When the applied force has the same periodic frequency as the natural frequency of the system, we say resonance occurs. When this happens, a large amount of energy is given by the force to the system. (You may have felt intense vibrations when in a car next to a large vehicle with a powerful engine running.)

In a spectacular case of resonance, vibrations set up in the Tacoma Narrows Bridge by strong winds led to its famous collapse (Fig 6.16). The amplitude of vibration of the bridge became larger and larger until the bridge broke up.

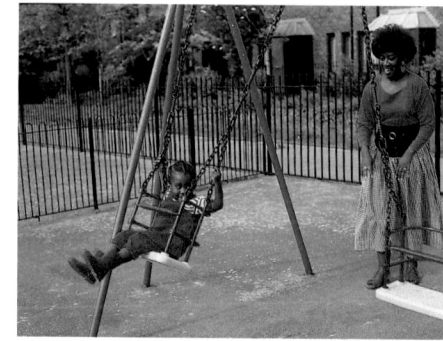

Fig 6.15 An adult pushing a child on a swing takes care not to reach a dangerous amplitude

Fig 6.16 Tacoma Narrows Bridge, known during its short life as Galloping Gertie because it oscillated in the wind. It took a wind of only 42 mph to make it collapse. (The newspaper reporter who owned the car crawled to safety)

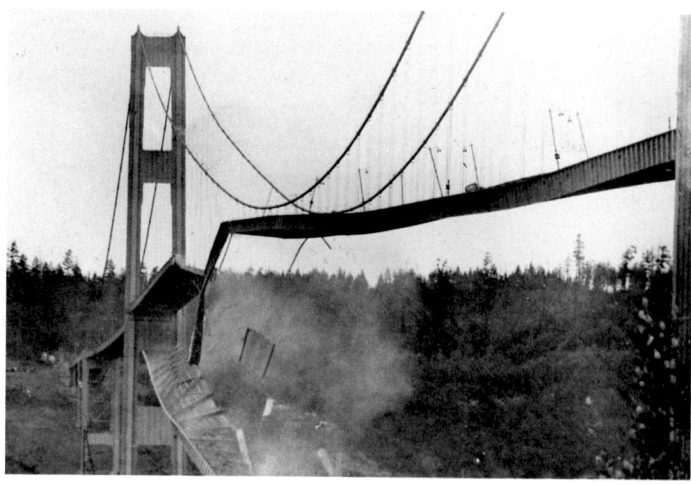

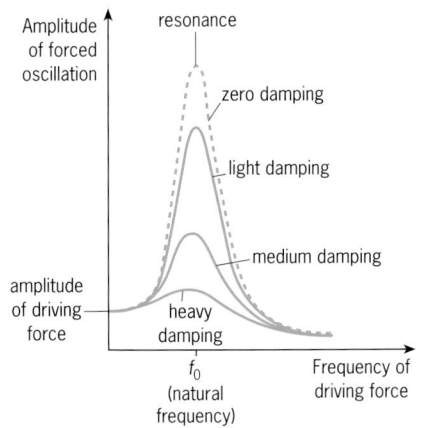

Fig 6.17 Resonance curves for a driven system with natural frequency f_0

Soldiers marching across a bridge can make it resonate. In 1850, 200 soldiers marching in step across a bridge in Angers, France, lost their lives when the resonance between the frequency of their steps and the natural frequency of the bridge caused the bridge to collapse. To avoid this, soldiers break step across bridges. It has proved necessary to damp out the oscillations set up by pedestrians when they walked across the Millennium Bridge built over the River Thames in central London.

In a car, you get uncomfortable vibrations due to resonance at particular speeds of either the engine or the vehicle itself. If resonance were set up in a turbine or a jet engine, it is possible that the engine would disintegrate. So we can see that it is important to avoid resonance in structures and vehicles.

Damping prevents the build-up of amplitude. Fig 6.17 shows how the amplitude of vibration of an oscillating system varies with the frequency of the driving force and also shows how damping affects the resonance curves. When the frequency of the driving force equals the natural frequency of the system being driven, the oscillations build up and can become totally uncontrollable.

Resonance can be used to advantage, however, and not only in pushing swings. Resonance is used to amplify the desired frequency when tuning an electrical circuit (see Chapter 12).

COUPLED PENDULUMS

If two identical oscillators can interact then they will exchange energy, just as the soldiers marching in Angers exchanged energy with the bridge with disastrous results.

A pair of pendulums of the same length can be connected to a common support and set swinging, as shown in Fig 6.18(a). It helps to lightly link the pendulums, but often enough energy can pass through the support itself. When pendulum 1 is set swinging, its energy gradually leaks through to pendulum 2 until all energy is transferred and it is stationary. Pendulum 2 has now achieved maximum amplitude and starts to pass the energy back to pendulum 1; and so on.

As a variation of this demonstration, the so-called Barton's pendulums are suspended from one length of string, as in Fig 6.18(b). There is one heavy pendulum (the driver), and a series of pendulums with bobs of smaller equal mass. The lengths of the pendulums differ but one is of equal length to the driver pendulum. It is this one which starts to vibrate with the largest amplitude.

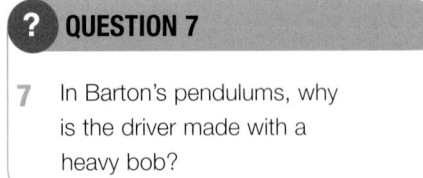

? QUESTION 7

7   In Barton's pendulums, why is the driver made with a heavy bob?

Fig 6.18 Two types of coupled pendulum systems

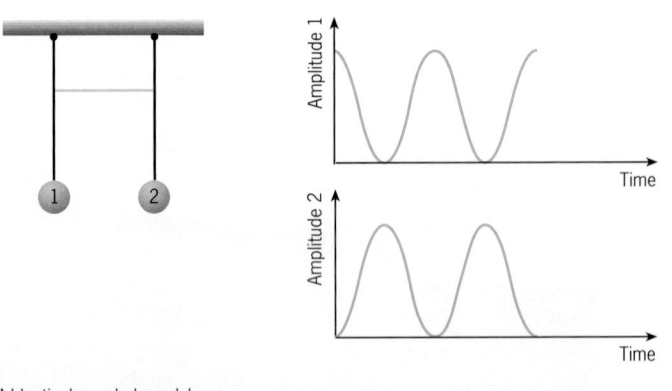

(a) Identical coupled pendulums. The graphs show how the amplitudes of the pendulums vary with time

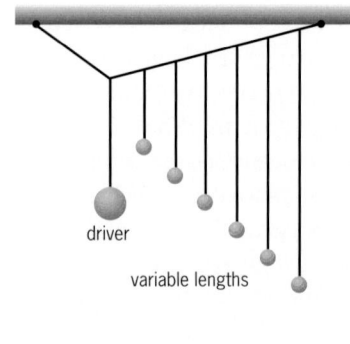

(b) Barton's pendulums

5 WAVES AS OSCILLATIONS

We have seen that oscillations are periodic. We know that waves are also periodic. Clearly there is a relationship between the two. In fact, an oscillating system can be used to set up waves in a mechanical system (Fig 6.19). Once the waves have been set off, they travel through the spring or other medium for long distances until the energy is dissipated.

There are different types of waves. Some need a substance to pass through – these are called mechanical waves. Such waves displace (i.e. move) the material which they pass through. However, there is no net motion of the material through which the waves travel, as displaced material has moved back into its original position by the time the wave has passed through.

Examples of mechanical waves are seismic waves in the Earth, water waves on the surface of ponds and oceans, and sound waves through air. Seismic waves are usually set up by earthquakes but can be caused by nuclear explosions. The speed with which they travel depends on the medium and the type of wave.

There are other waves, called electromagnetic waves, which require no medium to travel in. These waves are covered in Chapter 15.

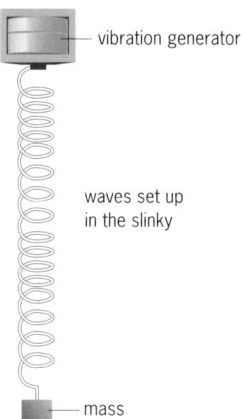

Fig 6.19 Setting off waves using a vibrating system

TRANSVERSE AND LONGITUDINAL WAVES

Mechanical waves can be classified as transverse or longitudinal according to how they travel (Fig 6.20). Both types of wave can be demonstrated using a slinky (a long steel spring). The transverse wave occurs when the coils move *at right angles* to the direction of motion of the wave, with the motion along the length of the slinky. To produce a transverse wave, the slinky is rested on a flat surface and one end is moved from side to side, setting up the oscillation and hence the travelling wave.

The end of the slinky can also be moved in and out along its axis. The coils undergo compression, followed by rarefaction when the coils open out. Displacement of the coils is now *along* the axis of the spring; this is a longitudinal wave.

Fig 6.20 Transverse and longitudinal waves in a slinky

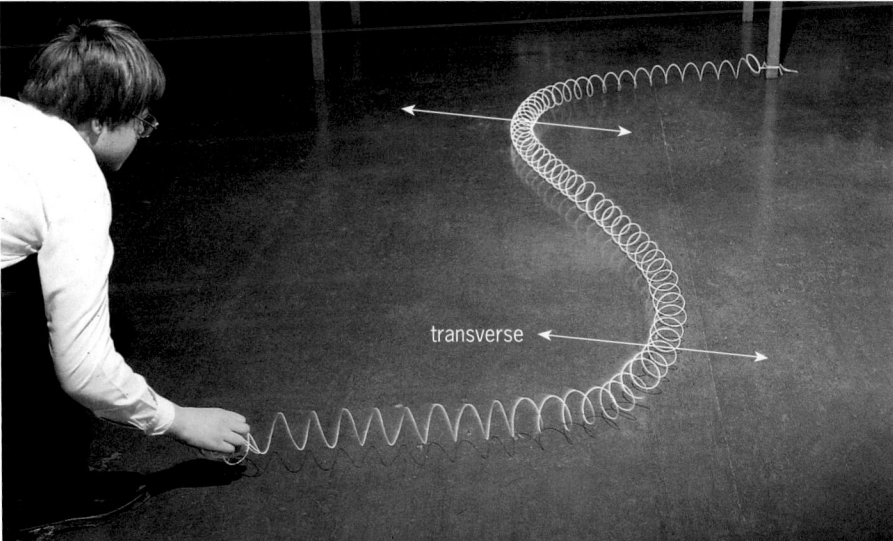

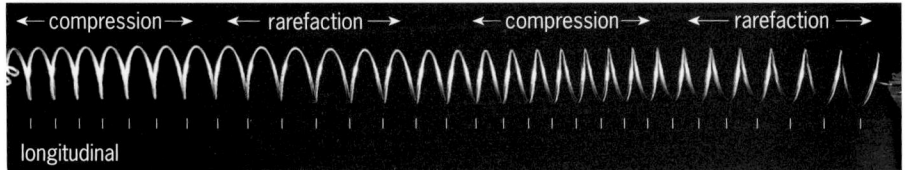

TRAVELLING AND STATIONARY WAVES

When we start a wave in the slinky, either transverse or longitudinal, we can watch it travel from one end to the other. Because it progresses along the slinky it is called a travelling (or alternatively a progressive) wave. However, if the far end of the slinky is fixed, waves are reflected back. These can combine with the next waves which are travelling forwards. At the right combination of frequency and speed, the waves travelling in opposite directions can produce a stationary or standing wave. In this chapter we shall consider both types.

6 SETTING UP TRAVELLING WAVES

In general, waves spread out once they are generated, like the ripples in a pond when a pebble is dropped into it. The spreading of waves, both transverse and longitudinal, is looked at in detail in Chapter 15. Here, we restrict ourselves to setting up linear waves such as along a slinky, in a string or in an organ pipe.

Transverse waves are easier to show, so let us look at transverse waves set up in a stretched string. With care, we can set up a single pulse in the string and watch it travel, as shown in Fig 6.21(a). Although the pulse maintains its shape, its amplitude is likely to decrease as it passes along the string. Such pulses can continue for long distances.

We can also set up in the string a wave train consisting of a number of waves. It too will travel down the string and preserve its shape – see Fig 6.21(b). Alternatively, by continuing to vibrate one end of the string, we can establish a continuous wave travelling along the string, as shown in Fig 6.21(c).

Fig 6.21 Transverse waves travelling along a stretched string

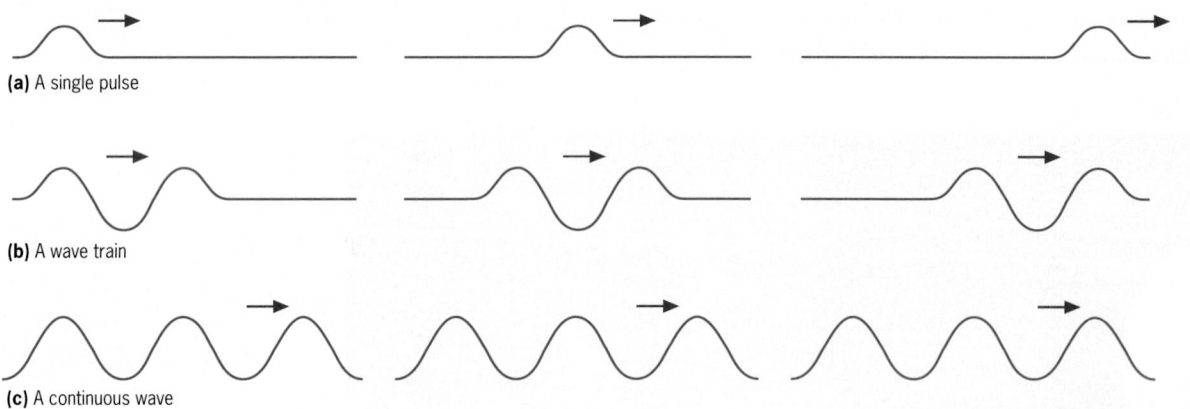

(a) A single pulse

(b) A wave train

(c) A continuous wave

There are a number of features of these waves to notice. First, the speed of the pulse, wave train or continuous wave passing down the string is independent of the frequency with which the end is vibrated, and is also independent of the amplitude of the waves established. The speed depends on the nature of the string only. It is because the speed is constant that the shape of the pulse or wave remains the same.

Fig 6.22(a) shows a single wave as it progresses along a string. Suppose the wave moves by exactly its own length during a time T, as shown in Fig 6.22(b). The wave has moved by a single wavelength λ. The velocity of the wave is the distance travelled divided by time and so we have:

$$v = \frac{\lambda}{T}$$

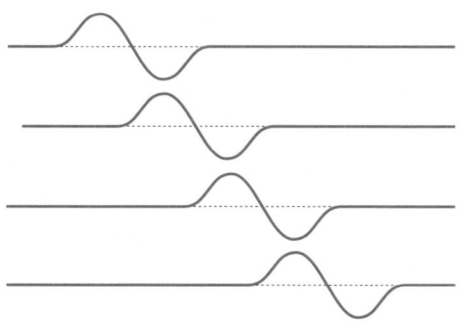

(a) A progressive wave moving along a string

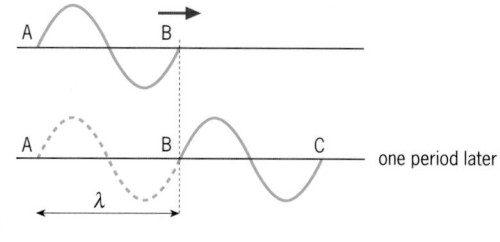

(b) Movement of the wave in time T

one period later

Fig 6.22 Travelling (progressive) waves

As the time T is the time of travel through one complete oscillation, the wave will have moved from AB to BC and a succeeding wave will have moved into position AB, as shown by the broken line in the drawing. T is the period of vibration. Also, the frequency of vibration f is given by:

$$f = \frac{1}{T}$$

so that we have:

$$v = \frac{\lambda}{T} = f \times \lambda$$

speed = frequency × wavelength

This simple wave formula applies to all waves. The frequency of the wave is the frequency of vibration used to set up the waves from the end of the string. As the speed is a characteristic of the string, wavelength in a given string will depend on the frequency of the oscillating source.

Another important property of the wave is its amplitude A, which is the maximum displacement of any point on the wave, or any point on the string, from the zero displacement position. The properties are summarised in Fig 6.23.

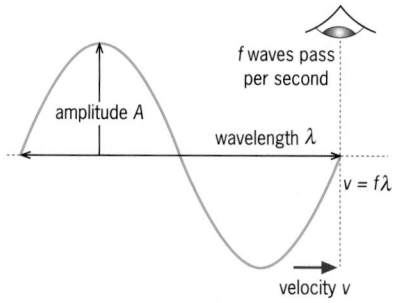

f waves pass per second

amplitude A

wavelength λ

$v = f\lambda$

velocity v

Fig 6.23 Properties that define a wave

? QUESTION 8

8   A wave moves along a string with velocity 0.60 m s^{-1}. Its wavelength is 20 cm. Calculate the frequency and period of the wave.

SCIENCE IN CONTEXT

Boat sets up a soliton

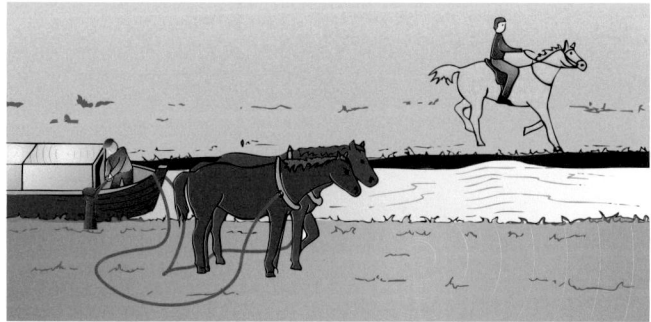

A single pulse has been given the special name of soliton. It is not easy to set one up in a string, but the transmission of solitons along optic fibres is important in optical signal communications.

In 1834, John Scott-Russell was walking by the Forth–Clyde canal when he saw a large-scale soliton and wrote this description of it.

'I was observing the motion of a boat which was rapidly drawn along a narrow channel by a pair of horses, when the boat suddenly stopped – not so the mass of water in the channel which it had put in motion; it accumulated round the prow of the vessel in a state of violent agitation, then suddenly leaving it behind, rolled forward with great velocity, assuming the form of a large solitary elevation, a rounded, smooth and well-defined heap of water, which continued its course along the channel apparently without change of form or diminution of speed. I followed it on horseback, and overtook it still rolling on at a rate of some eight or nine miles an hour, preserving its original figure some thirty feet long and a foot to a foot and a half in height. Its height gradually diminished, and after a chase of one or two miles I lost it in the windings of the channel. Such, in the month of August 1834, was my first chance interview with that singular and beautiful phenomenon.'

If one could set up a wave machine across the canal in order to establish continuous waves down the canal of a wavelength comparable with the separation of the canal banks, then these waves would keep going over a long distance without disruption. This is what happens on a much smaller scale when light pulses are sent long distances down a monomode optical fibre.

Wave equation and phase angle

When a vibration generator causes a wave train to travel along a string, there is a sideways displacement to the string given by:

$$y = A \sin \omega t \quad \text{where} \quad \omega = 2\pi f$$

Note that y is varying with time t and so we can write it as $y(t)$ to mean that y depends on t. We can use x for distance along the string. The generator is at the end where $x = 0$. So we can write the displacement of the end of the string connected to the generator as:

$$y(0,t) = A \sin \omega t$$

On page 122 we said that the displacement y of an oscillating trolley could be represented by $A \cos \theta$ where θ is the angular displacement around a circle. However, this time we need to start from the zero displacement position so that $y = A \sin \theta$. We can write:

$$y(0,t) = A \sin \theta$$

Further along the string, the displacement will be out of step by an amount which depends on how far one goes along the string. It is as if we have moved by an additional angular displacement corresponding to a distance x along the string. With phase angle Φ, we have:

$$y(x,t) = A \sin(\theta + \Phi)$$

As $\theta = \omega t$, we can rewrite this as:

$$y(x,t) = A \sin(\omega t + \Phi)$$

9 At time $t = 0$, the maximum transverse displacement for a small segment of a vibrating string is 2 cm. What is the displacement for a segment of the string which is vibrating out of phase by 35°?

SHOWING THE MEANING OF PHASE ANGLE

Consider a shadow arrangement similar to that shown in Fig 6.4 (page 122), but this time with *two* spheres mounted on the turntable. The spheres are both at the same distance from the centre, with an angular separation Φ. In Fig 6.24 we use the example $\Phi = 90°$.

Sphere A is shown in line with the lamp and the screen. This means that at time $t = 0$, the displacement x_A of the sphere is zero, that is $x_A = 0$ at $t = 0$.

We now consider a later time t when sphere B has come directly into line between the lamp and the screen. The displacement of the shadow of sphere A is now given by:

$$x_A = A \sin \omega t$$
$$= A \sin(\pi/2)$$

as the turntable has moved through 90°.

Meanwhile, the displacement of the shadow of B is given by:

$$x_B = A \sin 0$$

since the sphere is directly between the lamp and the screen. If we write the displacement of B in the form:

$$x_B = A \sin(\omega t + \Phi)$$
$$= A \sin(\pi/2 + \Phi)$$

then:

$$0 = \pi/2 + \Phi \quad \text{or} \quad \Phi = -\pi/2$$

The phase angle for B is the angle that it lags A around the turntable. Displacements for A and B are plotted in Fig 6.24 for Φ equal to $-\pi/2$.

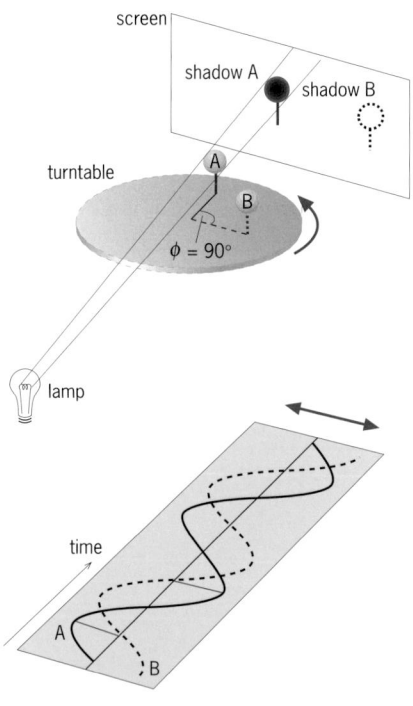

Displacement of the shadows on the screen
B lags A by an angle ϕ (=90° here)

Fig 6.24 Demonstrating phase angle

7 SETTING UP STATIONARY WAVES

Stationary waves are set up in stringed instruments such as a guitar (Fig 6.25). What we see is the string vibrating from side to side. At the moment that the string is plucked, a progressive transverse wave is set up travelling out from that point. It meets the fixed end of the string and is reflected back. The amplitudes of the two waves add together as they meet.

The string vibrates naturally at certain frequencies because it is fixed at both ends. When the outgoing and reflected waves are added together subject to this condition, a stationary wave is set up in the string. If the string is plucked centrally we get the fundamental mode (shape of wave). In this case, the string vibrates with maximum displacement at the central position (called the antinode) and the displacement falls away to zero at the two ends (called nodes).

We can investigate stationary waves in the laboratory using a stretched string or a long rubber band. The string is stretched from a fixed support over a pulley and is held taut by a suspended mass (Fig 6.26). A vibration generator is tied to the string near one end.

The frequency of vibration is altered starting from a low value, usually with little effect on the stretched string. As the frequency increases, the vibration generator reaches a particular frequency at which the string suddenly starts vibrating strongly, see (a). Resonance is occurring. The natural frequency of the string is now equal to that of the vibration generator. This resonance frequency is the fundamental frequency f_0 of the string, sometimes called the first harmonic.

As we increase the frequency of the vibration generator further, oscillation of the string is rapidly reduced. We notice little movement until the generator frequency has doubled to $2f_0$. Now the envelope of the string (the shape the vibrating string encloses) has altered. There are three nodes, one at each end and one in the middle, see (b). This means that there are two antinodes positioned a quarter of the string length from each end. These two antinodes are vibrating out of phase and there is a phase difference of π. This frequency of vibration is referred to as the second harmonic or the first overtone.

If we increase the frequency further, we identify other resonant frequencies. The next is $3f_0$ with three antinodes on the string, see (c), and so on.

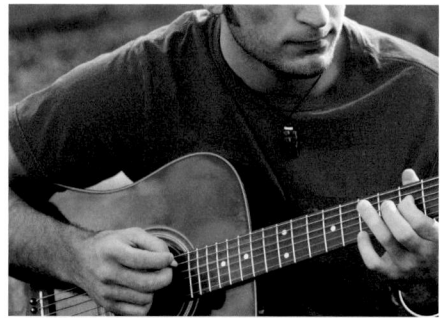
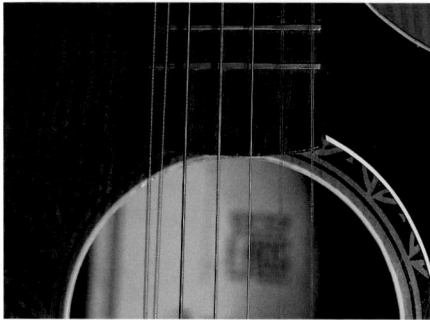

Fig 6.25 The high-speed lower photograph shows the bass and two top strings vibrating. The tension is least in the bass string, hence the amplitude of the wave is greatest

? QUESTION 10

10 A string vibrates with a fundamental frequency of 350 Hz. What is the frequency of
a) the first overtone and
b) the fourth harmonic?

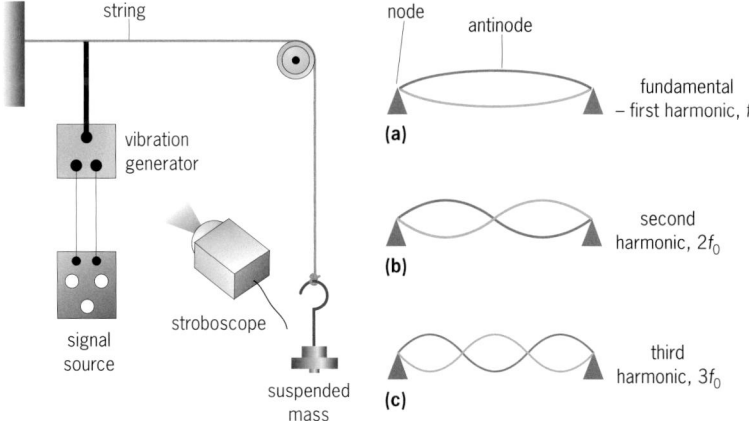

Fig. 6.26 Stationary waves on a stretched string (or rubber band)

REFLECTED WAVES

Let us look in more detail at how to set up standing waves. We set off a short wave on a slinky which has been firmly fixed at its far end. Assume that the wave consists of one and a half wavelengths, as in Fig 6.27(a). The wave travels along the slinky until it reaches the far end.

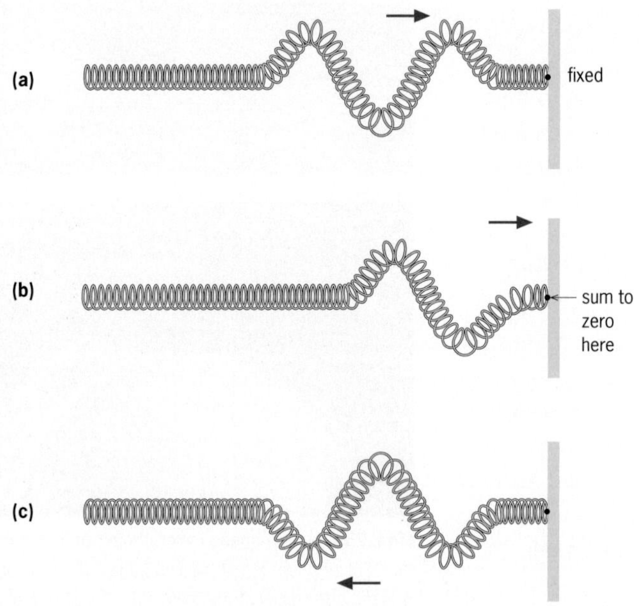

At this point, the wave can travel no further forwards and is reflected back, as in (b). This means that the velocity has changed sign. In addition, the phase of the wave has changed. If the displacement of the forward wave is upwards at the instant of time when it reaches the far end, then its displacement is downwards on reflection. This makes sense. At the fixed end, the displacements (note) of the incoming and outgoing waves sum to zero. This must be so because there can be no displacement of the string at the fixed point. The reflected wave is out of phase by π. It passes back 'through' the forward wave (think how ripples can pass through each other on the surface of a pond). Where the two waves overlap, the displacement of the slinky is the sum of the two waves. But, eventually, we see the reflected wave emerge complete and pass back along the slinky, as in (c).

The frequency, velocity and wavelength of the wave all remain the same in reflection. If no energy is lost at the far end, the amplitude of the reflected wave equals that of the incoming one. The phase difference of π which we have identified and which is illustrated by Figs 6.27(a) and (c) is crucial to the setting up of standing waves.

When waves pass through each other, the displacement at any point is the sum of the individual displacements of the two waves passing in opposite directions. Fig 6.28(a) shows the relative positions of two waves travelling in opposite directions. Work out for yourself what pattern you will see. The answer is given in Fig 6.28(b).

STANDING WAVES ON A STRING

Let us consider a progressive transverse wave on a string with an exact number of complete wavelengths in its length.

It is not easy to see what happens at all times, so let us select certain special times. We start with $t = 0$ when the displacement of the *forward* wave is maximum at both the initial and far ends, though of course this displacement will be modified by the reflected wave. Fig 6.29 shows the situation with the forward, reflected and summed waves at this time $t = 0$, and at a series of times during the first half-period. We could go on to show the waves for the second half-period in a similar way in order to complete the overall pattern. The envelope for all possibilities is shown in the final diagram.

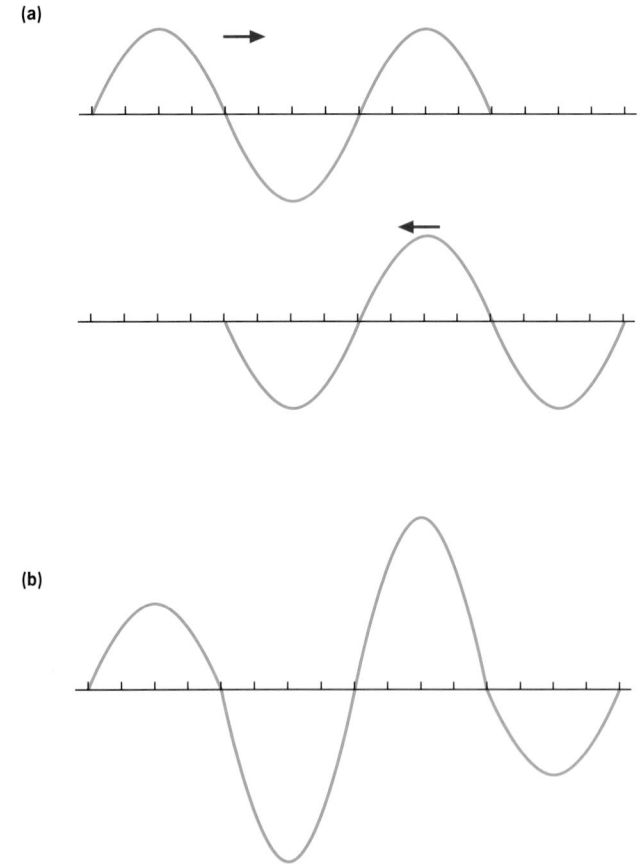

(a) fixed

(b) sum to zero here

(c)

Fig 6.27 Forward and reflected waves on a slinky

(a)

(b)

Fig 6.28 (a) Relative positions of two waves travelling in opposite directions.
(b) Sum of the displacements of the two waves in **(a)**

Frequency of standing waves on a string

We have seen that, as there are always nodes at the ends of the string, there must be a whole number, n, of half-wavelengths between each end. With a string length l, this means that:

$$n\frac{\lambda}{2} = l$$

or:

$$\lambda = \frac{2l}{n}$$

It can be proved that, if T is the tension in the string and μ is the mass per unit length, the velocity c of a wave down a string is given by:

$$c = \sqrt{\frac{T}{\mu}}$$

(The derivation of this formula is beyond the scope of this book.)

We already know that $c = f\lambda$, where f is the frequency of vibration. So:

$$f = \frac{c}{\lambda} = \frac{n}{2l}c = \frac{n}{2l}\sqrt{\frac{T}{\mu}}$$

STANDING WAVES USING SOUND WAVES OR MICROWAVES

Sound waves are longitudinal waves in air (or another medium) similar to longitudinal waves in a slinky. They consist of compressions and rarefactions in the air. By sending sound waves from a loudspeaker and reflecting them from a *hard* surface, standing waves are established in the air. There will be regions where the air molecules are vibrating back and forth strongly (antinodes) and other regions where there is no movement of the air (nodes). By moving a microphone between the loudspeaker and the reflecting surface (Fig 6.30), the variation of displacement can be shown on an oscilloscope.

Instead of a loudspeaker, we can use a microwave transmitter. In this case, instead of a microphone and oscilloscope we then use a microwave receiver and ammeter. A metal plate acts as reflector. Although the experiment is similar, the nature of the waves themselves is very different. Microwaves are electromagnetic waves, which you will meet in Chapter 15.

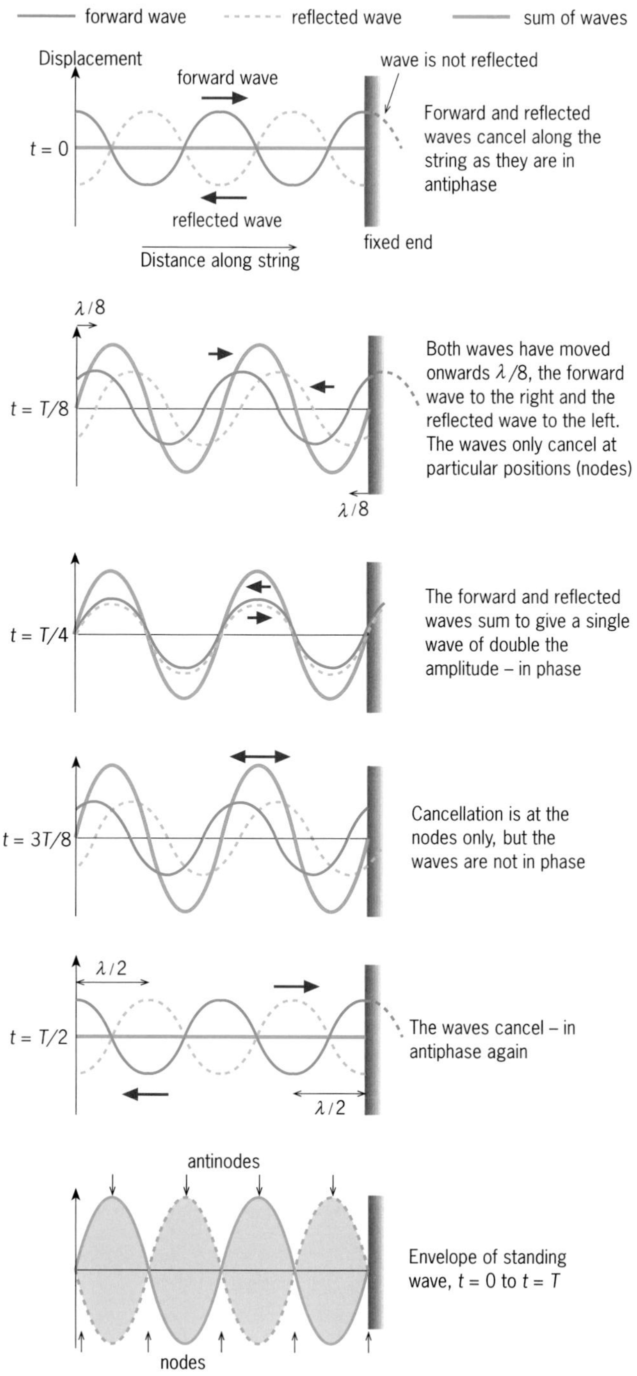

Fig 6.29 How a standing wave is set up from the combination of forward and reflected waves

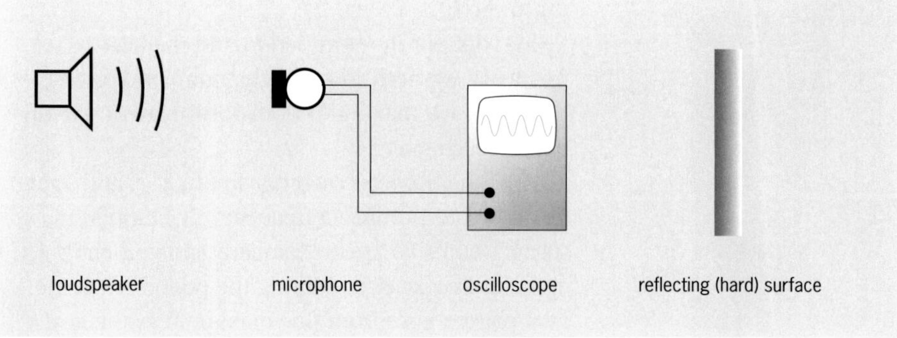

Fig 6.30 Demonstration of standing waves using sound waves

? QUESTION 11

11 Show that the units of $\sqrt{T/\mu}$ are the same as those of c.

STANDING WAVES IN AN ORGAN PIPE

These are sound waves and therefore longitudinal waves. They are set up by the compression and rarefaction of the air within the pipe. Nodes and antinodes occur just as they do for a vibrating string. But there is a difference. In the case of a string, both ends are effectively held fixed in order to establish the standing wave. In an organ pipe, vibrations can be set up either with both ends of the pipe open or with one end closed and the other open. At a closed end there must be a node present, and at an open end there must be an antinode (the air vibrates freely back and forth). The two situations are summarised in Fig 6.31.

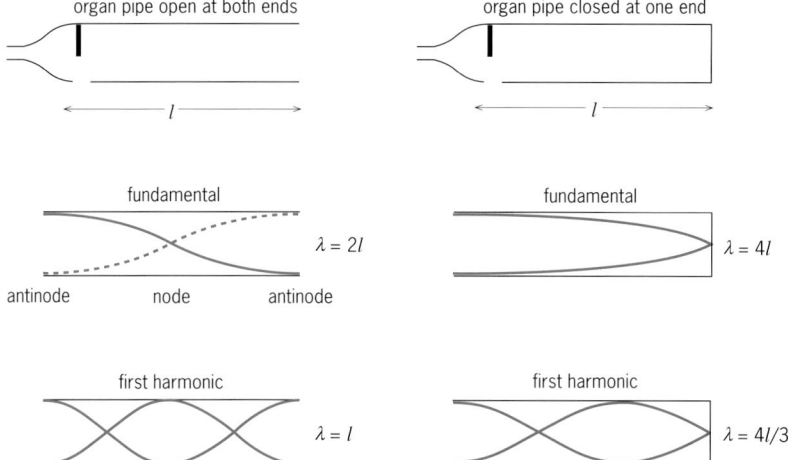

Fig 6.31 Modes of vibration for standing waves in an organ pipe

? QUESTION 12

12 a) An organ pipe is open at both ends. Calculate the length required such that the lowest frequency of vibration is 512 Hz.
b) What would be the required length for an organ pipe closed at one end?
Take the velocity of sound in air as 330 m s^{-1}.

BEATS

Suppose we tune two strings of a guitar to vibrate at almost, but not quite, the same frequency. Plucked simultaneously, the volume of the sound produced by them appears to rise and fall continuously. This rise and fall has a fixed frequency called the beat frequency. What is happening is that the sound waves produced by the two guitar strings interfere and our ears detect the variation of the resultant intensity. Maximum intensity is heard when the waves add together (interfere constructively) and minimum intensity is heard when the waves cancel each other out (interfere destructively).

We can see what is happening by adding together the two separate waves as shown in Fig 6.32(a). The resultant, obtained by the principle of superposition, is shown in Fig 6.32(b).

To work out the beat period and the beat frequency we need to know the number of cycles between each maximum of the beat pattern. We do this for each string.

The time between each maximum is T, and string 1 is tuned to produce a frequency f_1. During time T, string 1 emits f_1T cycles. Similarly, string 2 emits f_2T cycles at frequency f_2. During the period when the beat pattern goes from one maximum to the next maximum there must be one cycle difference

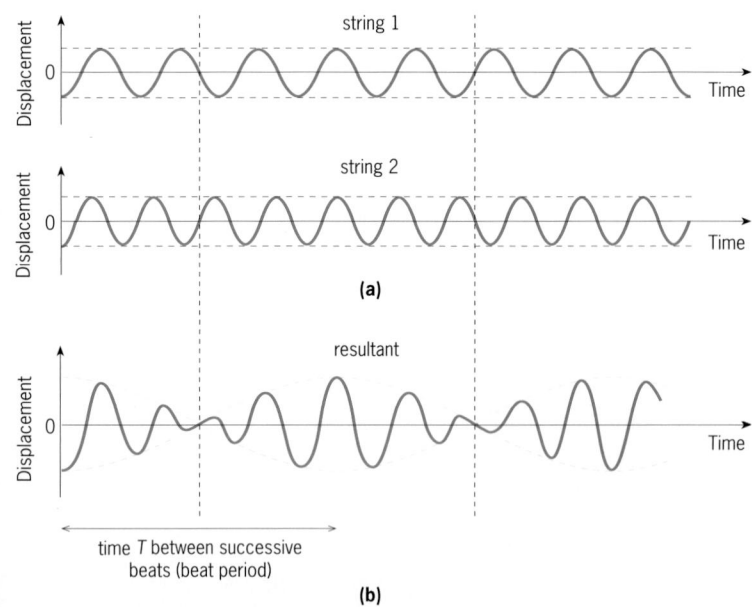

Fig 6.32 Setting up beats. Check that string 2 goes through one more cycle than string 1 during the beat period

between the waves from the two strings. The waves start in phase at the maximum, gradually go out of phase, and come back into phase, with a difference of one cycle (and only one cycle).

So:

$$f_2 T - f_1 T = 1$$

This gives:

$$T(f_2 - f_1) = 1$$

$$T = \frac{1}{f_2 - f_1}$$

The beat frequency f_B is given by:

$$f_B = \frac{1}{\text{beat period}} = \frac{1}{T}$$

Therefore:

$$f_B = f_2 - f_1$$

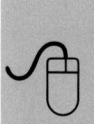

QUESTION 13

13 A tuning fork vibrating at 256 Hz and a vibrating guitar string produce beats at a frequency of 2.5 Hz. Obtain two possible values for the frequency of vibration of the guitar string. Suggest how you might determine experimentally which value is correct.

Sinusoidal waves can be added together to produce other wave shapes. This is explored in the How Science Works assignment for this chapter at www.collinseducation.co.uk/CAS

8 THE DOPPLER EFFECT

So far we have talked about setting up waves and the need to observe or detect them. In the case of transmitted sound waves we can use a microphone connected to a loudspeaker or oscilloscope to detect them. We are assuming that when we do this both the emitter of the sound waves and the detector are stationary. But what happens if one is moving relative to another? Is what we observe changed in any way? In Chapter 1 (pages 7–8) we saw that there were changes in the case of radar waves and that the police use the effect to determine the speed of motorists. Here we look at the effect, called the **Doppler effect**, in more detail. The effect is not restricted to electromagnetic waves, as you will realise if you listen to the siren on a police car or ambulance as it approaches and then travels away. The Doppler effect is the change in frequency produced when a source of waves moves relative to the observer, although there must be a component of the movement directly towards or away from the observer or source.

STATIONARY SOURCE AND STATIONARY OBSERVER

Fig 6.33 shows the sound waves emitted by a source S at a speed v and a frequency f. This is the frequency heard by the observer O when both are at rest. We also assume that the medium is air and that it is not moving. In fact, we shall assume that the air is not moving in all cases we consider. Below the figure, the *observed* wavelength λ' is denoted and here this is the same as the wavelength of the sound emitted.

STATIONARY SOURCE AND MOVING OBSERVER

Now we consider a stationary source with an *observer moving towards it* at speed v_o, as in Fig 6.34. The wavelength of the sound is not affected by the movement of the observer. But the observer crosses more wave crests per second than would a stationary observer. This means that the speed of the waves relative to the observer has increased. The relative speed will now be $v + v_o$. This increase of speed, but with the wavelength the same, means an increase in observed frequency. If this observed frequency is f', the wave formula gives us:

$$v + v_o = f'\lambda \quad \text{or} \quad f' = \frac{v + v_o}{\lambda}$$

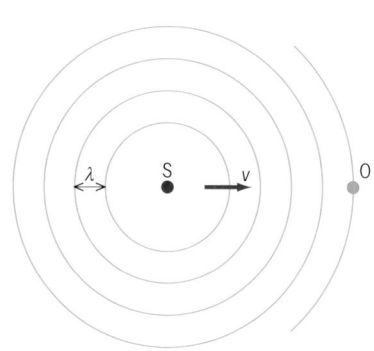

For observer: $f' = f$

Wave speed = v

$\lambda' = \lambda = \dfrac{v}{f}$

Fig 6.33 Source and observer are stationary

REMEMBER THIS

period is the inverse of frequency

$$T = \frac{1}{f}$$

wave speed

= wavelength × frequency

$$v = f\lambda$$

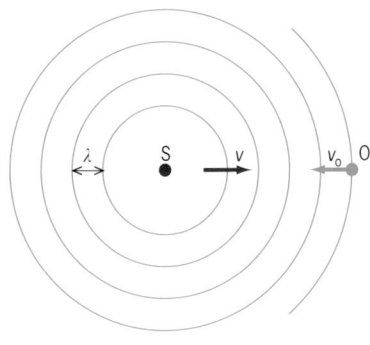

For observer: $f' > f$

Wave speed $= (v + v_o)$

$f'\lambda = (v + v_o)$

Fig 6.34 A stationary source with an observer moving towards it

The frequency as emitted by the source is $f = v/\lambda$, so the ratio of frequencies is:

$$\frac{\text{observed frequency}}{\text{source frequency}} = \frac{f'}{f} = \frac{v + v_o}{v} = 1 + \frac{v_o}{v}$$

If the observer is moving *towards* the source the observed frequency *increases*.

Also, the change of frequency is

$$f' - f = \Delta f = \frac{fv_o}{v}$$

If the observer is moving *away* from the source then fewer crests are crossed per second. The formula becomes

$$\frac{f'}{f} = \frac{v - v_o}{v} = 1 - \frac{v_o}{v}$$

If the observer is moving *away* from the source the observed frequency *decreases*.

The formulae for the two cases are often combined as:

$$f' = f(1 \pm \frac{v_o}{v}) \quad \text{or alternatively} \quad \Delta f = \pm \frac{fv_o}{v}$$

STATIONARY OBSERVER AND MOVING SOURCE

Fig 6.35 shows what happens when the *source* is moving towards a stationary observer at a steady speed v_s.

The effect is to *reduce* the wavelength, because in a given time more waves fill the space between source and observer than when both are at rest, as in Fig 6.33. The observed frequency thus increases – the observer is passed by more crests in that time. But the waves pass at the same speed. The observed frequency is f' and there is, as a consequence, an observed wavelength λ', which is different from the actual wavelength at the emitter:

$$\lambda' = \frac{v}{f'}$$

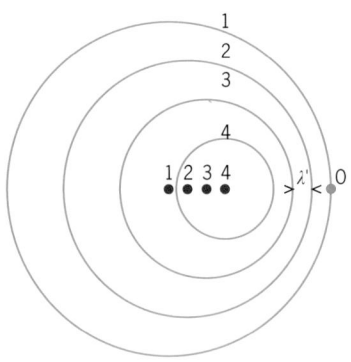

● = position of moving source S

The numbered waves correspond to the changing positions of the source

$$f' = f\left(\frac{1}{1 - \frac{v_s}{v}}\right)$$

Fig 6.35 A source moving towards a stationary observer

How the value of this new wavelength and hence the observed frequency is found is shown in the Stretch and Challenge box opposite. This frequency is

$$f' = f\left[\frac{1}{1 - v_s/v}\right]$$

This confirms that:

when the source moves *towards* the observer the observed frequency *increases*.

If the speed of the waves is very large, as in the case of electromagnetic waves (i.e. $v \gg v_s$), then the formula again becomes $\Delta f = fv_o/v$.

If the source is moving *away* the formula becomes:

$$f' = f\left[\frac{1}{1 + v_s/v}\right]$$

When the source moves *away* from the observer the observed frequency *decreases*.

BOTH SOURCE AND OBSERVER MOVING

One can now deduce from the above analysis that if both the source and the observer are moving then the observed frequency will be

$$f' = f\left[\frac{v \pm v_o}{v \pm v_s}\right]$$

where we use:

$+v_o$ when observer is approaching source
$-v_o$ when observer is receding from source
$-v_s$ when source is approaching observer
$+v_s$ when source is receding from observer

You may wish to check that this formula reduces to the appropriate earlier equations.

Motion towards each other increases frequency; motion away decreases frequency.

POSTSCRIPT: THE DOPPLER EFFECT WITH ELECTROMAGNETIC WAVES

On page 8 you saw the application of the police radar gun. This uses electromagnetic waves, so that the approximation of $v \gg v_s$ applies. Here there was reflection of waves off a moving vehicle so that the relative change of frequency was doubled ($\Delta f = 2fv_o/v$).

The main application of the Doppler effect in A-level concerns the shift of frequency of light waves, the so-called **red shift**, as observed from distant objects in the Universe that are receding as a consequence of the Big Bang. A full *relativistic* derivation of the Doppler effect formula would not be appropriate at A-level. Red shift and what it tells us will be considered in more detail in Chapter 26.

? QUESTION 14

14 Imagine you are standing on a railway bridge as a train approaches, passes underneath, and goes into the distance. As it does so, its siren is sounding. Describe what changes you notice to the sound of the siren.

STRETCH AND CHALLENGE

Deriving the observed frequency from a moving source

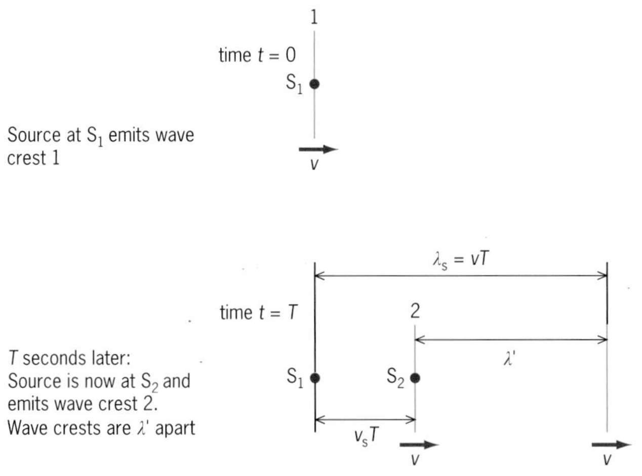

Fig 6.36 Doppler effect due to a moving source

Fig 6.36 helps us to find the value of the new wavelength. In the time T, where T is the period of the oscillation, the wave crest moves a distance vT. But in that time, the source has moved a distance v_sT, so the next crest is just λ' behind its predecessor, and as the diagram shows:

$$\lambda' = vT - v_sT$$

Now, period $T = 1/f$, and $\lambda' = v/f'$, so that we can express this as:

$$\frac{v}{f'} = \frac{v}{f} - \frac{v_s}{f} = \frac{1}{f}(v - v_s)$$

which may be rewritten as:

$$f' = f\left[\frac{v}{v - v_s}\right]$$

or, as usually quoted:

$$f' = f\left[\frac{1}{1 - v_s/v}\right]$$

This confirms that when the source moves towards the observer (v_s is positive) the observed frequency *increases*.

SUMMARY

After studying this chapter you should understand the following concepts and be able to use the following equations:

- The meaning of amplitude A, period T and frequency f of a wave and the relationship $T = 1/f = 2\pi/\omega$.

- The meaning of speed v and wavelength l of a wave and the relationship $v = f\lambda$.

- A mechanical wave needs a medium through which to pass. Waves may be longitudinal or transverse.

- The period of a simple pendulum is given by

$$T = 2\pi\sqrt{l/g}$$

  and the period of a mass–spring system is given by

$$T = 2\pi\sqrt{m/k}$$

- In simple harmonic motion (s.h.m.), acceleration is directly proportional to displacement from a fixed point and directed towards this point: $a = -\omega^2 x$.

- The velocity of a mass m under s.h.m. is given by

$$v = \pm\omega\sqrt{\left(A^2 - x^2\right)}$$

- The meaning of the terms: oscillator, displacement, node, antinode, harmonic, overtone, phase difference, damping.

- There is a transfer of energy between kinetic and potential forms during s.h.m.

- The difference between stationary (standing) and progressive (travelling) waves.

- A progressive wave can be represented by $y(x,t) = A \sin(\omega t + \Phi)$ where Φ is the phase angle.

- Energy can be exchanged between a driving system and a driven vibrating system. Resonance occurs when their frequencies are equal.

- The superposition of two waves of almost equal frequencies f_1 and f_2 where $f_2 > f_1$ produces beats of frequency $f_2 - f_1$.

- If the source of a wave and an observer are moving relative to each other, there is a Doppler shift of frequency. Motion towards increases the frequency; motion away decreases the frequency.

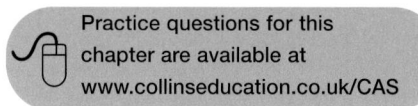

Practice questions for this chapter are available at www.collinseducation.co.uk/CAS

7

Ordinary matter

7 ORDINARY MATTER

Dry ice used for cleaning objects

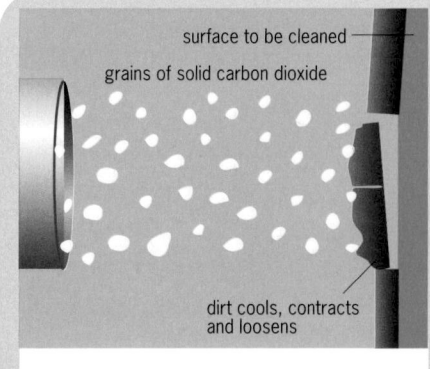

surface to be cleaned

grains of solid carbon dioxide

dirt cools, contracts
and loosens

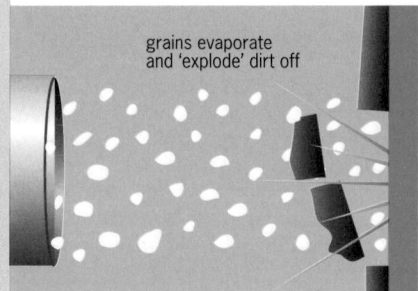

grains evaporate
and 'explode' dirt off

Cleaning machinery with dry ice

Solid carbon dioxide, called dry ice because it vaporises at −78 °C without first melting, is now being used as a cleaning agent to strip paint, oil and grime from machinery parts.

Equipment like a sandblaster sprays grains of dry ice at the parts. If paint is being removed, the number of layers that come away depends on the strength of the jet. The jet is controlled so that the material underneath will be undamaged.

The dirt is removed in two ways. First, since the temperature of the ice is −78 °C, the dirt cools rapidly and contracts, breaking its contact with the underlying material. Second, the hard grains of carbon dioxide chip away at the grime. Grains manage to pass through the dirt to the surface being cleaned. The impact heats the grains and they vaporise instantly, increasing their volume by 800 times. The gas forms little explosions behind the dirt and so strips it off.

The dry ice evaporates completely in the cleaning process, so it generates no waste, apart from the material it removes. So it merely returns a small amount of carbon dioxide to the environment, in contrast to the use of solvents in more conventional cleaning methods.

The ideas in this chapter

Every day, we see water pouring from a tap or moving in a river. We say it is **liquid**. Although water keeps the same volume as it moves, it does not keep its shape.

When water is cooled below 0 °C, it loses its ability to flow and turns to ice. Ice retains its shape as well as its volume. Before the days of refrigerators, blocks of ice were cut in winter (Fig 7.1) and stored in special ice-houses for keeping food cool in summer. The properties of ice are so different from those of water that we say that water changes its 'state of matter' (or 'phase') when it transforms to ice. It has become a **solid**.

When we heat water in a kettle to 100 °C, we get yet another state of matter – it becomes a **gas**. Most other materials exhibit these different states of matter, although they often do not change their phase under ordinary conditions of temperature and pressure.

There is a fourth state of matter (called **plasma**) which requires very high temperatures for its existence; see the Science in Context passage on page 147.

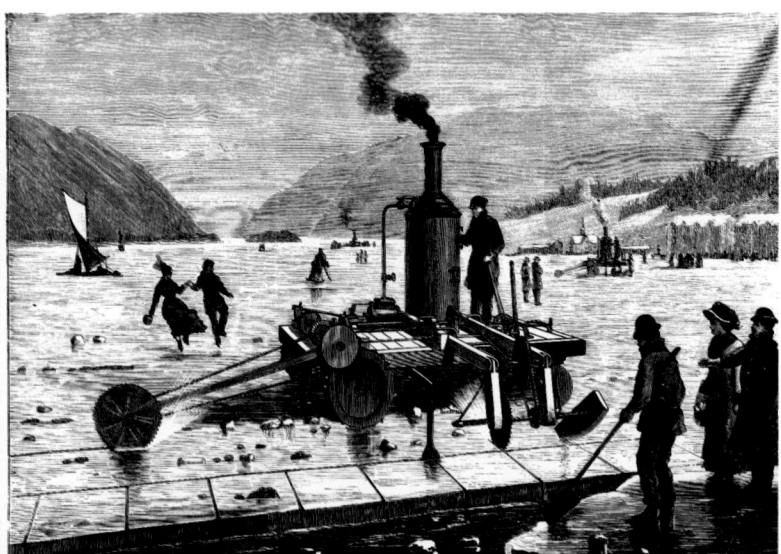

Fig 7.1 Cutting blocks of ice on the St Lawrence River in the nineteenth century

1 THE STATES OF MATTER

Liquid water is composed of molecules that are constantly moving. During the heating of water in a kettle these molecules begin to move around so rapidly that they leave the kettle and join the molecules of air in the room. The water is **evaporating** and becoming a gas. To some extent this would happen to the water even if it were not heated – heating simply speeds up the process. A gas does not keep to a fixed volume – the molecules disperse throughout the room.

Note that the 'steam' you see coming from a boiling kettle is not a gas. In fact, this 'steam' is made up of tiny droplets of water, produced when water vapour (gas) **condenses** in the cooler air. These droplets are then carried along in the gas flow.

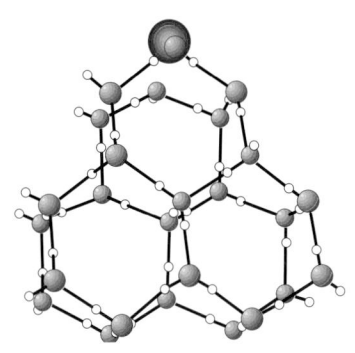

(a) ice

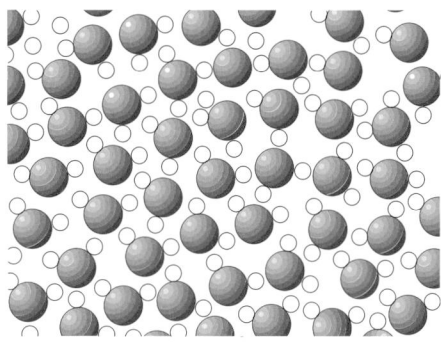

(b) water

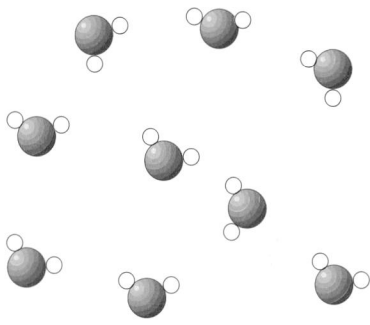

(c) water vapour (gas)

Fig 7.2 Pattern of atoms in ice, liquid water and water vapour (gas)

The main difference between the different states of matter is how the individual atoms or molecules are held (bound) together.

In a solid they are held so tightly that little movement is possible. The atoms or molecules can vibrate back and forth – the higher the temperature, the more they vibrate. But it is very difficult for them to push past each other. They take up a specific pattern in ice, for example, as shown in Fig 7.2(a).

In a liquid, the atoms or molecules are attracted but cannot move past each other easily. Water consists of molecules composed of two atoms of hydrogen and one of oxygen (Fig 7.2(b)), although a minute proportion of the molecules (1 in 10^7) may separate into oppositely charged particles called **ions**.

When the water becomes a gas, the gas molecules travel freely at high speeds, as we shall see later. The molecules are spaced wide apart (Fig 7.2(c)) – a gas is nearly one thousand times less dense than a solid.

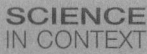

SCIENCE IN CONTEXT

Evaporation

When water evaporates the gaseous molecules have much more energy than the liquid water molecules. Only those molecules with enough energy can escape – that is why heating a liquid increases the rate of evaporation. The rate at which the liquid evaporates can also be increased by increasing the surface area of the liquid: the rate of evaporation is proportional to the surface area. The rate can also be increased by blowing a stream of air across the surface. This reduces the opportunity for the molecules to condense back again.

Evaporation is the method by which the human body controls its temperature. Sweat glands produce water on the surface of the body. When this water evaporates, energy is taken up by the water molecules and there is less energy left at the surface of the skin. Ultimately this produces a cooling effect on the body. A balance can be created between energy being produced by the body and energy being lost by evaporation such that a constant body temperature is maintained.

Table 7.1 Densities of common materials at room temperature (20 °C)

Substance	Density/kg m^{-3}
Solids	
Aluminium	2 700
Copper	8 930
Gold	19 300
Ice (0 °C)	917
Plastic (PVC)	1 300
Platinum	21 500
Uranium	19 000
Liquids	
Glycerol	1 260
Mercury	13 500
Olive oil	9200
Water	998
Gases	
Air	1.29
Carbon dioxide	1.98
Helium	0.177
Hydrogen	0.089 9
Oxygen	1.43

? QUESTION 1

1   What would happen to pond life if ice were denser than water?

So, the different states of matter have very different properties. One important property is density, usually labelled ρ (Greek 'rho'). Density is the mass per unit volume. That is, if M is the mass and V is the volume:

$$\text{density} = \frac{\text{mass}}{\text{volume}}$$

$$\rho = \frac{M}{V}$$

If we look at the densities of common materials at room temperature we should be able to identify their states. Table 7.1 gives this information for a selection of materials. The table also gives us some surprises.

There are large differences in density between gases and liquids and between gases and solids. The difference in density between a solid and a liquid is much less clear cut and there are some anomalies (peculiarities). For instance, the density of mercury at room temperature is higher than the density of copper – but mercury is a liquid because it can flow and copper is a solid because it is hard and can be cut. As another instance, glycerol as a liquid has a similar density to a typical plastic.

Most substances are denser as a solid than as a liquid. Yet compare water and ice: at 0 °C ice must be less dense than water, since ice forms on the surface of ponds and icebergs float on the surface of the sea. If the ice in the pond did not form on the surface but sank to the bottom, the entire pond would eventually freeze. We go to considerable lengths to insulate water pipes in winter because water expands as it freezes. When the water becomes ice its volume increases, so it breaks open the pipes. Because the ice cannot flow, a householder knows there is a problem when water doesn't flow – or when the ice turns back to water!

2 CHANGING THE STATE OF A SUBSTANCE

Let us continue to consider water. In order to turn it into ice we must reduce its temperature to 0 °C (zero Celsius) and then take away more energy thermally so that freezing begins. The usual method of extracting this heat is to cool the surroundings to below 0 °C so that the water loses energy to these surroundings.

The energy that water at 0 °C must lose so that it turns to ice at 0 °C is called the **latent heat of fusion**. It is energy that must be taken away from the molecules to reduce their ability to move around; its removal does not actually go towards reducing the temperature. The temperature at which this takes place is called the **temperature of fusion**. For water, the temperature of fusion is 0 °C. If we go in the other direction, that is, if we warm ice to turn it to water, this critical temperature is called the **temperature of melting**. Temperatures of fusion and melting are commonly called **melting points**.

To turn water into its gaseous state, we first heat it to 100 °C, the boiling temperature. We continue heating to provide the **latent heat of vaporisation**. This is the energy we must give to the water molecules to increase their separation and provide them with the kinetic energy they need to achieve the gaseous form. This kinetic energy is large, and the latent heat of vaporisation is greater than the latent heat of melting.

Fig 7.3 shows the change in temperature of a substance over time as it is heated at a constant rate through its different phases. During the periods of melting and

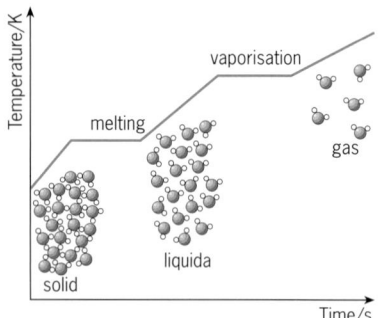

Fig 7.3 Variation of temperature of a substance as it is heated at a constant rate through its states of matter

vaporisation the temperature remains constant. The energy input provides the required latent heat.

Table 7.2 shows the latent heats required to convert 1 kg of some materials from one state to another. This is called *specific* latent heat. As latent heat is measured in joules, specific latent heat is measured in joules per kilogram ($J\ kg^{-1}$).

For a substance of total mass m and specific latent heat L, we shall need an amount of energy E given by:

$$\text{energy} = \text{mass} \times \text{latent heat for 1 kg}$$
$$E = mL$$

Table 7.2 Specific latent heats and melting and boiling points of common substances

Substance	Melting point /°C	Specific latent heat of fusion/MJ kg⁻¹	Boiling point/°C	Specific latent heat of vaporisation/MJ kg⁻¹
Aluminium	661	0.38	2520	10.8
Copper	1085	0.21	2590	4.7
Gold	1065	0.07	2850	1.7
Mercury	−39	0.016	357	0.29
Oxygen (O₂)	−219	0.014	−183	0.22
Water	0	0.333	100	2.257

? QUESTIONS 2–3

2 For water, find the ratio of the latent heats of fusion and vaporisation. Compare this ratio with the ratio for other substances. Comment.

3 An electric kettle contains three litres (3×10^{-3} m³) of water at 100 °C.
a) Calculate the amount of energy required to boil the kettle dry assuming that all the energy is used in the boiling process and none is lost to the kettle or its surroundings.
b) Given that electrical energy costs 7.5p per kilowatt-hour, find the cost of boiling all the water.
(Take the density of water to be 10^3 kg m⁻³.)

SCIENCE IN CONTEXT

Plasma – a fourth state of matter

If we heat gas molecules to a very high temperature, we obtain a fourth state of matter, a **plasma**. It has been known for hundreds of years that chemical reactions are not sufficient to produce the energies emitted by stars, including the Sun. In the Sun, temperatures are so high that the outer electrons of the atoms are separated from the protons and neutrons of the nuclei. The resulting positively and negatively charged particles move around separately and rapidly as a plasma.

This is how plasmas form. Because stars consist of large amounts of matter, the gravitational force tends to compress the particles into a smaller volume. The pressure increases and the electrons and protons move faster and faster. The temperature rises further and energy is radiated as electromagnetic rays (photons). Energy can only continue to be emitted if a nuclear reaction takes place. With fusion of the nuclei of elements at the low end of the Periodic Table, a minute proportion of their mass is converted to very large quantities of energy. Thus the high temperature is sustained.

Plasmas do not normally occur on Earth, outside the laboratory. A lot of research is carried out on them in the hope of producing large quantities of energy through nuclear fusion for the twenty-first century. It is difficult to produce sufficiently high temperatures to sustain high-energy plasmas (although a plasma is produced by argon-arc welding equipment). In an attempt to create fusion conditions, small capsules of hydrogen or helium are bombarded by laser beams from several directions to create high temperatures that will produce a plasma, and magnetic fields hold the charged particles of the plasma at high density. But sustained nuclear fusion is yet to be achieved.

There is more about nuclear fusion and the processes in stars in Chapter 25.

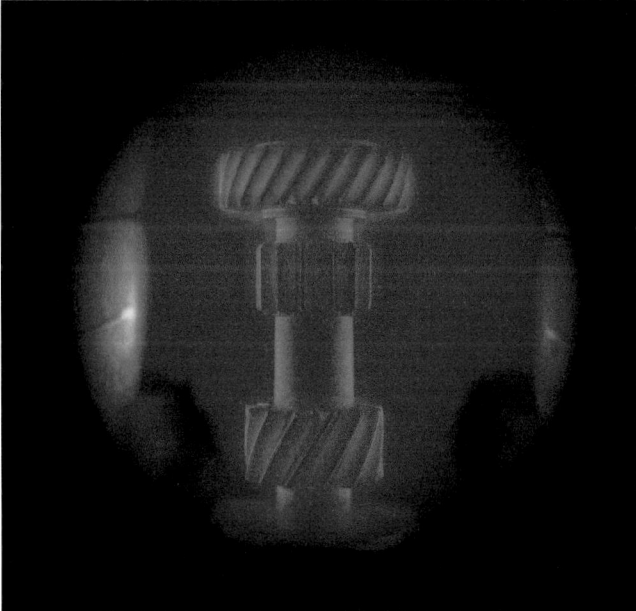

Fig 7.4 A plasma chamber in which a vehicle transmission gear is being hardened: ions from the plasma 'dissolve' into the steel surface (which is given a negative charge to attract them), and a modified, harder surface is formed

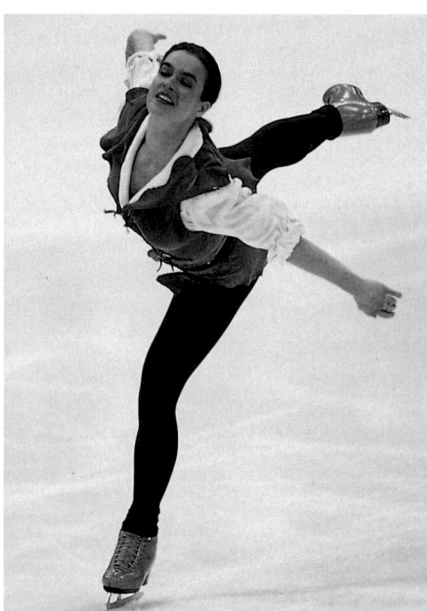

Fig 7.5 Skating on ice. The pressure under the blade causes the ice to melt

DEPENDENCE OF MELTING AND BOILING TEMPERATURES ON PRESSURE

So far, we have assumed that the water is at standard pressure. In fact the temperatures of melting and boiling alter if there is a change in pressure of the surroundings. The change in pressure needs to be large for us to notice the effect, but we do commonly meet it.

If we increase the pressure on a block of ice, the freezing temperature of the ice decreases. This is what happens when we ice-skate. The sharp blades of the skates apply a large force to the ice over a small area (Fig 7.5). There is a very large pressure under the blades which helps the ice to melt under the blades. The water effectively lubricates the skating surface.

The temperature of the ice and the width of the blades both need to be carefully controlled. If the skates were designed with very broad blades, they would not apply enough pressure. Even using narrow blades, it is not possible to skate on ice that is at too low a temperature.

The temperature of vaporisation of water is lowered by a *decrease* in pressure, so that water boils at a lower temperature on a mountain top, where the atmospheric pressure is lower, than at sea level. High up a mountain is not the best place to make a good cup of tea. Though the boiling temperature is not lowered much, the drop is enough to reduce the amount of flavour extracted from the tea leaves! You may also notice this on a plane flight.

Sublimation

Some substances can change directly from the solid state to the vapour state. This process is called **sublimation**. The temperature and pressure may need adjusting for this to happen. For example, solid carbon dioxide (dry ice) remains solid up to −78 °C, then it changes directly into the gas. Dry ice is used in research laboratories for keeping equipment and samples cold. It is also used in the theatre for creating an artificial fog – the evaporating carbon dioxide molecules cool the air and water in the air condenses out as droplets.

3 ATOMS AND MOLECULES

Solids can form many different structures at the microscopic level. In all cases, the solids consist of atoms held closely together, though the arrangements of these atoms can differ considerably. Here we are going to look at some of these patterns, especially those that are regular. For this, we use a very simple model in which the atoms are considered to be identical hard spheres. Bringing the atoms close together is similar to packing marbles or polystyrene spheres next to each other.

If we push the marbles or polystyrene spheres together, they resist compression once their outer surfaces touch. Since marbles are hard, they resist compression more than the polystyrene spheres. In both cases, there is a force opposing the movement.

In a similar way, there will be a force of repulsion when two atoms are brought together. Here it is due to the outer electrons repelling each other as the atoms become close. The force of repulsion, shown by the red curve in Fig 7.6, gets much larger as the separation between atoms is reduced.

We have no difficulty in separating the marbles or polystyrene spheres – there are no attractive forces to overcome. However, atoms do resist separation, because there is an attractive force. It has a negative value. But this attractive force must get rapidly smaller as the separation of the atoms increases – the blue curve in Fig 7.6

shows approximately how the force of attraction varies with distance. It will be zero at large separations. Similarly, the force of repulsion falls off as distance increases. Note that this fall-off is more rapid than for the attractive force, so atoms still attract each other after the repulsion has approached zero.

We must add together the attractive and repulsive forces to find the net force at any separation. This is the same as adding the two curves together. The resulting force–separation curve will depend on the relative sizes of the repulsive and attractive forces. In Fig 7.6, the final force–separation curve, the purple curve, is a good representation of the force between a pair of adjacent atoms.

What can we tell from this curve?

- At a separation d_0 the net force between the two atoms is zero. At this separation, the repulsive force exactly balances the attractive force. This will be the *equilibrium* position of the two atoms. At this separation, they remain stable.
- At very large separations the force between the atoms approaches zero. But the force of attraction does start to have an effect when approaching particles are relatively far apart.
- There is a large force of attraction for separations slightly greater than d_0. This attractive force must be overcome if we wish to separate the atoms.
- If the two atoms are brought closer together than d_0, the force of repulsion becomes very large.

Pulling atoms apart or pressing them closer together is similar to extending or compressing a spring. This is why we can apply Hooke's law (page 98) both to extending springs and to deforming solids.

If we pull the atoms apart against the attractive force trying to hold them together, we must do work. This is like doing work to raise a mass upwards in a gravitational field. Just as the mass being raised in the gravitational field gains potential energy, so these two atoms **gain potential energy** as they separate.

We can plot the potential energy gained by these atoms as their separation changes. As is usual (see page 50 in Chapter 3), we set the potential energy to be zero for very large separations. When the atoms are moved closer together, the potential energy drops, just as the potential energy of a mass decreases as it falls to Earth. Since it decreases from a zero value, the potential energy must become more negative (see Fig 7.7). The equilibrium position d_0, where the net force on the

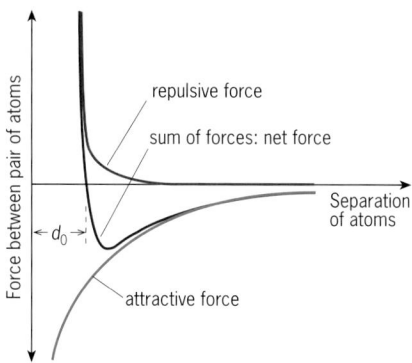

Fig 7.6 Forces of repulsion (red) and attraction (blue) between two atoms and also their sum (purple)

? QUESTION 4

4 Redraw the three curves shown in Fig 7.6 for a pair of atoms in which the force of repulsion is weaker and the force of attraction is stronger.

✔ REMEMBER THIS
Energy change equals force multiplied by distance moved.

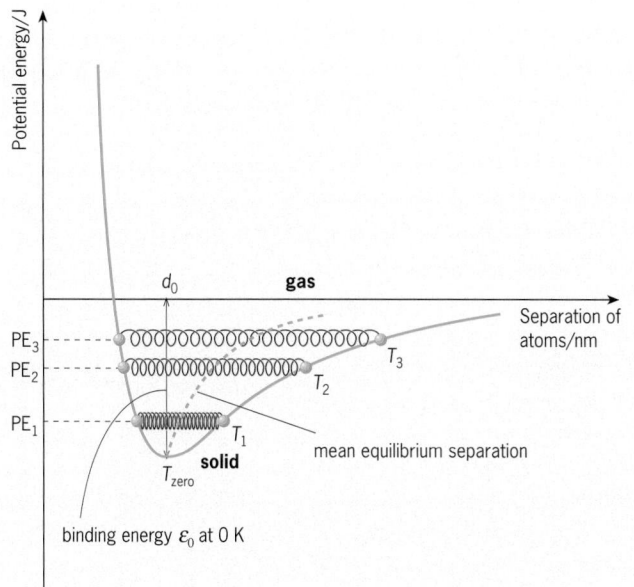

Fig 7.7 Variation of potential energy with separation for two neighbouring atoms

atoms is zero, corresponds to the minimum in the potential energy curve. For a very small change of separation from d_0 the potential energy does not change.

Take care – the potential energy minimum in Fig 7.7 does not correspond to the minimum on the resultant purple force curve in Fig 7.6. The minimum on the force curve corresponds to the separation where there is the biggest net attractive force, not zero net force.

To decrease the separation further, the atoms must now be moved against the force of repulsion. The potential energy starts to rise again. Eventually it reaches a very large positive value.

The type of force–separation curve we have looked at is very helpful for describing the interaction between atoms. Atoms in solids bond together in different ways, and the precise form of the interaction will vary according to the type of bonding involved. How the form of the potential energy curve can be related to the properties of materials and a summary of the main types of bonding found in solids are given in the following Stretch and Challenge boxes.

STRETCH AND CHALLENGE

The potential energy curve and properties of materials

We have seen that at equilibrium the separation of two atoms corresponds to the position of minimum potential energy. The atoms will remain at separation d_0 provided the temperature is at absolute zero. (Later in your studies you will discover that reaching absolute zero is not *quite* possible because of the 'uncertainty principle'.)

If we give the atoms some energy by heating them to a finite temperature T_1, the potential energy (PE) increases to a value PE_1 – see Fig 7.7. The atoms are bound together by a potential energy ε_0 equal to the maximum depth of the curve. The energy that heating gives to the atoms makes them vibrate towards and away from each other, in response to the repulsive and attractive forces. We have pictured the distance between the atoms as a spring between two points on the curve at T_1. These two points represent the minimum and maximum separations of the atoms at that temperature.

Alternatively, we can think of a marble oscillating backwards and forwards in a bowl within a gravitational field, as in Fig 7.8. The more energy we give the marble, the bigger the oscillations as it rises further up either side of the bowl. It is quite helpful to think in terms of an oscillating marble in a bowl that has the same shape as the potential energy curve for our two atoms in Fig 7.7.

Increasing the temperature of the atoms, say to T_2 and then T_3, giving total potential energies PE_2 and PE_3 respectively, makes them vibrate relative to each other by larger amounts. This is shown on the diagram as stretched springs at T_2 and T_3. The higher the energy of the atom pair, the wider their range of separations.

The mean separation of the atoms is the midpoint of these lines of vibration. We immediately see that, because the potential energy curve is not symmetrical about the minimum, the mean separation increases as the temperature increases. Look at the marble oscillating in the similarly shaped bowl. When this happens for many atoms, the average separation of all the atoms has increased. Our solid has *expanded* with increase in temperature.

If the temperature of the atoms is raised until their potential energy is zero, the atoms can fly apart – the gaseous state has been reached. Somewhere between the gaseous state and the solid state (and we cannot be sure where this is on our figure), there is sufficient movement for the atoms to be in the liquid state. The depth (ε_0) of the potential energy curve will be related to the sum of the specific latent heats of the substance.

equilibrium

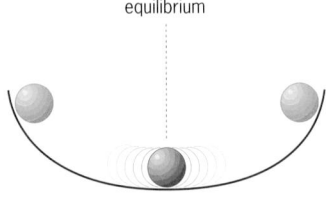

Marble spends equal time on left and right

equilibrium

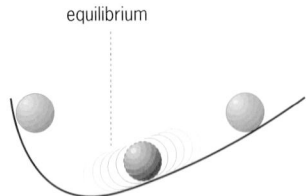

Marble spends longer time on gentler slope, so average position is to right of rest position

Fig 7.8 Model for the potential energy of a pair of atoms

Types of bonding 1: ionic and covalent

IONIC BONDING

This is found in many crystalline materials that consist of at least two different types of atom, such as sodium chloride – common salt. Atoms try to fill their outer shell of electrons. For example, one type of atom, the sodium atom in the case of sodium chloride, loses an electron and the other, chlorine, gains an electron. Once the sodium has lost an electron it becomes positively charged and is said to be a positive ion; by gaining an electron the chlorine becomes a negative ion. The crystal of sodium chloride must be electrically neutral everywhere. The only way this is possible is for the sodium and chloride ions to alternate in nearest-neighbour directions, as shown in Fig 7.9.

Electrical forces act over a relatively long distance, so bonding is not directional but it is strong. It is difficult for ions of opposite charge on different planes to slip past each other, so ionic crystals are not plastic (see page 107). They usually fracture before reaching their elastic limit.

Ionic crystals are poor conductors of electricity as neither the ions themselves nor individual electrons are free to move. When put into water, ionic crystals dissolve: the water reduces the electrical forces between the ions and so the ions can separate. They now move around and can conduct electricity (they move, carrying charge).

COVALENT BONDING

In this case atoms share, rather than exchange, electrons in the region between the two atoms. Unlike the ionic bond, the covalent bond is highly directional. Molecules produced by such bonding retain a definite shape. Oxygen, O_2, is a covalently bonded molecule. Both oxygen atoms would like two more electrons in their outer shells and, as shown in Fig 7.10(a), they achieve this by each providing two electrons for sharing (making a total of four shared electrons).

Covalent bonding can lead to highly extended 'molecules'. Diamond is such an example, as shown in Fig 7.10(b). Carbon has four electrons in its outer shell and by sharing a further four electrons, one from each of four other carbon atoms, it forms a continuous structure. The four bonds are symmetrically arranged in space and are called tetrahedral bonds.

Silicon and germanium also have four electrons in their outer shells (carbon, silicon and germanium are all from Group IV of the Periodic Table, see Table 17.4), and so they bond in the same way. The arrangement of the outer electrons of silicon and germanium gives rise to their semiconducting property. This property has been the basis of the development of semiconductor devices and the advance of much of the electronics industry. Unlike ionic compounds, covalent materials do not conduct in aqueous solution.

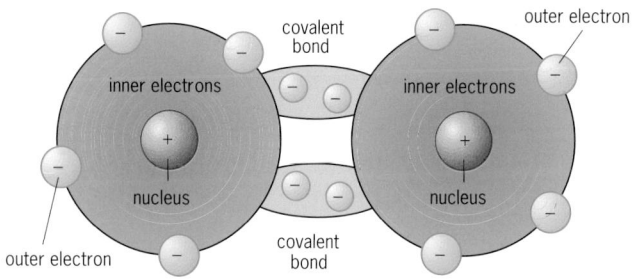

(a) Covalent bonds of the oxygen molecule showing the sharing of the outer electrons

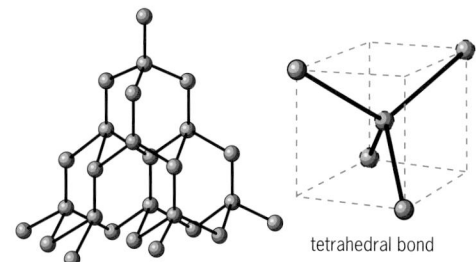

tetrahedral bond

(b) The tetrahedral covalent bonding in diamond.
Notice the similarity with the structure of ice, Fig 7.2(a)

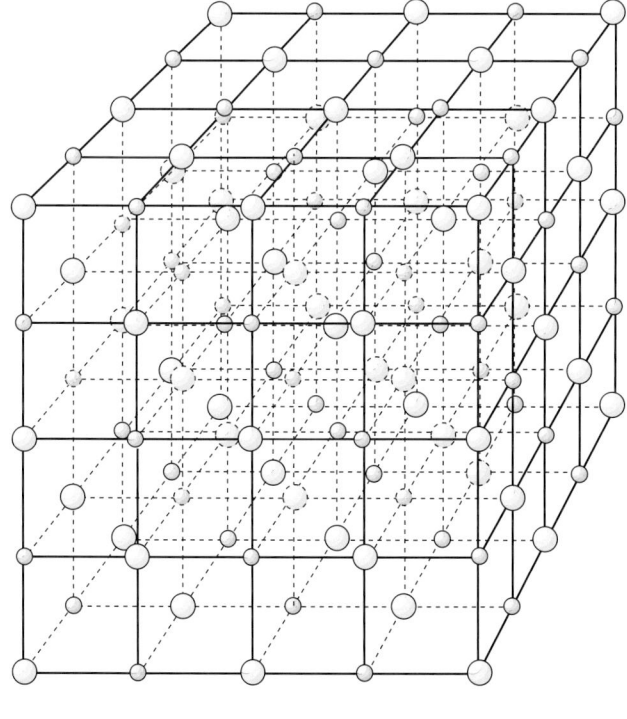

○ positive sodium ion

◌ negative chloride ion

Fig 7.9 Sodium chloride, a typical ionic structure

Fig 7.10 Examples of covalent bonding

Types of bonding 2: metallic and Van der Waals

METALLIC BONDING

In metals, each atom has one or more outer **delocalised** electrons that are free to move between atoms. The metal can be pictured as a giant structure of positively charged ions in a sea of electrons, as in Fig 7.11. We might expect these ions to repel each other and fly apart. Not so. The interaction between the electrons and the ions sets up a counteracting attractive force. Why this should happen was not properly understood until physicists came up with a new theory called quantum physics (see Chapter 16).

The fact that the electrons can move freely around accounts for the good electrical conductivity of metals. The interaction between the large number of ions and the 'sea' of electrons is not directional. The ions, though, stay fixed, often close packed together. If a tensile or shearing force is applied to the metal, it is easy for the planes of ions to move past each other. So metals exhibit plasticity as we saw in Chapter 5 (page 107).

VAN DER WAALS BONDING

Even neutral atoms attract each other weakly. The atoms are composed of both positively charged protons in their nuclei and moving electrons in a surrounding cloud that constantly changes shape. In a pair of like atoms, the positive and negative charges from one atom and the positive and negative charges from the other produce a small instantaneous force, as in Fig 7.12. Although the force changes as the electrons move, it averages over time to produce an attraction that is called van der Waals bonding and occurs between all atoms and molecules.

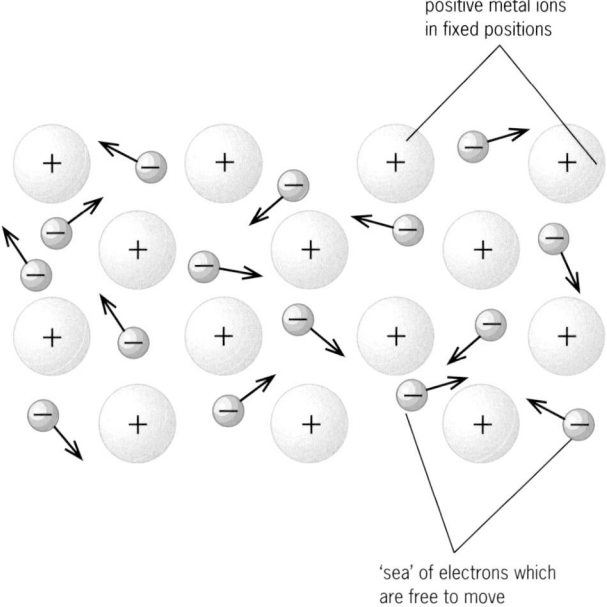

Fig 7.11 Metallic bonding, showing metal ions and surrounding electrons

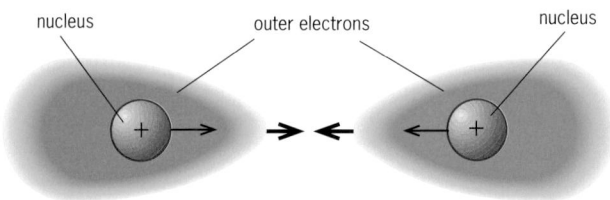

Fig 7.12 Van der Waals bonding between two neutral atoms

4 CRYSTAL STRUCTURES

Adding together layers of spheres is similar to adding together layers of atoms. The final structure will depend on how we build up the layers and whether these layers themselves are made up of identically sized spheres or spheres of different sizes. Substances that are built from an ordered stacking of atoms are called crystals. These often possess flat faces that match regular planes of atoms. Most crystals can be **cleaved**. This means that a hard blow with a sharp edge will split the crystal along a plane to create a pair of flat surfaces. Because they can be cleaved, diamonds and other gemstones have attractive, shiny surfaces and are valuable for jewellery.

SIMPLE CUBIC STRUCTURE

Let us continue to think of atoms as hard spheres. They can be arranged so that they touch in a single layer as a square array – see Fig 7.13(a). Note that there are four atoms round a hollow. Next we can arrange another layer of spheres vertically above the first, and so on – see Fig 7.13(b). Such a three-dimensional arrangement is called **simple cubic**.

Taking eight atoms from the arrangement in Fig 7.13(b), and reducing their size, their centres are shown joined by lines in Fig 7.13(c). Note that each atom will also be at the corners of eight cubes, the one in (b) and a further seven cubes. Alternatively, look at Fig 7.13(d) with the atoms (spheres) as in (b). It is clear that the part of an atom at each corner is an eighth of an atom.

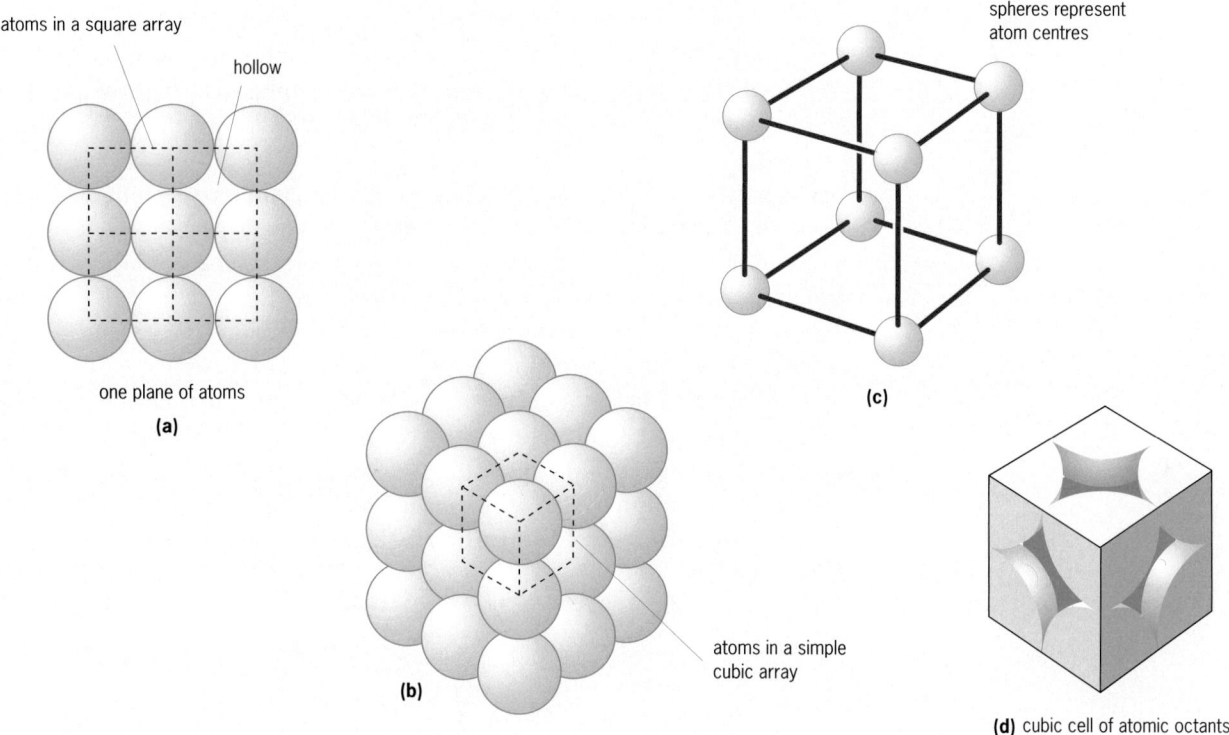

(a) atoms in a square array / hollow / one plane of atoms

(b) atoms in a simple cubic array

(c) spheres represent atom centres

(d) cubic cell of atomic octants

Fig 7.13 Different ways of representing a simple cubic structure

CLOSE PACKING STRUCTURES

The spheres in Fig 7.13(a) are not packed together as closely as possible. Fig 7.14 shows a different arrangement of spheres in a single layer. Here, a second row of touching atoms is displaced relative to the first one. The third row is a repeat of the first row. Comparing with Fig 7.13(a), note that there are only three atoms at a hollow but that the closest separation of centres of the atoms remains the same, equal to the diameter of the atom. The result is that in Fig 7.14 there are more atoms per unit area.

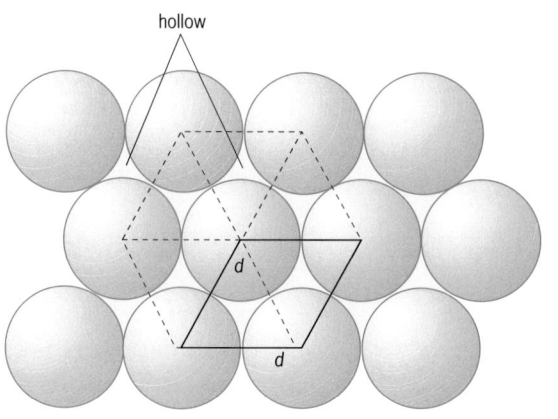

hollow

layer A

Fig 7.14 Close packing spheres in a single layer

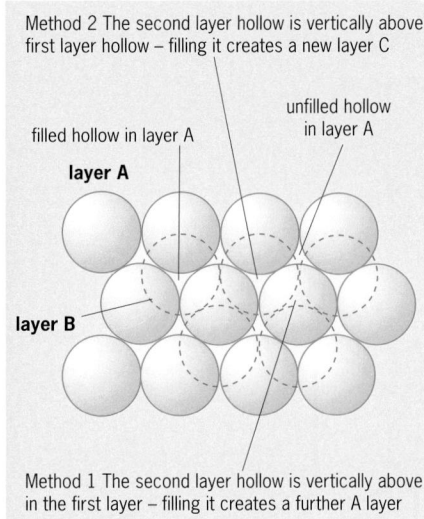

Method 2 The second layer hollow is vertically above first layer hollow – filling it creates a new layer C

filled hollow in layer A

unfilled hollow in layer A

layer A

layer B

Method 1 The second layer hollow is vertically above th in the first layer – filling it creates a further A layer

Fig 7.15 Two different ways of adding the third layer for close packing of spheres

Building close packed structures: hcp and fcc

We can build a regular close packed structure on the Fig 7.14 layer in two different ways, as follows:

Method 1

● We call our first layer of close packed spheres (atoms) layer A. Notice that each sphere touches six others (nearest neighbours) and is surrounded by six hollows (Fig 7.15).

● Now we start to build up a three-dimensional structure. We place the next plane of spheres into hollows. Notice that, even if we make the next plane of spheres close packed, we can only centre spheres in half the hollows. At this stage it doesn't matter which half-set of hollows we use. We label this second layer B.

● Next we add the third layer of spheres and again we can only fill half the hollows. This time the choice makes a difference.

● By filling one set of hollows, we can place all the spheres in this third layer vertically above spheres in the first layer. So we label this layer as another A layer. Note the hollows in layer B of Fig 7.15 in which the third-layer spheres are placed.

We can picture a hexagonal cell made up within these three layers, as shown in Fig 7.16(a). Fig 7.16(b) shows the conventional picture of the hexagonal cell with the spheres (atoms) shrunk to a small size. It is easy to see that we can continue with this ABABAB... arrangement of the layers. We call this pattern a **hexagonal close packed (hcp) structure**.

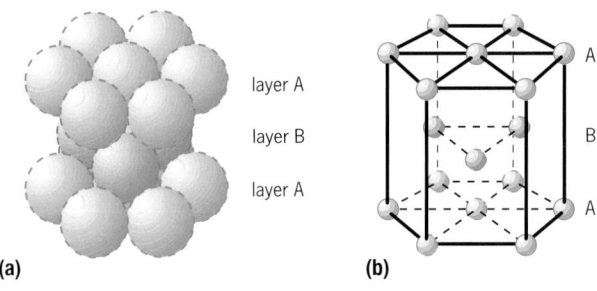

layer A

layer B

layer A

(a)

A

B

A

(b)

Fig 7.16 Hexagonal close packing (hcp)

Method 2

Let us return to packing our third layer and look again at Fig 7.15. We already have layers A and B. We now choose the alternative half-set of hollows to the set we chose previously. The spheres of the third layer no longer lie vertically above the spheres of layer A, nor do they lie above the spheres of layer B. So we label this third layer C. We go on to consider a fourth layer.

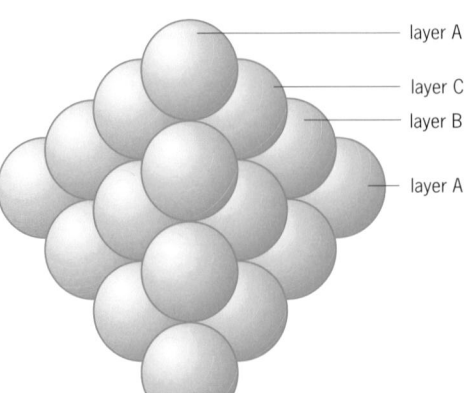

layer A

layer C

layer B

layer A

Again there is a choice of hollows, but we choose to place the spheres in hollows such that they lie vertically above the spheres in layer A. This produces another A-type layer. Packing on upwards produces an ABCABCABC... pattern. Fig 7.17 shows such layers packing in a pyramidal form starting from a triangular base. The structure is still close packed and the arrangement is called **face-centred cubic (fcc) close packing**.

Fig 7.17 Face-centred cubic packing (fcc) within a pyramid with a triangular base

But why cubic? As the name suggests, a face-centred cube has atoms at the corners of a cube and atoms at the centres of each face, as shown in Fig 7.18(c). The close packing structure that we have described can be related to a series of face-centred cells by tilting the close packed planes. It is tricky to see but you should be able to work out the relationship in Figs 7.18(a) and (b). The close packing planes link up three diagonally related corners of a cube. Try to identify how an atom in such a plane will be surrounded by six nearest neighbours within the same plane, and by three atoms in each of the two adjacent planes. All the outer surfaces of the pyramid shown in Fig 7.18(b) are of close packed planes of atoms.

> **? QUESTION 7**
>
> 7 By considering sharing of atoms between adjacent cubic cells, work out the number of atoms per cubic cell for the face-centred cube.

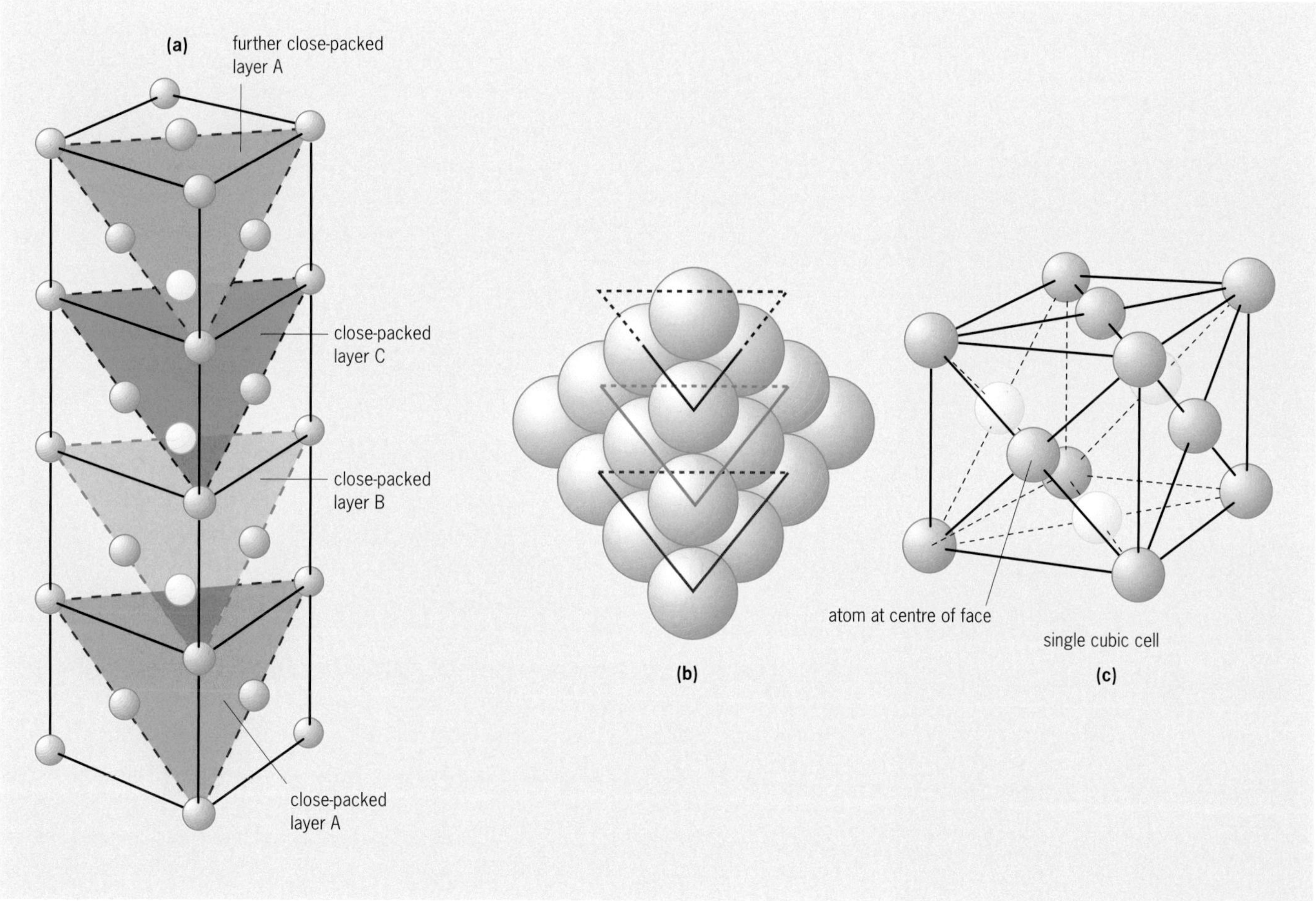

(a) further close-packed layer A

close-packed layer C

close-packed layer B

close-packed layer A

(b)

atom at centre of face

single cubic cell

(c)

Fig 7.18 Face-centred cubic (fcc) packing structure showing the close packed layers

BODY-CENTRED CUBIC STRUCTURE

Another common crystal structure is called **body-centred cubic (bcc)** because there is an atom at the centre of the cube (that is, at the centre of its 'body') in addition to the atoms at the corners (Fig 7.19). Iron has this structure up to 800 °C, at which temperature it changes to fcc. This is an example of a solid changing its phase but remaining a solid. Heating iron to above 800 °C and quenching it in water prevents the iron from returning to a bcc structure. The face-centred form of iron has different properties from the body-centred form – in particular it is very brittle. Iron containing carbon as an impurity gives steel. Such variations in the properties of iron are immensely important for the science of metallurgy and for the iron and steel industry.

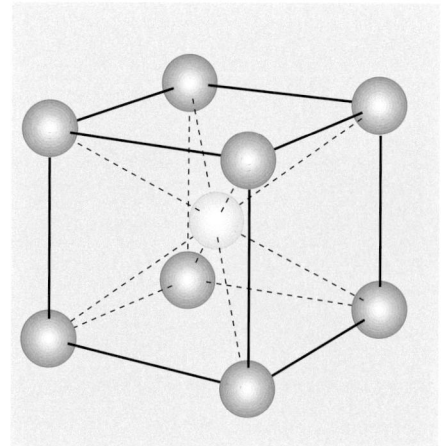

Fig 7.19 Body-centred cubic (bcc) structure

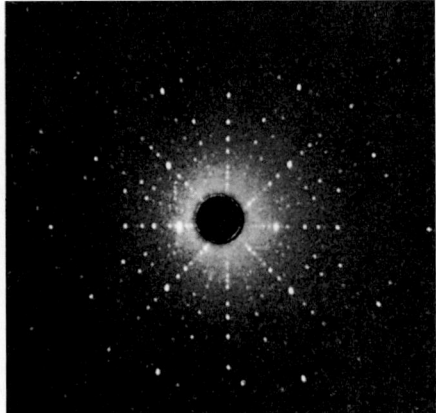

Fig 7.20 A von Laue diffraction pattern, above. Compare it with the diffraction pattern for two gratings crossed at right angles, below

DETERMINING THE STRUCTURES OF CRYSTALS

We find out about the structure of crystals by probing them with radiation. The spacing of the layers of atoms is about 0.5 nm, so we need radiation with a wavelength of similar size. X-rays are electromagnetic waves with a wavelength of about 1 nm. When the X-rays hit the crystal, they are diffracted by the planes of atoms, just as light is diffracted by a narrow slit or by a diffraction grating (see Chapter 15).

Max von Laue in 1912 was the first to observe this effect. Photographic film is used to detect the diffraction pattern (Fig 7.20), seen as a series of dots on the film. We can see a similar pattern when we pass a beam of light from a laser through two diffraction gratings crossed at right angles. In a crystal, it is the many parallel planes of atoms that produce the diffraction effect, just like the large number of rulings of the gratings. By measuring the distances between spots on the film, the spacing of the planes can be calculated.

Nowadays, we use solid state detectors, not film, to detect the X-rays. Measured intensities are digitised to store as a computer record, and computer software packages calculate the crystal structures and the positions of the atoms in the planes. Even the molecular structures of complex molecules such as DNA have been worked out from X-ray analysis.

We can use electrons instead of X-rays for studying crystal structures. Electron microscopes give pictures similar to those from an optical microscope. Alternatively, electron microscopes can be set to produce diffraction patterns, because electrons can behave as waves (see Chapter 16).

THE STRUCTURES OF OTHER SOLIDS

Although many materials have a regular crystalline structure, others do not. Such materials are described as **amorphous**, which means 'without form'. Alternative descriptions used are **glassy** and **solid liquid**. So, not surprisingly, ordinary glass is an amorphous material. It is made from silica (SiO_2) with added oxides.

A diffraction pattern for **glass** does not show spots. Instead, it shows a couple of very diffuse rings (Fig 7.21) that arise because the separations of nearest and next nearest atomic neighbours have different average values. But there is no order at longer range.

Glass is hard and brittle and surface cracks weaken it considerably (see also page 115). Glass cutters use this property extensively. They scratch the surface and break the glass along this scratch. As a demonstration, a glass rod is supported at its ends and loaded centrally (Fig 7.22); the load is increased until the rod breaks. The procedure is repeated, but using a glass rod with a small scratch on the under-surface. The rod now breaks, but with a much smaller load.

Glass softens when heated and then it is possible to shape it, as glass blowers do. It can be drawn out into the very fine fibres that carry light waves in fibre optic communications. Although not a liquid in the true sense, glass flows very slowly. Very old glass windows are thicker at the bottom than at the top as a result of slow flow in the Earth's gravitational field.

Polymers are made up of long chains of atoms forming long molecules. The backbone of the molecule is usually a series of carbon atoms covalently bonded together with other types of atoms attached. There are many examples of polymers in the home – polythene (made from polyethene molecules), nylon, PVC and Perspex are a few examples. The molecular chains can bend and become tangled. Some regions of the polymer may be entirely amorphous, while other regions may be composed of molecules arranged in a regular (crystalline) form. Rubber is such a polymer – Chapter 5 (page 116) describes how the molecules of rubber are more

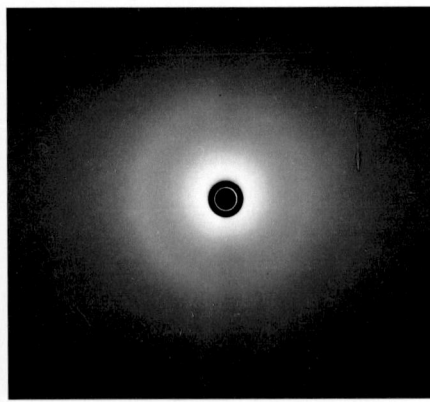

Fig 7.21 X-ray diffraction photograph for glass (an amorphous material)

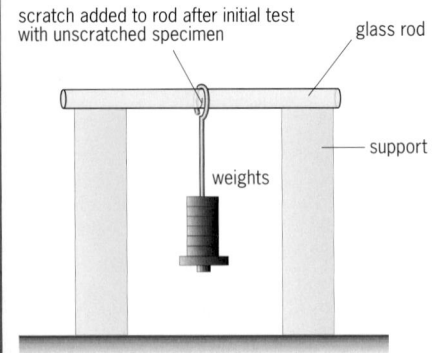

scratch added to rod after initial test with unscratched specimen

glass rod

support

weights

Fig 7.22 Testing the strength of a glass rod

tangled in its original shape than when stretched. Some polymer chains may have actual cross-links.

There are various other types of polymer. Thermosetting polymers can be moulded: they change to the required shape when heated through the so-called 'glass transition temperature' and then retain this shape when cooled. If reheated, they decompose rather than soften and distort. Such a material is melamine which can be used for kitchen utensils. Other polymers, called thermoplastics, soften on reheating, become flexible and then melt. Shaped articles can be made from the thermoplastic by moulding or by extruding the material through a tube.

5 LIQUIDS

We have seen that there is no long-range order between molecules within a liquid. An X-ray picture of a liquid is similar to that for an amorphous solid such as glass. Molecules move around relative to each other and do not keep the same molecules as neighbours. This ability of the molecules to move easily past each other allows liquids to flow. A liquid does not maintain its shape if shear forces are exerted on it, although a liquid can withstand compressive (hydrostatic) forces, because it maintains its volume.

We can see that liquid molecules move easily by observing **Brownian motion**. The botanist Robert Brown first noticed the effect in 1827 when looking at pollen grains suspended in water. The pollen grains have sufficiently small mass to be buffeted around by the unseen water molecules. A similar arrangement is shown in Fig 7.23. Smoke particles can be seen moving in air, demonstrating that gas molecules also collide with their neighbours.

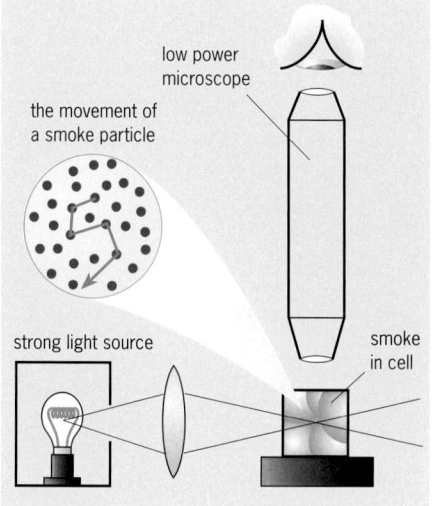

Fig 7.23 Demonstration of Brownian motion

SURFACE TENSION

Liquids behave as if there is a very delicate skin over their surface. For example, a pin can be balanced on the 'skin' of a water surface, and some insects can walk on the surface of ponds. This is possible because of **surface tension**: surface molecules tend to be further apart than underlying molecules, and attractive forces between neighbouring liquid surface molecules are stronger than forces between underlying molecules, as shown in Fig 7.24.

We shall return to liquids again to study other properties. We have already seen the importance of buoyancy and fluid flow to forms of transport (Chapter 4) and we shall learn more about the passage of thermal energy through a liquid in Chapter 13.

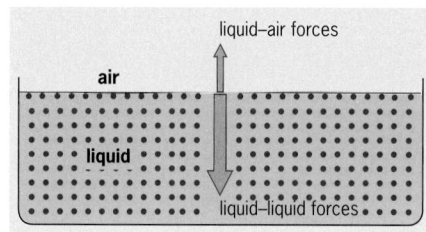

Fig 7.24 The surface of a liquid acts like a skin

6 GASES

We have seen that the atoms in a solid vibrate but do not move around. In a liquid, atoms or molecules are able to drift around, but they only alter their mean positions slowly. In contrast, the atoms or molecules in a gas move around rapidly over large distances. There is no pattern to the movement.

As they speed around, the molecules (or atoms) of a gas keep colliding with the walls of their container (Fig 7.25). As the molecules rebound off the walls, there is a change in their momentum.

Each molecule exerts a small force on the walls during a very small interval of time (Fig 7.26). All these small forces add up so that a large number of such collisions produce a total average force on the walls that is measurable.

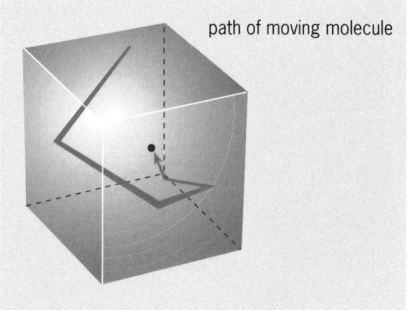

Fig 7.25 Molecules of a gas speed around and collide with the walls of their container

Assuming that the molecules are moving *equally in all directions*, the force per unit area of wall will be the same over all the walls of the container. This force per unit area is the **pressure** exerted by the gas and it is equal in all directions.

THE IDEAL GAS EQUATION

Fig 7.26 Averaging the forces from a number of impacts of gas molecules on the walls of the container

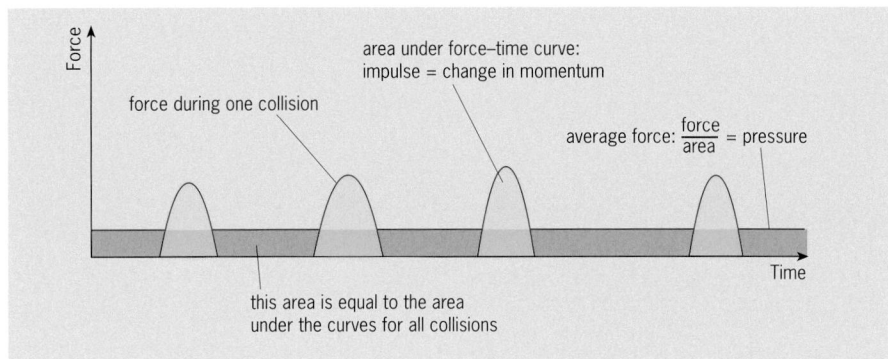

In the middle of the seventeenth century, Robert Boyle showed experimentally that:

> **The volume of a fixed mass of gas is inversely proportional to the pressure applied to it if the temperature is kept constant.**

That is, at constant temperature and mass:

$$\text{volume} \propto \frac{1}{\text{pressure}} \quad \text{or} \quad \text{pressure} \propto \frac{1}{\text{volume}}$$

If p is the pressure and V the volume of the gas, for constant temperature T and constant mass we have:

$$p \propto \frac{1}{V} \quad \text{or} \quad pV = \textbf{constant} \qquad \text{[Law 1]}$$

The law is known as **Boyle's law** and applies provided the pressure of the gas is low. In addition to Boyle's law, there are two other gas laws.

The **pressure law** states that:

> **The pressure of a fixed mass of gas at constant volume is proportional to temperature as measured on the Kelvin scale.**

That is, for constant volume and mass:

$$\text{pressure} \propto \text{temperature}$$

$$p \propto T \quad \text{or} \quad \frac{p}{T} = \textbf{constant} \qquad \text{[Law 2]}$$

This is a fundamental relationship for an ideal gas (real gases need to be at a low pressure). Note that we have not so far said precisely what we mean by temperature. The Stretch and Challenge box on pages 160–161 describes how a temperature scale is obtained.

The other law is called **Charles' law**:

> **The volume of a fixed mass of gas at constant pressure is proportional to temperature as measured on the Kelvin scale.**

That is, for constant pressure and mass:

$$\text{volume} \propto \text{temperature}$$

$$V \propto T \quad \text{or} \quad \frac{V}{T} = \textbf{constant} \qquad \text{[Law 3]}$$

Putting the three laws together we obtain the combined gas law. For a constant mass of **ideal gas**:

$$\frac{pV}{T} = \text{constant}$$

or:

$$\frac{p_1 V_1}{T_1} = \frac{p_2 V_2}{T_2}$$

Subscript 1 refers to the initial conditions for the ideal gas and subscript 2 refers to a later set of conditions.

If a real gas obeys the combined gas law equation, then it is behaving ideally. The equation assumes that there is no attraction, no repulsion and no collisions between the atoms or molecules of the gas. Real gases usually cool if allowed to expand – this property is exploited, for example, to liquefy helium from the gaseous phase at very low temperatures. But an ideal gas will not cool down if it is allowed to expand freely (that is, if it is allowed to expand into a vacuum) and an ideal gas cannot be turned into a liquid.

Finally, we need to know the constant of proportionality in the combined gas law equation. From experiment we find that the constant depends on the mass of gas involved. If we double the mass of gas (this means doubling the number of moles of gas) at constant pressure and temperature, then the volume of gas doubles. So pV/T is proportional to the amount of gas enclosed, that is, proportional to the number of moles n:

$$\frac{pV}{T} = nR \quad \text{or} \quad pV = nRT$$

where R is the constant of proportionality and is called the **molar gas constant**. It is a fundamental quantity that can be measured to high accuracy and it has units. The constant can be found from the fact that 1 mole of an ideal gas at standard temperature (273.16 K) and pressure (1.014×10^5 Pa) occupies 0.0224 m³:

$$R = \frac{1.014 \times 10^5 \times 0.0224}{1 \times 273.16} \frac{\text{Pa m}^3}{\text{mol K}} = 8.31 \text{ J K}^{-1} \text{ mol}^{-1}$$

(Note that Pa m³ ≡ N m⁻² m³ = N m ≡ J.)

This equation, $pV = nRT$ for n moles of gas, or the alternative form,

$$pV_m = RT$$

for one mole of gas, where V_m refers to molar volume, is called the **universal gas law equation**.

SCIENCE IN CONTEXT

Boyle and Charles – originators of the gas laws

Robert Boyle (1627–1691) was the youngest child of the Earl of Cork. He was privately taught and then went to Eton College before going on a Grand Tour of Europe. His main work was as a chemist, and he is known as the scientist who established chemistry as a separate science.

While working at Oxford, he improved an air pump made by Hooke and showed that objects in a vacuum fall at the same velocity under gravity. Besides publishing his gas law, he proposed the idea of chemical elements. He incorrectly believed that base metals could be transformed into gold and his attempts to convert metals led to the repeal of an English law against producing gold and silver from other substances.

Jacques Charles (1746–1823) was originally a clerk in the civil service. The French physicist became interested in gases from his experience of ballooning. In 1783 he made the first ascent in a hydrogen balloon. A few years later he formulated his famous law, and sent it to Gay-Lussac who made more accurate measurements to support it. Hence, in France, the law is called Gay-Lussac's law.

Demonstrating the gas laws

BOYLE'S LAW

As shown in Fig 7.27, a small amount of air is trapped at the closed end of a glass tube by an oil column. The tube is calibrated for volume. The other end of the tube connects with a chamber containing air. The air pressure in the chamber, and hence the pressure applied to the oil column, can be varied using a foot-pump. Whenever an adjustment is made to the pressure, time must be allowed for the gas to achieve thermal equilibrium with its surroundings at constant room temperature. To show Boyle's law, it is necessary to plot p against $1/V$, or pV against V.

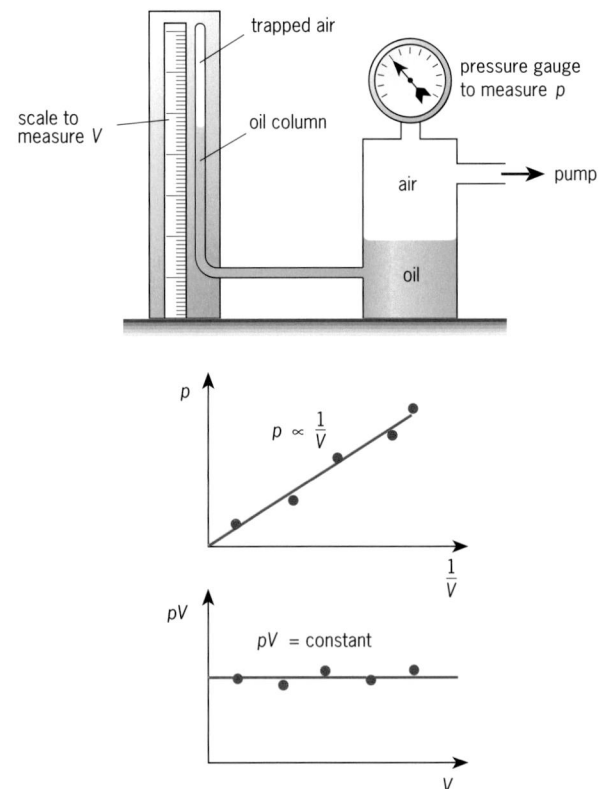

Fig 7.27 Demonstrating Boyle's law

THE PRESSURE LAW

As shown in Fig 7.28, a volume of gas is trapped in a flask that is connected to a pressure gauge. The flask is inserted in a water bath (or oil bath for higher temperatures) and the variation of pressure with temperature is measured.

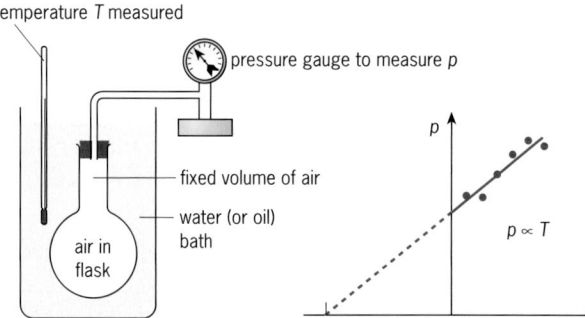

Fig 7.28 Demonstrating the pressure law

CHARLES' LAW

A small amount of gas (air is suitable) is trapped in a calibrated capillary tube, usually by a bead of concentrated sulphuric acid to ensure that the gas remains dry (Fig 7.29). The capillary tube is inserted in a water bath. The length of the gas column (proportional to the volume of the gas) is measured as the temperature of the water bath is varied.

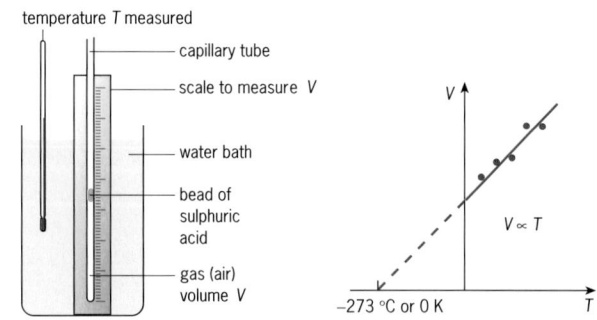

Fig 7.29 Demonstrating Charles' law

Ideal gas temperature scale – Kelvin temperature scale

We have seen that we can put $p_1V_1/T_1 = p_2V_2/T_2$, where subscripts 1 and 2 refer to two sets of conditions for our ideal gas. Alternatively, pV is proportional to T. On a molecular scale temperature is a measure of the average kinetic energy of the molecules of a substance. The following explains how the accurate calibration of temperature can be made so that we can define temperature for a large system.

We measure pV as we vary T (using a thermometer) over a range in which the gas behaves ideally. We get a straight line, showing this proportionality, as in Fig 7.30. The plot is that of a linear equation:

$$y = mx + c$$

where m is the gradient and c is a constant.

To establish the calibration line we use straight proportionality to extend the line through to the origin $pV = 0$, $T = 0$. This sets $c = 0$ and defines one fixed point.

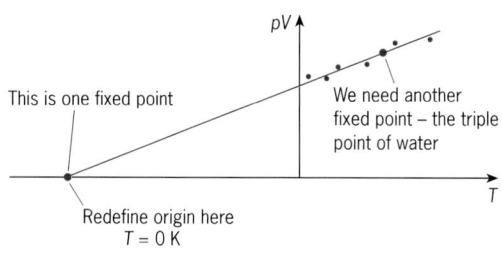

Fig 7.30 *pV* is proportional to *T* for an ideal gas

We now need only fix one other point to define the calibration line. This second fixed point must be reproducible by any scientist anywhere on Earth. The fixed point is chosen as the triple point of water, a unique temperature at which water vapour, liquid water and ice coexist in equilibrium, see Fig 7.31(a). To obtain this point experimentally, a triple point cell, shown in Fig 7.31(c), is used. Air has been removed, leaving a pressure due to water vapour alone. This pressure is 0.61 kPa, which is, of course, very much lower than atmospheric pressure (101.4 kPa). For historical reasons related to earlier definitions of the Celsius and centigrade scales, this triple point is defined as 273.16 on the Kelvin scale, temperature unit **kelvin** (K). With the Celsius values of −273.16 °C for absolute 'zero' and 0 °C for the triple point, this makes the interval between kelvins the same as between degrees Celsius.

Note that the negative slope of the pressure–temperature boundary line between ice and water (Fig 7.31(a)) is very unusual; the typical curve for most other substances is shown in Fig 7.31(b).

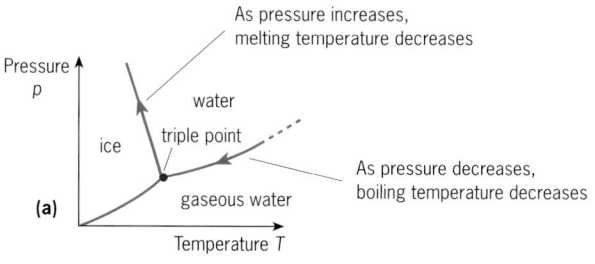

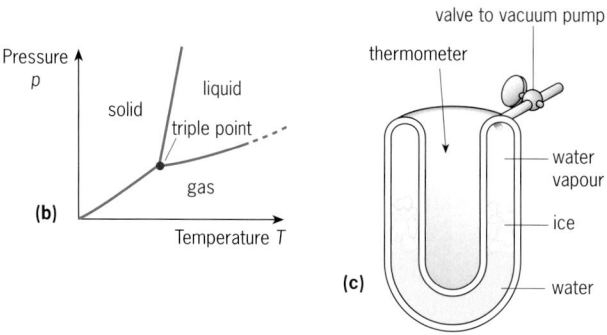

Fig 7.31 Phase diagrams for **(a)** water, **(b)** a more typical substance. **(c)** A triple point cell: temperature = 273.16 K, pressure = water vapour pressure (0.61 kPa)

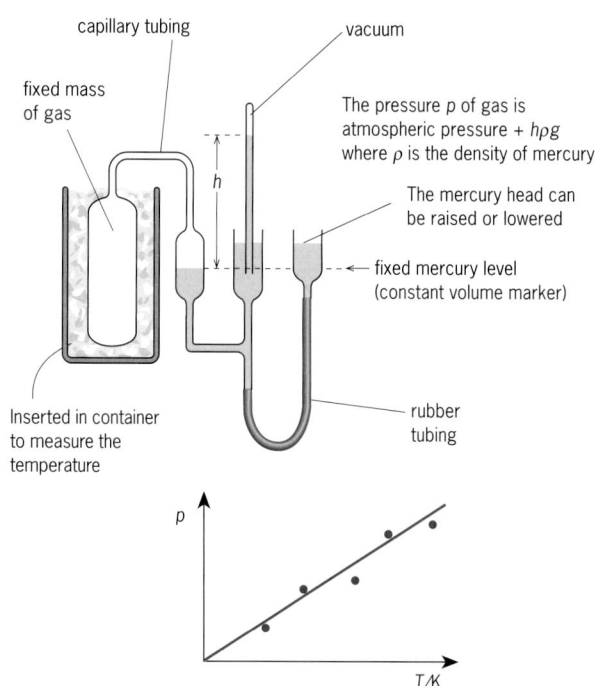

Fig 7.32 A constant volume gas thermometer

We now have, for a particular mass of ideal gas:

$$\frac{(pV)_{\text{at unknown temperature}}}{\text{unknown temperature}} = \frac{(pV)_{\text{at triple point temperature}}}{273.16}$$

If we call the unknown temperature *T* and rearrange the equation we get:

$$T = \frac{(pV)_T}{(pV)_{\text{tr}}} \times 273.16 \text{ K}$$

where the subscript 'tr' refers to the triple point. This gives us a primary scale of temperature.

We could go on to show that this scale is identical to a thermodynamic scale defined by the use of a reversible heat engine (see Chapter 14). But, while the thermodynamic scale is a theoretical concept, here we have a practical method of measuring temperature. We use a gas thermometer containing a small mass of a gas and calibrate the product *pV* to obtain temperature. To simplify, we keep the gas volume constant and change only the pressure: see Fig 7.32.

Once we have obtained our primary scale, we can cross-check it using other physical properties to measure temperature, such as the expansion of mercury with temperature, the variation of the resistance of a metal or the electromotive force (e.m.f.) set up between the junctions of two different metals at different temperatures (as in a thermocouple). We return to practical aspects of temperature measurement in Chapter 13.

EXAMPLE

Q A constant-volume gas thermometer shows a difference in height in its mercury column of 8.00 cm at the triple point of water.

a) What difference in height does it read at
  i) the boiling point of water and
  ii) the melting point of lead (327 °C)?

b) With the density of mercury 1.35×10^3 kg m^{-3}, convert the readings to values of pressure in kPa.

A

a) We have:

$$\frac{p}{T} = \frac{p_{tr}}{T_{tr}}$$

where p and T are the pressure and temperature read by the thermometer when in thermal contact with a substance, and p_{tr} and T_{tr} are the pressure and temperature when it is in contact with water at its triple point of 273 K. (Remember to convert temperatures to kelvin.) As the difference in height of the mercury column is proportional to pressure, we can obtain height differences for **i)** and **ii)** by direct proportionality:

i) p (of boiling water) $= \dfrac{8.00 \times 373}{273} = 10.9$ cm Hg.

ii) p (of melting lead) $= \dfrac{8.00 \times 600}{273} = 17.6$ cm Hg.

b) A 1 cm column of mercury creates a pressure given by:

mass of column per unit area $\times g$ = density $\times g \times$ height
$= (1.35 \times 10^3) \times 9.8 \times (1 \times 10^{-2}) \times 1 = 132$ Pa
$= 0.132$ kPa

(The 10^{-2} above is a value which converts to cm.)

Hence:

	Pressure/cm Hg	Pressure/kPa
Triple point water	8.0	1.06
Boiling point water	10.9	1.44
Melting point lead	17.6	2.32

7 THE KINETIC THEORY OF GASES

The behaviour of gases is related to the microscopic movement of the atoms or molecules, and we use kinetic theory to give a model of this behaviour.

From the model it is possible to obtain an expression for the pressure of an ideal gas, and to go on to find out how the speeds of the gas molecules vary. We use the model of a large number of molecules moving around in a closed box, making many collisions with the walls. There are a number of underlying assumptions.

SIMPLIFYING ASSUMPTIONS USED

- The gas consists of a very large number N of molecules.
- The molecules are moving rapidly and randomly.
- The motion of the molecules can be described by Newtonian mechanics.
- Collisions between the molecules themselves and between the molecules and the walls are perfectly elastic.
- There are no attractive intermolecular forces.
- The only intermolecular forces that act are those during collisions and these are effectively instantaneous (that is, of small duration compared with the time interval between collisions).
- Molecules have negligible volume compared with the volume of the container (the molecules are, in effect, points in space).

If the collisions were not elastic, the kinetic energy of the molecules would be converted to other forms of energy and the gas pressure would decrease with time. Attractive intermolecular forces would, in particular, affect collisions at the walls by pulling molecules away from the walls. To assume no attractive intermolecular forces, we must have a gas at a low density.

MAIN RESULTS OF THE KINETIC THEORY

The mathematics of the model are given in the Stretch and Challenge passage that follows but the main results are shown below.

Pressure

The pressure ρ exerted by the gas is given by

$$p = \frac{1}{3}\frac{mN\overline{c^2}}{V} = \frac{1}{3}\rho\overline{c^2}$$

where the gas of density ρ occupying a volume V has N molecules each of mass m and with mean square velocity $\overline{c^2}$.

Internal energy

The internal energy U of the gas arising from the kinetic energy of all the molecules is

$$U = \frac{3}{2}nRT$$

where the gas consists of n moles and R is the molar gas constant. The average kinetic energy per molecule is given by

$$U_{\text{one molecule}} = \frac{3}{2}\frac{RT}{N_A} = \frac{3}{2}kT$$

where N_A is the Avogadro constant, $k = R/N_A$ is the **Boltzmann constant** and $\frac{1}{2}kT$ can be associated with each degree of freedom (see page 165).

The derivation assumes ideal gases with negligible forces between molecules that have negligible size. In real gases, the molecules have a finite size and small forces act between them. But, under suitable conditions, gases do match the behaviour of ideal gases very closely.

We have emphasised that the gas laws apply best at low pressures. It is important that our real gas is not close to the conditions for liquefaction. So its temperature should be well above the critical temperature and its pressure well below the critical pressure at which liquefaction takes place. The real test of kinetic theory is that it gives satisfactory results for gases in most practical circumstances.

SCIENCE IN CONTEXT

EXAMPLE

Q The density of air at 20 °C is 1.20 kg m^{-3}. Assuming atmospheric pressure of 1.01×10^5 Pa, calculate the root-mean-square velocity of molecules in air.

A $p = \frac{1}{3}\rho c^2$ and hence:

$$\overline{c^2} = 3p/\rho = \frac{3 \times 1.01 \times 10^5}{1.20} = 2.53 \times 10^5 \text{ m}^2\text{ s}^{-2}$$

$$\sqrt{\overline{c^2}} = 502 \text{ m s}^{-1}$$

? QUESTION 9

9 The passage of sound through air relies on movement of the air molecules. Look up the speed of sound in air and comment on the value compared with the value calculated for $\sqrt{\overline{c^2}}$.

STRETCH AND CHALLENGE

Pressure of an ideal gas

Let us consider a cubic box with sides of length l containing N molecules of mass m (Fig 7.33). We start by working out the pressure that the molecules exert on the right-hand wall (points **1–6**), then the total pressure of all the molecules (points **7–9**).

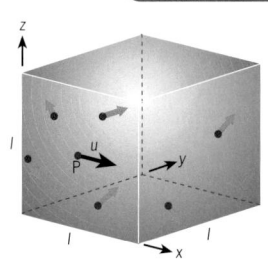

Fig 7.33 Cubic box containing molecules of an ideal gas. Molecule P is moving with speed u in the $+x$ direction

Pressure of an ideal gas

1 First consider molecule P moving in the $+x$ direction with speed u. The momentum when it approaches the right-hand wall is mu. The momentum after an *elastic* collision is $-mu$. So, the total change of momentum $= mu - (-mu) = 2mu$ (Fig 7.34).

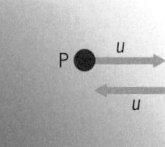

Fig 7.34 When molecule P collides elastically with the wall of the container:

change of momentum = $mu - (-mu) = 2mu$

2 Now consider the interval of time until the molecule makes another collision with the *same* wall. This is the time for the molecule to travel across the box, bounce off the opposite wall, and return. The distance travelled by the molecule is $2l$ at speed u. The time between collisions at the same wall is therefore $2l/u$. So the molecule makes one collision with the right-hand wall in each interval of time $2l/u$. The number of such collisions per unit time (i.e. per second) is $u/2l$ (which is the inverse of the time interval).

3 We are now able to find the *rate of change* of momentum for the molecule by multiplying the change of momentum for one collision by the number of collisions in unit time (i.e. the number in 1 s). The rate of change of momentum is:

$$2mu \times \frac{u}{2l} = \frac{mu^2}{l}$$

4 By Newton's second law, the rate of change of momentum of the molecule equals the force which the wall exerts on the molecule to cause it to rebound. This is equal and opposite to the force the molecule exerts on the wall. The force on the wall is mu^2/l. This is of course an averaged force, as Fig 7.26 showed.

5 We now find the overall force on the right-hand wall by adding forces from the impacts of all N molecules. The total force on the wall is:

$$\frac{mu_1^{\,2}}{l} + \frac{mu_2^{\,2}}{l} + \frac{mu_3^{\,2}}{l} + \dots$$

where u_1 is the velocity in the $+x$ direction of molecule 1, u_2 of molecule 2, and so on.

Hence the total force is:

$$\frac{m}{l}(u_1^{\,2} + u_2^{\,2} + u_3^{\,2} + \dots) = \frac{mN\overline{u^2}}{l}$$

where: $\quad \overline{u^2} = \dfrac{u_1^{\,2} + u_2^{\,2} + u_3^{\,2} + \dots}{N}$

is the average over the square of all the velocities in the $+x$ direction. (It is called the *mean square velocity* for molecules moving in the x direction.)

6 The pressure exerted on the walls by these molecules is given by:

$$\text{pressure} = \frac{\text{force}}{\text{area}} = \frac{mN\overline{u^2}/l}{l^2} = \frac{mN\overline{u^2}}{l \times l^2} = \frac{mN\overline{u^2}}{V}$$

where V is the volume of the box.

The total mass of the gas is mN and the density ρ of the gas is mN/V. This enables us to express the pressure as $p = \rho\, \overline{u^2}$.

7 The molecules are moving with components of velocity in the y and z directions in addition to a component in the x direction. We find the overall velocity c_1 for molecule 1 using Pythagoras' theorem:

$$c_1^{\,2} = u_1^{\,2} + v_1^{\,2} + w_1^{\,2}$$

where u_1 is the velocity component of molecule 1 in the $+x$ direction as previously, and v_1 and w_1 are the velocity components of molecule 1 in the $+y$ and $+z$ directions (Fig 7.35).

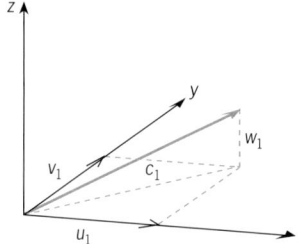

Fig 7.35 Resolving velocity c_1 into x, y and z components u_1, v_1 and w_1

8 Just as we obtained an average value of mean square velocity $\overline{u^2}$ for the velocity components of the molecules moving in the x direction, we can also obtain mean square velocities for the components in the y and z directions:

$$\overline{v^2} = \frac{v_1^{\,2} + v_2^{\,2} + v_3^{\,2} + \dots}{N} \qquad \overline{w^2} = \frac{w_1^{\,2} + w_2^{\,2} + w_3^{\,2} + \dots}{N}$$

This gives us an overall mean square velocity of:

$$\overline{c^2} = \overline{u^2} + \overline{v^2} + \overline{w^2}$$

9 We now obtain the final expression for pressure. The molecules on average are moving uniformly in all directions. So we can write:

$$\overline{u^2} = \overline{v^2} = \overline{w^2}$$

This gives:

$$\overline{c^2} = \overline{u^2} + \overline{v^2} + \overline{w^2}$$
$$= 3\overline{u^2}$$

or:

$$\overline{u^2} = \frac{\overline{c^2}}{3}$$

Hence:

$$p = \rho\overline{u^2} = \tfrac{1}{3}\rho\overline{c^2}$$

No account has been taken of collisions between molecules. However, provided these collisions are elastic, both total momentum and total kinetic energy are conserved. Exchange of momentum and kinetic energy between molecules has no overall effect on the pressure.

We can compare our expression for pressure from kinetic theory with that for pressure in the ideal gas equation. The first expression for pressure is based on the microscopic movement of the molecules and the second is based on the macroscopic quantities volume and temperature:

$$p = \frac{1}{3}\frac{mN\overline{c^2}}{V} \quad \text{and} \quad p = \frac{n}{V}RT$$

 REMEMBER THIS

$$\rho = \frac{Nm}{V}$$

Equating the two expressions for pressure gives:

$$\frac{1}{3}\frac{Nm}{V}\overline{c^2} = \frac{n}{V}RT$$

That is: $\frac{1}{3}Nm\overline{c^2} = nRT$

This equation creates a bridge between the small-scale and the large-scale models.

We know that $\frac{1}{2}m\overline{c^2}$ is the kinetic energy of one molecule and $\frac{1}{2}Nm\overline{c^2}$ is the total kinetic energy E_k of all the molecules. By using the bridging equation we see that the kinetic energy of the molecules is given by:

$$E_k = \frac{3}{2}nRT$$

This shows us that the kinetic energy of all the molecules is directly proportional to temperature. The energy must be the internal energy U of the gas. So:

$$U = \frac{3}{2}nRT$$

Remember that the above equation refers to n moles of gas. To obtain the

kinetic energy of the molecules in one mole we must divide by n. One mole of gas contains N_A molecules, where N_A is the Avogadro constant. We divide by N_A to obtain the energy for one molecule. These two steps give us:

$$U_{\text{one molecule}} = \frac{3}{2}\frac{nRT}{nN_A} = \frac{3}{2}\frac{RT}{N_A}$$

Here R/N_A is the **Boltzmann constant**, k, the gas constant for a single molecule. Its value is 1.380×10^{-23} J K^{-1}, and it is a fundamental constant that is very important in physics.

We now see that

average kinetic energy per molecule = $\frac{3}{2}kT$

and that we can associate kinetic energy $\frac{1}{2}kT$ with each degree of freedom – that is, with the freedom to move in each of the x, y and z directions.

Avogadro's hypothesis

This states:

Equal volumes of a gas under the same conditions of temperature and pressure have an equal number of molecules.

We consider two gases A and B and use subscripts A and B to identify them.

For gas A we have: $p_A V_A = \frac{1}{3} N_A m_A \overline{c_A^2}$

For gas B we have: $p_B V_B = \frac{1}{3} N_B m_B \overline{c_B^2}$

For the gases to be at the same pressure and volume, these expressions must be equal:

$$N_A m_A \overline{c_A^2} = N_B m_B \overline{c_B^2} \qquad [1]$$

Also, as they are at the same temperature:

$$\frac{1}{2}m_A\overline{c_A^2} = \frac{3}{2}kT \quad \text{and} \quad \frac{1}{2}m_B\overline{c_B^2} = \frac{3}{2}kT$$

giving: $\qquad m_A\overline{c_A^2} = m_B\overline{c_B^2}$

From equation 1, we can see that we must have:

$$N_A = N_B$$

which is the justification for Avogadro's hypothesis.

8 DISTRIBUTION OF MOLECULAR SPEED IN AN IDEAL GAS

In the calculation of the pressure of an ideal gas we used $\overline{c^2}$, the *mean* of the squared velocities. However, there will be wide variation in speed among the molecules. The situation is analogous to cars travelling along a motorway. A few will be travelling slowly. There will be many travelling close to the speed limit, others faster and some at an excessive speed. In a gas, too, there will be fast and slow molecules with a large proportion moving somewhere near the mean speed. This speed is determined by the temperature of the gas. Change the speed limit on a motorway and the distribution of the speed of the traffic changes. Alter the temperature of the gas and the speed (velocity) distribution alters.

For more on the Maxwell Boltzmann speed distribution please see the How Science Works assignment for this Chapter at www.collinseducation.co.uk/CAS

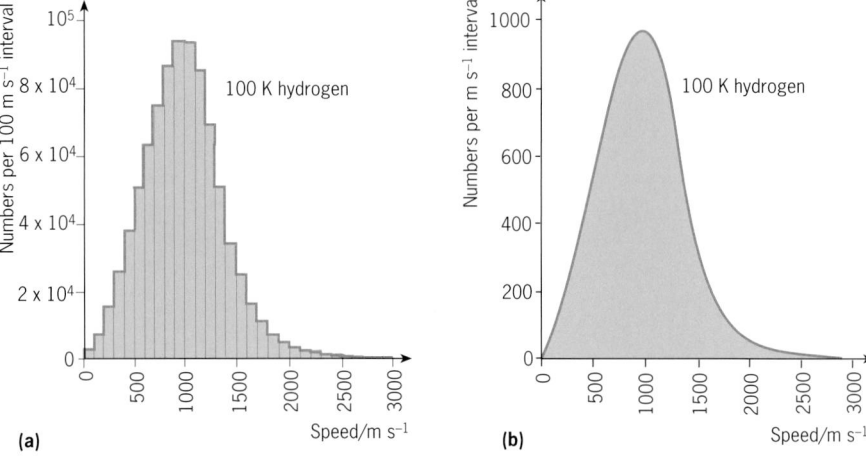

Fig 7.36 Typical speed distribution for 1 million molecules of hydrogen at 100 K shown **(a)** as a histogram at 100 m s^{-1} intervals and **(b)** as a continuous curve

Fig 7.36 shows a typical speed distribution for the molecules of a gas. Fig 7.36(a) shows the distribution as a histogram and Fig 7.36(b) shows it as a continuous plot. In both figures, the x axis shows the spread of speeds of the molecules. But what is plotted on the y axis needs more explanation.

The histogram shows the number of molecules moving within specific ranges of speed. Histogram intervals are set at 100 m s^{-1} so that the histogram represents the number of molecules with speeds 0 to 99 m s^{-1}, 100 to 199 m s^{-1} and so on. We can draw a curve to represent the outline of the histogram but it will not be very accurate.

If we take much smaller intervals we obtain more columns to the histogram and can draw a more precise curve. If we make the intervals of width 1 m s^{-1}, we obtain a distribution where the y axis is the number of molecules per unit interval of speed (that is, per m s^{-1}) and we obtain the continuous curve of Fig 7.36(b). The calibration of the y axis depends on the quantity of gas involved. This quantity is arbitrary, but a million molecules is assumed in Fig 7.36, so that the area under the graph is one million.

The graph shows distribution of *speed*. However, in calculating pressure, it is *speed squared* that is important and this means that the molecules at the upper end (right-hand side) of the distribution have the largest influence. Similarly, on a motorway, the seriousness of an accident usually depends on the kinetic energy of the vehicles as well as their mass. Kinetic energy is proportional to speed squared and accidents become proportionately more serious as speed rises. This is an important reason why speed restrictions are imposed.

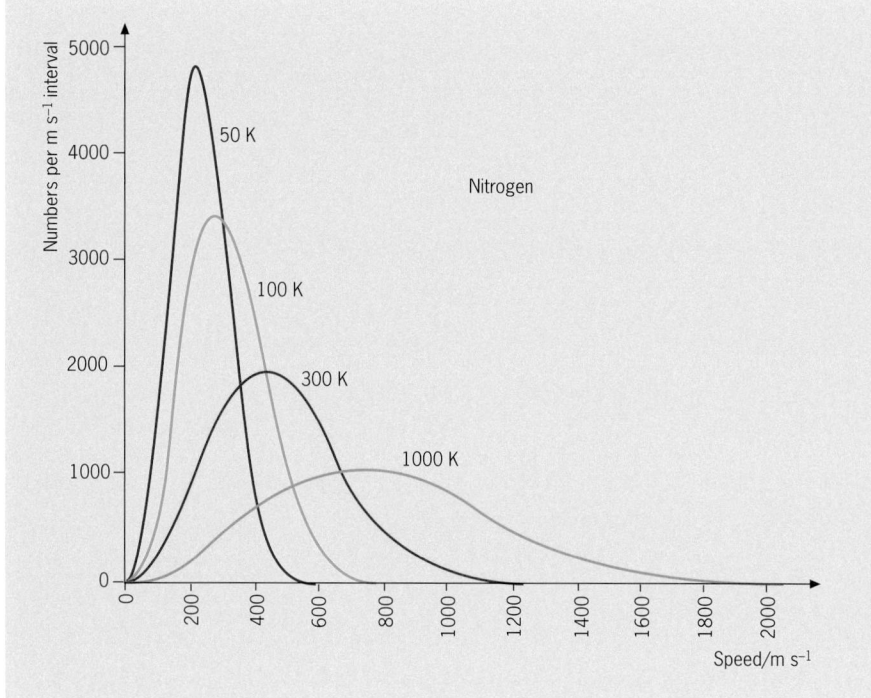

Fig 7.37 Variation of speed distribution for 1 million molecules of nitrogen as the temperature of the gas changes

? QUESTION 10

10 Using Fig 7.36(b):
a) State the most probable speed of the gas molecules.
b) Estimate what fraction of the molecules travel between 500 m s^{-1} and 1000 m s^{-1}.
c) Estimate what fraction of the molecules of the gas travel at twice the most probable speed or more.

If the gas is heated, the curve showing the distribution of speeds spreads out horizontally (Fig 7.37), but the area under each curve remains constant. The total area under the curve has to remain the same as the area represents the total number of molecules. Because the curve spreads out horizontally, it is clear that the number of molecules at the peak speed must decrease with increase in temperature.

SUMMARY

After studying this chapter you should be able to:
- Describe qualitatively the differences between states of matter.
- Describe different types of bonding between atoms.
- Explain the term latent heat and use values of specific latent heat in calculations.
- Draw and interpret force against separation and potential energy against separation curves for adjacent atoms in a solid or liquid.
- Describe simple cubic crystal structures in terms of packing of spherical atoms and carry out simple calculations of atomic spacing.
- Describe Brownian motion.
- State the gas laws:

$$pV = \text{constant} \quad \frac{p}{T} = \text{constant} \quad \frac{V}{T} = \text{constant}$$

and outline how they are proved experimentally.
- Be aware of the relation between the Kelvin temperature scale and the ideal gas equation and describe the use of the constant-volume gas thermometer to measure Kelvin temperature.

- Use the ideal gas equation:
$$\frac{pV}{T} = \text{constant} \quad \text{or} \quad \frac{p_1 V_1}{T_1} = \frac{p_2 V_2}{T_2}$$
to make simple calculations of pressure, volume and temperature of a gas.
- Understand that in an ideal gas the equation of state is given by $pV = nRT$, where R is the molar gas constant and n is the number of moles of gas.
- State the main assumptions used in the kinetic theory of an ideal gas and carry out simple calculations using the theory.
- Understand the relation between the Avogadro constant N_A and the mole.
- Know that the average kinetic energy per molecule is $3kT/2$, where k is the Boltzmann constant R/N_A.

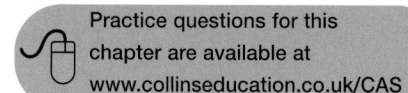

Practice questions for this chapter are available at www.collinseducation.co.uk/CAS

8

Charge and current

8 CHARGE AND CURRENT

Electricity in medicine

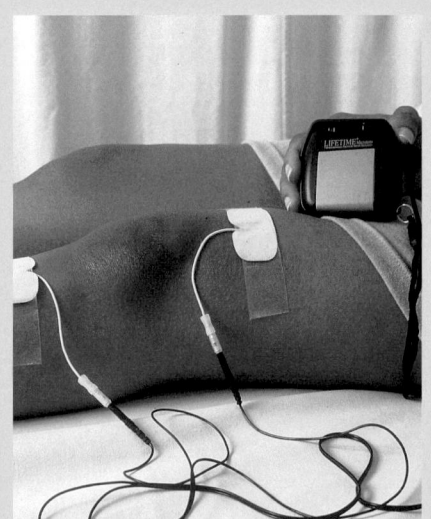

When you visit the dentist or have treatment in hospital for an accident, the chances are that you will be given drugs to combat the pain. Modern drugs are very effective for treating short-term pain. But some people suffer from conditions that give them continuous pain, and the prolonged use of pain-killing drugs can cause unwanted side effects.

One of the more effective methods of dealing with continuous pain is called transcutaneous electric nerve stimulation, or TENS for short. (Transcutaneous means 'across the skin'.) Users of TENS carry a box the size of a personal stereo on a belt. It runs from a 9 V battery and has two electrodes which the user can tape to the area of the body that has pain. The TENS unit supplies short pulses of current at low voltage through the electrodes to the painful area and the user can adjust the strength of the current and the length of the pulse time. The pulses of current stimulate nerve endings and this inhibits the sensation of pain.

Many pain sufferers find TENS to be very effective in treating acute pain, such as the pain in the stump of a limb after it has been amputated.

Pulses of current from a TENS unit can help relieve continuous pain and avoid the side effects of pain-killing drugs

The ideas in this chapter

Electricity was the development in physics during the twentieth century that has perhaps had the greatest effect on the largest number of people. Electric current to the homes of many millions of people has given them energy at the flick of a switch. In the United Kingdom, electricity is distributed on the national grid – a complex circuit connected to every home, factory, school and hospital.

Countless time- and labour-saving devices are run on electricity: examples range from our vast modern communications systems to the electric sensors that allow doctors to monitor the vital functions of the human body. Hundreds of amperes of current are needed to run our railway systems; it takes a current of only a microampere to keep a wristwatch working.

The basic ideas described in this chapter are relevant to these and many other circuits. To begin with, there are some basic facts about circuits that can be established easily by experiment.

1 CIRCUITS

The simplest electric circuit is a closed path starting from a battery (or cell) and returning to the battery, as in Fig 8.1. The fact that this complete loop is required suggests that something is moving round the circuit. We call what moves an **electric charge**, and the rate of flow of the charge an **electric current**. The size of a current is measured by an **ammeter** in **amperes**, symbol A. (Later in the chapter, we shall look in more detail at the nature of current, and of resistance and conductance.)

It is easy to show by experiment how currents behave in circuits. The simplest circuit is a **series** circuit. The charge has only one path to follow, and it passes through each component placed in the circuit, such as the bulbs in Fig 8.1.

REMEMBER THIS

A battery consists of a stack of several cells. Each cell has two electrodes, one positive and one negative. The word 'battery' is used to describe a single cell as well as a collection of cells.

For a simple series circuit, the current is the same at every point in the circuit. A component has a **resistance** which determines the current: when a component is added to the circuit, the current decreases as the resistance of the circuit increases. Each component, such as each of the bulbs in Fig 8.1, then receives the same lower current, as recorded by the ammeter.

Instead of wiring components in series, we can connect them in **parallel**, as shown in Fig 8.2. Each bulb offers a different path for the charge to flow through. As each bulb is switched on, the total current drawn from the power source increases. The total current I is equal to the sum of the currents in the parallel arms, that is:

$$I = i_1 + i_2 + i_3$$

A **voltmeter** measures a quantity called a **voltage**. (We shall see later in this chapter exactly what a voltage is.) In a series circuit, the voltage across the battery is equal to the sum of voltages across all parts of the circuit, as shown in Fig 8.3(a). When components are connected in parallel, the voltage across one component is the same as the voltage across any other component, Fig 8.3(b).

Parallel circuits are very important in everyday life. In the home, there is probably one circuit for lighting, and one with sockets in the wall for electrical equipment (known as the power circuit or ring main). The components – lights or equipment – are connected in parallel to their circuit.

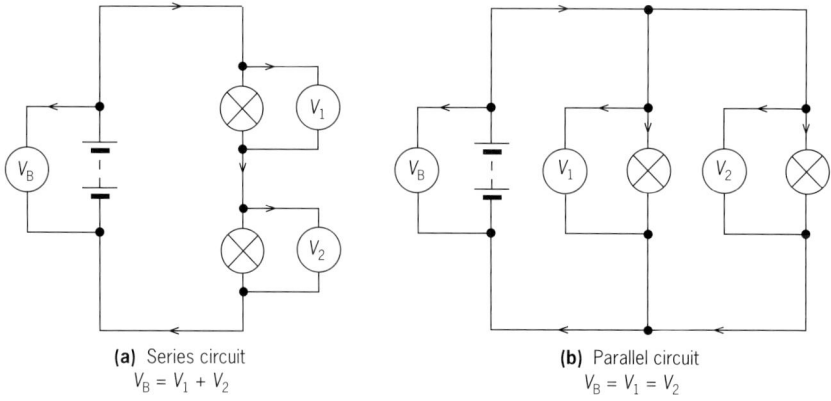

(a) Series circuit
$V_B = V_1 + V_2$

(b) Parallel circuit
$V_B = V_1 = V_2$

Fig 8.3 Measuring voltage in series and in parallel circuits. The voltmeters are connected across the battery and across each bulb

2 WHAT IS AN ELECTRIC CURRENT?

An electric current is a flow of electric charge; any moving charge is a current. Charge is carried by particles such as **electrons** or **ions**. When these particles are electrons, they usually travel in a wire. When they are ions, they are moving usually in a water solution. If charged particles are moving, a current exists. If the charged particles do not move, there is no current.

Electrons are negatively charged. When they move in a circuit they go from the negative terminal to the positive one. In spite of this, the *direction of the current* in a circuit is taken as being from *positive to negative* (look back at Fig 8.1). This is the conventional way to represent current, agreed by early experimenters working on current electricity. As we know, they were wrong about current in a wire, but it doesn't matter, as we shall see later.

The unit of electrical charge is the **coulomb**, symbol C, and it relates to amperes in this way:

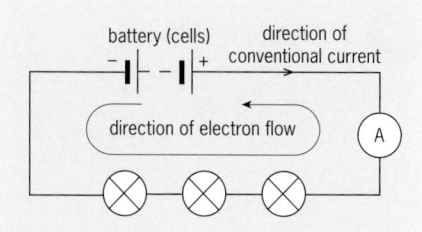

Fig 8.1 A simple circuit with a battery and three bulbs connected in series. The convention is that the direction of the current is from the plus to the minus side of the battery

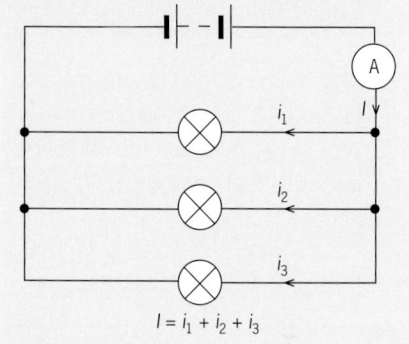

$I = i_1 + i_2 + i_3$

Fig 8.2 A simple circuit with three bulbs connected in parallel

? QUESTION 1

1 **a)** Sketch a circuit for a hair-dryer and a TV plugged into the power supply.
   b) One of the light bulbs in the lighting circuit of a house fails. What effect has this on the rest of the light circuit, and why?

? QUESTION 2

2 State whether or not a current exists in the following situations.
   a) Your hair stands on end after you comb it on a dry day.
   b) You are eating chocolate with a small piece of metal foil attached to it. The foil touches a filling and you feel pain.
   c) A bolt of lightning flashes through the sky.
   d) A gardener has cut through a cable of a lawnmower while mowing the lawn. The ends of the cable are lying apart on the ground while the gardener goes to switch off at the mains plug.

REMEMBER THIS

Common units used for electric currents include:

1 A = 1000 mA = 1 000 000 µA

'µA' means microampere

1 mA = 10^{-3} A

1 µA = 10^{-6} A = 10^{-3} mA

? QUESTION 3

3 The charge carried by one electron is 1.6×10^{-19} C. If the current in a wire is 1 A, calculate the number of electrons that pass any point each second.

REMEMBER THIS

When the current varies, the total charge that flows can be found by taking the area under the graph in small strips (one strip is seen in Fig 8.4(b)) and adding the areas of all the strips together. This is done using calculus and integrating:

$dQ = I\,dt$

$Q = \int I\,dt$

? QUESTIONS 4–5

4 Calculate the current in each of the following:
a) 2 C flows through a bulb in 10 s.
b) 2 µC flows through a light-emitting diode in 1 ms.
c) 20 nC flows into an integrated circuit in 500 ms.
(1 nC = 10^{-9} C)

5 How much charge flows in the following examples?
a) 5 A for an hour.
b) 50 mA for a day.
c) 5 µA for 20 s.

A coulomb is the amount of charge that flows when there is a current of one ampere for one second.

So, for example, if an ammeter in a circuit measures a current of 1 A, a charge of 1 C will pass through it during each second. Since the measured current I is the rate of flow of charge Q, the amount of charge that flows in a circuit can be calculated. Since:

$$I = Q \div t$$

then:

$$Q = I \times t$$

where t is in seconds and Q is in coulombs.

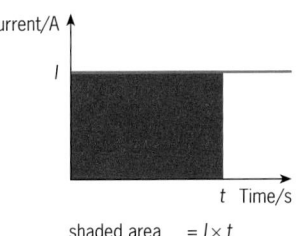

shaded area $= I \times t$
charge flowing $= Q$ (coulombs)

(a) Current does not change with time

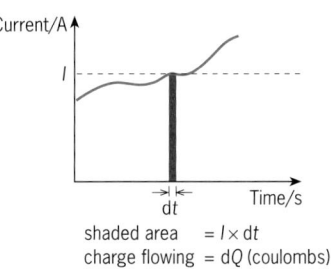

shaded area $= I \times dt$
charge flowing $= dQ$ (coulombs)

(b) Current changes with time

Fig 8.4 Graphs of current against time

Fig. 8.4(a) is for a constant current. The area under the graph is equal to the charge flowing in the time shown. Fig. 8.4(b) shows a changing current. The shaded area indicates the charge flowing in a small period of time, dt. Only a small amount of charge flows; we call it dQ. Even though the current is changing, we can consider it to be steady over the short time dt. Therefore we can. write:

$$dQ = I \times dt$$
$$I = \frac{dQ}{dt}$$

We can now give a general definition of current:

Current is equal to the rate of flow of charge.

We shall use this definition later in the chapter when we examine the behaviour of capacitors.

3 CURRENT AND FREE ELECTRONS

The current in a material (such as a wire) is due to the movement of **free electrons**. Copper, used for wires connecting components, is a good **conductor** of electrons. (So are other metals.) A copper wire consists of millions of identical copper atoms. Each atom has electrons. Most of them are tightly bound to the atomic nucleus by the electrical attractive force between the positive nucleus and the negative electrons.

One or two electrons on the outside of the atom are less tightly bound; being furthest from the nucleus, the attractive force on them is lowest. In a solid, the atoms are closely packed and each atom may have up to twelve other atoms next to it. An electron on the outside of an atom may be the same distance from a neighbouring nucleus as from its own nucleus. So which atom does it belong to? Such electrons can move between atoms and are known as free electrons. They behave like an electron 'cloud' and move inside the metal in random directions.

Derivation of the transport equation

Fig 8.5 shows a section of wire carrying a current of I amperes. As you read on, write down an expression for each step, and note the units.

Each electron carries a charge of e coulombs and travels with an average drift speed of v metres per second. There are n free electrons per cubic metre of wire, and its cross-sectional area is A square metres.

Suppose it takes t seconds for an electron to pass from X to Y. The distance from X to Y is vt metres and the volume of wire between X and Y is Avt cubic metres.

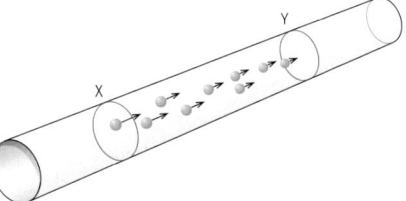

Fig 8.5 Current in a wire: the flow of free electrons carrying negative charge. (Conventionally, the current is in the opposite direction)

The number of electrons between X and Y is equal to the volume between X and Y multiplied by n, that is, $nAvt$. If each electron carries a charge of e coulombs, then the total charge that passes across point Y in t seconds is $nAevt$.

Now, the current is equal to the charge flowing per second, that is, $nAevt/t$. Therefore $I = nAev$ in coulombs per second.

The expression applies to a single electron of charge e. We can use Q to represent any charge, when the flow of charge $I = nAQv$.

When the wire is in a circuit and a voltage is placed across it, the free electrons are attracted towards the positive side of the power supply and there is a net drift of the electron 'cloud' in that direction. This is a **current**. Each electron carries an electric charge of 1.6×10^{-19} C.

Materials with many free electrons are good conductors; those with few are poor conductors. The number of free electrons per cubic metre – the number of *charge carriers per unit volume* – indicates how good a conductor a material is.

The current also depends on the speed at which the electron 'cloud' travels in a particular material – the **drift speed**. The cross-sectional area of the conductor also has an effect on the current: a thick wire offers an easier path for the electrons than a thin one. The way that the current depends on these factors is described by the **transport equation**, as explained in the Stretch and Challenge box above.

4 POTENTIAL DIFFERENCE AND ENERGY IN CIRCUITS

? QUESTION 6

6 Two wires X and Y are made from the same material. X has twice the cross-sectional area of Y and the current in X is twice that through Y. Work out the ratio of the average drift speed of electrons in X to the average drift speed of electrons in Y.

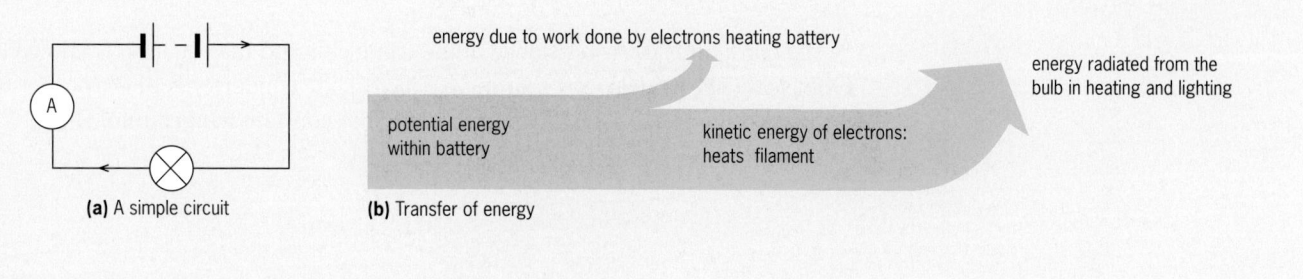

(a) A simple circuit

(b) Transfer of energy

energy due to work done by electrons heating battery

energy radiated from the bulb in heating and lighting

potential energy within battery

kinetic energy of electrons: heats filament

Fig 8.6 (a) A circuit with a light bulb. **(b)** The transfer of energy in circuit **(a)**

All circuits deliver energy from their source (a battery or power supply) to the components in the circuit. The amount of energy transferred depends on the current. In a circuit containing a bulb, as in Fig 8.6, electrons pass through the bulb filament. The electrons collide with filament atoms, work is done on these atoms, energy is transferred to them and they heat up and give out light. (Electrons can flow more easily through the copper connecting wire – there are fewer collisions – and so it does not get hot.)

We measure the energy delivered to the filament (the work done in it) in terms of **joules per coulomb** of charge passing through it. This is the **potential (energy) difference (p.d.)** across the filament, sometimes called the **voltage**. Now we can give this definition of a **volt**:

1 joule per coulomb = 1 volt

If the p.d. across a bulb is 6 V, this means that, for each coulomb that passes through the bulb, 6 J is the amount of energy transferred from the current to do work heating and lighting the bulb.

5 RESISTANCE

Why is energy transferred when charge flows through a bulb or through a motor? Why does the current get smaller when bulbs are connected in series? Why is the current from the supply greater when bulbs are connected in parallel?

The answers to all these questions are best understood if we use the idea of **resistance**:

Resistance is the electrical property of a material that makes the moving charges dissipate energy.

Resistance restricts the flow of charge, so a resistance makes the current smaller. Connection wires have very low resistance; the wires used in lamp filaments have higher resistances. But they are all conductors. Insulators like the plastic round the wires in a cable have very much higher resistance – ideally an infinite resistance.

Some very useful materials are both poor conductors and bad insulators. They are semiconductors. There is more about **semiconductors** on page 186 and in Chapter 20.

Resistance is measured in **ohms**. The symbol is Ω (the Greek letter omega) and the ohm is named after Georg Simon Ohm who found the relationship between current and p.d. He measured the current through wires as he changed the voltage across the wires. He discovered a very important relationship which he published in 1826. At a steady temperature:

p.d. across a conductor = current through conductor × a constant

$$V = I \times R$$

The constant R is the resistance of the conductor and the equation is known as Ohm's law. We can also say that the p.d. across the conductor is directly proportional to the current flowing through it at constant temperature. The equation can be rearranged as:

$$R = \frac{V}{I}$$

where V is the p.d. across the conductor and I is the current through it. From this equation it is clear that:

$$1\Omega = \frac{1\,V}{1\,A}$$

The graphs in Fig 8.7 show the behaviour of two types of conductor. Not all obey Ohm's law. Those that do are called **ohmic conductors**. At a constant temperature their resistance is constant over a wide range of currents, so their p.d.–current graphs are straight lines.

QUESTION 7

7 **a)** Explain why conductors are designed to have very low resistances.
b) Give an example of an insulator and its purpose in an electrical circuit in the home.

QUESTION 8

8 Calculate the resistance of a 6 V bulb that takes a current of 0.06 A.

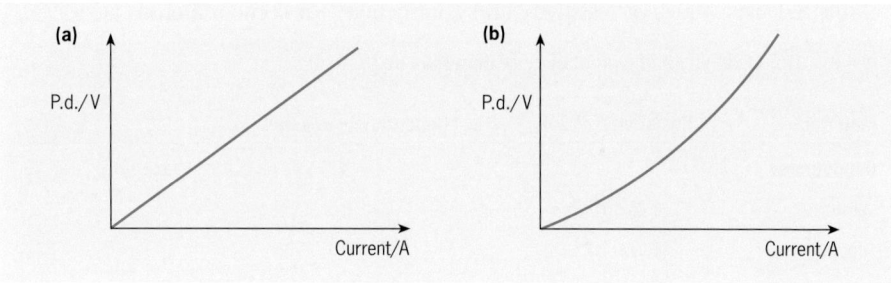

Fig 8.7 Graphs of p.d. against current for
(a) a conductor material that obeys Ohm's law and
(b) a conductor material that does not obey
Ohm's law

But many non-ohmic conductors are useful. Their resistance depends on p.d., even at a constant temperature, so their p.d.–current graphs are not a straight line and often show sharp changes in gradient. The semiconductor diode is a good example of a non-ohmic component, which we shall look at in Chapter 20.

RESISTIVITY

Ohm also investigated how the resistance of a conductor depends on its dimensions and the material that it is made of. For the same p.d. across a wire, its resistance increases with length l (so $R \propto l$), and decreases with cross-sectional area A (so $R \propto l/A$). If you increase the length of a wire in a circuit, the current will decrease. If you increase the thickness of the wire, the current will increase.

The resistance of a wire at constant temperature depends on its length, its cross-sectional area and its **resistivity**, symbol ρ (the Greek letter rho). The resistivity is a constant for the particular material of a wire and has the unit ohm metre (Ω m). The three factors give the following equation for resistance:

$$R = \rho \frac{l}{A}$$

The resistivity of a material can be altered by adding impurities that affect the structure of the crystal lattice. Resistivity changes with temperature for most materials. The resistivity of good conductors such as metals increases with temperature while, in general, the resistivity of semiconductors decreases with temperature.

> **? QUESTION 9**
>
> 9 Two wires, A and B, are made of the same material. A is twice as long as B but has twice its diameter. Which wire has the greater resistance?

CONDUCTANCE AND CONDUCTIVITY

The resistance of a sample of material tells us how difficult it is for charge to flow. Sometimes it is more convenient to look at how *easily* charge can flow. Then we talk about the **conductance**, G, of the sample. Quite simply,

$$\text{conductance} = \frac{1}{\text{resistance}} \quad \text{or} \quad G = \frac{1}{R}$$

Conductance is measured in **siemens** (S).

Similarly, instead of resistivity, the **conductivity** of a material may be a useful comparative property; this has the symbol σ (Greek sigma). Again the relation is:

$$\text{conductivity} = \frac{1}{\text{resistivity}} \quad \text{or} \quad \sigma = \frac{1}{\rho}$$

The unit of conductivity is S m^{-1}.

Table 8.1 lists values of resistivity and conductivity for some materials at 20 °C.

Table 8.1 The resistivity and conductivity of materials at 20 °C

Material	Resistivity ρ/Ω m	Conductivity σ/S m^{-1}
Conductors:		
silver	1.6×10^{-8}	6.3×10^{7}
copper	1.7×10^{-8}	5.9×10^{7}
aluminium	2.8×10^{-8}	3.6×10^{7}
iron	8.9×10^{-8}	1.1×10^{7}
mild steel	14×10^{-8}	7.1×10^{6}
constantan	49×10^{-8}	2.0×10^{6}
graphite	3000×10^{-8}	3.3×10^{4}
Semiconductors:		
germanium	0.6	1.7
silicon	2300	4.4×10^{-4}
Insulators:		
porcelain	10^{11}	10^{-11}
glass	10^{12}	10^{-12}
PVC	10^{12}	10^{-12}
PTFE	10^{16}	10^{-16}

? QUESTIONS 10–11

10 A 40 W, 240 V mains bulb has a filament that is the same length as the filament in a 40 W, 12 V car headlamp bulb. The filaments are both made from tungsten. Compare their thicknesses.

11 If two identical lengths of copper and iron wire of equal diameter are connected in series to a power supply, the iron wire reaches a higher temperature. When they are connected in parallel, the copper wire reaches the higher temperature. Compare the resistances of the two wires and explain these observations.

6 ENERGY AND POWER IN CIRCUITS

The energy transferred to a component in a circuit, such as a bulb, depends on the current in it and the p.d. across it. The current in amperes is the number of coulombs passing through the bulb per second, and the p.d. in volts is the amount of energy in joules transferred by each coulomb as it passes through the bulb. If we multiply the two quantities, p.d. and current, we get an interesting result:

joules per coulomb × coulombs per second = joules per second

Joules per second is the power, or rate of energy transfer, measured in watts.

We now have a very useful equation for electrical circuits:

power (watts) = p.d. (volts) × current (amperes)
$$W = V \times I$$

Energy is transferred when a current passes through something with electrical resistance. We can think of the energy transferred as the **work** done to overcome the resistance.

ENERGY TRANSFERRED IN A PARTICULAR TIME

If we know the power (the rate of energy transferred) by a motor, for example, then it is easy to calculate the amount of energy that is transferred in a particular time:

energy transferred = power × time
$$= IV \times t$$

? QUESTION 12

12 Calculate the energy radiated by a 6 V, 0.3 A torch bulb in half an hour.

Other forms of the power equation

For purely resistive components, it is often convenient to use other forms of the power equation, which we can derive from $V = IR$ or $I = V/R$.

If the *current* and resistance are known, then:

$$W = V \times I = IR \times I = I^2R$$

So: $W = I^2R$

Engineers refer to wasteful energy transfers (e.g. energy wasted in a power cable or in the windings of the rotor in a dynamo) as I^2R losses.

If the *voltage* and resistance are known, then:

$$W = V \times I = V \times V/R$$

So: $W = \dfrac{V^2}{R}$

7 INTERNAL RESISTANCE AND E.M.F.

In circuit (a) of Fig 8.8, the switch is open and there is no current through the bulb, but the reading on the voltmeter is 12.1 V. In circuit (b), the switch is closed and there is a current through the bulb. The voltmeter shows the p.d. across the bulb *and* across the battery. The reading on the voltmeter is now slightly less, at 11.8 V.

In the first case, the only current is a few microamperes through the voltmeter. This current is negligible compared with the current in the bulb in the second circuit. Why does the voltage decrease? The difference in voltage can be explained by considering the **internal resistance** of the battery.

When the circuit is complete and charges move, there are energy transfers within the battery. As chemical changes occur, potential energy is transferred to the charged particles: they move and a current is generated. Energy is also transferred to overcome resistances inside the battery – some 'joules per coulomb' are lost across the internal resistance, indicated by r in Fig 8.9. This resistance is due to collisions between charged particles and other atoms in the battery. The fact that a battery heats up is evidence for this. You may only notice this when currents of several amps are drawn.

A good battery has a low internal resistance, typically about 1 Ω or even less. When charge flows through the bulb, the current is quite high. For a 24 W bulb it would be about 2 A. Using $V = IR$, the voltage across an internal resistance of 0.5 Ω is 1 V. We have to consider the *whole* circuit, with the internal resistance in series with the load resistance (the total resistance outside the battery).

ELECTROMOTIVE FORCE, E.M.F.

The rate at which energy is transferred within the battery is measured in joules per coulomb, that is, volts. The battery voltage is responsible for forcing the current round the whole circuit, including through the battery, and is called the **electromotive force** or **e.m.f.** ($\mathcal{E}$).

Since energy must be conserved, the total energy transferred in the circuit must be equal to the energy transferred in the battery, so:

energy transferred per second within the battery	=	energy transferred in the circuit and in overcoming the internal resistance every second

So: $\qquad \mathcal{E}I = I^2R + I^2r$

Where r is the internal resistance of the battery and R is the resistance of the load which in this case is a bulb. I is the current when the switch is closed. Dividing both sides by the current I:

$$\mathcal{E} = IR + Ir$$

or: $\qquad IR = \mathcal{E} - Ir$

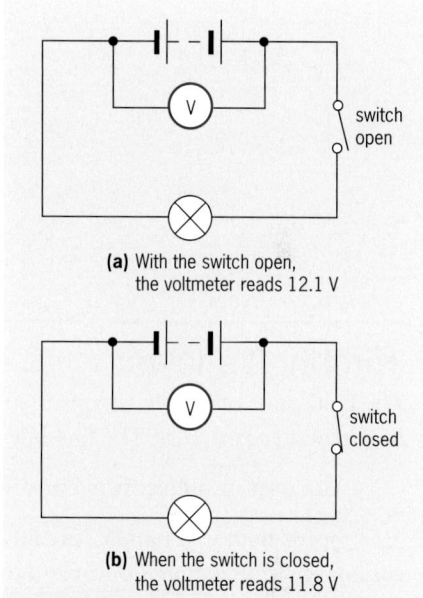

(a) With the switch open, the voltmeter reads 12.1 V

(b) When the switch is closed, the voltmeter reads 11.8 V

Fig 8.8 Reading voltage with the switch open and closed

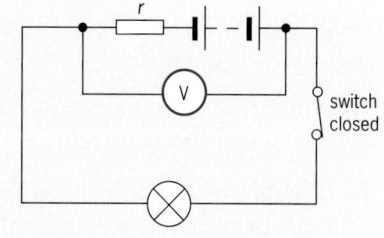

Fig 8.9 The circuit of Fig 8.8 with the internal resistance of the battery represented by r

REMEMBER THIS

Volts: p.d. and e.m.f.

The e.m.f. is a measure of the rate at which energy is transferred per coulomb from an energy source such as a battery or a dynamo, in the kinetic energy of the moving charge.

The p.d. is a measure of the rate at which energy is transferred per coulomb from the kinetic energy of the charge to do work in a circuit. Both are measured in joules per coulomb, that is, in volts.

Putting this in words:

p.d. across load = battery e.m.f. – voltage across internal resistance

Note that the word equation refers to voltage across internal resistance, rather than p.d. This is to distinguish p.d. as a voltage that can be measured with a voltmeter, from the p.d. across the internal resistance which cannot be measured directly.

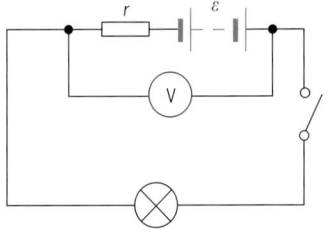
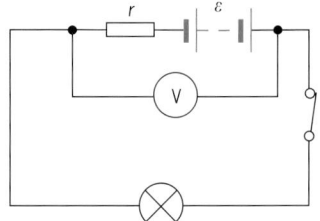

(a) Switch open: voltmeter reading = 12.1 V   **(b)** Switch closed: voltmeter reading = 11.8 V

Fig 8.10 Looking at the e.m.f. (ε) of a battery

In Fig 8.10(a), with the switch open, the voltmeter measures IR. I is small because the voltmeter has a large resistance. Also, r is very small compared with R. Therefore, Ir is small and the voltmeter reading IR is close to the e.m.f. ε.

STRETCH AND CHALLENGE

Kirchhoff's laws

The behaviour of simple circuits is summarised in Kirchhoff's two laws. The first law states:

Current in a circuit is conserved.

This means that, in a parallel circuit, all the current entering a junction leaves the junction, as shown in Fig 8.11(a). Kirchhoff's first law effectively says that charge does not collect at the junction.

The second law is the law of conservation of energy applied to circuits and is shown in Fig 8.11(b). The law states that:

The sum of the e.m.f.s is equal to the sum of the IR products.

The IR products are the p.d.s across each load in the circuit, including any internal resistances in the battery. The sum of the p.d.s is the total energy transferred as each coulomb does work around the circuit. The sum of the e.m.f.s is the total energy transferred to each coulomb within the current sources.

Accepting that e.m.f.s are positive and p.d.s are negative, then an alternative statement is:

The sum of the voltages around a circuit is zero.

(a)

$I = i_1 + i_2 + i_3$

(b)

$\varepsilon_1 + \varepsilon_2 = IR_1 + IR_2 + IR_3$

Fig 8.11 (a) The circuit junction, illustrating Kirchhoff's first law. **(b)** E.m.f.s and resistances in a circuit, illustrating Kirchhoff's second law

? **QUESTION 13**

13 Battery A has an e.m.f. of 2.0 V and an internal resistance of 1 Ω. For battery B, the values are 1.0 V and 2 Ω. A and B are connected to a 2 Ω resistor as shown. Using Kirchhoff's laws, calculate the current through the 2 Ω resistor.

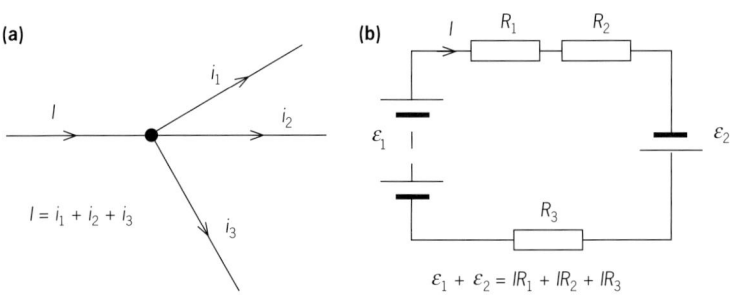

A 2.0 V, 1 Ω

2 Ω

B 1.0 V, 2 Ω

In Fig 8.10(b), with the switch closed, resistance R is small, so the current I is high. (For a bulb of 12 V and 24 W, R would be 6 Ω.) Ir is small, but significant, compared with IR.

If you think about it, we cannot measure the battery e.m.f. absolutely. The voltmeter itself will always require some current, however tiny, and some voltage will be lost across the internal resistance. As we use voltmeters of higher and higher resistances, the reading gets closer and closer to the actual e.m.f., but it never quite gets there.

? QUESTION 14

14 An extra high tension (e.h.t.) power supply for use in a laboratory is designed to provide very high voltages and is set to give 6000 V. A voltmeter capable of measuring this voltage is connected to measure the p.d. across the output of the supply. When a milliammeter is connected across the output it shows a current of 6 mA and the reading on the voltmeter drops to almost zero. What can you deduce about the internal resistance of the power supply?

HOW SCIENCE WORKS

Professor Georg Simon Ohm [1789–1854]

Today we can confirm Ohm's law by experiment with modern apparatus. We have reliable ammeters and voltmeters and stable sources of electrical energy. Ohm had none of these.

In the 1820s when he did his experiments, batteries were unreliable – their e.m.f.s changed unpredictably. To overcome this problem, he used an effect discovered in 1822 by another scientist called Thomas Johann Seebeck.

Seebeck had demonstrated that an e.m.f. is set up between two junctions where two unlike metals join. This is known as a thermocouple. So, as in Fig 8.12(a), a voltage is produced between the two junctions in the circuit made from copper and bismuth wires. When one copper/bismuth junction is in freezing water and the other is in steam, a voltage is produced that is proportional to the difference in temperature between the two: the greater the temperature difference, the larger the voltage. Ohm was therefore able to use a thermocouple as a source of e.m.f. that could be accurately controlled.

Thermocouples are used extensively in industry to measure temperature. Their great advantage is that the active junctions are very small and little energy is needed to produce the thermo-e.m.f. This is ideal when the temperature of very small bodies is being measured. In the home, a gas central heating boiler has a thermocouple to detect water temperature. It regulates the system for turning off the gas when the water is hot enough.

In his investigations, Ohm passed a current through copper wires of different lengths, and also used another recent discovery to measure the current. In 1819, the Danish scientist Hans Christian Oersted had discovered that a small magnet suspended near a wire was deflected when a current was passed through the wire. Ohm used this deflection to measure the current accurately. With these apparently crude techniques, he discovered the law named after him, one of the principal experimental laws in physics.

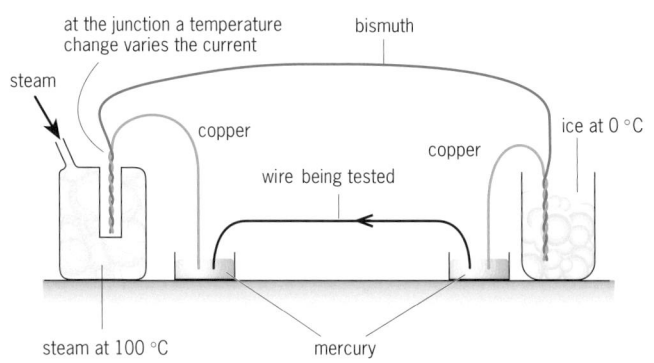

Fig 8.12 (a) The thermocouple apparatus which Seebeck devised and which Ohm used in his investigations. The arrow indicates the direction in which charge flows

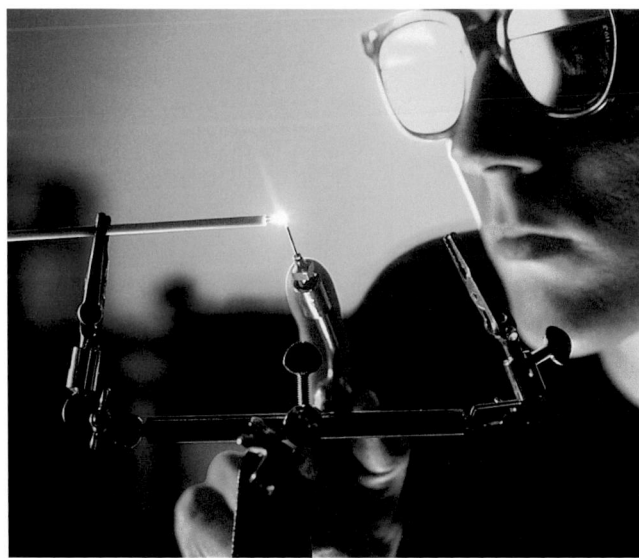

Fig 8.12 (b) Making a thermocouple: two wires, in this case one of platinum and the other of rhodium–platinum alloy, are being welded together to form one junction of the thermocouple. When the two junctions are at different temperatures, there is a current between them. When joined to a suitable meter, the thermocouple can be used as a thermometer or a thermostat

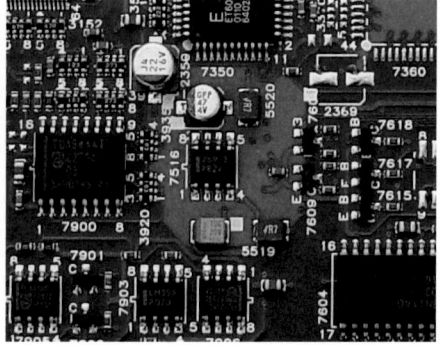

Fig 8.13 Modern electronics circuits use miniature 'chip' components. This section of the board shows several different components including chip resistors. There are three on the right, one each under the numbers 7615,7617 and 7618. The 'three-legged' components to the left of each resistor is a transistor.

8 SIMPLE CIRCUITS WITH RESISTORS

A resistor is a component designed to have a stated resistance. Resistors are manufactured to preferred values, from ohms to megohms, and to a specified accuracy or **tolerance**. They are made from a variety of materials, such as carbon, metal film on a ceramic base, or wound wire. Modern electronic microcircuits have resistors that are painted on to a circuit board using resistive paint. Some of the uses of resistors are now described.

RESISTORS USED TO LIMIT CURRENT

Some devices require only a small current. A good example is the **light-emitting diode** (LED), used as an on/off indicator on many electronic devices such as televisions, video players and computers. An LED shines brightly with a voltage of only 2.0 V across it and the maximum current through it should be 20 mA, so as not to overload it.

EXAMPLE

Q We want to use an LED with a 9 V supply and so we use a resistor in series with the LED to limit the current. What is the value of the resistor?

A The circuit is shown in Fig 8.14(a). The voltage across the resistor is:

$$9.0\text{ V} - 2.0\text{ V} = 7.0\text{ V}$$

and the current in the circuit needs to be 20 mA. Using $V/I = R$, the resistance of the limiting resistor should be:

$$7.0\text{ V}/20\text{ mA} = 350\ \Omega$$

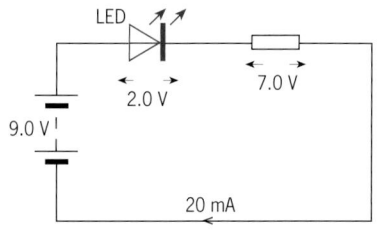

Fig 8.14(a) A circuit showing an LED in series with a limiting resistor

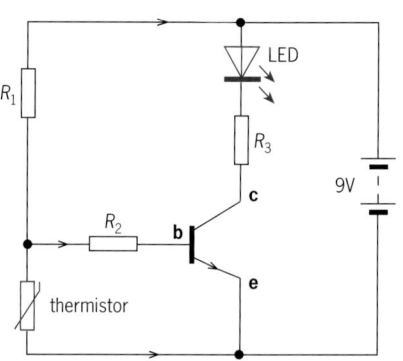

Fig 8.14(b) The circuit for a simple temperature-sensitive switch. When the temperature of the thermistor increases, the transistor is 'switched on'. Then, the p.d. across the transistor (contacts c and e) drops to nearly zero. The p.d. across R_3 and the LED is then nearly 9 V, just as in Fig 8.14(a) – the LED comes on when the temperature increases

---

Resistors are available in preferred values, the nearest values to 350 Ω being 330 Ω or 390 Ω. The use of 330 Ω in the Example above would mean the current would exceed 20 mA and therefore may damage the LED. The 390 Ω should therefore be used. This means that the LED may be a little dim but can be used without danger of being damaged.

COMBINATIONS OF RESISTORS (OR CONDUCTORS)

Resistors/conductors in series

To find the overall resistance of several resistors in series, called the **equivalent resistance**, we *add* the individual resistances together. The total resistance R_T of three resistors with resistances R_1, R_2 and R_3 connected in series is given by:

$$R_T = R_1 + R_2 + R_3$$

If, instead, we think in terms of their corresponding conductances, G_1, G_2 and G_3, the **equivalent conductance** G_T is given by:

$$\frac{1}{G_T} = \frac{1}{G_1} + \frac{1}{G_2} + \frac{1}{G_3}$$

For serial arrangements it is probably easier to think in terms of resistance.

Resistors/conductors in parallel

The total resistance R_T of three resistors with resistances R_1, R_2 and R_3 connected in parallel is given by:

$$\frac{1}{R_T} = \frac{1}{R_1} + \frac{1}{R_2} + \frac{1}{R_3}$$

But this time when we think in terms of their conductances, G_1, G_2 and G_3, the equivalent or total conductance G_T is given by:

$$G_T = G_1 + G_2 + G_3$$

When we combine conductors in parallel the total conductance increases. This means that the 'total' resistance gets smaller. In fact R_T will be smaller than any of the resistances used in the parallel combination.

? **QUESTION 15**

15 Three resistors of 10 Ω, 100 Ω and 1000 Ω are connected in parallel. Calculate the equivalent resistance of this arrangement.

STRETCH AND CHALLENGE

Deriving equation for resistors

RESISTORS IN SERIES

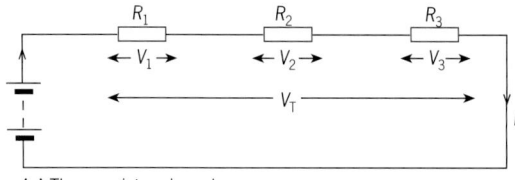

(a) Three resistors in series

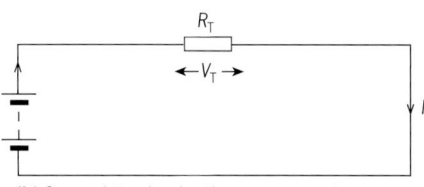

(b) One resistor drawing the same current

Fig 8.15 Resistors in series

Fig 8.15(a) shows three resistors in series with a battery. The total voltage across the three resistors is V_T and the current in the circuit is I amperes. Now, if the p.d.s across the resistors are V_1, V_2 and V_3 respectively, we can write:

$$V_T = V_1 + V_2 + V_3$$

We also know that the p.d. across one resistor is given by IR (current same everywhere in the circuit).

Therefore: $V_T = IR_1 + IR_2 + IR_3$

We now wish to replace the three resistors in this circuit with one that draws the same current, as in Fig 8.15(b). Call its value R_T. It follows that:

$$V_T = IR_T$$

or: $IR_T = IR_1 + IR_2 + IR_3$

The current I can be eliminated to give:

$$R_T = R_1 + R_2 + R_3$$

RESISTORS IN PARALLEL

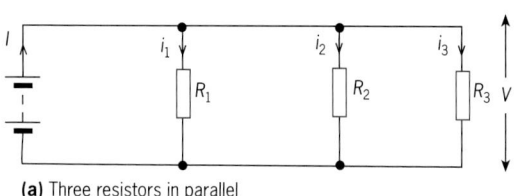

(a) Three resistors in parallel

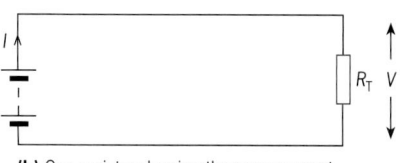

(b) One resistor drawing the same current

Fig 8.16 Resistors in parallel

Fig 8.16(a) shows three resistors R_1, R_2 and R_3 in parallel with a battery that is assumed to have zero internal resistance. This time, the p.d. across each resistor is the same: call it V. The current I from the battery splits so that:

$$I = i_1 + i_2 + i_3$$

where i_1, i_2 and i_3 are the currents through R_1, R_2 and R_3 respectively. Suppose we replace the three resistors by one, with resistance R_T, that draws the same current from the battery and will have the same p.d. V across it, Fig 8.16(b). Then:

$$I = \frac{V}{R_T} = \frac{V}{R_1} + \frac{V}{R_2} + \frac{V}{R_3}$$

This time we can eliminate the p.d. V to give:

$$\frac{1}{R_T} = \frac{1}{R_1} + \frac{1}{R_2} + \frac{1}{R_3}$$

? QUESTION 16

16 **a)** Write down equations to show that, for the circuit in Fig 8.17,

$$V_2 = V_B \frac{R_2}{R_1 + R_2}$$

b) Show that the p.d. across the 3 kΩ resistor in the circuit below is 6 V. How would you rearrange the resistors so that the p.d. between points A and B is 6 V?

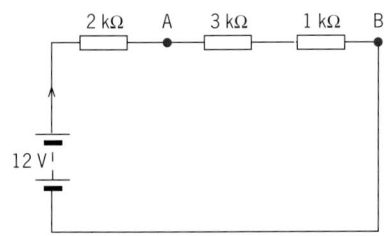

THE POTENTIAL DIVIDER

The circuit in Fig 8.17 shows two resistors connected in series to a battery. With this little circuit, we can obtain any voltage between zero and the supply voltage at the point between the two resistors (the p.d. across R_2). This voltage turns out to depend on the size of the two resistors and the supply voltage.

The voltage, or e.m.f., across the battery is V_B. The circuit is a simple series circuit, so that:

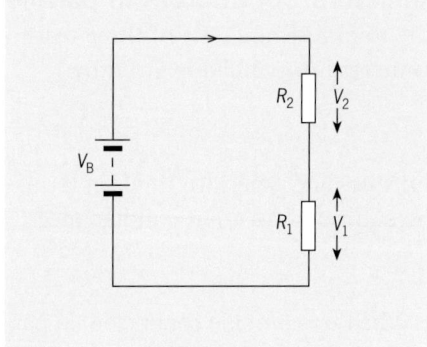

Fig 8.17 Two resistors are used in a potential divider to divide the voltage

$$V_B = V_1 + V_2 = IR_1 + IR_2 = I(R_1 + R_2)$$

The p.d. across R_1 is given by:

$$V_1 = IR_1$$

If we take the ratio of the p.d.s across R_1 and the battery, then:

$$\frac{V_1}{V_B} = \frac{IR_1}{I(R_1 + R_2)} = \frac{R_1}{R_1 + R_2}$$

or:

$$V_1 = V_B \times \frac{R_1}{R_1 + R_2}$$

This arrangement is called a **potential divider** since it can divide the supply voltage V_B in any ratio that is required. In the Science in Context box on the comparator below, for example, a potential divider is used to 'set' the voltage at one of the two inputs into the op-amp. This voltage is set by choosing appropriate values of the two resistors.

The comparator

A comparator is an electronic switch. It compares two voltages. The circuit in Fig 8.18 turns the light-emitting diode on when a changing voltage V_{in} is equal to or greater than a reference voltage. The op-amp (operational amplifier) in the comparator circuit has two inputs called the 'inverting' (–) and 'non-inverting' (+) inputs. The reference voltage is fixed at the non-inverting input by using a potential divider. The circuit in the diagram uses a 0 to 12 V supply, so the reference voltage at the non-inverting input will be given by:

$$V_{ref} = 12 \times \frac{R_2}{R_1 + R_2}$$

So, suppose we want the reference voltage to be 4 V. (This would mean that the LED would light when the input voltage is equal to or greater than 4 V.) We now have:

$$4 = 12 \times \frac{R_2}{R_1 + R_2} \quad \text{or} \quad \frac{R_2}{R_1 + R_2} = \frac{1}{3}$$

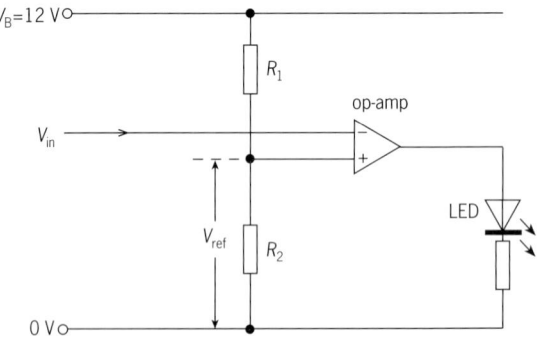

Fig 8.18 A comparator circuit

Comparators require very small currents, typically less than a microampere. This means that the current in the resistors will be very small, so their values should be high. In this circuit, values of R_1 = 200 kΩ and R_2 = 100 kΩ would be suitable.

The light-dependent resistor

The potential divider is widely used in electronics to fix the voltage at a point in a circuit. It can be used when one of the two resistors is a special resistor such as a light-dependent resistor (LDR).

The resistance of an LDR depends on the intensity of the light falling on it. In the dark, its resistance is very high, typically tens of kilohms. In bright light, its resistance drops to about 300 Ω. So, as the light changes, the p.d. across the fixed resistor with a value of 1 kΩ will vary. But whatever the resistance of the LDR, the p.d.s across it and the fixed resistor must add up to the supply voltage.

In Fig 8.19, the supply voltage is 6 V. When the resistance of the LDR is high (in the dark), the p.d. across it will be higher, probably about 5.5 V, with only about 0.5 V across the other resistor. In bright light, the situation is reversed, with only 1 V across the LDR and so about 5 V across the fixed resistor.

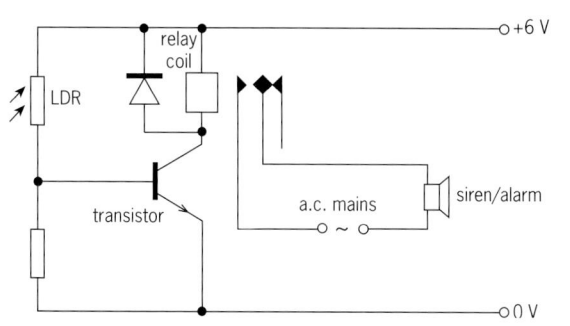

Fig 8.19 A potential divider circuit serving as a burglar alarm. It uses a light-dependent resistor and fixed-value resistors

When light falls on the LDR, the increase in voltage across the fixed resistor switches the transistor on, which in turn energises the relay. A mains-operated alarm is switched on by the relay.

VARIABLE RESISTORS – RHEOSTATS AND POTENTIOMETERS

Variable resistors differ from fixed resistors. Variable resistors usually have three connections, one at each end of the resistance element, the third as a slider (Figs 8.20 and 8.21). Variable resistors can be used in two ways: to control current or to control voltage.

In the circuit of Fig 8.21(a), the simple variable resistor is used as a **rheostat** to control current. The sliding (adjustable) contact is used, with one of the end connectors; the third terminal is not used. As the sliding contact moves, the current in the circuit varies and is measured on the ammeter.

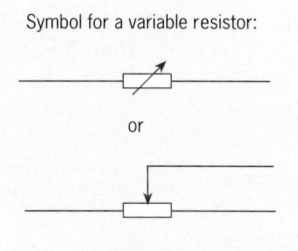

Symbol for a variable resistor:

or

Fig 8.20 Variable resistors

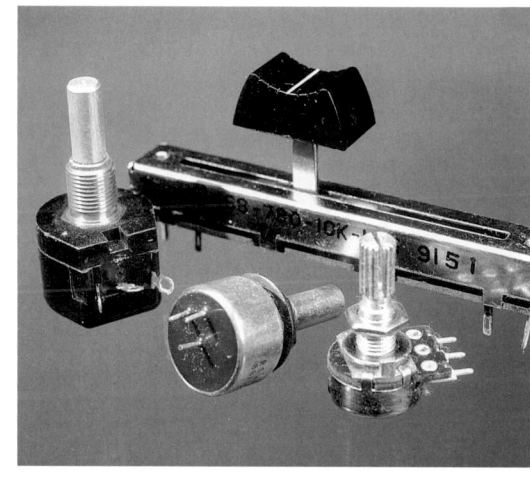

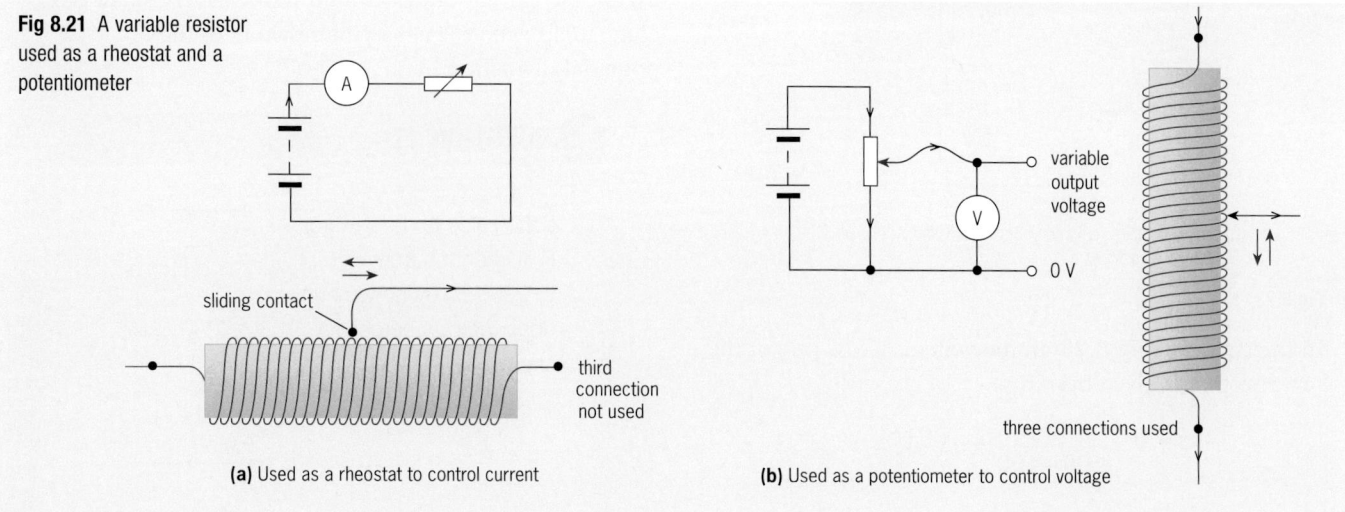

Fig 8.21 A variable resistor used as a rheostat and a potentiometer

sliding contact

third connection not used

(a) Used as a rheostat to control current

variable output voltage

0 V

three connections used

(b) Used as a potentiometer to control voltage

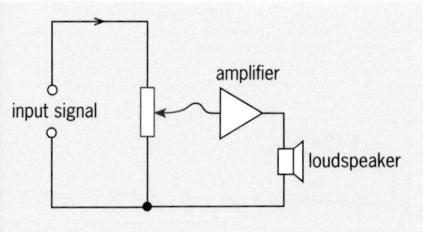

Fig 8.22 A potentiometer used as a volume control

The variable resistor in Fig 8.21(b) is used to control voltage. It is a **potential divider** (or **potentiometer**), and uses all three connections. The sliding contact effectively divides the variable resistor into two parts. The output voltage from a potentiometer can be any value from zero to the supply voltage as the variable contact is moved, and so the resistance is varied from its maximum to zero. Again, this is a very useful circuit to use in experimental work when you need a variable voltage supply. In electronics, such a circuit is used as a simple **volume control** in audio amplifier circuits (see Fig 8.22). When you adjust the volume control, you are moving the slider.

More on potential dividers

Circuits with potential dividers are very useful – but, be careful. So far we have made the assumption that the potential divider and the potentiometer do not provide any current. In Fig 8.17, we assumed that the current is the same in both resistors. In Fig 8.21(b), we assumed that there is a very small current in the wire from the slider of the variable resistor.

In practice, of course, some current passes from the potential divider to whatever is connected to it. Suppose you want to light a 3 V, 0.2 A bulb and you only have a 6 V battery. The circuit shown in Fig 8.23(a) might be thought a solution, but it is not.

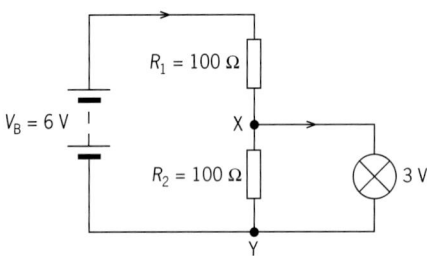

(a) A potential divider used in a circuit with a 6 V supply and a 3 V bulb. Will the bulb light up?

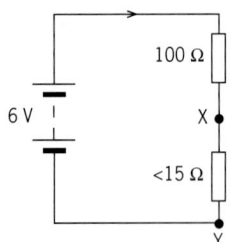

(b) The equivalent resistance between X and Y is less than 15 Ω.

Fig 8.23

In the circuit of Fig 8.23(a), the voltage across one of the two resistors is given by:

$$6\,\text{V} \times \frac{100}{100 + 100} = 6\,\text{V} \times \tfrac{1}{2} = 3\,\text{V}$$

When the bulb is connected across one of the resistors, we might expect it to light. But the bulb itself also has a resistance that affects the current. When it lights normally with 3 V across it, the current through it will be 0.2 A. Therefore the resistance of the bulb is 3 V/0.2 A = 15 Ω.

When the bulb is connected it changes the circuit. The effective resistance between X and Y is reduced since the bulb is in parallel with one of the 100 Ω resistors. Without doing an accurate calculation, we do know that the resulting resistance between X and Y will now be *less* than 15 Ω. The p.d. *V* across XY will therefore be much less than 3 V. Using:

$$V_2 = V_B \frac{R_2}{R_1 + R_2}$$

the p.d. is approximately:

$$6 \times \frac{15}{100 + 15} = 0.8\,\text{V}$$

With 0.8 V across it, there will not be enough current to light the bulb. In this application, the potential divider does not work. Also, the available current is limited by R_1 to be less than 0.06 A. A simple rheostat would be better, although not the ideal solution to this problem.

What we learn is that for a potential divider to be useful, the current drawn from it must be very small compared to the current in the resistors of the potential divider.

? QUESTION 17

17 If the value of the resistor R is changed from 500 Ω to 2000 Ω, by how much does the p.d. across XY change?

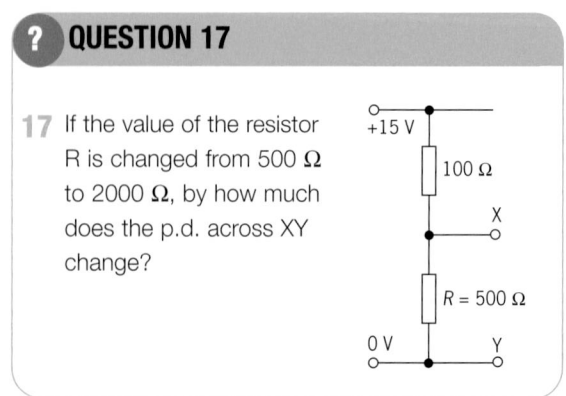

9 USING AMMETERS AND VOLTMETERS

It is an important principle that, when we take measurements, the act of measuring should not change what is being measured. But we sometimes have to compromise. In electrical measurements, for example, it is usually impossible to measure current without changing it a little. Provided the change is small enough to be negligible, we accept the change. The question to ask in any experiment is: how small is negligible? As a rule of thumb, anything of one per cent or less is acceptable. We may have to put up with larger errors in some circumstances, so it is important that we are aware of the error.

AMMETERS

Ammeters measure current. The ideal ammeter should have zero resistance so that, when connected correctly in series in a circuit, it will not affect the current but will just measure it. However, real ammeters always do have a resistance, which should be as small as possible – small compared with the resistance in the circuit as a whole.

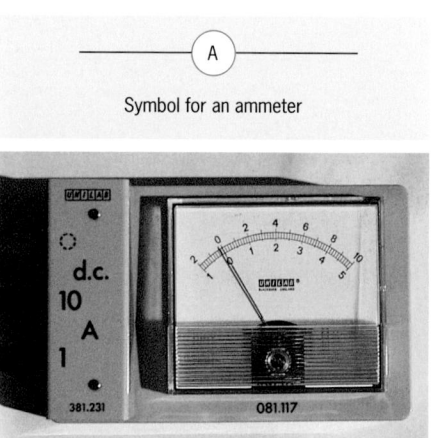

Symbol for an ammeter

Fig 8.24 An ammeter

EXAMPLE

Q The circuit in Fig 8.25(a) shows a 12 V battery connected to a powerful motor. With no load, this motor draws a current of about 10 A. Estimate the resistance of the motor.

A Assuming the internal resistance of the battery is negligible:

resistance = voltage/current
= 12/10 = 1.2 Ω

Q An ammeter in the circuit should have a resistance of about one-hundredth of this for the error to be acceptable. Calculate the resistance of a suitable ammeter to measure the current in the circuit of Fig 8.25(a).

A Resistance of ammeter = 1.2/100 = 0.012 Ω.

Q The motor is replaced with a 12 MΩ resistor, see Fig 8.25(b). What is the current now?

A 'New' current = $12/(12 \times 10^6) = 1.0 \times 10^{-6}$ A = 1 μA.

Q The resistance of an ammeter to measure the current in this circuit can be larger. How large?

A The resistance of the 'new' ammeter = $(12 \times 10^6)/100$
= 120 000 Ω = 120 kΩ.

(a)
12 V | A motor M
~10 A

(b)
12 V | μA 12 MΩ

Fig 8.25

For more information on how to take electrical measurements please see the How Science Works assignment for this chapter at www.collinseducation.co.uk/CAS

VOLTMETERS

A voltmeter is connected to a circuit in parallel to measure the p.d. across a part of the circuit. The ideal voltmeter would have such a high resistance that it would draw no current at all. The very high resistance electronic digital voltmeters approach this, using a negligible current. In practice, however, a voltmeter must draw some current; otherwise it wouldn't work.

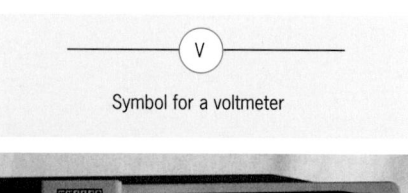

Symbol for a voltmeter

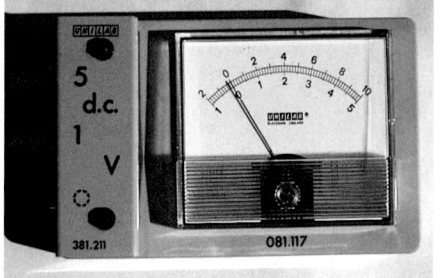

Fig 8.26 A voltmeter

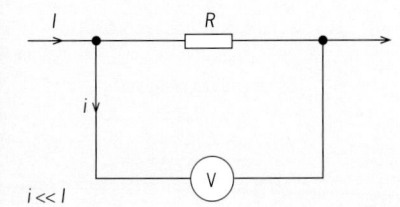

Fig 8.27 A voltmeter across a resistor

The current drawn by the voltmeter in Fig 8.27 must be very small compared with the current in the resistor. In practice, we ensure that the resistance of the voltmeter is much bigger than that across the part of the circuit for which the p.d. is being measured. A typical moving coil voltmeter has a resistance of 100 kΩ, while a digital voltmeter's resistance is typically 10 MΩ – a hundred times greater.

10 MORE ABOUT CONDUCTORS

The ideas about free electrons discussed at the start of this chapter give us a simple model that we can use to explain resistance. These ideas also explain why the resistance of good conductors tends to increase with temperature.

When there is a current in a wire, some electrons move 'freely'. A force acts on an electron due to the electric field created by the applied voltage. This accelerates it and it gains kinetic energy. It is not likely to travel very far before it collides with an atom, which itself has vibrational kinetic energy. In the collision, the electron loses some of its kinetic energy to the atom. After the collision, it will again be accelerated until it collides once more, losing energy and so on. The collisions with atoms provide the resistance that prevents an electron from accelerating along a clear path. With the energy transferred from the electrons, the atoms vibrate more (the wire gets hotter) and collisions are more likely. This increases the resistance.

Most metals behave in this way – their resistance decreases as the temperature decreases. Titanium behaves in a similar way, but when the temperature becomes very low (0.39 K, –272.8 °C) the resistance becomes zero. At this temperature, titanium becomes what is called a **superconductor**.

In recent years, materials have been discovered that become superconductors at much higher, more attainable temperatures than 0.39 K. Materials based on oxides of bismuth become superconductors at about 77 K, –196 °C, a temperature that can be obtained quite easily using liquid nitrogen as a coolant. These are called high-temperature superconductors.

SEMICONDUCTORS

Semiconductor materials include the best known, silicon. Others are germanium, lead sulphide, selenium and gallium arsenide. At ordinary temperatures, pure silicon is not a good insulator but not a good conductor either, because at these temperatures silicon has few free electrons in it. But when silicon is heated, the energy gained frees more electrons.

Semiconductor materials, then, are not much use at ordinary temperatures in their pure state. To make a semiconductor that is useful, the pure material is 'doped' by adding tiny amounts of impurity atoms. Semiconductors are dealt with in greater detail in Chapter 20.

11 CHARGE AND CAPACITORS

The flash on a camera takes time to store enough energy for the high intensity bulb to give a flash. To store this energy, the flash unit uses a **capacitor**, a component designed to store a particular amount of charge and release it when required. A capacitor consists simply of two conducting plates separated by an insulating layer, sometimes called a dielectric. Its circuit symbol is shown in Fig 8.28. Some capacitors are shown on page 202.

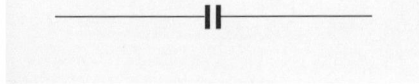

Fig 8.28 Symbol for a capacitor

CHARGING AND DISCHARGING

A capacitor in a simple d.c. circuit is shown in Fig 8.29 and its behaviour during charging and discharging is shown in Figs 8.30(a) and (b). In each, centre-zero microammeters record any current. Read the captions to these carefully, and then read on.

The current is a flow of charge. In each case, the flow of charge is high to begin with, and quickly gets less and less. In Fig 8.30(a), the battery drives a current round the circuit. One plate becomes positively charged and the other becomes negatively charged. When the free wire is moved (Fig 8.30(b)) to point A, the capacitor is 'discharged'. The charge on the plates returns to where it came from.

Looking again at Fig 8.30(a), the battery redistributes the charge around the circuit. Electrons move away from one plate of the capacitor and on to the other plate, but **not** by crossing between the plates: the electrons reaching the negative plate in Fig 8.30(a) come from the adjacent wire; those that leave the positive plate move into the wire connected to it.

The changing current is a consequence of the forces between charges. When the capacitor is charged, electrons flow to the plate that becomes negative. At first this is easy, so the current is large. The electrons spread out and the repulsive forces between them are small. As more electrons arrive, these forces increase, making it harder for more electrons to get on to the plate (the current decreases), until eventually there are so many electrons that repulsive forces prevent more from arriving. The capacitor is now fully charged.

(At the same time, there is a similar process on the positive plate, except that here electrons leave the plate and the forces are attractive.)

The battery does work moving the charge, and energy is stored in the capacitor. When the capacitor is discharged, the stored energy 'does work' moving the charge back.

CAPACITANCE

When fully charged, the potential difference across the capacitor plates is the same as that across the battery. So the maximum amount of charge that a capacitor can store is proportional to the battery voltage:

$$Q \propto V$$

where Q is the magnitude of charge on the plates measured in **coulombs**, and V is the voltage across the capacitor.

Therefore the ratio of Q/V is constant and is a measure of the amount of charge that is stored on the capacitor per volt. This is called **capacitance**, symbol C, and is a constant value for any particular capacitor. That is:

$$C = \frac{Q}{V}$$

Capacitance C is measured in **farads**, and one farad is one coulomb per volt:

$$1 \text{ F} = 1 \text{ C V}^{-1}$$

Be careful to distinguish between the italic C for the variable value of capacitance, and the upright C, the symbol for the unit the coulomb.

One farad (1 F) is a very large amount of capacitance, and most practical capacitors have much smaller values measured in microfarads (μF), nanofarads (nF) and picofarads (pF):

$$1 \text{ F} = 1\,000\,000 \text{ μF} = 10^6 \text{ μF} \quad \text{so} \quad \mathbf{1 \text{ μF} = 10^{-6} \text{ F}}$$
Also: $\quad 1 \text{ μF} = 1000 \text{ nF} = 10^3 \text{ nF} \quad \text{so} \quad \mathbf{1 \text{ nF} = 10^{-9} \text{ F}}$
and: $\quad 1 \text{ μF} = 1\,000\,000 \text{ pF} = 10^6 \text{ pF} \quad \text{so} \quad \mathbf{1 \text{ pF} = 10^{-12} \text{ F}}$

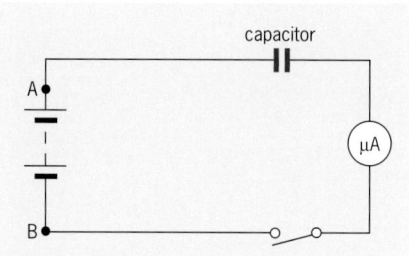

Fig 8.29 A capacitor in a d.c. circuit

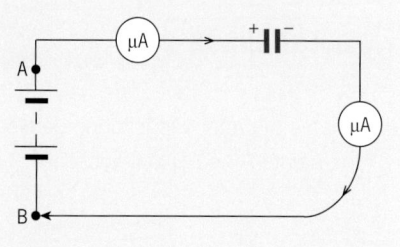

Fig 8.30(a) Charging: A current is shown on both meters when the free wire is touched to side B of the battery to complete the circuit. The needle on both meters moves sharply to one side and quickly returns to zero. After this, no further current flows. The capacitor has been 'charged'

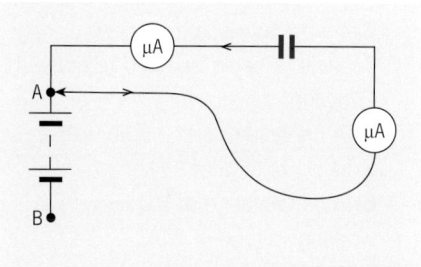

Fig 8.30(b) Discharging: When the wire is moved from point B to point A, both meters show a current, but this time in the opposite direction. Again, the readings on the meters fall quickly to zero. The capacitor has now been 'discharged'

Working voltage

If the voltage across a capacitor is too high, the insulator between the plates breaks down, and charge passes between the capacitor plates. This is why capacitors are marked with a working voltage, the maximum voltage that should be placed across the capacitor. A good rule of thumb is to make sure that the potential difference across a capacitor is never bigger than about two-thirds of the working voltage, especially in alternating current circuits. (See Chapter 12 for a more detailed description of peak voltages and r.m.s. voltages to understand why this is so.)

CAPACITORS IN PARALLEL AND SERIES

For capacitors connected in parallel, the total capacitance can be found by adding the individual capacitances:

$$C_T = C_1 + C_2 + C_3$$

So, as the number of capacitors connected in parallel increases, so does the total capacitance.

When capacitors are connected in series, the equivalent capacitance can be found from the equation:

$$\frac{1}{C_T} = \frac{1}{C_1} + \frac{1}{C_2} + \frac{1}{C_3}$$

This means that when capacitors are connected in series, the total capacitance is reduced. (Look at the similarities between these equations and those for resistors given earlier in the chapter.)

ENERGY STORED IN A CAPACITOR

Getting more charge on to an already charged capacitor requires you to do work against the repulsive forces between the charges. Adding a charge Q (measured in coulombs, C) will increase the p.d. across the capacitor by, say, ΔV joules per coulomb. This requires an amount of energy in joules given by:

$$\text{energy} = \text{joules/coulomb} \times \text{coulombs}$$
$$E = \Delta V \times Q$$

Charge on a capacitor is proportional to the voltage across it, so a graph of charge against voltage is a straight line through the origin, as shown in Fig 8.31. This means that adding the same amount of charge to a capacitor requires more work to be done. The total work done in charging the capacitor from 0 V is given by the shaded area under the graph. This is also the energy (in joules) stored in the capacitor:

$$\text{area} = \tfrac{1}{2}QV$$

But from the capacitance equation:

$$Q = CV$$

So: **energy stored** $= \tfrac{1}{2}QV = \tfrac{1}{2}CV.V = \tfrac{1}{2}CV^2$

Compare this equation with that for the energy stored in a spring that obeys Hooke's law:

$$E = \tfrac{1}{2}Fx = \tfrac{1}{2}kx^2$$

where x = extension of spring in metres produced by a force of F newtons, and k = force constant of the spring.

Fig 8.31 Graph of charge on a capacitor against voltage

18 What is the total capacitance between the points A and B in this circuit?

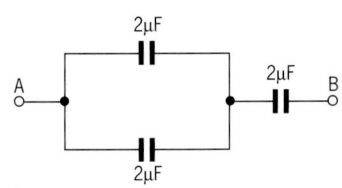

19 Some capacitors are marked '5.0 μF, 12 V'. What does this mean? Describe how some of these capacitors could be used to make the following:
a) A capacitance of 2.5 μF with a working voltage of 24 V.
b) A capacitance of 5.0 μF with a working voltage of 24 V.

20 The diagram shows four arrangements, A to D, of three 1 μF capacitors.
Which arrangement has:
a) the smallest capacitance?
b) the largest capacitance?

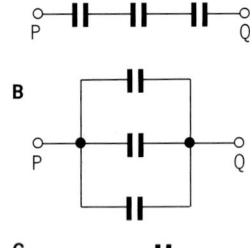

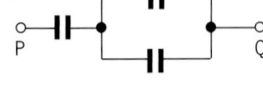

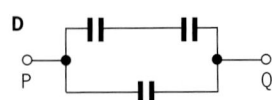

Deriving equations for capacitors

CAPACITORS IN PARALLEL

Fig 8.32(a) shows three capacitors with capacitances C_1, C_2 and C_3 connected in parallel with a battery. The p.d. across each capacitor is the same: call it V. The capacitors will have charges of Q_1, Q_2 and Q_3 respectively. The total charge on the three is simply:

$$Q = Q_1 + Q_2 + Q_3$$

In Fig 8.32(b), the three capacitors are replaced with one of value C_T, which stores the same charge, Q, when there is V volts across it.

Therefore, since $Q = CV$:

$$C_T V = C_1 V + C_2 V + C_3 V$$

The p.d. across all the capacitors is the same and can be eliminated:

$$C_T = C_1 + C_2 + C_3$$

CAPACITORS IN SERIES

Fig 8.33 shows three capacitors of capacitances C_1, C_2 and C_3 in series with a battery. At any time while they are charging, the current in the circuit will always be the same at all points in the circuit, and it will take the same time for each capacitor to charge. This means that the charge on each capacitor will be the same – call it Q.

Since charge does not ordinarily cross between plates in a capacitor, you may be wondering how the middle capacitor becomes charged. Electrons leave the left plate of capacitor 1. This 'induces' the movement of electrons from the left plate of capacitor 2 on to the right plate of capacitor 1. This in turn induces electron flow from the left plate of capacitor 3 on to the right plate of capacitor 2. Electrons move on to the right plate of capacitor 3 to complete the process. The end result is that each left plate becomes positively charged and each right plate is negatively charged.

The p.d. across each capacitor will be V_1, V_2 and V_3 respectively. Suppose we replace the three capacitors with one of size C_T that will carry the same charge, Q, and have a p.d. of V across it. Now this p.d. V will equal the sum of the p.d.s across the three capacitors:

$$V = V_1 + V_2 + V_3$$

Also:

$$V = \frac{Q}{C}$$

Therefore:

$$\frac{Q}{C_T} = \frac{Q}{C_1} + \frac{Q}{C_2} + \frac{Q}{C_3}$$

The charge Q can be eliminated to give:

$$\frac{1}{C_T} = \frac{1}{C_1} + \frac{1}{C_2} + \frac{1}{C_3}$$

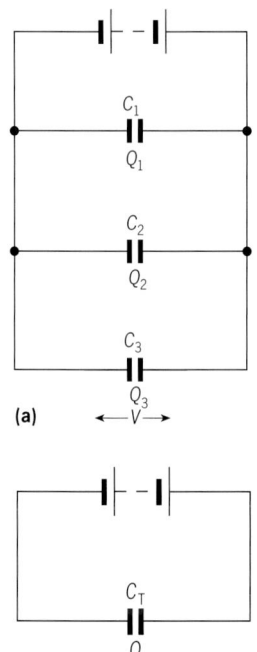

(a)

(b)

Fig 8.32 Voltage across capacitors in parallel

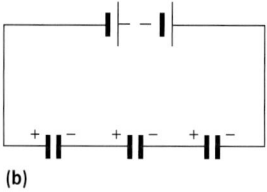

(a)

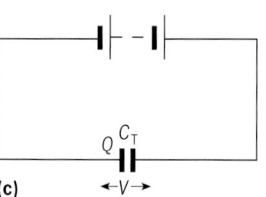

(b)

(c)

Fig 8.33 Voltages across capacitors in series

? QUESTIONS 21–22

21 The batteries in the circuits shown are all the same and all the capacitors are identical. Which arrangement stores the greatest amount of energy when the capacitors are all fully charged?

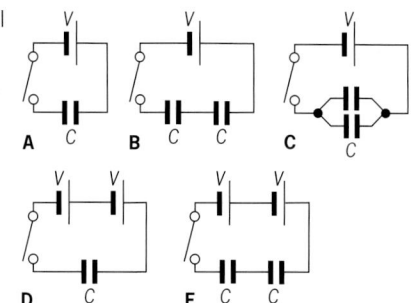

22 Some portable computers use capacitors as a short-term power backup. The circuits are designed so that the capacitor can discharge at a constant current. A 4 F capacitor charged to 5 V is required to supply 50 μA to a memory board. For how long would it be able to do this?

The mathematics of the exponential decay of a capacitor

Imagine a capacitor of capacitance C farads that is initially charged to a p.d. of V volts and then discharged through a resistor of R ohms. Although we know that the current decays, we shall assume that the average current over a small interval of time, Δt, is I amperes. The amount of charge, ΔQ, that flows in this time is given by:

$$\Delta Q = -I\Delta t$$

The current can also be given in terms of the resistance and the p.d. across it from Ohm's law ($V = IR$) so:

$$\Delta Q = -\frac{V}{R}\Delta t$$

The p.d. is also related to the charge on the capacitor from $CV = Q$, so:

$$\Delta Q = -\frac{Q}{RC}\Delta t$$

Another way of writing the equation is as:

$$\frac{\Delta Q}{\Delta t} = -\frac{Q}{RC}$$

If Δt is very small, the equation becomes:

$$\frac{dQ}{dt} = -\frac{Q}{RC}$$

or:

$$\frac{1}{Q}dQ = -\frac{1}{RC}dt$$

This is a first-order differential equation. To solve it we have to integrate both sides:

$$\int_{Q_0}^{Q}\frac{1}{Q}dQ = -\int_{0}^{t}\frac{1}{RC}dt$$

which gives:

$$\ln\left(\frac{Q}{Q_0}\right) = -\frac{t}{RC}$$

$$\frac{Q}{Q_0} = \exp\left(-\frac{t}{RC}\right)$$

$$Q = Q_0\exp\left(-\frac{t}{RC}\right)$$

A graph of charge Q against time t is an exponential decay curve. The rate of decay, or the steepness of the curve, depends on the initial charge Q_0 and on the values of R and C. This is shown in Fig 8.34(a).

If we substitute the time t in the equation with RC, then Q will be the charge after RC seconds:

$$Q = Q_0\exp\left(-\frac{t}{RC}\right) \quad Q_0 = \exp\left(-\frac{RC}{RC}\right)$$

$$= Q_0\exp(-1) = Q_0e^{-1} = Q_0\frac{1}{e}$$

So:

$$\frac{Q}{Q_0} = \frac{1}{e} = \frac{1}{2.718} = 0.37$$

That is, in RC seconds the charge on a capacitor decays to 37 per cent of the initial charge.

TESTING FOR EXPONENTIAL CHANGE – METHOD 1

If a quantity decreases in an exponential manner, then over equal intervals of time there is a *constant ratio* between the starting and finishing values. For example, if you record a quantity x at equal intervals, then consecutive readings (x_1, x_2, x_3, x_4, ...) should be in the same ratio to one another ($x_1/x_2 = x_2/x_3 = x_3/x_4 = ...$).

TESTING FOR EXPONENTIAL CHANGE – METHOD 2

The following equation was derived above:

$$\frac{Q}{Q_0} = \exp\left(-\frac{t}{RC}\right)$$

Taking the log of both sides, we get:

$$\ln\left(\frac{Q}{Q_0}\right) = -\frac{t}{RC}$$

or:

$$\ln Q - \ln Q_0 = -\frac{t}{RC}$$

A graph of $\ln Q$ against time t will therefore be a straight line (see Fig 8.34(b)) – a distinctive mark of an exponential change over time. The slope of the graph will be $-1/RC$.

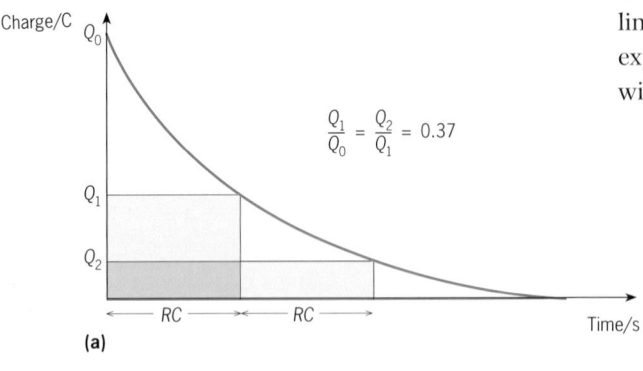

(a)

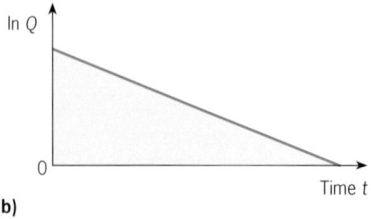

(b)

Fig 8.34 (a) Exponential decay curve for a discharging capacitor. **(b)** Plotted as ln Q against time

CAPACITORS AND RESISTORS

When a resistor is placed in series with a capacitor, as in Fig 8.35(a), the time taken for the capacitor to charge and discharge is increased because the current in the circuit is decreased. In the circuit in Fig 8.35(b), the oscilloscope (CRO) shows how the p.d. across the resistor changes as the capacitor discharges. The p.d. across the resistor is proportional to the current through it, so the trace on the oscilloscope (Fig 8.35(c)) shows how the current in the circuit changes.

The curve is an *exponential* decay curve. It has an interesting property: the current in the circuit decays by the same ratio in successive equal intervals of time. This kind of curve appears frequently in nature. You may be familiar with it in the radioactive decay curve. The constant ratio we measure in that case is called the **half-life**, that is, the time taken for the activity of the radioactive source to halve. In the case of capacitor discharge shown in Fig 8.35(c), the sizes of both the resistor and the capacitor determine the rate of discharge. If we consider the units of the product of resistance and capacitance, we can see that the result is a time measured in seconds:

$$R \times C = \text{ohms} \times \text{farads}$$

$$= \frac{\text{volts}}{\text{amperes}} \times \frac{\text{coulombs}}{\text{volts}}$$

$$= \frac{\text{amperes} \times \text{seconds}}{\text{amperes}} = \text{seconds}$$

The product RC is called the **time constant** and is used to measure the rate of decay of current from a charged capacitor.

See the Stretch and Challenge box on the opposite page for the mathematics of the exponential decay curve.

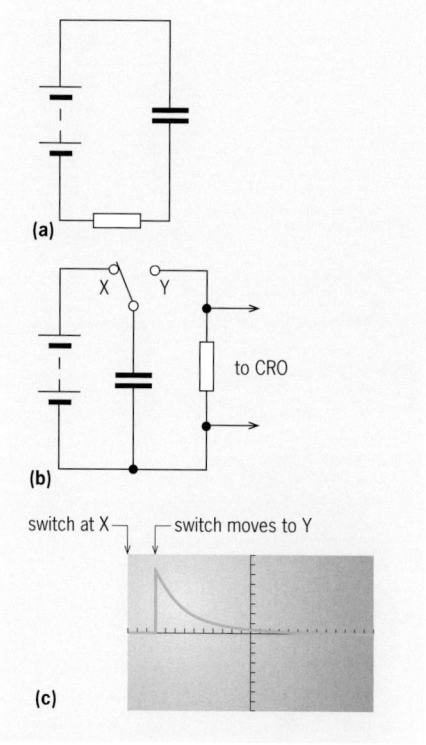

Fig 8.35 (a) A resistor and a capacitor in series. **(b)** With the switch at X the capacitor charges. With the switch at Y, it discharges and produces the CRO trace shown in **(c)**

SUMMARY

In studying this chapter, you should have learned and understood the following:

- An electric current is the flow of electric charge and can be described by the equations:
  $$I = dQ/dt \quad \text{and} \quad I = nAQv$$
- Energy is transferred when a charge flows through a circuit. The potential difference is the energy transferred per coulomb as charge passes through a component or device. This can be described as 1 volt = 1 joule/coulomb.
- The size of the current in a circuit depends on the resistance in the circuit.
- Resistance $R = \rho l/A$, where ρ is the resistivity, which depends on the material.
- Conductance $G = 1/R$ or $G = \sigma A/l$, where σ is the conductivity, and $\sigma = 1/\rho$.
- Ohm's law states that resistance = p.d./current for a conductor at constant temperature.
- The power in a circuit is given by $P = IV$. In a purely resistive circuit this equals I^2R or V^2/R.
- Electromotive force (e.m.f.) is the energy transferred per coulomb in a source of current. Some of the energy gained by each coulomb is transferred in

doing work against the internal resistance of the power supply.
- Potential dividers and potentiometers can be used to control voltages in circuits.
- The availability of free electrons decides whether materials are conductors, semiconductors or insulators. At low temperatures, some materials become superconductors.
- Capacitors store charge Q when there is a p.d. V across them. The capacitance C of a capacitor is given by $Q = CV$.
- Energy can be stored in capacitors. The energy stored E is given by $E = \frac{1}{2}QV = \frac{1}{2}CV^2$.
- The rate at which a capacitor discharges (or charges) depends on the time constant RC.
- The decay of charge on a capacitor is exponential.

Practice questions for this chapter are available at www.collinseducation.co.uk/CAS

9

Charge and field

9 CHARGE AND FIELD

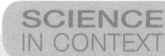
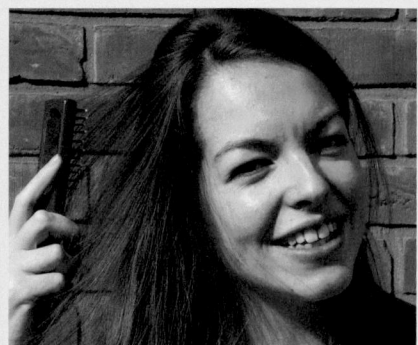

Brushing hair in a dry atmosphere produces
electrostatic charges

Shocks and sparks

The spark that jumps across a gap of 5 cm or so in a Van de Graaff generator
is the dramatic effect of static electricity. Less conspicuous, but the cause of
many problems in microelectronic circuits, are the tiny quantities of charge that
build up and jump only a few micrometres.

Many items of equipment that we rely on every day are controlled by
microelectronic devices – just think of telephones, radio and television, traffic
lights, domestic appliances such as washing machines and freezers, control
systems in all forms of transport systems, railway signalling and aircraft control.
On top of this there is all the computer equipment in use. It is very important
that these devices are not made unreliable by electrostatic effects.

The amount of charge that can damage circuits is very small – fractions of a
microcoulomb are enough. The relatively small voltages
that do damage are easily reached with everyday
activities. Shifting position on a foam-filled chair can
generate 1500 volts in a humid atmosphere and up to
18 000 volts if it is very dry. Just walking on some carpets
can generate up to 35 000 volts: that's why you may feel
a shock when you touch a metal door handle!

Voltages of this size would certainly destroy sensitive
microelectronic circuits. So, built into the design of
equipment are means to protect their delicate
microelectronics from static electricity. It is no wonder
that microelectronics engineers earth themselves before
going near a circuit board!

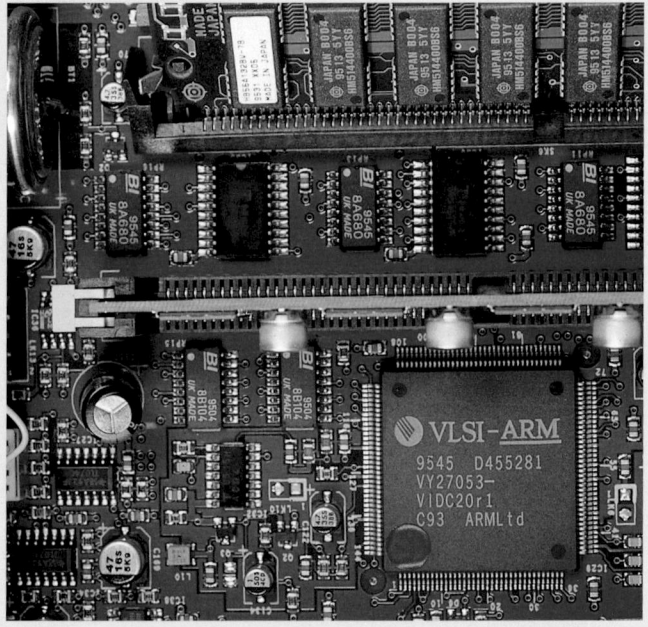

Sensitive microelectronic devices need to be
protected from everyday electrostatic charges

The ideas in this chapter

Most objects in the world around us consist of matter in which charge is
balanced, and to the surroundings such matter is electrically neutral. However,
the forces between the charges within materials are responsible for the
strength of the materials and all their mechanical and electrical properties.

Charged bodies exert forces on each other: some are pulled towards each other
and some are pushed away from each other. This is because there are two types of
charge – we call them positive and negative. Their action can be summarised as:

Like charges repel, unlike charges attract.

In this chapter we consider these charges in more detail. Of particular
importance are the electric fields that charge produces, and the movement of charge
from one place to another. We then go on to consider capacitors and finally we
show the similarity between the equations for an electric field and the equations for
a gravitational field.

1 ELECTROSTATIC FORCES

Atoms are made from tiny negatively charged particles called electrons, and larger positively charged particles called protons. Each carries the same (yet opposite) quantity of charge. The charges are responsible for the electrostatic behaviour of materials. Atoms (except hydrogen) also contain neutral particles called neutrons. When two materials rub together, a few atoms of one material lose electrons, becoming positively charged. These electrons 'stick' to atoms on the other material, giving it a net negative charge. (In a television, a beam of electrons strikes the screen. You are aware that negative charge has built up if you touch the screen and hear a crack.)

A very important property of electrostatic forces is that they act at a distance. Hair or fur can be raised if a charged object (such as a comb) is brought near. Any charged body in the space around another charged body is acted on by an **electric field**, and will 'feel' a force. (Compare with gravitational fields and magnetic fields – see Chapters 3 and 10.) The direction of the force depends on whether the charges are alike or unlike. The size of the force depends on the size of the charges and their distance apart.

The behaviour of electric fields is very similar to that of gravitational fields. It is easiest to begin with **uniform** fields.

2 UNIFORM ELECTRIC FIELD

The field between two parallel charged plates is uniform. When a charged body such as charged foil on an insulated handle (Fig 9.1) is held in the space between such plates, the foil is deflected, since a force acts on the foil to make it move. The amount of the foil's deflection is a measure of the field strength, and is the same at any point between the plates: the field is uniform.

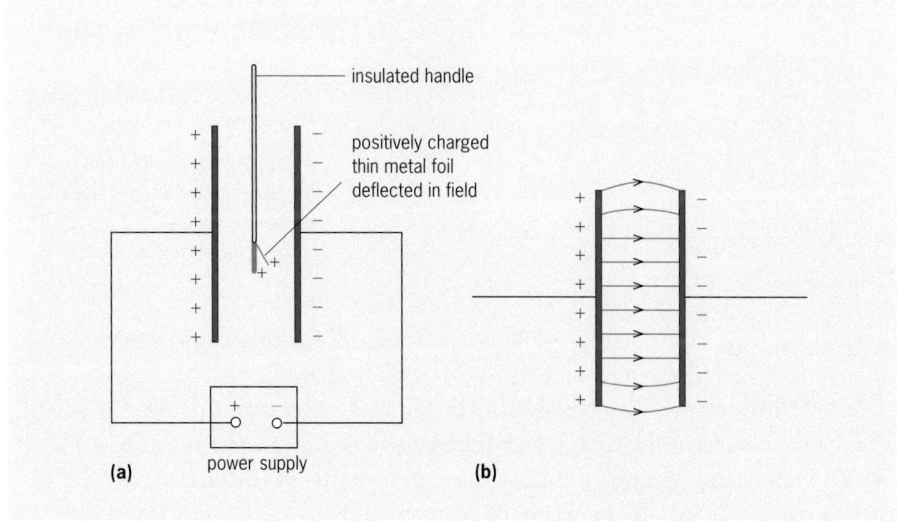

(a)

(b)

Fig 9.1 (a) Investigating the field between two parallel plates. **(b)** The electric field pattern between the plates. In the centre the even spacing of the field lines indicates a uniform field. Near the edges of the plates the field is no longer uniform

The strength of the field is defined as the force on each coulomb of charge:

$$\text{electric field strength} = \frac{\text{force in newtons on a charge of one coulomb}}{}$$

Electric field strength is measured in newtons per coulomb (N C^{-1}).

If a charged body is free to move, then it will move in the field – the field does work on the body and the charged body gains energy as it accelerates between the plates.

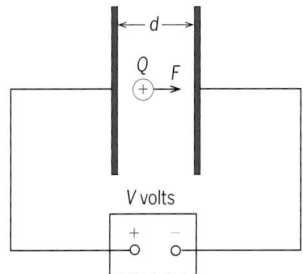

Fig 9.2 Calculating the electric field strength between two parallel plates

1   The beginning of this chapter described the problems static electricity can cause in micro-electronic circuits. Within such a circuit, the insulating property of the material (usually a layer of glass) between the layers of conducting track breaks down in an electric field of 10^6 V m^{-1}. If the insulation is 10 μm thick, what size voltage will cause this field?

2   A volt is 1 joule per coulomb. Show that V m^{-1} is equivalent to N C^{-1}.

When the separation of the plates is d metres, then the work done by a force of F newtons in moving the charge from one plate to the other will be:

$$F \times d \text{ (joules)}$$

The work done by the field is equal to the energy gained by the charge. If the potential difference (p.d.) across the plates is V volts (Fig 9.2), then the energy gained by Q coulombs will be:

$$Q \text{ coulombs} \times V \text{ joules per coulomb} = QV \text{ joules}$$

Therefore: $$Fd = QV$$

Rearranging this gives: $$\frac{F}{Q} = \frac{V}{d}$$

We now have an alternative and very useful way of measuring the strength E of an electric field:

E is measured in newtons per coulomb *or* volts per metre.

EXAMPLE

Q Estimate the electric field between the 'points' of a spark plug.

A First, estimate the distance between the points. This is usually very small, say 0.5 mm. The voltage across the points will be about 3000 V. So,

electric field strength:

$$E = \frac{V}{d}$$

$$= \frac{3000 \text{ volts}}{5 \times 10^{-4} \text{ m}}$$

$$= 6 \times 10^6 \text{ V m}^{-1}$$

THE ELECTRON GUN AND ELECTRONVOLTS

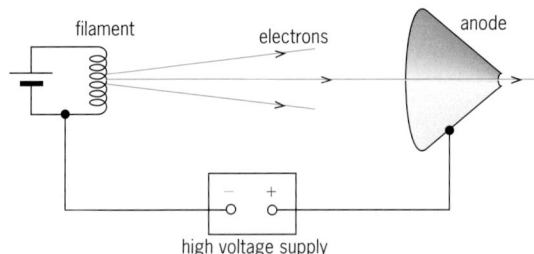

Fig 9.3 An electron gun. Electrons are emitted from the heated filament and attracted to the positive anode

Television tubes, cathode-ray oscilloscope tubes, X-ray tubes and electron microscopes are all devices that use beams of electrons.

The electrons come from the heated wire filament of an electron gun. Fig 9.3 shows a simple electron gun in which the filament is also the cathode. Electrons with enough energy escape from the surface of the wire, in **thermionic emission**. The large p.d. between the filament and a cone, the positive anode, generates an electric field, and the electrons are attracted to the anode. Between the filament and the anode, they accelerate, gaining kinetic energy from the electric field. If m and e are the mass and charge of the electron, then:

$$\text{kinetic energy gained} = \text{energy from electric field}$$

$$\tfrac{1}{2}mv^2 = eV$$

where v is the speed of the electron after it has been accelerated through a p.d. of V volts.

 REMEMBER THIS

Charge on an electron,
$e = 1.6 \times 10^{-19}$ C.
1 electronvolt (1 eV) = 1.6×10^{-19} J
1 keV = 1000 eV
1 Mev = 1000000 eV

The energy gained by the electron is eV joules or V electronvolts. One electronvolt is the energy gained by a particle carrying a charge of 1.6×10^{-19} coulombs after it has been accelerated through a p.d. of one volt. The electronvolt is a more convenient unit of energy than the joule when we are dealing with the energies of particles on an atomic scale.

? QUESTION 3

3 Calculate the energy gained by an electron in **a)** joules and **b)** eV, when accelerated through a p.d. of **i)** 1 V, **ii)** 1000 V, **iii)** 1 000 000 V.

EXAMPLE

Q Calculate the velocity of a 5 MeV alpha particle, which has a mass of 6.646×10^{-27} kg.

A The energy of the alpha particle is all kinetic energy. Therefore:

$$\tfrac{1}{2} mv^2 = 5 \text{ MeV}$$

To carry out this calculation the energy must be in joules:

$$5 \text{ MeV} = (1.6 \times 10^{-19}) \times (5 \times 10^6) = 8.0 \times 10^{-13} \text{ J}$$

We can now write:

$$0.5 \times (6.646 \times 10^{-27}) \times v^2 = 8.0 \times 10^{-13}$$

$$v^2 = \frac{8.0 \times 10^{-13}}{0.5 \times (6.646 \times 10^{-27})}$$

$$= \frac{8.0}{0.5 \times 6.646} \times 10^{14} = 2.4 \times 10^{14} \text{ m}^2 \text{ s}^{-2}$$

Therefore: $v = \sqrt{\left(2.4 \times 10^{14}\right)} = 1.6 \times 10^7 \text{ m s}^{-1}$

STRETCH AND CHALLENGE

The charge on the electron – Millikan's experiment

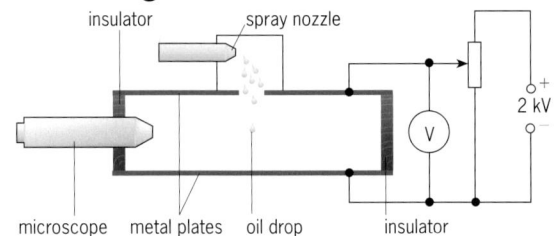

Fig 9.4 Apparatus for Millikan's oil-drop experiment

In 1917, Robert Millikan, an American physicist, devised a clever way of measuring the charge on the electron. He sprayed tiny oil droplets between two parallel charged plates and watched their motion carefully through a microscope (Fig 9.4).

We find with Millikan's apparatus that many of the oil droplets become charged as they are forced through the tiny hole of the spray. Most of the charged droplets are negative and these experience a force in the electric field between the plates. All the oil droplets are acted upon by gravity and by the buoyancy force of the air.

By carefully adjusting the voltage across the plates, Millikan was able to make some of the charged droplets stand still. Then, he knew that the resultant force on such a droplet was zero. The weight of the droplet and the resistance due to air molecules

were balanced by the electric force on the droplet.

According to Stokes' law (see page 86), the force F acting on a spherical oil droplet of radius r which is moving with velocity v through a medium of viscosity η is given by:

$$F = 6\pi r \eta v$$

For oil of density ρ, the mass of the drop will be:

$$\text{mass} = \tfrac{4}{3} \pi r^3 \rho$$

and its weight:

$$\tfrac{4}{3} \pi r^3 \rho g$$

There is an upthrust acting on the droplet equal to the weight of the air displaced:

$$\text{upthrust} = \tfrac{4}{3} \pi r^3 \rho_A g$$

where ρ_A is the density of air.

The apparent weight W of the oil droplet is therefore given by:

$$W = \tfrac{4}{3} \pi r^3 g(\rho - \rho_A)$$

Now, if the droplet is moving at a terminal velocity of v_t, then the apparent weight is:

$$W = \tfrac{4}{3} \pi r^3 g(\rho - \rho_A) = 6\pi r \eta v_t$$

The electric field strength E between the plates d metres apart is given by:

$$E = \frac{V}{d}$$

If an electric force F_E is applied so that the droplet with charge Q moves at constant velocity, then:

$$F_E = QE = W = \tfrac{4}{3} \pi r^3 g(\rho - \rho_A)$$

Millikan observed many droplets, carefully measuring the voltage required to give a constant velocity for each droplet. From his measurements he was able to calculate the smallest charge on a droplet. This was 1.6×10^{-19} C. He also discovered that other charged droplets carried either the same amount of charge or a whole-number multiple of this charge. He concluded that 1.6×10^{-19} C was the smallest possible charge and that it must be the charge on one electron.

Fig 9.5 Examples of some electric fields

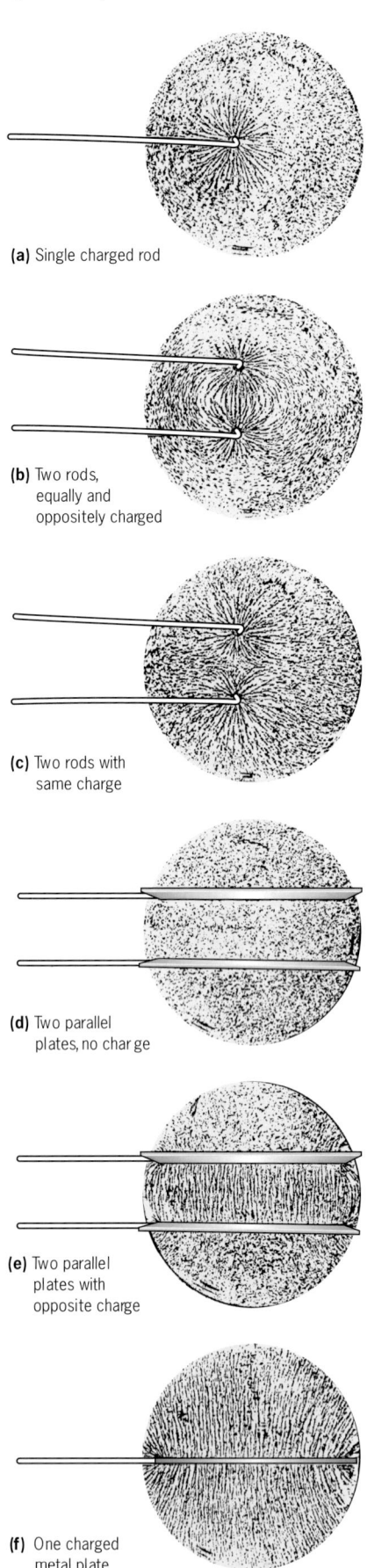

(a) Single charged rod

(b) Two rods, equally and oppositely charged

(c) Two rods with same charge

(d) Two parallel plates, no charge

(e) Two parallel plates with opposite charge

(f) One charged metal plate

DIRECTION OF THE ELECTRIC FIELD

A charged foil between two parallel plates is deflected in the same direction wherever it is placed between the plates – that is, the electric field has a direction. If the p.d. across the plates were reversed, the direction of the field would also be reversed and the foil would be deflected in the opposite direction.

The direction of the electric field between the plates is the direction of the force on a positive charge, that is, from positive to negative. The direction of any electric field is the same; the idea can even be used to describe the field around an isolated charge.

We use lines to describe the field, as indicated by small particles in Fig 9.5 and drawn as in Fig 9.6. A field line represents the orientation of the force and the arrow shows the direction of the force (positive to negative). The strength of the field is shown by the spacing of the lines – the closer they are, the stronger the field. Between the parallel plates they are evenly spaced, indicating a field of uniform strength.

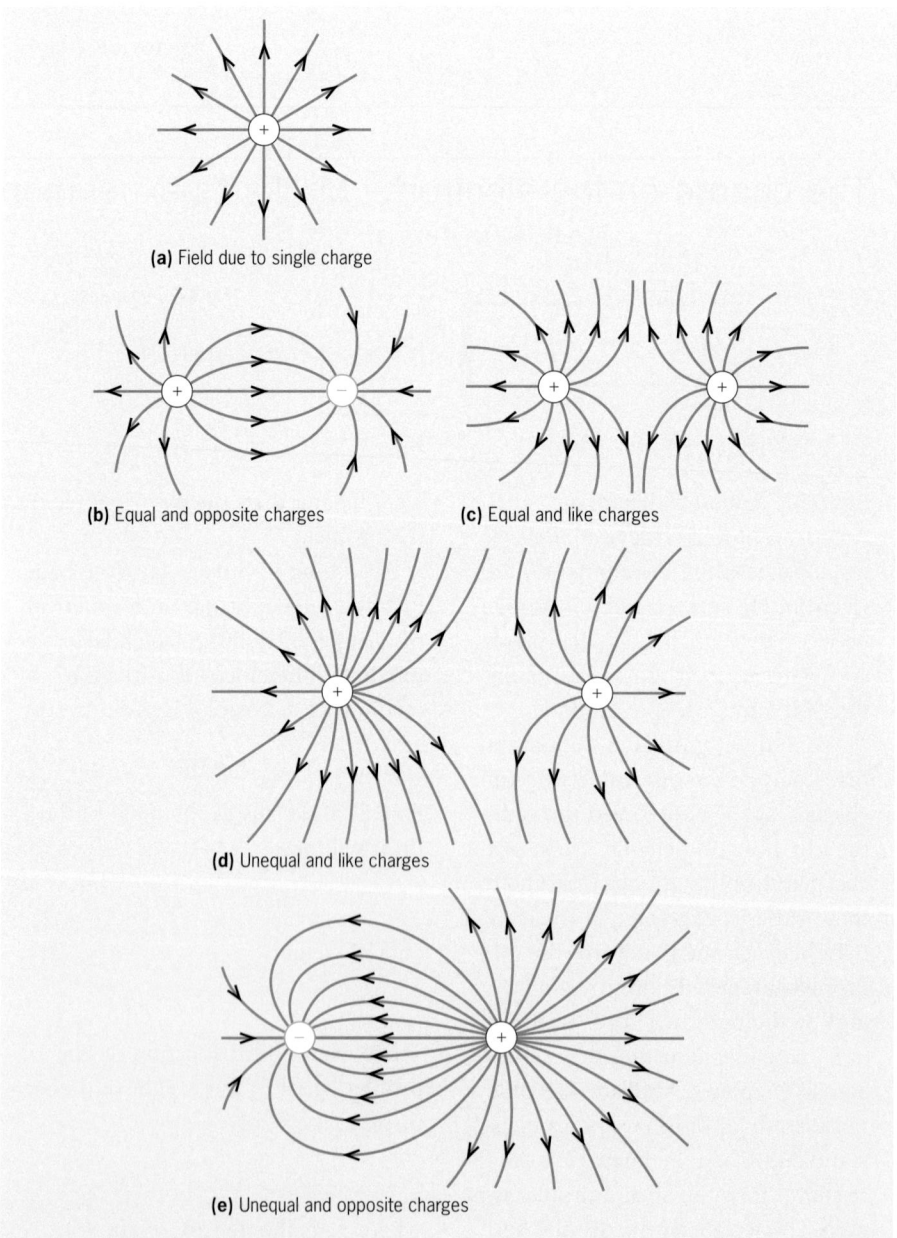

(a) Field due to single charge

(b) Equal and opposite charges

(c) Equal and like charges

(d) Unequal and like charges

(e) Unequal and opposite charges

Fig 9.6 Diagrams of some electric fields

3 ELECTRICAL POTENTIAL AND EQUIPOTENTIALS

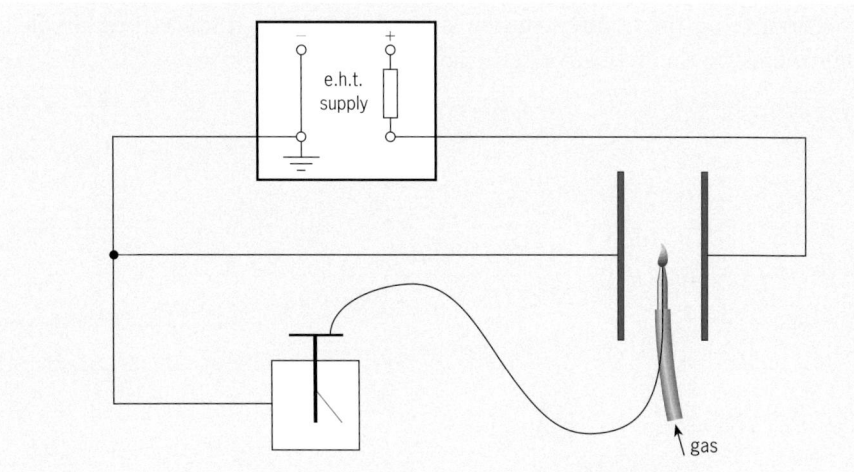

Fig 9.7 A flame probe for investigating the potential between two parallel plates

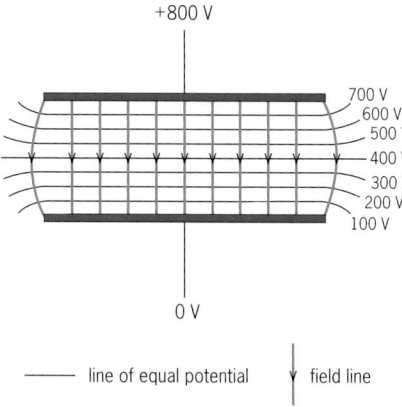

Fig 9.8 Equipotentials and field lines between two parallel plates. The field lines always cut the equipotentials at right angles

A voltmeter measures the p.d. across the parallel plates. A flame probe is used to measure voltage at points in the space between the plates (Fig 9.7): the voltage increases as the probe is moved from the left plate, which is at 0 V, to the right plate. More precisely, the probe measures a voltage *in the field between the plates*. This voltage is called the **electric potential**. The potential can be defined as the p.d. between the plate at 0 V (or zero potential) and the probe.

When the probe is moved parallel to the plates the potential remains the same: the probe is moving along an **equipotential**, that is, a plane of equal voltage or potential. The equipotentials are always at right angles to the field lines (Fig 9.8). Notice that at the edges of the plates where the field is no longer uniform, the equipotentials are still perpendicular to the field lines.

The potential changes gradually in a uniform field. Fig 9.9 is a graph of potential against distance between the plates. The plot shows that the potential gradient is constant and negative. Thus, where r is the distance, the field strength (the force on unit charge) is given by the equation:

field strength = −(potential gradient)

$$E = -\frac{dV}{dr}$$

Although this relationship has been derived for a uniform field, we shall see later that it is true for all fields.

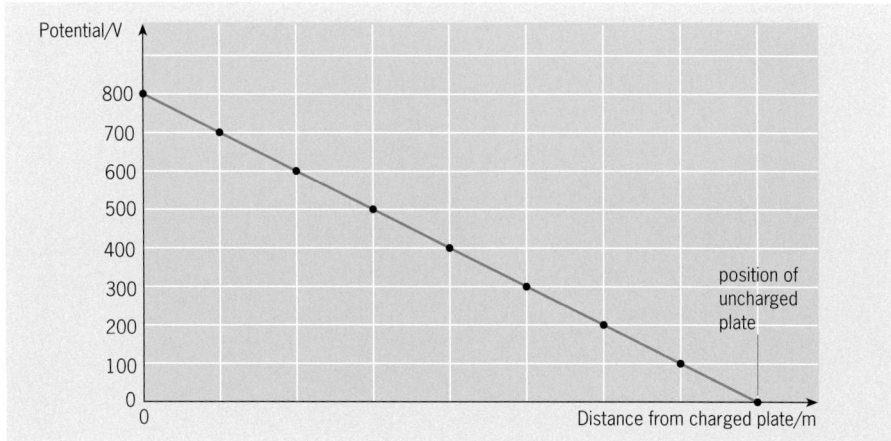

Fig 9.9 Potential between two charged parallel plates plotted against distance from positive plate

? QUESTION 4

4   Copy the four diagrams of the electrodes and sketch the electric fields between them. Show the direction of the fields. Add equipotentials to your diagrams.

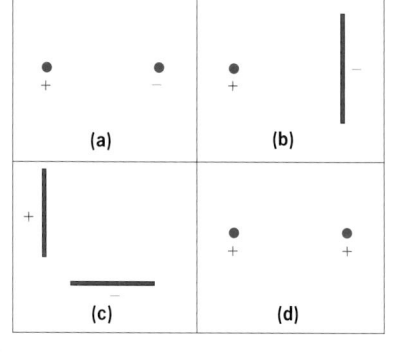

NON-UNIFORM FIELDS

In non-uniform fields the potential gradient varies. Fig 9.10(a) shows the electric field below a thundercloud. Notice how the potential gradient increases around the pointed church spire. The pointed spire distorts the field pattern, making the field stronger around the point.

Fig 9.10 (a) Equipotentials below a typical thundercloud. Notice how the equipotentials are closer around the pointed spire of the church **(b)** Rapid discharge of a thundercloud

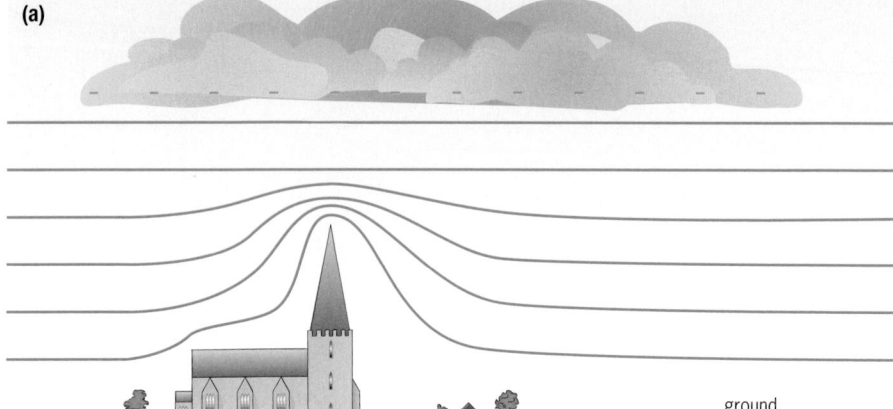
(a)

ground

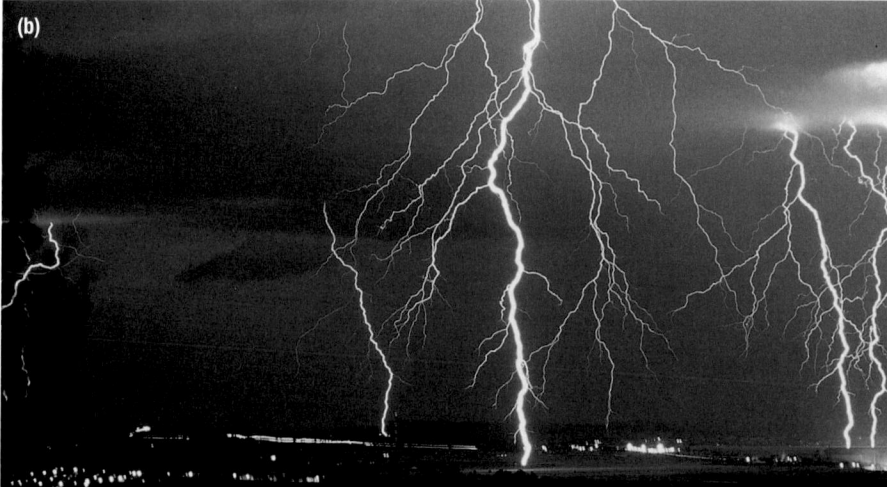
(b)

? QUESTION 5

5 On a dry day, over flat country, measurements taken above the ground show that the electric potential can increase by about 100 volts per metre.
a) What is the p.d. between the ground and a distance 1.8 m above it?
b) A person is 1.8 m tall. Why isn't there such a voltage between that person's nose and feet?
c) Sketch the equipotentials around the person standing in the open.

For more on the charge distribution of a thunder cloud, and the propagation of lightning please see the How Science Works assignment for this chapter at www.collinseducation.co.uk/CAS

This property is used in a lightning conductor, which is basically a pointed metal rod. One end is earthed and the pointed end extends above the top of the building to which it is attached. A thundercloud often has a concentration of negative charge at its base. This generates an electric field between the base and the ground. Below the thundercloud, the field at the point of the lightning conductor is strong enough to ionise air molecules around the point.

The resulting charged molecules – ions – move in the field: positive ions go towards the cloud base and electrons go to earth through the lightning conductor. This mechanism allows the thundercloud to discharge slowly before enough charge builds up to cause lightning.

Electrostatic paint spraying

Particles of paint are given a positive charge as they leave the nozzle of a spray gun (Fig 9.11). The object to be painted is earthed so that there is an electric field between the nozzle and the object. The charged paint droplets follow the field lines and are deposited evenly over the surface of the object.

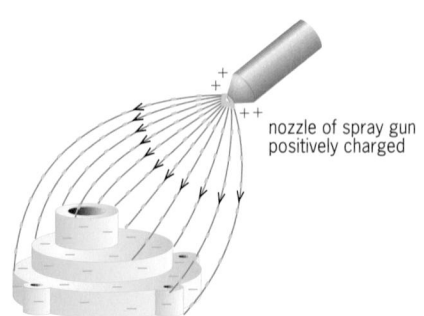
nozzle of spray gun positively charged

Fig 9.11 Electrostatic paint spraying: the charged droplets follow the field lines to the object to be painted, which is earthed

4 PARALLEL PLATE CAPACITOR

So far, we have been looking at the electric field between two parallel plates. This arrangement can in fact *store electric charge*, which makes it a capacitor. We have seen that the field between the capacitor plates depends upon the p.d. across them and the distance between them. Let us now look at other factors that affect the strength of a field.

There is a p.d. across the plates when they are charged (see page 189). In fact, the charge on the plates is proportional to the p.d. ($Q = CV$). The quantity of charge on the plates also depends on the area of the plates. If the area of the plates is doubled, the quantity of charge the capacitor can store is doubled. So:

$$Q \propto A$$

The ratio of charge to area (Q/A) is called the charge density (σ). Since the charge density is proportional to p.d., it is proportional to the field strength:

charge density $\propto$ field strength

$$\sigma \propto E$$

$$\frac{Q}{A} \propto \frac{V}{d}$$

There is one other factor that affects the field strength. This is the medium between the plates, the **dielectric**. The dielectric is an insulator, the simplest being a vacuum. Often, the insulating material is air, oil or paper. For a vacuum between the plates:

$$\frac{Q}{A} = \varepsilon_0 \frac{V}{d}$$

where ε_0 is a constant called the **permittivity of free space** (or of a vacuum) which links charge density and field strength. Its units are farads per metre and it tells us how good a vacuum is at allowing an electric field to be established.

The value of ε_0 is 8.85×10^{-12} F m^{-1}, or alternatively 8.85×10^{-12} C^2 N^{-1} m^{-2}.

Another way of arranging the equation gives expressions for capacitance, symbol C:

$$C = \frac{Q}{V}$$

$$= \varepsilon_0 \frac{A}{d}$$

The second line of the equation gives the capacitance in terms of the physical dimensions of the dielectric medium and the capacitor.

In practice, different dielectric materials are used for capacitors, depending on their size (see Table 9.2 in the Science in Context box on page 202).

The equation for the capacitance is slightly modified to account for the dielectric:

$$C = \varepsilon_0 \varepsilon_r \frac{A}{d}$$

where ε_r is called the **relative permittivity** of the dielectric used. Table 9.1 gives values of relative permittivity for some common materials.

The plates of a capacitor are covered with a 'blanket' of charge. The charge spreads out evenly over most of the plates – only at the edges is the distribution more uneven with more charge concentrated at any 'sharp' edges and corners.

 REMEMBER THIS

The farad, symbol F, is the unit of capacitance: a 1 farad capacitor charged by a p.d. of 1 volt carries a charge of 1 coulomb. In practice, capacitors have much smaller values, ranging between microfarads and picofarads.

? QUESTION 6

6 **a)** An air-spaced capacitor of 1 µF is needed. Estimate the size of the plates if they are 1 mm apart.

b) Mica has a relative permittivity of 6. What would be the size of the plates with mica as the dielectric?

Table 9.1 Relative permittivity for some common materials

Substance	Relative permittivity
air	1
paper	between 2 and 3
water	about 80

Practical capacitors

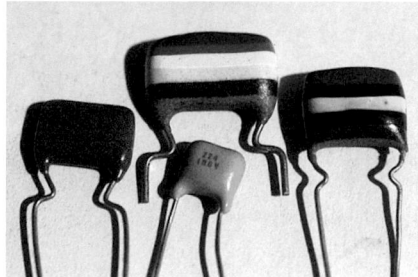

Fig 9.12 (a) Small value ceramic capacitors

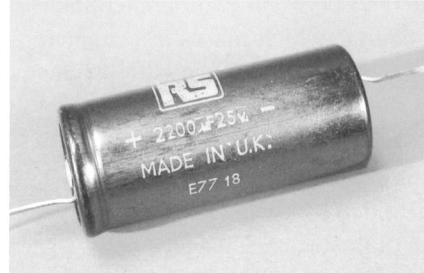

(b) Aluminium electrolytic capacitor

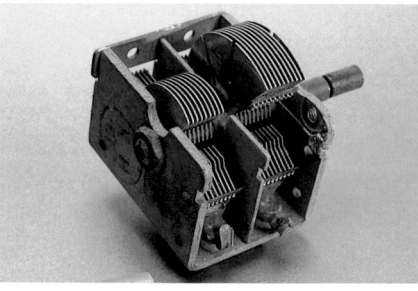

(c) Variable capacitor

There are many different types of capacitor available, made from different materials and suitable for different applications. They come in a range of shapes and sizes, in values from picofarads up to farads. Capacitors are used to store charge (and energy), to 'smooth' a fluctuating voltage (see Chapter 12) or to allow high frequency signals to 'bypass' parts of a circuit. They are essential in circuits designed to respond to certain frequencies.

Examples are the 'tuned circuit' (see Chapter 12) in radio receivers used to select a signal of a particular frequency, and 'filters' which use the fact that the behaviour of a capacitor in a.c. circuits depends on frequency. With accurate capacitors, filters will respond to very narrow bands of signal frequencies, which can be either filtered out or allowed to pass.

Sometimes very accurate capacitors are needed, usually of

low value, typically pF or nF. Capacitors of very high value are used, such as in 'smoothing', where accuracy is not important.

All capacitors lose charge over time, that is, they 'leak'. Most capacitors have a fixed value, but others vary over a range of values, as in tuned circuits. Table 9.2 shows some of the common types of capacitor that are used.

Table 9.2

Type	Capacitance range	Maximum voltage	Accuracy	Leakage	Comments
mica	1 pF–10 nF	100–600 V	good	good	very useful at radio frequencies
ceramic	10 pF–1 μF	50–30 000 V	poor	fair	cheap, small
polystyrene	10 pF–2.7 μF	100–600 V	excellent	excellent	high quality, used in accurate filters
polycarbonate	100 pF–30 μF	50–800 V	excellent	good	high quality, small
tantalum	100 nF–500 μF	6–100 V	poor	poor	high capacitance, polarised
electrolytic (aluminium)	100 nF–2 F	3–600 V	horrible	awful	smoothing power supply filters, polarised

EFFECT OF THE DIELECTRIC

Placing an insulating material between the plates of a capacitor increases the capacitance. That means that more charge can be stored for the same voltage across the plates, and this effect is greater when materials with greater values of ε_r are used. For more about dielectrics, see Chapter 20.

5 NON-UNIFORM ELECTRIC FIELD – COULOMB'S LAW

In 1785, Coulomb measured the forces between small charged bodies and summarised his results in the form of an equation that is now known as Coulomb's law. He discovered that force F depends on the size of the charges Q_1 and Q_2 on the bodies, and on the distance r between them. As the distance increases, the force decreases – in fact, if the distance doubles, the force decreases by a factor of four. That is, the force obeys an inverse square law:

$$F = k\frac{Q_1 Q_2}{r^2}$$

where k is a constant.

This equation is almost identical in form to Newton's law of gravitation:

$$F = -G\frac{m_1 m_2}{r^2}$$

Unlike gravity, which is always attractive, the electric force can be either attractive or repulsive. See Fig 9.13: when the charges are opposite, the force is attractive and defined as negative, like gravity; when the charges are of the same sign, the force is repulsive and defined as positive.

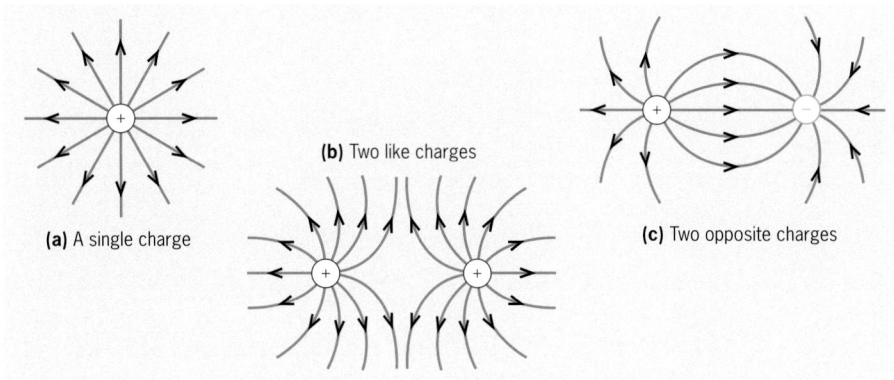

(a) A single charge

(b) Two like charges

(c) Two opposite charges

Fig 9.13 The electric fields around point charges

Fig 9.14 shows the field around an isolated charge. Fig 9.14(a) is a two-dimensional representation, but the field around the charge is three-dimensional. Fig 9.14(b) attempts to show this. The field lines spread out radially from the centre. Yet again, this 'map' of field lines helps us visualise the field, but it is limited. It is very difficult to show on such a 'map' the precise way that the magnitude of the field changes. The equations below help solve this problem.

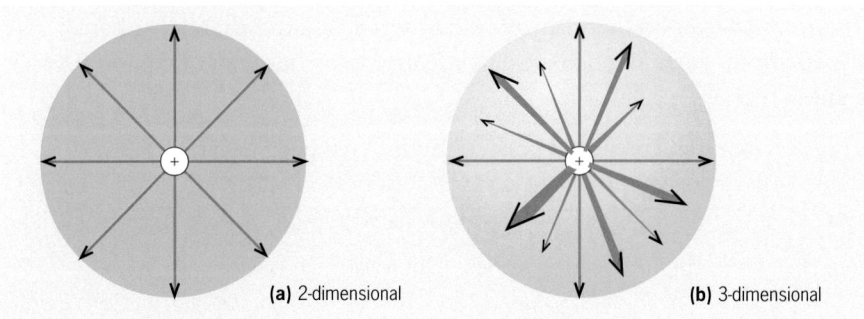

(a) 2-dimensional

(b) 3-dimensional

Fig 9.14 The field around an isolated charge

FIELD STRENGTH

The strength E of the electric field can be measured by considering the force on a second 'test' charge, Q_2, at a distance r from a charge Q_1:

$$\text{field strength} = \text{force per unit charge}$$

$$= \left(\frac{kQ_1 Q_2}{r^2}\right) \div Q_2$$

$$E = \frac{kQ_1}{r^2}$$

That is, the field strength in a non-uniform electric field also obeys the inverse square law.

? QUESTIONS 7–8

7   Two spheres of equal size and mass carry identical charges. Explain what would happen to the repulsive force between them if:

a) the charge on one of them is doubled,

b) the charge on both of them is doubled,

c) the charge on both of them is doubled and the distance between them is doubled.

8   In a hydrogen atom the electron and proton are about 10^{-10} m apart. Calculate the attractive force between them.

EXAMPLE

Q The electric field strength 50 cm from the centre of a small charged sphere is 18 N C^{-1}. Calculate the charge on the sphere.
($k = 9 \times 10^9$ N m^2 C^{-2})

A The field strength is:

$$E = k\frac{Q}{r^2} = 18\text{ N C}^{-1}$$

Rearranging:

$$Q = \frac{Er^2}{k} = \frac{18 \times (5 \times 10^{-1})^2}{9 \times 10^9}\text{ C}$$

$$= \frac{18 \times 25 \times 10^{-2}}{9 \times 10^9}\text{ C}$$

$$= 5 \times 10^{-10}\text{ C}$$

POTENTIAL IN A RADIAL FIELD

The flame probe used to investigate the potential between parallel plates was described earlier (see Fig 9.7). As shown in Fig 9.15, it can also be used to investigate the way electrical potential varies around an isolated charged body, in this case a sphere. The potential decreases, but it follows a $1/r$ law.

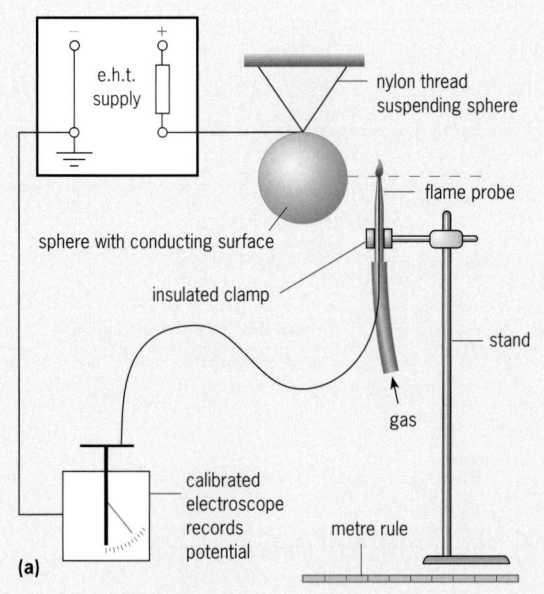

(a)

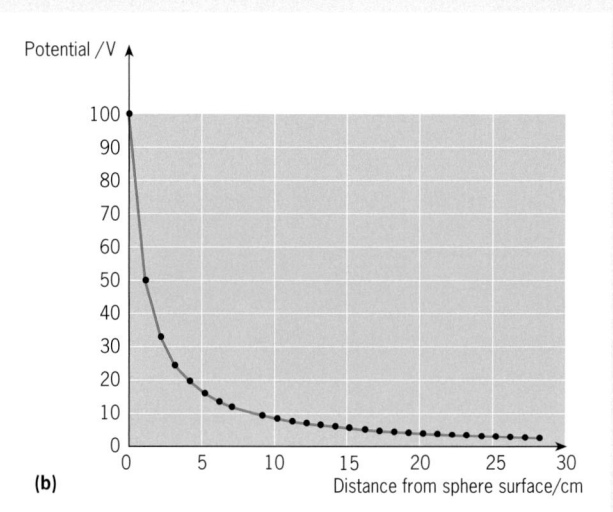

(b)

Fig 9.15 (a) A flame probe used to investigate the electrical potential around a charged sphere
(b) Potential plotted against distance from sphere surface

The potential again depends on the charge:

$$V = k\frac{Q_1}{r}$$

The constant k can be found by considering an isolated charged sphere. Fig 9.16 shows such a sphere, radius r, carrying a charge of Q coulombs. We know that:

charge density $= \varepsilon_0 \times$ field strength   (see page 201)

$$\frac{Q}{A} = \varepsilon_0 \frac{kQ}{r^2}$$

where $A = 4\pi r^2$, the area of the sphere. Therefore we have:

$$\frac{Q}{4\pi r^2} = \varepsilon_0 \frac{kQ}{r^2}$$

The charge and radius squared cancel, leaving us with:

$$k = \frac{1}{4\pi\varepsilon_0}$$

Fig 9.16 An isolated charged sphere

RELATIONSHIP BETWEEN FIELD AND POTENTIAL

Earlier in this chapter, on page 199, we found that for a uniform field the field strength E was equal to minus the potential gradient:

$$E = -\frac{dV}{dr}$$

? QUESTION 9

9 Fig 9.15(b) shows how potential varies around a charged sphere. Sketch a graph to show how potential varies **a)** close to a flat surface, and **b)** far away from that surface.

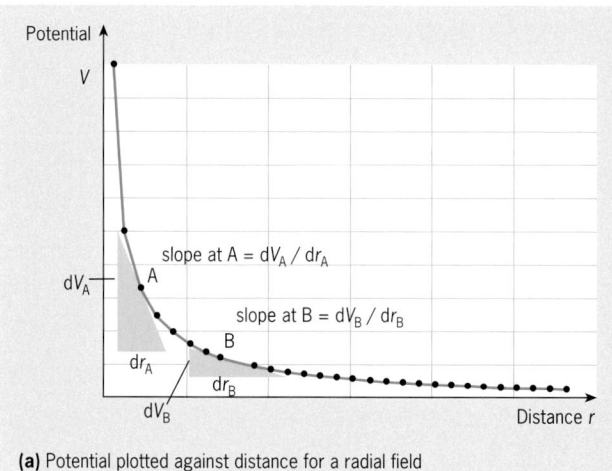

(a) Potential plotted against distance for a radial field

(b) Electric field plotted against distance for a radial field

The same is still true for fields that vary by an inverse square law. We can show this mathematically:

$$V = \frac{1}{4\pi\varepsilon_0}\frac{Q}{r}$$

$$E = -\frac{dV}{dr}$$

$$= -\frac{Q}{4\pi\varepsilon_0}\frac{d(1/r)}{dr}$$

Therefore:

$$E = \frac{1}{4\pi\varepsilon_0}\frac{Q}{r^2}$$

This means that the slope of the potential–distance graph of Fig 9.17(a) gives the value of the field strength at that point.

The equations for inverse square electric fields are summarised in Table 9.3, together with the equivalent gravitational field equations.

Fig 9.17 The relationship between potential and electric field. The gradient of the potential–distance curve gives the field strength at any point

Table 9.3 Comparison of electric field and gravitational field equations

Gravitational field	Electric field
$F_G = -G\dfrac{m_1 m_2}{r^2}$	$F_E = \dfrac{1}{4\pi\varepsilon_0}\dfrac{Q_1 Q_2}{r^2}$
$g = -G\dfrac{m}{r^2}$	$E = \dfrac{1}{4\pi\varepsilon_0}\dfrac{Q}{r^2}$
$V_G = -G\dfrac{m}{r}$	$V_E = \dfrac{1}{4\pi\varepsilon_0}\dfrac{Q}{r}$

SUMMARY

By the end of this chapter you should know and understand the following:

- The field between charged plates is uniform.
- Electric field strength is the force per unit charge measured in newtons per coulomb.
- The equations for uniform fields are $E = F/Q = V/d$.
- The work done in moving a charge of Q coulombs through a p.d. of V volts is QV joules.
- The kinetic energy of an electron emerging from an electron gun is given by $\frac{1}{2}mv^2 = eV$.
- The electronvolt is the energy gained by a particle carrying a charge of 1.6×10^{-19} coulombs when it has been accelerated through a p.d. of 1 V.
- The potential at a point in an electric field is the work done per coulomb in moving a unit charge from zero or earth potential to that point.

- Equipotentials can be thought of as surfaces in space of equal potential which cut electric field lines at right angles.
- Field strength E is equal to (minus) the potential gradient, $-dV/dr$.
- Charge density = permittivity × field strength of free space, and capacitance $C = \varepsilon_0 A/d$.
- The force between two charges is given by Coulomb's law, $F = kQ_1Q_2/r^2$, and field strength $E = kQ/r^2$, where $k = 1/4\pi\varepsilon_0$.
- The potential around a charge Q is given by $V = kQ/r$.

Practice questions for this chapter are available at www.collinseducation.co.uk/CAS

10

Electromagnetism

10 ELECTROMAGNETISM

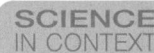

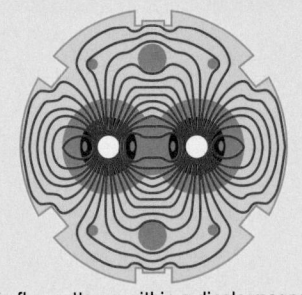

Magnetic flux patterns within a dipole magnet used in the LHC

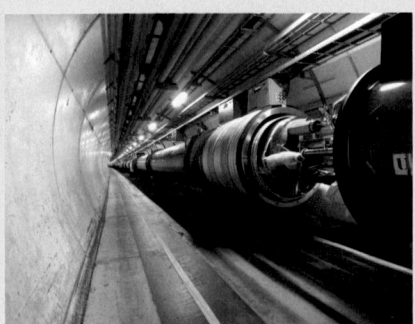

The Large Hadron Collider at CERN

Our electromagnetic world

Nikola Tesla has been described as the man who invented the twentieth century because of his understanding of electromagnetism and the applications he evolved that led to the large-scale generation and distribution of electricity.

Now in the twenty-first century scientists study the interaction of the magnetic field of the Sun with that of the Earth using data from the Cluster satellites. Not only does this help us understand better the physics of our nearest star but it also helps us predict some of the more damaging effects of large solar flares on the Earth and its near environment.

In 2008 the Large Hadron Collider (LHC) will start its search for the Higgs boson and a deeper understanding of the fundamental nature of matter. The LHC accelerates beams of protons around a synchrotron ring of 27 km circumference until they reach energies of 7 TeV. To bend protons around this path requires dipole magnets that produce a magnetic field of 8.4 Tesla (that's about 100 000 times the magnetic field of the Earth). These magnets use superconductors and draw currents of about 11 700 amps. They are 14.3 metres long and 1232 of them are needed. The LHC uses over 2500 other magnets to guide and collide the proton beams.

This is just a tiny fraction of the billions of electromagnetic devices, including motors and drives, and even down to magnetically controlled nano-rods of gold, nickel and platinum, that require an understanding of electromagnetism.

The ideas in this chapter

In this chapter you will learn about the inextricable link between moving charges and magnetic fields. When charges move in a circuit the current is surrounded by a complete loop of magnetic field – a loop of electric current surrounded by a loop of magnetic field – each linked with the other. This chapter looks at the way current loops create magnetic fields; the next chapter will look from the other direction, at how changing magnetic loops can create currents.

1 FIELDS AROUND CURRENTS

If we pass an electric current along a wire and then bring a compass near to it, the compass needle (which is a strong magnet) will be deflected (Fig 10.1). This is because the current has a **magnetic field** around it, as first demonstrated by Hans Christian Oersted in 1820.

What do we mean by a magnetic field? The compass needle is deflected because it experiences a force. With a constant current, the size of the force depends only on how far the needle is from the wire: the closer it is, the greater the force on the needle – but the needle does not have to touch the wire. The effect, then, acts at a distance. So we describe the space around the wire as containing a magnetic field.

A magnetic field can be represented by 'field lines' that show the shape of the field. We draw the lines close together if we want to show a strong field, and further apart for a weaker field.

The field has a **direction of action**. We define the direction of the field at a point as the direction of the force that would act on an isolated north pole placed there. (So far no-one has ever found such a thing as an isolated north pole – magnetic poles always occur in pairs – but it is a useful idea to help define field directions.) The direction of the magnetic field is from north to south, as shown in Fig 10.2(a). The Earth has its own magnetic field, which has been used for hundreds of years in navigation – see Fig 10.2(b). Magnetic field is a vector quantity.

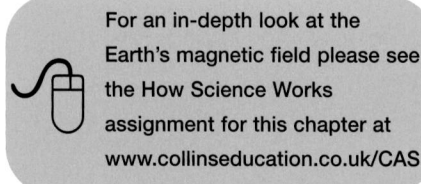

For an in-depth look at the Earth's magnetic field please see the How Science Works assignment for this chapter at www.collinseducation.co.uk/CAS

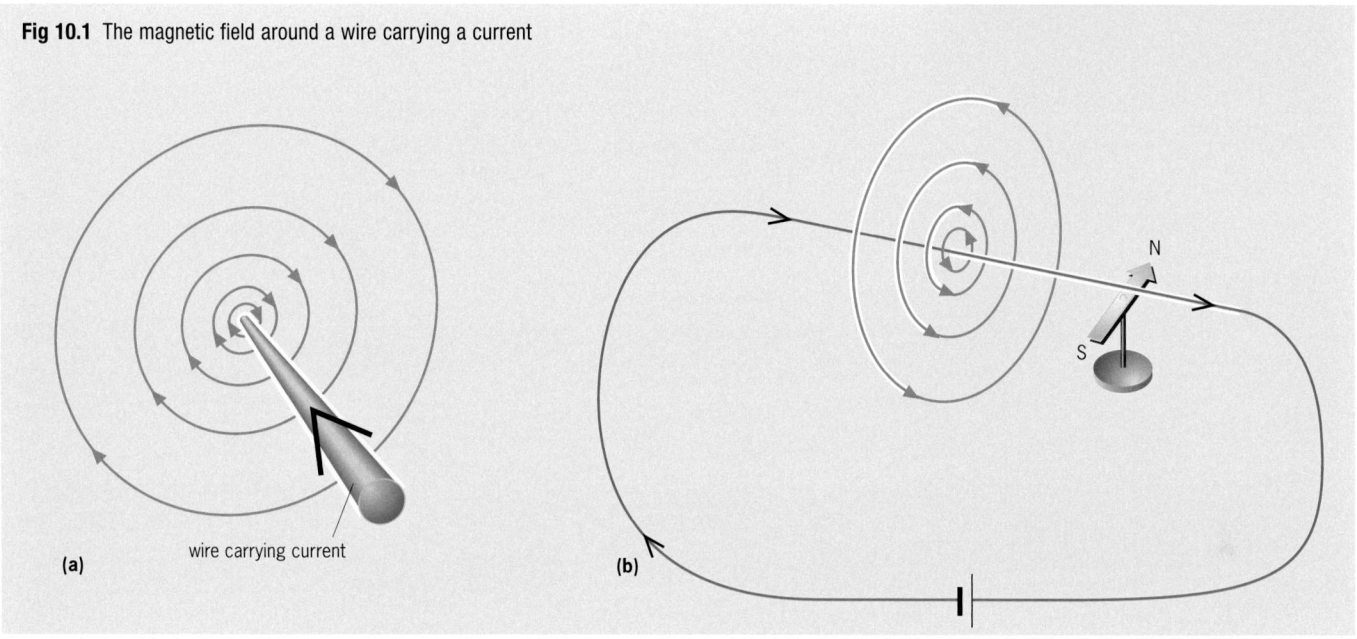

Fig 10.1 The magnetic field around a wire carrying a current

(a)   wire carrying current   (b)

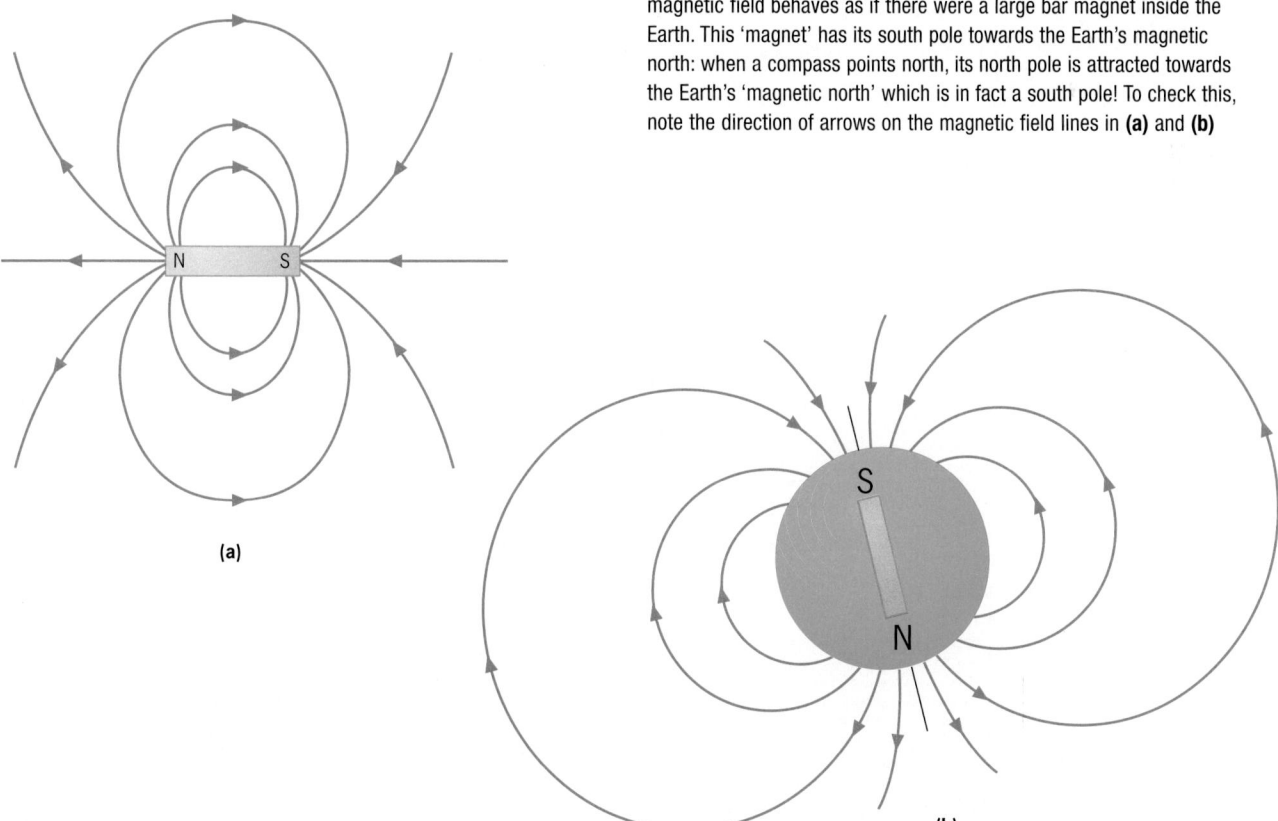

Fig 10.2 (a) The magnetic field around a bar magnet. **(b)** The Earth's magnetic field behaves as if there were a large bar magnet inside the Earth. This 'magnet' has its south pole towards the Earth's magnetic north: when a compass points north, its north pole is attracted towards the Earth's 'magnetic north' which is in fact a south pole! To check this, note the direction of arrows on the magnetic field lines in **(a)** and **(b)**

(a)

(b)

2 MAGNETIC FIELD AND FLUX

The idea of field lines was one of Faraday's important contributions to physics. The patterns we draw around magnets and coils to describe the shape and variation in strength of fields were first used by him. He imagined the field lines passing through a surface as shown in Fig 10.3, and he called this **'flux'**.

The flux Φ is defined as:

$$\text{flux} = \text{field strength} \times \text{the area it passes through}$$
$$\Phi = BA$$

If the field is not perpendicular to the area, then the equation becomes:

$$\Phi = BA \sin \theta$$

Flux is measured in **webers** (Wb).

The strength of the magnetic field can be defined in terms of flux and is correctly termed the **flux density**:

$$\text{flux density, } B = \frac{\Phi}{A}$$

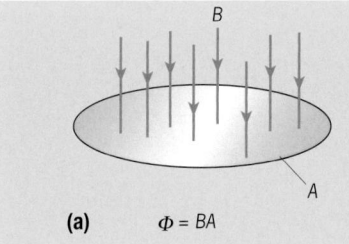 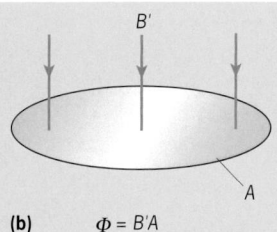 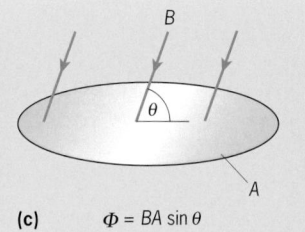

(a) $\Phi = BA$ (b) $\Phi = B'A$ (c) $\Phi = BA \sin \theta$

Fig 10.3 In **(a)** and **(b)** the magnetic field is perpendicular to the area it is passing through, where field B' is less than B. In **(c)** the field is not perpendicular to the area and must be resolved into components – only the component perpendicular to the area is used in calculating the flux

Field lines or flux paths are always in complete loops. This is not always obvious when we look at fields around permanent magnets. If we could see the field lines inside the magnet we would be convinced.

Just as we are used to the idea of electric circuits being complete paths or loops (we call them 'circuits'), we can use the idea of **magnetic circuits**.

3 MAGNETIC CIRCUITS

In the examples shown in Fig 10.4, the flux is set up by a current flowing through a coil, or **solenoid**. The flux, represented by the field lines, is in complete loops. This is always the case. In some cases, as in Fig 10.4(a), the loops are set up in the space around and through the coil, while in others, as in (b), they are contained within a solid core such as 'soft iron'. We can think of these complete loops as 'magnetic circuits'.

Fig 10.4 The flux **(a)** around a solenoid and **(b)** in a transformer core

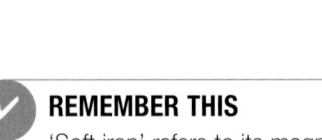

REMEMBER THIS

'Soft iron' refers to its magnetic properties – not to its hardness. See page 214.

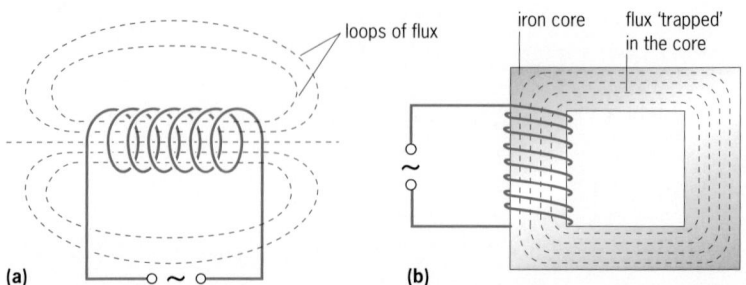

(a)   (b)

We saw in Chapter 8, page 173, that the physical dimensions of the wire (cross-sectional area and length) in a simple electric circuit affect the current. Similarly, we shall see here that the dimensions of a magnetic circuit affect the flux that can be set up.

The flux also depends on the size of the current and the number of turns on the coil. Without current and turns of the coil there would be no flux. We say the flux is 'generated' by the current turns. If N is the number of turns, I is the current and Φ is the flux, then:

$$NI \propto \Phi$$

To understand how the dimensions of the magnetic circuit can affect the flux it is probably easier to think about a transformer. The flux is generated by a primary coil. The iron core has the interesting and useful property of confining nearly all the flux within the core. The physical dimensions of the core, its cross-sectional area and the length all affect the flux, as shown in Fig 10.5.

? **QUESTION 1**

1 Describe clearly how the physical dimensions of the core affect the flux.

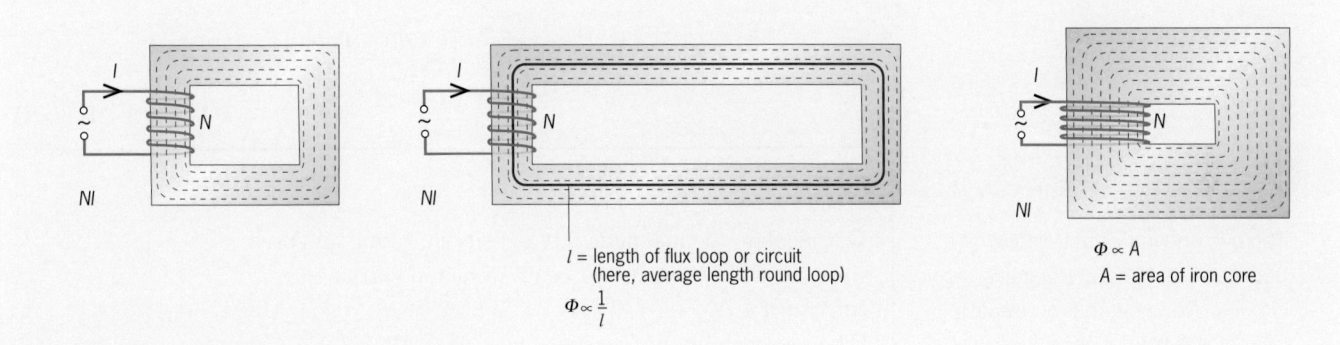

l = length of flux loop or circuit (here, average length round loop)

$\Phi \propto \dfrac{1}{l}$

$\Phi \propto A$
A = area of iron core

Fig 10.5 These diagrams illustrate how the characteristics of a magnetic circuit affect the flux created by NI current-turns. Taken together we can combine them to give $\Phi \propto NIA/l$

MAGNETIC CIRCUITS COMPARED WITH ELECTRIC CIRCUITS

At this point it is worth comparing magnetic circuits with simple electric circuits.

A voltage V causes a current I in a circuit that has electrical resistance. The resistance depends upon the physical dimensions of the wire and the material of the wire. When A is the cross-sectional area, l is the length of the wire and ρ is the resistivity of the material of the wire, then:

$$V = IR$$

$$= I\frac{\rho l}{A}$$

Looking at Fig 10.5, we can write a similar equation for a magnetic circuit:

$$NI = \Phi \times \text{constant} \times \frac{l}{A}$$

Just as the current is 'set up' by a voltage in the electric circuit, the flux Φ is set up by the current-turns, NI.

The constant is $1/\mu$, where μ is the **permeability** of the medium within which the flux is set up.

The quantity $l/\mu A$ is the magnetic circuit equivalent to resistance. It is called the **reluctance** of the magnetic circuit (R_{mag}).

If the magnetic field is set up in air (which is very similar to a vacuum – free space – free space – for magnetic fields) then the constant is $1/\mu_0$, where μ_0 is the **permeability of the vacuum** (free space), with units N A^{-2}. In any other medium, the constant is $1/\mu_0\mu_r$, where μ_r is the **relative permeability** of the medium. That is:

$$NI = \Phi \frac{l}{\mu_0 \mu_r A}$$

We think of permeability as a kind of 'magnetic conductivity' – it tells us how good a medium is at allowing a magnetic field to be established in that medium. The relative permeability tells us how much better that medium is compared to a vacuum.

In electric circuits, instead of *resistance* we often find it more convenient to think of *conductance*:

$$\text{conductance, } G = \frac{\text{current}}{\text{potential difference}} = \frac{\sigma A}{l}$$

(Remember from Chapter 8 that σ is electrical conductivity, where $\sigma = 1/\rho$.)

We can similarly define a *magnetic conductance*, which we call **permeance**:

$$\text{permeance, } \Lambda = \frac{\Phi}{NI} = \frac{\mu_0 \mu_r A}{l}$$

? QUESTION 2

2   There is one important difference between electric and magnetic circuits. We know that an electric current is a flow of charge – coulombs per second – but what 'flows' in a magnetic circuit? Is there anything?

✔ REMEMBER THIS

Magnetic flux density, or the strength of a magnetic field is measured in tesla (T) in honour of Nikola Tesla (1856–1943) who was responsible for many developments in electricity which led to the widespread use of electricity as a means of distributing energy.

EXAMPLE

Q Calculate the magnetic flux density in a long air-cored solenoid with 10 turns per centimetre and carrying a current of 1 A.
(The permeability of free space $\mu_0 = 4\pi \times 10^{-7}$ N A^{-2}.)

A Use the equation for current-turns:

$$NI = \Phi \frac{l}{\mu_0 A} = \frac{\Phi}{A}\frac{l}{\mu_0}$$

$$= B \frac{l}{\mu_0} \quad (\text{since } B = \frac{\Phi}{A})$$

Rearranging:

$$B = \frac{N}{l} I \mu_0 \quad (10 \text{ turns cm}^{-1} = 1000 \text{ turns m}^{-1})$$

$$= 1000 \times 1 \times 4\pi \times 10^{-7}$$

$$= 12.6 \times 10^{-4} \text{ T}$$

Magnetic flux density in the solenoid = 1.26 mT.

In Table 10.1 we compare electrical and magnetic quantities.

Table 10.1

Electrical quantity	Magnetic quantity
Voltage V	Current-turns NI
Resistance R	Reluctance R_{mag}
Conductance G	Permeance Λ
Conductivity σ	Permeability $\mu_0\mu_r$
Current I	Flux Φ

4 FLUX DENSITIES IN SOME USEFUL MAGNETIC CIRCUITS

FLUX DENSITY DUE TO A LONG SOLENOID

Imagine a solenoid of length l metres with N turns, forming a circle as in Fig 10.6. Therefore, when there is a current the flux forms an enclosed loop inside the coil, also of length l. The cross-sectional area of the solenoid, and so of the tube of flux, is A m^2. We shall assume that the medium in the solenoid is air.

Start with the equation for the flux:

$$NI = \Phi \frac{l}{\mu_0 A}$$

Now, since $\Phi = BA$ (flux density × area), we can write:

$$NI = \frac{BAl}{\mu_0 A} = \frac{Bl}{\mu_0}$$

We can rearrange this to obtain an equation for the flux density B in a solenoid:

$$B = \mu_0 \frac{N}{l} I = \mu_0 nI$$

where $n = N/l$, the number of turns per metre.

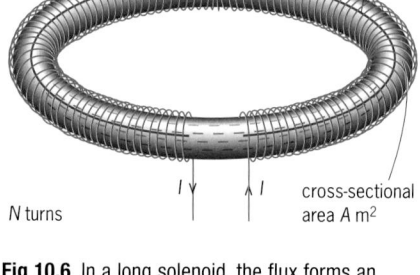

Fig 10.6 In a long solenoid, the flux forms an enclosed loop inside the coil

FLUX DENSITY DUE TO A LONG STRAIGHT WIRE

As in Fig 10.7, imagine a ring of flux of cross-sectional area A, around the wire at a distance r from the wire. The wire can be considered as part of a very large single-turn coil, that is, $N = 1$. Therefore current:

$$I = \Phi \frac{l}{\mu_0 A}$$

The length l of the ring of flux is $2\pi r$ and, since $\Phi = BA$:

$$I = BA \frac{2\pi r}{\mu_0 A}$$

Rearranging, we get:

$$B = \frac{\mu_0 I}{2\pi r}$$

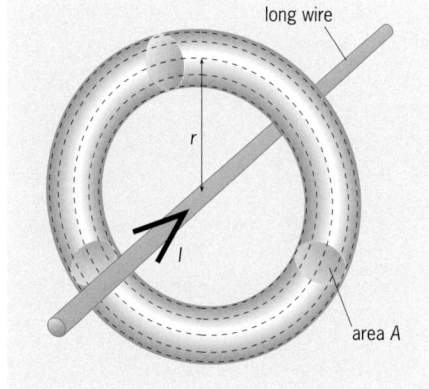

Fig 10.7 The flux due to a long straight wire

EXAMPLE

Q Calculate the magnetic flux density around a straight wire carrying a current of 10 A at a distance of **a)** 10 cm, **b)** 20 cm, **c)** 100 cm. (The permeability of free space $\mu_0 = 4\pi \times 10^{-7}$ N A^{-2}.)

A

a) We use the equation for magnetic flux density:

$$B = \frac{\mu_0 I}{2\pi r}$$

$$= \frac{4\pi \times 10^{-7} \times 10}{4\pi \times 10} \text{ T}$$

Magnetic flux density at 10 cm
$= 2 \times 10^{-5}$ T

b) Since r is inversely proportional to B, and since r doubles here, B will halve to 1×10^{-5} T.

c) With a value for r of 100 cm, the field strength is 2×10^{-6} T.

THE EFFECT OF IRON

Iron has a very large relative permeability, which is why it is useful for making electromagnets, for example. When a coil is wound on a soft iron core, the magnetic field produced is about a thousand times stronger than it would be if the iron were not there. Iron also has the property of losing most of the magnetism as soon as the current stops flowing. This is why it is described as 'soft'. A magnetically 'hard' metal such as steel would retain much of the magnetism if it were used in the same coil. The magnetic flux density in a solenoid with an iron core is:

$$B = \mu_r \mu_0 \frac{N}{l} I$$

where N = number of turns and l = length of flux loop. The value of μ_r for iron is about 1000.

We can say that iron is a 'good conductor' of magnetism. Many other magnetic materials have high relative permeabilities but are less dense than iron. These find uses where light weight is an advantage, such as in miniature earphones and the small motors used inside CD and DVD drives.

5 MAGNETIC CIRCUITS AND SOME ELECTROMAGNETIC DEVICES

Many simple electromagnetic devices can be understood by using the idea of magnetic circuits. One is the **electromagnetic relay**, which allows remote switching of several circuits at once. If we examine the flux path in a relay we see that there is a 'high reluctance' air gap between the core of the electromagnet and the armature (Fig 10.8). The flux in this magnetic circuit is weak. When the electromagnet is 'energised' by a current in it, the armature is attracted towards the electromagnet core. This reduces the reluctance of the magnetic circuit and a strong flux is established. It should also be noted that the force between the core and the armature is in a straight line and that the armature moves in the same direction.

Many simple motors also produce rotation when the *rotor* moves to make a magnetic circuit with a lower reluctance. They are called **reluctance motors** and are used in disk drives and fans in computers. The *stepper motor* found in all computer printers is also a more sophisticated relative of the reluctance motor.

Fig 10.9 shows a simple reluctance motor. The rotor can be a permanent magnet or an electromagnet (or even a soft iron bar). When the coils are energised so that one pole becomes a north pole and the other a south pole, the rotor experiences a sideways *alignment* force. In trying to line up, the rotor is reducing the 'high reluctance' gap in a magnetic circuit so that a stronger flux path can be established. The coils could be connected to an a.c. source as shown. As the rotor turns it is in turn attracted to and repelled from the changing poles, continually trying to produce the lowest reluctance path for the flux. (The rotational speed of this motor will depend on the frequency of the a.c. supply. These are often also called *synchronous* motors.)

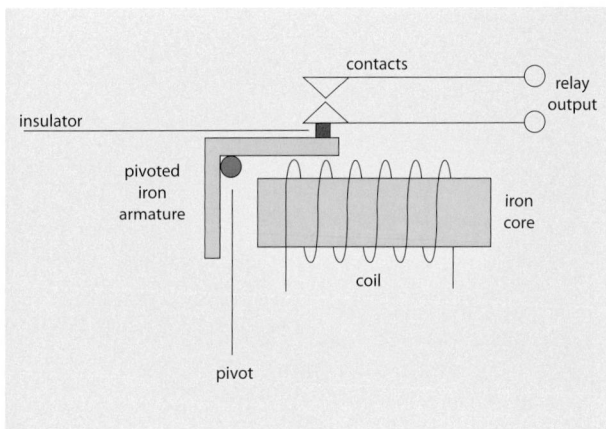

Fig 10.8 Principle of an electromagnetic relay

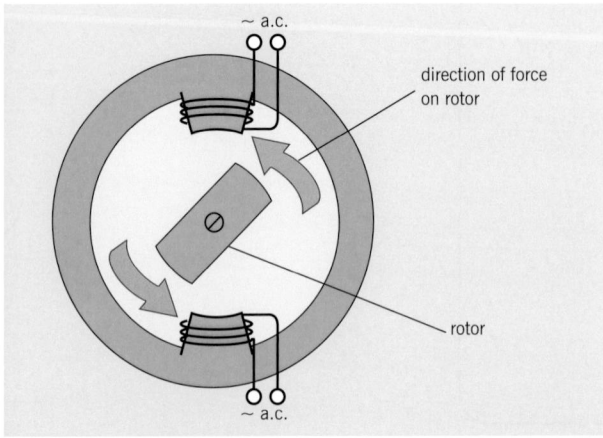

Fig 10.9 The reluctance motor

6 FORCES ON WIRES CARRYING CURRENTS

Fig 10.10(a) shows a wire carrying a current and placed at right angles to a magnetic field. As shown in Fig 10.10(b), we can predict the direction of the force on the wire by using **Fleming's left-hand rule**. The wire will tend to move in the direction of the force. This link between a wire carrying a current and its movement in a magnetic field is used in the moving coil electric motor, as Fig 10.10(c).

The size of the force F depends upon the current I in the wire of length l in the magnetic field of strength B. That is:

- $F \propto I$, the current in the wire
- $F \propto l$, the length of wire in the field
- $F \propto B$, the magnetic flux density

Taken together, these can be expressed as:

$$F = kIlB$$

where k is a constant.

We choose the units of B to make $k = 1$, as follows. Suppose the magnetic field is such that a wire 1 metre long carrying a current of 1 ampere feels a force of 1 newton. We shall define the flux density B as 1 newton per ampere metre (N A^{-1} m^{-1}). Therefore we have:

$$1 \text{ N} = k \times (\text{N A}^{-1}\text{ m}^{-1}) \times 1\text{ A} \times 1\text{ m}$$

The newton per ampere metre is called a **tesla**, symbol T. Small magnetic fields are measured in µT (micro-tesla). The magnitude of the Earth's magnetic field varies between 24 µT and 66 µT. In the UK it is about 49 µT.

Under these conditions $k = 1$. So we have:

$$\boldsymbol{F = IlB}$$

By writing the equation for the force like this we are being consistent with other 'forces in fields':

- In a uniform electric field, force = charge × electric field strength ($F = q \times E$)
- In a gravitational field, force = mass × gravitational field strength ($F = m \times g$)

the general idea being:

force = magnitude of quantity feeling the force × field strength

The 'thing' feeling the force in a magnetic field is a current-carrying wire (Il). So:

$$\text{magnetic force} = Il \times B$$

The force on a coil of N turns would be N times greater than on a single wire, namely $N \times IlB$.

Force F is a maximum when the field and current are perpendicular (with magnetic field constant). If the angle is smaller, the force is reduced (Fig 10.11):

$$F = Il \times B \sin \theta$$

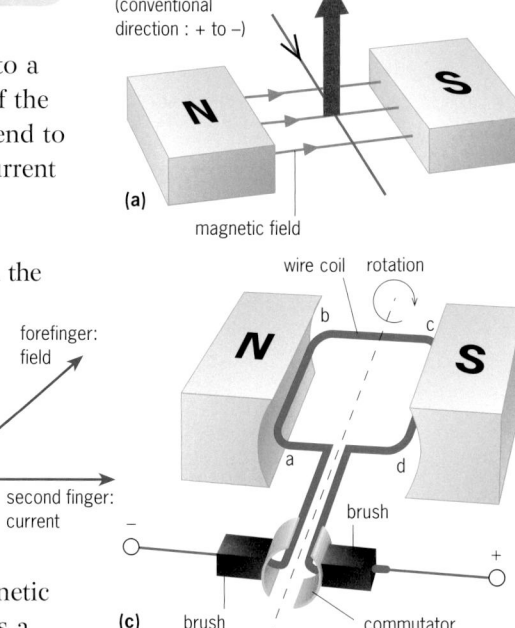

(a) magnetic field

(c) brush   commutator

Fig 10.10 Fleming's left-hand rule.
(a) A wire carrying a current in a magnetic field.
(b) Direction of force predicted by Fleming's rule. The thumb and second finger are in the plane of the page – the forefinger is pointing into the page.
(c) A simple d.c. motor

thumb: motion force   forefinger: field

(b)

second finger: current

✔ **REMEMBER THIS**
Note that the tesla can also be expressed as weber m^{-2} since B is the flux *density*, $B = \Phi/A$.

EXAMPLE

Q Calculate the flux density of the magnetic field that will apply a force of 0.01 N per metre to a wire carrying a current of 5 A.

A $F = IlB$ or $B = F/Il$

$$B = \frac{0.01\text{ N}}{5\text{ A} \times 1\text{ m}}$$

$$= 0.002\text{ N (A m)}^{-1}$$

Flux density = 2 mT

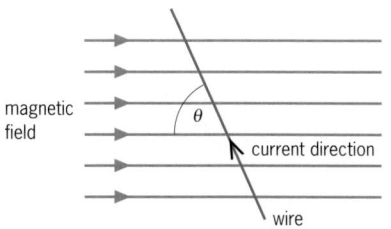

magnetic field

current direction

wire

Fig 10.11 A current-carrying wire placed at an angle θ to a magnetic field

? QUESTIONS 3–4

3 Calculate the force on a 100 m power cable carrying a current of 10 A in a magnetic field of 50 μT.

4 Look at Fig 10.10 (c). Use Fleming's left-hand rule to check the movement of sections a–b and c–d of the wire. Hint: see also drawing (a).

THE CURRENT BALANCE

The current balance, shown in Fig 10.12(a), is used to measure magnetic flux density. The force on a known length of wire carrying a known current in an unknown magnetic field is measured and is used to determine B, the magnetic flux density, using the equation $F = IlB$ in the form:

$$B = \frac{F}{Il}$$

The force can be measured using a counterweight and scale as in (a), or directly using a sensitive top-pan balance as in Fig 10.12(b).

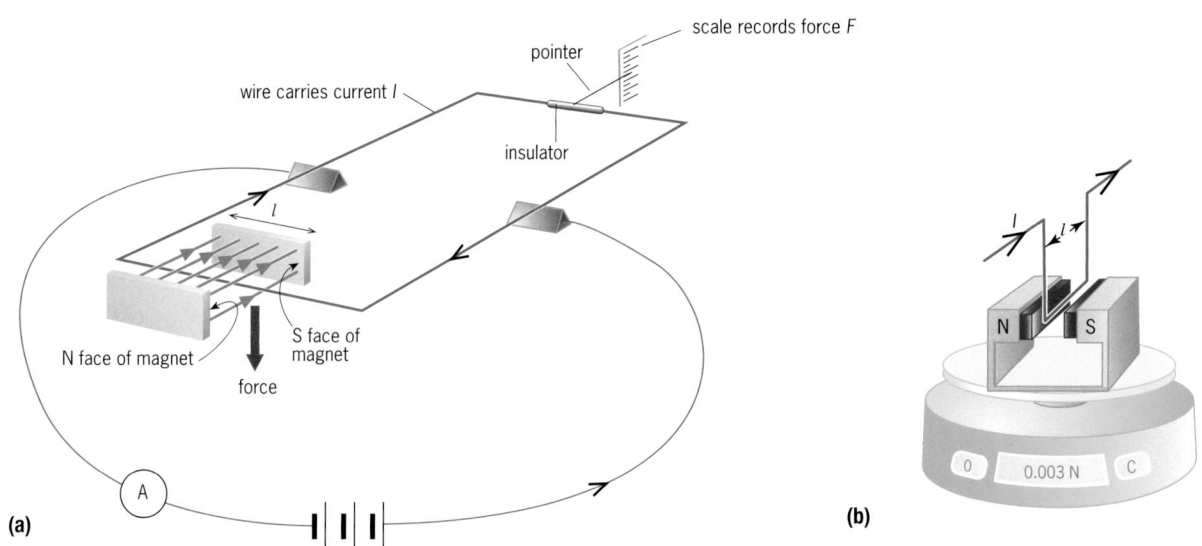

(a)

(b)

Fig 10.12 (a) A current balance for measuring the field between two magnets and **(b)** a top-pan balance for measuring the field between two magnets. The force on the wire is measured as the weight shown on the balance

The ampere

Two wires carrying currents also exert forces on each other, as shown in Fig 10.13.

The unit of electric current, the ampere, is defined in terms of its magnetic effect, that is, the force between two wires each carrying a current of 1 A (Fig 10.14). When the wires are parallel and 1 m apart, the force between them should be 2×10^{-7} N (in theory, if they are infinitely long). This is the force used to define the ampere.

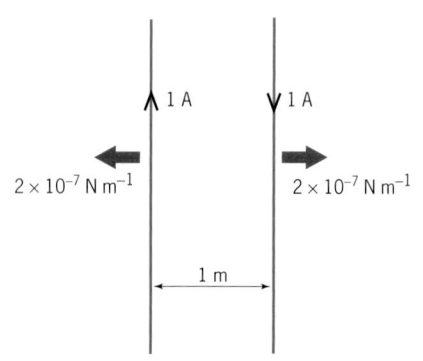

Fig 10.14 The definition of the ampere

? QUESTION 5

5 Examine the magnetic fields in Fig 10.13 carefully and use Fleming's left-hand rule to show that the directions of the forces on the wires are correct.

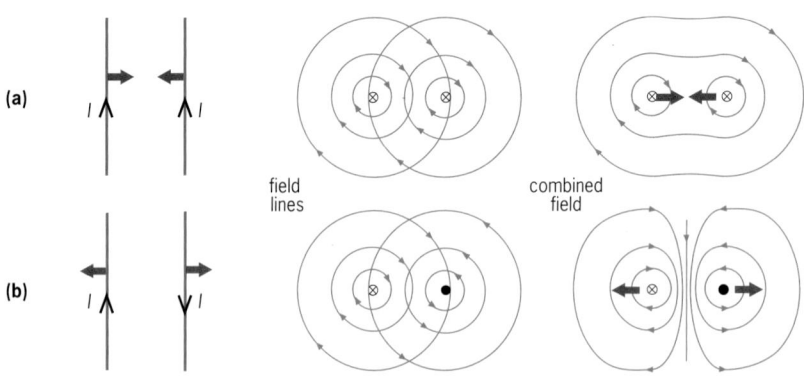

Fig 10.13 Two wires carrying current exert forces on each other: **(a)** like currents attract, **(b)** unlike currents repel (direction of current in lower right wire: out of page)

7 FORCES ON CHARGED PARTICLES IN BEAMS

A television picture is produced from an electron beam controlled by magnetic fields. The beam scans across the television screen at high speed. The cathode ray oscilloscope also uses an electron beam. In fact, J.J. Thomson investigated 'cathode rays' in 1897 and observed how electric and magnetic fields affected them. Thomson showed that the cathode rays were tiny negatively charged particles. It was several years before they were called 'electrons' but Thomson is credited with their discovery.

Fig 10.15 shows a beam of identical charged particles, each with a charge q coulombs and moving with an average velocity of v metres per second. The beam is moving at right angles to a uniform magnetic field of flux density B tesla. We can work out the force exerted by the field on each particle in the beam. When the length of beam in the field is l and it takes t seconds for a particle to move this distance, then:

$$l = vt$$

If the length l of the beam contains N particles, then the number of particles passing a point in the field is also N, and therefore the total charge passing through any point in the field in t seconds is Nq coulombs. Therefore the current is given by:

$$I = \frac{Nq}{t}$$

If we now treat the beam like a wire, then using $F = IlB$ we get:

$$
\begin{aligned}
F &= IlB \\
&= \frac{Nq}{t} \times vt \times B \\
&= NqvB
\end{aligned}
$$

This is the force on a beam of N particles. Therefore the force on a single particle is given by:

$$F = \frac{NqvB}{N}$$

So, force on one particle is:

$$\mathbf{F = QvB}$$

(This time the 'thing' feeling the force is a moving charged particle, qv.)

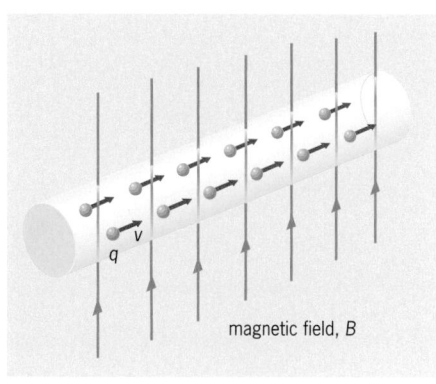

Fig 10.15 A beam of charged particles in a magnetic field

magnetic field, B

✔ **REMEMBER THIS**

An electric current in a wire is a flow of charged particles confined in the wire. A beam of charged particles is also a current – for example, a beam of electrons is a current.

SCIENCE IN CONTEXT

EXAMPLE

Q Television tubes use magnetic fields to deflect the beam of electrons. Electrons are emitted from the electron gun in the tube at a speed of 2×10^7 m s^{-1}. They travel a horizontal distance of 20 cm to the screen and are deflected sideways by the magnetic field a distance of 10 cm.

Calculate an approximate value for the flux density of the magnetic field required to do this. (Mass of an electron = 9.1×10^{-31} kg.)

A
Time taken to reach screen

$$= \frac{0.2 \text{ m}}{2 \times 10^7 \text{ ms}^{-1}} = 1 \times 10^{-8} \text{ s}$$

In this time the electrons are accelerated sideways a distance s of 10 cm with an acceleration a, given by:

$$s = \tfrac{1}{2} at^2$$
$$a = 2 \times 0.1 \text{ m}/(1 \times 10^{-8} \text{ s})^2$$
$$= 0.2 \times 10^{16} \text{ m s}^{-2}$$

The force required is:

$$F = ma = (9.1 \times 10^{-31}) \times (0.2 \times 10^{16})$$
$$= 1.8 \times 10^{-15} \text{ N}$$

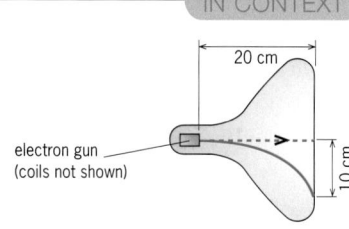

From $F = evB$, the flux density is given by $B = F/ev$. Therefore:

$$
B = \frac{1.8 \times 10^{-15}}{(1.6 \times 10^{-19}) \times (2 \times 10^7)}
$$
$$= 5.6 \times 10^{-4} \text{ tesla}$$

Approximate magnetic flux density
$$= 0.56 \text{ mT}$$

Measurement of *e/m* for electrons

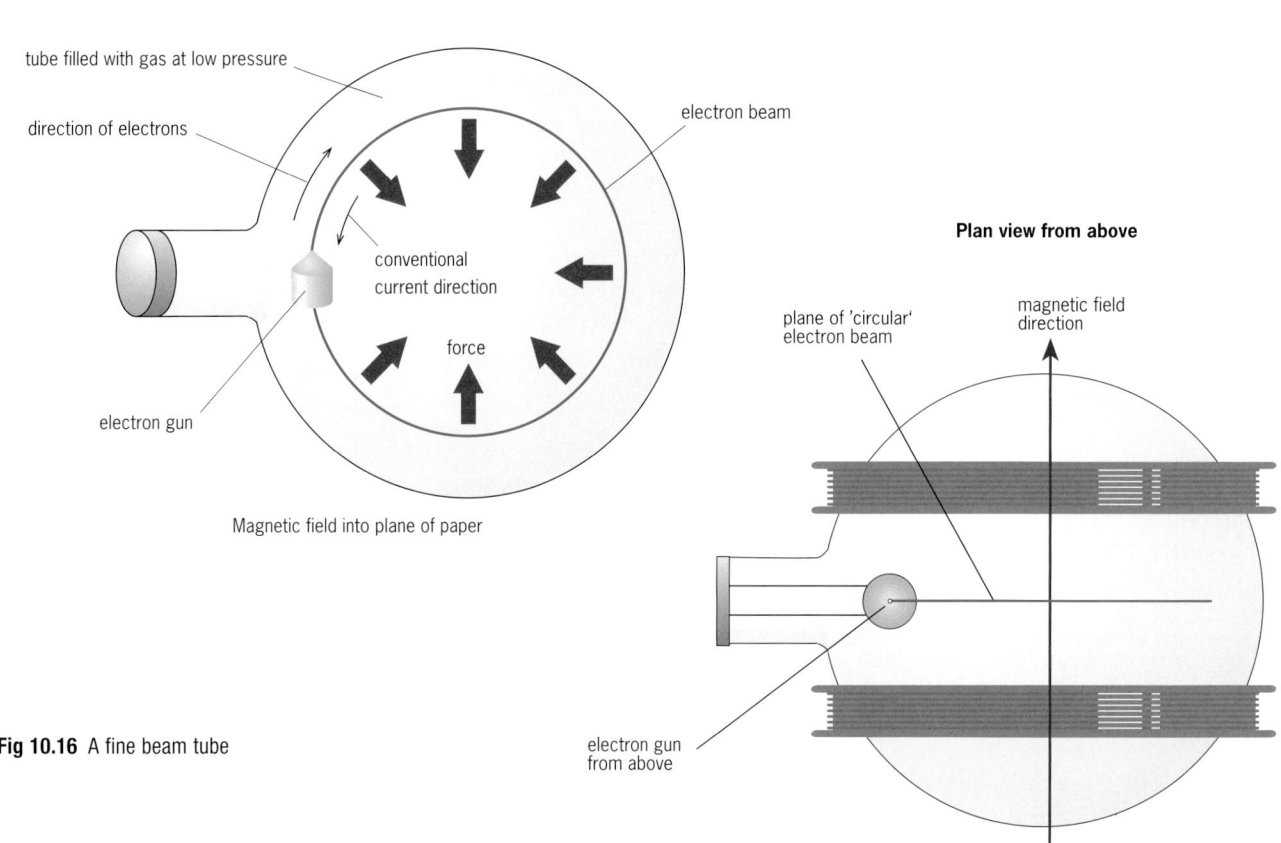

Side view

tube filled with gas at low pressure

direction of electrons

electron beam

conventional
current direction

force

electron gun

Magnetic field into plane of paper

Fig 10.16 A fine beam tube

Plan view from above

plane of 'circular'
electron beam

magnetic field
direction

electron gun
from above

The apparatus in Fig 10.16 is called a fine beam tube, though it has a bulb rather than a tube. It includes an electron gun that fires a beam of electrons vertically into the spherical cavity of the bulb. As the drawing shows, the bulb is mounted between two coils (called **Helmholtz coils**). The coils produce a uniform magnetic field that is horizontal and at right angles to the path of the electron beam.

When the electrons emerge from the electron gun, the magnetic force is at right angles to both their direction of travel and the direction of the magnetic field. With the directions shown in Fig 10.16, the force is towards the centre of the tube. As the electron beam turns, its direction of travel is always perpendicular to the field and the force is always directed towards the centre of the tube. This

results in the electrons moving in a circular path, with the magnetic force providing the centripetal force. So, using the equation $F = QvB$, derived on page 217 (in this case Q is the charge on the electron for which we use the symbol 'e'):

$$evB = \frac{mv^2}{r}$$

where r is the radius of the circular path.

The electron gun provides us with more information about the energy of the electrons (see Chapter 9, page 196):

$$eV = \tfrac{1}{2}mv^2$$

Apart from e, m and v, all the other quantities in these two equations, that is B, r and V, can be measured by experiment.

The two equations can be rearranged to give the velocity v and the ratio e/m:

$$v = \frac{2V}{Br}$$

and:

$$\frac{e}{m} = \frac{2V}{(Br)^2}$$

e/m for electrons is 1.76×10^{11} C kg^{-1}. With accelerating voltages of about 100 to 200 V, the velocity of the electrons is about 10^7 m s^{-1}. The apparatus described above gives results similar to these, using very ordinary laboratory equipment to make measurements. An ammeter and top-pan balance are needed to measure B, a voltmeter to measure the accelerating voltage V and a ruler to measure radius r of the beam.

8 THE HALL EFFECT

An easy way to measure magnetic fields is to use a Hall probe. The probe is based on a small integrated circuit that produces an output voltage proportional to the magnetic flux density. This 'chip' depends on the effect discovered in 1879 by E.H. Hall. The Hall effect allows us to gain some important information about conduction in solids, including the speed of charge carriers and the number of charge carriers per unit volume.

If charged particles are moving in a solid placed in a magnetic field, then the magnetic force will affect their motion. Fig 10.17 shows a slice of conducting material carrying a current. A magnetic field is applied at right angles to the direction of the current. The current shown is the *conventional* current. We should remember that electrons move in the opposite direction, as shown. The moving electrons are pushed by a force towards the back edge of the block. They are unable to leave the block and therefore gather at the edge.

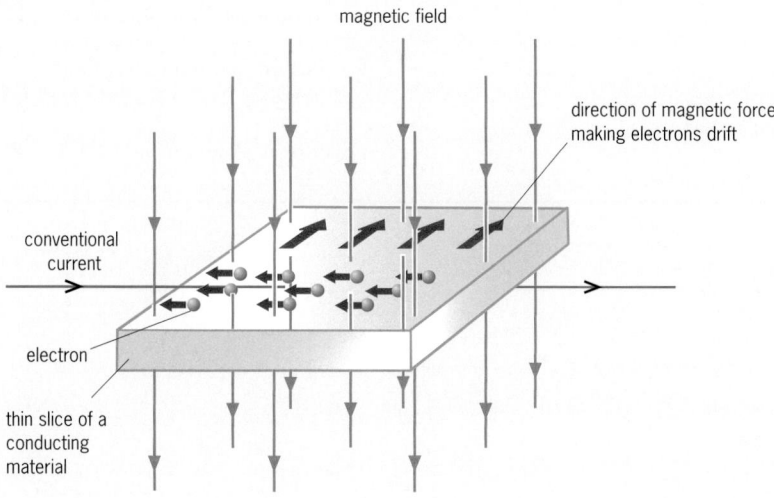

Fig 10.17 The Hall effect

So, in Fig 10.17 the magnetic force causes electrons to drift from the front edge towards the back edge. This makes the back edge negative and the front edge positive with a gradient in between. Like charges repel, so as the electrons, each of charge e, build up at the back, an electric field of strength E develops that opposes this sideways movement of electrons. Eventually the force from the electric field (Ee) on each electron exactly balances the magnetic force (evB), as shown in Fig 10.18.

As the charges gather at the back edge, a voltage develops across the slice. This voltage is called the **Hall voltage**. The Hall voltage is largest for semiconductor materials like silicon and germanium. Good conductors have much smaller Hall voltages (the Stretch and Challenge box on page 220 explains the reason for this).

So far, we have considered the charge carriers to be electrons. In n-type semiconductors, current is certainly due to the movement of (negative) electrons. However, in p-type semiconductors, current is due to the movement of positive 'holes' (see Chapter 20). Electrons move into holes in one direction, making the holes effectively move in the opposite direction. Therefore, the description above is correct for an n-type semiconductor, but for a p-type semiconductor the polarity of the Hall voltage is reversed.

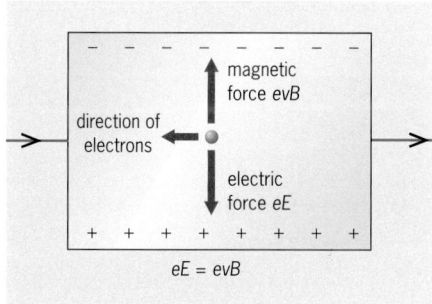

Fig 10.18 The balance of forces in the Hall effect, as viewed from above

? QUESTION 6

6 Apply Fleming's left-hand rule to show that the movement of the electrons in Fig 10.17 is correct. If the current (in the same direction) were due to positive holes, which way would they move in the field? Why is the Hall voltage reversed?

Factors affecting the Hall voltage

An equilibrium is quickly reached when the magnetic force on the electrons is exactly balanced by the electric force:

$$eE = evB$$

But the electric field strength E can be expressed as the Hall voltage V_H divided by the width d of the block of material. Therefore:

$$e\frac{V_H}{d} = evB$$

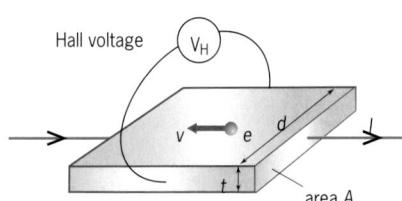

Hall voltage

This gives:

$$V_H = Bvd$$

The velocity of the electrons can be derived from the transport equation (see Chapter 8, page 173):

$$v = \frac{I}{nAe}$$

where n is the number of charge carriers per cubic metre.

The equation for the Hall voltage now becomes:

$$V_H = \frac{BId}{nAe}$$

Fig 10.19 The variables affecting the Hall voltage

This can be simplified further because $A/d = t$, the thickness of the block. So the final expression is:

$$V_H = \frac{BI}{nte}$$

We can now see why semiconductor materials are used for Hall probes. The number of carriers n in a semiconductor is many magnitudes smaller than for a good conductor, but is still large enough to allow for a significant current I. A small value of n produces a large Hall voltage V_H. Insulators have a very low value of n, but allow very little current to flow:

For doped semiconductors, $n \approx 10^{22}$ m^{-3}.

For a typical metal, $n \approx 10^{28}$ m^{-3}.

? QUESTION 7

7   A sample of aluminium 10 mm wide and 0.01 mm thick has 2×10^{29} free electrons per cubic metre. A current of 5 A flows through the sample and a magnetic field of flux density 2 T acts at right angles to the surface of the sample. (The resistivity of aluminium is 2.7×10^{-8} Ω m.) Calculate:
   a) the drift velocity of the electrons in the sample,
   b) the Hall voltage between the edges of the sample.
   Why is it important that the Hall voltage is measured between two points which are exactly opposite each other? What would be the effect if the two contact points were misaligned by 0.1 mm?

SUMMARY

By the end of this chapter you should be able to:
- Describe a magnetic field in terms of its shape and direction.
- Describe the magnetic field around a wire carrying a current.
- Define magnetic flux as the product of the vertical component of flux density and the area it is passing through.
- Use the unit weber (Wb) for magnetic flux.
- Describe examples of magnetic circuits and compare magnetic circuits with electric circuits.
- Explain the action of some simple electromagnetic devices using the ideas of magnetic circuits.
- Use magnetic circuits to calculate the magnetic flux density in a solenoid and around a long wire.
- Measure magnetic flux density in tesla (N A^{-1} m^{-1}).

- Use the equation $F = IlB$ to calculate the force on a wire carrying a current.
- Describe the use of a current balance to measure magnetic flux density.
- Describe the application of magnetic forces in the moving coil d.c. motor.
- Use the equation $F = qvB$ for the force on a moving charged particle in a uniform magnetic field.
- Describe the Hall effect and use the Hall voltage to measure magnetic flux density.

 Practice questions for this chapter are available at www.collinseducation.co.uk/CAS

11

Electromagnetic induction

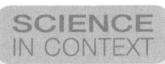

Applications of electromagnetic induction

In 1831, Michael Faraday discovered electromagnetic induction, which enabled him to transfer electrical power from one circuit to another by varying the magnetic linkage. Faraday's discovery led to the large-scale generation and distribution of electrical energy that transformed society and industry, as this energy could now be delivered to homes, hospitals, schools and factories many miles from the source. Over 150 years later, new applications of electromagnetic induction are still being developed.

Induction cooking is faster and more energy efficient than more traditional hobs, with the added advantage that less heat is lost to the surroundings and it's fairly simple to monitor changes in resistance so that cooking rings can be turned off automatically if pans boil dry or spill over.

Tiny currents induced in brain tissue can be used to monitor brain activity and this offers a non-invasive way of treating many disorders including depression. It's called Transcranial Magnetic Stimulation.

Linear induction motors have become established in some of the fastest train systems on Earth. Magnetic levitation enables near-frictionless motion, and the Japanese MLX-01 reached a speed of 581 km h^{-1} in 2003. There are plans to link Edinburgh and Glasgow with a Maglev link, which would make it possible to travel from city centre to city centre in 15 minutes.

'Induction Loop Systems' are now widely used to enable people with hearing impairment to hear more clearly. These systems are used in the home and in public places such as theatres and cinemas.

These are just some examples of how Faraday's discovery in 1831 has been applied in today's world.

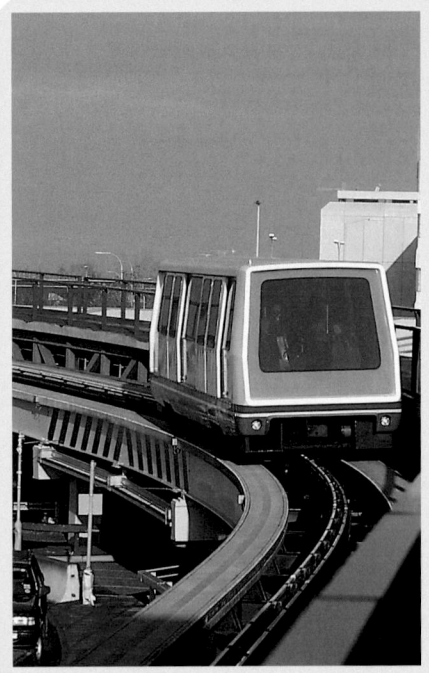

The Gatwick Airport monorail, which transports passengers between terminals. This train 'floats' above the single track because of magnetic forces, and the force that drives it along is due to induced currents

The ideas in this chapter

This chapter is about **electromagnetic induction**. This was Michael Faraday's amazing discovery on the 29 August 1831, which led to the birth of the electrical industry.

Today we are surrounded by devices and gadgets that use electricity. Try to imagine life without 'electricity'. Many devices use batteries as a source of energy but most rely on 'mains' electricity. That is, electricity that is **induced** or generated in power stations. By the start of the twenty-first century Britain's power stations were producing nearly 60 gigawatts (6×10^9 W) to cope with the demands of modern society and industry.

Induced currents have many other applications, ranging from car speedometers to domestic cookers that induce currents in the base of cooking pans. **Induction heating** is extensively used in industry, while the most common motor used for driving all sorts of machinery is the **induction motor**.

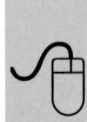

For a detailed analysis of the economic, environmental and social repercussions of electromagnetism in action please see the How Science Works assignment for this chapter at www.collinseducation.co.uk/CAS

1 WHAT IS ELECTROMAGNETIC INDUCTION?

Michael Faraday's discoveries early in the nineteenth century have made the large-scale production of electrical energy possible. The date 29 August 1831 is acknowledged as the 'birth of the electrical industry' – the day on which Faraday discovered electromagnetic induction. He made the link between electricity and magnetism when he showed that an electric current was produced when a magnet was moved near to a conductor (a metal wire).

Simple experiments provide the evidence. A magnet is moved into and out of a coil connected to a galvanometer, as shown in Fig 11.1(a), and a current is observed whenever the magnet moves (or, if the magnet is kept stationary, whenever the coil moves). A wire moved through a magnetic field produces the same result, as in Fig 11.1(b).

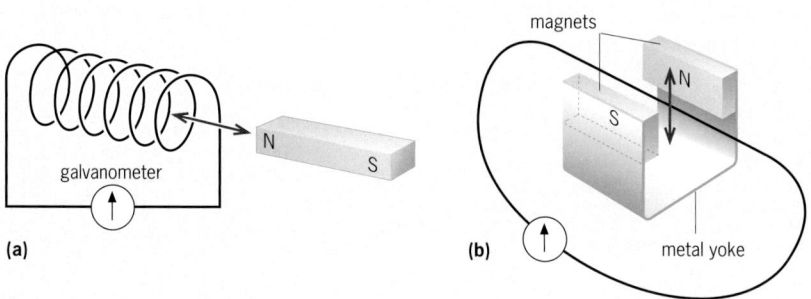

(a)

Fig 11.1 (a) A current is recorded when a magnet is moved into and out of a coil. **(b)** The same result is recorded when a wire is moved through a magnetic field

Faraday's experiments also led to the first simple transformer. He wound two coils on an iron ring (Fig 11.2). One, the primary coil, was connected to a battery and the other, the secondary coil, to a galvanometer. The galvanometer showed a current in the secondary coil only when the current from the battery was switched on or off; that is, only when the current from the battery, and hence the magnetic field, was *changing*.

So, a current is induced whenever a wire in a closed circuit moves through a magnetic field *or* when the field changes through the wire.

The following helps to explain the important ideas in more detail (refer to Fig 11.3):

- The rigid straight wire XY moves with a velocity v perpendicular to a uniform magnetic field of strength B tesla. The wire is l m long.
- There is a force on the electrons in the moving wire (evB, where e is the charge on a charge carrier, see page 217), and free electrons will move towards end X of the wire. As they build up at X, so does an electric field that opposes the movement of electrons (just as in the Hall effect, page 219).
- Eventually the electric force is equal to the magnetic force:

$$eE = evB$$

where E is the electric field strength (see page 196). We can also write:

$$E = \frac{V}{l}$$

where V is the final voltage induced across the ends of the wire.

- This 'voltage' is an induced e.m.f., since it is the movement of the wire through the field that produces charge separation.
- Putting this together we have:

$$e\frac{V}{l} = evB$$

or:

$$V = Blv$$

- Thus the induced e.m.f. V is proportional to the magnetic flux density B, the length of the conductor and the speed at which it moves.
(Note that if the conductor is at an angle θ to the field the induced voltage is $V = Blv \sin \theta$.)

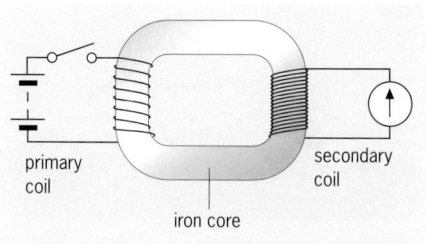

Fig 11.2 When the current in the primary coil is switched on or off, the galvanometer shows a current in the secondary coil

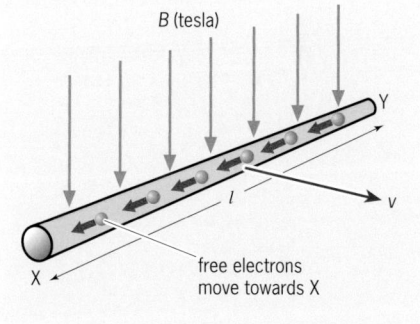

Fig 11.3 A rigid straight wire XY moving with velocity v in a magnetic field of flux density B tesla

? QUESTION 1

1   A wire of length 10 cm moves at 5 m s^{-1} through a magnetic field of 1 T, cutting the field at right angles. Calculate the e.m.f. induced across the wire.

THE INDUCED CURRENT

Once the e.m.f. is established, no more charge flows because the electric force is equal to the magnetic force. What happens when the wire is part of a complete circuit?

To answer that, suppose the wire XY shown in Fig 11.4 runs along two rails that are part of a simple circuit with a total resistance of R ohms and a uniform magnetic field B. The induced e.m.f. will drive a charge around the circuit. The direction of the 'conventional' current is shown.

Fig 11.4 When the wire of Fig 11.3 forms a complete circuit, the induced e.m.f. drives a current round the circuit

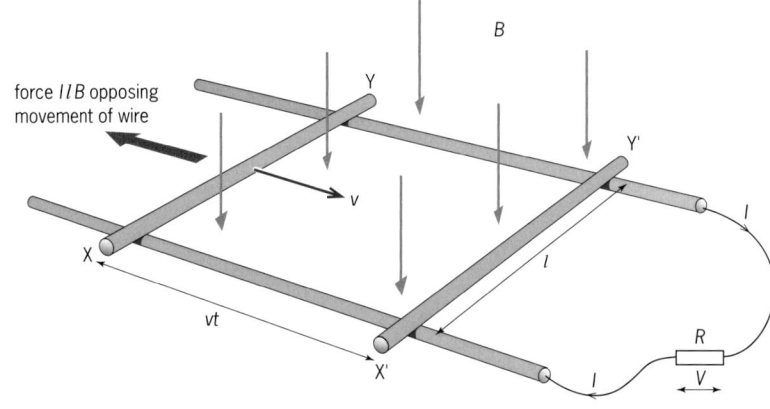

REMEMBER THIS

The direction of the conventional current is opposite to the direction in which the electrons move.

For the derivation of *F = ILB* see Chapter 10.

Now that there is a current (charge flowing), a force (*IlB*) affects the wire because it is in a magnetic field. This force acts in the opposite direction to the way the wire is moving. To keep the wire moving at a constant velocity v, a force equal to this must be applied in the direction of the movement. In t seconds the wire moves to X'Y' a distance of vt metres.

The work done in moving the wire is given by:

$$\text{work done} = \text{force} \times \text{distance moved}$$
$$= IlB \times vt$$

Since energy must be conserved, the work done is equal to the electrical energy transferred in the circuit:

$$\text{electrical energy supplied} = \text{power} \times \text{time}$$
$$= IV \times t$$

where V is now the p.d. across the load R. Therefore, we can write:

$$IVt = IlBvt$$

or:

$$V = Blv$$

This is the same as the formula obtained on page 223. What this tells us is that V, the induced e.m.f., is the same, whether a current is drawn or not.

TOWARDS A MORE GENERAL LAW

With the help of Fig 11.4, we can look at this result in a slightly different way. When the wire XY moves it sweeps through an area of ($vt \times l$), so vl is the area swept through per second:

$$\frac{vt \times l}{t} = vl = \frac{dA}{dt}$$

where dA/dt is the rate of change of area.

We can now write the equation for the induced e.m.f. as:

$$V = B\frac{dA}{dt}$$

That is, the induced voltage is equal to the flux density of the field multiplied by the rate at which the area swept through changes.

Faraday reached the same result, but he used the idea of **flux**, as explained in Chapter 10.

REMEMBER THIS

Flux Φ is defined (in Chapter 10) as the B field, or magnetic flux density, multiplied by the area through which the field passes, A:

$$\Phi = BA$$

EXAMPLE

Q A 10 cm wire is moved perpendicular to a steady magnetic field of flux density 5 mT at a speed of 0.5 m s^{-1}. Calculate

a) the rate of change of the area that the wire sweeps through, and

b) the induced e.m.f.

A

a) Speed of wire $\times$ length $= \dfrac{dA}{dt} = vl$

$$= 0.5 \text{ m s}^{-1} \times 0.1 \text{ m}$$

So rate of change of area $= 0.05$ m^2 s^{-1}

b) $V = B\dfrac{dA}{dt}$

$$= 5 \times 10^{-3} \times 0.05 = 0.25 \times 10^{-3} \text{ V}$$

So induced e.m.f. $= 0.25$ mV

---

2 FARADAY'S LAWS OF ELECTROMAGNETIC INDUCTION

After careful experiment, Faraday set out his laws of electromagnetic induction. For a wire moving through a magnetic field he found that the size of the induced e.m.f. is proportional to:

- the strength of the magnetic field,
- the speed at which the wire cuts the field,
- the number of turns of wire (as part of a coil, for example).

FLUX CUTTING AND FLUX LINKING

The action of a wire being passed through a field is often referred to as 'flux cutting'.

Faraday's 'transformer' experiments, however, do not involve moving wires. Look back at Fig 11.2: a current is induced in a secondary coil when the current in the primary coil changes. The current in the primary produces a magnetic flux which links with the secondary coil. When this flux changes, a current is induced in the secondary coil. This is called 'flux linking'. The induced current is proportional to:

- the strength of the field,
- the rate of change in the flux produced by the primary coil,
- the number of turns, N, on the secondary coil.

To induce a continuous current in the secondary, then, the current in the primary must continually change. For instance, if it is an alternating current (a.c.), then the induced current will also alternate.

The induced current will also depend on the a.c. frequency. An increase in frequency means that the flux is changing over a shorter time; that is, the rate of change of flux increases and the induced current is larger.

? QUESTION 2

2 To induce a current in a secondary coil, does the current in the primary coil have to change? Explain your answer.

Conversely, if the frequency of the a.c. in the primary is reduced, the flux changes over a longer time, so this reduces the rate of change of flux and the induced current:

the size of the induced current in the secondary coil is proportional to the frequency of the alternating current in the primary coil.

Faraday's laws can be summarised in one statement:

the induced e.m.f. is proportional to the rate of change of flux.

Or, if ε is the induced e.m.f.:

$$\varepsilon = N\frac{\mathrm{d}\Phi}{\mathrm{d}t}$$

where N is the number of turns of wire.

The equation could also be written as:

$$\varepsilon = \frac{\mathrm{d}(N\Phi)}{\mathrm{d}t}$$

The quantity $N\Phi$ is called the **flux linkage** and is used when a particular coil with N turns is considered.

3 LENZ'S LAW

? QUESTIONS 3–4

3   Explain why energy would not be conserved if Lenz's law were not true.

4   When a magnet is pushed into a coil as in Fig 11.1(a), the galvanometer needle moves to one side and back to zero. When the magnet is removed, the needle moves the other way and back to zero. Use Lenz's law to explain this.

When the north pole of a magnet is pushed into a coil, the direction of the induced current creates another 'north pole' at the end of the coil because the current 'opposes' the approaching north pole. When the magnet is removed, the direction of the induced current is reversed, changing the end of the coil to a south pole. This again opposes the north pole, which is now leaving the coil (Fig 11.5).

Lenz's law states:

The direction of the induced current opposes the change that causes it.

Lenz's law is the 'electromagnetic' version of the law of conservation of energy. If Lenz's law were not true, energy would not be conserved.

To show that the effects are opposed, we introduce a negative sign. The equation for the induced e.m.f. then reads:

$$\varepsilon = -N\frac{\mathrm{d}\Phi}{\mathrm{d}t}$$

Fig 11.5 Demonstrating Lenz's law

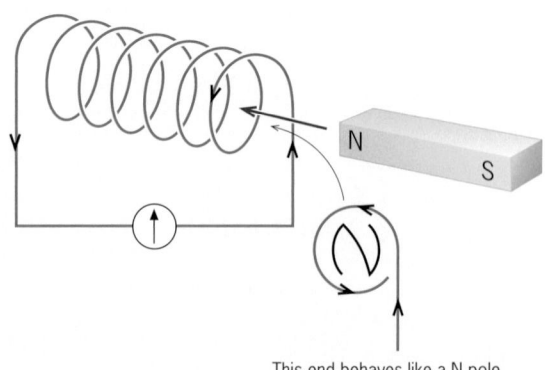

This end behaves like a N pole

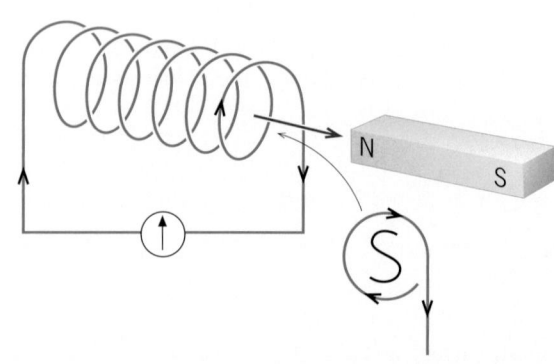

Now it behaves like a S pole

Mathematical treatment of Faraday's laws

The induced e.m.f. ε is given by:

$$\varepsilon = -N\frac{d\Phi}{dt}$$

$$= -N\frac{d(BA)}{dt}$$

$$= -N\left(B\frac{dA}{dt} + A\frac{dB}{dt} \right)$$

$$= -\left(NB\frac{dA}{dt} + NA\frac{dB}{dt} \right)$$

flux cutting term   flux linking term

The flux cutting term describes the induced e.m.f. produced by a wire *moving* through a *constant* magnetic field such as in a dynamo. The rate at which the wire sweeps out an area as it passes through the field determines the e.m.f.

The flux linking term describes the induced e.m.f. produced by a *changing* flux linking with a *fixed* wire as in the transformer. The flux produced by one coil 'links' with a second coil. The rate at which the field changes, which often depends on the current in the primary coil, determines the induced e.m.f.

4 THE TRANSFORMER

We have seen in Chapter 10 that loops of current create loops of magnetic flux. Faraday showed us that loops of changing flux can create loops of current. Magnetic circuits link with electric circuits. The **transformer** is an example where the magnetic circuit links two electric circuits (Fig 11.6).

Faraday's original experiments demonstrated the action of the transformer. If the current in the primary coil is continually changing, then the flux it produces will also change continuously.

The flux path, through the transformer core, is at right angles to the primary current path. The flux path also cuts the secondary coil at right angles. The changing flux induces a continually changing current in the secondary.

If the voltage applied to the primary is sinusoidal then the e.m.f. induced in the secondary will also be sinusoidal; that is an **alternating voltage**.

An alternating voltage of V_p is applied to the primary which has N_p turns and resistance R_p ohms. The alternating voltage drives a current I_p which creates a flux in the core. The flux induces an e.m.f. in the secondary, but it also induces an e.m.f. in the primary. The 'primary' e.m.f. opposes the applied voltage so that:

$$V_p - N_p\frac{d\Phi}{dt} = I_pR_p$$

If the core is short and fat then a small current will produce a large flux, and if the resistance of the primary coil is low then:

$$V_p \approx N_p\frac{d\Phi}{dt}$$

If there are N_s turns on the secondary then the voltage induced in it, V_s, will also be linked to the changing flux:

$$V_s = N_s\frac{d\Phi}{dt}$$

If we divide V_s by V_p,

$$\frac{V_s}{V_p} \approx \frac{N_s\, d\Phi/dt}{N_p\, d\Phi/dt}$$

The flux and its rate of change through each coil is the same. This leaves us with a very useful relationship for transformers:

$$\frac{V_s}{V_p} \approx \frac{N_s}{N_p}$$

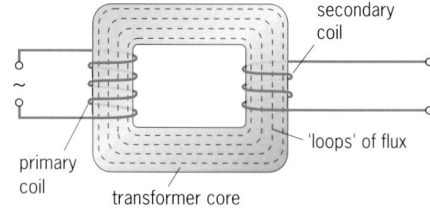

Fig 11.6 Loops of flux in a transformer

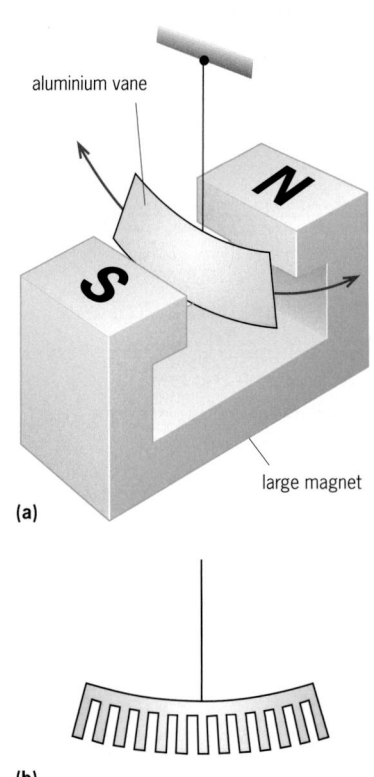

(a)

(b)

Fig 11.7 (a) The oscillations of an aluminium vane in a magnetic field illustrate the damping effect of eddy currents. **(b)** When a slotted vane replaces the solid vane, it oscillates for longer

 REMEMBER THIS

Permeance is a measure of how well a material allows a flux to be set up in it. **Reluctance** is the reciprocal of permeance. See Chapter 10 for more on magnetic circuits.

❓ QUESTIONS 5–6

5   A magnet allowed to fall freely down a plastic pipe accelerates to the ground. When the same magnet falls down a copper pipe of the same dimensions it takes longer to reach the ground. The magnet does not touch the sides of either pipe. Why does it take longer to fall down the copper pipe?

6   Give some practical examples of the use of magnetic braking.

The ratio N_s/N_p is called the **turns ratio** of the transformer and the equation shows it is approximately equal to the ratio of the secondary and primary voltages. This is very useful if you are designing transformers.

Transformers have many applications over a wide range of a.c. frequencies. They are used to **step-up** and **step-down** voltages in power supplies and they are essential in the **National Grid**, which is discussed in the next chapter.

5 EDDY CURRENTS

The flux in the core of a transformer induces currents in the coils at right angles to it. Why doesn't the flux induce currents in the core itself? After all, the core is made from iron or some similar magnetic material, which is also a good conductor.

The answer is it does, and if the core were solid the currents induced would make the core very hot and the energy transferred to the secondary coil would be far less. Currents induced in conductors like this are called **eddy currents**. The term 'eddy currents' came about because the charge moves in a swirling pattern, rather like the eddy currents we see in river water.

Eddy currents can be useful. Fig 11.7 shows a simple demonstration of eddy currents. The pendulum in (a) has an aluminium vane. When it swings between the poles of a magnet its motion is very heavily damped – it slows down and stops after a few swings.

This effect, sometimes called 'magnetic braking', is due to the currents induced in the aluminium as it cuts through the magnetic field. The currents flow in loops within the aluminium and, like all induced currents, they obey Lenz's law. That is, they flow in the direction that opposes the change that causes them.

As the vane enters the field (and B is getting stronger), an eddy current is induced in the vane. The moving electrons in the eddy current experience a force in the field of the magnet that opposes the motion of the vane, so slowing the vane. The force on the moving electrons is the same as the 'motor effect' (page 215).

When the vane moves out of the field (and B is now getting weaker) the direction of the induced current reverses, and so does the 'motor effect' force. This slows the vane down more. After a few swings it comes to rest.

If the solid vane is replaced by one with slots cut into it, Fig 11.7(b), the oscillating vane is affected far less and continues to swing for longer. The slots restrict the possible paths for eddy currents and effectively reduce the size of any currents induced.

Magnetic braking can be useful where damping is required. But eddy currents are a nuisance in many practical situations, because they dissipate energy due to electrical resistance of the material. This dissipation of energy can itself sometimes be useful, for example in induction heating, but in transformers and motors the heating is not only wasteful but potentially dangerous.

In practice, transformers are very efficient devices. Very little energy is lost in heating the core because eddy currents are reduced by careful design. The core in low frequency transformers is not made from a solid block of material but it is **laminated**. That means it is made up of many thin, lacquer-coated slices of the material, each insulated from its neighbour, which are bound together to make a high *permeance* (or low *reluctance*) core. The *electrical* resistance at right angles to the flux is very high so eddy currents are very small.

Modern ferrite materials are made from a paste of small iron oxide particles baked into a solid shape. The particles are close enough to produce good magnetic properties (high μ_r) but eddy currents are reduced to a minimum.

The dynamo

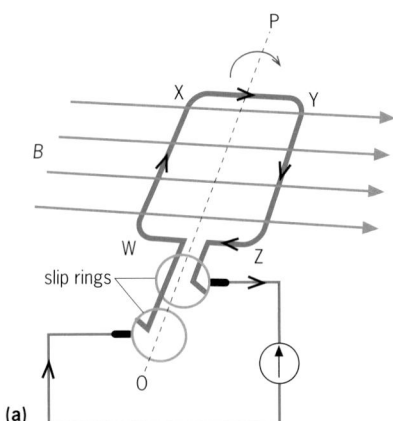

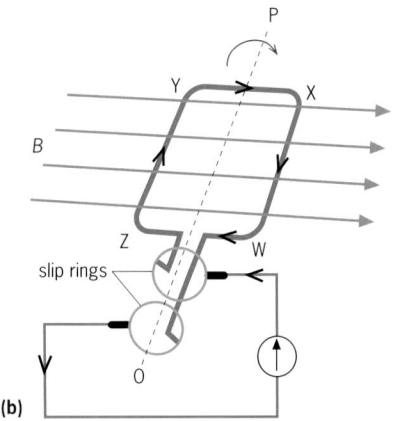

Fig 11.8 How a dynamo works, and the definition of a

(a)   (b)   (c)

We have seen that the large-scale production of electrical energy has developed from Faraday's experiments. Power stations all over the world, whether burning fossil fuels or using wind power, produce induced currents. In the UK, electricity is generated as an **alternating current**. The equation for an alternating current is:

$$I = I_0 \sin 2\pi ft$$

where I_0 is the peak current. The simple bicycle dynamo and the generators used in power stations are basically the same.

Fig 11.8(a) shows a simple rectangular loop that is rotating about an axis OP in a uniform magnetic field of flux density B tesla. Because the sides of the loop WX and YZ are moving at right angles to the field but in opposite directions, the e.m.f.s induced in each side will drive a current in the same direction around the loop.

After half a cycle, WX and YZ will have changed places: Fig 11.8(b). The current passes out of the loop through slip rings. Each end of the circuit is always in contact with one slip ring, allowing for a continuous current. The current in the galvanometer will now be reversed. After another half-cycle the loop is back where it started and the current

will be in the same direction as in the first half-cycle.

During each half-cycle the size of the current rises and falls. In Fig 11.8(c), suppose the plane of the loop makes an angle a with the magnetic field and that the sides WX and YZ have a length y and are moving at a speed v. The induced e.m.f. in each side will be given by:

$$\varepsilon = Byv \sin(90° - a) = Byv \cos a$$

Now suppose the angular velocity of the loop is ω and it takes t seconds to move through an angle a. Then:

$$a = \omega t$$

and the velocity v is related to ω and the width of the coil x by:

$$v = \omega \frac{x}{2}$$

So the total e.m.f. due to both sides is given by:

$$\varepsilon_{tot} = 2By\omega \frac{x}{2} \cos \omega t$$
$$= Bxy\omega \cos \omega t$$

But $xy = A$, the area of the loop, and $\omega = 2\pi f$, where f is the frequency of rotation. Therefore, for a coil of N turns:

$$\varepsilon_{tot} = 2\pi f NBA \cos 2\pi ft$$

This is the equation of an alternating voltage of peak value:

$$\varepsilon_0 = 2\pi f NBA$$

so that:

$$\varepsilon_{tot} = \varepsilon_0 \cos 2\pi ft$$

The output of the dynamo is shown in the graph of Fig 11.9.

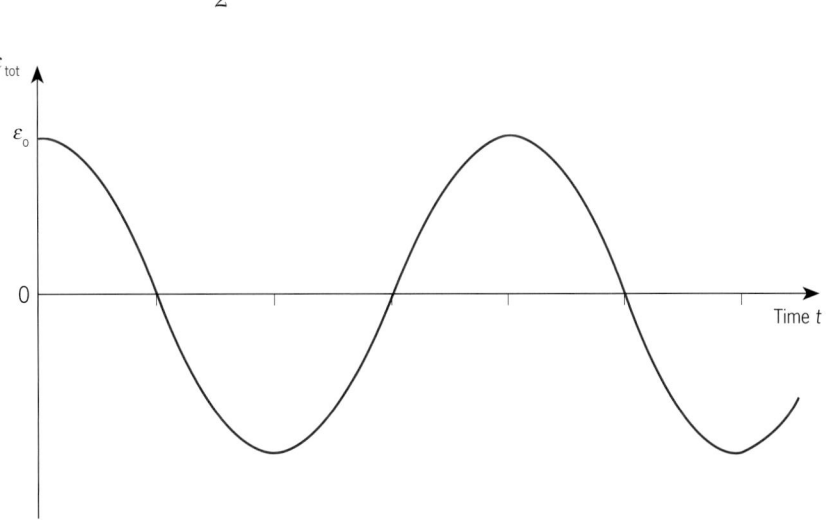

Fig 11.9 The output of the dynamo

6 BEHAVIOUR OF THE SIMPLE D.C. MOTOR

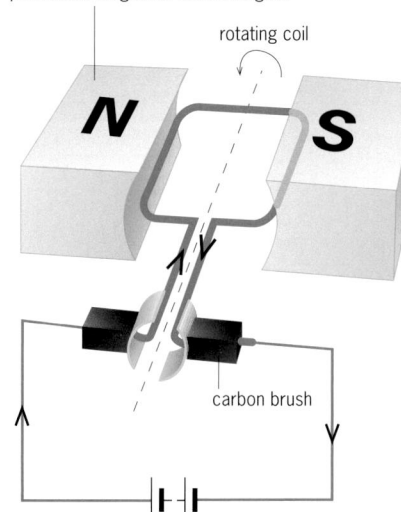

permanent magnet or electromagnet

rotating coil

N S

carbon brush

Fig 11.10 (a) A simple d.c. motor (no load attached)

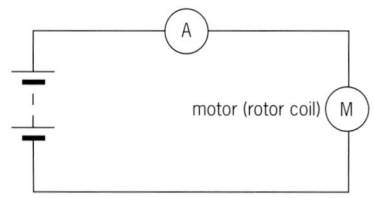

A

motor (rotor coil) M

Fig 11.10 (b) Circuit diagram for a simple motor

? **QUESTION 7**

7   What will be the effect on **a)** the resistance and **b)** the current if the coil heats up considerably?

The current drawn by a simple motor (Fig 11.10(a)) varies in an interesting way. When a motor with no load is switched on, the initial current drawn by the rotor coil from its power supply is very high, but it quickly drops to a much lower value. If the motor is then loaded, the current drawn by the motor gradually increases. Another important fact is that when the motor does work its speed decreases.

The motor rotates because of the force on a wire carrying a current, IlB. Current I is driven by an applied e.m.f. ε_s (from the supply).

As the coil rotates, an e.m.f. ε_i is induced in the coil. This e.m.f. tends to drive a current in the opposite direction to the current from the power supply (Lenz's law). The size of this induced e.m.f. depends on the speed of rotation of the coil. The faster the coil rotates, the larger the induced e.m.f. The resultant current as measured by an ammeter arises from the sum of the two e.m.f.s. Fig 11.10(b) shows a circuit diagram for a simple motor.

When the motor starts from rest there is no induced current. Therefore the initial current measured on the ammeter is high. As the motor's speed increases, so does the induced e.m.f., and the total current measured on the ammeter drops. If the motor does work and it slows down, the induced e.m.f. decreases and the measured current increases, delivering more energy to the motor.

If we consider the resistance in the rotor circuit (this includes any internal resistance of the power supply), we can say:

$$\text{total resistance} = \frac{\text{e.m.f. of supply} - \text{induced e.m.f.}}{\text{current}}$$

or:

$$R = \frac{\varepsilon_s - \varepsilon_i}{I}$$

We can rearrange this to give the current:

$$I = \frac{\varepsilon_s - \varepsilon_i}{R}$$

I is the current that is measured by the ammeter.

Assuming the resistance stays constant, which is a reasonable assumption if the coil does not get hot, then we can see that the current depends on the difference between the applied and induced e.m.f.s. The induced e.m.f. ε_i is often referred to as the **back e.m.f.**

The following equation also helps us understand the energy balance of the motor:

$$IR = \varepsilon_s - \varepsilon_i$$

or:

$$\varepsilon_s = \varepsilon_i + IR$$

Multiplying both sides by the current, I, we get:

$$\varepsilon_s I = \varepsilon_i I + I^2 R$$

Put in words, this says:

power from supply = useful power + power lost in heating rotor coil

Power lost in heating the rotor coil is also known as 'copper losses'.

This is a rather simplified picture of a real motor. In order to make the magnetic field as strong as possible, the coil in most motors is wound on a soft iron 'former'. This introduces the possibility of some eddy current losses, even though the

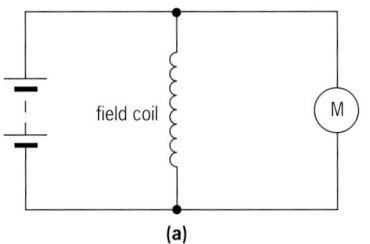 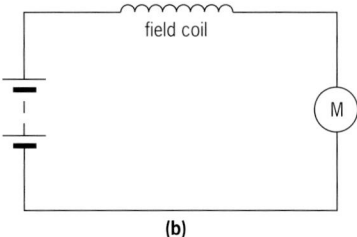

Fig 11.11 Circuit diagrams for a practical motor:
(a) shunt wound; **(b)** series connection

material will be laminated to minimise them. Another source of energy loss is called 'flux loss': the inevitable gap between the rotor and the poles of the magnet (or electromagnet) is a low permeance (or high reluctance) section in the magnetic circuit. This reduces the flux linking them as some of the flux spreads out or 'escapes' at the gap.

Instead of permanent magnets, most practical motors use electromagnets, usually called 'field coils': several coils are wound on a high permeability former to provide a strong field with the desired shape. Such a motor then has field coils and the rotor coil. These can be connected in parallel (shunt wound) or in series (Fig 11.11).

7 INDUCTANCE

In the simple demonstration circuit of Fig 11.12 the two bulbs are identical and the resistance of the variable resistor R is the same as the resistance of the coil L. The coil should have a soft iron core for the effect to be noticeable.

When the switch is closed, the bulbs both light up but do not come on together. There is a noticeable lag between the time when the bulb in series with the resistor lights up and when the other bulb lights up. When both are lit they have the same brightness. The effect of slowing down the growth of the current is described as the **inductive effect** of the coil. Hence such coils are also called **inductors**.

When the circuit in Fig 11.12 is first switched on, charge begins to flow in the inductor. This current creates a magnetic field in the coil where none existed before, that is, there is a changing magnetic field. The changing magnetic field induces a voltage that opposes the change (Lenz's law). It does this by creating an e.m.f. in the opposite direction to the e.m.f. from the applied voltage. As a result, the current in the coil builds up more slowly than in the simple resistor. However, eventually the current in the coil reaches a maximum (Fig 11.13). This maximum current is determined by the applied voltage and the total resistance in the circuit.

Fig 11.12 A simple circuit to demonstrate self-inductance. The value R for the resistor is adjusted so that both bulbs are equally bright when the current is steady. When the circuit is switched on, the bulb in series with the resistor lights before the bulb in series with the inductor, L

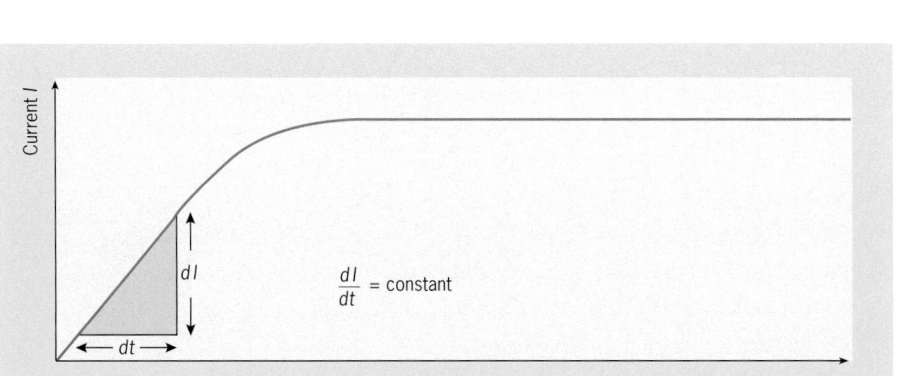

Fig 11.13 Graph of current against time for the inductor circuit of Fig 11.12

231

The final steady current depends on the supply and the resistance of the inductor:

$$I = \frac{\text{applied e.m.f.}}{\text{total resistance}}$$

Although the build-up of current may take only a small fraction of a second, we can see from the initial gradient of the curve in Fig 11.13 that the rate of change of current (dI/dt) at the start is constant.

This rate of change of current depends on two factors: the applied voltage and the inductive effect of the coil. Experiment shows that the initial rate of increase of current is directly proportional to the applied voltage:

$$V \propto \frac{dI}{dt}$$

The constant of proportionality is a property of the coil called the **self-inductance** of the coil and is given the symbol L:

$$\mathbf{V = L\frac{dI}{dt}}$$

The unit of self-inductance is volt second per amp (V s A^{-1}) or the **henry** (H).

EXAMPLE

Q A 50 mH inductor is connected to a 3 V d.c. supply. By how much does the current increase in the first 10 ms?

A We can use the equation: $V = L\dfrac{dI}{dt}$

Assuming the rate of change of current is constant in this time interval, the increase in current ΔI is given by

$$\frac{V}{l}\, dt = \frac{3 \times 10 \times 10^{-3}}{50 \times 10^{-3}} = 0.6\text{A}$$

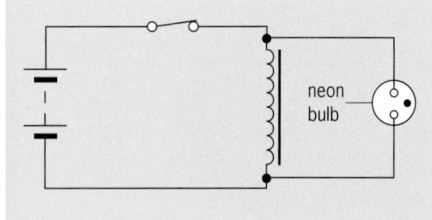

Fig 11.14 When the circuit is opened, the neon bulb lights up, illustrating the high induced e.m.f. of about 80 V or more

When the switch in the circuit of Fig 11.12 is opened, the inductor current collapses much more quickly. This reducing current induces a large e.m.f. in the opposite sense to the applied e.m.f.

We can demonstrate the size of this e.m.f. by connecting a neon bulb across the inductor as shown in Fig 11.14. A neon bulb requires a voltage of at least 80 V across it for it to light. When the switch in this circuit is opened the bulb will light.

Induction coils

The motive force of a petrol engine is supplied when a mixture of petrol and air explodes. This explosive mixture is ignited by the spark from a spark plug, and the spark itself is produced when about 2 to 3 kV are applied across the spark gap.

Using induction, this high voltage comes from the 12 V car battery. The rotating cam in the distributor opens the 'points', and so cuts off the current in the primary coil. The sudden drop in the primary current means that the strong magnetic field due to that current also suddenly collapses. The rapid change then induces a very high voltage in the secondary coil. This voltage is applied to one of the spark plugs through the rotor arm. In one cycle of the cam, a high voltage is induced four times and is applied to each of the four plugs in turn.

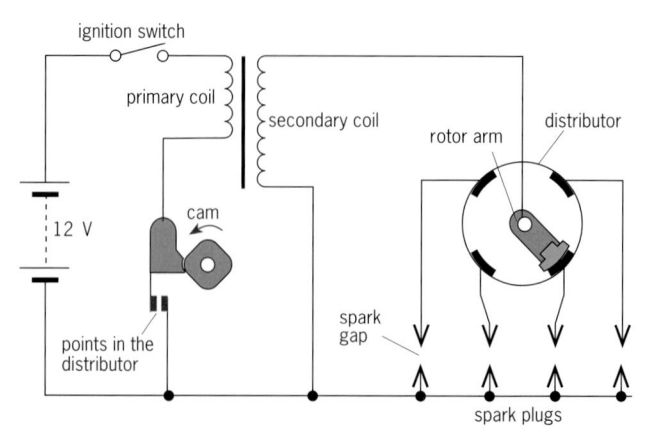

Fig 11.15 The ignition system for a car

Current variation in circuits containing inductance

We can treat the inductor as being similar to the motor we described on page 230. Like the motor, the e.m.f. of the supply is opposed by the e.m.f. induced in the inductor. The current in the circuit is given by:

$$\text{current} = \frac{\text{e.m.f. of supply} - \text{e.m.f. of inductor}}{\text{total resistance of circuit}}$$

or, in symbols:

$$I = \frac{V - L\dfrac{dI}{dt}}{R}$$

which can be rearranged as:

$$\frac{dI}{dt} = \frac{V - IR}{L}$$

This is a first-order differential equation which can be solved using calculus. The solution to this equation is another equation, which describes the exponential growth of the current shown in the graph in Fig 11.16.

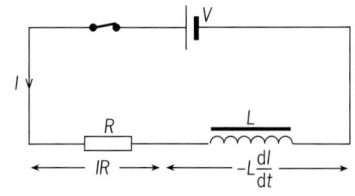

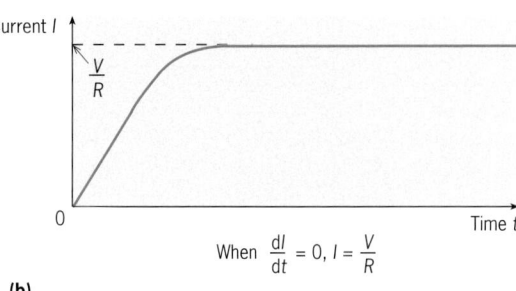

(a)

(b)

When $\dfrac{dI}{dt} = 0$, $I = \dfrac{V}{R}$

Fig 11.16 (a) A circuit containing an inductor;
(b) variation of current in the circuit

SUMMARY

By the end of this chapter you should be able to:
- Describe Faraday's experiments on electromagnetic induction.
- Understand Faraday's laws of electromagnetic induction, leading to: $\varepsilon = -N(d\Phi/dt)$.
- Use the equation $V = vlB$ to calculate the e.m.f. induced in a moving wire.
- Use Lenz's law to predict the direction of an induced current.
- Describe the behaviour of a simple transformer.
- Describe the behaviour of a simple moving coil dynamo.

- Describe how eddy currents are induced and give examples of their effects.
- Describe the behaviour of a simple d.c. motor under variable loads.
- Describe the self-inductance of a coil, $V = L\,(dI/dt)$, and the behaviour of inductors in d.c. circuits.

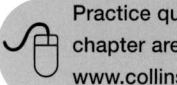

Practice questions for this chapter are available at www.collinseducation.co.uk/CAS

12

Alternating currents and electrical power

Electricity generation in the UK

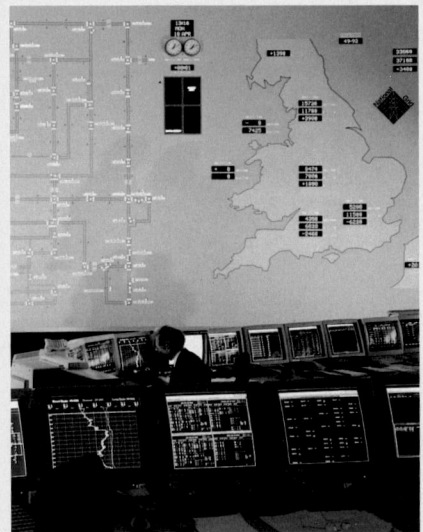

Continual monitoring and maintenance of the National Grid.
Above: an operations room
Below: repairing transmission lines

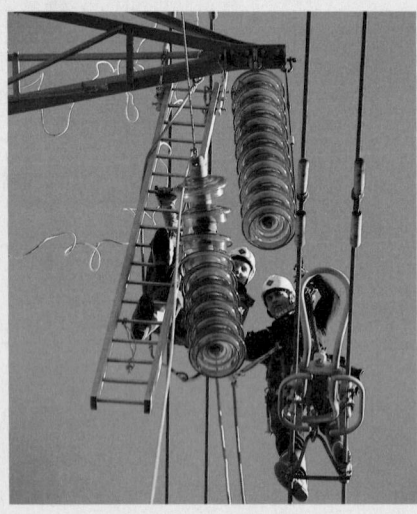

In 2006/7 the UK's electricity consumption reached 348 000 GWh or about 1.3×10^{18} joules of energy. This energy is supplied to about 28 million consumers, factories, hospitals, schools and homes over the National Grid.

The National Grid is a huge assembly of equipment: cables, pylons and transformers connecting the power stations to the consumer. There are over 7000 km of overhead, high voltage cable supported by about 20 000 pylons plus over 500 km of underground cable.

The UK has a diverse range of power stations providing a total 'installed' capacity of 76.4 GW. In recent years the peak demand has reached about 60 GW. This can still stretch the system because, at any time, some generators will be off line being serviced. Large power stations may have three or four generators, but at any time one may be out of use for servicing, or just on standby.

Managing the distribution of energy on the Grid is a complex business. Prediction of demand is essential. Daytime demand is twice as high as at night, and the maximum demand in winter is four times the minimum in the summer. Major events such as international sporting events can increase demand by 10%. Extreme weather conditions can also create extra demands and are often difficult to predict.

Today, the UK Grid is connected to the continent via France. This offers extra flexibility for the planners and a market to sell our excess energy when we have it. In 2007/8 about 2000 MW of capacity was used in this way.

As non-renewable sources run out and because burning fossil fuels adds to greenhouse gases, there will be more emphasis on using renewable energy sources. Although some of these sources, such as wind, have increased in recent years, they are still unreliable and have not proved that they can provide energy on the scale our society demands. In the UK we have some large-scale renewable sources in the 'pumped storage' schemes such as Dinorwig in North Wales and Ben Cruachan in Argyll. These have the advantage that they can be switched on when demand is high and can be used to store the excess energy produced by other power stations at other times.

In all, there are over 250 power stations, large and small, 'plugged' into the National Grid. These range from large coal and nuclear stations to small wind farms and biofuel plants. Together, these are managed so that the system can deliver energy by alternating current with a frequency of 50 Hz (± 1%) and a voltage of 230 V (± 6%); that is, between 216 and 244 volts.

The system is designed to do this as efficiently as possible. In 2007/8 the total energy losses came to a mere 2.16% of the demand, or put another way, the system was very nearly 98% efficient.

The ideas in this chapter

Alternating currents play a very important role in electronic and physical systems. A microphone converts sound, caused by vibrations in the air, into an alternating current signal. When a loudspeaker is connected to an alternating current supply, it converts the signal back into sound. The electromagnetic waves radiated from a transmitting aerial are created by alternating currents and the signal picked up by a receiving aerial is converted into an alternating current. The speed at which a computer carries out instructions is determined by the frequency of alternating current created by the vibration of a tiny quartz crystal.

On an average day the output of power stations in the UK is over 50 gigawatts and the energy generated is carried by alternating currents to the consumer. The nature of alternating current circuits is important to our understanding of the National Grid distribution system.

In this chapter we also consider how basic components like capacitors and inductors behave in a.c. circuits, so that we can understand the role they play in communications systems such as radio, in separating information from the 'carrier'.

1 ALTERNATING VOLTAGES AND CURRENTS

The 'voltage' from a battery is direct – that is, it drives a steady or **direct current** (**d.c.**) around a circuit. This means that the charge flows in one direction. Fig 12.1 shows that the current (or voltage) does not change with time. This is an idealised situation, since in reality the current from a real battery would gradually get smaller as the battery 'runs down'.

The electrical energy we get from the 'mains' is an alternating voltage. It drives an **alternating current** (**a.c.**) around a circuit.

An alternating current is continually changing direction: see Fig 12.2, which shows a typical current in a mains circuit in the UK.

Alternating current shows a distinctive **waveform** that is continually repeated: the graph shows three complete cycles of the pattern. The pattern of the a.c. mains is repeated 50 times every second – it has a **frequency** of 50 Hz. One cycle takes one-fiftieth of a second or 0.02 s. This time is the **period** of the waveform. Another important characteristic of the waveform is that each cycle has a positive half-cycle and a negative half-cycle. During the positive half-cycle the current is in one direction; during the negative half-cycle the current direction is reversed.

The alternating current produced by a dynamo or generator varies in a very precise way – the current varies as a sine wave because of the way it is made by a spinning coil (see page 229). That is, where I_0 is the maximum current and f is the frequency of the current:

$$I = I_0 \sin 2\pi f t$$

2 POWER IN A.C. CIRCUITS

Fig 12.3 shows two simple circuits in which a bulb is lit from an a.c. supply and from a d.c. supply. In each case the supply delivers energy to the bulb; the bulb gets hot and emits light.

In the d.c. circuit the energy transferred in the bulb each second (the power) can be found easily by using the equation:

power = p.d. × current

Energy is also transferred in the a.c. circuit. However, there is a problem if we try to use the same equation. If the current and voltage are continually changing, which value of current and voltage do we use? The peak values are reached only twice each cycle. What about the average value? What is the average value of current or voltage over a complete cycle? Look at Fig 12.4 and decide.

The answer is zero! The positive half-cycle is cancelled by the negative one.

There is a solution: instead of current, we consider power. In a simple circuit like this, the current and voltage vary together, increasing and decreasing in time with each other. We say they are **in phase** with each other. If we multiply the value of the current at any instant by the corresponding voltage, we get the power at that same instant in time. The result is as shown in Fig 12.5.

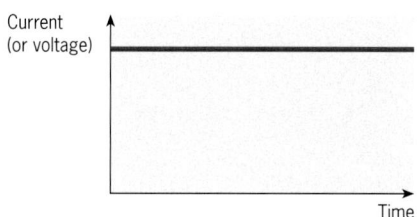

Fig 12.1 A direct current does not change with time

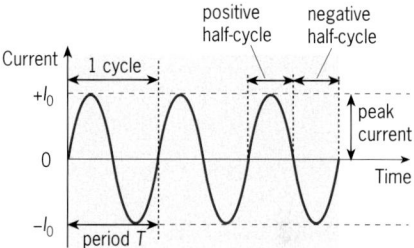

Fig 12.2 An alternating current. This current varies sinusoidally, with alternate positive and negative half-cycles

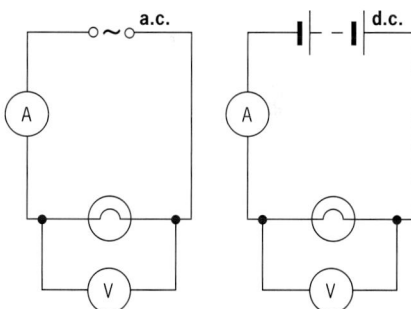

Fig 12.3 Simple a.c. and d.c. circuits. In both cases the bulb lights: there is an energy transfer from the power supply to the bulb

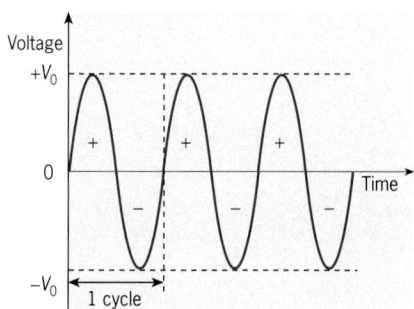

Fig 12.4 Three complete cycles of alternating voltage. The average over a complete number of cycles is zero

Fig 12.5 Change in current, voltage and power over three cycles for a resistor. The power is always positive

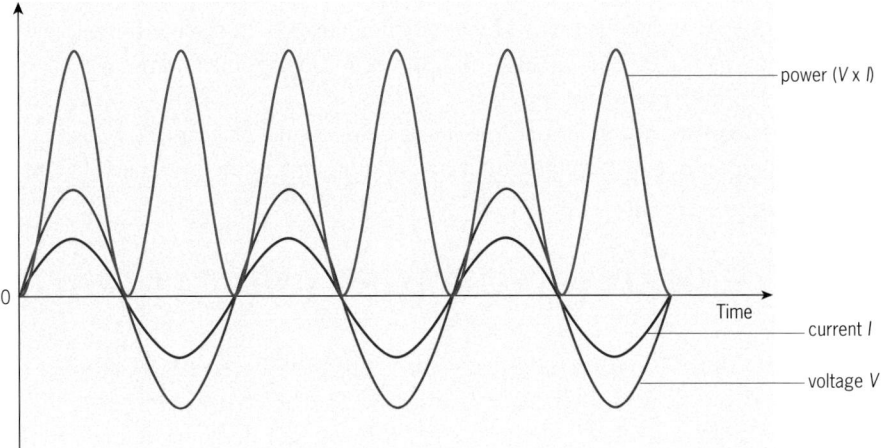

Since the current and voltage shown are sine waves, the corresponding power is a sine-squared wave. Notice that when the current and voltage are both negative the power is positive – the power is always positive, even though it is still varying.

You can see from the graph that the average value for power is not zero. In fact, it works out that the average value of sine-squared is half of the maximum or peak value:

$$\text{average power} = \tfrac{1}{2} \times \text{peak power}$$
$$= \tfrac{1}{2} \times (\text{peak current} \times \text{peak voltage})$$
$$= (\tfrac{1}{\sqrt{2}} \times \text{peak current}) \times (\tfrac{1}{\sqrt{2}} \times \text{peak voltage})$$
$$= \text{r.m.s. current} \times \text{r.m.s. voltage}$$

where:

$$\text{r.m.s. current} = \tfrac{1}{\sqrt{2}} \times \text{peak current}$$
$$\text{r.m.s. voltage} = \tfrac{1}{\sqrt{2}} \times \text{peak voltage}$$

The 'r.m.s.' alternating current and voltage are actually equal to the steady, direct current and voltage which transfer the same amount of energy in the bulb. The abbreviation r.m.s. stands for **root mean square**. It refers to the square **root** of the **mean** of the **squares** of the current or voltage at every instant.

Also:

$$\text{peak current or voltage} = \sqrt{2} \times \text{r.m.s. value}$$
$$= 1.4 \times \text{r.m.s. value}$$

R.M.S., CAPACITORS AND WORKING VOLTAGES

The voltage stated for power supplies is usually the r.m.s. voltage. When using a capacitor we have to be sure not to exceed the working voltage of the capacitor (see page 188). In d.c. circuits it is wise not to use voltages over about two-thirds of the rated working voltage of the capacitor. With a.c. supply we have to be even more careful.

For example, suppose a capacitor has a working voltage of 16 V. If such a capacitor were used in a circuit operated from a 9 V d.c. supply we could be confident that it would behave well as a capacitor. However, if we have a 9 V *alternating* voltage across the same capacitor, the peak voltage across it would be (9 × 1.4) or 12.6 V. This is still below 16 V but is about 2 V over two-thirds of 16 V, which is 10.7 V. It would be better to use a capacitor with a higher rated working voltage.

✔ **REMEMBER THIS**

Remember: minus × minus = plus

✔ **REMEMBER THIS**

The mathematical idea used here is:

$$\tfrac{1}{2} = \tfrac{1}{\sqrt{2}} \times \tfrac{1}{\sqrt{2}}$$

? **QUESTION 1**

1 In the UK the mains voltage is 230 V. This is in fact the r.m.s. value of the voltage. What is the peak value?

? **QUESTION 2**

2 What r.m.s. alternating voltage has a peak voltage which just exceeds 16 V?

---

3 DISTRIBUTION OF ELECTRICAL ENERGY – THE NATIONAL GRID

The National Grid is the system used for distributing electrical energy around the country. It is a large and very complex circuit through which the power stations feed energy into every home, factory, hospital and school.

The size of the circuit creates problems. In more remote parts of the British Isles, consumers may be up to a hundred miles from the nearest power station. Cables of that length have substantial resistance. A current in these cables heats them – there is **resistive heating**. This unwanted heating is lost energy, wasted energy that does not reach the consumer.

These energy losses are often called I^2R **losses** since, in a cable of resistance R carrying a current I, the resistive power loss is I^2R (see Chapter 8, page 177). The fact that the power loss is proportional to I^2 is significant: it means that halving the current reduces the power lost by a factor of four. This fact plays an important part in the design of the National Grid (Fig 12.6) – electricity is transferred at high voltages so that currents can be kept small for a given power load. Transformers are used to increase and decrease voltages (see Chapter 11, page 227).

The largest modern generators produce electricity at 25 000 V. Heavy industries use electricity at 33 000 V while lighter industries use it at 11 000 V. Smaller users such as our homes use electricity at 230 V. Electricity is transmitted around the country at much higher voltages – 132 kV, 250 kV and 400 kV.

One of the advantages of generating electricity as an alternating current is that transformers change a.c. voltages easily and efficiently (large transformers are typically about 99 per cent efficient). Step-up and step-down transformers are used throughout the system to change voltages to obtain the required voltage.

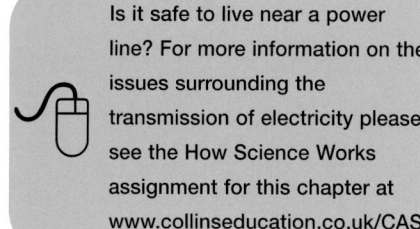

Is it safe to live near a power line? For more information on the issues surrounding the transmission of electricity please see the How Science Works assignment for this chapter at www.collinseducation.co.uk/CAS

 REMEMBER THIS
'Step-up' and 'step-down' refer to voltage and not current.

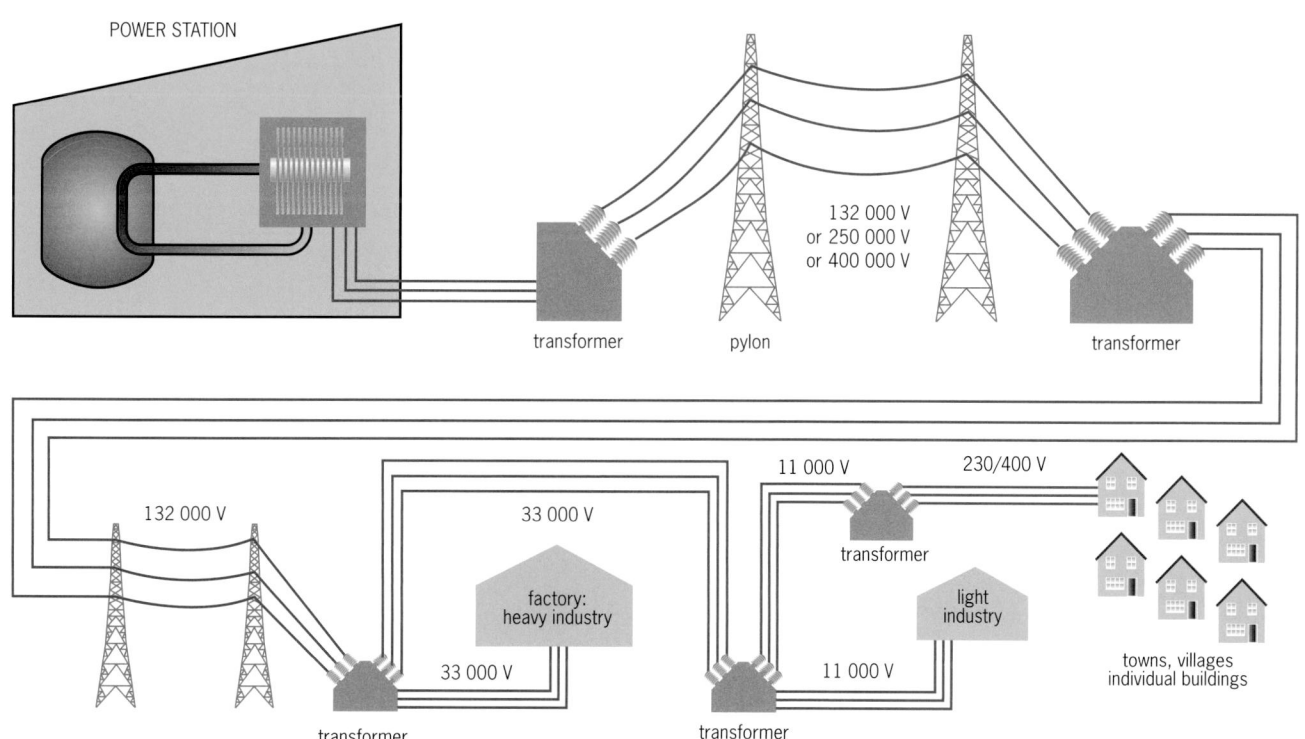

Fig 12.6 The National Grid, a large complex circuit which delivers energy from the power stations to the consumer. Different consumers require energy to be delivered at different voltages

EXAMPLE

Q A power station generates a current of 100 A at 25 kV. The electricity is transferred along 100 km of power line to a chemicals factory. The power line has a total resistance of $50\,\Omega$. Calculate the power lost in the power line and the percentage efficiency.

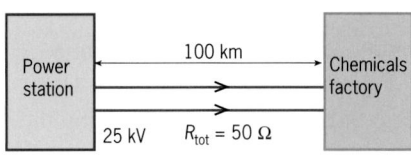

Fig 12.7 The system described in the question

A Power output of power station

$= I \times V$

$= 100\ \text{A} \times 25\,000\ \text{V}$

$= 2\,500\,000\ \text{W}$

$= 2.5\ \text{MW}$

Power lost in heating power line

$= I^2R$

$= 100^2 \times 50$

$= 500\,000\ \text{W}$

$= 0.5\ \text{MW}$

That means that only 2.0 MW is available at the factory. The system is only 80 per cent efficient.

Q The system is improved by adding two transformers, one to step up the voltage to 125 kV and a second to step it back down at the factory. The first transformer has a turns ratio of 1:5; the second has a turns ratio of 5:1. By how much does this reduce the power losses? What is the percentage efficiency? (Assume both transformers are 100 per cent efficient.)

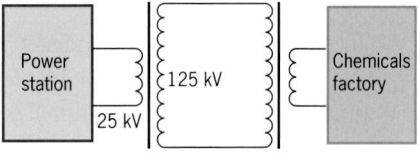

Fig 12.8 Two transformers added to improve the system shown in Fig 12.7

A The voltage is stepped up by a factor of 5, therefore:

Current along power line

$= 100/5$

$= 20\ \text{A}$

Power lost in heating power line

$= I^2R$

$= 20^2 \times 50$

$= 20\,000\ \text{W}$

$= 0.02\ \text{MW}$

A loss of 0.02 MW is smaller than 0.5 MW by a factor of 25 or 5^2. This means that 2.48 MW is now available at the factory. The system is now 99.2 per cent efficient.

? QUESTION 3

3   **a)** What is the turns ratio required to step up the 25 000 V from a generator to 250 000 V?

b) By how much will the current be changed in this transformer? (Assume the transformer is 100 per cent efficient.) How will this affect the power losses in the cable carrying current from the transformer?

Electricity in industry

Many industries that depend on electricity require vast amounts of energy. Take, for example, the large-scale production of aluminium, which is produced electrolytically from molten aluminium oxide obtained from the ore bauxite. The process requires a d.c. supply at nearly 1000 V and currents of 70 000 A. The d.c. voltage is derived from the secondary coil of a step-down transformer, which we will assume gives a secondary voltage of 1000 V. We can make some estimates of the turns ratio and primary current in the primary coil of the transformer.

Let us assume 100 per cent efficiency. The factory is connected to the National Grid via a local substation that gives an output voltage of 33 000 V. The required turns ratio would be:

$$\frac{1000}{33\,000} = 1{:}33$$

(a step-down transformer)

While the voltage is being stepped down, the current will be stepped up in the same ratio. That is:

$$\frac{\text{secondary current}}{\text{primary current}} = \frac{33}{1}$$

This gives:

primary current $= 70\,000/33$
$\qquad\qquad\qquad = 2121.2\ \text{A}$

This is still a large current, but far smaller than the 70 000 A needed to produce the aluminium.

This example is quite typical of many heavy industries that need electricity supplied at such large voltages.

4 RECTIFICATION – CHANGING A.C. TO D.C.

Many electronic devices require a d.c. power supply. This means that, despite the advantages of transmitting electrical energy as an alternating current, the first thing that most devices need to do is to convert the a.c. to d.c. This process is called **rectification**. One of the simplest ways of rectifying current is to use a diode.

Diodes allow current to pass easily in one direction only (Fig 12.9). The two leads of the diode are called the **anode** and the **cathode**.

Examine the circuit in Fig 12.10a. The diode will conduct only when the anode is positive – that is, during positive half-cycles. Fig 12.10(b) shows the alternating voltage from the supply and (c) shows the voltage (p.d.) across the resistance R_{load}. The voltage can be shown on an oscilloscope connected across the resistor.

The voltage across the load and the current in it are not steady, but are direct. That is, they are always positive and the charge flows in one direction – it does not alternate. This simple circuit satisfies the aim of turning a.c. into d.c., but we do lose half the energy. For obvious reasons, this process is called **half-wave rectification**.

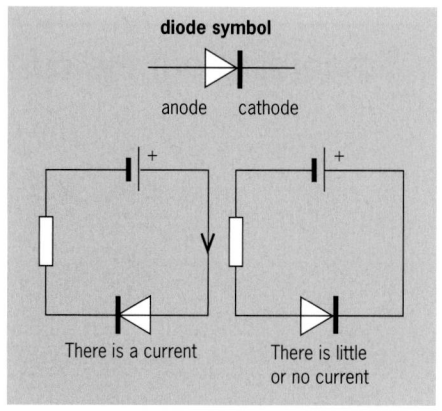

Fig 12.9 The two circuits illustrate the action of a diode. The diode conducts only when the anode is positive

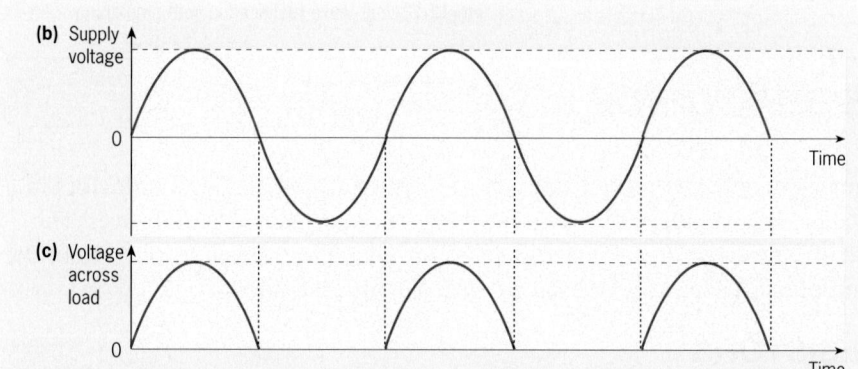

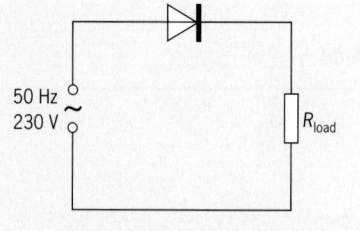

(a) The circuit with one diode

Fig 12.10 Half-wave rectification using a single diode: as **(c)** shows, the diode conducts and allows a current through the load only during positive half-cycles

The circuit in Fig 12.11(a) goes one step further. The arrangement of four diodes is called a **bridge rectifier** and it achieves **full-wave rectification**. The diodes are arranged so that a charge goes through the load in the same direction on each half-cycle. During the positive half-cycle the diodes D1 and D4 conduct; during the negative half-cycle the diodes D2 and D3 conduct.

The current is now direct. It is not steady but the current is in the same direction through the load during the whole cycle of applied a.c. As Fig 12.11(c) shows, the voltage has a 'ripple', with the ripple frequency being twice the frequency of the original alternating voltage shown in (b).

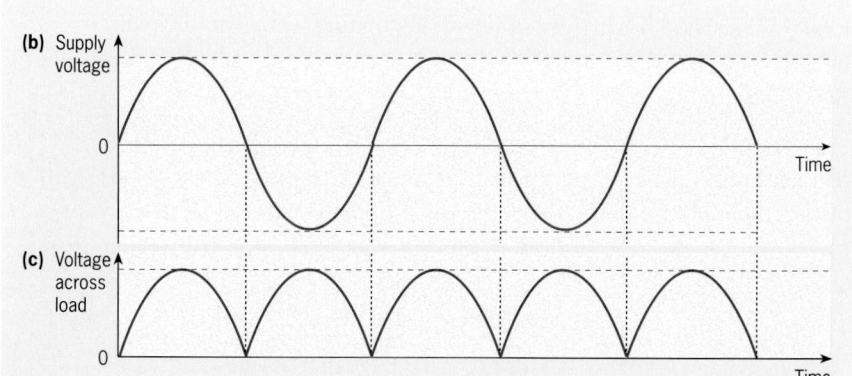

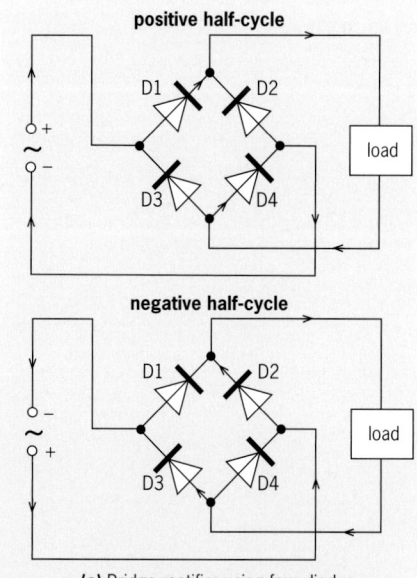

(a) Bridge rectifier using four diodes

Fig 12.11 Full-wave rectification using a bridge rectifier. This time, the current through the load is the same for positive and negative half-cycles

Smoothing out the current from a full-wave rectifier

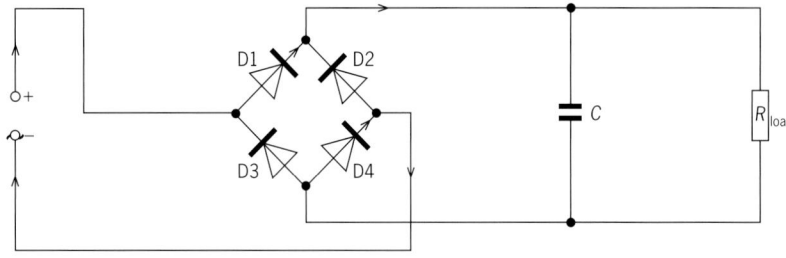

(a) Circuit with bridge rectifier and large-value capacitor

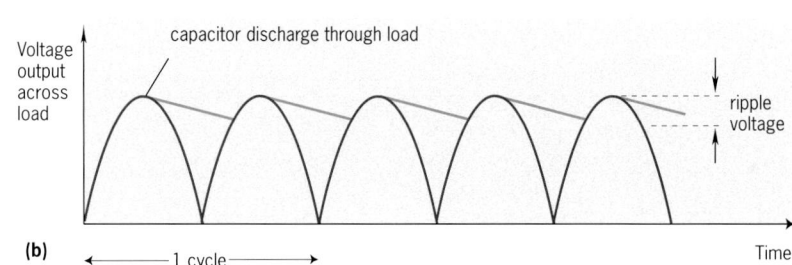

(b)

The varying d.c. can be smoothed out by placing a large-value capacitor across the load, as in Fig 12.12(a).

Fig 12.12(b) shows that during the first quarter of the cycle the capacitor charges. During the second quarter the voltage from the bridge rectifier drops and the capacitor starts to discharge. The rate of discharge depends on the capacitor and the resistance of the load – the RC constant (see Chapter 8, page 191).

If RC is large compared with the period of the ripple (1/ripple frequency), then the ripple will disappear and the voltage will be smooth.

Fig 12.12 Full-wave rectification with smoothing

5 REACTANCE

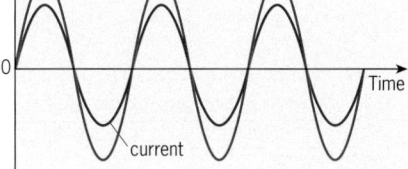

Fig 12.13 The graphs show how the current in the resistor and the voltage across it vary with time. They are in phase

The behaviour of components such as resistors, capacitors and inductors in circuits carrying alternating current is the basis of many useful devices. The size of the current turns out to depend on frequency as well as the size of the component, which can be used to make circuits like filters.

RESISTORS

Ohm's law is obeyed for a.c. just as it is for d.c. The alternating current in a resistor is in phase with the alternating potential difference across it (that is, they vary together as shown in Fig 12.13). The resistance in ohms is the same for d.c. and a.c.

CAPACITORS

In d.c. circuits we say that a capacitor 'blocks d.c.'. In other words, there is no current after the initial brief charging period. The space between the plates contains an insulator – charge does not flow from one plate to the other.

Similarly, charge does not flow between the plates when an alternating voltage is applied. However, charge flowing to and from one plate does induce a flow of charge on the other. That means that there are currents in the rest of the circuit.

So what does happen when we apply an alternating voltage to a circuit containing a capacitor? We can work this out from first principles. For a capacitor we know that:

$$Q = CV$$

where V is the p.d. at any instant in time across a capacitor of C farads and when there is a charge of Q coulombs on the plates.

Now, current is the rate of flow of charge, so the current at this instant is given by:

$$I = \frac{dQ}{dt} = \frac{d(CV)}{dt} = C\frac{dV}{dt}$$

This says that the current at any time is proportional to the rate of change of voltage.

If the p.d. across the capacitor changes sinusoidally, that is, if it is a standard alternating voltage, then:

$$V = V_0 \sin 2\pi ft$$

so:

$$I = C\frac{dV}{dt} = C\frac{d}{dt}\left(V_0 \sin 2\pi ft\right) = 2\pi f\, CV_0 \cos 2\pi ft$$

That is, if the p.d. is a sine wave then the current will be a cosine wave, as shown in Fig 12.14.

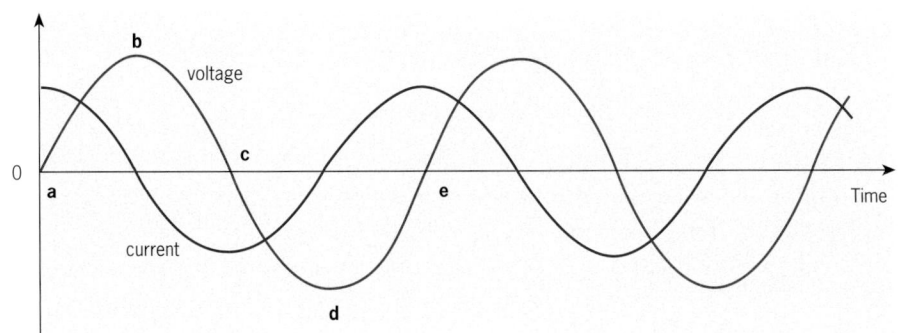

Fig 12.14 The graphs show how the current in the capacitor and the voltage across it vary with time. Notice that the current 'leads' the voltage by 90°

The first thing to notice is that the voltage and current are not in phase – they do not vary up and down together. Let us look carefully at what is going on as the applied voltage changes, referring to the letters in Fig 12.14.

- *From **a** to **b*** At the start, when time $t = 0$, the voltage is zero, but at the same instant the current is a maximum value. As the voltage across the capacitor increases, the current decreases until it reaches zero when the voltage is a maximum. At this point the capacitor is fully charged.

- *From **b** to **c*** The voltage now decreases and the current increases in the opposite direction – that means that charge is flowing in the opposite direction, discharging the capacitor. By the time the voltage reaches zero the current is a 'negative' maximum. The capacitor is now fully discharged.

- *From **c** to **d*** Charge continues to flow in the same direction as the direction of the voltage changes and gradually increases to a negative maximum. At this point the current is again zero and the capacitor is again fully charged but the charge on the plates is now reversed.

- *From **d** to **e*** As the voltage returns to zero the capacitor discharges as charge now flows in the opposite direction again until at **e** the capacitor is uncharged.

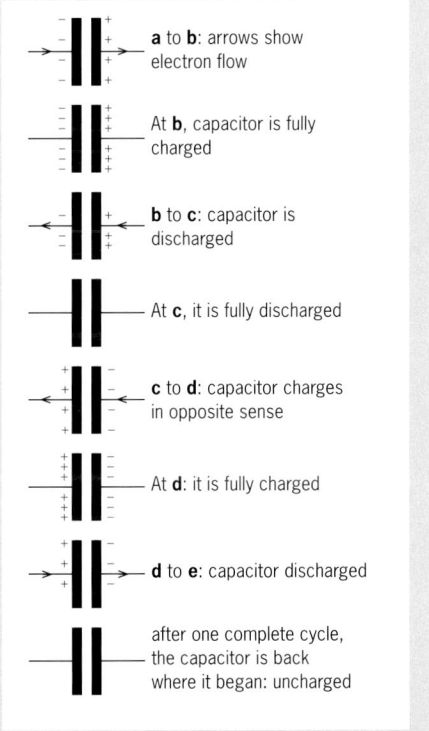

Look back to Fig 12.14: the current is always a quarter of a cycle ahead of the voltage. (Remember: events to the left of the graph happen before events to the right.) A quarter of a cycle is equivalent to 90°, so we say that the current **leads** the voltage by 90°. The current is a maximum when the p.d. across it is zero. As the p.d. increases, the current drops.

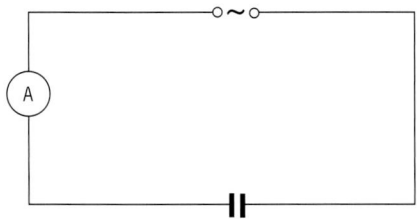

Fig 12.15 The simple capacitive circuit has a variable frequency supply connected to a capacitor

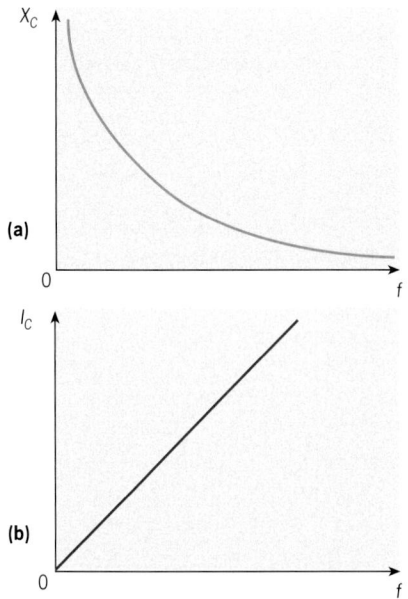

(a)

(b)

Fig 12.16 The graphs show how the reactance of the capacitor and the current in the circuit vary with frequency

? QUESTION 4

4 Calculate the reactance of a 1 μF capacitor at **a)** 1 kHz, **b)** 100 kHz and **c)** 1 MHz.

In simple circuits the ratio of voltage to current tells us something important – which is the resistance of the conductor. Although it is a bit trickier, a ratio of voltage to current is also useful in circuits with capacitors, also known as **capacitive circuits**.

A simple ratio of voltage to current will not make much sense – when the voltage is zero the current is a maximum, giving a ratio of zero, and when the voltage is a maximum the current is zero, giving a ratio of infinity.

However, the ratio of maximum voltage to maximum current is useful. Let the maximum value of voltage be V_0. The maximum value of the current will be when the cosine term is 1. That is:

$$I_{max} = 2\pi f V_0 C$$

So the ratio of maximum voltage to maximum current is given by:

$$\frac{V_{max}}{I_{max}} = \frac{V_0}{2\pi f V_0 C} = \frac{1}{2\pi f C} = X_c$$

This ratio X_C is called the **reactance** of the capacitor. As reactance is a ratio of voltage to current, it is measured in volts per ampere, V A^{-1}, or ohms, Ω.

The equation shows that in a simple capacitive circuit (Fig 12.15) the reactance decreases as frequency increases, as shown in Fig 12.16(a). Or, put another way, as frequency increases, the current in the circuit will increase, as seen in Fig 12.16(b).

It appears as though the capacitor 'conducts' better at high frequencies. Remember, though, that charge does not move directly from one plate to the other.

INDUCTORS

A continually changing current in an inductor will create a continually changing magnetic field. This changing magnetic field induces an e.m.f. that opposes the current. The equation that defines inductance (see page 232) gives us a relationship between the current and the voltage:

$$V = L\frac{dI}{dt}$$

where V is the applied voltage across the capacitor and I is the current in the inductor.

If the current is sinusoidal, that is:

$$I = I_0 \sin 2\pi ft$$

then:

$$V = L\frac{d}{dt}\left(I_0 \sin 2\pi ft\right) = 2\pi f L I_0 \cos 2\pi ft$$

As with the capacitor, the current and voltage are not in phase. Again, voltage and current are out of phase by a quarter of a cycle or 90°. This time, as Fig 12.17 shows, the voltage leads the current by 90°.

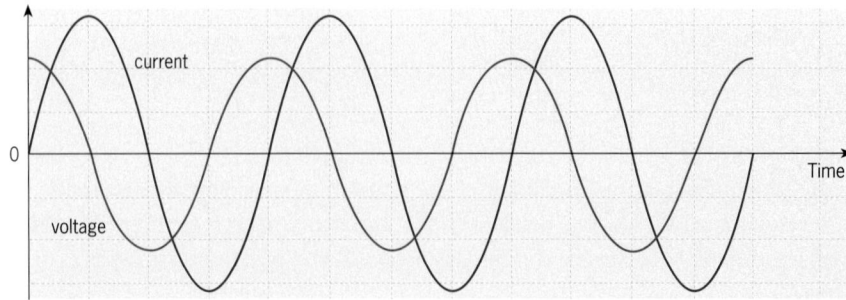

Fig 12.17 The graphs show how the current in an inductor and the voltage across it vary with time. Notice this time that the voltage leads the current by 90°

We can define an **inductive reactance** Ω in the same way as for a capacitor:

$$X_L = \frac{V_{max}}{I_{max}} = \frac{2\pi f L I_0}{I_0} = 2\pi f L$$

Inductive reactance is proportional to frequency. As frequency increases, the current in an inductor in a simple inductive circuit (Fig 12.18) will get smaller; see Fig 12.19.

Phase differences of exactly 90° are found only in purely capacitive or purely

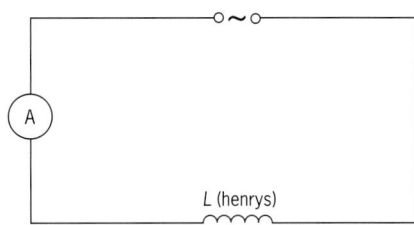

Fig 12.18 The simple inductive circuit has a variable frequency supply connected to an inductor of inductance L

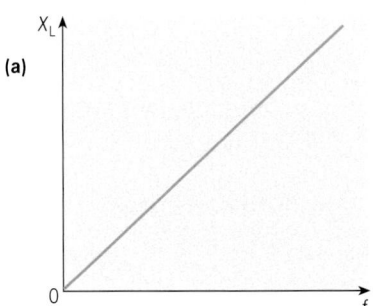

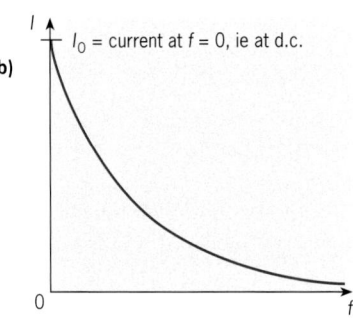

inductive circuits. In reality, it is almost impossible to get a 'purely inductive' circuit as the wire in the coil always has some resistance.

Most practical circuits contain combinations of resistance and reactance. The combined effect of the two is called **impedance** (see Chapter 22, page 443). It is also measured in ohms and is dependent on frequency.

Fig 12.19 The graphs show how the reactance of the inductor and the current in the circuit vary with frequency. The maximum current is equal to the applied voltage divided by the resistance of the coil

? QUESTION 5

5 Calculate the reactance of a 1 μH inductor at **a)** 1 kHz, **b)** 100 kHz and **c)** 1 MHz.

6 IMPEDANCE

Many circuits contain a combination of resistance and reactance (Fig 12.20). Such circuits pose a slightly more complicated problem.

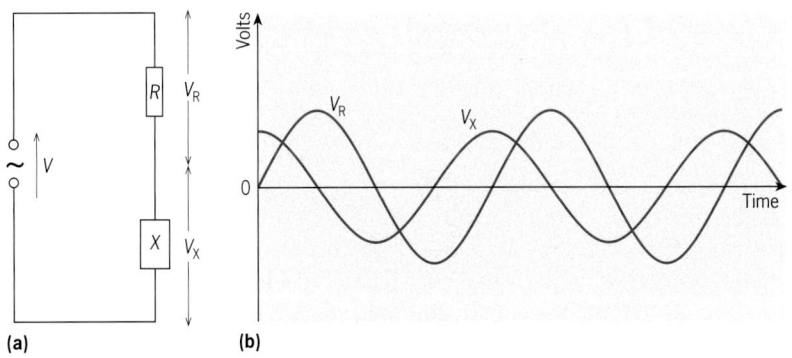

Fig 12.20 (a) A circuit containing a combination of resistance and reactance.
(b) The graph shows that the peak voltages across each component are not in phase

When an alternating voltage of fixed frequency is applied across a circuit that includes resistance and reactance in series, the current is the same at any point in the circuit. However, the relationship between the voltages is a little more complex.

Conservation of energy leads us to say, correctly, that the supply voltage at any instant is equal to the sum of the voltages across the resistance and the reactance at that instant. However, the peak voltages across each component are not in phase, so their sum cannot be equal to the peak voltage of the supply.

? QUESTION 6

6 **a)** Calculate the impedance of a 100 ohm resistor in series with a 10 μF capacitor at **i)** 1 kHz, **ii)** 1 MHz.
b) Repeat the calculations replacing the capacitor with a 1 mH inductor.

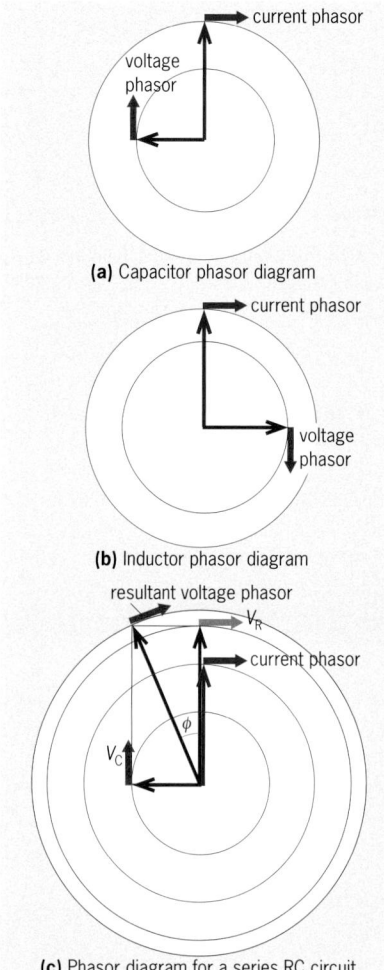

(a) Capacitor phasor diagram

(b) Inductor phasor diagram

(c) Phasor diagram for a series RC circuit

Fig 12.21 Phasors are rotating vectors. They are very useful when analysing a.c. circuits containing capacitors and inductors. The phasor in the diagram is rotating clockwise. It rotates at the frequency of the supply. Note that for a capacitor, the current phasor is 90° ahead of the voltage phasor. For an inductor, the voltage leads the current by 90°.

In **(c)**, the resultant voltage lags the current by an angle ø

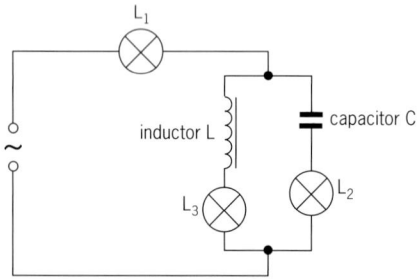

Fig 12.22 An inductor and capacitor in parallel connected to a variable frequency supply

Fig 12.23 Graphs showing how the currents change as frequency increases in the circuit in Fig 12.22

The combination of resistance and reactance is called the **impedance**, measured in ohms. Impedance can be calculated by treating the voltages across the different components in a similar way to vector quantities. We use vector diagrams to add together two forces that act in different directions, as shown in Fig 12.21(a). The voltages in Fig 12.20 may have different magnitudes but they also differ in phase. (The reactive voltage phasor is always 90° out of phase with the resistive voltage phasor.) Fig 12.21(b) is called a phasor diagram. The voltage phasors can be added in a similar way to vectors.

The impedance Z (in ohms) is defined by the equation:

$$Z = \frac{V}{I}$$

Resultant voltage: $\qquad V = \sqrt{V_R{}^2 + V_X{}^2}$

where V_R is the p.d. across the resistor, and V_X is the p.d. across any reactance, capacitive or inductive. Therefore

$$Z = \frac{\sqrt{V_R{}^2 + V_X{}^2}}{I}$$

$$= \sqrt{\left(\frac{V_R}{I}\right)^2 + \left(\frac{V_X}{I}\right)^2}$$

$$Z = \sqrt{R^2 + X^2}$$

7 LC CIRCUITS

LC circuits include combinations of inductance (L) and capacitance (C).

The circuit in Fig 12.22 is of great importance in electronics in general, and in radio in particular. It is called a **tuned circuit**. One of its uses is to select radio stations in a radio receiver (see Chapter 21).

As the frequency of the supply in Fig 12.22 is increased, the brightness of bulb L_1 gradually decreases until it reaches a minimum level of brightness. It then increases in brightness as the frequency is increased further.

The appearance of the two other bulbs also changes. Bulb L_2, which is in series with the capacitor, is unlit to start with, and gradually gets brighter as the frequency increases. L_3, which is in series with the inductor, starts off bright and gradually gets dimmer. This is shown graphically in Fig 12.23.

The capacitor and inductor are in parallel so that the voltage across each component is always the same. The voltage across the capacitor lags the current by 90° but it leads the current in the inductor by the same amount. This means that the current in the inductor is 180° out of phase with the current in the capacitor arm (see Fig 12.24).

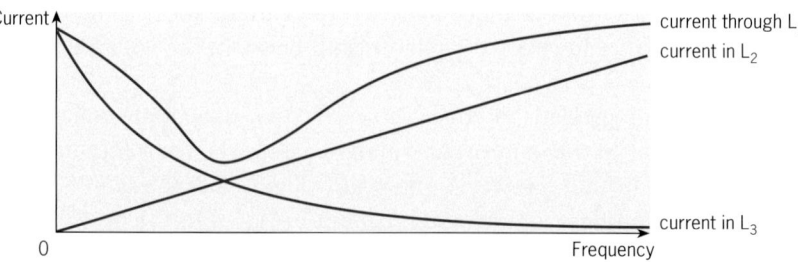

As the frequency of the supply changes, there will be a frequency when the reactances of the capacitor and the inductor are the same:

$$X_L = X_C$$

That is:

$$2\pi f L = \frac{1}{2\pi f C}$$

This can be rearranged as:

$$f^2 = \frac{1}{4\pi^2 LC}$$

and so:

$$f = \frac{1}{2\pi\sqrt{LC}}$$

At this frequency the current drawn from the supply is a minimum, yet the currents in the capacitor and inductor are quite high. The currents in each arm are equal but they are also in antiphase (180° out of phase). They cancel out so that the actual current drawn from the supply is a minimum – see the curves of Fig 12.25 – and also explains why the bulb L_1 in Fig 12.22 reaches a minimum brightness.

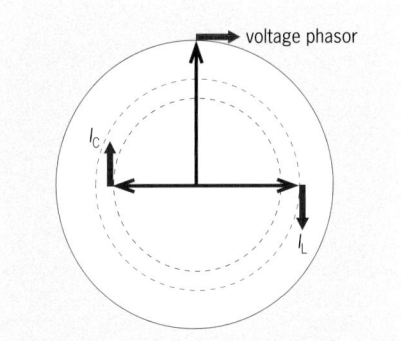

Fig 12.24 The phasor diagram for a parallel LC circuit. The voltage is the same across both L and C. The currents in L and C are 180° out of phase. What happens when the currents are the same size?

Fig 12.25 Graphs of the current I_C in the capacitor and the current I_L in the inductor when the reactances X_C and X_L are the same. The currents are the same size but are 180° out of phase

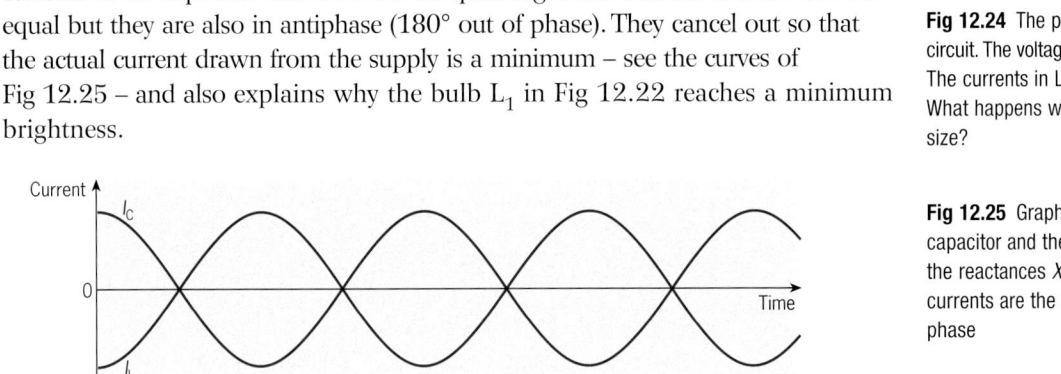

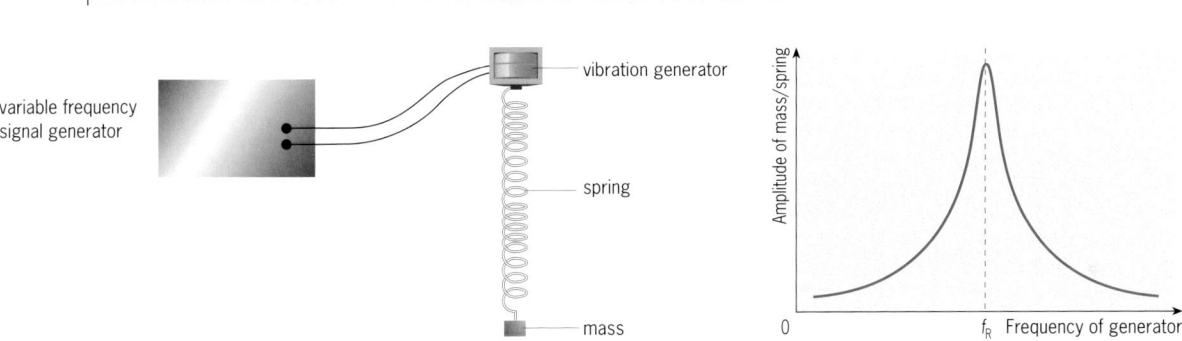

Fig 12.26 A mass on a spring has a natural frequency of vibration. When it is driven by a variable frequency vibration generator, the amplitude of the oscillating mass/spring changes (see graph) and is a resonance curve. The amplitude of the mass–spring system is a maximum when the driver frequency is the same as the natural frequency of the system

The behaviour of this circuit can be compared to the behaviour of mechanical oscillating systems. Fig 12.26 shows a mass and spring which is made to oscillate by means of a vibration generator. The graph shows how the amplitude of the oscillating mass changes as the frequency of the vibration generator is varied.

The characteristic peak on the graph shows resonance. When the frequency of the vibration generator is the same as the natural frequency of the mass–spring system, the energy transferred from the generator to the mass–spring is a maximum (see Chapter 6).

The frequency at which the capacitive reactance is equal to the inductive reactance is called the **resonant frequency** of the circuit. This frequency can also be described as the **natural frequency** of the parallel LC circuit, when the 'amplitudes' of the currents in the capacitor and inductor are at a maximum, and the energy transferred from the signal source to the LC circuit is a maximum.

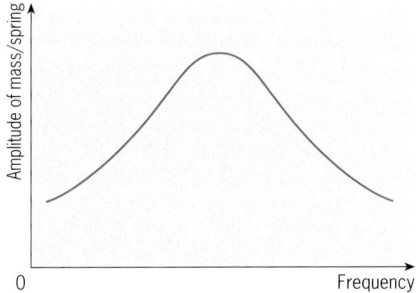

Fig 12.27 If the mass–spring oscillator in Fig 12.26 is damped, the resonance curve is broadened. Adding resistance in a parallel LC circuit has the same effect on its resonance curve

> **? QUESTION 7**
>
> 7 Calculate the resonant frequency of a parallel LC circuit made from a 1 mH inductor and a 500 pF capacitor. (1pF = 10^{-12} F.)

There is always some resistance in the circuit, so the minimum current drawn from the supply at resonance is not zero. Resistance also has the effect of broadening or 'damping' the resonance (Fig 12.27).

8 IMPEDANCE OF A SERIES LCR CIRCUIT

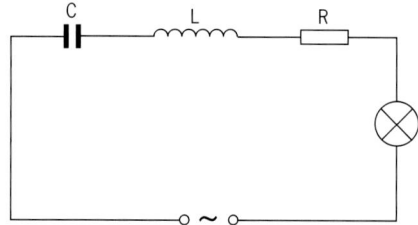

Fig 12.28 A circuit with a capacitor, inductor and resistor in series to a variable frequency supply

In the circuit shown in Fig 12.28, as the frequency is increased the brightness of the bulb increases to a maximum and then decreases again. To analyse this circuit we need to know its impedance.

As with all series circuits, the current is always the same at any point in the circuit. The voltage across the inductor will lead the current by 90° and the voltage across the capacitor will lag the current by 90°. The voltage across the resistor will be in phase with the current. The phasor diagrams in Fig 12.29 show these voltages and how we can find their resultant.

The resultant voltage is given by:

$$V = \sqrt{(V_R)^2 + (V_L - V_C)^2}$$

The impedance is given by V/I, which gives:

$$Z = \sqrt{\frac{V_R^2}{I^2} + \frac{(V_L - V_C)^2}{I^2}}$$

$$Z = \sqrt{R^2 + (X_L - X_C)^2}$$

At resonance, $X_L = X_C$ and $X_L - X_C = 0$. This means that the impedance is a minimum and that $Z = R$.

Fig 12.29 Phasor diagrams for the series LCR circuit. **(a)** All the voltage phasors relative to each other. **(b)** The voltage phasors in isolation. **(c)** The resultant of the voltage phasors. **(d)** The resultant voltage in relation to the current. The current lags the voltage by angle ø. ø is called the 'phase angle'

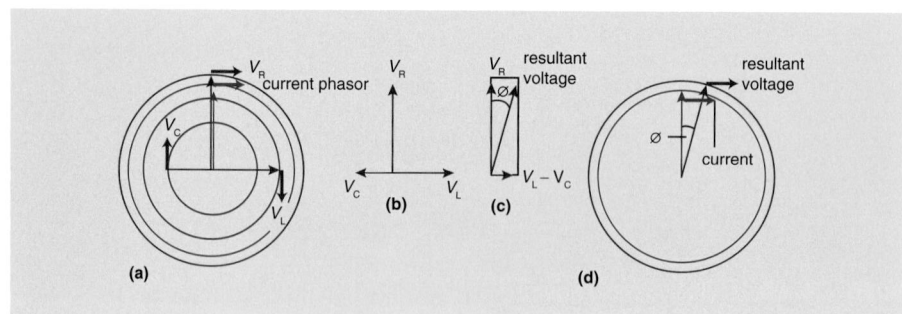

The resonance curve for this circuit is shown in Fig 12.30. At the resonant frequency the current is a maximum.

As $X_L = X_C$ at resonance, the resonant frequency is given by the same equation we derived for the parallel LC circuit:

$$f_0 = \frac{1}{2\pi \sqrt{LC}}$$

Fig 12.30 The resonance curve for the series RCL circuit of Fig 12.28. In the series circuit the current from the supply is a maximum at resonance

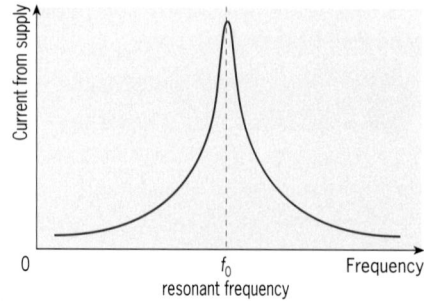

From Fig 12.29(c), the phase angle ø is given by:

$$\tan \varnothing = (V_L - V_C)/V_R = I(X_L - X_C)/IR = (X_L - X_C)/R$$

Tuned circuits

LCR circuits are very useful for filtering out signals at particular frequencies. They are often called 'tuned circuits' and have found application in a wide range of devices, especially for 'tuning' radio frequencies in radios and televisions. Their ability to pick out or select a narrow band of frequencies – the station you want to listen to or watch – is called their *selectivity*. If the selectivity is poor, you will hear several stations at the same time or there will be a lot of interference from other stations. The selectivity is measured using the *magnification factor* or *quality* (Q) factor.

Let's go back to the resonant frequency for a series LCR circuit. At resonance, the impedance of the circuit simplifies to

$$Z = \sqrt{(R^2 + X^2)} = \sqrt{(R^2 + 0)} = R$$

So the size of the maximum current at resonance is given by

$$I = V/R$$

where V is the applied voltage across the circuit. There are still voltages across L and C, although they will be the same size at resonance but 180° out of phase. V_C and V_L effectively cancel each other so that the applied voltage is that across R. It is quite possible that these voltages could be larger than the applied voltage. The voltages across L and C will be given by:

$$V_L = IX_L \qquad \text{and} \qquad V_C = IX_C$$

where I is the current at resonance (Fig 12.31).

The *magnification factor* or Q of the circuit is defined as the ratio of the voltage across L (or C) to that across R:

$$Q = V_L/V_R = IX_L/IR = X_L/R = 2\pi fL/R$$

or

$$Q = V_C/V_R = X_C/R = 1/2\pi fCR$$

If R is small, then Q will be large and the circuit is very selective. When R is large, then Q is smaller. Increasing R is analogous to more damping in a mechanical resonant system (Fig 12.32).

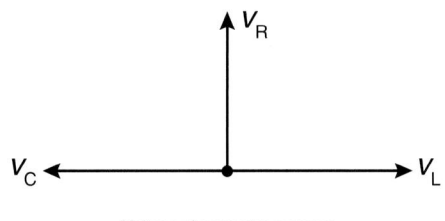

Voltage phasor at resonance

$$V_C = V_L$$

Fig 12.31

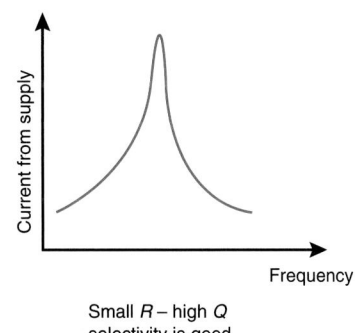

Small R – high Q
selectivity is good

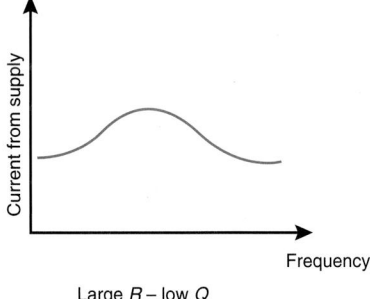

Large R – low Q
selectivity is poor

Fig 12.32

Filter circuits

Audio systems are designed to reproduce sound signals in the range of 20 Hz to 20 kHz. Basic systems use two loudspeakers – one called a **woofer**, designed to reproduce low frequency or bass sounds, and a second called a **tweeter**, which reproduces the higher frequency or treble sounds. The output signal from the audio amplifier contains the whole range of frequencies. Filters are used to direct the 'correct' frequencies to the appropriate loudspeaker. Fig 12.33 shows a simple filter circuit called a **crossover** using capacitors and inductors.

Low frequency signals find a lower reactance path through the inductor to the woofer and the higher frequency signals find it easier to pass through the capacitor.

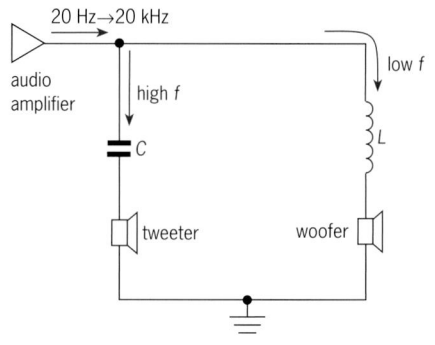

Fig 12.33 Crossover circuit

SUMMARY

By the end of this chapter you should be able to:
- Describe the characteristics of alternating voltages and currents: peak voltage, frequency and period.
- Use the relationships for r.m.s. and peak currents and voltages.
- Describe the use of transformers in the National Grid and the advantages of transmitting electrical energy at high voltages.
- Describe the use of diodes for rectifying alternating currents.
- Describe the behaviour of resistors, capacitors and inductors in a.c. circuits.

- Use the equations $X_C = 1/2\pi f C$ and $X_L = 2\pi f L$ for the reactance of capacitors and inductors in calculations.
- Calculate the resonant frequency of a parallel LC circuit.
- Calculate the impedence and phase angle of a series LCR circuit.
- Calculate the Q value for a resonant circuit using the equations $Q = X_L/R$ or $Q = X_C/R$.

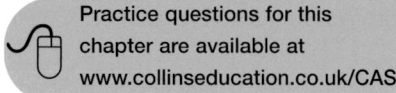

Practice questions for this chapter are available at www.collinseducation.co.uk/CAS

13

Energy and temperature

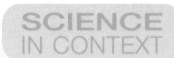

Freeze drying coffee granules

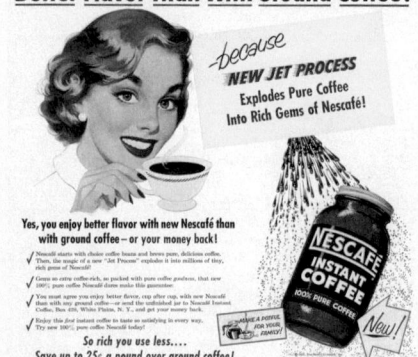

Like most books, this book was written only after a lot of late nights and numerous cups of coffee – usually 'instant' coffee!

The instant coffee industry has developed into a multi-million pound market since it first began in the late 1930s. And the latest development is 'freeze-dried' granules, which give the coffee a much better flavour than all the earlier versions.

Once the coffee beans have been roasted and ground, the soluble solids and flavour compounds are extracted. This mixture contains a lot of water, which would make granules stick together. The problem is to remove the water without removing the flavour.

In freeze drying, the mixture is cooled to just below 0 °C (it is still sticky) and air is added to make a 'foam' that is of the right density. This foam is then deep frozen and broken into the familiar airy granules we see in the coffee jar. The granules are then heated very rapidly in a drying cabinet at very low pressure so that the ice converts immediately to vapour without passing through the liquid stage, leaving behind almost all of the aroma and flavour of the original coffee.

The largest modern freeze-drying plants can produce up to 7 million cups of coffee each day – more than enough for several more physics books!

The ideas in this chapter

When we switch on an electric fire in the home, a current passes through the element – usually a coiled wire. The electrical energy for this is provided at the power station by the chemical change when gas, oil or coal is burned. This energy is then transferred via the resistive coil of the fire to air molecules in the room. The air molecules in the room start to move around faster in every direction. This increased movement constitutes the so-called 'heating' of the air.

We can transfer energy quite efficiently from the fire to the air molecules. But we cannot easily reuse the energy and change back this increased movement of the air molecules to energy that can be returned along our electrical circuit. There are certain restrictions on the transfer of energy. **Thermodynamics** is the science that describes how systems alter when their energy content changes. It describes and explains the transfer processes.

We can define heating as a process in which energy transfers from one body at a higher temperature to another body at a lower temperature. We saw how to obtain a temperature scale in Chapter 7 (pages 160–161) and we shall look at practical methods of measuring temperature in this chapter.

Different forms of energy are so important in physics that they are discussed and explained in Appendix 1. When we heat a substance we transfer energy from some outside source (as we have indicated) and this energy goes to the atoms or molecules of that substance. The kinetic energy of these atoms or molecules increases. So, often, does the separation of the atoms or molecules. If the separation changes, so does the force between them. Essentially, then, this extra energy given by heating is an increase in both the kinetic energy and the potential energy of the components. For this reason many scientists do not like to use the term 'heat', which would appear to describe a unique form of energy.

The energy of the atoms or molecules inside the substance (the internal energy) can be increased not only by flow of energy but also by doing work. It is therefore usual in advanced physics to refer to these two contributions as heat and work. It is not until the next chapter that we shall look at the first law of thermodynamics, which states how these contributions change the internal energy and hence why a so-called form of energy called heat is in fact often used. The energy flow referred to as heat (or thermal) flow is a random process, whereas when we do work we exchange energy in some ordered manner. Order and disorder are also discussed in more detail in Chapter 14.

1 ENERGY AND WORK

Historically, the nature of heating greatly puzzled scientists. This is because they did not know then what we now understand about the structure of matter – that it is made up of atoms. Count Rumford in the late eighteenth century became interested in the way thick metal rods became hot when bored out to make cannons. But a great step forward came when Joule showed that mechanical work could be transferred to thermal energy, which resulted in an increase in temperature of water in a cylinder (see page 48).

We can demonstrate the transfer of mechanical work to thermal energy (as internal energy) using lead shot in a closed cylindrical tube. The tube is repeatedly inverted so that the lead shot falls from end to end each time. When the lead shot weighs 150 g (0.15 kg) and each fall is 0.75 m, we can calculate the rise in temperature of the lead shot after 100 falls.

- As the masses fall, work is done as a result of the gravitational force. This work is given by:

$$\text{work done} = \frac{\text{mass of}}{\text{lead}} \times \frac{\text{acceleration due}}{\text{to gravity}} \times \frac{\text{length}}{\text{of fall}} \times \frac{\text{number}}{\text{of falls}}$$

$$= 0.15 \times 9.8 \times 0.75 \times 100 \text{ J} = 110 \text{ J}$$

- The work is transferred to kinetic energy as the lead shot is falling.
- But the lead shot is brought to a sudden halt at the bottom of the tube. Now the energy transfers to internal energy within the shot. As a result, the amount of movement and the potential energy of the lead atoms are increased. Overall, the work done has been used to raise the temperature of the lead by ΔT.
- The specific heat capacity (see page 258) for lead is 129 J kg^{-1} K^{-1}. The amount of energy given to the lead shot is given by:

$$\text{energy (in J)} = \text{mass of lead} \times \frac{\text{specific heat}}{\text{capacity of lead}} \times \text{temperature rise}$$

$$= 0.15 \times 129 \times \Delta T = 19.4 \times \Delta T$$

- Equating work and energy (in J):

$$110 = 19.4 \times \Delta T$$

So the temperature rise is:

$$\Delta T = 110/19.4 = 5.7 \text{ K}$$

This temperature rise will be detectable even when there are some energy losses to the surroundings. Note that the mass of the lead shot is used twice, once for the work done and once for the energy transferred to the lead shot. This means that the temperature rise does not depend on the mass of the

? **QUESTION 1**

1 Calculate the work done and the amount of energy produced after 100 falls if 250 g of lead shot are used in the same tube. Show that the temperature rise is again 5.7 K.

Joule's work on thermodynamics

James Prescott Joule came from a family of wealthy brewers in Salford and conducted his early experiments in a laboratory at the brewery. He was wealthy enough to fund his own experiments (see page 56). He devised an accurate thermometer and on his honeymoon he spent time measuring the temperature difference between the top and bottom of a scenic waterfall.

Joule's first thermometers measured to within ±0.02 °C and later ones to ±0.005 °C. It was a great achievement to measure temperatures so accurately, and necessary for Joule's study of the conversion of mechanical work to energy.

Joule had been educated privately at home, with no formal education in mathematics, so that he could not on his own keep up with the new science of thermodynamics. However, he won the support of William Thomson (Lord Kelvin) and together they made great advances in thermodynamics, Joule providing the practical ability and Thomson the theory.

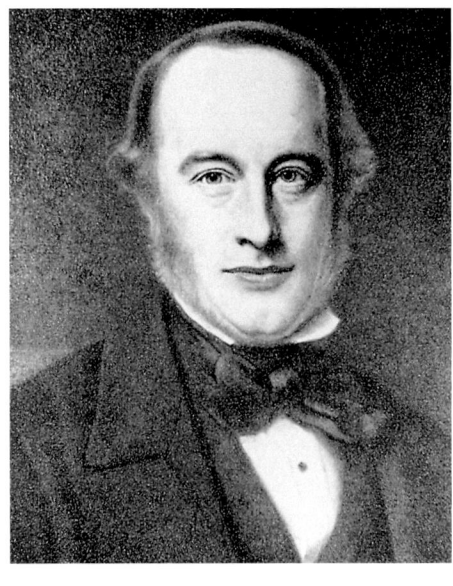

Fig 13.1 James Prescott Joule (1818–1889)

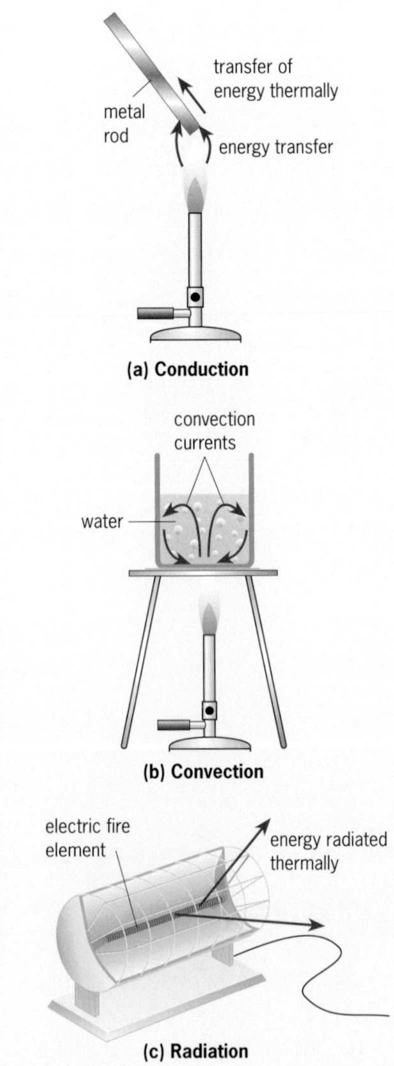

shot used and need not have been given in the overall calculation. Increasing the mass of shot increases the amount of required work but also increases the mass to be heated. In the calculation we could use a symbol for mass and then cancel mass on either side of the equation.

2 THERMAL TRANSFER OF ENERGY

There are three types of thermal transfer of energy: **conduction**, **convection** and **radiation** (Fig 13.2).

CONDUCTION

Energy is transferred within solids by the process called **thermal conduction**. The atoms in a solid vibrate, and as the temperature increases, the amplitude of vibration increases. The energy of the atoms increases and the internal energy of the solid is increased. The vibration of the atoms is rather like that of a set of masses connected to a lattice of springs.

Energy travels through a solid by way of vibrations through the system. Neighbouring atoms are set into increased vibration one after another. In metals, 'free' electrons travelling among the atoms also gain extra energy and travel a little faster as the temperature increases. Importantly, they are the means of energy transport through the metal and they pass on energy to more distant atoms.

CONVECTION

There is movement of internal energy in a fluid (a liquid or a gas) by the process of **thermal convection** (conduction also occurs). The fluid particles, usually molecules, are free to move around independently. Their kinetic energy increases as more thermal energy is added to the fluid. Heating the fluid causes it to expand and become less dense. Because of the effect of gravity, the less dense (higher temperature) fluid rises up through the more dense fluid, which then falls to take its place. This movement is a very effective way of transferring those molecules that have been given extra kinetic energy. Currents of molecules are set up called convection currents.

transfer of energy thermally

metal rod

energy transfer

(a) Conduction

convection currents

water

(b) Convection

electric fire element

energy radiated thermally

(c) Radiation

Fig 13.2 Thermal conduction, convection and radiation

Convection currents cause thermal energy to circulate in kitchen ovens. Cooks know that less dense hotter air rises to the top of the oven. When cooking more than one item of food, they choose the appropriate shelf for each item. Many modern ovens include an electric fan, which both increases the circulation rate and produces a more uniform temperature distribution. This is called forced convection, whereas if the thermal energy is left to distribute itself, the process is called natural convection.

RADIATION

Energy can be transferred in the form of **electromagnetic radiation** (see Chapter 15). All objects emit and reflect electromagnetic radiation. We are aware of the radiation in the form of light waves. However, as the temperature of an object increases, both the range of frequencies and the quantity of radiation given out increase.

An electric fire radiates much of its energy in the visible region – we see the element glowing orange or red. Stars are much hotter and radiate much of their energy in the ultraviolet region.

On the other hand, thermal imaging cameras can pick up infrared radiation at longer wavelengths and smaller frequencies than the visible range. This means that hot bodies can be detected against a cooler background. Imaging cameras are used by the fire service to detect people overcome by smoke in buildings on fire. When slung from police helicopters, these cameras can detect suspected criminals on the run at night.

Black body

An object that completely absorbs thermal radiation at all wavelengths is called a **black body**. It reflects none of the radiation falling on it, yet it can emit radiation at all wavelengths. Fig 13.3 shows the radiation curves for a black body.

A furnace with a very small opening and thick, insulating walls approximates to a black body. Radiation directed into the furnace through the opening is absorbed by the inside walls. However, the furnace walls will be very hot (they will be at the temperature of the furnace) and so will be emitting radiation at all wavelengths, a small amount of which will escape through the opening.

Fig 13.3 shows that, as the temperature increases, the amount of radiation from the black body also increases (corresponding to the area under the curve). The wavelength at which peak emission occurs falls as the temperature increases. This is why when a piece of metal such as steel is heated, it first appears to be a dull red but, as it gets hotter and the peak in the emitted light moves to smaller wavelengths, its appearance becomes more orange. See also Chapter 15, page 285 and Chapter 16, page 307.

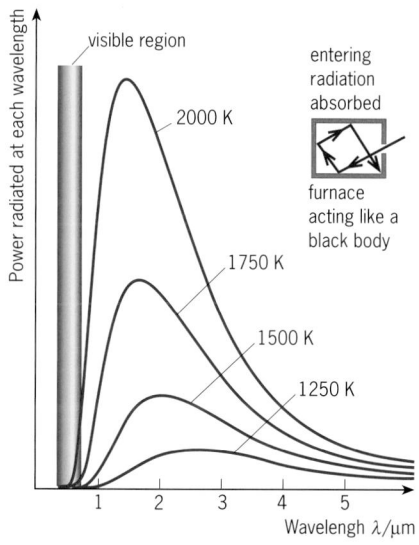

Fig 13.3 Black body radiation and diagram of a black body

3 MEASURING TEMPERATURE

In Chapter 7 (pages 160–161) we saw how to use the properties of an ideal gas to define a temperature scale that is reproducible anywhere. This scale is the Kelvin scale. We also saw that a constant-volume gas thermometer measures temperature. But such a thermometer is not easy to carry around and to use.

Temperature can be measured using *any physical property that varies with temperature in a reproducible way*. But we must be able to calibrate the variation against our standard Kelvin scale as obtained with the gas thermometer. We do not have to stay with the Kelvin scale itself, but the only other scale now in common use is the Celsius scale (discussed shortly).

Examples of physical properties that we might use are:
- **length**, such as the length of a column of alcohol in a liquid-in-glass thermometer,
- **voltage**, such as that produced with a thermocouple,
- **electrical resistance** of a wire (often platinum) or semiconductor (thermistor),
- **pressure**, as in a gas thermometer,
- **thermal radiation** (using a pyrometer).

TEMPERATURE SCALES

The thermodynamic scale (or absolute scale or Kelvin scale)

This is the scale already discussed in Chapter 7. A single fixed point is taken at the triple point of water and defined as 273.16 K. The unit of temperature, the kelvin, is 1/273.16 of this triple point temperature. The size of the unit then determines at what stage we get down to the zero of the scale. There is no negative temperature and we can never quite reach zero in the laboratory.

Because scientists need to make measurements over a very wide range of temperatures, they have defined some additional fixed points for calibrating thermometers. However, only the triple point is fundamental to all scales.

The Celsius scale

The Celsius scale is derived from the thermodynamic (Kelvin) scale using the same single fixed point as the thermodynamic scale. But, in Celsius, the ice point is 0.01 °C (usually assumed 0 °C for practical purposes) and the steam point is 100.00 °C.

The relationship is:

$$t = T - 273.15$$

where t is the temperature on the Celsius scale and T is the temperature on the thermodynamic scale.

Physical properties to calibrate temperature

Calibration is easy if we are measuring a change of length. More generally, though, we need to know the value of the property (here, length) at the fixed points and calibrate using a proportionality.

Let us see this in action for a **mercury-in-glass thermometer**:
- l_{100} is the length of mercury thread at 100 °C.
- l_0 is the length of mercury thread at 0 °C.
- l_θ is the length of mercury thread at θ °C.
- Each degree interval will have a length $(l_{100} - l_0)/100$.
- The change of length due to a temperature rise from 0 °C to θ °C is $(l_\theta - l_0)$.
- The temperature θ in degrees is given by change of length divided by length per degree interval:

$$\theta = \left[\frac{l_\theta - l_0}{(l_{100} - l_0)/100} \right] \text{(degrees)} = \frac{l_\theta - l_0}{l_{100} - l_0} \times 100°$$

We could also use a **platinum resistance thermometer** to measure the resistances R_0 at 0°C, R_{100} at 100°C and R_θ at an unknown temperature θ °C:

$$\theta = \frac{R_\theta - R_0}{R_{100} - R_0} \times 100°$$

? **QUESTION 2**

2 Describe what you expect to happen at zero temperature.

All mercury-in-glass thermometers should agree precisely if they are calibrated correctly. So should platinum resistance thermometers. Also, all thermometers of either type should also agree with each other. However, we cannot assume that, for every degree change in temperature, the length of the mercury thread or the resistance of the platinum changes by exactly the same value. For example, the changes in length of the mercury column between 9°C and 10°C and between 40°C and 41°C may differ. Similarly, resistances at different degree intervals may vary. So the two types of thermometer may not give precisely the same temperature readings between fixed points. Hence our need for the absolute scale.

Mercury-in-glass thermometers are not often used in modern laboratories in case of breakage. Mercury has a significant vapour pressure and is slightly toxic.

USE OF THERMOMETERS

The choice of a thermometer will depend on the temperature range and where it is used. Mercury thermometers are no use below –39°C, which is the freezing point of mercury. But they can be used over a wider range of temperature than the alcohol-in-glass thermometer. A large thermometer is not suitable for measuring the temperature of small amounts of material. This is because, while the thermometer achieves thermal equilibrium, energy could be transferred to or from the material and so the temperature being measured could change. A resistance thermometer is a likely choice if high accuracy is required. Table 13.1 summarises the main types of thermometer, together with their advantages and disadvantages.

> ## ? QUESTION 3
>
> 3 Readings using a resistance thermometer are 40.0 Ω at the ice point, 86.3 Ω at the steam point and 77.8 Ω at an unknown temperature θ. Calculate this unknown temperature as measured on the Celsius scale. What is the temperature on the Kelvin scale?

Table 13.1 Different types of thermometer

Thermometer		Thermometric property	Main advantages	Main disadvantages	Temperature range
Liquid-in-glass		Volume change (i.e. changing length of thread of mercury or alcohol)	Simple to use, cheap, portable	Fragile, limited range, not suitable for small objects	Mercury: 234–723 K; Ethanol: 173–323 K
Constant-volume gas thermometer		Pressure of fixed mass of gas at constant volume	Absolute scale given, accurate, wide range	Bulky and inconvenient, slow response, not suitable for small objects directly	3–500 K
Resistance		Resistance of platinum wire	Accurate, wide range, useful for small temperature differences	Slow to respond, not suitable for small objects	15–900 K
Thermocouple		E.m.f. across junction of two dissimilar metals	Can measure small differences, fast response, wide range, can be read remotely	Small voltages, so need electronic amplification	25–1400 K (depending on metals)
Thermistor		Changing resistance of semiconductor	Provides electrical signal suitable for computer circuits	Calibration necessary, not very accurate	200–700 K
Optical pyrometer		Adjustment of current through lamp filament to match colour of object	No contact with hot object, simple to use, portable	Calibration necessary, not very accurate	Above 1250 K

4 HEATING AN OBJECT

We know from everyday experience that some things need more energy than others to raise their temperatures by the same amount. For instance, it takes more energy to heat water by one kelvin than the same mass of copper requires. The water molecules require more energy in order to move around fast enough to record a one kelvin rise than do the copper atoms, which mainly vibrate. The **heat capacity**, C, of an object is the amount of energy required to raise its temperature by one kelvin. The unit is kJ K^{-1}.

SPECIFIC HEAT CAPACITY, MOLAR HEAT CAPACITY AND LATENT HEAT

Heat capacity refers to a particular object of any mass. A more general quantity would be more useful. This is **specific heat capacity**, c, which refers to *unit mass* of a single substance. Each pure substance has its own particular value of specific heat capacity at a given temperature (though this value may change as the temperature of the substance varies). In heating a substance energy is given to its molecules, and unit masses of different substances have different numbers of molecules of different mass.

We can compare expressions for heat capacity C and specific heat capacity c. Let's say we heat an object of mass m (kilograms) of a single substance by giving it energy ΔQ (kilojoules) so that the temperature rises by ΔT (kelvin or Celsius), then:

$$C = \frac{\Delta Q}{\Delta T} \quad \text{and} \quad c = \frac{\Delta Q}{m \Delta T}$$

? QUESTION 4

4 The kettle in the Example will transfer energy to the water with less than 100 per cent efficiency. List ways in which energy from the kettle is lost when increasing the temperature of the water.

SCIENCE IN CONTEXT

EXAMPLE

Q A 3.0 kW electric kettle is used to bring 1.50 kg of water to the boil from a starting temperature of 18.0 °C. Assuming all the energy goes into heating the water, calculate the amount of energy and the time required to boil the water. Specific heat capacity of water = 4.20 kJ kg^{-1} K^{-1}.

A Energy required = specific heat × mass × temperature rise
$$= 4.20 \times 1.5 \times 82 \text{ kJ}$$
$$= 517 \text{ kJ}$$

Time required $= \dfrac{\text{energy required}}{\text{rate of heating}}$

$$= \frac{517 \text{ kJ}}{3.0 \text{ kJs}^{-1}}$$

$$= 172 \text{ s, or 2 min 52 s}$$

We can use another thermal quantity, the **molar heat capacity**, particularly for gases. As the name suggests, this is the energy required to heat one mole of the substance through one kelvin.

We have already seen on page 174 that when a substance changes from one state to another, for example from solid to liquid, energy called **latent heat** is required to produce the change. The latent heat does not cause any change in temperature. The ordering (arrangement) and the spacing of the molecules is changed but not the temperature. Also, most substances have different specific heat capacities depending on whether they are solid, liquid or gas. If we add energy to

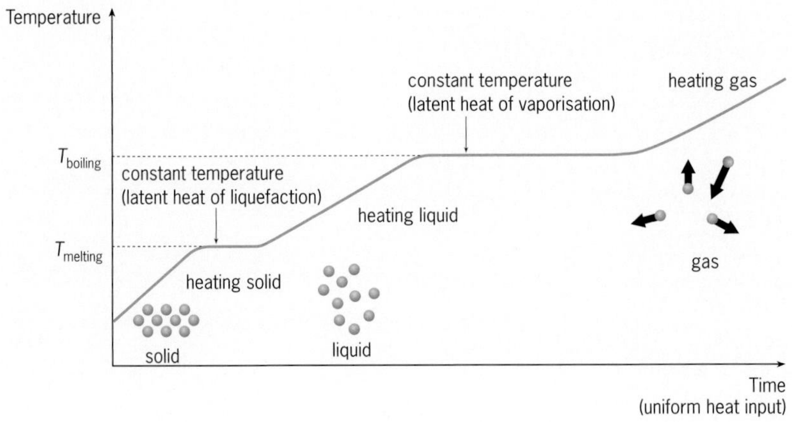

Fig 13.4 Heating a substance uniformly to show effects of thermal capacities and latent heats

Temperature

constant temperature (latent heat of vaporisation)   heating gas

$T_{boiling}$ constant temperature (latent heat of liquefaction)

heating liquid

$T_{melting}$

heating solid   gas

solid   liquid

Time (uniform heat input)

the substance at a constant rate, we can see how these differences in heat capacity affect the rate of heating, and we can identify the temperatures where changes of state occur (Fig 13.4). We assume no energy loss to the surroundings.

THERMAL CONDUCTIVITY

When one side of a body is heated, it takes time for the internal energy to spread (by thermal conduction) to the other side. That is, there is a time lag between the heated side of the body changing its temperature by a significant amount and a corresponding change occurring on the far side.

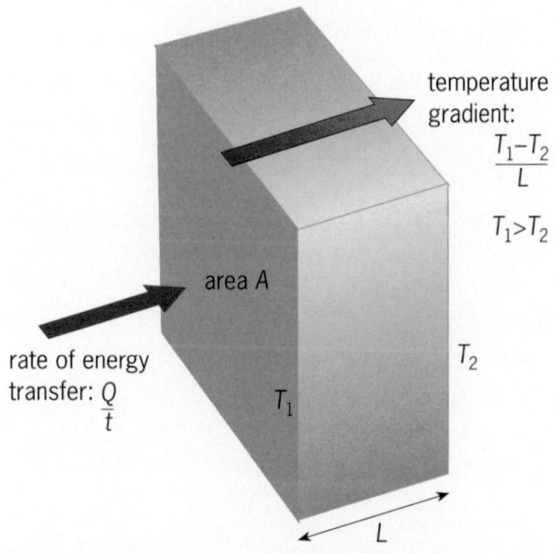

Once thermal equilibrium has been reached, a temperature difference will be maintained through the object, assuming that heating continues and that energy can escape from the far side. The ease with which energy can transfer through the object depends on a property called **thermal conductivity**. However, as well as thermal conductivity, other factors determine how much energy passes through the object. We now consider all these factors.

Fig 13.5 Thermal energy flow through a block of material

temperature gradient:
$\dfrac{T_1 - T_2}{L}$

$T_1 > T_2$

area A

rate of energy transfer: $\dfrac{Q}{t}$

T_2

T_1

L

Take the flow of energy through a block of material with a thickness of L metres (Fig 13.5). For energy to flow, there has to be a temperature difference between opposite faces of the block.

- Assuming the block is of exactly the same material throughout, the temperature gradient at any point between the opposite faces will be the same. We have:

$$\text{temperature gradient} = \frac{\text{temperature difference}}{\text{thickness of block}}$$

$$= \frac{T_1 - T_2}{L}$$

The larger the temperature gradient, the greater the rate of flow of energy.

259

**Thermal conductivity
(energy flow)**

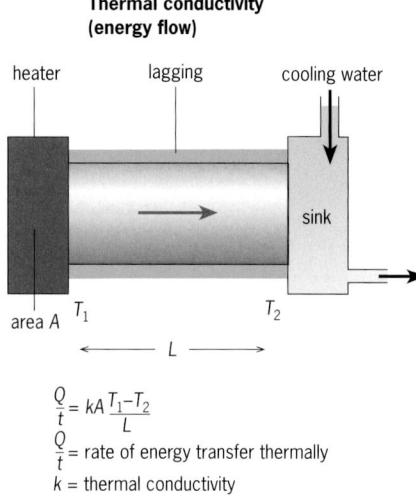

$$\frac{Q}{t} = kA\frac{T_1 - T_2}{L}$$
$\frac{Q}{t}$ = rate of energy transfer thermally
k = thermal conductivity

Fig 13.6 Flow processes compared

**Electrical conductivity
(charge flow)**

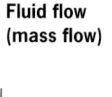
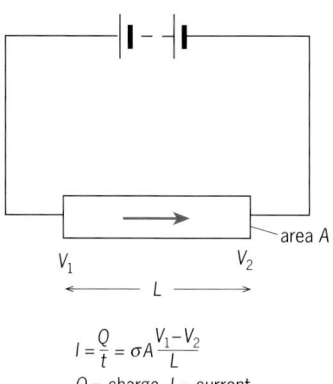

$$I = \frac{Q}{t} = \sigma A\frac{V_1 - V_2}{L}$$
Q = charge, I = current

σ = electrical conductivity, V = voltage (potential)

**Fluid flow
(mass flow)**

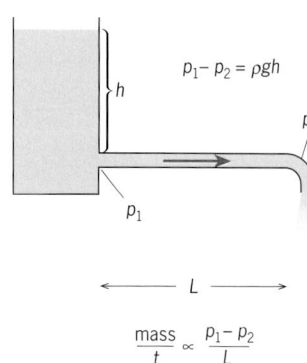

$$\frac{\text{mass}}{t} \propto \frac{p_1 - p_2}{L}$$

REMEMBER THIS
Units of k

k will have units which we work out from the equation.

Q/t has units of energy/time, that is J s^{-1} or W.

$A(T_1 - T_2)/L$ has units of length^2 × temperature/length, that is m^2 K m^{-1}, equal to m K. (Note the space between m and K as otherwise the symbols would represent one thousandth of a kelvin.)

So:

W = (units of k) × m K

So the units of k must be W divided by m K which equals W m^{-1} K^{-1}.

- The flow will also depend on the area of cross-section A (m^2) of the block. This is very similar to water passing through a pipe – the quantity of water flowing depends on the area of cross-section of the pipe and the pressure difference between the two ends. Transfer of thermal energy is also similar to flow of charge in an electrical conductor – electrical current is proportional to the cross-sectional area of the conductor and to the electric field (potential gradient) along the conductor (Fig 13.6).

- The amount of energy that flows will depend on how well the material conducts it. Copper is a good conductor, while glass is a poor conductor. The rate of energy flow is proportional to the thermal conductivity, k, of the material. This dependence is the same as the way in which flow of electric charge depends on the electrical conductivity of a conductor. The rate of flow of energy is the quantity of thermal energy Q (kilojoules) transmitted, divided by time t (seconds). We have:

$$\frac{Q}{t} \propto \frac{T_1 - T_2}{L}$$

$$\frac{Q}{t} \propto A$$

$$\frac{Q}{t} \propto k$$

So far, k has not been fixed, so we can make it the constant of proportionality for the combined expression:

$$\frac{Q}{t} = kA\frac{(T_1 - T_2)}{L}$$

Note that, in this equation, T_1 is greater than T_2 and that energy goes *down* a temperature gradient from the side of higher temperature to the side of lower temperature.

5 THERMAL FLOW OF ENERGY: CONDUCTION

FLOW ALONG A ROD

Suppose we heat one end of a long rod that is thermally lagged (i.e. surrounded with insulation). We assume that energy flow is the same at all points along the whole length. We can represent this flow by a series of parallel lines (Fig 13.7), just as we can illustrate the uniform flow of water through a pipe.

What is happening on the atomic scale? We have already said that we can think of the atoms as solid spheres connected in all directions by springs (see pages 177 and 254). When we heat one end of the rod, the atoms at that end vibrate with increasing amplitude. Energy from the vibrations of these atoms is passed on to neighbouring atoms. Eventually the amplitude of vibration of all the atoms in the solid increases.

After a time, the rod reaches a state of equilibrium, with just as much energy leaving the far end as enters the heated end. Energy is transferred thermally through the rod, which means that, as you would expect, there is a temperature gradient in the rod. The far end is cooler than the heated end. We can think of the difference in temperature as driving the energy through the rod, just as a difference in voltage drives an electric current through a wire.

As already seen (pages 172–173 and 254), some of the energy in a metal is carried by free electrons. They move around faster at the hot end than at the cold end. By colliding with the lattice of ions (the spheres in our ball-and-spring model) they help rapid transfer of energy through the rod. We have already noted that copper, a typical metal, has a large thermal conductivity. This is because of its free electrons.

The vibrations of the atoms in the metal rod are transmitted as waves along the rod. However, just as sometimes light is described as the passage of particles called photons with no rest mass, so the passage of these vibrations can be also considered as the movement of particles with no rest mass, this time called 'phonons'.

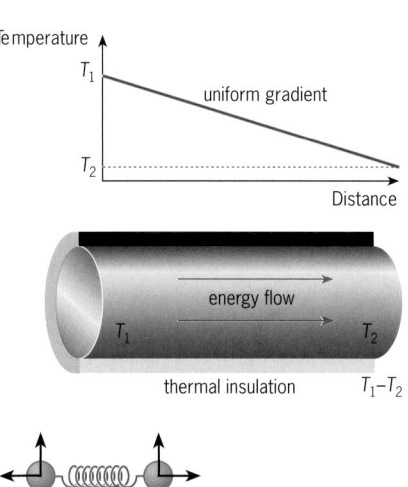

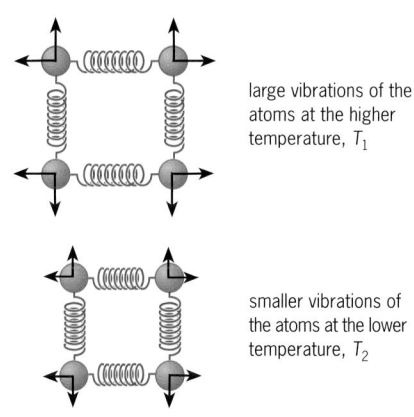

large vibrations of the atoms at the higher temperature, T_1

smaller vibrations of the atoms at the lower temperature, T_2

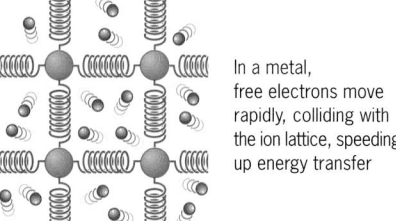

In a metal, free electrons move rapidly, colliding with the ion lattice, speeding up energy transfer

Fig 13.7 Thermal energy flow in a lagged conductor

EXAMPLE

SCIENCE IN CONTEXT

Q An iron bar 0.50 m long and a copper bar 1.2 m long are joined end to end. One end of the iron bar is kept at 80 °C while the far end of the copper bar is maintained at 0 °C by a mixture of ice and water. The outer surfaces of the bars are lagged so that there are no thermal energy losses. Both bars are of circular cross-section, diameter 0.16 m. At thermal equilibrium the temperature at the junction of the metals is T_j. Calculate T_j and the rate of energy flow. Thermal conductivity of iron = 75 W m⁻¹ K⁻¹; thermal conductivity of copper = 390 W m⁻¹ K⁻¹.

A The rate of energy flow through each conductor is the same.
Rate of energy flow through the iron bar is:

$$\frac{Q}{t} = k_{iron} A \frac{(T_{80} - T_j)}{0.5} \text{ (watts)}$$

$$= \frac{75 \times \pi \times 0.08^2}{0.5} \times (80 - T_j)$$

$$= (3.02)(80 - T_j) \text{ W}$$

Rate of energy flow through the copper bar is:

$$\frac{Q}{t} = k_{copper} A \frac{(T_j - T_0)}{1.20} \text{ (watts)}$$

$$= \frac{390 \times \pi \times 0.08^2}{1.20} \times (T_j - 0)$$

$$= (6.53)(T_j - 0) \text{ W}$$

Equating gives:

$$(3.02)\,(80 - T_j) = 6.53(T_j - 0)$$
$$242 = 9.55 T_j$$
$$T_j = 25.3 \text{ °C}$$

Hence, $\dfrac{Q}{t} = 165 \text{ Js}^{-1}$

Fig 13.8

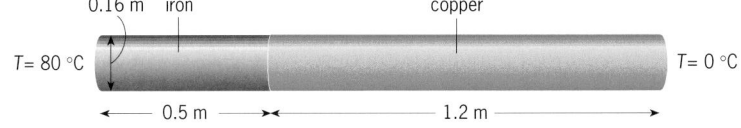

0.16 m   iron

copper

T = 80 °C

T = 0 °C

0.5 m

1.2 m

? QUESTION 5

5 Why is the energy flow the same in each conductor in the Example?

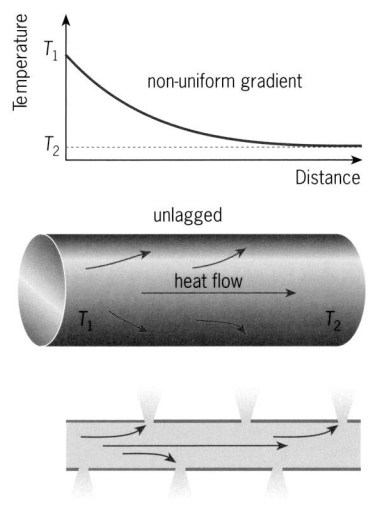

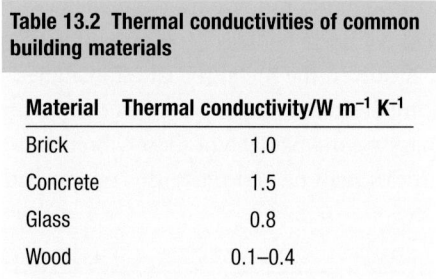

garden hose with holes
to sprinkle water

Fig 13.9 Thermal energy flow in an unlagged conductor – similar to water flow in a garden hose with holes, though the conductor loses energy uniformly at all points on its surface

Suppose that the rod in the Example on the previous page is not lagged. In this case, energy is lost by thermal processes along the sides of the rod.

This is similar to water escaping from holes in the side of a hosepipe (as often used for watering gardens or orchards). The flow lines will no longer be parallel (Fig 13.9). More importantly, we can no longer assume a constant temperature gradient.

FLOW THROUGH A GLASS WINDOW

The thermal energy flow through glass windows is of great practical importance. Glass has a low thermal conductivity (Table 13.2), comparable to that of brick. But because the thickness of glass in a window is so much less than the thickness of a typical house brick, it is important to reduce the loss of energy through windows. The most common way is to use double glazing.

Table 13.2 Thermal conductivities of common building materials

Material	Thermal conductivity/W m^{-1} K^{-1}
Brick	1.0
Concrete	1.5
Glass	0.8
Wood	0.1–0.4

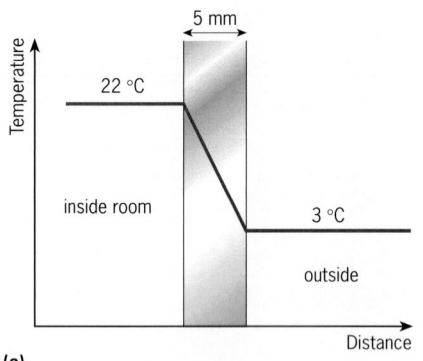

(a)

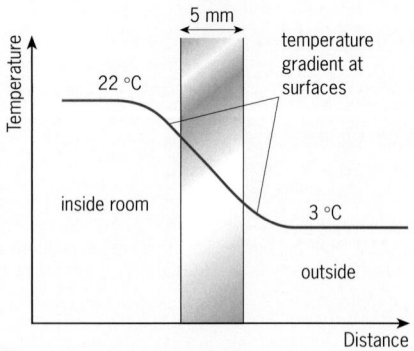

(b)

Fig 13.10 Temperature profiles close to and through a glass window:
(a) profile assumed in the calculation;
(b) a more realistic profile

EXAMPLE

Q A room has a single glass window of length 2.2 m, height 1.2 m and thickness 5 mm. Assuming that the temperature in the room at the surface of the glass is 22 °C and that outside it is 3 °C, calculate the loss of energy from the room.
Thermal conductivity of glass is 0.8 W m^{-1} K^{-1}.

A We use the equation:

$$\text{rate of energy flow} = \frac{Q}{t} = kA\frac{(T_1 - T_2)}{L} \text{ (watts)}$$

$$= 0.8 \times (2.2 \times 1.2) \times \frac{(22 - 3)}{0.005}$$

$$= 8026 \text{ W}$$

(Note that it is not necessary to convert °C to K because the equation involves a temperature difference and one degree Celsius has the same magnitude as one kelvin.)

At this point we should question the model. We are losing over 8 kW of thermal energy from the room, and would need a very large heater to maintain the temperature at 22°C. Something must be wrong. Yet the numbers we have put in seem reasonable.

The error is that we have not allowed for layers of still air on either side of the window. The thermal conductivity of air is very low (approximately 0.025 W m^{-1} K^{-1}). Part of the temperature drop will be just inside the window and part will be just outside. Therefore the temperature difference between the opposite sides of the glass and the temperature gradient through the pane of glass will be rather less than we used in the calculation. The overall temperature profile is not as we have assumed in Fig 13.10(a) but is as shown in Fig 13.10(b).

Note that there has to be some temperature gradient at the two glass surfaces; otherwise, energy would be unable to enter or leave. We would need to take measurements to find the actual profile close to the window pane. Away from the windows of the room, energy is transferred mainly by convection.

Double glazing and thermal resistance

Most new windows in Britain are now double glazed. The glass is commonly 4 mm thick, though the distance between the panes is less standard, perhaps 5 mm for windows or now, more usually, at least 10 mm for patio doors. Using the analogy of flow of charge through a conductor, we can see that our double-glazed unit can be modelled as three resistances in series: the resistances of glass, air and glass. So the thermal resistance R of double glazing will be the sum of the thermal resistances of the three layers. The thermal resistance R for one layer is defined as t/kA where t is the layer thickness, A its area and k the thermal conductivity. With the three layers present, the summation is represented by:

$$\Sigma \frac{t}{kA}$$

where the symbol Σ (capital Greek letter sigma), meaning 'sum of', refers to the three layers – glass, air and glass.

Now $k_{air} = 0.025$ W m^{-1} K^{-1} and $k_{glass} = 0.8$ W m^{-1} K^{-1}. Therefore with windows of thickness 4 mm, separation 10 mm and area 1 m^2 we obtain:

$$\text{thermal resistance} = \frac{4 \times 10^{-3}}{0.8} + \frac{10^{-2}}{0.025} + \frac{4 \times 10^{-3}}{0.8} \text{ K W}^{-1}$$
$$= 0.41 \text{ K W}^{-1}$$

For a single pane of glass, the thermal resistance will be 0.005 K W^{-1}, but remember that there will be some convection in the air gap also.

U-VALUES

U-values are quantities used by architects and heating engineers for working out thermal energy flows within buildings – in particular, energy losses through the windows and walls. The U-value of a particular thickness of material is its thermal transmittance, that is, the thermal energy flow through the material per unit area for a temperature difference of one degree. Hence it is given by:

$$U\text{-value} = \frac{\text{rate of energy flow}}{\text{area} \times \text{temperature difference}}$$

Its units are W m^{-2} K^{-1}. U-values are available for different types of walls, windows, floors and roofs. The values have been obtained by *direct measurement* rather than theoretical calculation. Thus thermal transmittance values are more realistic than thermal conductivity values as they take account of the actual composition of the building material and allow for any convection within hollow components.

The thermal transmittance from a room or building can be calculated by multiplying the U-value for each component of the surface structure by the corresponding area.

? QUESTION 6

6 Use the formula for thermal resistance to check that the units K W^{-1} are correct.

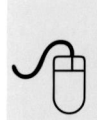

For an investigation on heat loss in the home please see the How Science Works assignment for this chapter at www.collinseducation.co.uk/CAS

SUMMARY

After studying this chapter you should be able to:

- Discuss the equivalence of work and energy and, in particular, the equivalence of work and the thermal energy required to heat a substance.
- Describe the thermal energy transfer processes of conduction, convection and radiation.
- State the advantages and disadvantages of different methods of measuring temperature.
- Describe the difference between the thermodynamic (absolute or Kelvin) and Celsius scales of temperature.
- Explain the terms: thermal capacity, specific heat capacity, thermal conductivity and U-value.

- Carry out calculations on the change of temperature of objects using thermal capacity or specific heat capacity.
- Calculate thermal resistance using t/kA for a single layer and $\Sigma\,(t/kA)$ for a number of layers.
- Use thermal conductivity (or U-value) for calculating thermal energy flow through materials.

 Practice questions for this chapter are available at www.collinseducation.co.uk/CAS

14

The laws of thermodynamics

THE LAWS OF THERMODYNAMICS

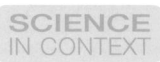

Obtaining the lowest temperature in the world

By this stage of your physics course, you will have spent a lot of time learning about properties of materials – conductors have resistance, fluids are viscous, and so on. But at very low temperatures we cannot take these properties for granted. At 4 K, for example, mercury loses all its electrical resistance and so can carry a current for ever without any reduction in the current. At very low temperatures, helium becomes a fluid that loses its viscosity and can flow freely. Oxygen even becomes magnetic.

Scientists are working to achieve lower and lower temperatures and trying to discover more unusual low-temperature properties in a wider range of materials.

The absolute zero of temperature has been defined as 0 K (about −273.16 °C), when the only remaining energy is 'zero point' energy that arises from the so-called uncertainty principle and can never be removed. We also know that we will never be able to reach absolute zero. But that doesn't stop scientists from trying to get as close to it as possible.

Eric A. Cornell, Wolfgang Ketterle and Carl E. Wieman of the United States shared the 2001 Nobel Prize for Physics for research that involved cooling a gas down to just above 1 nK (1 billionth of a degree above absolute zero). The technique involved slowing down alkali atoms by colliding photons head-on with them and then skimming off the faster atoms by evaporative cooling to obtain a condensate. But competition continues. At the Low Temperature Laboratory in Helsinki, Finland, a piece of rhodium metal has since been cooled to 100 pK (0.1 nK).

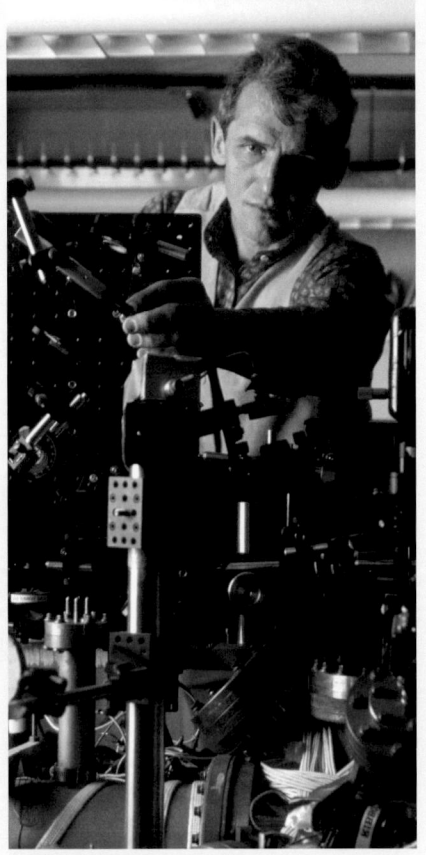

Wolfgang Ketterle with his low-temperature apparatus

The ideas in this chapter

Ever since physicists knew about absolute zero temperature, they have been trying to reach it. This is a problem of **thermodynamics**, that is, the study of energy transfer processes including work and heating, and how these two processes are connected.

But thermodynamics is a lot more than trying to reach absolute zero. Thermodynamics explains why we can heat and expand a gas to drive internal combustion engines: most vehicles rely on some form of thermodynamic (heat) engine. It explains the limits to transferring energy, and shows, for example, that we can never build a totally efficient power station to supply electricity. In the home, thermodynamics explains the operation of refrigerators and other equipment that we use to do work for us.

1 THE ZEROTH LAW

When physicists first began to study thermodynamics, they identified three laws. Logically enough, they called these laws the first, second and third laws of thermodynamics. However, in the 1930s they realised that there was a much more fundamental law than these, so, rather than change the names of

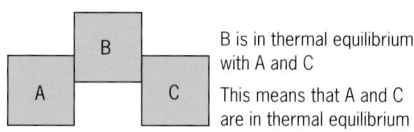

Fig 14.1 The zeroth law

the others, they called the new one the **zeroth law of thermodynamics**. This states:

> **If two bodies are in thermal equilibrium with a third body, then they must be in thermal equilibrium with each other.**

If two or more bodies are in this kind of equilibrium, as in Fig 14.1, they must have the same temperature because thermal energy is not transferred between bodies that are at the same temperature. As we saw in the previous chapter, for energy to be transferred thermally, a *temperature gradient* is required. Without the zeroth law a practical thermometer would not be possible.

We use the zeroth law in calibrating a thermometer. A practical thermometer (such as a mercury thermometer) and a gas thermometer are both placed in a liquid or similar reservoir of thermal energy, as in Fig 14.2. The gas thermometer is an 'ideal' thermometer used to define temperature (see page 161). Both thermometers reach thermal equilibrium with the liquid. Then the two thermometers are also in equilibrium with each other and so they are at the same temperature. This means that the practical thermometer can be calibrated against the gas thermometer for a fixed temperature. Further points can be established by altering the temperature of the liquid as measured using the gas thermometer.

- The practical thermometer A is in thermal equilibrium with the liquid B

- The gas thermometer C is in thermal equilibrium with the liquid B

- Therefore the practical thermometer A and the gas thermometer C are in thermal equilibrium

- The thermometers will read the same temperature

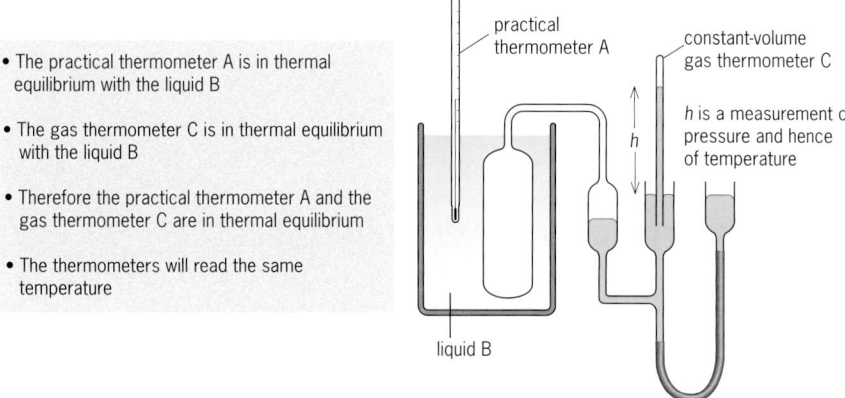

Fig 14.2 Calibrating a practical thermometer is possible as a consequence of the zeroth law

2 THE FIRST LAW

We saw (pages 56 and 254) that Joule found he could increase the temperature of water by doing work on it. He kept the water thermally insulated from the surroundings so that no energy was thermally transmitted to the water from outside. But the internal energy of the water changed.

We use the symbol U for **internal energy** (measured in joules) and represent a small change by ΔU. We assume that a small amount of **work** ΔW is done to produce this change of internal energy. So the change of internal energy in joules is:

$$\Delta U = \Delta W$$

Alternatively, the internal energy of the water could be increased by allowing energy to enter from the outside, usually by thermal processes (such as conduction). We often call this energy 'heat' or 'thermal energy'. Assume that this amount of energy (in joules) entering the water is small, represented by ΔQ. The change of internal energy is given by:

$$\Delta U = \Delta Q$$

This assumes no work has been done.

> ✔ **REMEMBER THIS**
> The internal energy is the sum of the potential and kinetic energy of the molecules in the substance.

> **REMEMBER THIS**
>
> Beware! We are considering here
> the work done *on* the water so we
> use a plus sign in the equation.
> Some books refer to work done
> *by* the system so the relationship
> is written with a minus sign:
>
> $$\Delta U = \Delta Q - \Delta W$$
>
> See Fig 14.3.

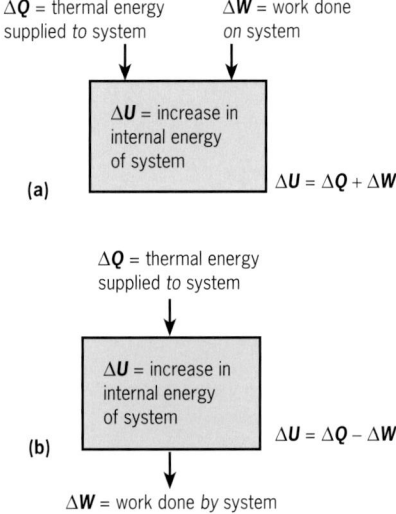

Fig 14.3 We write the expression for increase in
internal energy differently depending on whether
we are considering **(a)** work done *on* the system or
(b) work done *by* the system

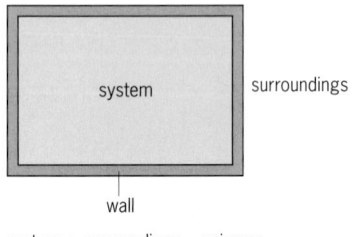

system + surroundings = universe

Fig 14.4 The system, the imaginary wall
and the surroundings

> **? QUESTION 1**
>
> 1 An athlete eats a bar of chocolate
> and then enters the high-jump
> event. Describe what energy
> transfers occur and how the first law
> is upheld.

But most changes in the internal energy of a body arise from a combination of
both thermal transfer and mechanical transfer of energy or work. So more generally
we write:

$$\Delta U = \Delta Q + \Delta W$$

We can use any combination of amounts of thermal energy or mechanical
energy (work) to produce a given change of internal energy ΔU. The equation is an
algebraic statement of the **first law of thermodynamics**. We can state the
law in words:

> **The increase in internal energy of a system is the sum of the
> work done on the system and the energy supplied thermally to
> the system.**

It is probably easier for us to remember the law as the equation
$\Delta U = \Delta Q + \Delta W$. Notice that in words, the law refers to a **system**. In our
example, the system is the mass of water whose temperature has been raised
by work or heating.

Sometimes we need to consider what happens to more than one object: we may
have to consider the behaviour of a number of components. We refer to them all
together as our system – we can think of the system as surrounded by an imaginary
wall. All things outside this wall are the surroundings. The system plus its
surroundings taken together make up its **universe** (Fig 14.4).

Although energy can be transformed in different ways, it is not possible to create
or destroy energy. (Later, in Chapter 17 (page 338), you will read about how mass
can be turned into energy and how energy can be transformed into mass. This is
possible only with nuclear interactions; it does not happen in everyday
thermodynamics.)

APPLYING THE FIRST LAW TO A GAS

Most real-life engines contain a gas which is heated and expands, and the gas
(which does the work) follows a cycle of changes before it ends up under the
same set of conditions as when it started the cycle. We shall look at the
expansion of a gas, and other changes, restricting ourselves to an *ideal* gas.

Because there are no forces of attraction or repulsion between the molecules of
an ideal gas, the only way that the internal energy and the temperature of the gas
can alter is by a change in the kinetic energy of the molecules. This makes an ideal
gas system easier to consider than many other systems.

Fig 14.5 Work done *by* a gas
on a piston

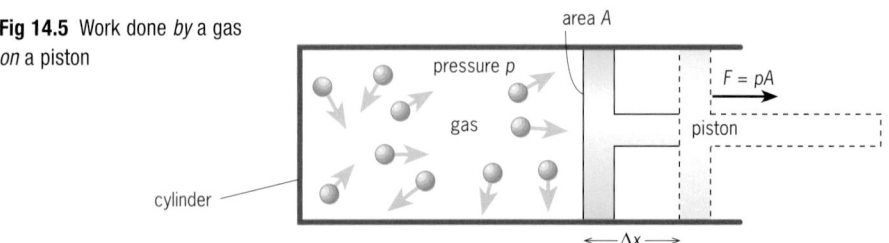

We look at what happens when work is done *by* the gas. Suppose the gas is
inside a cylinder with one end closed. At the other end is a piston (Fig 14.5). The
molecules move around inside the cylinder, colliding with the walls, rebounding
elastically off the walls and piston. This results in a pressure p on the walls and
piston. The pressure acts on the piston of area A, producing an overall force:

$$F = pA$$

Suppose that, as a result of this force, the piston moves outwards slightly so that the volume of the gas increases. We then make the following assumptions:

- There is negligible friction between the piston and the walls of the cylinder.
- The force F exerted by the gas is balanced almost exactly by an external force F.
- But the external force is reduced by a very small amount.

This very slight imbalance of forces allows the piston to move. We assume it travels a small distance Δx so that there is negligible change of pressure of the gas. The volume of the gas changes by a small amount ΔV. The gas does work ΔW in expanding against the external force. We therefore have:

$$\text{work} = \text{force} \times \text{distance}$$
$$\Delta W = F\Delta x$$
$$= pA\Delta x$$

The product $A\Delta x$ is the increase in volume ΔV of the gas. So the work done *by* the gas is:

$$\Delta W = p\Delta V$$

Note that if we consider the work done *on* the gas, the equation must have a minus sign:

$$\Delta W = -p\Delta V$$

? QUESTION 2

2 Explain clearly why we must make each of the three assumptions.

EXAMPLE

Q A circular cylinder and piston of diameter 52 mm contains a gas at 2 atmospheres. Calculate the work done by the gas when the piston moves outwards a small distance (compared with the length of the cylinder) of 3 mm.
1 atmosphere $= 1.01 \times 10^5$ Pa.

A Work done = pressure × change of volume = $pA\Delta x$
$$= 2 \times 1.01 \times 10^5 \times [\pi \times (26 \times 10^{-3})^2 \times 3 \times 10^{-3}] \text{ J} = 1.3 \text{ J}$$

ISOTHERMAL CHANGES IN A GAS

When the volume of a sample of gas changes, there is often a change of pressure. A common situation is for a gas to change its volume at constant temperature, that is, under **isothermal** conditions. Here we can use the equation of state for an ideal gas (see page 159):

$$pV = nRT$$

where R is the gas constant and n is the number of moles in the sample.

Experimentally, we can achieve an isothermal change by changing the volume slowly so that the gas remains in thermal equilibrium (that is at the same temperature) with the surroundings. With temperature constant, the pressure is related to volume by:

$$p = \frac{\text{constant}}{V}$$

This inverse dependence is shown on the pV diagram in Fig 14.6.

To find the work done by the gas when it expands, we plot the curve for actual values of p and V and measure the area under the curve. Remember: work done = $p\Delta V$. We measure the area by adding up the areas of the large number of strips (each a $p\Delta V$) making up the total area. Alternatively, we can obtain a mathematical expression for the work done. This does not require values of p to be calculated (see the Stretch and Challenge passage overleaf).

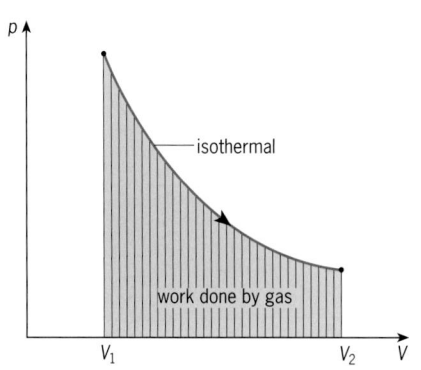

Fig 14.6 The variation of p with V of an ideal gas during an isothermal expansion. The area under the curve equals the work done by the gas in joules

Calculation of the work done by a gas during an isothermal expansion

For a small change in volume, the work done is given by:

$$\Delta W = p\Delta V \qquad [1]$$

Also we use the ideal gas equation:

$$p = \frac{nRT}{V}$$

Substituting for p from equation 1 we get:

$$\Delta W = \frac{nRT}{V}\Delta V$$

Instead of adding strips of width ΔV, we use calculus to integrate $dW = \frac{nRT}{V}\,dV$ between the initial volume V_1 and the final volume V_2:

$$dW = \int_{V_1}^{V_2} \frac{nRT}{V}\,dV = nRT \int_{V_1}^{V_2} \frac{dV}{V}$$

As the integral of dV/V is $\ln V$, we obtain:

$$dW = nRT[\ln V]_{V_1}^{V_2}$$
$$= nRT(\ln V_2 - \ln V_1)$$
$$= nRT \ln \frac{V_2}{V_1}$$

CHANGE OF PRESSURE OF A GAS AT CONSTANT VOLUME

Rather than changing the volume of a gas at constant pressure, we might choose to alter the pressure at constant volume.

Suppose the gas is in a container with fixed walls and we change the temperature by either heating or cooling. Because the volume is fixed, the gas equation tells us we can expect the pressure to rise with a temperature increase: the kinetic energy of the gas molecules increases, their momentum increases, they make greater impacts as they collide with the walls, and so *pressure* on the walls increases.

Although we change the internal energy, no work is done. We can confirm this on the pV diagram of Fig 14.7 where the change is represented by a vertical line: below this line there is no area.

How much energy is required to raise the temperature of the gas by 1 kelvin? The amount will depend on the quantity of gas involved. We usually take one mole of gas and quote the **molar heat capacity**, which is the amount of energy in joules required to heat 1 mole by 1 kelvin. The symbol for this is C_V.

The amount of energy needed to increase the temperature of the gas by a small amount ΔT is $C_V\Delta T$. The subscript V tells us that this is the **molar heat capacity at constant volume**. No work is done on the gas (it does not change volume). All the thermal energy Q_V supplied goes to changing the internal energy of the gas. For 1 mole of gas:

$$\Delta U = \Delta Q_V = C_V\Delta T$$

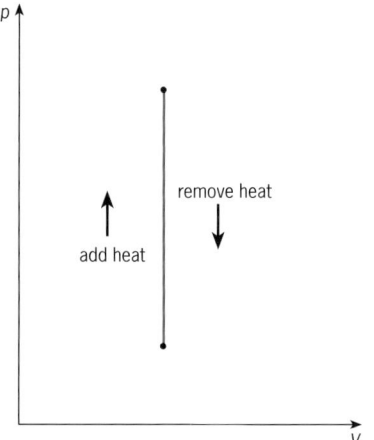

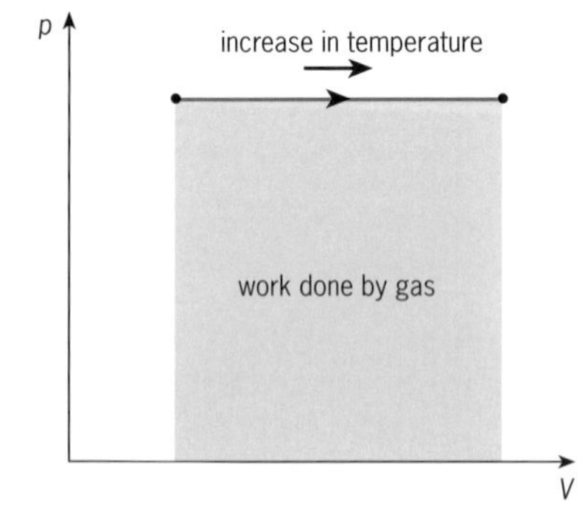

Fig 14.7 Change of pressure at constant volume of an ideal gas. No work is done, but energy must be removed thermally for a reduction in pressure and added for an increase in pressure

CHANGE OF VOLUME OF A GAS AT CONSTANT PRESSURE

We have seen that the work done by an ideal gas in expanding by a small amount ΔV is $p\Delta V$. If the expansion is large, the only way in which the pressure can remain constant (from the gas equation) is for the temperature to increase. The pV diagram of Fig 14.8 tells us that work done is still pressure × volume change, as this is the area under the horizontal line representing the change.

Again, we need to be able to work out by how much internal energy is increased. This time, we use the **molar heat capacity at constant pressure**, C_p. It is defined as the amount of energy in joules required to heat 1 mole of gas by 1 kelvin at constant pressure. For gases, the molar heat capacities at constant pressure and constant volume are not the same. When an ideal gas is heated at constant pressure its volume increases. It must do work against its surroundings as

Fig 14.8 Change of volume at constant pressure. The work done by the gas is the area under the line for p = constant. The temperature of the gas must be increased

well as increase its internal energy (kinetic energy of the molecules). As a result, we expect the molar heat capacity at constant pressure to be significantly larger than that for constant volume for a gas. For liquids and solids, the difference is very small because they expand very little on heating at constant pressure.

SUMMARY OF MOLAR HEAT CAPACITIES FOR AN IDEAL GAS

Assume that Q_V is the thermal energy added to the ideal gas at constant volume, Q_p is the thermal energy added at constant pressure, and ΔT is the temperature change in each case. Then, for n moles of the gas:

$$\Delta Q_V = nC_V\Delta T \quad \text{and} \quad \Delta Q_p = nC_p\Delta T$$

that is:

$$C_V = \frac{\Delta Q_V}{n\Delta T} \quad \text{and} \quad C_V = \frac{\Delta Q_V}{n\Delta T}$$

It can be shown (but the proof will not be given here) that there is a simple relationship between the two molar heat capacities for an ideal gas:

$$C_p - C_V = R$$

? QUESTION 3

3 Use the equation of state for an ideal gas to show that the temperature of a gas must increase for the pressure to remain constant as its volume increases. Suggest why this is so.

SCIENCE IN CONTEXT

EXAMPLE

A two-step process: isobaric plus isothermal change

Q A vessel contains 0.5 mol of an ideal gas which is taken through an isobaric (constant pressure) change AB, followed by an isothermal (constant temperature) change BC, as shown in Fig 14.9. At A, the gas has a pressure of 2.0×10^5 Pa (2 atmospheres) and volume 5.0×10^{-3} m^3 (5 litres). The gas volume changes to 1.0×10^{-2} m^3 at B, and to 1.5×10^{-2} m^3 at C.

Calculate the work done by the gas.

A

Stage AB

The work W_{AB} done by the gas will be the area under the path AB:

W_{AB} = pressure (constant) × change of volume
$= 2.0 \times 10^5 \times (1.0 - 0.5) \times 10^{-2}$ J = 1000 J

Temperature **T** at the isothermal

We need the temperature T_A at A to find the temperature T_B at B.

$$T_A = \frac{p_A V_A}{nR} = \frac{2.0 \times 10^5 \times 5.01 \times 10^{-3}}{0.5 \times 8.31} = 240 \text{ K}$$

At B the volume is twice as large, and as the pressure remains constant the temperature doubles to $2T_A$, that is, 480 K.

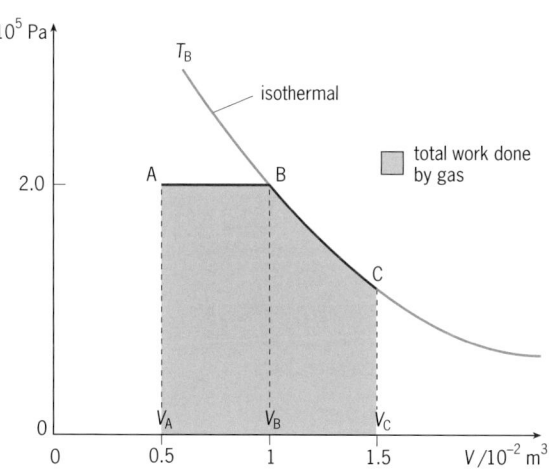

Fig 14.9 pV diagram for a two-step process (isobaric plus isothermal change)

Stage BC

To calculate the area under BC we need either to plot a graph and work out the area under the curve or we use calculus. Here we use calculus:

$$W_{BC} = \int_{V_B}^{V_C} p \, dV = nRT \int_{V_B}^{V_C} \frac{dV}{V} = nRT \ln\left(\frac{V_C}{V_B}\right)$$

$$= 0.5 \times 8.31 \times 480 \times \ln\left(\frac{1.5 \times 10^{-2}}{1.0 \times 10^{-2}}\right) \text{ J}$$

$$= 810 \text{ J}$$

The total work done by the gas in expanding from A to C is 1810 J.

CHANGE OF VOLUME OF A GAS WITH NO THERMAL ENERGY TRANSFER – AN ADIABATIC CHANGE

When a gas is compressed *very rapidly*, there is no time for energy to leave the gas by thermal processes and go to the surroundings. But the temperature changes because work is done – temperature increases for a compression. The change is caused by an external force, so there will be an increase in pressure. This rapid change of volume is called an **adiabatic** change (no thermal transfer of energy). It is the opposite case to compressing very slowly where the gas remains at a constant temperature.

A common example of a process that is almost adiabatic is the compression of air in a bicycle pump (Fig 14.10). The mechanical work done in compression increases the internal energy of the air and so its temperature rises. If this is done very quickly, the energy does not have time to escape thermally through the walls of the pump.

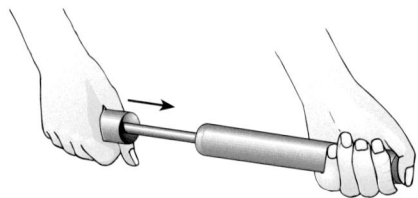

Fig 14.10 The rapid compression of air in a bicycle pump is an example of adiabatic change

There is also an adiabatic change when the gas is thermally isolated from its surroundings by an insulated wall preventing all thermal transfer. This contrasts with the isothermal case where the gas is contained by a wall that is a good thermal conductor of energy.

Zero thermal transfer is a very precise state, so what happens to an ideal gas in an adiabatic change is also precise. It is that:

$$pV^\gamma = \text{a constant}$$

where γ is the ratio of the principal specific heats of the ideal gas, C_p/C_V; γ is a constant.

This equation provides an important relationship between p and V during the change. In addition, it can be used with the ideal gas equation $pV = nRT$, so that it also provides relationships between T and p and between T and V during the change. It is an example of an exceptionally useful result in physics, used by practising physicists who take for granted the derivation. We do not need to prove the equation here.

We have now looked at different changes of volume that can occur to an ideal gas: change of volume at constant pressure, change of volume at constant temperature and change of volume with no thermal transfer. These are compared on a pV diagram in Fig 14.11 for a decrease in volume from the same starting volume.

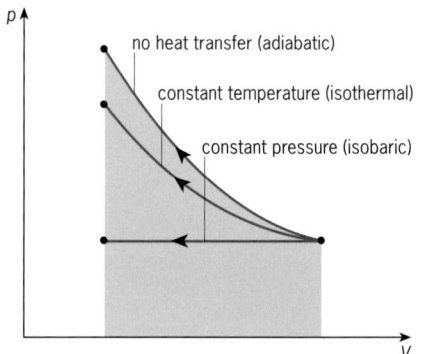

Fig 14.11 Decrease in volume of an ideal gas compared on a pV diagram for adiabatic, isothermal and constant pressure changes. Note that adiabatic changes are steeper on the pV diagrams than isothermal changes

3 THE SECOND LAW

We saw from the first law that the change of internal energy of a system is related to the sum of the energy transferred to it thermally and to the work done on the system. We have also seen how work can increase internal energy.

So far, we have avoided discussing how to transfer internal energy to work. We find that we can transfer *some* of the energy to work, *but not all of it*. This gives rise to the **second law of thermodynamics**. One of several alternative statements for the law is:

Version 1 of the second law
It is impossible for thermal energy to transfer from a high temperature source to do an amount of work equivalent to that amount of thermal energy.

The industrial importance of this version of the second law is immediately obvious. Coal, gas or oil is burnt in a boiler in a power station to provide large quantities of thermal energy. This energy is transferred to energy within turbines and finally to energy used in the home. It is not possible for all the energy from the fuel to be transferred completely into work via the turbines.

It is a consequence of the second law that some energy is transferred to a reservoir of energy at a lower temperature than the temperature of the boiler. This reservoir may be the surrounding atmosphere or the water in a cooling system such as a river. There is no way of avoiding this transfer of lost thermal energy. Engineers have put a lot of effort into designing more and more efficient engines to do work but, as we shall see, there is an efficiency limit that arises from the second law.

There is an important alternative statement of the law:

Version 2 of the second law
It is not possible to have a thermal transfer of energy from a colder to a hotter body without doing work.

If the law did not apply, it would be very easy to take thermal energy from our garden and use it to heat the house in winter, and to do this without limit. We *can* transfer energy from a colder to a hotter body (or reservoir) but it is necessary to do some work. Both refrigerators and heat pumps do this.

4 HEAT ENGINES

THE INTERNAL COMBUSTION ENGINE
Engines are designed to do work. The type of engine with which we are most familiar is the car engine, which uses the thermal energy produced by igniting petrol. It is called an **internal combustion engine** (See Fig 14.12).

Air and fuel are mixed during the intake stroke (Fig 14.13). After the intake valve is closed, the air and fuel mixture is compressed as the piston goes through the compression stage of the cycle. The spark plug ignites the mixture and this produces the expansion, which is the part of the cycle producing the power. Finally, spent gases are expelled through the engine's exhaust.

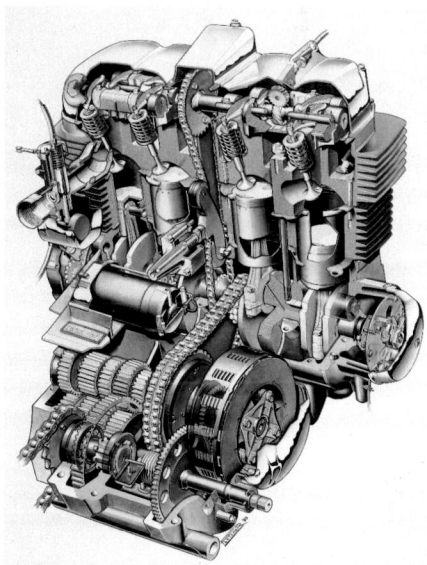

Fig 14.12 A Honda 750cc motorcycle engine – an example of an internal combustion engine

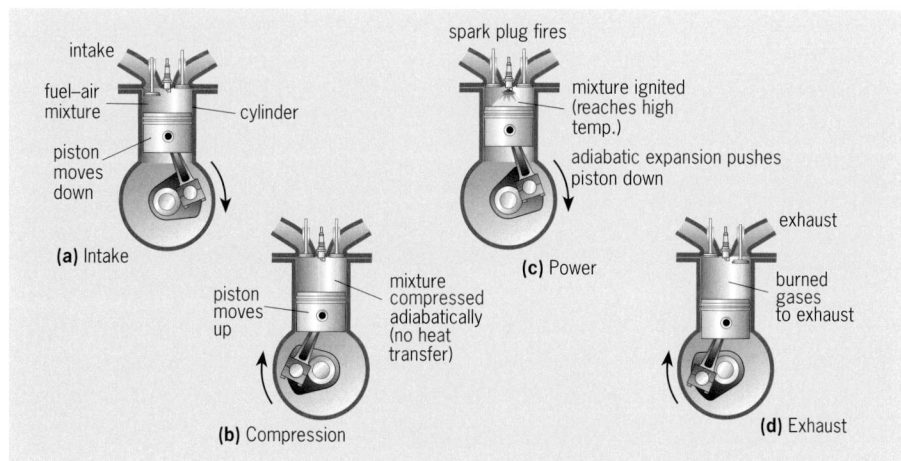

(a) Intake

(b) Compression

(c) Power

(d) Exhaust

Fig 14.13 The internal combustion engine. The up and down motion of the piston is converted to rotatory motion to drive the car or motorcycle

The motion is kept going by having a number of pistons connected together at different stages in the cycle. The straight-line piston motion becomes a rotation in the wheels.

The internal energy of the engine is unchanged at the end of the cycle compared with that at the beginning. However, energy is lost to the surroundings and in the exhaust gases. So the energy supplied thermally by igniting the petrol equals the work done plus the thermal losses that heat the surroundings. See Fig 14.16 on page 276.

Entropy – a way of describing disorder

The second law is fundamental to what is happening to the Universe and to the direction of time, and is related to a measure of disorder called **entropy**.

Some events cannot go backwards in real life. They are events in which disorder sets in. For instance, a waiter drops a stack of plates and they shatter: you know that shattered plates cannot rise up and reassemble themselves in the waiter's hands (Fig 14.14).

As the Universe develops, the ordering of its constituents gets less and less. The second law may also be expressed as:

Version 3 of the second law
It is not possible to have a process in which there is an overall decrease in the entropy of the Universe.

From our everyday experience we know that some changes can occur and others cannot.

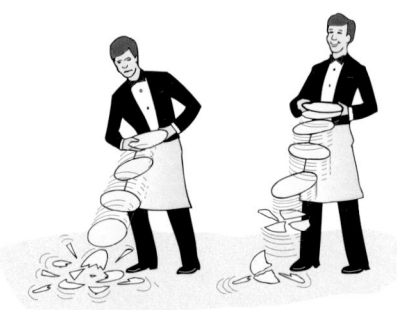

Fig 14.14 Some events happen in everyday life; others do not

We can understand why some events are so unlikely as to be impossible, by considering arrangements of molecules in a container. First, let us imagine a few molecules of a gas held in one half of the container by a partition. We then see what happens when we remove the partition. The molecules move around rapidly and very soon disperse throughout the container (Fig 14.15).

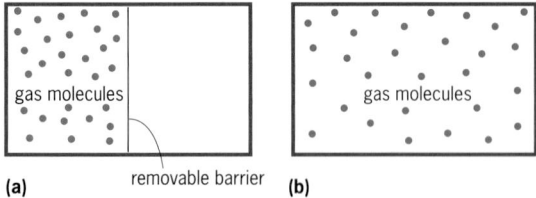

gas molecules   gas molecules

(a)   removable barrier   **(b)**

Fig 14.15 Molecules of a gas in one half of a container **(a)** rapidly diffuse throughout the container **(b)** when the central barrier is removed

In the laboratory we can demonstrate this effect with a coloured gas such as bromine.

As they move around, the molecules will on average spend half their time on one side of the container, half the time on the other. What is obvious is the extreme unlikelihood of the molecules all simultaneously returning to the original side. Let us use some numbers to try and see why this is so.

Suppose we start with 10 molecules only.

- When the molecules have had a chance to spread out, each molecule has a 50 per cent chance of being on the left side, that is, probability 1/2.
- For all the molecules to exist on the left-hand side there is a probability of:

$$\tfrac{1}{2} \times \tfrac{1}{2} \times \tfrac{1}{2} \times \tfrac{1}{2} \times \tfrac{1}{2} \times \tfrac{1}{2} \times \tfrac{1}{2} \times \tfrac{1}{2} \times \tfrac{1}{2} \times \tfrac{1}{2} \text{ or } \left(\tfrac{1}{2}\right)^{10}$$

This is 1 in 1024 – not a likely event, but one that can easily happen for a brief moment as the molecules speed around.

- But now suppose we increase the number of molecules to 10^{23} (less than the Avogadro number). We replace the 10 as used previously by 10^{23}. The chance of all the molecules being on the left-hand side becomes:

$$\left(\tfrac{1}{2}\right)^{10^{23}} \text{ or 1 in } 1024^{22} \text{ or 1 in } 1.7 \times 10^{66}$$

(To show that $1024^{22} = 1.7 \times 10^{66}$, use the x^y key on your calculator.)

? QUESTION 4

4   Show that $\left(\tfrac{1}{2}\right)^{10^{23}}$ is the same as 1 in 1024^{22}.

The likelihood of all the molecules being on the left side is therefore very small indeed:

- Suppose we want all the molecules to exist on the one side for a time t.
- For this to happen for total time t, there must be a time of $1.7 \times 10^{66}t$ when the molecules are dispersed on both sides.
- On average, we expect to wait for half of this time before a given situation occurs.
- So we can expect to have to wait for a time of the order of magnitude $10^{66}t$ for the atoms to all be on the left side.
- So for all the molecules to exist on the left side for a time t of one microsecond we must wait $(10^{66} \times 10^{-6})$ seconds or approximately 10^{60} seconds. This is over 3×10^{52} years, which is many billions of times longer than the age of the Universe.

All this arises because there are approximately 1.7×10^{66} ways of arranging the molecules between the two sides of the container. For all of them to be on one particular side is one special arrangement.

Relation between entropy and number of arrangements

We say that entropy is a measure of the number of ways in which a system can exist. Whereas there is only one way of choosing all the molecules to be on one side, there are many ways in which we can select out half the molecules to exist in one half of the container, leaving the remainder in the other half. So a distribution with the molecules arranged either side of the barrier has a high entropy (lots of ways of choosing the molecules), and all molecules on one side has a low entropy (one way).

This was understood by Boltzmann, and the idea was developed much later by Planck. It became known as the **Boltzmann–Planck hypothesis**, expressed as:

$$S = k \ln W$$

where W is the number of ways in which an arrangement can be set up (for instance an arrangement of molecules in a box), k is the Boltzmann constant and S is the value of the entropy measured in the same units as k (that is, J K^{-1}).

As a system becomes more disordered, there is an increase in the number of ways its molecules or components can be arranged; the equation shows directly how the entropy increases. The equation eventually made an important contribution to quantum theory, which is covered in Chapter 16.

Life on Earth and entropy

At this point, you might wonder about the implications of entropy for biological life and its complexity. For instance, DNA is a very complex, ordered biological molecule, built from atoms and molecules that were arranged in a more random way. This seems to represent a reverse of the process of increasing entropy. Is it an example of overall negative entropy?

Certainly there is a local decrease in entropy as the arrangement of a biological molecule builds up. However, the entropy version of the second law makes it clear that there must be an overall increase in entropy of the molecule's universe – its surroundings. So where exactly is the expected increase in entropy, an increase that should more than balance the local biological decrease?

On the wide scale, a rapid increase in entropy is taking place in the Sun, the source of energy that sustains Earth's life. The Sun's nuclear reactions produce huge amounts of thermal energy as random movements of particles and radiation. More locally, many biological processes involve a breakdown (reduction in complexity and order) in the material of their surroundings and, in so doing, give off thermal energy as a by-product.

It is rather as if the Sun and the Earth are acting as components of a heat engine (which is discussed next). Just as in a heat engine, so, in life processes, energy is dissipated and the overall entropy of the surroundings is increased.

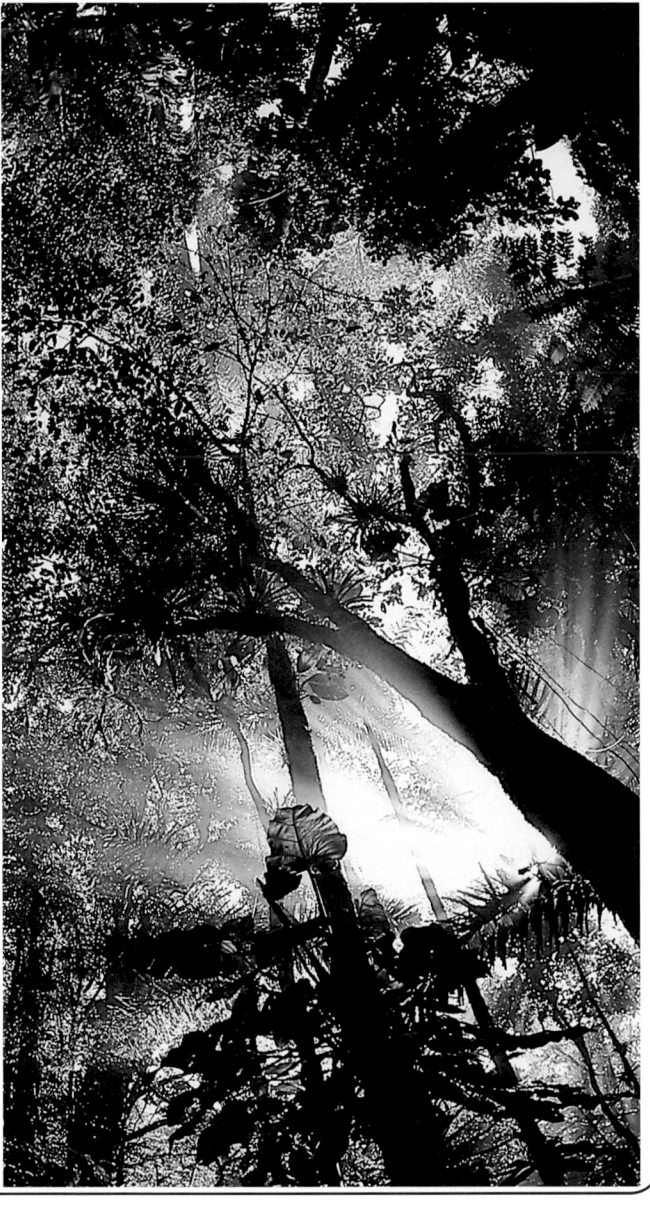

? QUESTION 5

5 Explain why living matter would be unable to develop on Earth without a source of energy arising from the formation of the Solar System.

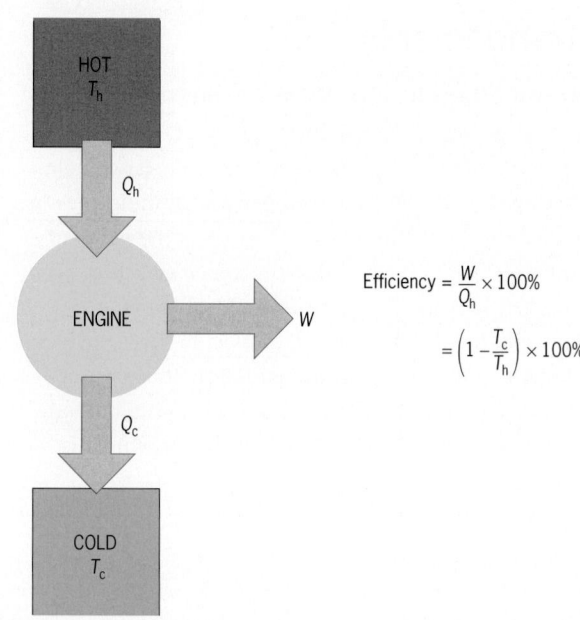

Fig 14.16 Schematic diagram of the energy transfer in a heat engine

$$\text{Efficiency} = \frac{W}{Q_h} \times 100\%$$

$$= \left(1 - \frac{T_c}{T_h}\right) \times 100\%$$

HEAT TRANSFER IS THE ENGINE

If Q_h = 'heat' input (from hot source), W = work done and Q_c = 'heat' output (thermal losses to cold sink), then:

$$\boldsymbol{Q_h = W + Q_c}$$

The amount of work done in a cycle equals the amount of energy actually used. However, it is not possible to do this work without a thermal loss of energy. That is, there must be a **thermal sink**. In Fig 14.16, we show transfer of energy thermally to a thermal sink.

THE CARNOT CYCLE

We can put together two isotherms and two adiabatics (the names given to the changes) to produce a closed cycle. This is called a Carnot cycle (Fig 14.17). In a closed cycle we finish at the same pressure, volume and temperature at which we started. The Carnot cycle is not the only cycle we can produce on a pV diagram, since we can also have changes at constant volume and constant pressure or other changes, as well as isothermal and adiabatic changes. If we follow the cycle in the clockwise direction shown, we see that the gas does net work on its surroundings equal to the area enclosed by the cycle. This is similar to finding the work done in Fig 14.6 by taking a series of strips of area $p\Delta V$ but here the strips go from a lower pressure to a higher pressure such that each strip has an area of $(p_{\text{higher}} - p_{\text{lower}})\Delta V$.

THE CARNOT ENGINE

Thermodynamics limits the amount of work that can be extracted between the hot source and the cold sink. An engine operating using the Carnot cycle (Fig 14.17) consisting of two adiabatics and two isothermals is the most efficient engine possible. It has an important feature: it can be operated in reverse. It is called a Carnot engine and is the standard by which other engines are compared. A Carnot engine cannot actually exist – it is just an imaginary ideal engine in which there are no energy losses, such as through friction and conduction.

The Carnot cycle is a special case of a **reversible cycle**. All ideal engines using a reversible cycle and working between the same two temperatures have the same efficiency, but the Carnot engine uses the simplest reversible cycle. Real engines do not use reversible cycles and so have a much lower efficiency.

The temperatures of the hot source and cold sink are crucial to the amount of work that can be extracted. We might expect this as we know from everyday experience that when engineers are designing an internal combustion engine or the operation of the turbines of a power station they try to achieve high temperatures on the input side.

It turns out that we can define the source temperature T_h and the sink temperature T_c in terms of the ratio of the thermal energies Q_h and Q_c transferred:

$$\frac{T_h}{T_c} = \frac{Q_h}{Q_c}$$

Note that the temperatures T_h and T_c are measured on the Kelvin scale – this is *very important*. Although we cannot go into details here, this relationship between the temperatures and energy inputs and outputs can be used for defining the thermodynamic scale of temperature, and the scale agrees completely with the scale defined by using a constant-volume gas thermometer and the triple point.

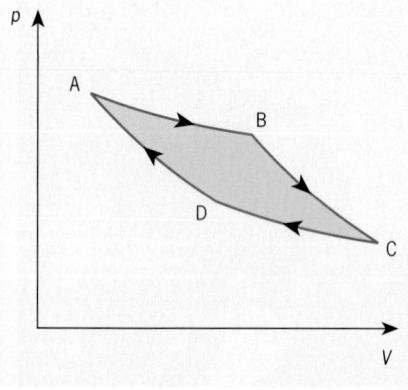

Fig 14.17 The Carnot cycle for an ideal gas consisting of two isotherms AB and CD and two adiabatics BC and DA

? QUESTION 6

6 Devise closed cycles on a pV diagram using isothermal, adiabatic, constant-pressure or constant-volume changes. Restrict yourself to either three or four sides for your cycles. Even with this restriction, there are a number of possibilities.

THE DIESEL ENGINE

The Diesel engine is similar to the internal combustion engine but there is no fuel in the cylinder at the beginning of the compression. Air is taken into the cylinder during an intake stroke AB (see Fig 14.18). When this point is reached, the inlet valve is closed. The air in the cylinder is next compressed adiabatically along BC such that there is a large compression ratio. This means that the volume at C is very small compared with that at B (more so than can be shown in Fig 14.18). This produces a high temperature at C. Fuel is sprayed into the cylinder at C and ignites because of this high temperature. The input of fuel can be carefully controlled such that there is an expansion CD at constant pressure (that is there is an isobaric expansion). Injection of fuel now stops and the cylinder continues to move such that there is an adiabatic expansion to E. The cylinder has at this stage moved fully, a valve opens, and the pressure immediately drops. This corresponds to returning to point B on the pV diagram. This is followed by an exhaust stroke of the cylinder back along BA to drive out the gases in the cylinder such that the cycle can begin again.

The higher efficiency of the Diesel engine compared with the internal combustion engine arises from the large compression ratio which can be typically as high as 20. However, even a Diesel engine cannot match the efficiency of the ideal, but hypothetical, Carnot engine.

EFFICIENCY

The **efficiency** of an engine is defined by:

$$\frac{\text{the work done by the engine}}{\text{the energy supplied by the engine}} \times 100\%$$

which we can express as:

$$\frac{W}{Q_h} \times 100\%$$

But the work done is the difference between the energy supplied and the energy given to the sink (conservation of energy), that is, $Q_h - Q_c$. So the efficiency of the engine is given by:

$$\frac{Q_h - Q_c}{Q_h} \times 100\% = \left(1 - \frac{Q_c}{Q_h}\right) \times 100\%$$

For an ideal reversible cycle such as a Carnot cycle this equals

$$= \left(1 - \frac{T_c}{T_h}\right) \times 100\%$$

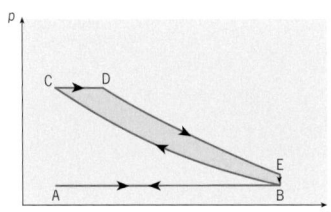

Fig 14.18 pV diagram for the Diesel cycle

 REMEMBER THIS

The Carnot cycle is a special case of a reversible cycle. All engines operating reversibly between the same two temperatures for source and sink have the same efficiency. This is referred to as **Carnot's theorem**.

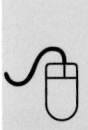

For more information on how to work out energies and efficiencies using a pV diagram and a graphical method please see the How Science Works assignment for this chapter at www.collinseducation.co.uk/CAS

? QUESTION 7

7   Internal combustion engines operate at high input and exhaust temperatures. Calculate the efficiency of an engine operating between 3000 °C and 1000 °C. How might the efficiency of the engine be improved? Why is 100 per cent efficiency not attainable?

SCIENCE
IN CONTEXT

EXAMPLE

Q A power station uses superheated steam (at high pressure) at approximately 500 °C. The cold sink corresponds to the temperature at which steam condenses at atmospheric pressure, that is, 100 °C. What is the maximum theoretical efficiency for the power station?

A Using the equation for the efficiency of an ideal cycle:

$$\text{efficiency} = \left(1 - \frac{T_c}{T_h}\right) \times 100\%$$

$$= \left(1 - \frac{373}{773}\right) \times 100\%$$

$$= (1 - 0.48) \times 100\%$$
$$= 52\%$$

SCIENCE
IN CONTEXT

Real engines

From the thermodynamics we can see that it is nowhere near possible to get 100% efficiency from an engine. But so far we have taken no account of the mechanical inefficiency of the engine itself. Modern technology has been gradually improving efficiencies but no engine can be produced with zero friction.

The nominal input power is given by

rate of fuel flow × calorific value of the fuel

On the other hand, the power we would obtain thermodynamically is given by

area contained within one *pV* loop × number of cycles per second × number of cylinders making the loops

Obviously an amount of work *pV* is done *every cycle* if there are no losses and most engines have a number of cylinders (four or six are common in car petrol engines).

The *actual* output power is often measured by the torque *T* that can be produced at angular frequency *ω* multiplied by this frequency *ω*, i.e. *Tω*, and is called brake power. (*Tω* is equivalent to a force multiplied by a distance divided by a time, which is power. The power brake consisting of a belt wrapped around a flywheel under tension *T* was invented by Lord Kelvin.)

The lost power or friction power is then

(thermodynamic power calculated) – (brake power)

REFRIGERATORS AND HEAT PUMPS

We mentioned that a Carnot engine is reversible. In real life, we operate cycles reversibly to remove energy from a cold source and get rid of this energy at a higher temperature. **Refrigerators** and freezers do this (Figs 14.19(a), (b)). Here the cooling cycle involves the evaporation of a low boiling point liquid in the refrigerator. The energy for this evaporation comes from the internal energy of the contents of the refrigerator, but we need a source of work.

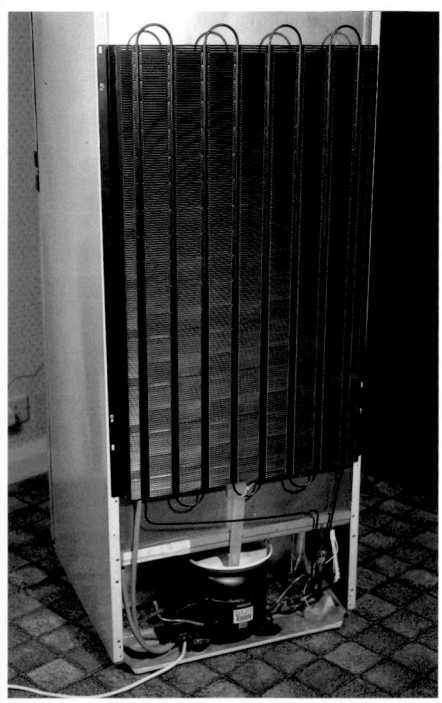

Fig 14.19 (a) The back of a domestic refrigerator, showing the compressor at the bottom, and the looped pipe in which the refrigerant circulates

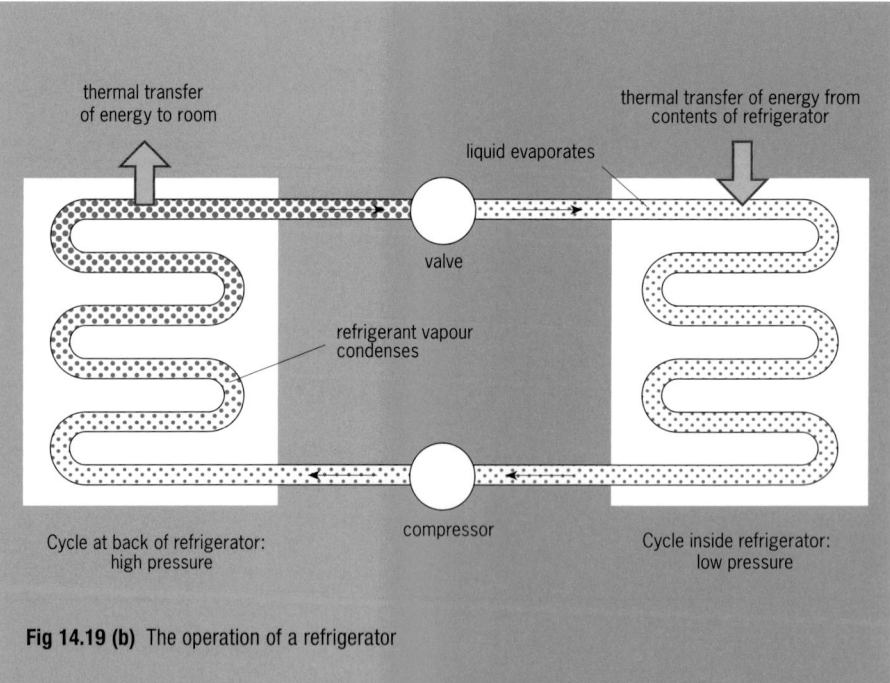

Fig 14.19 (b) The operation of a refrigerator

The vapour is condensed using a compressor. This compressor, of course, does work using energy from the electrical mains. As the vapour is compressed and condensed, it gets hotter and loses (dissipates) its energy thermally through a long metal pipe at the back of the refrigerator. So, overall, internal energy extracted from the food is dissipated by the element which becomes warm at the rear of the cabinet. Hence, a refrigerator will warm the room it is in.

We show the energy transfer in a refrigerator in Fig 14.20(a) in the same way as we did for the heat engine. The efficiency, or more appropriately the

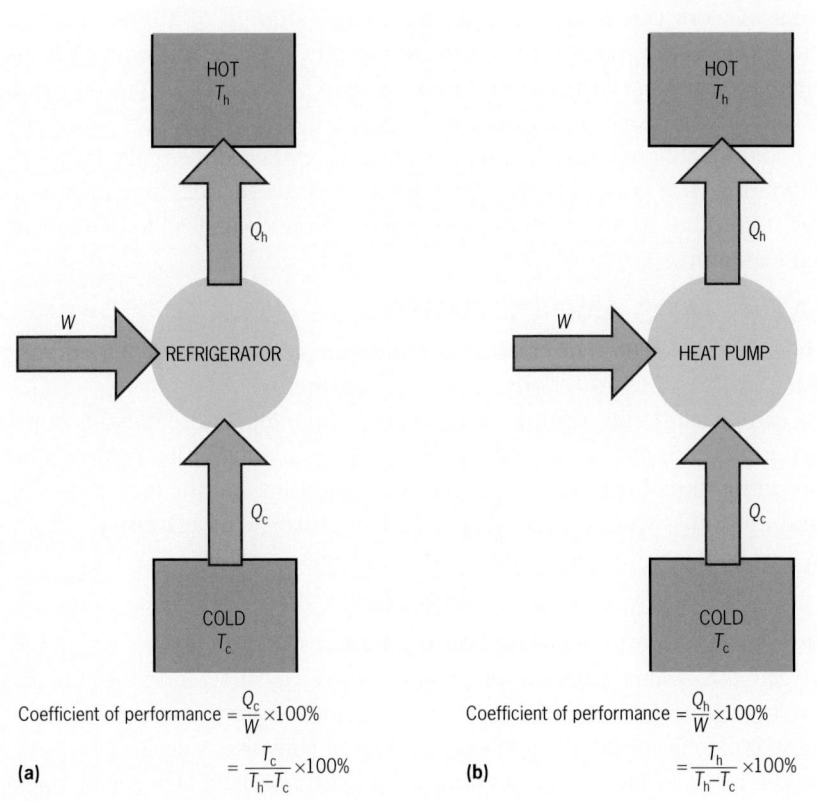

Coefficient of performance $= \dfrac{Q_c}{W} \times 100\%$

(a) $\qquad\qquad = \dfrac{T_c}{T_h - T_c} \times 100\%$

Coefficient of performance $= \dfrac{Q_h}{W} \times 100\%$

(b) $\qquad\qquad = \dfrac{T_h}{T_h - T_c} \times 100\%$

Fig 14.20 The energy transfer in **(a)** a refrigerator and **(b)** a heat pump

coefficient of performance, as values can be greater than 100 per cent, is defined by:

$$\frac{\text{energy extracted from the cold source}}{\text{work done by the compressor}} = \frac{Q_c}{W} \times 100\%$$

$$= \frac{Q_c}{\left(Q_h - Q_c\right)} \times 100\%$$

$$= \frac{T_c}{\left(T_h - T_c\right)} \times 100\%$$

(Again the temperature relationship refers to an engine operating reversibly, such as one with a Carnot cycle.)

A **heat pump**, as shown in Fig 14.20(b), operates in a similar way to a refrigerator by extracting energy thermally from a cold source such as a river and delivering it into a body such as a house at a higher temperature. Here we are interested in the amount of internal energy added to the house rather than the amount extracted from the river, so we define the percentage coefficient of performance by:

$$\frac{\text{energy added to the hotter body}}{\text{work done by the pump}} = \frac{Q_h}{W} \times 100\%$$

$$= \frac{Q_h}{\left(Q_h - Q_c\right)} \times 100\%$$

$$= \frac{T_h}{\left(T_h - T_c\right)} \times 100\%$$

(again assuming an ideal reversible cycle)

> **? QUESTION 8**
>
> 8 Obtain appropriate temperatures found in a typical kitchen and in a kitchen refrigerator, and estimate the theoretical coefficient of performance of the refrigerator.

On the basis of this equation, heat pumps look very attractive. A small amount of work can be used to transfer a large amount of thermal energy. In practice, real heat pumps turn out to have a much lower efficiency than the efficiency of an ideal heat pump based on the Carnot cycle. Heat pumps also have high capital cost, partly because they are not made in large numbers.

In addition, although energy can be continually extracted thermally from a neighbouring river (assuming the river does not freeze up), extracting internal energy from other sources such as neighbouring ground can lead to permanent frozen conditions.

HEAT PUMPS AND ENTROPY

We have already seen that entropy is a measure of disorder. When energy is transferred thermally to a body, this increases the disorder.

We can measure the entropy change best if the temperature remains constant. For example, suppose we add energy thermally to a solid at its melting point. The resulting liquid is more disordered than the solid and the molecules move around randomly with a range of speeds. The **change of entropy** ΔS can be shown to be related to the change of thermal energy ΔQ by:

$$\Delta S = \Delta Q/T$$

where T is temperature measured on the Kelvin scale.

We can also assume constant temperature when we extract from, or put energy into, a large reservoir. When the temperature is not constant, working out the entropy change becomes more difficult (and usually involves calculus).

We can consider the change of entropy that occurs when a heat engine operates. Here we can assume that the hot source and the cold sink remain at constant temperature. See the Example below.

EXAMPLE

Q A heat engine operates between 373 K and 300 K and has an efficiency of 18 per cent. What is the change of entropy when work of 1000 J is done by the engine?

A First we find the transfer of energy from the hot source.

1000 J of work is done with 18 per cent efficiency. Therefore, $(100/18 \times 1000)$ J must be transferred from the hot source. That is:

$Q_1 = 5560$ J

Loss of entropy of the hot source
   $= Q_1/T$
   $= 5560/373$ J K^{-1}
   $= 14.9$ J K^{-1}

Gain of energy by the heat sink
   $= Q_2 = Q_1 - W$
   $= (5560 - 1000)$ J
   $= 4560$ J

Gain of entropy of the heat sink
   $= Q_2/T$
   $= 4560/273$ J K^{-1}
   $= 16.7$ J K^{-1}

Net change in entropy $= 1.8$ J K^{-1}

As we have come to expect, there is a net increase in entropy.

---

5 POSTSCRIPT – THE THIRD LAW

There is a third law of thermodynamics. It states:

The entropy of a system approaches a constant value (zero in a simple system) as the temperature approaches absolute zero.

To achieve zero temperature requires an infinite number of steps – we have to extract a bit of energy, and a bit more, and a bit more and so on. A practical statement of the law is:

It is impossible to achieve absolute zero temperature for a system by a finite number of steps.

At the start of this chapter we saw that a temperature less than 1 billionth of a kelvin has been reached. This statement of the third law tells us that we shall never get to 0 K.

SUMMARY

After studying this chapter you should be able to:
- Provide a statement of the zeroth law and indicate its application to temperature measurement.
- Provide a statement of the first law and apply the equation $\Delta U = \Delta Q + \Delta W$.
- Carry out calculations for isothermal (constant temperature) and isobaric (constant pressure) changes of an ideal gas.
- Use the relationship between C_V and C_p for an ideal gas in calculations.
- Use the relationship $pV^\gamma = $ constant in calculations for an adiabatic change of volume of an ideal gas.

- Provide a statement of the second law and explain its importance.
- Have an understanding of the concept of entropy, $S = k \ln W$, and change of entropy, $\Delta S = \Delta Q/T$, and calculate ΔS values for simple applications.
- Understand the principles underlying heat engines, refrigerators and heat pumps and carry out simple calculations, including those for efficiencies (or coefficients of performance).

 Practice questions for this chapter are available at www.collinseducation.co.uk/CAS

15

Electromagnetic radiation

15 ELECTROMAGNETIC RADIATION

A healing light

Life on Earth depends on one chemical in particular – chlorophyll. It can interact with red light in sunlight; in a photochemical reaction, its electrons become more energetic. A chain of reactions forms sugar from water and carbon dioxide in the surroundings, with oxygen as a useful by-product.

A photochemical reaction is now being applied to the treatment of cancers, in a procedure called photodynamic therapy (PDT). Its key process parallels the action of chlorophyll. A patient is given a harmless drug designed to build up in cancerous tissue. The drug is a small part of the very complex chlorophyll molecule and acts as a light-absorbing dye. Dyes absorb certain frequencies from white light directed at them, so the light they reflect lacks those frequencies, which is why a dye looks coloured: leaves look green because green light is, roughly, white minus the red.

In PDT, light comes from a laser tuned to a frequency absorbed by the drug. The laser produces a low-energy dose of red light which penetrates quite deeply into the body and causes no harm to ordinary tissue. The important thing is what happens to the energy carried by the absorbed radiation.

In typical laser treatment, absorbed radiation heats up target tissue enough to kill the cells, both ordinary and cancerous. In PDT, the less energetic radiation that the drug absorbs triggers a photochemical reaction which releases a poison consisting of single atoms of oxygen. In contrast to the harmless diatomic oxygen molecules we breathe from the air, single oxygen atoms are highly reactive and are able to kill living cells. Photodynamic therapy is effective because, since the poison only forms at the point where the dye accumulates, only the diseased cells are killed.

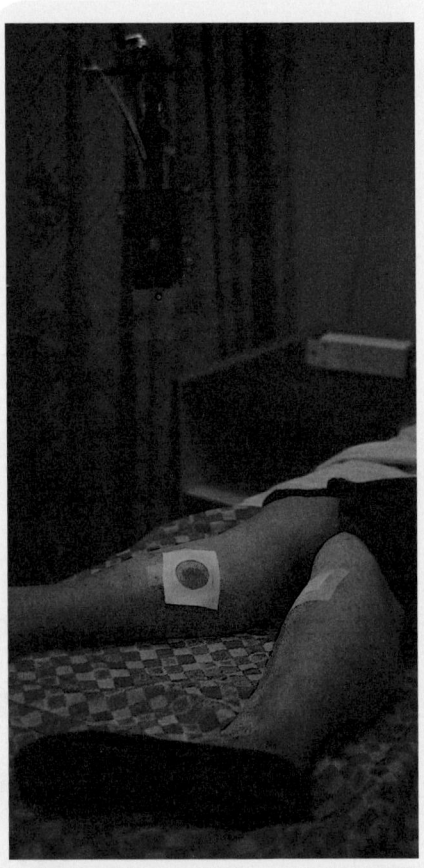

Photodynamic therapy treatment: the cancerous tissue in the patient's leg has accumulated the dye that is being illuminated with laser light. As a result, the cancer cells are killed

The ideas in this chapter

We can say that the Universe consists of matter – in one form or another – and electromagnetic radiation. Light is just one small part of the range of electromagnetic radiation that exists. It has just the right character to get through the Earth's atmosphere – a useful property that living things have taken advantage of. It is visible because our eyes are adapted to respond to it.

Electromagnetic radiation can fool us into thinking that it can be both a **wave** and a **particle**, though maybe not at the same time. The particle – **photon** – aspect of electromagnetic radiation is discussed in the next chapter, which deals with quantum theory; Chapter 24 also features the photon, as one of the family of particles making up the Universe of matter. This chapter covers the **wave** aspect of the range of radiations observed in the **electromagnetic spectrum**, their **speed** of propagation, how they are produced and detected, and how we make use of the wave nature of the radiations. So we deal here with **diffraction, interference** and **polarization**. (Chapter 21 covers the use of electromagnetic radiations as information carriers.)

1 THE ELECTROMAGNETIC SPECTRUM

A very hot object such as a star produces a range of radiation; the **spectrum** of the Sun is shown in Fig 15.1. **Visible light** is the tiny fraction that we detect with our eyes. White light can be separated into a range of colours to form a visible spectrum, from violet with a wavelength of about 4×10^{-7} m, to red of about 7×10^{-7} m (Fig 15.2).

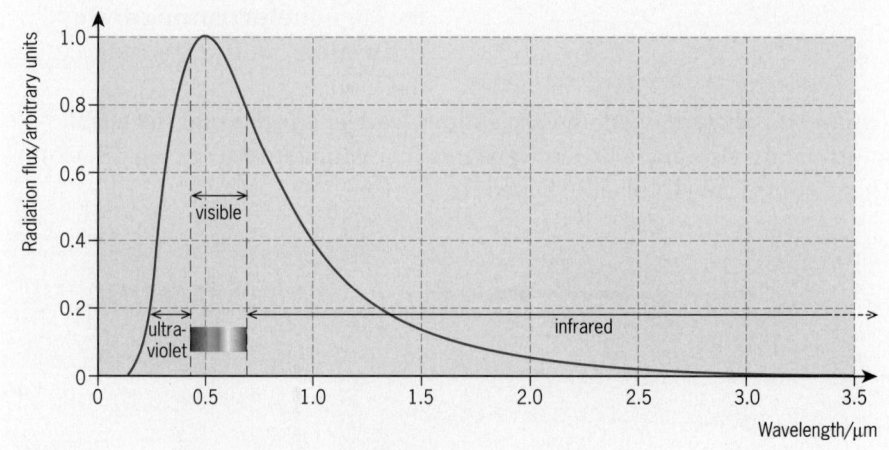

Fig 15.1 Graph showing the continuous spectrum of solar radiation

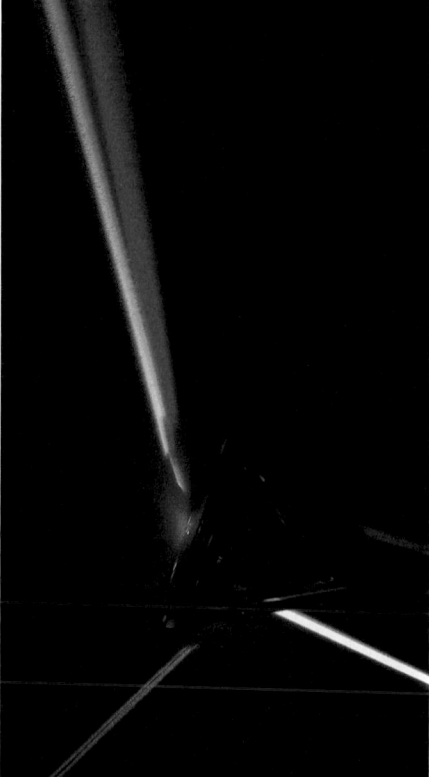

Fig 15.2 A prism splits white light into the colour spectrum that we can see

WHY 'ELECTROMAGNETIC'?

The radiations are produced and detected by the *acceleration* or *sudden movement of electrons* (or occasionally of other charged particles). For example, a **radio signal** is produced by electrons as they oscillate to and fro in an aerial, as in Fig 15.3. The result is an interlocked pair of fields, electric and magnetic, oscillating at the frequency of the electron current. We can think of the **electric field** as being produced by the *charge* on the electrons.

A **magnetic field** is produced whenever charges move, and is proportional to the size of the current (see Chapter 10).

What is surprising (and hard to explain) is that the interlocking fields move away from the aerial at a speed which in a vacuum is the same for all electromagnetic radiations, whatever their frequency. This is the **speed of light**, labelled with the standard symbol c. These moving fields *behave like waves*: they can be *diffracted*, they *interact* with each other to show *interference*, and they can be *polarised*. These terms are explained later.

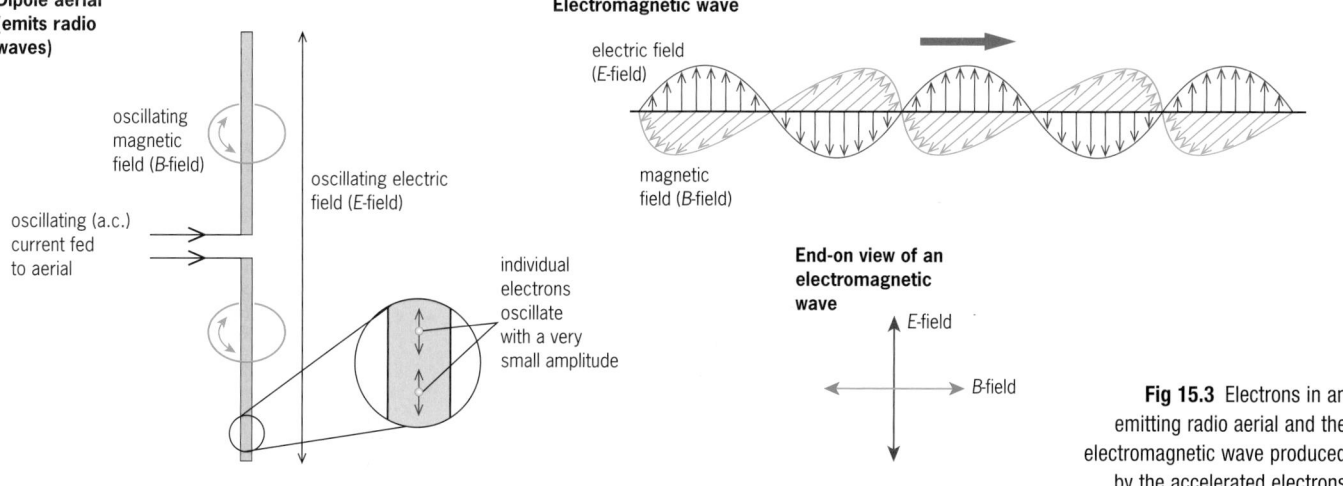

Fig 15.3 Electrons in an emitting radio aerial and the electromagnetic wave produced by the accelerated electrons

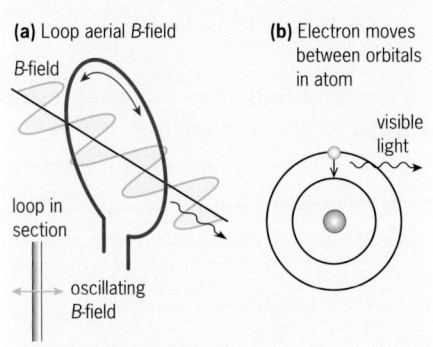

Fig 15.4 (a) A loop aerial detects electromagnetic waves because the varying *B*-field induces an electric current in the loop. **(b)** Electrons in atoms move from higher to lower energy orbits and produce light

(a) Loop aerial *B*-field
B-field
loop in section
oscillating *B*-field

(b) Electron moves between orbitals in atom
visible light

When the waves reach another metal rod, the electric field component exerts a varying *electric* force on the electrons in the metal which oscillate in time with the variations of the field. A loop-shaped metal aerial – as in Fig 15.4(a) – encloses the varying magnetic field of the waves and, by the laws of **electromagnetic induction**, an e.m.f. is induced in the loop.

Infrared radiation, light and the shorter wavelengths beyond the visible spectrum are also made by electrons moving within atoms, see Fig 15.4(b). There is more about this in Chapter 16.

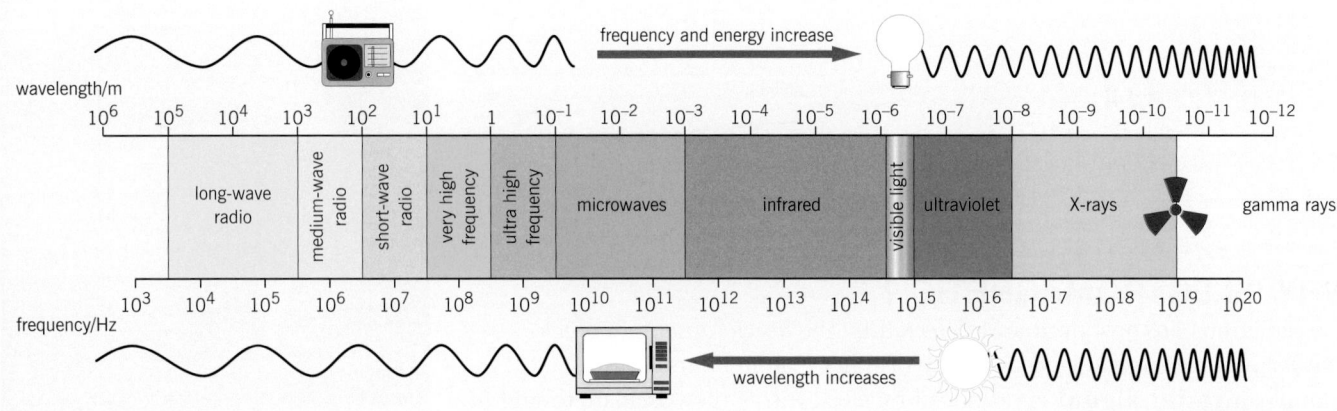

frequency and energy increase

wavelength/m
10^6 10^5 10^4 10^3 10^2 10^1 1 10^{-1} 10^{-2} 10^{-3} 10^{-4} 10^{-5} 10^{-6} 10^{-7} 10^{-8} 10^{-9} 10^{-10} 10^{-11} 10^{-12}

long-wave radio | medium-wave radio | short-wave radio | very high frequency | ultra high frequency | microwaves | infrared | visible light | ultraviolet | X-rays | gamma rays

frequency/Hz
10^3 10^4 10^5 10^6 10^7 10^8 10^9 10^{10} 10^{11} 10^{12} 10^{13} 10^{14} 10^{15} 10^{16} 10^{17} 10^{18} 10^{19} 10^{20}

wavelength increases

Fig 15.5 The electromagnetic spectrum

? QUESTION 1

1 How do the two common designs of TV aerials (loop and rod) support the idea that TV signals are somehow both electric and magnetic?

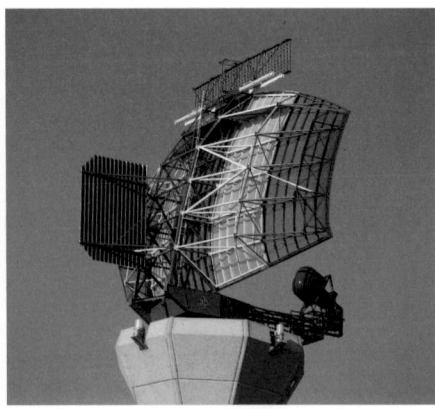

Fig 15.6 A radar aerial at Heathrow airport for ground–air control

PRODUCING AND DETECTING ELECTROMAGNETIC WAVES

Radio waves

Radio waves are produced by the *accelerated* motion of free electrons as explained above, and are used mainly in communication systems – see Chapter 21.

A process was developed in the 1930s to provide short-wavelength radio waves – **microwaves** – to help in the medical treatment of damaged tissue. Most school laboratories now have low power microwave sources for experiments on the nature of electromagnetic waves. Microwaves are still used in physiotherapy, as well as in cooking (see page 287) and as message carriers (see Chapter 21).

Radar

The potential of these very short radio waves for the **ra**dio **d**etection **a**nd **r**anging of aircraft in the Second World War was quickly exploited with the development of **radar**. In radar transmitters (Fig 15.6), electrons oscillate in small metal cavities called *magnetrons* which contain a strong magnetic field.

The waves produced have a frequency determined by the size of the cavity and the strength of the magnetic field, depending on how long it takes an electron to complete an oscillation. The waves are led out of the cavity through a metal tube called a *waveguide*. The metal walls reflect the waves and keep them moving in the right direction, towards a small aerial at the focus of a metal mirror. They are then emitted as a beam. The transmitting aerial and mirror can also act as the main *receivers* of the radiation, with a detector at the focus.

Microwave ovens

Similar magnetrons are used in **microwave ovens**. The frequency of the microwaves is selected to match the resonance frequency of water molecules so that energy from the waves is transferred efficiently to the kinetic energy of the molecules. This raises the temperature of any food containing water.

Infrared radiation

Infrared radiation (IR) overlaps with short microwaves in the electromagnetic spectrum (Fig 15.5), but in practice the term describes the (invisible) hot body emissions that have wavelengths just beyond the visible red. Infrared is readily absorbed by matter, by giving its energy to cause movement in the molecules of a body, thus raising the body's temperature. This is why IR is often called 'heat rays' or **thermal radiation**.

Being sensitive to near (i.e. short wavelength) infrared, the human skin is a simple detector – we feel the 'heat'. A thermometer with a blackened bulb (or sensor surface) will show a rise in temperature when placed in the red region of a white-light spectrum. But it shows a greater temperature rise when placed in the dark region just outside the red – as was first shown in 1800 by the astronomer Sir William Herschel (Germany/Britain, 1738–1822).

Special film takes photographs in infrared, but is difficult to use and has largely been replaced by electronic detecting methods. Modern infrared detectors use solid state (electronic) detectors which act rather like TV cameras. In industry, they monitor processes that cause temperature differences. They are used in Earth satellites both for military purposes and to observe the growth of crops, measure surface temperature, etc. (see page 55). Infrared detectors can be made sensitive to a narrow wavelength band: in the rescue cameras used to find fire or earthquake victims, the detectors are most sensitive to the infrared radiation that is characteristic of body temperature (see Fig 15.7).

Electronic devices (e.g. semiconductor light-emitting diodes) also emit infrared, and are widely used in the remote controls of household electronic systems such as TV sets, DVD players/recorders and hi-fi systems.

Light

Light is emitted from matter when it is made hot enough – as in the Sun, in flames and in filament lamps. It is also emitted in certain chemical changes – in the **photoluminescence** of fireflies and glow worms, for example – and as a result of electron movements in stimulated atoms – as in lasers and ordinary fluorescent lighting. Visible radiation is detected by both human and animal eyes and also by a range of devices including ordinary photographic film, photoelectric cells of various types and by very sensitive 'charge-coupled devices' (CCDs). There is more about light-sensitive devices and the control of light in Chapter 18.

> **? QUESTION 2**
>
> 2 Suggest reasons why
> **a)** food in metal containers cannot be cooked in a microwave oven;
> **b)** an empty glass or plastic container doesn't get hot in a microwave oven.

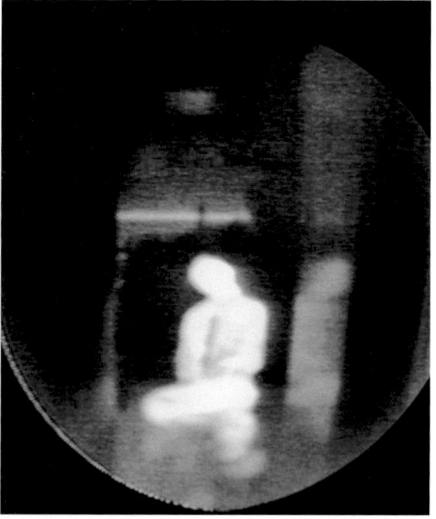

Fig 15.7 Left: Rescuers using body-sensing equipment
Right: The infrared image of a disaster victim

Short wave and ionising radiation

Ultraviolet radiation (UV) is produced by changes in the energy levels of atomic electrons, as we shall see below, which happens in very hot bodies. UV was discovered during early photochemical experiments in which it was found that light blackened silver chloride. Studying the effects of a spectrum of white light in 1801 Johann Ritter (Germany, 1776–1810) found that a type of radiation beyond violet in the visible spectrum had even more effect on silver chloride than visible light. As explained below, the *shorter* the *wavelength*, the *more energetic* the *radiation*, so UV is very effective at exposing photographic film. UV is good at making chemicals called *phosphors* glow, and low-intensity UV is used for special stage effects. Ordinary fluorescent ('daylight') tubes and compact ('low-energy') lamps emit light from a phosphor coating, stimulated by UV light from excited mercury atoms (Fig 15.8). UV is also energetic enough to ionise atoms and so can harm living tissue, causing sunburn and skin cancers.

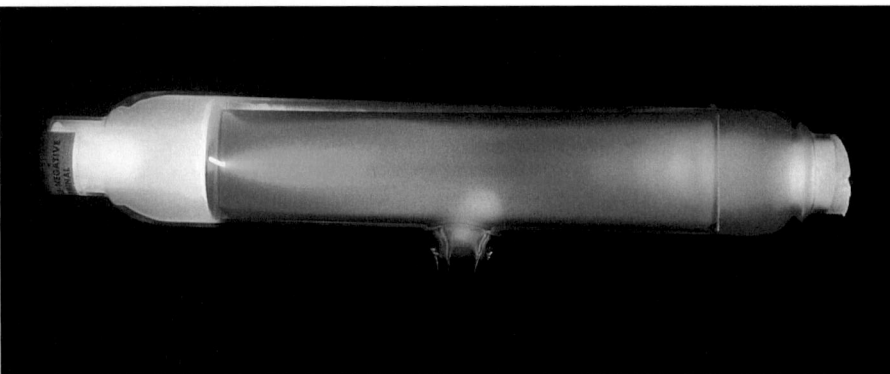

Fig 15.8 In fluorescent tubes UV from mercury atoms makes a phosphor coating glow

X-rays have shorter wavelengths than ultraviolet. They are produced when electrons decelerate very rapidly, such as when high-speed electrons are stopped by colliding with a metal target. They were first discovered, accidentally, by William Röntgen (Germany, 1845–1923). He was experimenting with cathode rays (electron streams in an evacuated tube) and noticed that they caused a phosphor screen some metres away to glow. He soon found that the rays could pass through soft tissue but were selectively absorbed by denser material such as metal and bone. Within weeks of the discovery, X-rays were being used in hospitals for diagnosis and treatment – rather too soon and too dangerously.

Nowadays carefully monitored doses of X-rays are used for medical diagnosis (see Chapter 19). They are also used to inspect metal objects for flaws, and they have played a significant role in the science of X-ray crystallography which, amongst other things, led to the discovery of the helical structure of DNA.

Gamma (γ) radiation is produced by changes in the internal energy of an atomic nucleus in radioactive decay (see Chapter 17). Gamma rays are very energetic and penetrating: photographic film and ionisation detectors such as Geiger counters will detect them.

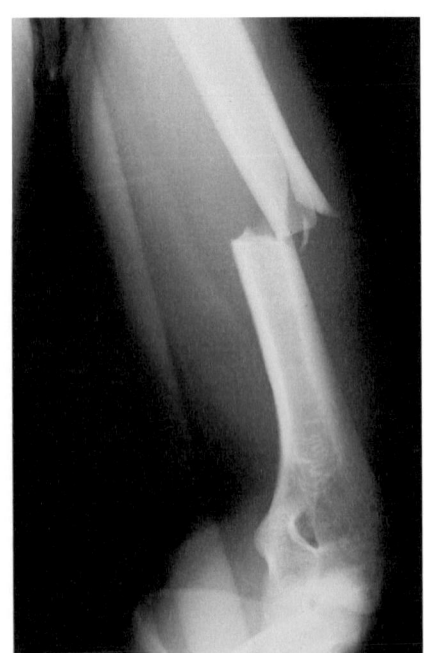

Fig 15.9 X-ray image of a broken arm bone

Damage caused by ionising radiation

Because of the high energy associated with photons of such short wavelength radiation, UV, X- and gamma radiation can all damage living tissue. These radiations **ionise** atoms and molecules in living cells and disrupt their biochemical processes. The cells may die, or worse, they may become cancerous. Small changes to the DNA in sperm or ovum cells are particularly dangerous since they may cause *genetic mutations* to appear in offspring.

2 THE CHARACTERISTICS OF AN ELECTROMAGNETIC WAVE

Electromagnetic waves have a frequency f and a wavelength λ related by the simple wave formula:

$$c = f\lambda$$

The amplitude of the wave is measured by either its electric or its magnetic component, depending on the instrument used. As with all waves, the energy carried by the wave is proportional to the square of the amplitude. As we shall see in the next chapter, when radiation has a wavelength of comparable size to atoms and molecules, we need to think of the energy as being carried as packets or **quanta**, in the form of particles or **photons**.

THE SPEED OF ELECTROMAGNETIC WAVES

The speed of electromagnetic waves travelling in a vacuum is the same for all frequencies and is defined as

$$c = 2.997\,924\,58 \times 10^8 \text{ m s}^{-1} \text{ exactly}$$

In 1983 it was found that measurements using radio waves gave the best results and the speed of light was defined at this value. The same year, this value was confirmed by a very careful experiment using a stabilised laser working with red light. It no longer makes sense to measure the 'speed of light' (see page 4).

What decides the speed of electromagnetic waves?

In 1864, James Clerk Maxwell was considering the speed of the alternating electric and magnetic fields that define an electromagnetic wave. From theory, he worked out that the speed of these fields is determined by the electric and magnetic constants of the medium in which the waves travel. These are the **force constants** ε and μ (see pages 201 and 211).

In a vacuum, the electric field (force) constant is ε_0 and is called the **permittivity of a vacuum**. If one charged particle is moving relative to the other, there is an additional force on both particles, the *magnetic* force. The magnetic field (force) constant for a vacuum is μ_0 and is called the **permeability of a vacuum** (see page 212). Air is near enough a vacuum for everyday calculations. Maxwell was able to prove from

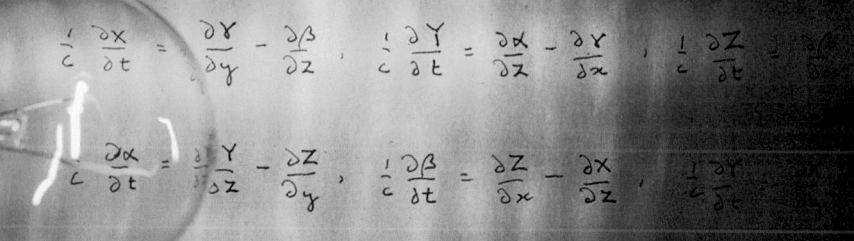

theory both that electromagnetic waves other than light should exist, and also that the speed of all such waves in empty space is given by the Maxwell formula:

$$c = \left(\varepsilon_0\mu_0\right)^{-\frac{1}{2}} \text{ or } c^2\varepsilon_0\mu_0 = 1$$

In a vacuum, the constants have the values:

$\mu_0 = 4\pi \times 10^{-7}$ H m^{-1}
(by theoretical definition)

$\varepsilon_0 = 8.854\,187\,82(7) \times 10^{-12}$ F m^{-1}
(calculated from c and μ_0)

? QUESTION 3

3   Use the Maxwell formula to check that these values agree with the value for c quoted above.

Fig 15.10(a) Some of Maxwell's equations as he recorded them

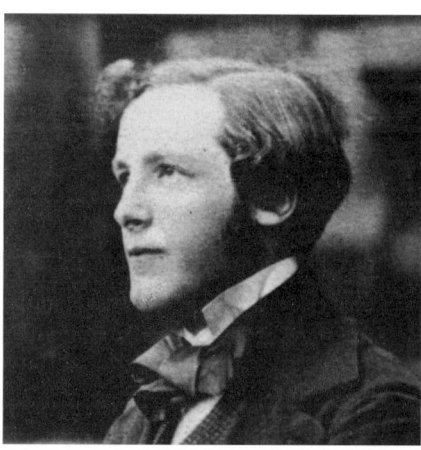

Fig 15.10(b) The Scottish physicist James Clerk Maxwell (1831–1879) whose equations brought together electricity and magnetism

ELECTROMAGNETIC WAVES IN MATTER

The speed of electromagnetic waves is a maximum in a vacuum and less in materials which are 'transparent' to the waves. As a general rule, electromagnetic waves cannot travel at all through 'opaque' materials containing free electrons (e.g. metals) as the waves lose so much energy to the electrons. *Bound* charged particles (including electrons) may also absorb energy from the waves, but do so at definite frequencies or bands of frequencies that depend on the atoms or molecules of the medium. Fig 15.11 shows, for example, that the transparency of the Earth's atmosphere varies in different regions of the electromagnetic spectrum.

Fig 15.11(a) The atmosphere acts as a filter for some electromagnetic frequencies. Radiation reaches the Earth's surface in two main bands: optical (with some UV and IR) and short-wave radio. There are also a few narrow windows in the near infrared and sub-millimetre microwave bands

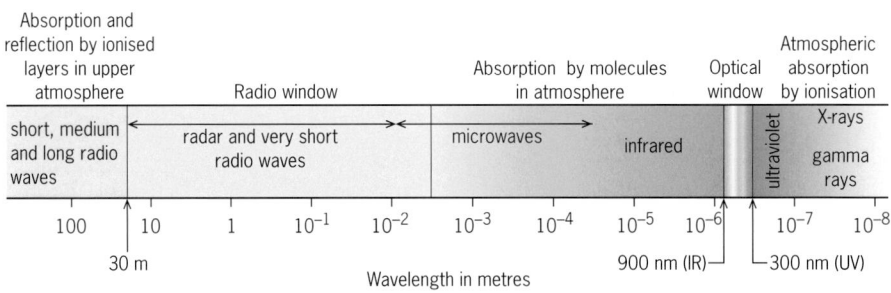

(a) Waves parallel to boundary

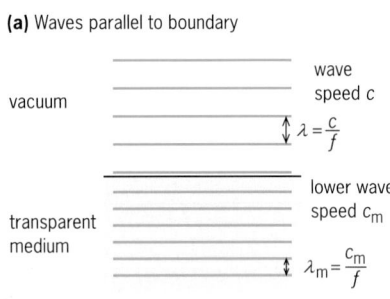

(b) Waves cross boundary at an angle

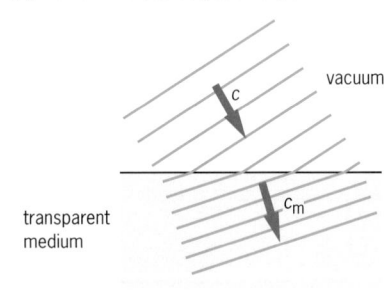

Fig 15.12 A change in wave speed produces a change in wavelength, but not frequency, and causes refraction

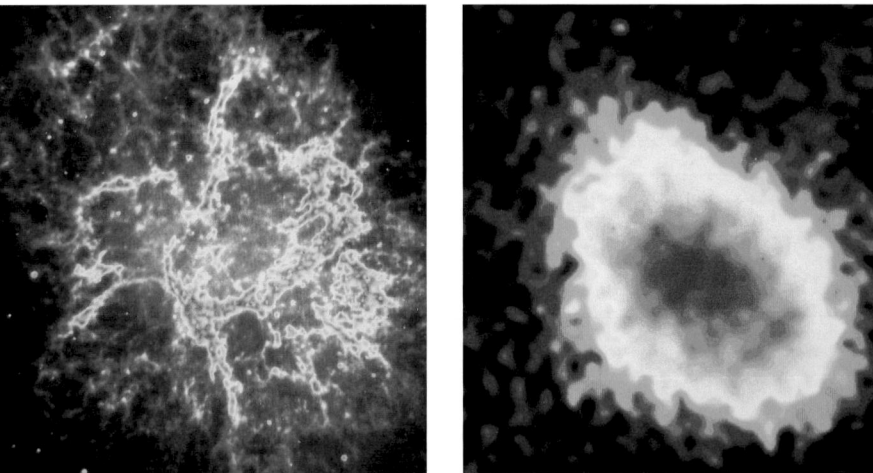

Fig 15.11(b) Astronomers use radiation that penetrates the atmosphere to produce images of stars. Images of the same objects differ according to the radiation used. For instance, the Crab Nebula is shown on the left as an optical telescope image and on the right as a radio telescope image

Refraction and the speed of electromagnetic waves

We have noted that electromagnetic waves travel more slowly in a transparent medium than in a vacuum. Fig 15.12(a) shows what happens as waves enter a transparent medium in which their speed is c_m. Their frequency stays the same but their wavelength gets less such that:

$$c_m = f\lambda_m$$

This change in speed also causes the **refraction** effect – the wavefronts change direction when they enter or leave the surface of the material at other than 90° (i.e. at an angle to the normal).

Fig 15.12(b) shows a set of parallel wavefronts of single-frequency radiation entering a transparent medium. As the leading edge enters the medium, the wave slows down but the 'outside' section of the front does not, so it catches up on the inside section. Inside the medium the distance between successive fronts is smaller and the direction of travel of the wave has changed. Snell's law of refraction follows directly from this effect.

? **QUESTION 4**

4 Sound waves travel more quickly in glass than in air. What should be the shape of a 'sound lens' that is meant to focus a beam of sound to a spot?

Snell's law

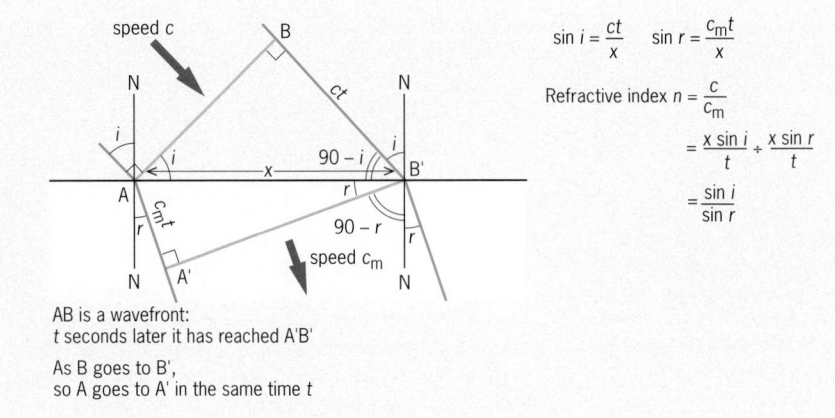

$$\sin i = \frac{ct}{x} \qquad \sin r = \frac{c_m t}{x}$$

$$\text{Refractive index } n = \frac{c}{c_m}$$

$$= \frac{x \sin i}{t} \div \frac{x \sin r}{t}$$

$$= \frac{\sin i}{\sin r}$$

AB is a wavefront:
t seconds later it has reached A'B'

As B goes to B',
so A goes to A' in the same time t

Fig 15.13 Snell's law of refraction: the geometry of wave refraction and proof of the sine formula

Fig 15.13 shows the geometry when the leading edge of a particular wavefront travels for a time t inside the medium before the rest of the front enters. Inside the medium the leading (left) edge A travels a distance $c_m t$, whilst the right edge B travels a distance ct. As the diagram shows, simple geometry gives the result that:

$$\frac{\sin i}{\sin r} = \frac{c}{c_m} = n \quad \text{(a constant)}$$

The constant n is the **refractive index** and is a property of *both* media since it involves the speeds of electromagnetic radiation in both media. Table 15.1 shows the refractive indices of light for some ordinary transparent materials with reference to air. The **absolute refractive index** is the value for light entering the medium from a *vacuum* ('free space'), and is the value quoted in most reference books.

Refractive index varies with wavelength

The speed of light in a given transparent medium is also likely to vary with frequency – the refractive index is different for different frequencies. Fig 15.14 shows how the refractive index of fused quartz and crown glass varies with the vacuum wavelength of radiation between short ultraviolet wavelengths (~200 nm) and near infrared (~750 nm). Fused quartz is widely used in optical devices as it is transparent over a wide range of wavelengths.

Note that glass has a higher refractive index for light of shorter wavelengths (higher frequencies) than for longer wavelengths: light of shorter wavelength is refracted more. This is why prisms produce a spectrum from white light, with blue light deviated more than red light (see Fig 15.2). This effect is called **dispersion**.

Dispersion is a serious problem that the makers of optical instruments with lenses have to solve. Dispersion means that red light is brought to a focus further away from a positive lens than blue light is (Fig 15.15). This blurs images, an effect called **chromatic aberration**. Newton solved the problem for telescopes by designing one in which the light was focused by a curved mirror (see Chapter 18).

An **achromatic** lens can be made – a combined *double lens* using two different types of glass (e.g. crown and flint glass). One lens is positive and stronger than the other, negative, lens. The overall combination is positive, but the negative lens is made from a more dispersive type of glass so that the total dispersion of the combination can be made very small.

Table 15.1 Refractive indices for light travelling between air and materials

Material	n (at λ = 589 nm)
diamond	2.419
fused quartz (SiO_2)	1.458
bottle glass	1.520
borosilicate (glass beakers)	1.474
ice	1.309
polystyrene	1.6
polythene (low density)	1.51
acrylic	1.49
Optical glass:	
light crown glass	1.541
dense crown glass	1.612
light flint glass	1.578
dense flint glass	1.613
Liquids:	
ethanol	1.361
glycerol	1.473
water	1.333
Gases (at 0 °C, 1 atm):	
air	1.000 293
carbon dioxide	1.000 45

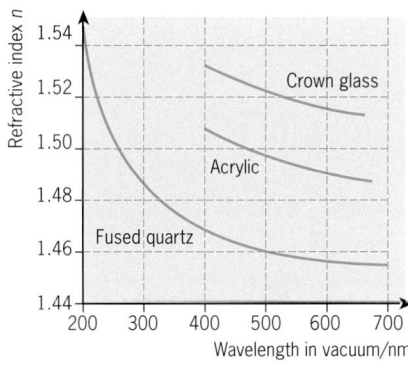

Fig 15.14 Graph of refractive index n against wavelength. Dispersion occurs because refractive index varies with wavelength *(after Serway)*

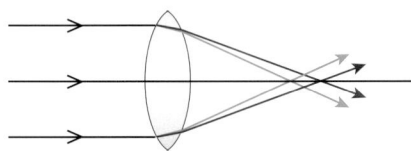

Fig 15.15(a) Chromatic aberration occurs because blue light moves more slowly than red light, and so is refracted more

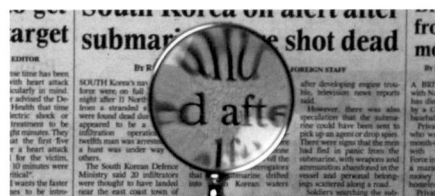

Fig 15.15(b) Chromatic aberration: the image has blurred colours at its edges

Competing models of light

Back in the seventeenth century, when Huygens proposed his wave model (see opposite), there was another model of how light travelled (as indeed there is today). This was a model proposed by Isaac Newton. He imagined light as being made up of particles, and he developed a mechanical model to explain what was then known about the behaviour of light. The big advantage of Newton's model was that it was easy to explain why light travelled in straight lines. It was quite easy to explain refraction too, by assuming that matter exerted a short-range force on light particles that accelerated them towards a surface, so changing their direction. It wasn't so easy to explain such things as diffraction, and the strange fringes that could be seen due to what we now know to be the interference of waves.

Fig 15.16 shows how both Newton's and Huygens' models explain reflection. Both work. The two explanations of refraction, however, lead to two contrasting conclusions, as shown in Fig 15.17. According to the wave theory, light slows down when it enters a transparent medium. According to Newton's theory, it speeds up. The critical test couldn't be made until better techniques for measuring the speed of light were developed in the nineteenth century. Then in 1850, Leon Foucault (France, 1819–1868) measured the speed of light in water and showed that it did indeed go slower than in air.

So, with care, Huygens' theory could explain everything – but at the time it wasn't too well worked out. In the next century Newton's prestige – and his careful reasoning – won the contest. By 1800, thinking of light as a wave was heresy in the scientific community. But then along came Thomas Young.

Thomas Young was a terrifyingly precocious child. He could read fluently at the age of two. He qualified as a doctor at the age of 19 and at 27 was appointed a professor at the new Royal Institution in London, later moving to

Fig 15.16 Newton's and Huygens' explanations of the reflection of light

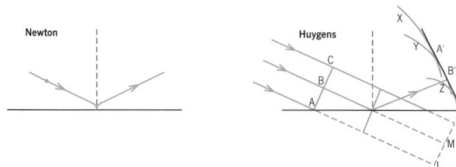

(a) Newton: the incoming particle speeds up as it gets attracted by the surface. It bounces away then gets slowed down by the same force so goes off at the same speed. The angle of incidence equals the angle of reflection. Comment: nice and simple!

(b) Huygens: the incoming wavefront is ABC. With no reflection it would get to the line LMN in a certain time. But the wavelet from A travels back into the air and spreads out along the arc labelled X. Similarly the wavelet from B forms the arc Y, and C forms the arc Z. Wavelets from the rest of the wavefront have not been shown, but they also make arcs and contribute to forming the reflected plane wavefront A'B'C'. The angle of incidence equals the angle of reflection. Comment: not easy to follow.

Fig 15.17 Newton's and Huygens' explanations of the refraction of light. According to Newton, light travelled faster in glass than in air; Huygens' model predicted correctly that light slowed down

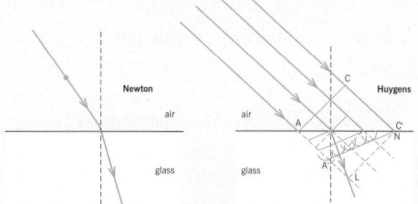

(a) Newton: the incoming particle is accelerated towards the surface and so changes direction. Inside it carries on along the same path. Comment: again, nice and simple!

(b) Huygens: the incoming wavefront is AC. A wavelet from A goes into the glass, spreads out in an arc but travels more slowly than in air. So the radius of the arc based on A is shorter than in air. Similarly the wavelet from C moves more slowly. Adding up all the contributions from the wavefront between A and C produces the new wavefront A'C'. If they didn't slow down they would make the wavefront LN. Comment: still tricky – but it predicts that light slows down in a transparent medium. And it does!

For more on competing models of light please see the How Science Works assignment for this chapter at www.collinseducation.co.uk/CAS

work at the Royal Society. He studied the eye and vision, and found that the best model for optics was to think of light as a wave. For example he used the principle of superposition to explain the colour effects seen in thin films of oil on water. He was jeered at for this, and went back to medical studies. In his spare time he showed how to decipher the Ancient Egyptian writing (hieroglyphs). But his wave theories gained support in France from younger physicists, and he returned

to the study of light. His experiments on the interference of light (page 294) provided firm evidence for its wave nature. However, evidence for a theory is often not enough. Even after the evidence for a wave theory became overwhelming it wasn't accepted until the older 'particle supporters' died out. This is not an uncommon way in which radical new theories get accepted!

Fig 15.18 The English doctor and scientist Thomas Young (1773–1829) who established that light behaved as a wave

3 ELECTROMAGNETIC RADIATION AS A WAVE

So far in this chapter we have thought of electromagnetic radiation as a wave. But physics in fact uses three main models of light – a straight line 'ray' model (see Chapter 18), a particle (photon) model (see Chapter 16), and the wave model which we shall develop in this chapter.

THE DIFFRACTION OF WAVES

Fig 15.19(a) shows a set of parallel water waves passing through a small gap in a barrier. The waves spread out after passing through. This spreading out is called **diffraction** and is a key to distinguishing *wave* behaviour from *particle* behaviour (Fig 15.19(b)).

HOW WAVES MOVE FORWARD

We see in Fig 15.19(a) that a wave crest such as a single ripple moves forward and keeps its direction. At the crest of the water wave there is a volume of water temporarily lifted above its normal level. Imagine raising just a small part of a water surface (e.g. by touching it and lifting your finger away). You would expect, correctly, that it would immediately collapse in all directions. The water surface then oscillates up and down and a circular pulse moves away from the site of the initial disturbance.

Why does the ring of raised water in the pulse (a circular crest) keep going with the same shape? To answer this – and to explain diffraction properly – we have to use two ideas proposed by Jan Christian Huygens (Holland, 1629–1695). One is known as **Huygens' principle**, the other is the **principle of superposition**.

HUYGENS' PRINCIPLE AND THE PRINCIPLE OF SUPERPOSITION

Huygens explained how water waves travelled by saying something quite original: *every point on the front of a wave gave rise to another wave centred on that point*. At first sight this looked as if the wave would descend into chaos, and Huygens' model skated over this possibility. He used his idea to explain two main effects: how light travels in a straight line, and why light spreads out after passing through a small aperture (diffraction). But to explain both effects properly another principle is needed: the principle of superposition.

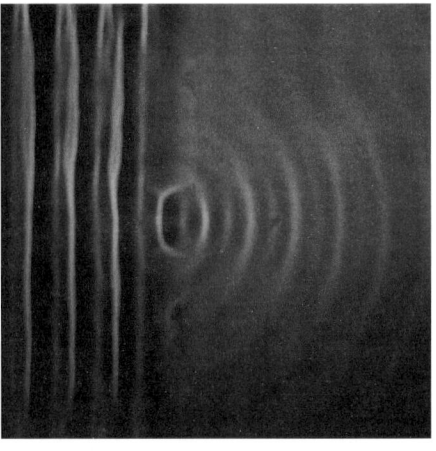

Fig 15.19(a) Water waves passing through a gap and diffracting

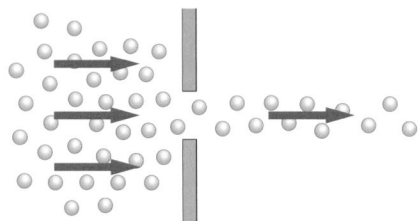

Fig 15.19(b) Particles streaming through a gap. They don't spread out. (But could they bounce off the edges?

Fig 15.20 The principle of superposition: what happens when wave pulses and continuous waves meet and interfere

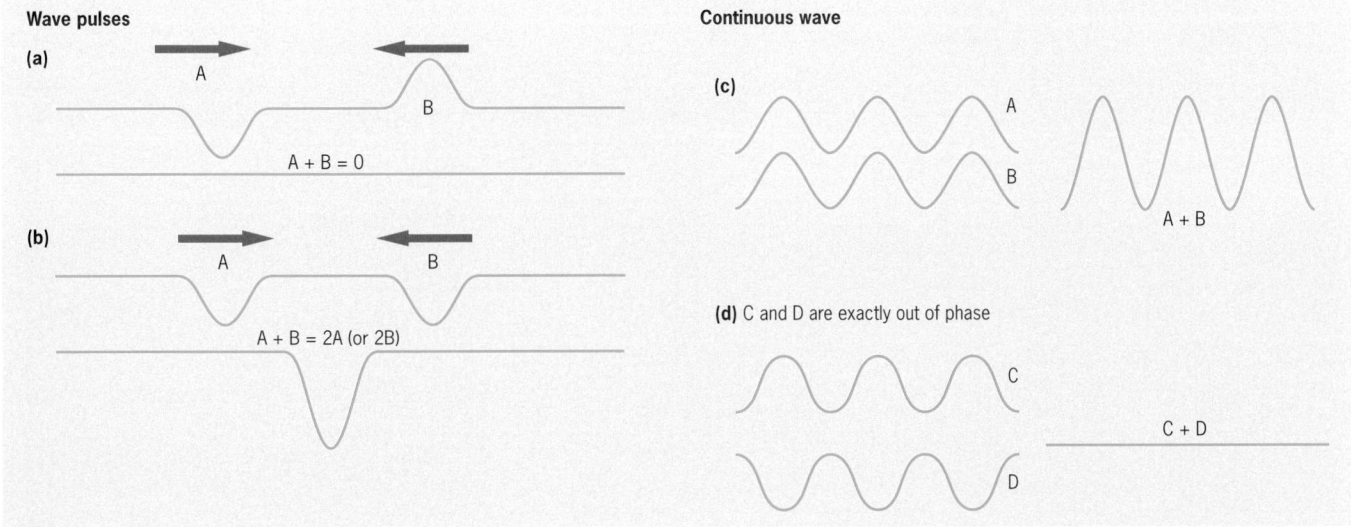

Wave pulses

(a)

A

B

A + B = 0

(b)

A

B

A + B = 2A (or 2B)

Continuous wave

(c)

A

B

A + B

(d) C and D are exactly out of phase

C

C + D

D

Fig 15.21 Huygens' wave model of light propagation

(a) Each point on a wavefront produces 'secondary wavelets'. For clarity, only a few points and wavelets are shown. For a very long wavefront, a plane wave reproduces itself as a plane wave, that is, 'light travels in straight lines'

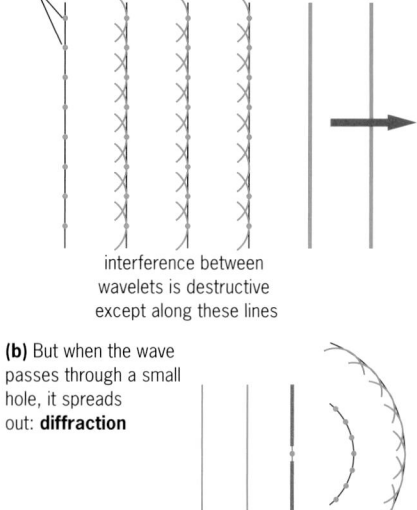

sources of wavelets

interference between wavelets is destructive except along these lines

(b) But when the wave passes through a small hole, it spreads out: **diffraction**

When two water wave pulses meet, they pass through each other. However, at the meeting point the wave amplitudes add: two crests produce a larger crest, and, similarly, two troughs make a deeper trough. A crest meeting an equal-sized trough produces an instant of completely flat water. See Figs 15.20(a) to (d) on the previous page, which illustrate the principle of superposition by which the amplitudes of two waves that occupy the same space at the same time simply add together. (See page 138 to compare with the superposition of mechanical waves.) This effect is called **interference**.

Huygens' wave model of light explains how waves propagate as follows. Imagine that each point on a straight wavefront (equivalent to the water wave crest) is the source of another wave (i.e. as the wavefront 'collapses'). Then the waves (or *wavelets*) from each of these point sources **interfere** with the wavelets from the other points in such a way that the only places where they add together is in the forward direction. Thus a plane (straight-fronted) wave would move forward as a plane wave and therefore light would travel in straight lines (see Fig 15.21).

But note that at the edges of the plane wavefront, the wavelets would have no supporting wavelets to interfere with. The waves here could propagate sideways, in other words **diffraction** would occur.

4 INTERFERENCE AND WAVELENGTH

YOUNG'S TWO-SLIT INTERFERENCE EXPERIMENT

This experiment is the best known of those designed by Thomas Young in 1801 in support of the wave theory of light.

Fig 15.22(a) shows a parallel beam of light (e.g. from a distant point object) reaching an opaque screen with two narrow slits in it. Light is diffracted at each slit and the spreading beams overlap. This means that, at any point along a line such as XY, light is received from both slits A and B (Fig 15.22(b)). The contributions from the slits reaching a point such as P may be **in phase** or **out of phase**, as in Fig 15.22(c), and the resulting intensity at P could be anything from zero to double the contribution from any one slit.

Fig 15.22 Light travelling through two slits and showing superposition at a screen

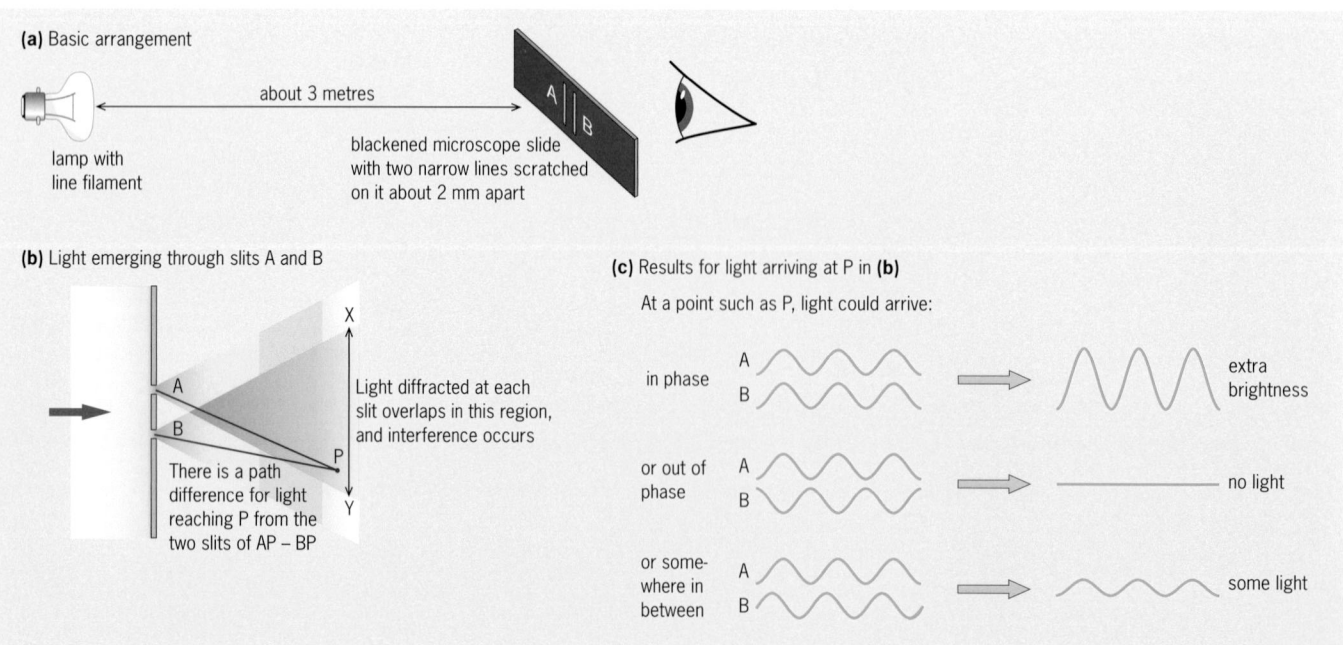

(a) Basic arrangement

about 3 metres

lamp with line filament

blackened microscope slide with two narrow lines scratched on it about 2 mm apart

(b) Light emerging through slits A and B

X

A

B

P

Y

Light diffracted at each slit overlaps in this region, and interference occurs

There is a path difference for light reaching P from the two slits of AP – BP

(c) Results for light arriving at P in **(b)**

At a point such as P, light could arrive:

in phase
A
B
extra brightness

or out of phase
A
B
no light

or somewhere in between
A
B
some light

What exactly happens at P depends on the geometry, in fact, on the *difference* in the path lengths AP and BP in Fig 15.22(b):

- If AP – BP is zero, a whole wavelength or a whole number of wavelengths, the contributions are in phase, and we have a brightness at P.
- If AP – BP is a half wavelength or an *odd* number of half wavelengths, the contributions are exactly out of phase, destructive interference occurs and there is a darkness at P.

You can imagine that as the point P in Fig 15.22(b) moves along XY, the path difference changes and P will be alternately in bright and dark zones, called **interference fringes**. These fringes are easy to see when you look at a distant lamp (say, 3 metres away) through two slits scratched about a millimetre apart in a blackened microscope slide. This is **Young's two-slit interference experiment**. This experiment can be used to measure the wavelength of light.

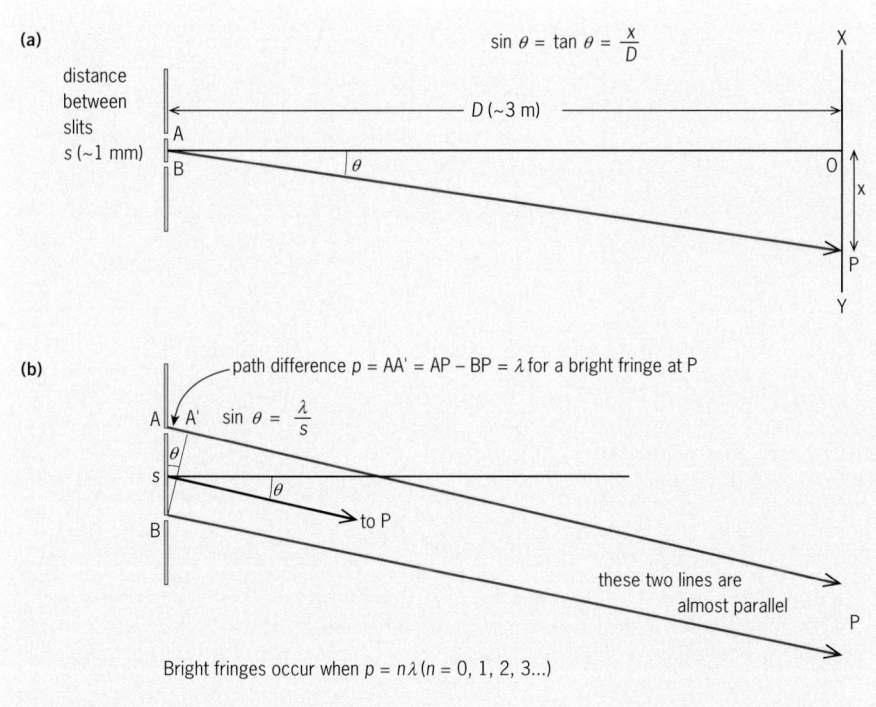

 REMEMBER THIS

Phase is short for *phase angle,* explained in Chapter 6 on page 134. When a wave travels one wavelength the phase angle changes by 2π radians or 360°.

Phase difference, Δ(phase), between two superposing waves depends on *wavelength* and the *difference* in path distance, Δ(path), travelled by the two waves coming from the same source via different paths. When the path difference is a whole wavelength there is no phase difference. For half a wavelength, the phase difference places crest over trough. Look at Fig 15.17. The phase relationship is

$$\Delta(\text{phase}) = \frac{2\pi}{\lambda}\,\Delta(\text{path})$$

Fig 15.23 Young's experiment. The difference in path length for light through the two slits causes phase differences and creates the fringes

MEASURING THE WAVELENGTH OF LIGHT

Fig 15.23 shows Fig 15.22(b) with angles drawn to a more realistic scale. The slit separation s is a millimetre or two, and the distance D from the slits to the plane of observation (XY) is several metres. O is a point equidistant from the slits A and B, so the path difference is zero and O is in the centre of a bright fringe. P is distance x from O, chosen so that P is in the centre of the next bright fringe.

Look at the triangle in Fig 15.23(a). The angle θ is very small, so that $\sin\theta = \tan\theta$, and we can write

$$\sin\theta = \tan\theta = \frac{x}{d}$$

Fig 15.23(b) shows the detail nearer the two slits. The path difference between light reaching P from A and B is p (AA'). As the waves add up to

? **QUESTIONS 5–6**

5 **a)** Why do we so rarely (if ever) notice the effects of light interference in everyday life?
b) Suppose that human eyes had evolved to detect a band in the electromagnetic spectrum that was different from the visible region. And suppose that in this different region of the spectrum, car headlamps generated interference patterns on the road in front of them that we could clearly see. Estimate a value for the wavelength of this 'light'.

6 The pattern produced by a pair of slits (and also a diffraction grating) consists of a set of light zones separated by dark zones. The dark areas are produced by light waves (which carry energy) meeting and 'destroying each other' because they are out of phase. Does this effect contradict the law of conservation of energy? As this law cannot be broken, suggest what has happened to the energy?

brightness this path difference must be one wavelength. The two lines AP and BP are almost parallel, since P is so far away. Thus the angle ABA' is also θ, and we can write:

$$\sin \theta = \frac{\text{path difference}}{\text{slit separation}}$$

$$\sin \theta = \frac{\lambda}{s}$$

which is usually rearranged as

$$\lambda = s \sin \theta$$

In general, bright fringes occur at all angles that involve whole wavelength path differences, i.e.

$$n\lambda = s \sin \theta$$

where n is a whole number.

The spacing between fringes

Look at Fig 15.23 again. Suppose that P is the position of the *first* bright fringe. OP is now Δx, the *spacing* between two fringes. As before,

$$\sin \theta = \frac{\Delta x}{D}$$

or

$$\Delta x = D \sin \theta$$

Looking at the angle θ near the slit, the path difference is now just one wavelength. So we have $\sin \theta = \lambda/s$ and putting in this value we can write the fringe separation as

$$\Delta x = \frac{\lambda D}{s}$$

This relationship applies with good accuracy to all the fringes close to the centre of the fringe system.

Taking measurements

The fringes produced by the arrangement shown in Fig 15.22 are viewed through either a microscope eyepiece with a micrometer scale (marked in millimetres) or a movable (travelling) microscope mounted on a vernier scale. The fringe separation is measured by counting a whole number n of fringes – as many as possible – and measuring the value of x shown in Fig 15.23(a).

D is measured with a good steel tape. A travelling microscope (or some optical imaging method) may be used to measure the small distance s. These values are then inserted in the equation

$$\lambda = \frac{xs}{Dn}$$

to calculate the wavelength of light, λ.

COHERENCE

We do not observe interference effects if the path difference between two interfering wavelets is longer than about 30 cm. Neither do we see the effects when light is combined from two *different* sources (two lamps or two stars, say). This is because the waves are emitted randomly, in short bursts, as in Fig 15.24(a). Interference still occurs, but the effect is so random and on such a short time scale (about 10^{-8} s) that it is impossible to observe. For all practical purposes, we can only observe interference when light from the same 'burst' is combined: such light is described as **coherent** (meaning 'belonging together'), see Fig 15.24(b). **Lasers** can emit continuous coherent light – particularly useful for applications of interference effects, such as making holograms. For more about lasers, see page 407, Chapter 20.

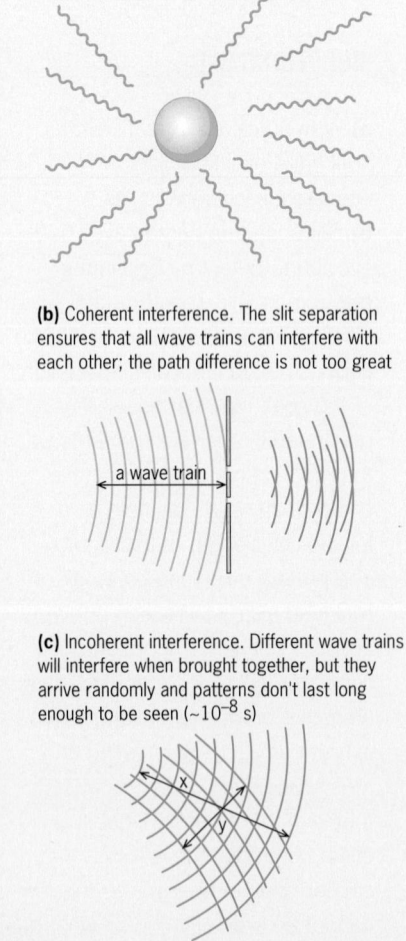

(a) A luminous object emits light randomly, as wave trains tens of centimetres long

(b) Coherent interference. The slit separation ensures that all wave trains can interfere with each other; the path difference is not too great

a wave train

(c) Incoherent interference. Different wave trains will interfere when brought together, but they arrive randomly and patterns don't last long enough to be seen (~10^{-8} s)

Fig 15.24 Random light emission, coherence and incoherence

5 DIFFRACTION AND IMAGE FORMATION

Diffraction becomes more noticeable when waves pass through a small hole (aperture). A greater fraction of the incident wave energy moves 'sideways', and interference effects occur which produce a **diffraction pattern** of the kind shown in Fig 15.25.

All optical instruments direct light to pass through apertures (or to reflect off mirrors) of finite size. So some diffraction will occur, and the images produced will tend to lack clarity. The image of a small source of light (effectively a point source) is no longer a point, and the diffraction pattern is a more or less inaccurate version of the point object. With larger objects, fine detail is lost as light from separate points on the object reaches the image as overlapping diffraction patterns. Diffraction affects the images made by telescopes, which is one reason why they have to be so large (see page 299).

DIFFRACTION THROUGH A SLIT

When light goes through a narrow slit it spreads out – just as water waves do. Think of a set of plane waves reaching a slit whose width is just a few wavelengths across, as in Fig 15.26. The light then spreads out in all directions and clearly does not consist of particles travelling in straight lines. When the spread-out light is focused on a screen the result, surprisingly, shows a pattern of light and dark fringes, similar to those in Fig 15.25. This happens because light waves from different parts of the wavefront that get through the slit *interfere* with each other. Using Huygens' principle (see Fig 15.21), we can think of the wavefront that fills the slit as a set of small point sources which produce circular wavelets spreading out in all directions.

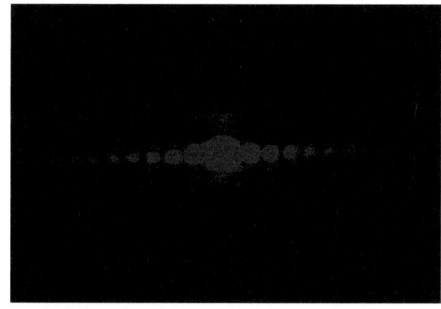

Fig 15.25 Diffraction image produced by light passing through a narrow slit. Waves interfere constructively in the bright regions and destructively in the dark regions

The effects of single-slit diffraction can be simulated by using Excel. See the How Science Works assignment for this chapter at www.collinseducation.co.uk/CAS

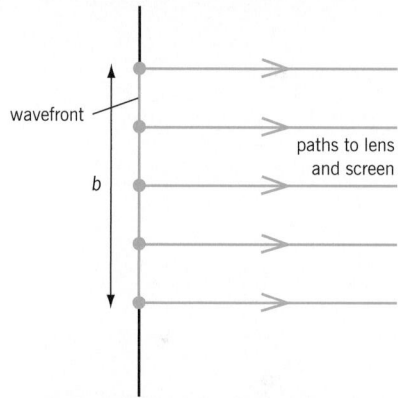

(a) All the wavelets are in phase (in step) all along the paths and travel the same distance to the screen. They arrive in phase with each other

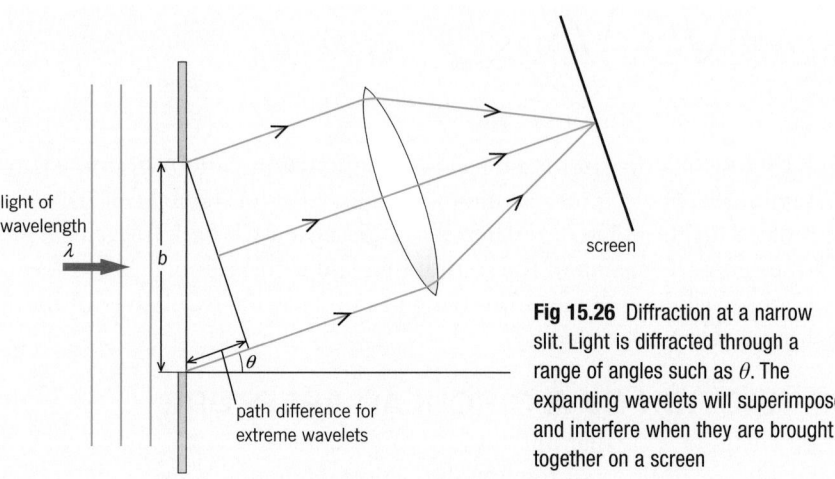

Fig 15.26 Diffraction at a narrow slit. Light is diffracted through a range of angles such as θ. The expanding wavelets will superimpose and interfere when they are brought together on a screen

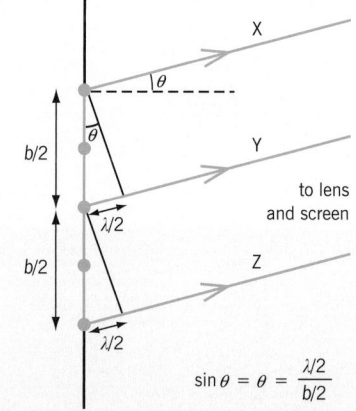

$$\sin \theta = \theta = \frac{\lambda/2}{b/2}$$

(b) Wavelet X arrives exactly out of phase with wavelet Y, and Y is out of phase with Z. Imagine all the other wavelets (not shown) between X and Y cancelling with mutually destructive partners between Y and Z

Fig 15.27 The geometry of diffraction. This explains why there are light and dark fringes

Directly ahead all wavelets travel the same distance to a screen and so arrive in step (in phase) – see Fig 15.27(a). But at *certain* angles each wavelet travelling gradually increasing distances will arrive at the screen exactly out of phase with at least one other wavelet. This is because each wavelet travels just one half-wavelength further than some other wavelet. This situation is shown in Fig 15.27(b). The result is darkness when wavelets in this direction are focused on the screen: the out-of-phase wavelets cancel.

Darkness is produced when the angle of the light is θ, such that each wavelet can find a 'partner' that is exactly out of phase, one that has travelled an extra distance $\lambda/2$. This happens when wavelet X pairs up with a central wavelet Y, say. The wavelet next to X can find a partner next to Y – and so on and so on until each wavelet between X and Y finds a mutually destructive partner between Y and Z. The slit has a width b, and the geometry shows that the sine of angle θ is given by

$$\sin\theta = \frac{\text{path difference } \lambda/2}{\text{half the width of the slit } b/2}$$

so

$$\sin\theta = \frac{\lambda/2}{b/2} = \frac{\lambda}{b}$$

Rather surprisingly, it seems that light from one half of the slit cancels out light from the other half.

Of course destructive interference will occur at other angles producing a path difference of an odd number of half-wavelengths, e.g. $3\lambda/2$, $5\lambda/2$, $7\lambda/2$,… etc. This means that there is a range of angles θ for destructive interference, given by the relationship

$$\sin\theta = \frac{n\lambda}{b}$$

which is usually written

$$b\,\sin\theta = n\lambda \quad \text{(where } n \text{ is a whole number)}$$

The angles θ are much smaller in practice than are shown on the diagrams. With such small angles $\sin\theta$ quite accurately equals θ in radians. The formula for the angular directions of dark fringes is thus often given as $b\theta = n\lambda$.

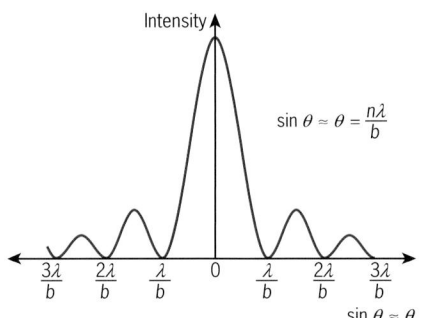

Intensity

$$\sin\theta \approx \theta = \frac{n\lambda}{b}$$

$\dfrac{3\lambda}{b}$ $\dfrac{2\lambda}{b}$ $\dfrac{\lambda}{b}$ 0 $\dfrac{\lambda}{b}$ $\dfrac{2\lambda}{b}$ $\dfrac{3\lambda}{b}$

$\sin\theta \approx \theta$

Fig 15.28 The diffraction pattern of parallel light passing through a narrow slit (width b). The central maximum has greater intensity than the side fringes

Fig 15.28 is a graph of the intensity of a diffraction pattern from a narrow rectangular slit. The central maximum contains most of the light. It has a width of 2θ for the value of θ when $n = 1$, because each dark fringe is θ away from the centre. The peak of the central maximum corresponds to $n = 0$, that is, all light reaching it comes from pairs of points in the two halves of the slit which have zero path difference.

DIFFRACTION BY A CIRCULAR APERTURE

The geometry of a circular aperture is more complex, but the equivalent result for the angular position of the first diffraction minimum is given by:

$$\sin\theta = \frac{1.22\lambda}{D}$$

Here, D is the *diameter* of the aperture. Fig 15.29 shows the diffraction pattern produced by light passing through a small hole. Most optical instruments – including the eye – have circular apertures and this relationship is more generally applicable than the one for a narrow slit – see the Example opposite.

Fig 15.29 Diffraction image caused by light passing through a small hole

EXAMPLE

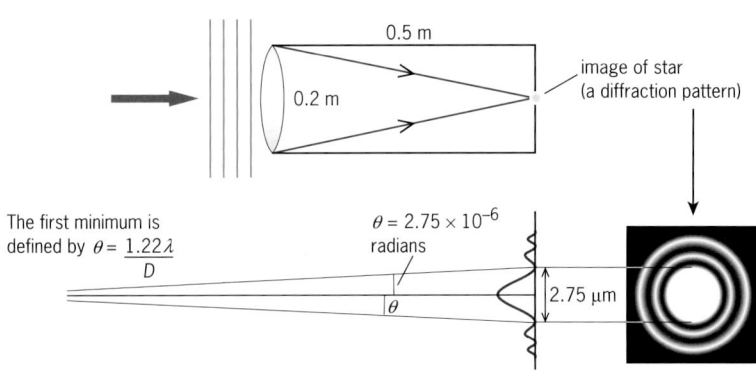

Fig 15.30 Geometry of the telescope system and image formation

Q **a)** What is the angular width of the central maximum of the image of a star when photographed in blue light of wavelength 450 nm? The image is produced by a telescope system with a circular aperture of diameter 0.2 m.

b) The image is formed 0.5 m from the prime focusing lens. What is the size of the central maximum on the photographic plate?

A **a)** Using the diffraction formula for a circular aperture:

$$\sin \theta = \frac{1.22\lambda}{D}$$
$$= \frac{1.22 \times 450 \times 10^{-9}}{0.2}$$
$$= 2.75 \times 10^{-6}$$

The angle is so small that we can write $\theta = 2.75 \times 10^{-6}$ *radians.* The image has a central maximum of angular width 2θ (see Fig 15.30), equal to 5.5×10^{-6} radians.

b) The angle calculated in a) produces a central maximum of width:

$$0.5 \times 5.5 \times 10^{-6} \text{ m} = 2.75 \times 10^{-6} \text{ m } (2.75 \text{ μm})$$

Comments on the Example

Stars are so far away that each star is effectively a point and its image on a photographic plate or other detector is a diffraction pattern.

Astronomers need to distinguish the diffraction pattern of any one star from those of its nearest apparent neighbours, as in Fig 15.32(b) in the next Example. So, for good **resolution** between images, the diffraction image should be made as small as possible. Astronomers do this by making D as large as possible for a given wavelength, that is, they use as large a telescope as possible. Also, light of smaller wavelength gives a smaller diffraction pattern. In practice, this tends to be blue light because the atmosphere absorbs the shorter UV wavelengths. The largest optical telescope (at the observatory of Mauna Kea in Hawaii, Fig 18.31) has a diameter of 9.82 m. A radio telescope uses much longer wavelengths – typically 6 cm compared with 6×10^{-7} cm for optical telescopes – and would need to be 10 million times larger to get the same kind of resolution!

RESOLVING POWER: THE RAYLEIGH CRITERION

Resolving power is the measure of how good an optical system is at clearly distinguishing detail, for example, of two stars close together, or two structures in a living cell. The standard measure of the resolving power of any image-making device is the **Rayleigh criterion** (due to Lord Rayleigh, Britain 1842–1919). This states that it is possible to separate the images of two point objects if the centre of the central maximum of one image lies on the first dark fringe of the other. This is illustrated in Fig 15.31, and shows that when the criterion is satisfied the central maxima are separated by an angle of θ given by the relationship:

$$\sin \theta = \frac{1.22\lambda}{D}$$

In most optical instruments the angles are so small that the criterion is usually written, with θ in radians, as:

$$\theta = \frac{1.22\lambda}{D}$$

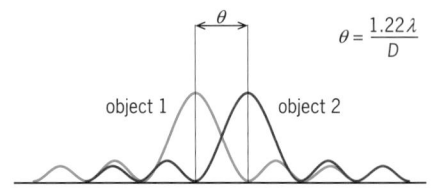

Fig 15.31(a) Graph of light intensity for two point sources with central maxima separated by angle $\theta = 1.22\lambda/D$

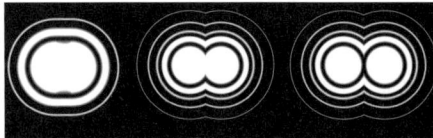

Fig 15.31(b) Illustrating the Rayleigh criterion: diffraction images for two point sources. Left: two unresolved sources; middle: two sources just resolved; right: two sources completely resolved

---

STRETCH
AND CHALLENGE

EXAMPLE

The Hubble space telescope

Q The mirror aperture of the Hubble space telescope has a diameter of 2.40 metres.

a) What is its theoretical resolving power in green light of wavelength 5.20×10^{-7} m?

b) At its closest approach Mars is 7.83×10^{10} m from Earth. What is the closest possible distance between two small objects on the Martian surface that would allow them to be distinguished as separate by the Hubble telescope?

A a) Resolving power

$$\theta = \frac{1.22\lambda}{D} = \frac{1.22 \times 5.20 \times 10^{-7}}{2.40}$$

giving: $\theta = 2.6 \times 10^{-7}$ radians

b) Let the separation be x metres. The angle subtended by this distance at the telescope must be equal to or greater than θ, so at the limit:

$$\frac{x}{7.83 \times 10^{10}} \geq 2.64 \times 10^{-7}$$

giving: $x \geq 20\,697$ m, or 20.7 km

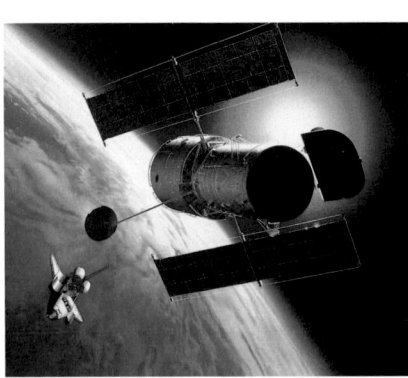

Fig 15.32(a) The Hubble space telescope: it detects objects 50 times fainter and 7 times further away than a ground-based telescope

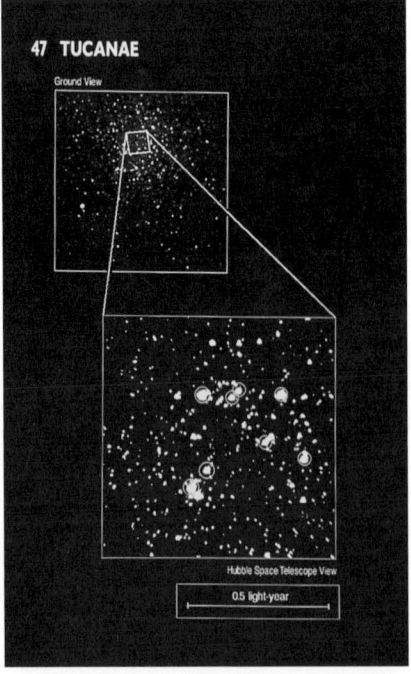

Fig 15.32(b) Comparing star pictures taken by a ground-based telescope (small box), and the Hubble telescope which has far better resolution and has led to the discovery of new stars

---

? **QUESTIONS 7–8**

7 Human eyes are quite good at resolving images formed in light of wavelength about 500 nm. Estimate how much bigger your eyes would have to be to get equivalent resolution if they worked at UHF TV wavelengths (λ about 1 m).

8 Two radio telescopes on different continents are linked to provide data on a radio star. The telescopes are separated by 4000 km and observe on a wavelength of 21 cm. What is the angular resolution (resolving power) of this arrangement?

6 THE DIFFRACTION GRATING AND SPECTRA

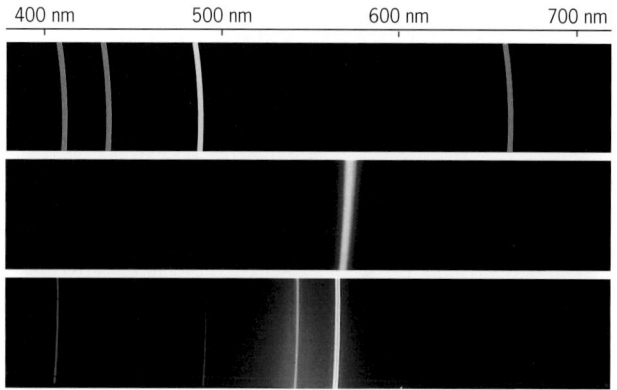

400 nm   500 nm   600 nm   700 nm

Fig 15.33 Line emission spectra of hydrogen (top), sodium (middle) and mercury (bottom) produced by a typical grating

The study of the electromagnetic spectra of radiation in and near the visible has produced some of the most important discoveries in science. The element helium is named after the Greek for Sun as it was first identified in the spectrum of sunlight before being discovered as a gas. Many other examples are given in Chapters 25 and 26.

Prisms were first used to produce spectra but glass absorbs ultraviolet and some infrared radiation. Prisms are useless for microwave and radio studies.

Modern spectroscopy relies heavily on the principle of the **diffraction grating**. A diffraction grating is a glass or metal sheet with a large number of very fine parallel lines ruled on it. These lines diffract radiation in such a way that a series of spectra is formed (as in Fig 15.33). If the grating lines are close enough together, the spectrum is spread over a very large angle compared to that produced by a prism and much more detail can be observed (see the Stretch and Challenge passage on the next page).

Diffraction gratings were used in astronomy to study the spectra of stars and of sunlight from early in the nineteenth century. In 1882, the American Henry Rowland made the first precisely engineered grating, ruling lines with an accuracy and constant separation much better than anyone else had managed.

A typical grating used in school laboratories today might have 5000 lines per centimetre. *Transmission* gratings are ruled on good optical glass and the radiation passes through the series of slits between grooves ruled on the glass. Cheaper gratings are made by copying these on to a plastic film. *Reflection* gratings are ruled on good metal mirrors and do not suffer from absorption problems. The mirrors may be curved, to focus the spectra without the need for lenses. The principles are shown in Fig 15.34.

Fig 15.34 Diffraction gratings

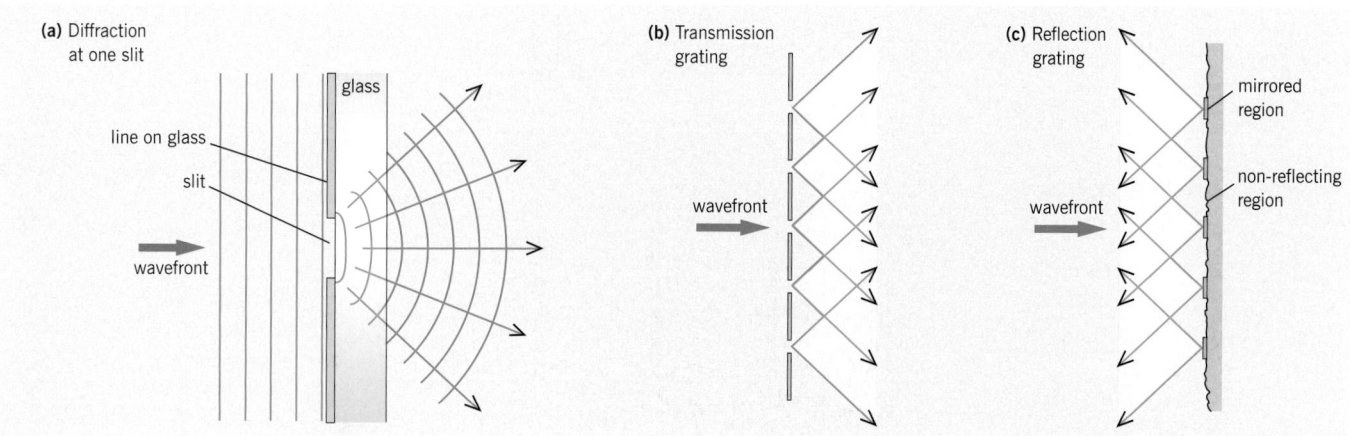

More about diffraction gratings

We can analyse the principle of the diffraction grating in a similar way to our analysis of the formation of a diffracted image by a narrow slit on pages 297–298. Fig 15.35 shows what happens when a plane beam of parallel light (e.g. from a distant point) passes through one slit of a diffraction grating.

Light is diffracted and travels in circular waves from the slit, as in Fig 15.34(a). Suppose the slits are a distance d apart and consider light diffracted at an angle θ. For light with wavelength λ, there is a series of angles θ at which the waves from successive slits reinforce each other by travelling paths that differ by whole numbers of wavelengths λ before they are combined by the lens. This will happen for light diffracted at an angle such that $\lambda = d \sin \theta$. Light with a slightly different wavelength will be diffracted at a slightly different angle. This causes the first order spectrum. Spectra will also occur at other angles for which the path difference for light from adjacent slits is 2λ, 3λ, 4λ, etc. In general, spectra occur at angles given by:

$$n\lambda = d \sin \theta$$

where $n = 2, 3, 4$, etc; $n = 2$ gives the second order spectrum.

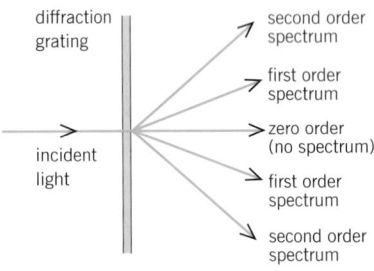

Fig 15.35 A diffraction grating produces several spectra for different values of θ

THE ENVELOPE OF THE GRATING DIFFRACTION PATTERN

The width b of *each slit* is also important. The diffracted light forming the spectra must obey the basic diffraction rules for waves passing through a narrow slit: this means that the envelope of the spectra fits into the diffraction pattern produced by a narrow slit of width b. Fig 15.36 shows the effect produced for a single narrow slit, two slits (Young's fringes of course) and more slits.

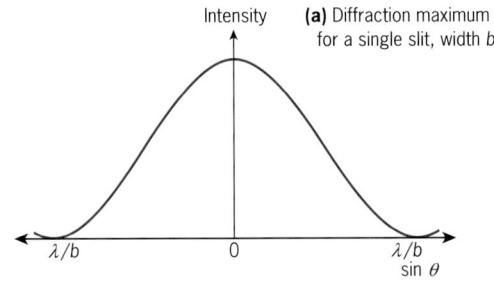

(a) Diffraction maximum for a single slit, width b

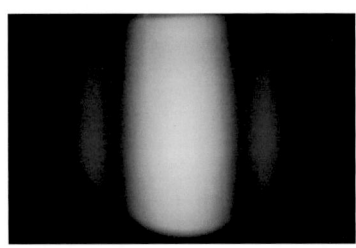

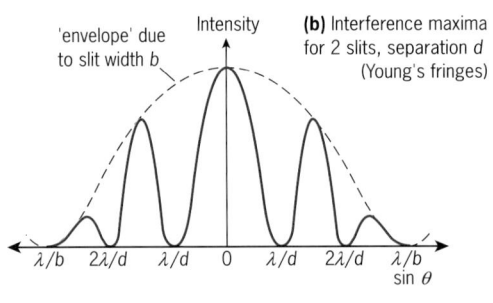

(b) Interference maxima for 2 slits, separation d (Young's fringes)

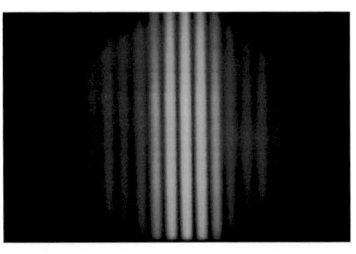

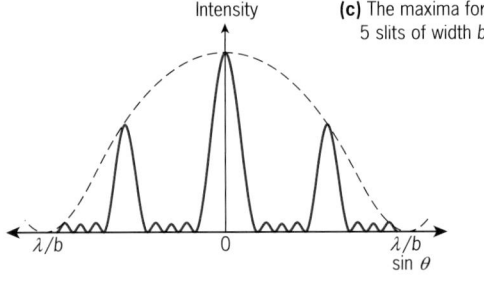

(c) The maxima for 5 slits of width b

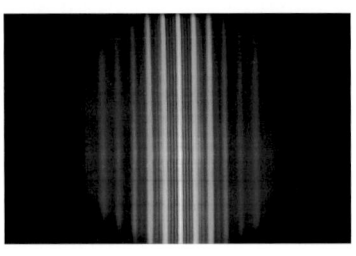

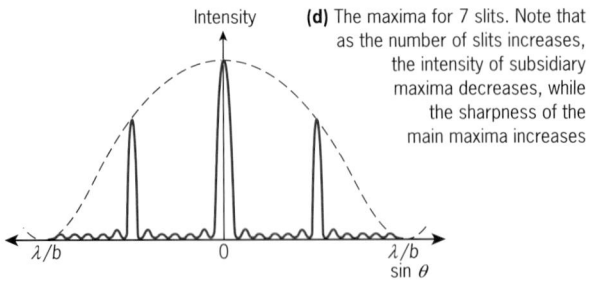

(d) The maxima for 7 slits. Note that as the number of slits increases, the intensity of subsidiary maxima decreases, while the sharpness of the main maxima increases

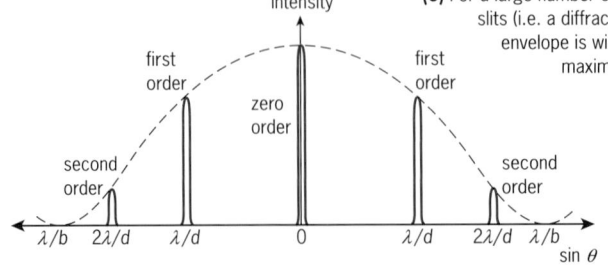

(e) For a large number of much narrower slits (i.e. a diffraction grating), the envelope is wider and principal maxima are very sharp

Fig 15.36 Envelope and fringes for 1, 2 and more slits
b = slit width
d = grating spacing

THE ADVANTAGES OF DIFFRACTION GRATINGS

If d is small, $\sin \theta$ can be large and so can angle θ. However, if the spectrum is to be detectable, θ must be less than 90°, which means that there is a limit to how widely spread a spectrum can be. The advantage of a diffraction grating, however, is that it can spread a typical spectrum of visible and near visible light over a large enough angle to show its fine detail. Note that although light appears to be 'destroyed' in the dark spaces between the orders of the spectrum, the original energy the incoming waves carried has to go somewhere. This means that the visible spectra can be very bright.

In fact for a diffraction grating with many slits, light emitted at angles close to θ will be cancelled out and the intensity graph of light of a single wavelength will be very sharp, as in Fig 15.36(e). Compare this with (b), the graph of intensity for two slits.

The sharpness of the peaks in Fig 15.36(e) means that the grating can distinguish between wavelengths that are very close together. In theory, if a grating has N slits it will produce a line at $\sin \theta$ for light of a given wavelength, such that the intensity falls to zero for values which differ from $\sin \theta$ by $\sin \theta / N$. This formula assumes a perfect grating. In practice, however, gratings cannot be ruled to the accuracy that would allow the results to be as good as the formula predicts.

7 POLARISATION

Electromagnetic waves are transverse: both the electric and magnetic components oscillate at right angles to the direction of travel (look back at Fig 15.3). If all the electric oscillations are made to lie in the same plane, the waves are said to be plane polarised (Fig 15.37).

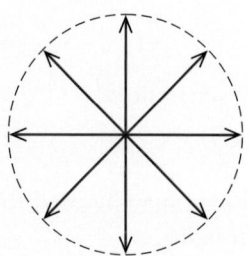 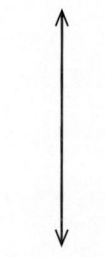

Unpolarised waves   Partly polarised   Plane polarised

Fig 15.37 Polarisation: the diagrams show the electric component of an electromagnetic wave only, as 'seen' end on

The easiest way to polarise a beam of light is to pass it through a sheet of polarised film, manufactured as Polaroid. This contains a large number of small aligned crystals which absorb light whose electric component is aligned along the long axes of the molecules. The emerging beam is thus plane polarised (Fig 15.38). This light will not pass through a Polaroid filter whose crystals are aligned perpendicularly to the first.

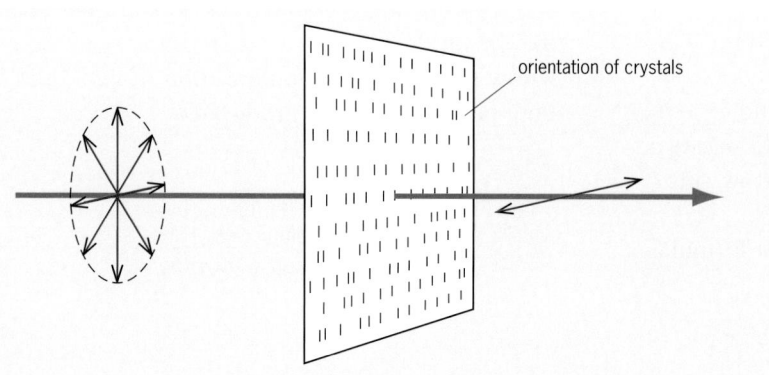

orientation of crystals

Fig 15.38 A Polaroid sheet transmits light waves with the electric field oscillating in one direction only

? **QUESTION 9**

9 Light reflected from a sheet of clear ice at an angle of 53° is found to be completely plane polarised. What is the refractive index of ice?

POLARISATION BY REFLECTION

When light is partially reflected by a transparent insulator, such as a sheet of glass, both the reflected and refracted light is always partly polarised. When the reflected and refracted beams are at right angles to each other, the reflected light is completely polarised (Fig 15.39). This occurs at an angle of incidence called the **Brewster angle**, B, where $\tan B = n$, the refractive index of the reflecting medium.

Fig 15.39 Polarisation by reflection is complete when the incident angle is given by tan $i = n$

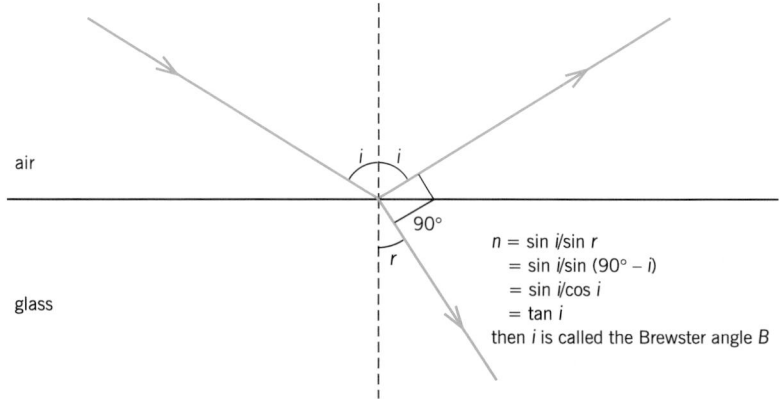

$$n = \sin i/\sin r$$
$$= \sin i/\sin (90° - i)$$
$$= \sin i/\cos i$$
$$= \tan i$$
then i is called the Brewster angle B

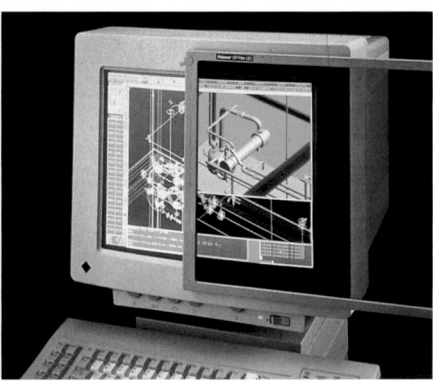

Fig 15.40 A Polaroid sheet removes reflection glare from the screen

Polarised light is now a common feature of everyday life. Many people use Polaroid sunglasses, and the liquid crystal displays (LCDs) on watches, calculators, PCs and laptops involve the use of polarised light. Polaroid sunglasses and filters reduce reflection glare because they absorb the polarised component (Fig 15.40).

SUMMARY

Having studied this chapter, you should be able to do the following:

● Understand the nature and production of electromagnetic waves.
● Know the properties of the main sections of the electromagnetic spectrum.
● Know what determines the speed of electromagnetic waves and use the formula:

$$c = \frac{1}{\sqrt{\varepsilon_0 \mu_0}}$$

● Understand how Huygens' principle is used to explain why light travels in straight lines, is reflected and refracted.
● Understand why a change in speed may produce refraction and dispersion of light.
● Understand the principle of superposition for waves.
● Understand the meaning of diffraction and interference and what happens when light passes through a single narrow slit and two narrow slits (Young's experiment).
● Know and be able to use Young's two-slit formula:
$n\lambda = s \sin \theta$

and the formula for fringe separation:

$$\Delta x = \frac{\lambda D}{s}$$

and know how the experiment may be used to measure the wavelength of light.

● Know the conditions for interference between two wave trains, especially the concept of coherence.
● Understand the meaning of resolution for an optical instrument and the significance of the Rayleigh criterion:

$$\sin \theta \approx \theta = \frac{1.22\lambda}{D}$$

● Understand how a diffraction grating works, why it is an improvement on prisms for use in spectroscopy and be able to use the grating formula $n\lambda = d \sin \theta$.
● Know the meaning of polarisation of light, and how polarised light is produced.

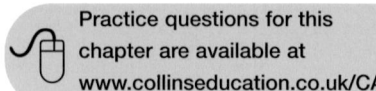
Practice questions for this chapter are available at
www.collinseducation.co.uk/CAS

16

Atoms, spectra and quanta

16 ATOMS, SPECTRA AND QUANTA

Wavy particles

The pictures on this page were taken using modern techniques which rely on the wave nature of particles, such as electrons, and the particle nature of light, which Chapter 15 should have convinced you 'is a wave'. This is the world of *quantum physics* – probably the most successful theory in physics at providing explanations and accurate predictions.

The pictures were made by extremely useful imaging devices that work because of the strange ability of the very small – atoms, electrons, light waves – to show quantum effects. These effects mean we have to think again about the meaning of 'real' – and be prepared to set aside some of the ideas which have worked so well in explaining and predicting the behaviour of everyday objects like cars, tennis balls and planets.

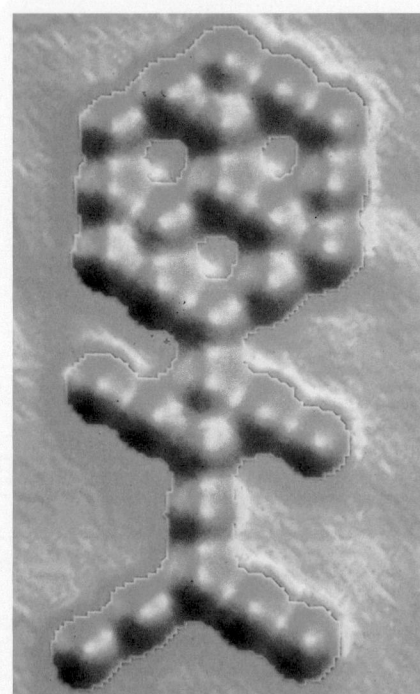

The small mounds in this picture are the outlines of atoms: they are images of the whirling cloud of particles that we call electrons. The picture was taken by a scanning tunnelling microscope (STM) which relies not only on the wave properties of electrons but also on the strange fact that electrons can 'tunnel' through an apparently impassable energy barrier

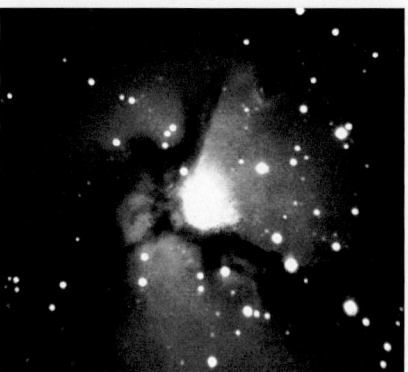

This picture of the Trifid Nebula was taken with a charge-coupled device (CCD) – an electronic light detector that relies on the fact that light sometimes behaves as a particle – although we normally think of it as a wave

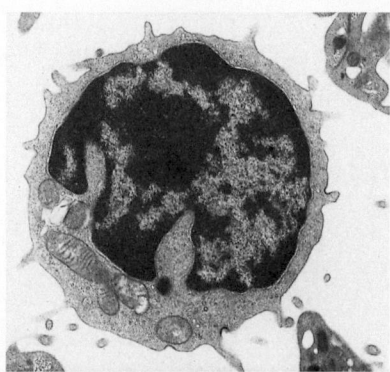

This picture, from an electron microscope, shows a white blood cell which helps the body fight disease. It is taken with a beam of electrons, which we normally think of as particles. Here, they are acting as waves

The ideas in this chapter

Physicists developed quantum theory during the twentieth century. Physics before 'the quantum' is called **classical physics**; after the quantum, it has become **modern physics**. Quantum theory originated from two apparently quite different areas of physics.

Firstly, there was a puzzle that seemed just a small fault in the otherwise superb theory developed in the nineteenth century to explain the nature of **electromagnetic radiation**. The spectrum of radiation emitted by a hot object – so-called **black body** (or **thermal**) radiation – didn't match the theory.

Secondly, there was the (accidental) discovery of **radioactivity**, described in Chapter 17. This led physicists to discover the nucleus, and to propose a new model of the atom. According to the theories at the time, a nuclear atom surrounded by orbiting electrons would immediately self-destruct as its orbital electrons spiralled into the nucleus. At the same time, they would radiate energy as electromagnetic waves. This doesn't happen, a fact which proved to be the link between the two unsolved problems.

The key ideas developed in this chapter also include: Einstein's insight that the photoelectric effect meant that radiation was quantised; how alpha particles from radioactive sources were used to probe atoms and so uncover the nucleus; the fact that electrons show both wave and particle properties; and, finally, why atoms can exist without self-destruction.

1 THE CONTINUOUS SPECTRUM OF A HOT BODY

Hot objects emit electromagnetic radiation and its intensity varies with wavelength in a pattern that depends on the temperature of the body. This radiation pattern is called by various names: **temperature radiation**, **thermal radiation** or **black body radiation**. Fig 16.2 shows the intensity of the radiation plotted against wavelength for a generalised object at several temperatures. The graphs are based on experimental results.

Real materials may not emit radiation in precisely these distributions, particularly at low temperatures, hence the notion of an ideal or 'perfect' radiator called a **black body radiator**. An argument (which we won't go into here) suggests that a perfect *radiator* must also be a perfect *absorber* of radiation. Anything that perfectly absorbs all the radiation falling on it will look black – hence the term *black body* (Fig 16.1).

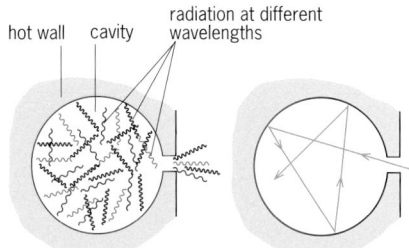

hot wall   cavity   radiation at different wavelengths

On entering, radiation is reflected so many times, losing energy each time, that it is eventually totally absorbed

Fig 16.1 Cavity or black body or temperature radiation. The radiation in the cavity of a mass of hot material settles down into a steady distribution of intensity at different wavelengths. The exact distribution depends only on temperature. A small hole lets out a sample of radiation to study

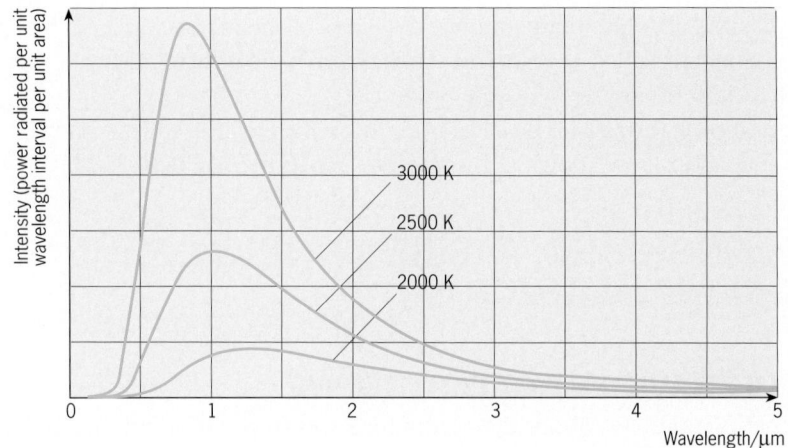

Fig 16.2 The graphs show how the distribution of the intensity of radiation from a hot object changes as the temperature is increased: the peak shifts to shorter wavelengths. Check that $\lambda_{max}T$ is a constant. The total energy emitted is represented by the area under the graph

The graphs in Fig 16.2 have a similar pattern. The intensity reaches a peak at a particular wavelength, say λ_{max}. The higher the temperature, the smaller λ_{max} becomes. It obeys a law discovered experimentally in 1893 by Wilhelm Wien (Germany, 1864–1928), known as **Wien's displacement law**:

$$\lambda_{max}T = \text{constant}$$

where T is the absolute temperature of the body (in kelvin). The constant has a value of 2.898×10^{-3} m K. The graphs also increase in area as the temperature increases, showing that the hotter the body, the more energy it radiates per second.

Cool objects emit entirely in the infrared. As they first become red hot, they start to emit visible radiation (at about 700 K). They then become

> **? QUESTION 1**
>
> 1 **a)** One of the brightest stars in the sky is Vega. It emits radiation with a peak wavelength of 240 nm. Use Wien's displacement law to calculate its surface temperature.
> **b)** What would be the peak wavelength of the radiation emitted by a red giant star with a surface temperature of 3000 K?

EXAMPLE

Q At what wavelengths do **a)** the Sun and **b)** the human body emit maximum intensity of radiation? (Assume Wien's constant is 2.9×10^{-3} m K, the surface temperature of the Sun is 6000 K, and the human body has a skin temperature of about 35 °C.)

A **a)** The Sun has a surface temperature of 6000 K, so by Wien's law:
$\lambda_{max} \times 6000$ K $= 2.9 \times 10^{-3}$ m K; $\lambda_{max} = 4.8 \times 10^{-7}$ m

b) The skin temperature of the body is 308 K, thus:
$\lambda_{max} \times 308$ K $= 2.9 \times 10^{-3}$ m K; $\lambda_{max} = 9.4 \times 10^{-6}$ m

white hot, then blue hot, as shorter wavelengths begin to dominate at even higher temperatures.

Comment on the Example

The wavelength of maximum energy emission for the Sun is 480 nm, which is in the visible range (green). At a λ_{max} of about 10 μm, the human body emits most energy in the infrared, hence the popularity of infrared burglar alarms and body-sensor light switches.

TOTAL ENERGY RADIATED BY A HOT OBJECT

Experiments showed that for a black body (a perfect radiator) emitting radiation, the total energy emitted per second (power P) increases very rapidly with temperature. This behaviour was investigated by Josef Stefan (Austria, 1835–1893). He showed that the total energy emitted *per second* (power, P) as radiation by such a black body is given by a simple formula:

$$P = \sigma A T^4$$

where T is the absolute temperature (in kelvin), A the surface area of the body and σ a constant called the **Stefan–Boltzmann constant**. It has a value of 5.6696×10^{-8} W m^{-2} K^{-4}.

This relationship was later deduced from theory by Stefan's student, Ludwig Boltzmann, and is now known as the **Stefan–Boltzmann law**.

2 PLANCK AND THE BEGINNING OF QUANTUM THEORY

THE ULTRAVIOLET CATASTROPHE

The experimental laws about the continuous spectrum of radiation emitted by hot objects were discovered during the nineteenth century. The British physicist Lord Rayleigh (1842–1919) and the young British astrophysicist Sir James Jeans (1877–1946) derived a theoretical relationship between temperature and intensity, the **Rayleigh–Jeans law**. This related the intensity I at a particular wavelength λ to the absolute temperature T of a black body by a formula:

$$I = \frac{2\pi c k T}{\lambda^4}$$

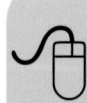

QUESTION 2

2 The adult human body has a surface area of about 1.8 m². A comfortable skin temperature is 33 °C and for all skin colours the skin is a fairly good 'black body' radiator, with about 85% of the body area as an effective radiator. Show that with an ambient (surrounding) temperature of 22 °C the unclothed body would radiate at a power of about 100 W.

For more information and an overview of the development of quantum theory please go to www.collinseducation.co.uk/CAS

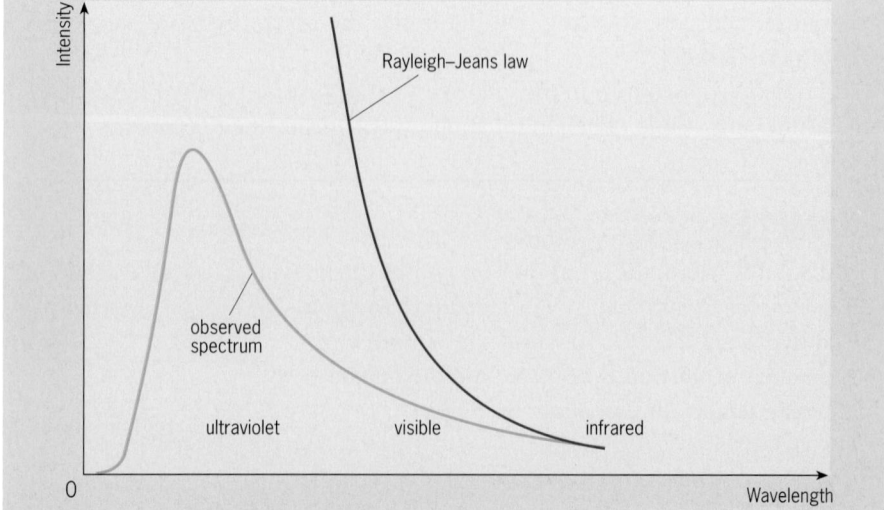

Fig 16.3 The Rayleigh–Jeans formula fitted observations only for very hot objects at the longer wavelengths

where c is the speed of light and k is a thermal constant (the Boltzmann constant, see page 163). I is the power emitted per unit area having wavelength λ in a small wavelength interval $\Delta\lambda$. The equation was based on the idea that electromagnetic radiation is emitted by oscillating charged particles (see page 285). The oscillators were taken to be the atoms in the wall of the black body.

But the formula had a serious flaw – it didn't work! The villain is the term λ^4. It means that the Sun, with $T = 6000$ K, should emit ever-increasing quantities of energy as the wavelength gets smaller (Fig 16.3). The energy emitted in the ultraviolet should be immense – and become infinite at even shorter wavelengths. In reality, as Fig 16.3 shows, the curve bends over at the Stefan maximum and less energy is radiated as wavelength decreases. This failure of nineteenth-century classical physics to account for the short-wavelength decrease became known as the **ultraviolet catastrophe**.

SHORT-WAVELENGTH ENERGY EMISSION AND THE PLANCK CONSTANT

The solution was eventually found in 1900 by the German physicist Max Planck (1858–1947). He saw the cause of the problem – it was an assumption that seemed to everyone else at the time to be perfectly sensible. As explained in Chapter 15, electromagnetic waves are produced when electrons or charged particles oscillate. The incorrect formula assumed that the charged particles in matter could oscillate at *any* frequency. But Planck thought that if the oscillators were more like the strings of a musical instrument, they would oscillate *only at definite fixed frequencies*. Fig 16.4(a) shows the natural modes of vibration of a stretched string – which can have an infinite number of frequencies, but they cannot vary continuously.

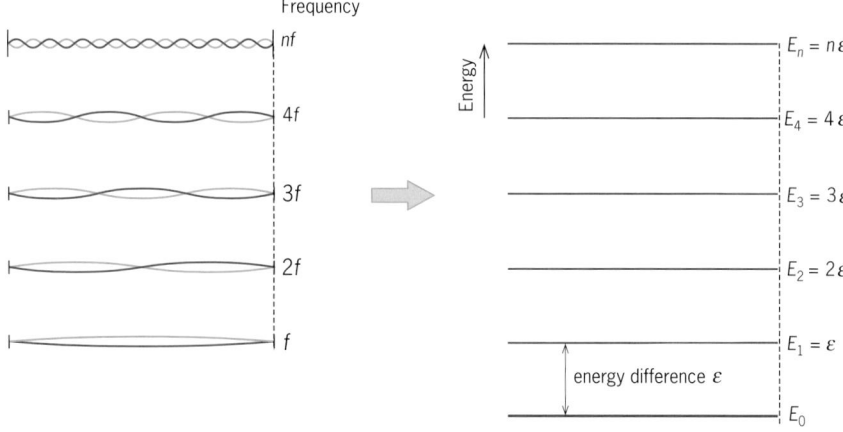

Fig 16.4(a) The natural vibrations of a stretched string can have only certain definite frequencies. Frequency is 'quantised'

Fig 16.4(b) The energy of a simple oscillator is also quantised with equal differences between the 'energy levels' or energy states

When Planck fed this idea into the mathematics, there turned out to be a natural limit to the short wavelength (high frequency) radiation. He produced a formula giving an intensity–wavelength curve that matched the experimental evidence.

He also showed that the energy E of the oscillators was proportional to their frequency f:

$$E = hf$$

where h is called the **Planck constant** and has a value of 6.626×10^{-34} J s.

Planck had used the idea that, as for a stretched string, the frequency of the oscillating charges in a hot object cannot change continuously. The frequency can have values of f, $2f$, $3f$, ..., nf, where f is a fundamental frequency and n is a whole

? **QUESTION 3**

3 Use the Rayleigh–Jeans formula to calculate the expected intensities of radiation for the Sun (temperature 6000 K) at wavelengths of 10^{-3} m (infrared) and 3×10^{-7} m (ultraviolet). Look up the data you need. Compare your answers with the graph of Fig 16.1 and comment on the differences.

number, now called a **quantum number**. Planck's formula relating energy to frequency means that the **energy** of an oscillator cannot change continuously either – it must change in small, discrete steps, called **quanta** (Fig 16.4(b)). In other words,

$$\text{oscillator energy} = hf, 2hf, 3hf, \ldots, nhf$$

Planck received the Nobel Prize for his theory in 1919.

EINSTEIN AND THE QUANTISATION OF LIGHT

Planck did not himself take the next step, which was to recognise that the *radiation itself is also quantised*, meaning it is in small packets. The step was made by an unknown young civil servant working in the Patent Office in Berne, Switzerland, the 26-year-old Albert Einstein. His argument was simple:

- An oscillating charge can accept or lose energy only in small quantities of value $\Delta E = h\Delta f$ where Δf is its change in frequency.
- It gains or loses the energy as electromagnetic radiation.
- Therefore the radiation must also be emitted in small packets, each carrying energy ΔE.

Einstein suggested that the emitted radiation should also obey the Planck rule, and have its own frequency f_{rad} such that the energy E_{rad} it carries is related by:

$$E_{rad} = hf_{rad}$$

This meant that the radiation from a hot object was no longer to be thought continuous. It had to consist of a set of radiation packets each carrying a bit of energy – *a quantum of energy*. This was difficult to imagine: radiation such as light was a packet of energy but was also a wave – it had a frequency. It is what we now call a **photon**.

Einstein used this idea to explain another effect that was puzzling physicists at the turn of the twentieth century – the photoelectric effect.

THE PHOTOELECTRIC EFFECT

Fig 16.6(a) in the Science in Context box opposite shows the arrangement used to investigate the photoelectric effect, together with typical results in Figs 16.6 (b) and (c).

When light is shone on a clean metal surface, the surface may become positively charged. This happens because energy carried by light waves is absorbed by free electrons in the metal, giving them enough kinetic energy to 'jump' out of the metal. But there are a number of puzzling features in the photoelectric effect which cannot be explained by the simple wave model of light – see Fig 16.5.

One is that electrons are not emitted unless the frequency of the incident light is greater than a certain threshold value. For example, blue light produces a photoelectric effect in sodium, but red light does not. Perhaps red light does not carry enough energy? The simple wave model suggests that even if the waves of red light are less energetic than blue light waves, eventually the beam of red light will transfer enough energy to liberate electrons from the metal atoms. *But this does not happen.*

Another strange fact is that when even a very weak beam of blue light is shone on sodium metal, electrons are released almost immediately. It is hard to explain why this happens using a wave theory in which the light is spread evenly all over the metal surface. How could it be concentrated enough to give even just a few electrons the energy to escape so quickly?

A third observation is also difficult to explain. The electrons leave the metal surface with kinetic energy, which must have been given to them by the light. Some have more kinetic energy than others, and experiments show that the *maximum* kinetic energy $E_{K,max}$ possessed by the emitted electrons depends on the *frequency* of the light, not on its *intensity* (see Science in Context box

? QUESTION 4

4 **a)** Calculate the energy of a photon of electromagnetic radiation with a wavelength of:
i) 200 nm **ii)** 600 nm **iii)** 2 mm
iv) 10 mm.
b) In which part of the electromagnetic spectrum is each of the above photons?

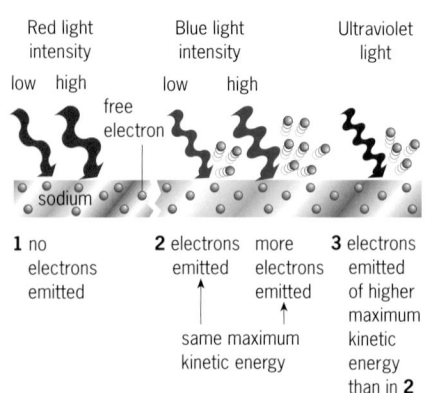

Red light intensity	Blue light intensity	Ultraviolet light
low high	low high	

1 no electrons emitted

2 electrons emitted   more electrons emitted

3 electrons emitted of higher maximum kinetic energy than in **2**

same maximum kinetic energy

Fig 16.5 Features of the photoelectric effect that need to be explained

The photoelectric experiments

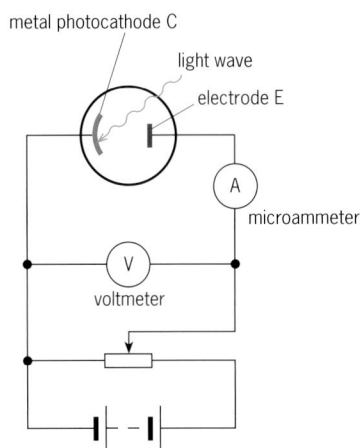

Fig 16.6(a) The circuit used

Light shone on the cathode C makes it emit electrons with a range of energies. The aim of the experiment is to measure, for a range of metals and a range of light frequencies and intensities:

- how the size of the current produced in the circuit by electrons moving from C to E changes,
- the highest energy that is gained by an electron for any given metal.

The emitted electrons move to the electrode E and form a current that is read by the ammeter A. To start with E is made positive and all the electrons emitted are captured. Then the voltage of E is reduced until it becomes negative with respect to the cathode. The current stays about the same until the electrode becomes negative. Then the slowest electrons are repelled and so the current falls. When the negative voltage is large enough, even the fastest electrons are repelled and the current becomes zero. It is this value of the negative potential difference between the emitter cathode C and collector E, the **stopping voltage** V_s, that measures the **maximum kinetic energy** of emitted electrons.

When the fastest, most energetic electrons are just stopped, their kinetic energy becomes zero: it has been used up in doing work against the repelling force from electrode E. The work done moving a charge e through a p.d. *V* is *eV* (see Chapter 9, page 196).

Equating energies: $E_{K,max} = eV_s$

where $E_{K,max}$ is the maximum kinetic energy of any emitted electron and *e* is the electronic charge.

In the series of experiments both the kind of metal used at C and the frequency (colour) and brightness of the light can be varied. The results are as follows.

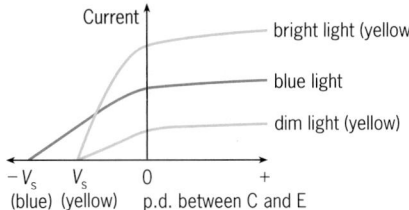

Fig 16.6(b) Graphs showing how the current in the circuit changes as the p.d. between C and E is reduced, for a given metal. For a given frequency of light falling on C, the current gets smaller when the light is less bright, but the stopping voltage stays the same. However, the stopping voltage V_s is different for different light frequencies

Keeping the metal of C the same

- With different brightnesses: the curr- ent is weaker for weaker light, but the stopping voltage (i.e. maximum electron energy) stays the same.
- With increasing light frequency the stopping voltage needed increases, showing that maximum electron energy increases with light frequency.

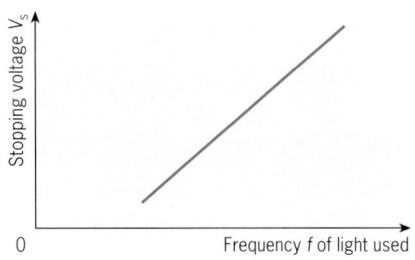

Fig 16.6(c) Graph of stopping voltage against frequency for a given metal: there is a linear relationship, explained by Einstein's theory

Changing the metal used

- The same pattern is observed, but the stopping voltage for a given frequency is different for different metals.

As explained in the main text, these results can be explained by using Einstein's model of light photons carrying energy quanta proportional to their frequency, $E = hf$. This leads to the relationship:

$$E_{K,max} = hf - W$$

where *W* is a constant for a given metal.

above). Weak ultraviolet light produces electrons with greater energy from sodium than, say, very bright blue light does.

Einstein's theory that light arrived in packets with energy proportional to frequency gives a simple explanation of all this. In the photoelectric effect, all of the energy carried by one light-packet (one photon) is given to one electron. There are forces that normally hold the electron inside the metal, and it needs some minimal energy to do work against these forces before it can escape. Suppose this minimal escape energy is *W*. If the electron gets energy *E* from a photon, then the *maximum* kinetic energy that an escaped electron can have is $E_{K,max}$ such that:

$$E_{K,max} = E - W$$

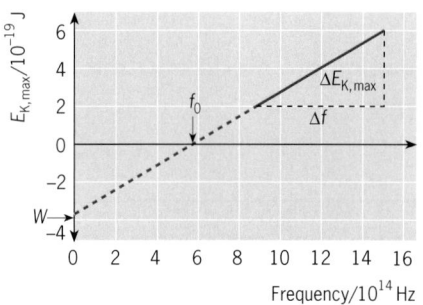

Fig 16.7 Graph of Einstein's photoelectric equation:
$$E_{K,max} = hf - W$$
No electrons are emitted for frequencies of light less than a threshold frequency f_0.
At intercept value f_0, $W = hf_0$.
The slope of the graph is the Planck constant h:
$$h = \Delta E_{K,max}/\Delta f$$

Table 16.1 Work functions of some metals

Metal	W/eV	W/10⁻¹⁹ J
sodium	2.28	3.65
aluminium	4.08	6.53
copper	4.7	7.52
zinc	4.31	6.9
silver	4.73	7.57
platinum	6.35	10.2
lead	4.14	6.62
iron	4.5	7.2
potassium	1.81	2.9

✔ **REMEMBER THIS**

An **electronvolt** (eV) is a unit of energy. It is the energy gained by an electron accelerated through a p.d. of 1 volt. See Chapter 9, page 196.

? **QUESTION 5**

5 Use Fig 16.7 to do the following.
   a) From its work function, identify the metal involved.
   b) Estimate a value for the Planck constant.

The Planck–Einstein formula gave $E = hf$, so we have:

$$E_{K,max} = hf - W \quad \text{or} \quad hf = E_{K,max} + W$$

See Fig 16.7 and compare this with Fig 16.6(c).

This model explains the experimental results. If hf is smaller than W, the electron cannot escape. The 'threshold frequency' f_0 is such that $hf_0 = W$. A graph of $E_{K,max}$ against f will be a straight line of slope h with the intercept on the energy axis being $-W$.

W is called the **work function** of the metal (see Table 16.1). It is a measure of how hard it is for an electron to escape from the metal. It is easy for electrons to escape from sodium, compared with platinum, for example.

Einstein's model also explains why there is a such a small delay between irradia- ting the metal and the escape of electrons. Just one photon might be enough to cause an electron to be emitted–there is no need to wait for the energy to 'build up'.

The model also explains why increasing the *intensity* of the radiation does not increase the maximum energy of the electrons emitted. *No electron can gain more than one quantum of energy.*

To summarise:

- Electrons are only emitted when light of a high enough frequency is used; there is a cut-off frequency, below which no electrons emerge, however bright the light.
- The electrons are emitted instantly.
- Brighter light means more electrons emitted, not electrons with more energy.
- The kinetic energy of the electrons is proportional to the frequency of the light.
- All these effects are explained by a photon (particle) model of light.

For many physicists, the Planck–Einstein quantum theory of light remained 'just a theory'. But in 1922, Arthur Compton (USA, 1892–1962) did experiments which showed that X-ray quanta behaved like particles when they bounced off electrons. The photons not only had *energy*, they also had *momentum*. This seems very odd, since momentum is defined as mass Δ velocity, and photons have no mass. But see Chapter 23 for an explanation of how all energy has an equivalent mass.

3 QUANTUM THEORY AND THE NUCLEAR ATOM

There are two main ways of finding what atoms or other small particles are like. One is to fire something even smaller at them and see either how they break up or how the projectile bounces off them. The other is to shake them about (give them some energy) and see what comes out. Both these methods were used to give physicists their first idea of what an atom is like.

PROBING THE ATOM WITH ALPHA PARTICLES

The first method was used for a very fruitful experiment in 1909. Alpha particles from a radioactive source were fired at a thin film of metal atoms: this was the **Geiger–Marsden experiment** (see Chapter 17). Some particles bounced back at angles that meant they had hit something small and with mass. From this, Rutherford worked out in 1911 that an atom has a positive nucleus surrounded by negative electrons. He suggested that the electrons could be orbiting round the nucleus like planets round the Sun. But such an atom would not be stable. An orbiting electron, like an orbiting planet, has an acceleration directed towards the attracting object. An accelerating electron continuously radiates electromagnetic waves, so should lose energy and spiral into the nucleus.

Rutherford's model was saved in 1913 by the Danish physicist Niels Bohr (1885–1962). He used the new quantum ideas of energy, saying that the electron could have only certain 'allowed' energy states, with definite energy gaps between them corresponding to definite orbits. So electrons could not lose energy continuously and spiral into the nucleus. Electrons could only move between orbits by gaining or losing definite, fixed quanta of energy.

This seemed a very far-fetched idea at the time – but Bohr backed it up with calculations of how much energy an atom could gain or lose, and matched this with the energy of the light quanta it emitted.

Bohr didn't explain why the electron couldn't fall into the nucleus – this had to wait for a later version of the quantum theory (see page 317).

LINE SPECTRA

The spectrum of the radiation emitted by a hot body is continuous because there are very many different kinds of oscillators in any real lump of matter, so that in practice quanta exist at all frequencies.

But there are discontinuous spectra called line spectra – the then mysterious pattern of radiation emitted by *pure* elements when they are heated or electrically 'disturbed'. See Fig 16.8 and Fig 15.33 (page 301) for examples of line spectra. The lines are differently coloured images of the slit that was illuminated by the original light. An arrangement for producing a line spectrum is shown in Fig 16.9.

Each element has a unique spectrum. The spectrum of the smallest atom, hydrogen, has four visible lines (see page 301), and a large number of invisible ones in the ultraviolet and infrared. Niels Bohr was able to explain the pattern of the spectral lines of hydrogen – and to calculate their wavelengths.

REMEMBER THIS
'Orbital' is the term that mainly chemists use to describe the modern quantum-theory fuzziness of an electron in an atom.

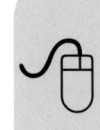

For an in-depth study of Bohr's atom model, please see the How Science Works assignment for this chapter at www.collinseducation.co.uk/CAS

Fig 16.8 Line spectra of helium (top), neon (centre), mercury (bottom)

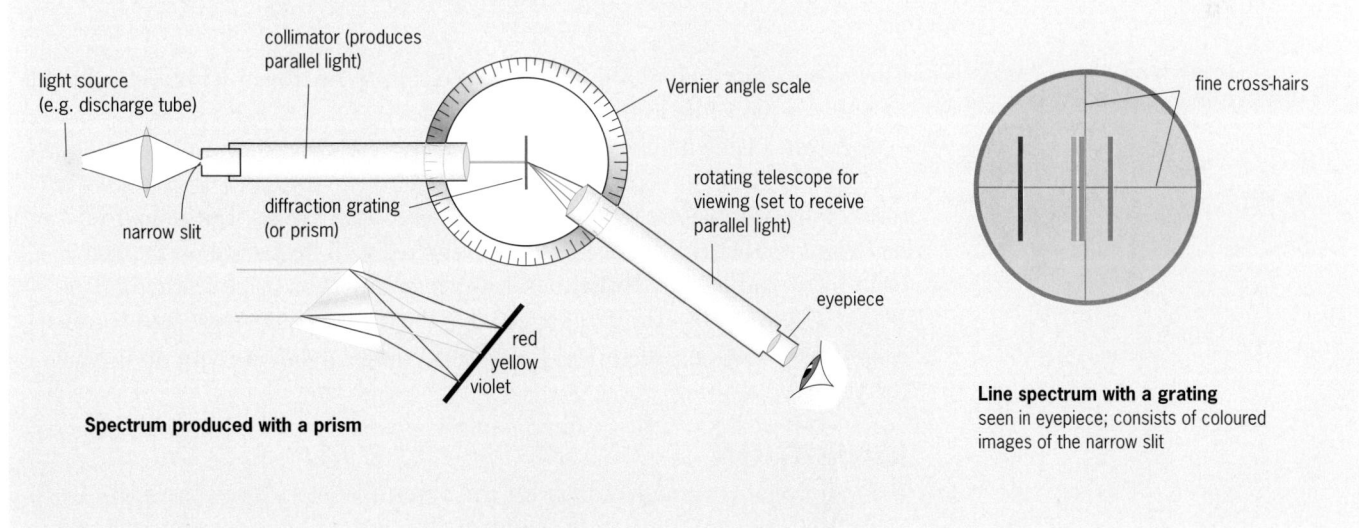

light source (e.g. discharge tube)

collimator (produces parallel light)

Vernier angle scale

rotating telescope for viewing (set to receive parallel light)

narrow slit

diffraction grating (or prism)

red
yellow
violet

eyepiece

Spectrum produced with a prism

fine cross-hairs

Line spectrum with a grating
seen in eyepiece; consists of coloured images of the narrow slit

The explanation is as follows. The single electron in the hydrogen atom could exist in a set of definite orbits, each associated with a definite quantity of energy. It was normally in the 'lowest orbit'. When you supply energy to a hydrogen atom, as in a discharge tube, the electron can move to an orbit further from the nucleus. Such *excited* atoms are unstable, and the electron quickly falls back to its normal orbit. As it does so, it emits a quantum of

Fig 16.9 A spectrometer is used to study spectral lines

Fig 16.10(a) In this early model of a hydrogen atom, its one electron was imagined as a particle in orbit around the positive nucleus. This was the Rutherford–Bohr model

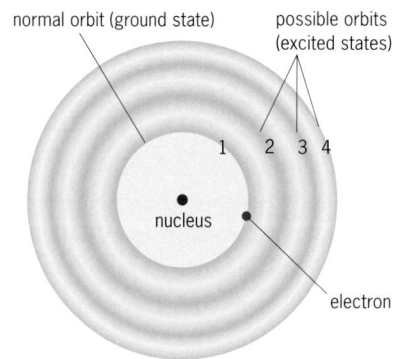

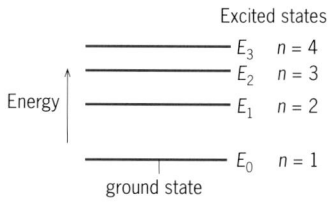

Fig 16.10(b) Energy level diagram corresponding to the simple Rutherford–Bohr model. n is the quantum number which defines the state of the atom

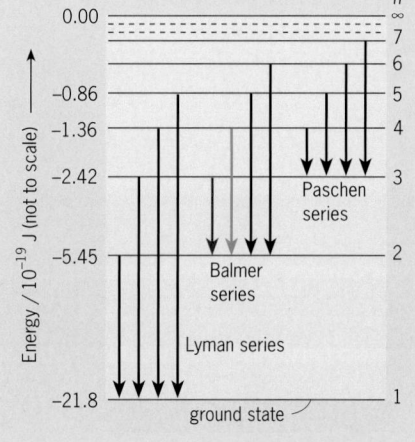

Fig 16.12 Hydrogen emits several series of lines in its spectrum. Each series is named after the scientist who discovered it. Each arrow corresponds to a different transition, and it is the transitions from higher excited states (energy levels) to lower ones that produce the spectral series

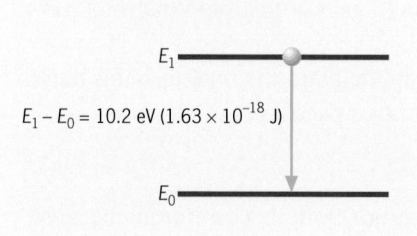

Fig 16.11 For a hydrogen atom, a photon of energy 1.63×10^{-18} J is emitted when an electron moves to the ground state from the first excited state

electromagnetic radiation. This is illustrated in Fig 16.10, which shows a simple (early) model of a hydrogen atom and a more modern energy level diagram.

For an electron to make the transition from energy level E_0 to level E_1 (Fig 16.10(b)), the hydrogen atom needs to be given exactly 10.2 eV (1.63×10^{-18} J) of energy. An electron in level E_1 is not stable: it quickly falls back to level E_0. In this transition, it then emits the energy difference ΔE as a photon of light, with energy 1.63×10^{-18} J (Fig 16.11).

Planck's formula allows us to calculate the frequency of this light:

$$\Delta E = E_1 - E_0 = hf$$

giving:

$$f = \frac{1.63 \times 10^{-18}}{6.63 \times 10^{-34}} = 2.46 \times 10^{15} \text{ Hz}$$

This is the frequency of a line in the spectrum of hydrogen with a wavelength of 122 nm, which is in the ultraviolet range.

There are a large number of 'orbits' or energy levels for an electron around the nucleus of a hydrogen atom. Some of these are shown in Fig 16.12. It shows just three of the possible sets of jumps from higher to lower levels. The jump from higher states to level 2 produces photons emitted with frequencies in the visible region. This is called the **Balmer series** after the Swiss schoolteacher Johann Balmer (1825–1898) who first spotted that the frequencies of these lines formed a simple mathematical pattern, or *series*. Bohr's simple model was able to explain this pattern.

IONISATION

If an atom gains enough energy for the outermost electron to leave it completely, the atom becomes **ionised**. The negative energy values shown in Fig 16.12 are in fact measured from the state in which the electron is a long way from the nucleus: the electron has escaped, and the atom is ionised. The energy required to ionise a hydrogen atom is 2.18×10^{-18} J (13.6 eV).

The success of the quantum theory – both to *explain* the simple Rutherford model of an atom and the pattern of lines in the hydrogen spectrum, and also to *predict* the values of the wavelengths – led to its acceptance.

? QUESTION 6

6 What is the frequency of the highest energy photon emitted in the Lyman series (see Fig 16.12)? In which part of the electromagnetic spectrum would it appear?

✔ REMEMBER THIS

The concept of negative potential energy is discussed in Chapter 2, in terms of the gravitational field.

Types of spectra

Disturbed atoms emit electromagnetic radiation when orbital electrons lose energy by falling to a lower energy state. Line spectra are images of the narrow slit that the light falls on in a spectrograph or spectrometer. Such spectra are most likely to be produced by elements and mixtures of elements in the gaseous form, for example in hot gases. Solids can be vaporised in a hot flame (the Bunsen burner was developed in the laboratory of Robert Bunsen (Germany, 1811–1899), probably by his chief technician, to produce a clean flame to make his spectroscopy easier). Spectra can also be made by disturbing atoms electrically, for example by firing electrons and ions through a low pressure gas in a 'discharge tube'. All of these methods produce **emission spectra**. Each line corresponds to a definite frequency (and so wavelength) of radiation.

A heated solid or a hot, highly disturbed mixture of many elements tends to produce a **continuous spectrum**, with no visible separate lines. This is because there are so many frequencies produced that the lines overlap. At first glance the spectrum of sunlight is continuous. But early in the nineteenth century Josef von Fraunhofer, a professional lens-maker, discovered that the spectrum of sunlight was crossed by a large number of **dark** lines (Fig 16.13). It was soon shown that the frequencies associated with these lines corresponded to the emission spectra of known elements. They were formed as illustrated in Fig 16.14. Highly disturbed atoms in hot regions in the Sun produced a continuous emission spectrum, but this light then had to travel through cooler regions. The atoms in these cool regions *absorbed* energy from the light, which lifted electrons from their normal energy levels to higher ones. This could only happen at the set

Fig 16.13 Fraunhofer lines in the solar spectrum

frequencies dictated by the quantum jumps needed to do this. The light thus travelled on weaker in intensity at those frequencies – so producing the **absorption spectrum** with the characteristic Fraunhofer dark lines. The light was weaker at these frequencies even when the disturbed electrons went back to normal, because they re-emitted the light in all directions – not just outward from the Sun.

Fraunhofer had discovered a way of finding out what elements were present in the Sun's atmosphere, and such absorption spectra are now used to find out what elements there are in stars and galaxies. The Doppler effect uses absorption spectra to measure the speeds of stars and galaxies; this has led to the discovery that the Universe is expanding (see Chapters 25 and 26).

Fig 16.14 How absorption spectra are produced

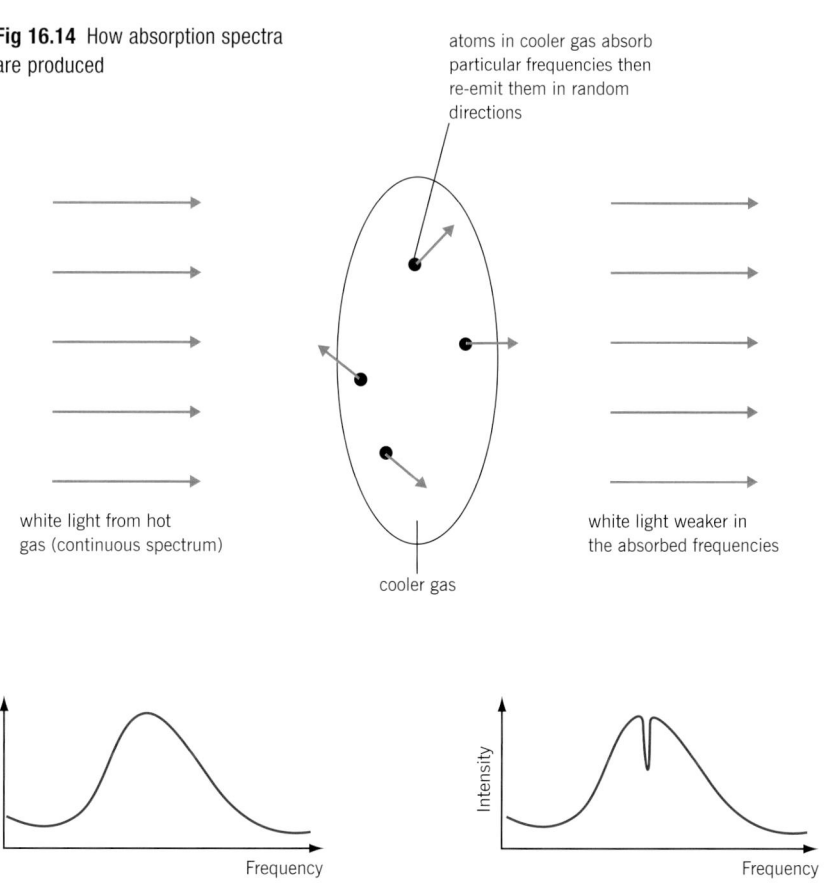

atoms in cooler gas absorb particular frequencies then re-emit them in random directions

white light from hot gas (continuous spectrum)

cooler gas

white light weaker in the absorbed frequencies

REMEMBER THIS

(See Chapter 23.)

In general, $\Delta E_k = v\Delta p$ for a particle.
And, for light of speed c,

$$E = pc \qquad [1]$$

where E is the photon energy.
But $E = hf = hc/\lambda$, giving

$$\lambda = \frac{hc}{E} = \frac{h}{p} \quad \text{from [1].}$$

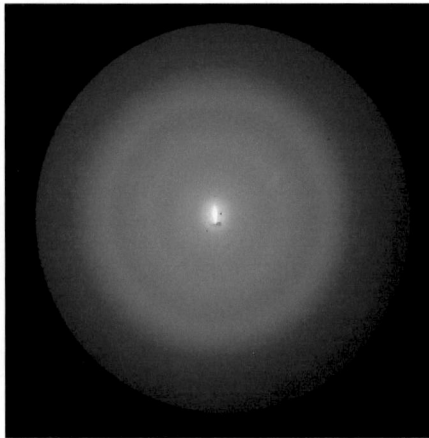

Fig 16.15 Diffraction rings for electrons formed by standard laboratory diffraction apparatus

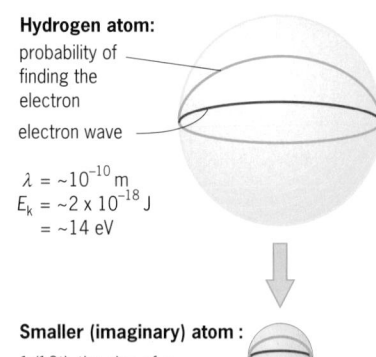

Hydrogen atom:
probability of finding the electron
electron wave
$\lambda = \sim 10^{-10}$ m
$E_k = \sim 2 \times 10^{-18}$ J
$\quad = \sim 14$ eV

Smaller (imaginary) atom :
1/10th the size of a hydrogen atom
$\lambda = \sim 10^{-11}$ m
$E_k = \sim 2 \times 10^{-16}$ J
$\quad = \sim 1.4$ keV
$\quad (= 100$ times greater)

Nucleus:
1/10 000th the size of a hydrogen atom
Required values:
$\lambda = \sim 10^{-14}$ m
$E_k = \sim 2 \times 10^{-10}$ J
$\quad = \sim 1.4$ TeV
$\quad (= 10^8$ times greater)

Fig 16.16 Squashing a wavy electron. As the wave gets smaller, its wavelength decreases, and its momentum and energy increase.
Energy is proportional to $1/\lambda^2$, so the increase is great. Even nuclear forces are too small to keep an electron in the nucleus: its escape velocity would be too great

4 WAVY ELECTRONS

'I suddenly got the idea, during the year 1923, that the discovery made by Einstein in 1905 should be generalised by extending it to all material particles and notably to electrons.'

Louis de Broglie, PhD thesis, 1924

Prince Louis de Broglie (1892–1987) first studied history and then turned to physics. In his PhD thesis he suggested that the formula $E = hf$ should apply to electrons as well as photons. There ought, he said, to be a 'fictitious wave' associated with electrons. If so, it should be possible to diffract electrons, just as you could diffract light.

THE WAVELENGTH OF AN ELECTRON

Relativity theory shows that a photon, although without mass, nevertheless has a momentum p related to its wavelength λ by the relation:

$$\lambda = \frac{h}{p}$$

By analogy with the photon, an electron should have a wavelength given by:

$$\lambda = \frac{h}{mv}$$

where m is the mass of the electron and v its speed. The wavelength of an electron therefore depends on its speed: the faster it goes, the smaller its wavelength.

The predicted diffraction of electrons was first shown to happen in 1925. C. J. Davisson was investigating the effect of bombarding a nickel target with low-energy electrons (54 eV). But the surface had been specially cleaned, causing the growth of large crystals of nickel on the target surface. The rows of atoms in the crystals acted as a diffraction grating so that the reflected beams showed regions of electrons or no electrons. Ordinary diffraction grating theory ($n\lambda = d \sin \theta$) allowed the wavelength of electrons to be calculated and showed that de Broglie's theory was correct.

EXAMPLE

Q Calculate the wavelength of an electron accelerated by a potential difference (V) of 8 kV (as in a TV tube).

The mass m of an electron $= 9.11 \times 10^{-31}$ kg,

the charge e on an electron $= 1.60 \times 10^{-19}$ C.

A Kinetic energy gained by electron
$$\tfrac{1}{2}mv^2$$
= change in electrical potential energy
$$= eV$$

Thus: $\quad v = \sqrt{\dfrac{2eV}{m}}$

$$v = \sqrt{\frac{2 \times 1.6 \times 10^{-19} \times 8000}{9.11 \times 10^{-31}}}$$
$$= 5.3 \times 10^7 \text{ m s}^{-1}$$

(This is about 18 per cent of the speed of light, but we ignore relativistic effects!)

Wavelength of electron

$$\lambda = \frac{h}{mv}$$
$$= \frac{6.63 \times 10^{-34}}{9.11 \times 10^{-31} \times 5.30 \times 10^7}$$
$$= 1.37 \times 10^{-11} \text{ m}$$

For comparison, the wavelength of light is of the order of 10^{-7} m.

Fig 16.15 shows the diffraction pattern of rings produced when a beam of electrons passes through a 'grating'. The grating consists of the regular rows of carbon atoms in a graphite crystal.

The pattern is exactly the same as is produced by light passing through a similar type of grating – although the grating spacing for electron diffraction is very much smaller. This is because the wavelength of an electron is far smaller than the wavelength of visible light. Now we shall calculate how much smaller.

WHAT DOES THE ELECTRON WAVE ACTUALLY MEAN?

De Broglie called the electron's wave 'fictitious'. The modern view is that the wave is linked to the **probability** of finding an electron at a certain point in space. We can write a *wave equation* for an electron, as for any other wave. And, just with any other wave, we see that the amplitude varies – with distance, say.

Theory and experiment both suggest that:

- The probability of finding an electron at a given point is proportional to the square of the amplitude of the wave at that point.
- The amplitude is given by a rather complicated wave formula, the **Schrödinger wave equation**, which was put forward in 1926 by Erwin Schrödinger (Austria, 1887–1961). There is more about this on pages 318–319).

NOW WE KNOW WHY ATOMS DO NOT SELF-DESTRUCT!

De Broglie's idea was the key to unlocking the last secret of the atom – why it didn't immediately collapse in a dramatic burst of electromagnetic radiation. The simple answer is this:

- The electron is a wave whose length decreases with energy.
- If you try to squash an electron wave closer to the nucleus, the wavelength must get smaller and its energy must increase.
- If its wavelength gets close to the size of a nucleus, its energy becomes so great that the attractive force of the nucleus isn't big enough to keep it there.

The (simplified) mathematics of this is shown in Fig 16.16, which illustrates how an electron wave fits into a hydrogen atom, together with the probability function, which is the square of the amplitude of the electron wave. This will always be positive. The diagram is based on a simple solution of the Schrödinger wave equation.

ELECTRON TUNNELLING

Solutions of the Schrödinger wave equation can exist only for certain definite values of the total energy of the electron: bear in mind that the energy determines the momentum, which in turn determines the wavelength. Solutions exist for excited states of the atom as well, and any valid solution (for the amplitude of the wave, and hence the electron probability) must reach a zero value at some reasonable distance from the nucleus – otherwise the electron has effectively escaped from the atom.

One of the unexpected consequences of the wave theory is that the successful wave solutions do *not in fact* become zero at the calculated boundary of the atom. This effect would be forbidden in classical theory, because the edge of the atom is the place where the electron has zero kinetic energy, so going further means that its kinetic energy is negative, which is a

EXAMPLE

Fig 16.7 shows waves trapped in an atom of width L. As the waves have to be complete, we associate a *whole* number n with each wave.

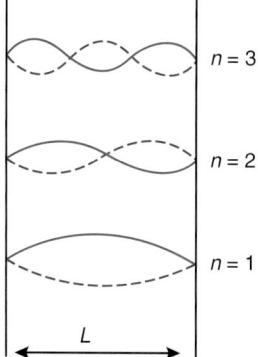

Fig 16.17 Waves trapped in an 'atom' of width L

The half wave has a wavelength of $2L$. This is the longest wave that could fit into the box. Give this a value of $n = 1$.

Wave 2 has $n = 2$ and a wavelength L.

Wave 3 has $n = 3$ and wavelength $(2/3) L$.

n is the quantum number associated with the electron of a particular wavelength, momentum and energy.

a) Check for yourself that, for any (whole number) value of n, the wavelength is $2L/n$.

b) The de Broglie connection h/λ between wavelength and momentum means that the momentum p of the electron is $hn/2L$.

c) The kinetic energy of a particle of mass m and momentum p is $E_k = p^2/2m$ (see page 47). Insert the p relationship from b) to show that $E_k = n^2h^2/8mL^2$.

This simple – but hard to believe – model of the electron as a wave shows why the electrons in an atom have definite quantised energy levels, and explains why excited atoms produce line spectra (page 223).

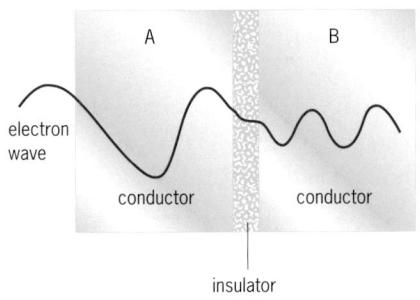

Fig 16.18 Electrons can 'tunnel' from A to B because the probability curve extends through a narrow insulator. There is more about this on page 343

physical impossibility. However, it seems to be allowed in quantum wave theory, so that there is a definite probability that electrons can exist outside the atom without breaking any energy rules. This gives rise to the phenomenon called tunnelling, which is used in the electron scanning tunnelling microscope (see the left-hand photo on page 306 and Fig 16.18).

The wave nature of electrons is thus more than just a convenient model for giving right answers about atoms. It is vital to the understanding of semiconductor materials (now so important in practical microelectronic devices), the nature of chemical bonds and the shapes of molecules.

A brief look at the real hydrogen atom – electron clouds and the Schrödinger wave equation

Fig 16.19 shows how the potential energy of the electron–proton system varies with separation of the particles in a hydrogen atom. Remember that the potential energy is negative. When the electron is at the edge of the atom its kinetic energy is zero. Closer to the nucleus it speeds up as the potential energy gets less. The total energy of the system stays constant at 2.18×10^{-18} J (13.6 eV).

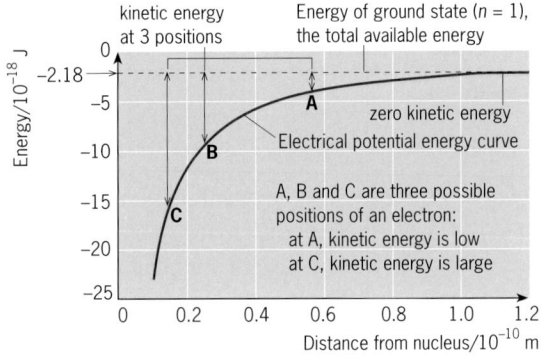

Fig 16.19 The 'potential well' of a hydrogen atom. As the electron gets closer to the nucleus, electrical potential energy gets less and kinetic energy increases

We can no longer assume that the electron is a simple particle, of course. What wave mechanics tells us is that the electron can be anywhere around the nucleus, with a probability of being at any particular *distance* which is given by a wave formula. The *probability* of the electron being at a particular *place* is given by the square of the electron wave's amplitude at that place. What is the shape of the basic electron wave?

We know that it depends on the electron's momentum, since we have $p = h/\lambda$ (de Broglie). But as the electron moves nearer to the nucleus, its speed and momentum increase, so its wavelength gets smaller. Fig 16.20 shows a possible shape for the wave of an electron in a hydrogen atom. It shows that the wave is curved more steeply nearer the nucleus. This means that it would have a smaller wavelength

there. We can't show it as a whole wavelength because it varies with distance, but the red and blue lines show waves with wavelengths that fit the curve at particular points.

The electron wave shown was calculated using a theoretical wave function called the Schrödinger wave equation.

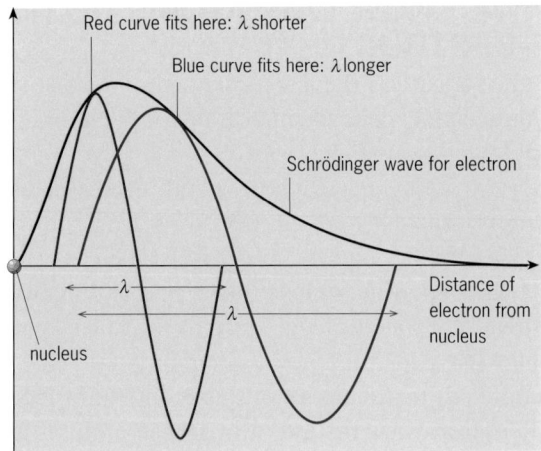

Fig 16.20 The shape of the electron wave could be fitted to a set of sine waves of changing wavelength, with shorter and shorter wavelengths the closer they get to the nucleus. As the wavelengths get shorter, their contributions reach a peak, but quickly go to zero as the distance from the nucleus approaches zero

(Note that Fig 16.22 shows *probability* waves, which represent the square of the changing amplitude of the electron wave.)

The diagram in Fig 16.21(a) shows the result for the lowest (stable) energy state of hydrogen with the atom drawn as a simple two-dimensional object, but of course it is three-dimensional, and Fig 16.21(b) gives a better picture. Chemists tend to think of the space the electron occupies as a sort of cloud and draw an atom with orbits showing the region where there is the greatest probability of finding an electron.

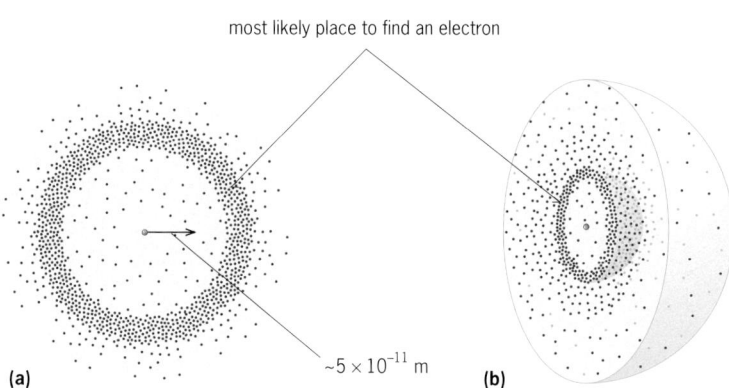

most likely place to find an electron

~5 × 10⁻¹¹ m

(a)   (b)

Fig 16.21(a) The electron moves so fast that all we observe is a 'cloud' of varying electron density, which is densest at about 0.5×10^{-10} m from the nucleus
(b) The electron occupies three-dimensional space

Fig 16.22 shows in orange the one-dimensional *probability* curve produced by plotting the square of values calculated from the Schrödinger wave equation against r for a value of total energy $E_0 = -2.18 \times 10^{-18}$ J. (This is the total energy of the atom in its normal (ground) state when the quantum number n is 1.) The electron wave values have been squared to give positive results for the probability of finding the electron at any place. The curve drops to zero, showing that the electron is enclosed inside the atom. In fact, we can get similar closed solutions only for values of E given by E_0/n^2. This satisfies Balmer-type formulae for energy levels in the hydrogen atom, as also explained by Bohr using a much simpler model. Fig 16.21 shows such curves, corresponding to higher energy states. In each case, the main peak corresponds to the most likely radius of the 'orbit' of the electron in the excited atom. The predictions match measured values.

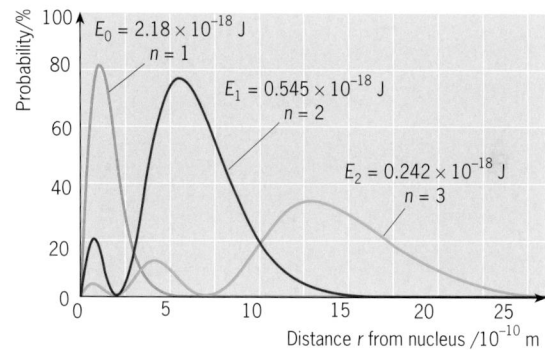

Fig 16.22 Probability curves for the electron in three energy states in a hydrogen atom

SUMMARY

After studying this chapter you should be able to do the following:
- Understand the nature of black body (temperature) radiation.
- Know Wien's displacement law and the Stefan–Boltzmann law relating wavelength, temperature and intensity in black body radiation.
- Understand how the classical theory of radiation had to be changed to a quantum theory in order to account for the experimental data.
- Understand that Planck's quantum theory explained black body radiation.
- Know about the photoelectric effect and how Einstein explained its strange results using quantum theory and the idea of the photon ($E = hf = W + E_k$).
- Know how Rutherford's nuclear model of the atom was linked to simple quantum theory (Rutherford–Bohr model).
- Understand how quantum theory explained the emission of light from an excited atom, using the idea of energy levels, and that it was able to explain the patterns in the line spectrum of hydrogen ($hf = E_1 - E_2$).
- Understand the idea that electrons have a wave nature, with a de Broglie wavelength $\lambda = h/p$.
- Know how wavy electrons produce a better model of the atom than particle electrons can – with the waves as an indicator of the probability of finding an electron.

 Practice questions for this chapter are available at www.collinseducation.co.uk/CAS

17

The atomic nucleus

17 THE ATOMIC NUCLEUS

Energy and politics

France produces 75 per cent of its electrical power from nuclear power stations and only 12 per cent from fossil fuels. This compares with just 28 per cent nuclear power in Britain, and 70 per cent from fossil fuels.

Fossil fuels contribute to the greenhouse effect and global warming. They also pollute the atmosphere, and most developed countries are searching for ways to reduce their dependence on fossil fuels. This suggests that making more use of nuclear power should be a good thing.

But in the United States (the world's largest producer of electricity from nuclear power), electricity suppliers decided in 1987 not to build any more nuclear power stations. Britain, too, cancelled plans in 1995 for building two large nuclear power stations. The main reason for these decisions was economic. In the debate on energy from nuclear or fossil fuel sources, economic and environmental arguments compete.

Since then, politicians have had to think harder about how we use and obtain energy. Looming on the not too distant horizon is global warming. The pollutants produced by burning fossil fuels make it easier for the atmosphere to trap solar thermal radiation. The main culprit seems to be carbon dioxide.

At the atomic level, the thermal energy we can get from a nuclear fission event is 200 MeV, compared with just a few eV from breaking up a molecule of a carbon-based fuel. It takes 1.5 tonnes of coal to produce as much energy as we can get from a piece of nuclear fuel about 15 mm long. For the UK, North Sea gas and oil are running out, so we are becoming more dependent upon foreign suppliers of fossil fuel.

Chernobyl Nuclear Power Station was badly designed and badly maintained. The first generation nuclear power stations were designed in the 1950s – they are now building Generation 3 power stations in Finland and in France, and Generation 4 designs are in the pipeline. The main benefits from these new designs are much increased efficiency for safer operation and much less radioactive waste.

People are scared of anything called nuclear, and of radiation. The utterly safe and effective medical diagnostic tool Magnetic Resonance Imaging (MRI) had to change its original name of Nuclear Magnetic Resonance (NMR) because of the N-word. People in general don't realise that the dangerous stuff is **ionising** radiation. You can sit in front of an electric fire without coming to much harm.

At the moment of writing, the UK government is taking a serious look at how new design power stations can be financed and built – and, if so, how they can be made politically acceptable to the voters.

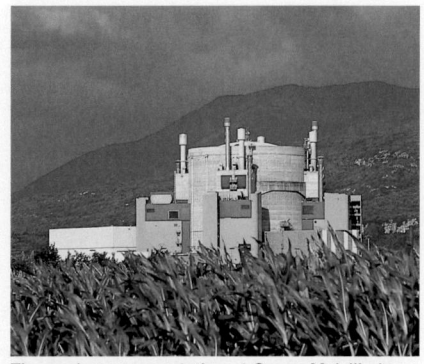

The nuclear power station at Creys–Malville in France: any radioactive pollution from nuclear power stations is invisible

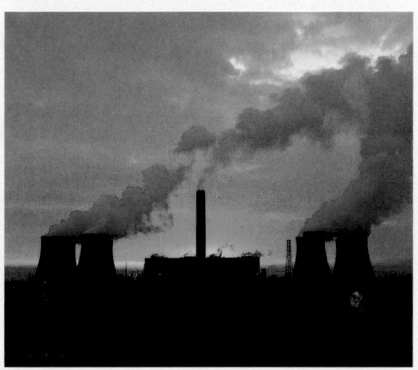

The Drax coal-fired power station in North Yorkshire. Its cooling towers give off steam which appears as clouds of water vapour, but the smoke from the central chimney includes sulphur and nitrogen oxides from burning the coal.

The ideas in this chapter

The atomic nucleus was not known about until the early twentieth century. Yet, only thirty years on, in 1945, two nuclear bombs were to kill an estimated 200 000 people in Japan, an event which ended the Second World War in a matter of days.

This chapter deals with the evidence we have about the nature and structure of the nucleus, and why some nuclei break up and others are **radioactive**.

It was the chance discovery of **radioactivity** at the end of the nineteenth century that began the series of investigations that led to an understanding of what an atom was like: a tiny but massive **nucleus** surrounded by a **cloud of electrons**. The evidence came from using the emissions that came from **unstable** nuclei: **alpha**, **beta** and **gamma** radiations.

The nucleus can provide useful energy through a process that occurs only with certain rare, very large nuclei, when they break up into two smaller nuclei – **nuclear fission**. Radioactivity itself is a minor source of energy, but the radiations are useful tools for industrial and medical use. The radiations are able to knock electrons from, or **ionise**, ordinary atoms. The ionisation effects allow the radiation to be easily detected – but also cause harm to living tissue.

Life on Earth depends on the energy from nuclear reactions in the Sun known as **nuclear fusion**, in which two hydrogen nuclei combine to form a helium nucleus. But attempts to use nuclear fusion as a steady, controlled source of cheap and almost pollution-free energy have so far been unsuccessful.

1 RADIOACTIVITY

Radioactivity was discovered in 1896 by Henri Becquerel (France, 1852–1908). He was investigating the property that some natural minerals have of glowing in the dark – fluorescence. He detected the faint light emitted by fluorescent substances using photographic plates. One day he found (by accident) that a salt of uranium emitted *invisible* radiation which blackened the photographic plates.

Soon, three types of radiation were discovered, and because they were then unidentified they were simply labelled **alpha** (α), **beta** (β) and **gamma** (γ) rays, after the first three letters of the Greek alphabet. Table 17.1 lists the nature and properties of the radiations.

Table 17.1 Properties of alpha, beta and gamma radiations

Radiation	Alpha	Beta	Gamma
Nature	helium nucleus (2n + 2p)	electron or positron	photon of electromagnetic radiation
Symbol	He	e	γ
Charge	$2e^+$	e^- or e^+	none
Range in air	1–5 cm	10–100 cm	infinite – obeys the inverse square law
Range in matter	stopped by e.g. a sheet of paper	stopped by e.g. a thin (1 mm) sheet of aluminium	intensity reduced to half by e.g. 1 or 2 cm of lead
Mass in atomic mass units (page 334)	4 u	5×10^{-4} u	zero
Relative ionising ability	very high: 1	high: 1/100	low: 1/10000

Marie Curie (Poland/France, 1867–1934) and her husband Pierre (France, 1859–1906) investigated radioactivity and developed ways for measuring the **activity** of sources, i.e. how much radiation a source emitted per second. In doing so they discovered other elements that also emitted energetic radiation, identifying completely new ones such as polonium and radium. Later, the physicist Ernest Rutherford (New Zealand/Britain, 1871–1937) and the chemist Frederick Soddy (Britain, 1877–1956) worked together to establish the nature of the radiations and track down the changes to the elements that were linked to them. Their results began to make sense when Rutherford's team discovered the nucleus in the years 1909–1911.

2 DETECTING THE RADIATIONS

THE GEIGER COUNTER

The most common device – and one of the oldest – for detecting and monitoring ionising radiation is the **Geiger counter**. The key part of the

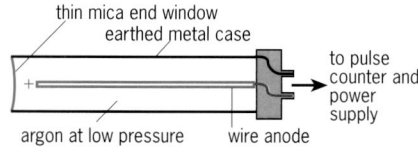

Fig 17.1(a) An end-window Geiger–Müller (GM) tube for the detection of alpha particles

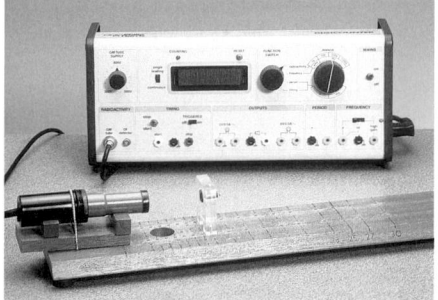

Fig 17.1(b) A GM tube attached to a ratemeter

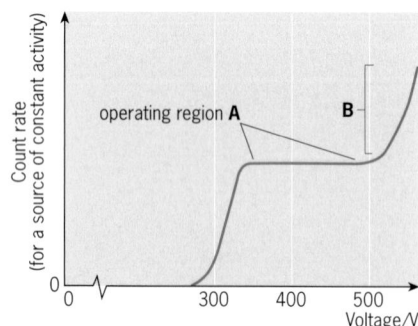

Fig 17.2 Characteristic curve for a GM tube

counter is the **Geiger–Müller tube**, the GM tube, as in Fig 17.1(a) overleaf. A sealed metal tube has a thin wire down the middle and is filled with a non-reactive gas (e.g. argon) at low pressure. The wire is kept at a voltage of about +400 V with respect to the metal case, which is earthed. The radiation enters the tube through a thin window in the front. Alpha particles are easily absorbed by matter so the window in an alpha detector is a thin film of mica – but strong enough to withstand the pressure difference between the atmosphere and the gas inside the tube.

Radiation entering the tube ionises argon atoms. The positive argon ions are attracted to the metal case and electrons to the central wire. These charged particles are accelerated by the voltage and will collide with other argon atoms. If they are moving fast enough, the collisions will ionise the atoms. The new particles are in turn accelerated and will cause further ionisation, producing an avalanche effect. The sudden large flow of charge in the tube causes a pulse of current in the central wire which is amplified electronically. The amplified pulses may be counted by a **scaler** or averaged out to give a current reading on a **ratemeter**, Fig 17.1(b). The pulses may also be fed into an audio circuit to give a series of clicks, so providing an audible indication of the radiation level.

The charge avalanche takes time to be cleared out of the gas, so there is a **dead time** (of about 200 ms) in which the tube cannot react to any incoming radiation.

Beta and gamma detectors are similar: windows for beta detectors can be made of glass, and gamma detectors can be made entirely of metal.

Working voltage of a GM tube

The voltage on the central rod has to be set high enough to accelerate ions and electrons and cause the avalanche effect. But the voltage should not be so high as to produce a continuous discharge, as at B in Fig 17.2. This happens when a continuous supply of ions hitting the metal walls have enough energy to eject electrons from it, which are then accelerated to cause further ionisation of the argon atoms.

Fig 17.2 is a plot of the count rate, which is proportional to the mean current in a GM tube, against voltage when the ionising radiation enters the tube at a constant rate. The **operating plateau** at A shows the range of applied voltage for which the tube works well. At plateau voltages, all ionising particles of the same type will produce the same size pulse of charge.

SOLID STATE DETECTORS

In industry and research laboratories, the most common kind of radiation detector is 'solid state'. The energy of the incoming radiation (particle or photon) liberates electrons from semiconductor material. This produces a pulse of current and so indicates the arrival of the radiation. Such detectors can both count individual events and also measure the energy of the radiation.

PHOTOGRAPHIC DETECTION

Photography works because photons of light have an ionising effect on certain chemicals – generally salts of silver such as silver nitrate. **Radiation badges**, described in Chapter 19, use this effect. Such a badge has to be worn by anyone who works in an area where they might be exposed to ionising radiation, such as a nuclear power plant, an X-ray department in a hospital, or a radioactivity laboratory. More advanced particle detectors are described in Chapter 24.

BACKGROUND RADIATION

A Geiger counter set up anywhere on Earth will always register a count. This count is due to **background radiation**, produced by tiny fragments of radioactive elements present in all rocks and soil, the atmosphere and even in living material itself. Also, the Earth is continuously bombarded by high-speed particles from outer space and from the Sun called **cosmic rays**. Cosmic rays smash up the nuclei of atmospheric molecules and produce other high-speed particles which can cause ionisation. Many of these reach ground level.

The background count varies considerably from place to place on Earth. As detected by a Geiger counter, it is typically one or two counts a second. It is a lot more where there are igneous rocks such as granite, which are relatively rich in minerals containing natural radioactive elements. Also, the radioactive decay of these elements produces a radioactive gas, radon, which may accumulate in buildings, so increasing the local background count.

3 ACTIVITY AND HALF-LIFE

The **activity** of a radioactive source is the number of ionising particles it emits per second. Each emission corresponds to a change in the nucleus of one atom and is also called the decay rate. The SI unit of activity (and decay rate) is the **becquerel** (Bq):

$$1 \text{ Bq} = 1 \text{ decay per second}$$

What we actually record is the reading on any radiation detector we use to monitor the effect of the radiation. Usually this is the count rate as measured by a Geiger counter. The count rate is simply the number of counts recorded per second, and in simple experiments it is taken to be directly proportional to the activity. Note that it is very unlikely that all the decays of a source will be recorded. Usually, some of the radiation is trapped inside the source, and in most measurements only a small fraction of the radiations actually enter the detector to be counted.

As time goes on, the activity of a source (and so the count rate) decreases in a consistent manner. Fig 17.3 shows a typical plot of the alpha particle count rate against time for a small sample of the radioactive gas radon (Rn-220).

? QUESTION 1

1 A GM tube has a detection area of about 3 cm². It shows an average background count of 1.5 per second in your home. Estimate how many ionising particles are likely to be hitting your body per second.

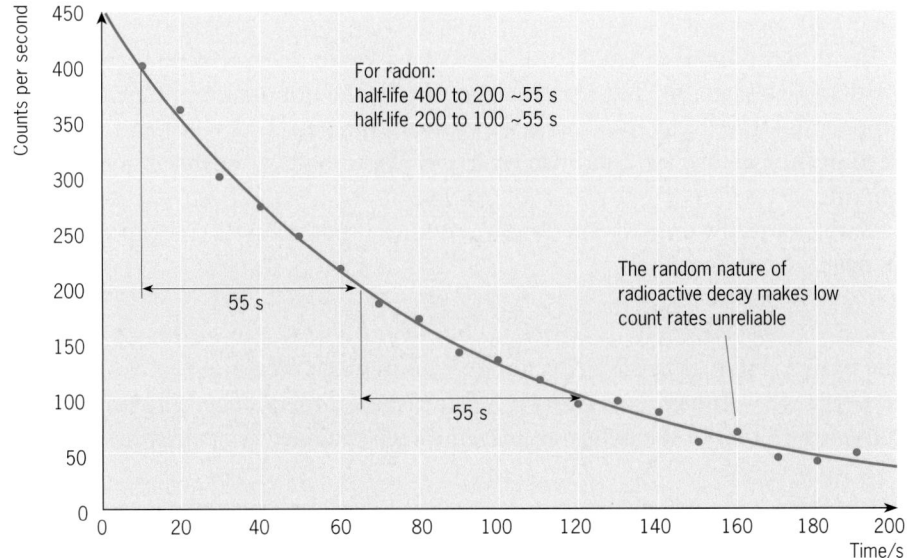

Fig 17.3 Activity curve for radon-220

The graph has been drawn as a 'best fit' through actual numbers recorded by a counter. The count rate in counts per second is calculated from the total number of counts measured at 10-second intervals.

There are two significant features of the graph. One is that the values aren't all on the line, so the measurements have some inbuilt uncertainty. Secondly, as the annotation shows, the time taken for the count rate to fall from 400 s^{-1} to 200 s^{-1} is the same as the time for the count rate to fall from 200 s^{-1} to 100 s^{-1}. That is, the graph suggests that:

the time taken for the activity of a radioactive sample to decrease to a half of any starting value is the same, whatever the starting value of the count rate.

This time is called the **half-life** of the radioactive substance. We return to this when looking at the shape of the curve.

RANDOMNESS OF DECAY

Both the uncertainty in measuring and the constancy of the half-life have the same cause: *the time at which any given radioactive nucleus emits its radiation cannot be predicted*. It is impossible to tell which one of a hundred radon nuclei will be next to emit its alpha particle. All the nuclei are identical, and all are equally liable to decay. But the breakdowns are completely *random*. However, if we have a sample of several hundred billion radon nuclei, a pattern would emerge. Bear in mind that ten billion (10^{10}) radon nuclei have a mass of a few thousandths of a billionth of a gram (about 4×10^{-12} g).

What is constant about the radioactive process is that each nucleus has a **definite probability** of undergoing decay. Starting with a large enough number of radon nuclei, we can be reasonably certain that a predictable number will emit an alpha particle in the next 10 seconds. Similarly, with a large enough sample, the values of count rate we measure will coincide closely with the smooth graph we draw between the values. Our estimate of half-life will be more reliable.

THE SHAPE OF THE ACTIVITY CURVE

We associate an exponential change with any system where the change is proportional to the quantity that is changing, either increasing or decreasing. An example of an *increase* is a biological population growth, where the number of young born is proportional to the number of organisms in the population. This property is also characteristic of many physical changes: on page 190 we saw it for the charging and discharging of capacitors.

The graph plotted in Fig 17.3 is a decay curve for an exponential change to a radioactive material, and here the *decrease* in the population of nuclei is exponential: the decay rate *decreases by equal fractions in equal times*. The fraction that we use for a radioactive material is a half, so we refer to its *half-life*.

Mathematically, if ΔN is the number of nuclei that decay in a small time Δt, then:

$$\Delta N = -kN\Delta t \qquad [1]$$

The minus sign is because ΔN is a *reduction* in N: as time goes on N decreases. The **decay constant** k is a measure of the *probability of a nucleus decaying in the following second*. (Each radioactive nucleus has its own value of k.)

The Stretch and Challenge passage overleaf gives the calculus version of deriving the exponential form of radioactive decay.

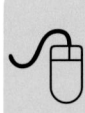

To simulate radioactive decay using a spreadsheet, please see the How Science Works assignment for this chapter at www.collinseducation.co.uk/CAS

THE DECAY CONSTANT AND HALF-LIFE

For a radioactive nucleus, the decay constant k indicates the probability that the nucleus will undergo decay. Its value is in terms of the *fraction* of the potentially active nuclei in a sample that do actually decay in any second of time. So, the larger the value of k, the higher the number of nuclei decaying in a given time – and the shorter the half-life. The Stretch and Challenge passage overleaf shows that the relation between half-life and the decay constant is:

$$\text{half-life (in seconds)} = \frac{\ln 2}{k} \qquad [2]$$

where ln 2 is the logarithm to base e of 2 (0.693).

Table 17.2 gives some values for the half-lives of selected nuclei.

? QUESTION 2

2   The half-life of radon-220 is 55.5 s. Use equation 2 to show that the decay constant for radon-220 is 0.0125 s^{-1}.

Table 17.2 Half-lives and types of emission of some nuclei

Nuclei	Comment	Emission	Half-life
uranium-238	Most common isotope of uranium	α, γ	4.51×10^9 y
thorium-232	100% of normal thorium found on Earth	α, γ	1.4×10^{10} y
radon-220	Radioactive gas – a decay product formed when thorium-232 decays	α	55.5 s
plutonium-239	Found naturally but in minute quantities; made artificially by bombarding uranium with neutrons. Fissile: used in nuclear reactors and nuclear bombs. The most dangerous component in nuclear waste: highly toxic and difficult to store, with a long half-life	α	24 360 y
americium	Formed by bombarding plutonium with neutrons; often used as a laboratory source of alpha particles	α, γ	433 y
carbon-14	Formed from nitrogen-14 by the action of cosmic rays; useful in archaeology for radioactive dating of organic materials (see the Science in Context box on page 351)	β$^-$	5730 y
potassium-40	Naturally occurring isotope (0.12% abundance); a significant source of internal (body) background radiation	β$^-$	1.3×10^9 y
radium-226	The first element to be discovered due to its radioactivity (Pierre and Marie Curie, 1898)	α, γ	1622 y

EXAMPLE

Q The half-life of bismuth (Bi-212) is 60.6 minutes. What is

a) its decay constant,
b) the activity of 1 g of bismuth-212?

The Avogadro constant is 6.02×10^{23}.

A a) Half-life of bismuth = (ln 2)/k, so:

decay constant k
   $= 0.693/(60.6 \times 60)$
   $= 1.91 \times 10^{-4}$ s^{-1}

b) 212 g of bismuth-212 contains 6.02×10^{23} atoms.

Therefore number of atoms in 1 g:

$N = (6.02 \times 10^{23})/212$
   $= 2.84 \times 10^{21}$

The probability of decay for bismuth-212 is k per second. Thus we would expect kN atoms to decay per second:

activity kN
   $= 1.91 \times 10^{-4} \times 2.84 \times 10^{21}$ Bq
   $= 5.4 \times 10^{17}$ Bq

Random decay and the exponential rule

Equation 1 on page 326 can be written in calculus notation as:

$$\frac{dN}{dt} = -kN$$

Rearranging this gives:

$$\frac{dN}{N} = -k\,dt$$

which can be integrated to give:

$$\ln N = -kt + A \qquad [3]$$

where A is a constant and ln is the logarithm to base e. Assume that we start at time zero with a number N_0 of radioactive nuclei. When $t = 0$, equation 3 gives:

$$\ln N_0 = A$$

so that we can rewrite equation 3 as:

$$\ln N = -kt + \ln N_0 \qquad [4]$$

Rearranging,

$$kt = \ln N_0 - \ln N$$

then using the rule of division using logarithms, we have:

$$kt = \ln \frac{N_0}{N} \qquad [5]$$

Equation 5 tells us that the number of nuclei has changed from N_0 to N in time t.

Equation 5 also gives rise to a simple connection between half-life and decay constant k: if $N = N_0$ when $t = 0$, and if after a time $t_{\frac{1}{2}}$ (the half-life) the number has decreased to $N_0/2$, then inserting values $t = t_{\frac{1}{2}}$ and $N = N_0/2$ in equation 5, we get:

$$kt_{\frac{1}{2}} = \ln \frac{N_0}{0.5N_0} = \ln 2$$

which can be rearranged to give the half-life:

$$t_{\frac{1}{2}} = \frac{\ln 2}{k} \qquad [6]$$

Also, equation 4 can be rewritten as:

$$\ln N - \ln N_0 = -kt$$

or:

$$\ln \frac{N}{N_0} = -kt \qquad [7]$$

and by converting logarithms to exponentials we get:

$$\frac{N}{N_0} = e^{-kt} \quad \text{or} \quad N = N_0 e^{-kt}$$

showing the *exponential* form of the relationship.

Fig 17.4 shows a logarithmic plot of a decay curve: $\ln N$ is plotted against time. As indicated in equation 7, the intercept on the $\ln N$ axis gives $\ln N_0$, and the slope of the line is $-k$.

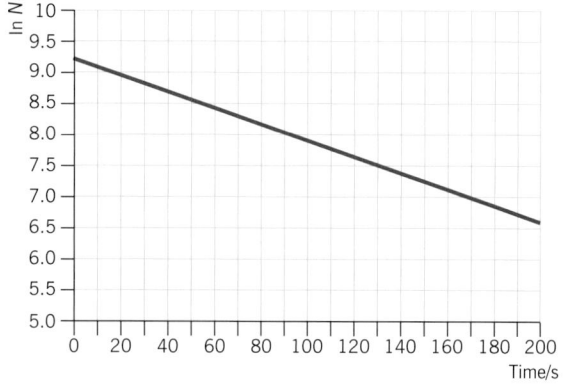

Fig 17.4 Log graph for the decay curve for radon-22 gas

4 THE ATOMIC NUCLEUS

Atoms are mostly empty space (Fig 17.5). We picture a hydrogen atom, as a very small central blob of matter surrounded by a single rapidly moving electron. The central nucleus contains 99.95 per cent of the atom's mass but only a ten-billionth part of its volume. The space surrounding the nucleus is occupied by the single electron, moving so rapidly that we can think of it as being everywhere in the space at once (see pages 318–319).

THE VERY FIRST NUCLEAR PROBE – ALPHA SCATTERING

The first evidence for the existence of the nucleus was the alpha scattering experiment of Geiger and Marsden in 1909 at the University of Manchester under the leadership of Ernest Rutherford.

At that time, most physicists' idea of an atom was of a round ball completely filled with a positive 'jelly' in which the newly discovered electrons were embedded, like currants in a currant bun. Rutherford told his assistants, the experienced Hans Geiger and a young undergraduate, Ernest Marsden, 'See if

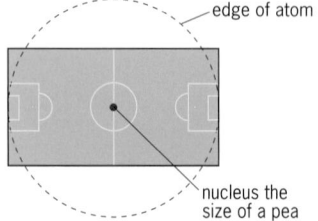

Fig 17.5(a) A modern view of an atom. It has a very definite size, but most of its volume is filled with 'non-localised' electrons forming a fuzzy cloud

nucleus ~10^{-14} m diameter

electron cloud ~10^{-10} m diameter

edge of atom

nucleus the size of a pea

Fig 17.5(b) A nucleus is very small compared with an atom. If it were the size of a pea, an atom would be as big as a football pitch

you can get some effect of alpha particles directly reflected from a metal surface.' A diagram of the apparatus they used is shown in Fig 17.6. It shows the main features of all such collision or scattering experiments:

- a source of high-speed particles,
- a vacuum to avoid unwanted collisions,
- a target, or more precisely the atomic or subatomic components of the target,
- a detector of the scattered particles or any fragments produced,
- a means of measuring the paths of scattered particles or fragments.

A radioactive source, contained in a lead box with a small hole in it, emitted alpha particles. The targets included thin gold foil only a few atoms thick. Most alpha particles went straight through the foil, and were detected by the faint glow (scintillation) that each particle produced when it hit a detecting glass screen coated with a phosphorescent chemical. The scintillations were so faint that Geiger and Marsden had to allow half an hour before each observation session for their eyes to become 'dark adapted'.

The detecting screen was fitted to a pivoted arm moved along a scale marked in degrees. About one alpha particle in 8000 was reflected back through a large angle. A typical distribution of particles by angle is shown in the graph of Fig 17.7.

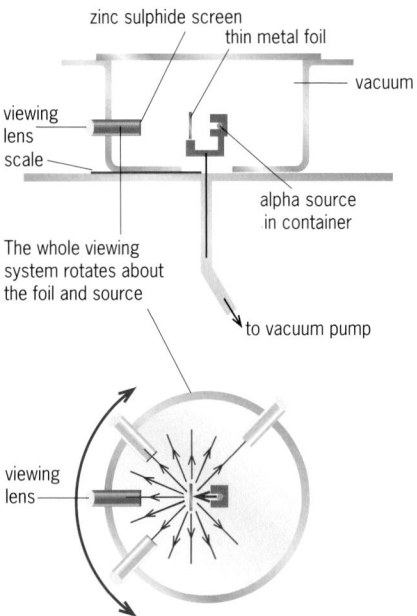

Fig 17.6 Geiger and Marsden probe the atom – and discover the nucleus

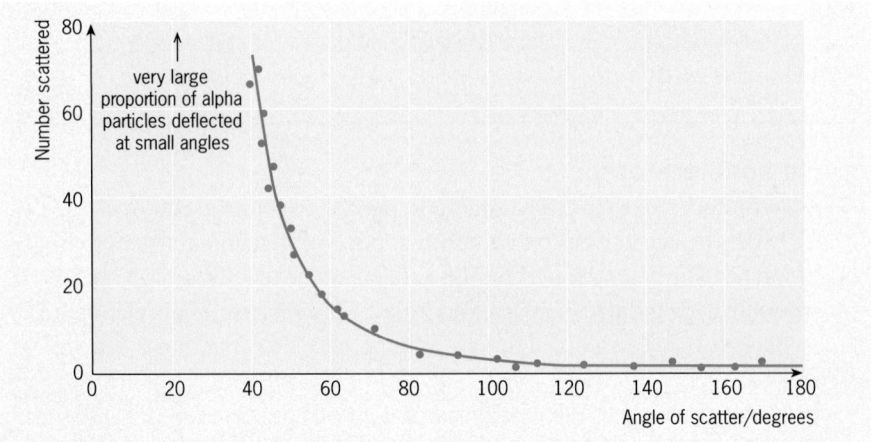

Fig 17.7 The results of the alpha particle scattering experiment

An alpha particle is deflected by repulsion from another positively charged object. The 'positive jelly' model proposed by J.J. Thomson (Fig 17.8(a)) would have provided a repulsion force far too small to deflect the massive alpha particle through a large angle – it predicted a deflection of 2° at most. Rutherford deduced that there must be a very much stronger electric field inside an atom, which could only be produced by a very high charge density, such as if all the charge were locked into one small volume.

For the fast and quite massive alpha particle to bounce back at all, most of the mass of the atom would also have to be squashed into this small space. Rutherford named this small space, in which all the positive charge and most of the mass of an atom is concentrated, the atomic **nucleus**. By comparison, the electrons had negligible mass but occupied most of the space.

Fig 17.8(b) illustrates Rutherford's idea of what was happening in the gold foil experiment. Alpha particle A passing some distance from the nucleus is hardly deflected at all – the electric field is too small. A closer approach such as B's produces a larger deflection. A (rare) head-on 'collision', C, stops the alpha particle dead in its tracks and repels it back along its own path.

Rutherford wasn't very keen on mathematics, and it took him nearly two years to produce a calculation which related his nuclear model of the atom to the distribution of the number of deflected particles and the angles they were deflected through.

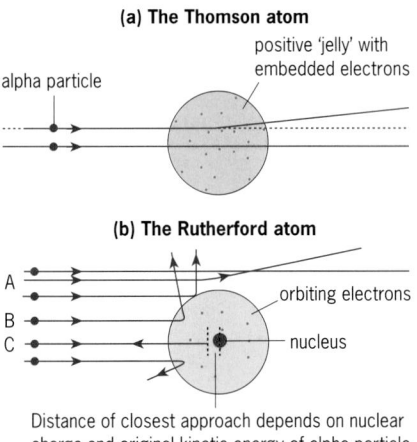

Fig 17.8 Alpha scattering: Rutherford saw that the only model that would produce large scattering angles required a massive, positive nucleus

EXAMPLE

Q An alpha particle with kinetic energy 5 MeV makes a head-on collision with a gold nucleus. How close to the centre of the nucleus does it get?

The charge Q on a gold nucleus is $79e$, where e is the electronic charge 1.6×10^{-19} C, an alpha particle has charge $q = 2e$, and the electric force constant k ($1/4\pi\varepsilon_0$) is 9×10^9 N m^2 C^{-2}.

A The alpha particle stops at a distance r from the centre of the nucleus, when all its kinetic energy has been converted to electrical potential energy in the field of the gold nucleus. So:

$$E_k = \frac{1}{4\pi\varepsilon_0} \frac{Qq}{r}$$

Rearranging gives:

$$r = \frac{1}{4\pi\varepsilon_0} \frac{Qq}{E_k}$$

and so, inserting values:

$$r = 9 \times 10^9 \times \frac{79 \times 1.6 \times 10^{-19} \times 2 \times 1.6 \times 10^{-19}}{5 \times 10^6 \times 1.6 \times 10^{-19}}$$

gives: $r = 4.6 \times 10^{-14}$ m

Particle accelerators

Early experiments used naturally energetic particles to probe the nucleus, but by the 1920s physicists were using 'atom-smashing machines' to accelerate charged particles in a controlled manner. Their main techniques are still used today, though with greatly increased energies. One technique accelerates charged particles in a straight line by applying an electric field – a **linear accelerator**. The other uses a combination of electric and magnetic fields to accelerate the charged particles in a circular path – leading to such devices as 'cyclotrons' and **synchrotrons**. See Chapter 24 for details of particle accelerators.

NUCLEAR PATTERNS

Practically all the mass of an atom is the mass of its nucleus, which consists of particles called **nucleons**. There are two kinds of nucleon with very slightly different masses (see Table 17.3). The **proton** is electrically charged: its positive charge is equal in size to the charge on an electron. It is slightly less massive than its partner, the uncharged nucleon called the **neutron**.

The Periodic Table of the chemical elements, shown in Table 17.4, arranges the elements in the order of the number of protons in the nucleus. This number is the **proton number** or the **atomic number**, symbol **Z** (Fig 17.9).

Table 17.3

Nucleon	proton	neutron
Mass/10^{-27} kg	1.672 623	1.674 929
Charge/e	1.00	0.00

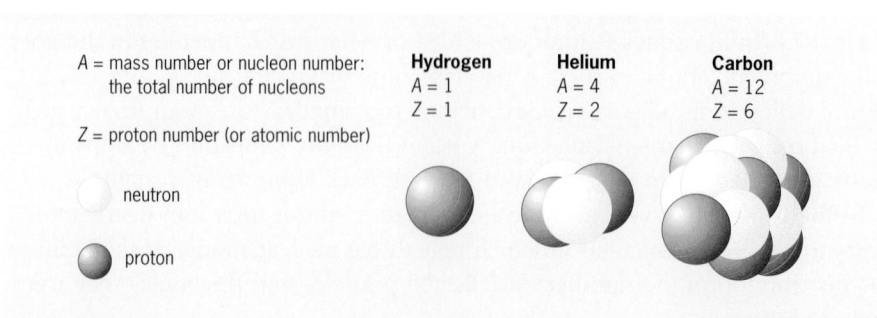

A = mass number or nucleon number: the total number of nucleons

Z = proton number (or atomic number)

○ neutron

● proton

	Hydrogen	Helium	Carbon
	$A = 1$	$A = 4$	$A = 12$
	$Z = 1$	$Z = 2$	$Z = 6$

Fig 17.9 Simple models of atomic nuclei

Adding the number of protons and neutrons gives the **mass number** or **nucleon number** of an element, symbol **A**. For the actual mass of a nucleus, see page 338. Fig 17.10 shows the conventional way of writing the proton and mass numbers of a nucleus.

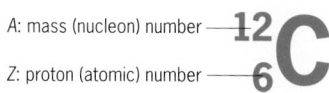

A: mass (nucleon) number ——**12**
Z: proton (atomic) number ——**6** C

Fig 17.10 Describing the carbon nucleus

Table 17.4 The Periodic Table

groups	I	II											III	IV	V	VI	VII	0
periods																		
1							1 **H** hydrogen 1											2 **He** helium 4
2	3 **Li** lithium 7	4 **Be** beryllium 9											5 **B** boron 11	6 **C** carbon 12	7 **N** nitrogen 14	8 **O** oxygen 16	9 **F** fluorine 19	10 **Ne** neon 20
3	11 **Na** sodium 23	12 **Mg** magnesium 24											13 **Al** aluminium 27	14 **Si** silicon 28	15 **P** phosphorus 31	16 **S** sulphur 32	17 **Cl** chlorine 35.5	18 **Ar** argon 40
4	19 **K** potassium 39	20 **Ca** calcium 40	21 **Sc** scandium 45	22 **Ti** titanium 48	23 **V** vanadium 51	24 **Cr** chromium 52	25 **Mn** manganese 55	26 **Fe** iron 56	27 **Co** cobalt 59	28 **Ni** nickel 59	29 **Cu** copper 64	30 **Zn** zinc 65	31 **Ga** gallium 70	32 **Ge** germanium 73	33 **As** arsenic 75	34 **Se** selenium 79	35 **Br** bromine 80	36 **Kr** krypton 84
5	37 **Rb** rubidium 85.5	38 **Sr** strontium 88	39 **Y** yttrium 89	40 **Zr** zirconium 91	41 **Nb** niobium 93	42 **Mo** molybdenum 96	43 **Tc** technetium 98	44 **Ru** ruthenium 101	45 **Rh** rhodium 103	46 **Pd** palladium 106	47 **Ag** silver 108	48 **Cd** cadmium 112	49 **In** indium 115	50 **Sn** tin 119	51 **Sb** antimony 122	52 **Te** tellurium 128	53 **I** iodine 127	54 **Xe** xenon 131
6	55 **Cs** caesium 133	56 **Ba** barium 137	57 **La** lanthanum 139	72 **Hf** hafnium 178.5	73 **Ta** tantalum 181	74 **W** tungsten 184	75 **Re** rhenium 186	76 **Os** osmium 190	77 **Ir** iridium 192	78 **Pt** platinum 195	79 **Au** gold 197	80 **Hg** mercury 201	81 **Tl** thallium 204	82 **Pb** lead 207	83 **Bi** bismuth 209	84 **Po** polonium 210	85 **At** astatine 210	86 **Rn** radon 222
7	87 **Fr** francium 223	88 **Ra** radium 226	89 **Ac** actinium 227	104 **Db** dubnium 261	105 **Jl** joliotium 262	106 **Rf** rutherfordium	107 **Bh** bohrium	108 **Hn** hahnium	109 **Mt** meitnerium									

58 **Ce** cerium 140	59 **Pr** praseodymium 141	60 **Nd** neodymium 144	61 **Pm** promethium 147	62 **Sm** samarium 150	63 **Eu** europium 152	64 **Gd** gadolinium 157	65 **Tb** terbium 159	66 **Dy** dysprosium 162.5	67 **Ho** holmium 165	68 **Er** erbium 167	69 **Tm** thulium 169	70 **Yb** ytterbium 173	71 **Lu** lutetium 175
90 **Th** thorium 232	91 **Pa** protactinium 231	92 **U** uranium 238	93 **Np** neptunium 237	94 **Pu** plutonium 242	95 **Am** americium 243	96 **Cm** curium 247	97 **Bk** berkelium 247	98 **Cf** californium 251	99 **Es** einsteinium 254	100 **Fm** fermium 253	101 **Md** mendelevium 256	102 **No** nobelium 254	103 **Lr** lawrencium 257

metal	non metal	atomic no. **symbol** name mass no.

Nuclides

The word **nuclide** is the name for atoms that have identical nuclei; this means they have the same proton number (atomic number) and the same mass number, so they have the same number of neutrons. Compare this with 'isotopes' (see page 333), whose nuclei have the same proton number but *different* mass numbers (because they have different numbers of neutrons).

5 FORCES IN THE NUCLEUS

THE ELECTRICAL FORCE

The positively charged protons exert an electrical force of repulsion on each other. The force between two protons, of equal charge $+e$, can be calculated from the formula:

$$F_E = \frac{ke^2}{r^2}$$

where k is the electric force constant (9×10^9 N m^2 C^{-2}) and r is a typical nuclear distance, about 10^{-14} m. (See also the equation on page 203.) So the force between the two protons in a helium nucleus is 2.3 N. This is a repulsive force and is immense on the nuclear scale because protons are so close together. The force would, on its own, cause the protons to fly apart at high speeds in a nuclear disintegration. But this doesn't happen!

? QUESTION 3

3 Use the data given in the Periodic Table to find the number of neutrons in the nuclei of calcium (Ca, $Z = 20$) and tellurium (Te, $Z = 52$).

? QUESTION 4

4 Check that the force between two protons in a helium nucleus is about 2.3 N. Use the data: $r = 10^{-14}$ m; force constant $k = 9 \times 10^9$ N m^2 C^{-2}; $e = 1.6 \times 10^{-19}$ C.

THE STRONG NUCLEAR FORCE

Nuclei do exist, and are quite hard to break apart. So there must be another force, stronger than this electrical repulsion force, to attract nucleons to each other and so keep the nucleus together. This is the **strong nuclear force**, about 100 times as strong as the electrical force in the nucleus. Unlike electrical and gravitational forces, the strong nuclear force has a very short range: it reaches only as far as from one nucleon to its next neighbours (Fig 17.11). This force affects both neutrons and protons. However, large nuclei have a problem: there comes a size when the long-range electrical force from a large number of protons will overcome the short-range nuclear force. Two things may then happen:

- A stable 'unit' of matter might escape – the unit is an **alpha particle**. Larger nuclei tend to be radioactive alpha emitters (e.g. Th-232, Th-228, Ra-224, Rn-220, etc.).
- The nucleus simply breaks apart into two roughly equal smaller nuclei – this is **nuclear fission**, which happens with uranium and is the main source of **nuclear power**.

There is more about this on pages 344–345.

Fig 17.11 Forces in the nucleus

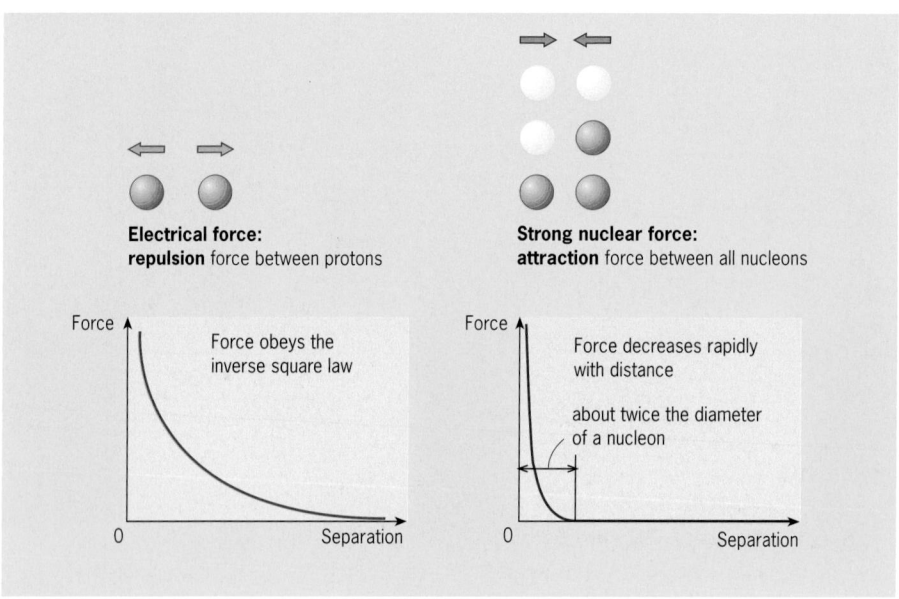

CHEMISTRY AND ATOMIC STRUCTURE

Fig 17.12 shows how the chemical behaviour of an element relates to its place in the Periodic Table. More and more nucleons join together to make larger and larger nuclei, and patterns emerge linking atomic structure and chemical behaviour.

Fig 17.12 Connection between atomic structure, chemical behaviour and Periodic Table position

1 An atom of an element is electrically neutral

equal numbers of electrons and protons

region of electrons

nucleus

Number of electrons
= number of protons
= order in Periodic Table
= Z

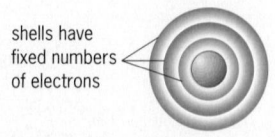

2 Electrons are arranged in shells

shells have fixed numbers of electrons

Shells (usually) fill up before the next shell is occupied

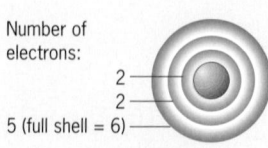

3 Electrons are added to the outer shell, one at a time ≡ sequence in Periodic Table, row by row

Number of electrons:

2
2
5 (full shell = 6)

This is fluorine, a halogen – which is very reactive

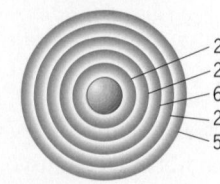

4 Elements in vertical columns of the Periodic Table have the same number of outer electrons

2
2
6
2
5

This is chlorine, also a very reactive halogen

QUESTION 5

5 Look at the Periodic Table on page 331 and identify four elements which have an equal number of protons and neutrons.

Table 17.5 Isotopes of carbon

Nucleon no. A	Proton no. Z	No. of neutrons (A − Z)
9	6	3
10	6	4
11	6	5
12 (98.89%)	6	6
13 (1.11%)	6	7
14	6	8
15	6	9

QUESTION 6

6 Draw diagrams to illustrate the structure of the nuclei of the following isotopes of carbon: carbon-9, carbon-13, carbon-15.

In chemical reactions, the outer electrons of atoms interact. Elements with the same number of outer electrons react similarly, and are arranged in columns in the Periodic Table called groups. Examples of groups include the alkali metals (lithium, sodium, etc.), the halogens (fluorine, chlorine, etc.), and the noble gases (helium, neon, etc.).

ISOTOPES

All nuclei except the hydrogen nucleus contain both protons and neutrons. For the smaller nuclei, the number of neutrons is about equal to the number of protons – but this is a very rough rule.

All atoms of an element have the same number of protons, but they may have different numbers of neutrons and are then called **isotopes** of that element. The mass of an atom of one isotope of an element will then be different from the mass of another isotope. For example, the nucleus in the most common atom of carbon has 6 protons and 6 neutrons. But we can find seven forms of carbon nuclei with different masses. So carbon has seven isotopes – as in Table 17.5. They all have the same number of protons (and electrons), so they occupy the same place in the Periodic Table and have identical chemical properties.

Only carbon-12 and carbon-13 nuclei are **stable**; the rest are unstable due to an imbalance of protons and neutrons (see Fig 17.13) and are radioactive.

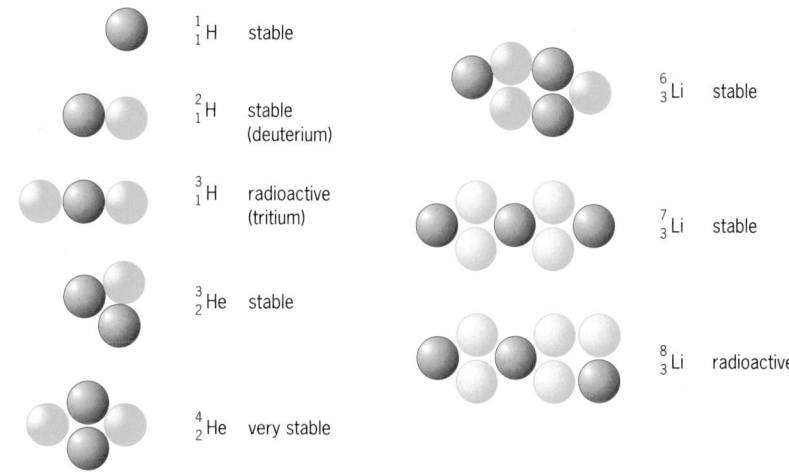

Fig 17.13 Nuclear composition of some light nuclei. A serious imbalance between protons and neutrons leads to instability

A **nuclide** is the name of a particular isotope and is shown by a 'formula' giving both its mass number and its proton number:

$$^{228}_{88}\text{Ra}$$

The formula tells us that this nuclide is an isotope of radium (Ra) with a mass number (protons + neutrons) of 228 nucleons, and a proton (or atomic) number of 88. Thus there are 88 protons and 140 neutrons in the nucleus, and the atom would be surrounded with a cloud of 88 electrons.

Relative atomic mass

The mass of an atom is very small. So it is usually given as a multiple of a standard unit, the **unified atomic mass unit**, u (see the Science in Context box overleaf). This multiple is called the **relative atomic mass** or **RAM**. This is usually quoted as the mean of the relative atomic masses of the naturally occurring isotopes.

The atomic mass unit is defined as one-twelfth of the atomic mass of the commonest isotope of carbon (carbon-12).

Measuring nuclear masses

The mass spectrograph

Accurate measurements of the masses of nuclei are made using the mass spectrograph, see Fig 17.14.

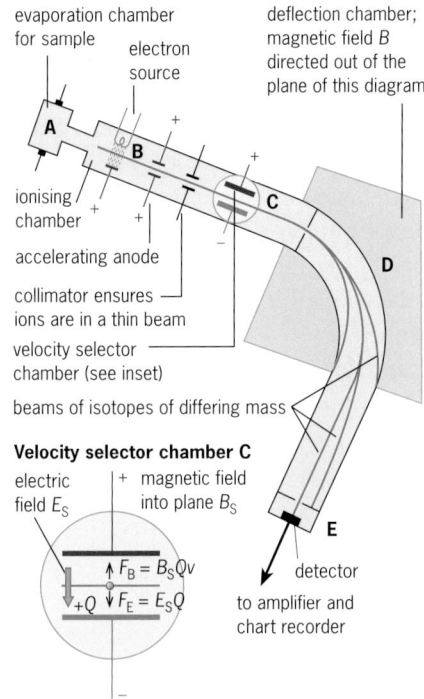

Velocity selector chamber C

electric field E_S + magnetic field into plane B_S

$F_B = B_S Qv$

$+Q$ $F_E = E_S Q$

E

detector

to amplifier and chart recorder

Fig 17.14 The mass spectrograph

This device vaporises atoms and then ionises them with a beam B of electrons. The ions are accelerated and enter the spectrograph chamber D which separates ions of different mass into different paths.

The *separation* is done using a magnetic field directed out of the plane of the diagram. The magnetic field exerts a force at right angles to the direction of motion of the ions – so providing a centripetal force to make the ions move in a circular path (see Chapter 10). A centripetal force F makes a mass m move in a circle of radius r at a speed v such that:

$$F = \frac{mv^2}{r}$$

F is a magnetic force of size $Qv \times B$ for a field of flux density B acting on a charge Q travelling with speed v:

$$F = QvB = \frac{mv^2}{r}$$

and so the radius of the path is given by:

$$r = \frac{mv}{BQ} \quad [1]$$

This simple theory assumes that all the atoms are ionised to the same degree, so that the charge Q is the same for them all, namely e, the electronic charge.

The velocity selector

Note that equation 1 involves the speed v. If we want all ions of the same mass and charge to follow the same path, they must also have the same speed. This is achieved by the *velocity selector* labelled C in Fig 17.14. Ions enter the selector with a wide range of speeds and are in both a magnetic field B_S and an electric field E_S (see diagram inset). These fields are at right angles to each other and to the direction of the ion beam, with the result that the electric force (QE_S) and the magnetic force (QvB_S) on the ions act in opposite directions. When these forces are equal, the ions are undeflected and carry on to go through the exit aperture into the *deflection chamber* D. But the forces only balance out at a particular value of v, when:

$$QvB_S = QE_S$$

so that:

$$v = \frac{E_S}{B_S} \quad [2]$$

Ions with different speeds are deflected out of the straight path, so do not pass into chamber D.

The strength of the deflecting field B in chamber D is varied, so bringing, in turn, ions of different mass into the detector E. The detector counts individual ions and so measures the relative quantities (abundances) of ions of different mass in the sample. By combining formulae 1 and 2 above:

$$r = \frac{mv}{BQ} \quad \text{and} \quad v = \frac{E_S}{B_S}$$

we get: $\quad r = \frac{mE_S}{BQB_S}$

and so: $\quad m = \frac{QrBB_S}{E_S}$

This boils down to:

$$m = kB \quad [3]$$

where k is a constant.

A typical readout from a mass spectrometer is shown in Fig 17.15.

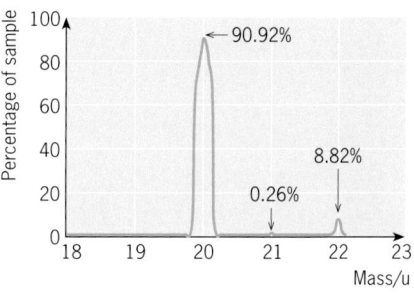

Fig 17.15 Readout from a mass spectrometer as a graph, showing the isotopes of neon

? **QUESTION 7**

7   An ion enters a mass spectrometer with a speed of 800 m s⁻¹. It passes between two plates, 5 mm apart, with a potential difference of 1000 V between them. What value of B-field (in tesla) must be applied in order that the ion is not deflected?

The unified atomic mass constant, u

It is hard to measure the constant k in equation 3 accurately, so values of m for different ions are measured by comparison with a *standard nuclear mass*. This is the nucleus of carbon-12, which is defined to have a mass of exactly 12 unified atomic mass constants (12 u), where u is $1.660\,540\,2 \times 10^{-27}$ kg. In energy terms this is equivalent to 930 MeV – see page 338 for more about the equivalence of energy and mass.

On this scale, the mass of a proton is 1.007 276 5 u.

The size of a nucleus

A SIMPLE THEORY

Protons and neutrons have almost exactly the same mass. Assuming that they also occupy the same space, volume v, the volume of a nucleus with A nucleons is Av.

If the nucleus is spherical with radius r, then we can write:

approximate volume of a nucleus $= Av$

$$= \frac{4\pi r^3}{3}$$

This result is usually written as:

$$r = r_0 A^{\frac{1}{3}}$$

where r_0 is an experimental constant of value 1.2×10^{-15} m.

THE EXPERIMENTAL EVIDENCE

When a metal is bombarded with a beam of charged particles, some of the particles bounce back almost exactly along the approach path. The first such experiment used alpha particles and led to the discovery of the nucleus. It is described on page 329.

What happens is shown in Fig 17.16. The approaching particle is repelled by the nucleus. Its kinetic energy E_k is converted to electrical potential energy E_p.

The point of closest approach occurs when all the E_k becomes E_p, that is:

$$\frac{1}{2}mv^2 = k\frac{qQ}{d}$$

$$= k\frac{2Ze^2}{d}$$

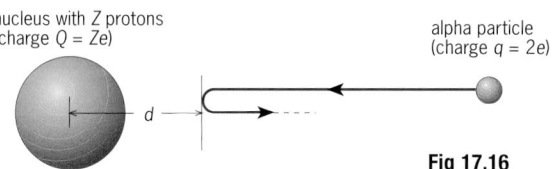

nucleus with Z protons
(charge $Q = Ze$)

d

alpha particle
(charge $q = 2e$)

Fig 17.16

where k is the electric force constant (which is 9×10^9 N m^2 C^{-2}) and the other quantities are as shown in Fig 17.16.

The energy of the approaching particle is known and so are the charges of the particle and the nucleus. This means that we can calculate d. A missile with high energy gets very close to the nucleus, so d is very nearly the same as the nuclear radius r.

Experiments similar to this in which electrons are scattered by nuclei have shown that most nuclei are approximately spherical with a size given by the relationship $r = r_0 A^{\frac{1}{3}}$ with the value of the constant r_0 as given above.

NUCLEAR DENSITY

The volume of a nucleus is $V = 4\pi r^3/3$ where $r = r_0 A^{\frac{1}{3}}$. Inserting this value gives

$$V = 4\pi r_0^3 A$$

For iron $A = 56$. Check that the volume of an iron nucleus is 1.22×10^{-42} m^3.

Each nucleon has a mass of 1 u or 1.67×10^{-27} kg, so the iron nucleus has a mass of 9.35×10^{-26} kg.

Thus the (approximate) density of an iron nucleus is

$$d_n = \text{mass/volume} = 7.7 \times 10^{16} \text{ kg m}^{-3}$$

This is a huge density: a matchboxful of nuclear matter would have a mass of 5 billion tonnes!

? QUESTIONS 8–9

8 The mass number of platinum is 195. Calculate the size of a platinum nucleus.

9 An alpha particle ($Z = 2$) collides with a platinum nucleus of $Z = 78$. The alpha particle has kinetic energy 8×10^{-13} J (5 MeV) and the charge on a proton is 1.6×10^{-19} C. Calculate how close the alpha particle gets to the centre of the nucleus. Is this value consistent with the size of the nucleus you calculated in **8**?

6 HOW NUCLEI CHANGE AS A RESULT OF RADIOACTIVE DECAY

When a nucleus emits an alpha particle it loses two neutrons and two protons. Its mass number decreases by 4 and its proton (atomic) number by 2. This means that it has become a *different element*. For example, thorium-232 emits an alpha particle and becomes an isotope of radium:

$$^{232}_{90}\text{Th} \rightarrow \,^{228}_{88}\text{Ra} + \,^{4}_{2}\alpha$$

The radium-228 then emits a negative beta particle (an electron), leaving its mass unchanged since the electron has negligible mass compared with a nucleon. What has happened is that a neutron has decayed and emitted an electron, so changing to a proton. The proton number increases by one to 89. This means that the new nucleus has approximately the same mass but becomes a new element – actinium:

$$^{228}_{88}\text{Ra} \rightarrow ^{228}_{89}\text{Ac} + ^{\ 0}_{-1}\beta$$

We have represented these changes as two **nuclear equations**. Note that they are doubly balanced: both the mass numbers and the proton numbers have the same totals on each side of the equation.

Many of the natural radioactive nuclides on Earth are the result of similar alpha and beta emissions from larger nuclei that were formed during the final explosion of a dying star, billions of years ago. This event formed some nuclides with such long half-lives that they still exist. Examples, and their half-lives, are:

$$\begin{array}{ll} \text{thorium-232:} & 1.41 \times 10^{10} \text{ y} \\ \text{uranium-238:} & 4.51 \times 10^{9} \text{y} \\ \text{uranium-235:} & 7.1 \times 10^{8} \text{ y} \end{array}$$

The decay of these nuclides and of their radioactive 'daughter' products provides a large amount of energy, which helps to keep the interior of the Earth hot enough to be molten.

Fig 17.17 shows the natural decay series for thorium-232. Look carefully at this to see how the changes described above result in the formation of successively different elements. Similar decay series exist for the large nuclei of the long-lived naturally radioactive elements that went to make up the Earth as it formed from the debris of dead, exploded stars.

Fig 17.17 The decay series of thorium

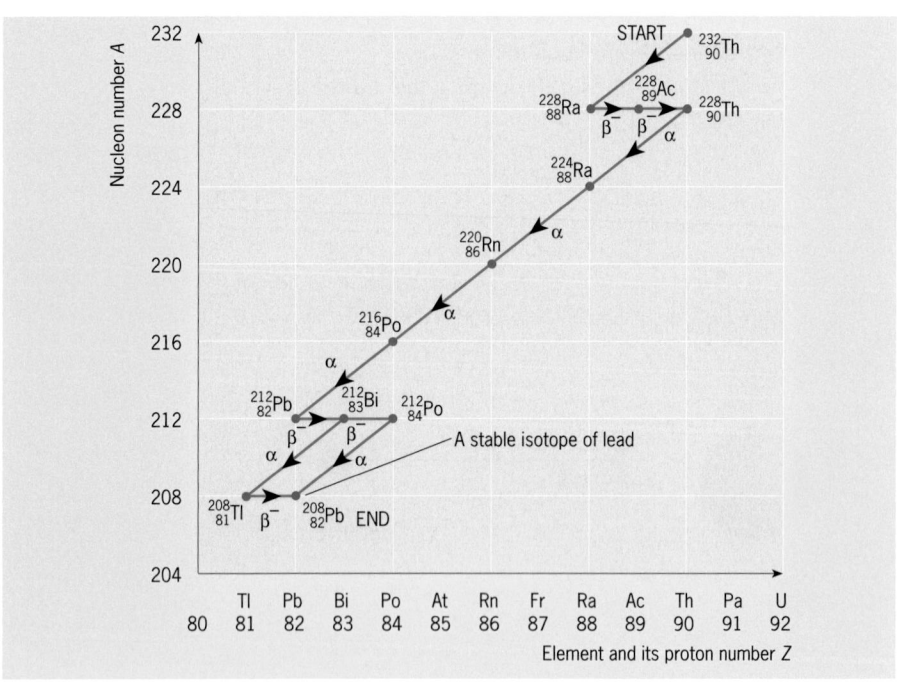

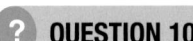

? QUESTION 10

10 Explain why:
   a) the emission of an alpha particle from thorium-232 results in a nucleus of radium-228,
   b) the emission of a beta particle (β^-) then changes the radium into an isotope of actinium.

GAMMA EMISSION

Gamma rays are photons of very short-wave electromagnetic radiation. Their wavelength is about 10^{-13} m, about a thousandth of the wavelength of X-rays. They have a photon energy some ten million times that of a photon of light. As gamma rays have neither mass nor charge, the nuclide stays the same (but in a more stable state) after emission of a gamma photon, so gamma emission does not feature in Fig 17.17.

The emission of gamma photons from an unstable nucleus can be explained by a model similar to that used to explain why low-energy photons are emitted from an atom in an excited state – that is, electrons move between energy levels so that the atom reaches its ground state. The energy of a gamma photon from a nucleus is very much greater than that of a photon from an excited atom, because the nuclear forces between nucleons are far greater than the electromagnetic forces between the nucleus and the electrons.

7 THE PROBLEMS OF BEING A LARGE NUCLEUS

Fig 17.18 is a graph of the elements, with proton number Z (on the x-axis) plotted against (nucleon) number A, for the most common isotope of each element. It has a slight curve which shows that A (protons + neutrons) increases more rapidly than Z (protons only). For example, the nucleus of lead (Pb-206) has 82 protons and 124 neutrons, whilst calcium (Ca-40) has 20 of each. We see this increase in the neutron–proton ratio more clearly in the graph of Fig 17.19.

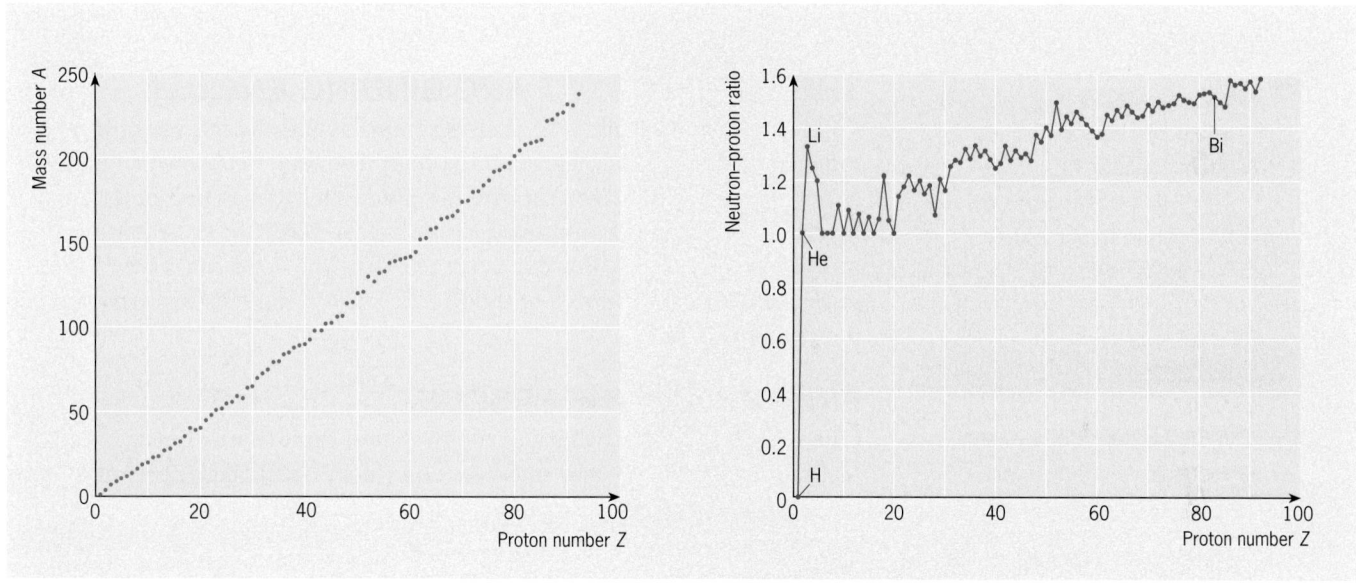

Fig 17.18 Graph of mass (nucleon) number against proton number   **Fig 17.19** Graph of neutron–proton ratio

Nuclei larger than those of bismuth (Bi) with more than 83 protons and 1.5 times as many neutrons, are unstable. They are all radioactive – which means that they break down (disintegrate) to emit:
- a group of two protons plus two neutrons as an **alpha particle**, *or*
- an electron (as a **beta particle**),
- then, for both, possibly a photon (a **gamma ray**).

BINDING FORCE AND BINDING ENERGY

A mass on the Earth's surface is held there by the force of gravity. When the mass is lifted above the ground, the Earth–mass system gains energy. Work has been done to separate the two bodies. This energy is the **gravitational potential energy** covered in Chapter 3. In that chapter, we calculated the gravitational potential energy per kilogram of a mass on the Earth's surface. Since the force is attractive, and since the potential energy when the mass is at infinity is zero, the potential energy at the surface is therefore negative. Although this value is calculated for the mass m, it is in fact the energy of the

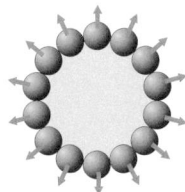

Fig 17.20(a) An unstable sphere: repelling particles have positive potential energy

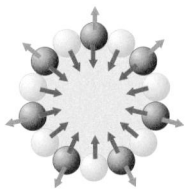

Fig 17.20(b) A mixture of attracting and repelling particles may or may not be stable. A stable arrangement has negative potential energy: a supply of energy is needed to break it apart

 REMEMBER THIS

Mass of proton m_p
  = $1.672\,623 \times 10^{-27}$ kg
Mass of neutron m_n
  = $1.674\,929 \times 10^{-27}$ kg
Mass of helium nucleus
  = $6.646\,782 \times 10^{-27}$ kg

? **QUESTION 11**

11 Use the Einstein mass–energy relationship to check that the binding energy of the helium nucleus is 4.349×10^{-12} J.

 REMEMBER THIS

To convert electronvolts to joules, multiply the value by the electronic charge e, 1.6×10^{-19} C.

? **QUESTION 12**

12 **a)** How many joules are equivalent to **i)** 2 eV, **ii)** 4 MeV?
(2 eV is the typical energy required to ionise an atom; 4 MeV is the typical energy acquired by an alpha particle when ejected from a nucleus.)
b) Convert the following to electronvolts: **i)** 1.09×10^{-12} J, **ii)** 25 J.

Earth–mass *system*, not of the movable mass alone. We could call it the binding energy of the Earth–mass system, which Chapter 3 shows to be:

$$-G\frac{Mm}{r}$$

where G is the gravitational constant, M the mass and r the radius of the Earth.

In the same way, we can think of the particles in the nucleus as making up a system which contains **binding energy**. The force here is not gravity, but the net sum of the attractive *strong nuclear force* and the repelling *electric force* (Fig 17.20). For nuclei that can actually exist, the strong force is greater than the electric force. The effect is much the same as for the Earth–mass system: it takes a supply of energy to break up the nucleons of a normally stable nucleus.

You cannot work out the binding energy of a nuclear system by summing the forces for the individual nucleons. The two main forces involved obey different laws, unlike the simple one-force gravitational system. But we can do it easily using a very simple, but quite amazing idea:

mass and energy are equivalent.

THE MASS DEFECT AND BINDING ENERGY
Physicists have measured the masses of nuclei, and the masses of the individual protons and neutrons to a high degree of accuracy using mass spectrography as explained above. A helium nucleus has two protons and two neutrons, and so we would expect it to have a mass of $2m_p + 2m_n$ totalling $6.695\,104 \times 10^{-27}$ kg. But this is *greater* than the acual mass of a helium nucleus. We seem to have lost $0.048\,322 \times 10^{-27}$ kg. This lost mass is called the **mass defect**.

EINSTEIN TO THE RESCUE
One of the major discoveries of the twentieth century was Einstein's realisation that energy and mass are equivalent: mass has energy and energy has mass. In the right circumstances they are interchangeable. Any energy change means a mass change. We explain the lost nuclear mass by saying that it represents the loss of energy that occurred when the particles combined to form the helium nucleus. Just as an Earth–mass system loses potential energy when a lump of matter falls to Earth, so a nucleon system loses potential energy when nucleons fall together to make helium nuclei. The energy loss appears as a mass loss according to the Einstein relation $\Delta E = c^2 \Delta m$.

Using the value of the speed of light c as 3×10^8 m s^{-1}, we can calculate the mass defect for helium as a **binding energy** of 4.349×10^{-12} J.

BINDING ENERGY PER NUCLEON
It is often more useful to consider the **binding energy per nucleon** (BEPN) in a particular nucleus. This is the energy needed to take one nucleon out of a nucleus, doing work against the net attracting force. For helium-4, the binding energy per nucleon is a quarter of the total binding energy calculated above from the mass defect: 1.0873×10^{-12} J.

Physicists also prefer to use the **electronvolt** (eV) as the unit of energy. The electronvolt is explained on page 196. The value of the binding energy per nucleon for helium-4 is –7.07 MeV.

The binding energy per nucleon is useful because it tells how strongly bound the nucleons are in different nuclei. Fig 17.21 is a graph of BEPN against proton number. The nucleus in which the particles are most strongly bound is that of iron ($Z = 26$, $A = 56$). This is because iron has the lowest value of BEPN – when they enter iron, nucleons have 'further to fall' than for any other nucleus. It means that more energy has to be supplied to get them out again. This means that iron (Fe) has the most stable nucleus.

The position of nucleons on this curve decides whether or not we can get energy by their **fission** (see section 9, page 344) or by **fusion** (see below and page 348).

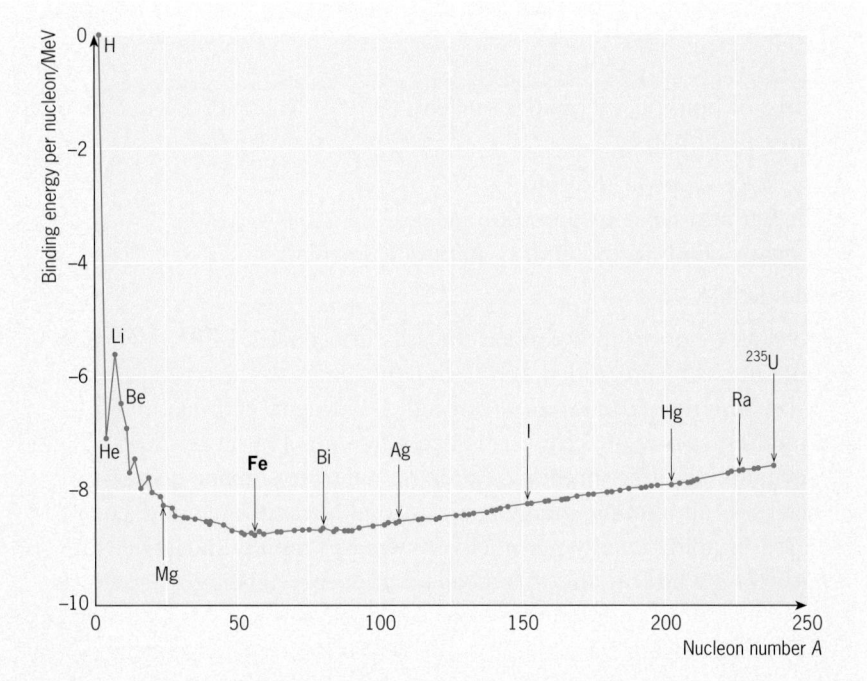

Fig 17.21 Graph of binding energy per nucleon (BEPN), with some of the elements identified

HOW BINDING ENERGY LEADS TO GETTING ENERGY FROM NUCLEAR FUSION

In theory, any two nuclei could be combined together to form a larger one. Consider adding a helium nucleus ($Z = 2$, $A = 4$) to a lithium nucleus ($Z = 3$, $A = 7$). We would end up with an isotope of boron ($Z = 5$, $A = 11$). Think of doing this the hard way, by breaking up the smaller nuclei into nucleons and then reassembling them into boron. This break-up would cost their binding energies (in MeV):

Binding energy for 4 nucleons of He/MeV @ 7.07 MeV per nucleon–28.30
Binding energy for 7 nucleons of Li/MeV @ 5.61 MeV per nucleon–39.25
Sum of this binding energy for all 11 nucleons/MeV   –67.55

If we now push the bits together to form boron, we would create a nucleus with a known binding energy per nucleon of –6.93 MeV. This gives a total binding energy of –76.21 MeV. This would produce an energy *gain* of 8.66 MeV (76.21 – 67.55) per nucleus of boron produced. In forming boron, the nucleons have fallen further into the energy well, so have less potential energy. This difference in energy would leave the nucleus as radiation, say. But lithium is a rare element, so this fusion is not a cost-effective source of nuclear energy (see Fig 17.22).

The formation of helium from four protons (by a complex route, see page 348 and Chapter 25) releases 26.7 MeV per helium nucleus formed. Look at the graph in Fig 17.21: the fall from hydrogen (one proton) to helium is large, and suggests a large energy release when hydrogen is converted to helium. The falls from helium + lithium to boron are smaller, so less energy is released.

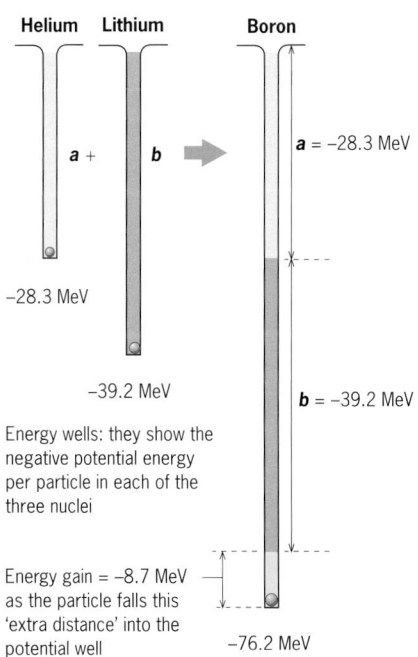

Fig 17.22 Fusing helium and lithium to make boron releases 8.7 MeV of binding energy

Even with smaller nuclei, it is not easy to produce fusion. The electric repulsion between positively charged nuclei is a long-range force and produces a barrier stopping nuclei getting close enough to each other for the strong nuclear force of attraction to come into play. So, for nuclear fusion, nuclei need to collide at speeds high enough to overcome the repulsion barrier. There can be nuclear fusion in stars because the very high temperatures in their cores (over 10 million kelvin) mean that the average speed of the particles is very high.

8 EXPLAINING THE BINDING ENERGY CURVE

The curve of binding energy per nucleon (BEPN) in Fig 17.21 can be divided into three main parts:

1. The steep slope at the start
2. The flat part close to the iron nucleus
3. A steady climb to the limit of natural elements

In more detail:

1. Here, as we go from hydrogen towards iron nuclei, BEPN increases as more nucleons are added and each contributes to the strong nuclear force, so binding the particles more strongly. Hydrogen with just one proton has a binding energy of zero; this is like a free mass far away from any other gravitational attracting body. Adding a neutron to make deuterium increases the binding energy as the strong nuclear force now comes into action. Binding energy per nucleon increases rapidly (negatively) as particles are added, and this means that energy is being released. As explained above, adding nucleons to a nucleus is not easy, but happens in the extreme conditions found in the very hot ultradense cores of stars. This **nuclear fusion** is of course the source of a star's energy output which keeps it hot and maintains the reaction. We can imagine nucleons and nuclei 'falling downhill' and converting potential energy (binding energy) to kinetic energy ('heat') and radiation as they do so.

2. Adding even more nucleons increases the binding forces but also increases the electrical repulsion effect as protons are added. This means that there comes a stage when adding more nucleons starts to decrease the BEPN. The turning point is iron, which has the greatest BEPN of all nuclides. No nucleons or nuclei can 'fall' further than iron. Just as it needs an input of energy to break up an iron nucleus into smaller nuclei (going up the steep initial slope), it also needs an input of energy to create nuclei larger than iron (going up the shallower slope to the right).

3. The shallow rising slope is the effect of electrical repulsion (protons) beginning to have an increasing effect on the net force holding the nucleus together. So it is sometimes called the **Coulomb slope**. There is a tendency here for nuclei to fall down the slope towards iron by emitting a very stable unit – the helium nucleus, which has a high BEPN. It is emitted as the familiar alpha particle. Very large nuclei with a weak net binding force (low BEPN) can reach stability by simply falling apart. This is rare but can happen in large nuclei with an excess of neutrons (e.g. U-235). It can be stimulated by adding neutrons to the nucleus – which is what happens in **nuclear fission** – in bombs and nuclear reactors. See page 345.

All the nuclides to the right of iron on the graph have been made when stars have collapsed and subsequently exploded: the huge amounts of energy released have caused nuclei to fuse into heavy nuclei. All the nucleons to the left of iron have been made as a consequence of the energy-producing nuclear fusion that keeps stars hot during their lifetime. There is more about this in Chapter 25.

FROM TWO TO THREE DIMENSIONS

The BEPN curve in Fig 17.21 is drawn as two-dimensional. In fact each point on it (representing an element) has partners with the same proton number (Z) – the element's isotopes. This is illustrated in Fig 17.23.

The slope looked at in three dimensions is like a valley with steep sides – like a canyon. At any point the isotopes of an element lying on either side of the most stable isotopes have smaller (negative) values of BEPN. This means that they can lose potential (binding) energy by falling down to the stable isotope at the bottom of the canyon. The isotopes tend to be unstable because of a faulty proton–neutron balance. On one side the isotopes have too many neutrons, on the other too many protons, for stability. Like electrons in atoms, these nucleons can't have the same energy level, so their nuclei are at higher energy states – higher up the canyon wall. They gain stability by converting neutrons into protons – or protons into neutrons – in other words by **beta decay**.

In 'ordinary' beta decay, a neutron changes to a proton and an electron is emitted (β^-):

$$^1_0n \rightarrow {}^1_1p + {}^{\ 0}_{-1}e$$

In **positron decay**, a proton changes to a neutron and a positive electron, called a positron, is emitted (β^+):

$$^1_1p \rightarrow {}^1_0n + {}^0_1e$$

Gamma emission

It is useful to think of the nucleus as a kind of onion having layers of nucleons – rather like a simple model of an atom with its 'layers' of electrons. Just as atoms can be in excited states because electrons are at higher levels, so neutrons and protons in a nucleus can be left at higher levels when nuclei change quite dramatically by alpha decay or by nucleons changing via positive and negative beta decay. Atoms achieve stability as electrons move, emitting electromagnetic radiation as they do so. Nuclei do the same, but because the nuclear force is so strong the radiation emitted is highly energetic – the gamma ray (see Fig 17.24).

A REGION OF STABILITY

Along a narrow band at the bottom of the 'canyon' of the three-dimensional binding energy curve are nuclei with a balance of protons and neutrons that keep them stable. In general as Z increases more neutrons than you might expect are needed to do this: the neutron–proton ratio (shown in Fig 17.19) increases for stable nuclei, from 1 for He to 1.6 for uranium. It is these stable nuclei that make up the ordinary chemical world. It is only the very long-lived unstable nuclei (like uranium-238, thorium-232) that still exist on Earth – unless they are fairly new nuclei formed by radioactive decay or artificially in nuclear reactors.

Fig 17.25 overleaf is a plot of neutron number against proton number which clearly shows that neutron number increases more rapidly than proton number for stable isotopes. If isotopes stray from this equilibrium line they tend to decay via beta$^+$ or beta$^-$ routes or, more rarely, by a nucleus capturing an electron from the nearest electron orbital shell – **electron capture**.

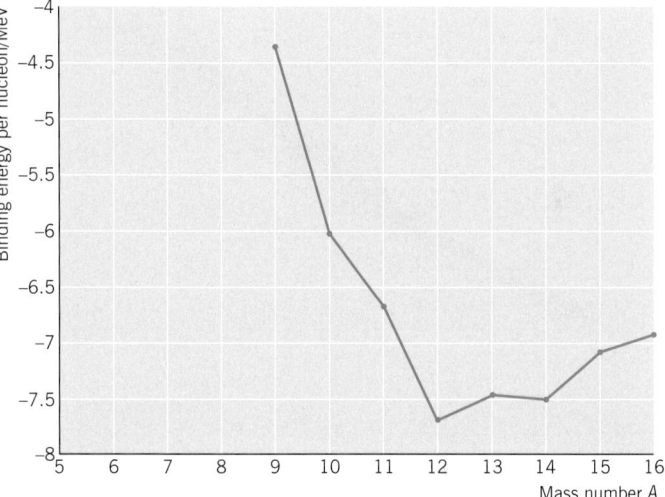

Fig 17.23 Cross-section of the binding energy curve for carbon isotopes. This shows that C-12 has the lowest binding energy per nucleon

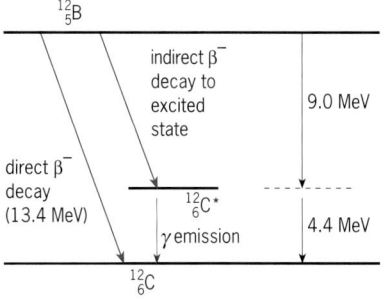

Fig 17.24 Gamma emission occurs when a nuclide is created with its nucleus in an excited state. The formulae for such nuclei are labelled with a star; here we have $^{12}_{6}C^*$

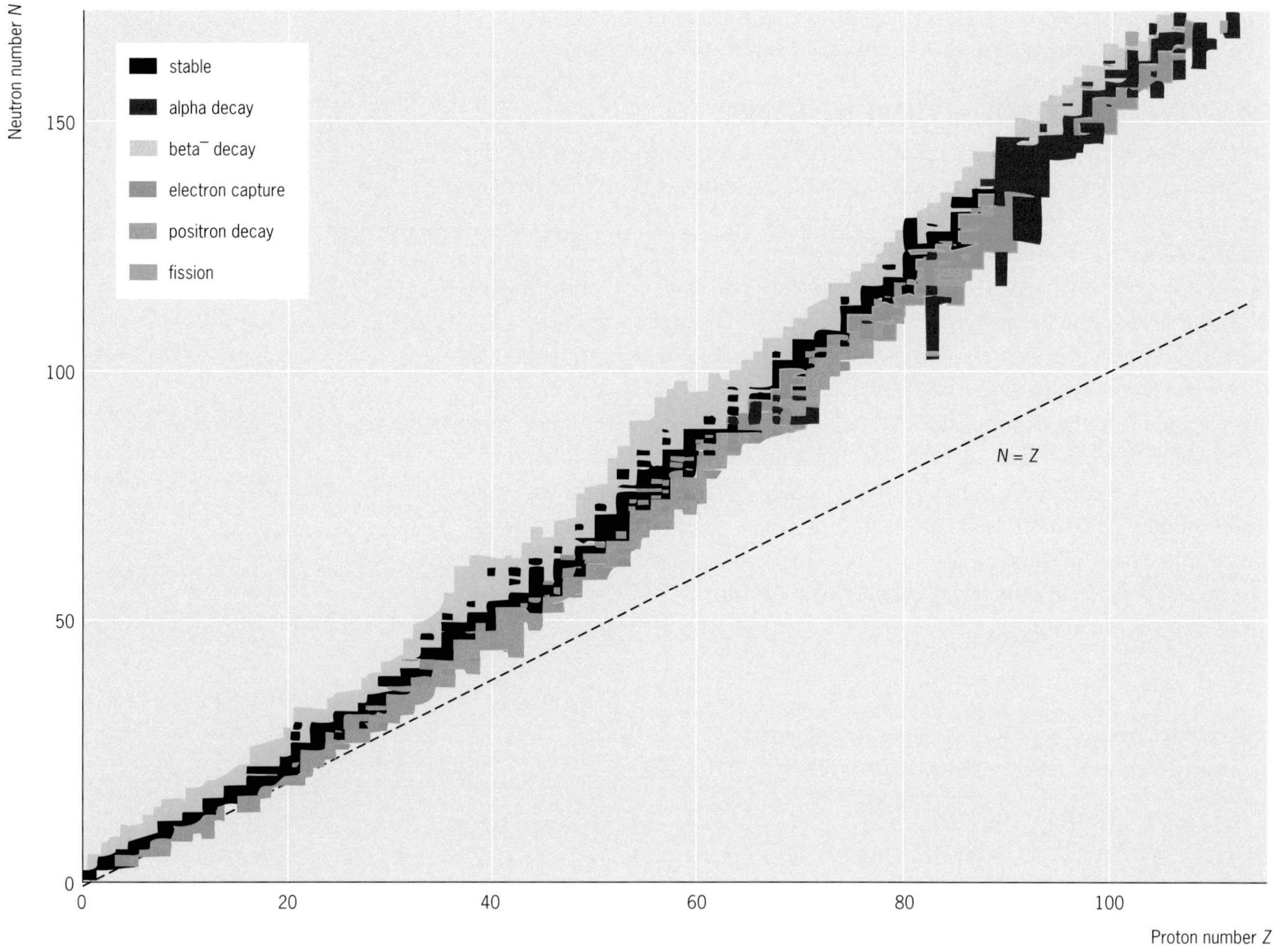

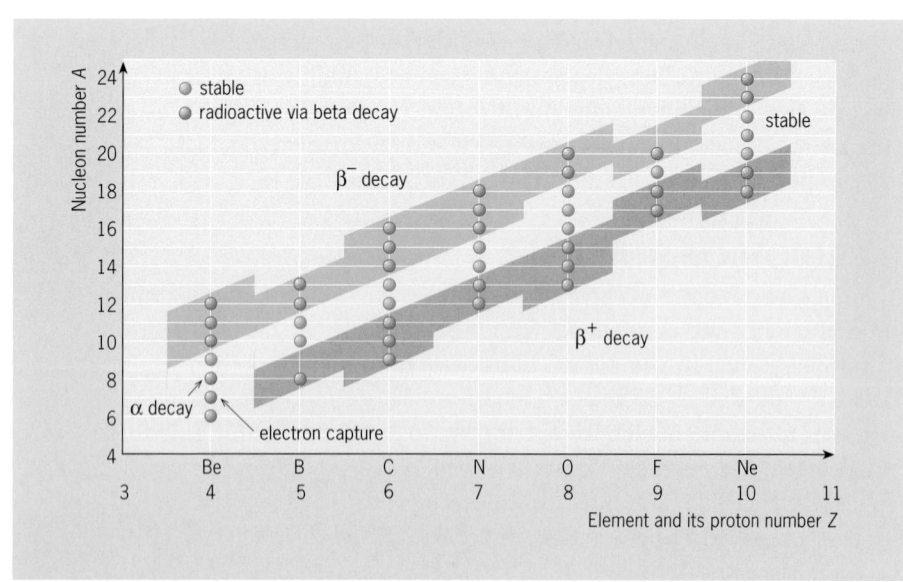

Fig 17.25 A plot of neutron number *N* against proton number *Z* for stable and unstable nuclides

Fig 17.26 shows a close-up of the region of stability for the isotopes of some of the lighter elements, surrounded by unstable isotopes liable to beta⁻ or beta⁺ decay.

Fig 17.26 Nucleon number *A* against proton number *Z*: close-up of the region of stability for lighter nuclides. Each vertical row shows isotopes of the same element

WHY DON'T ALL UNSTABLE NUCLEI DECAY IMMEDIATELY?

Some radioactive nuclei decay so slowly that it takes billions of years for half of them to decay (e.g. U-238 with a half-life of 45 billion years). Others decay in fractions of a microsecond. What causes even the shortest delay? The answer is to do with the facts of quantum behaviour. As an example, consider alpha decay.

An alpha particle is so stable that it behaves as a single object inside a large nucleus. We can think of this particle in a nucleus as being at the bottom of a potential energy well. This is similar to picturing a mass on the Earth's surface at the bottom of the Earth's 'gravitational well', see Fig 17.27. In both cases, there has to be some energy input for the object to reach an 'escape speed' and get away from the well.

But how does the alpha particle 'escape' from the well? Fig 17.27(a) suggests that it needs to be given kinetic energy to get away from the other particles in the nucleus. It does have some kinetic energy – the nuclear particles are imagined as joggling about inside the nucleus like gerbils in a bag – but not enough to allow a particle to escape. Fig 17.27(a) shows a typical alpha particle with an energy of 5 MeV inside a nucleus. But the nuclear force is so strong that an energy of some 30 MeV is needed for the particle to escape. You can compare this with the idea of escape speed for a rocket leaving the Earth.

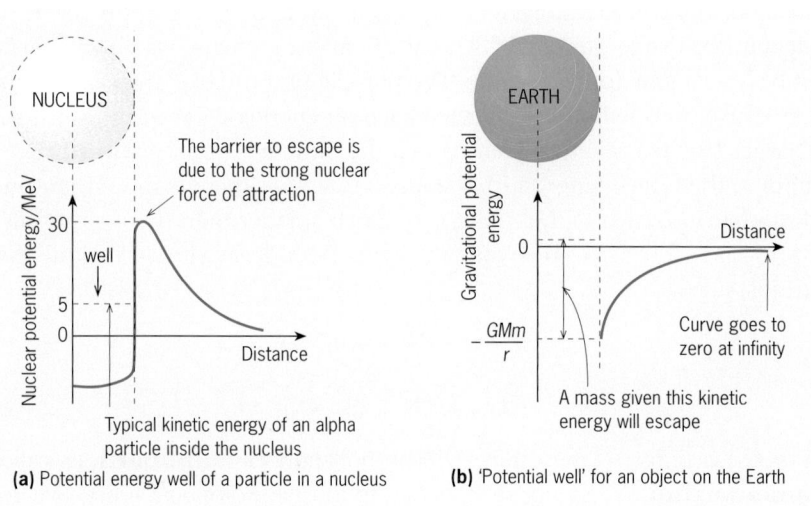

(a) Potential energy well of a particle in a nucleus   **(b)** 'Potential well' for an object on the Earth

Fig 17.27 Potential energy wells for a nucleus and the Earth. According to classical theory, the alpha particle does not have enough kinetic energy to escape

This is where the quantum theory of matter comes in. This says that, like a gerbil that eats through the side of the bag, an alpha particle could 'tunnel' its way out. A quantum view of the alpha particle is shown in Fig 17.28.

In this theory, the position of an alpha particle is represented by a probability wave of a size that fits into the nucleus. Compare this with an electron inside an atom, as discussed in Chapter 16. But, as Fig 17.28 shows, the probability wave doesn't end *inside* the nuclear potential energy barrier; there is a small but finite probability that the alpha particle is outside the nucleus, where the electric repulsion force alone acts and returns the alpha particle's kinetic energy as it accelerates away. The probability of decay – essentially the decay constant k (page 327) which determines the half-life – is different for different nuclei and as it is a probability the resulting decay is random.

Similar quantum behaviour decides the decay probabilities for beta and gamma emission.

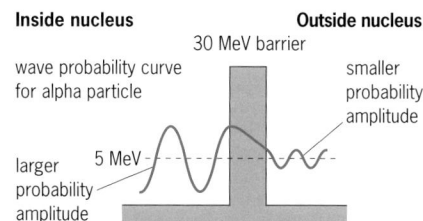

Fig 17.28 The quantum explanation for alpha decay: 'tunnelling' occurs, making it possible for an alpha particle with a kinetic energy of only 5 MeV to exist outside the nucleus. This is not a certainty, hence radioactive decay is random

A RADIOACTIVE PUZZLE – AND ITS SURPRISING SOLUTION

Energy conservation and beta decay – the neutrino

In radioactive decay, both alpha particles and gamma radiation are emitted from a given nuclide with a definite energy which is characteristic of the nuclide. This however does not happen for beta particles. Measurements show a range of energies for the beta particles emitted from a given radioactive substance (Figs 17.29(a) and (b)).

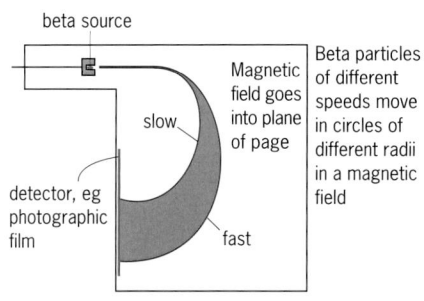

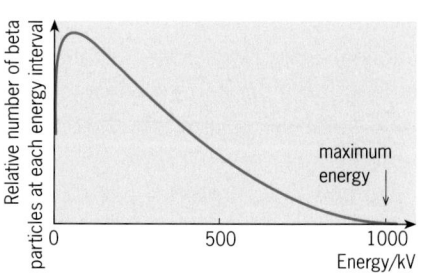

Fig 17.29(a) Experiments on the deflection of beta particles from a pure source show that they are emitted with a range of speeds

Fig 17.29(b) The beta particle spectrum of bismuth-210

> ### ✔ REMEMBER THIS
>
> In summary, there are six main ways in which unstable nuclei decay or change:
>
> **alpha decay** (mostly very large nuclei; A and Z change),
> e.g. $^{232}_{90}\text{Th} \rightarrow ^{228}_{88}\text{Ra} + ^{4}_{2}\alpha$
>
> **negative beta decay** (nuclei that have too many neutrons; Z changes),
> e.g. $^{14}_{6}\text{C} \rightarrow ^{14}_{7}\text{N} + _{-1}\beta^- + \bar{\nu}$
>
> **positive beta decay** (nuclei with too many protons; Z changes),
> e.g. $^{10}_{6}\text{C} \rightarrow ^{10}_{5}\text{B} + _{1}\beta^+ + \nu$
>
> **electron capture** by nucleus of an electron in innermost shell (some nuclei that have too many protons; Z changes),
> e.g. $^{54}_{25}\text{Mn} + _{-1}e^- \rightarrow ^{54}_{24}\text{Cr} + \gamma$
>
> **gamma emission** (nuclei left in an excited state after decay; no change in A or Z but a change in energy level)
>
> **nuclear fission** (some very large nuclei, particularly after neutron capture),
> e.g. $^{235}\text{U} \rightarrow ^{100}\text{Ru} + ^{133}\text{Cs} + 2\ ^{1}\text{n}$

This spread of energies posed a serious problem to nuclear physicists. Why did some emerge with less energy than others? It seemed to contradict the principle of the conservation of energy. To avoid this appalling prospect, Wolfgang Pauli suggested in 1930 that the missing energy was being carried away by a *new* subatomic particle. The particle had to have a very small mass, and, because no one had detected such an energetic particle, it must carry no charge. This particle has been named the 'little neutron', or **neutrino** (symbol ν, the Greek letter 'nu'). We also know that there is more than one kind of neutrino, each with a mass very much smaller than the mass of an electron – possibly zero. Reactions involving beta decay should include the neutrinos, e.g.

$$^{14}_{6}\text{C} \rightarrow ^{14}_{7}\text{N} + _{-1}\beta^- + _{0}\bar{\nu}$$

$$^{15}_{8}\text{O} \rightarrow ^{15}_{7}\text{N} + _{1}\beta^+ + _{0}\nu$$

In these reactions ν is the 'ordinary' neutrino, and $\bar{\nu}$ is its **antiparticle**, called the **antineutrino**. When a neutron decays to form a proton and a negative beta particle, the antineutrino is involved:

$$^{1}\text{n} \rightarrow ^{1}\text{p} + \beta^- + \bar{\nu}$$

Note that the beta decays shown on page 341 are incomplete: neutrinos are also emitted.

In the C-14 decay above, a neutron has changed to a proton; in the O-15 decay a proton has changed to a neutron. Deeper inside the nucleus *quarks* are changing to cause these effects – see Chapter 24.

9 NUCLEAR REACTORS

The binding energy curve per nucleon of Fig 17.21 shows that for nuclei larger than the iron nucleus at the low point of the curve, energy might be generated by splitting a nucleus into two parts. For this to work, both new nuclei must be near the bottom of the curve. The best-known fissionable nucleus is of uranium-235. The nucleus can split spontaneously, a very rare event, but one that can be triggered by the nucleus absorbing a neutron (see Fig 17.31).

A simple but workable model for this is to imagine a large nucleus to be a drop of liquid (Fig 17.30), with the net nuclear attracting force acting like the surface tension that keeps a water drop together. A neutron entering this

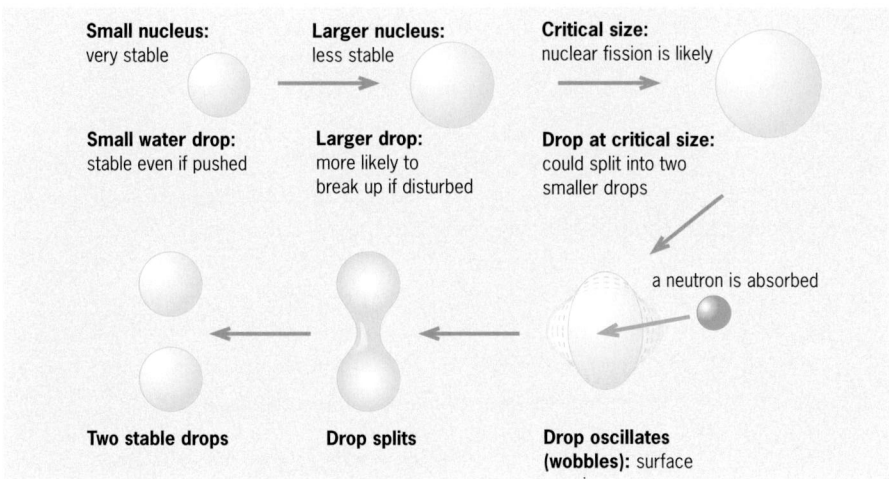

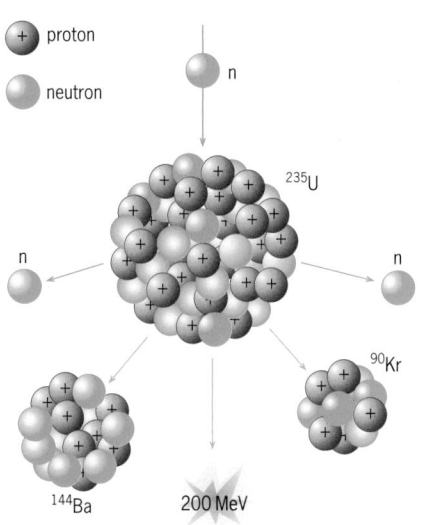

Fig 17.30 The liquid drop model of nuclear fission

Fig 17.31 Nuclear fission. Adding a neutron to a potentially unstable nucleus induces fission, a process used in nuclear fission reactors

nucleus will set it oscillating like a disturbed drop of mercury in a dish, say. If the nucleus forms a dumb-bell shape it may split into two parts. Like the liquid drops, two smaller nuclei have less energy than the single drop or nucleus. Both new nuclei are nearer the bottom of the nuclear valley described earlier.

The fission (disintegration) products shown in Fig 17.31, barium and krypton, are just two of many possibilities. Note that two neutrons are also released. This means that a nuclear disintegration may cause a **chain reaction** (Fig 17.32) in which more nuclei split as they absorb the released neutrons.

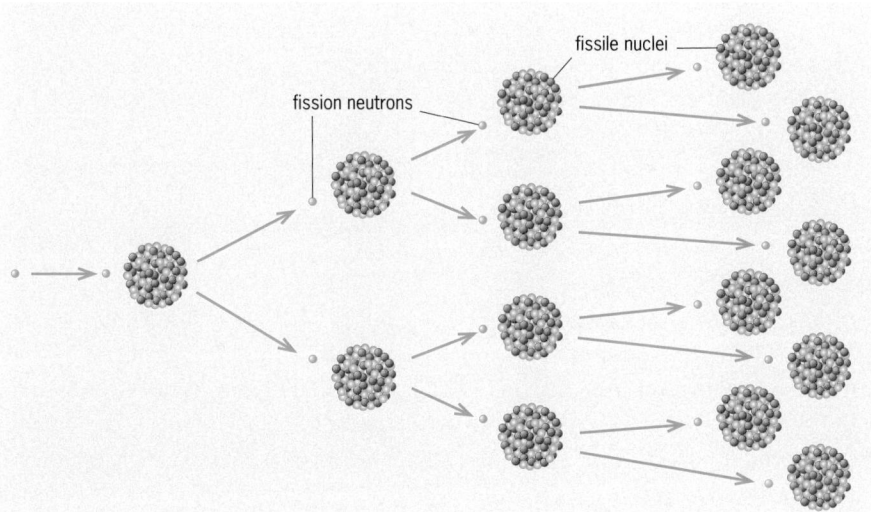

Fig 17.32 A chain reaction. If each fission releases two or more neutrons, each of which triggers a fission, we get an uncontrolled nuclear process (fission products not shown)

CRITICAL MASS

In a small mass of fissile material – such as uranium enriched with uranium-235 – some natural (spontaneous) fission occurs all the time, producing neutrons. Most of them escape from the mass completely, and so do not cause fission of other nuclei. This is because any lump of matter is mostly empty space, and the chance of a neutron colliding with the tiny nucleus of an atom is very small.

But suppose the mass, and so the size of the fissile material, is increased. There are more neutrons released and there is also an increase in the total 'target area' of nuclei for each neutron. So there will be more *induced* fission, and more energy will be released in the mass – it will get hotter.

? QUESTIONS 13–14

13 A nucleus of uranium-235 splits spontaneously into two smaller nuclei and three neutrons. Identify two of the smaller nuclei that could be produced, apart from barium and krypton.

14 The total binding energies of the nuclei in the nuclear reaction described are:
uranium-235–1736.8 MeV
barium-144–1161.5 MeV
krypton-90   –754.6 MeV
a) Show that the energy released in this example of fission is about 180 MeV per event.
b) One gram of uranium-235 contains 2.5×10^{21} nuclei. Estimate how much energy (in joules) would be released when 1 gram of U-235 is split in a nuclear reactor.

Explosion or meltdown?

This is a classic case of **positive feedback**: the more fission, the more neutrons are released, so there is even more fission. In a large enough mass of the fissile material, induced fission produces a runaway chain reaction: a very large number of nuclei will disintegrate in a very short time. There is a sudden very large release of energy – an explosion. For a given composition of material, the mass at which this will occur depends on its shape. But for a sphere, it is called the **critical mass**.

In practice, simply putting lumps of enriched uranium in a container will not have this effect. Before the critical mass is reached, the energy generated will melt (indeed, vaporise) the uranium. This is a 'meltdown', as happened in the worst nuclear reactor accident of all time at Chernobyl in 1986.

STRUCTURE OF A NUCLEAR REACTOR

In a nuclear reactor, energy is generated in **fuel rods** contained in thin non-corrosive tubes inserted into the reactor core. Around the core is a gas or water under pressure. The fuel rods contain either plutonium or uranium oxide, made with an 'enriched' mixture of 97 per cent uranium-238 and 3 per cent uranium-235. The core of a typical reactor contains about 80 tonnes of uranium oxide. Only the uranium-235 nuclei are likely to undergo fission, the ultimate energy source in the fuel rod.

Increasing induced fissions by using slow neutrons

The neutrons from spontaneous random fission of U-235 are emitted at high speeds. Fast neutrons have a much smaller probability of entering a nucleus than slow ones; they tend to bounce off.

To slow down the neutrons, the fuel rods are surrounded by a **moderator**. This used to be graphite, but modern pressurised water reactors use the water which also acts as a coolant. The fast neutrons collide with coolant molecules and gradually lose kinetic energy until they are slow enough to have a much greater chance of causing induced fission when they reach the next fuel rod.

Controlling the reactions

Once induced fission starts, too many neutrons could be produced and the reaction could start 'running away'. Therefore, excess neutrons must be removed, so that the fission rate is controlled and energy is released at a steady rate. To do this, cylindrical **control rods** are inserted into the reactor core near the fuel rods. The material of the control rods, for example boron or cadmium, absorbs neutrons.

USING THE ENERGY FROM A NUCLEAR REACTOR

The fission products are large nuclei which separate at high speed. They collide with other nuclei and their kinetic energy is shared out, so that the reactor core containing the fuel rods, moderator and control rods becomes very hot. Nowadays, the reactor core contains and is surrounded by a fluid, most commonly water under pressure, as in **pressurised water reactors** (PWRs); see Fig 17.33.

The energy is carried from the core by superheated water at a temperature of 325 °C kept from vaporising by a pressure of 150 atmospheres. This water heats a secondary loop of water in a 'heat exchanger', and produces steam to drive a turbine that produces electricity.

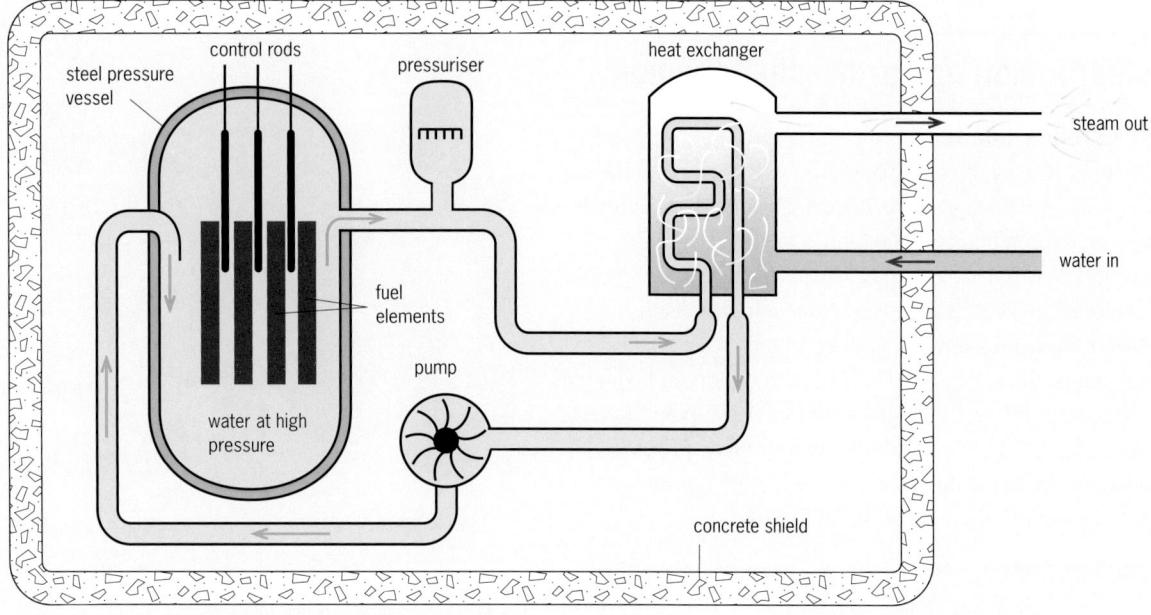

Fig 17.33 Scheme of a pressurised water reactor (PWR)

The first, and so far only, pressurised water reactor (PWR) in Britain is Sizewell B in Suffolk, which came on stream in 1995. Worldwide, it is the most popular type being built today. PWRs have a compact core because water is the most effective moderator for slowing down the neutrons. This means that the cores can be prefabricated in a factory and transported to the site. Any new reactors built in the UK are likely to be improved versions of the PWR, which need less fuel, have little need for mechanical pumps, which might break down, and are easier to maintain. In case of an accident, reactor safety relies on passive features such as gravity and convection.

THE TROUBLE WITH NUCLEAR POWER

It seems that nuclear power avoids many of the problems we associate with the most common UK energy source, fossil fuel. Nuclear power does not add to the greenhouse effect, which is mainly due to carbon dioxide from burnt fuel, and its raw material will not run out as quickly as, say, oil reserves. Nor does it produce the gases from burning coal and oil which affect health and cause acid rain.

But nuclear power has its own problems. There is the risk of accidents in which radioactive materials can escape into the environment. Also, even for perfectly managed systems, there are the problems of **nuclear waste** and of closing down (decommissioning) power stations at the end of their useful life. These are problems because they may expose people (and other forms of life) to harmful ionising radiations, as described below.

Nuclear waste

Nuclei of the non-radioactive material in the core may become radioactive isotopes when they absorb neutrons. Also, the spent fuel rods contain the fission products which tend to be radioactive, as well as the unused uranium-238. The uranium can be recycled, but eventually the main components of the reactor core become radioactive waste and have to be taken out.

Radioactive waste includes both short-lived isotopes which are highly active, and isotopes with very long half-lives (such as plutonium-239, half-life 24 000 years, formed from uranium-238). The waste is kept in storage tanks for years to allow the 'high-level' wastes to decay to less active or stable isotopes.

? **QUESTION 15**

15 What costs are ignored in the current use of fossil fuels, compared with nuclear fuels?

Nuclear fusion on Earth – the tokamak

The hydrogen bomb

Small nuclei can combine to make larger nuclei with the release of energy, as explained in the main text. This happens naturally in the extreme conditions in the centres of stars. On Earth, nuclear fusion was achieved artificially in the 'hydrogen bomb', first exploded in 1952. This used the uncontrolled chain reaction of nuclear fission (a fission bomb) to create a high enough temperature for isotopes of hydrogen (normal hydrogen and deuterium, ^2_1H) to fuse together to form helium and release enormous energy. This is called a **thermonuclear process**. Such bombs are many thousands of times more destructive than the first nuclear bombs used on Japan in 1945.

Controlled fusion – the ultimate energy source?

Russia, the United States and the European Union have for many years tried to develop a working version of a controlled thermonuclear energy source. The main problems are to produce and maintain a high enough temperature for the process to begin, whilst at the same time keeping the very hot particles close enough together for fusion to continue, and in a controlled way.

The working gases are a mixture of two hydrogen isotopes, deuterium and tritium (^2_1H and ^3_1H). At high temperature, the gas molecules separate into atoms and then into electrons and nuclei, so forming a **plasma**. The plasma is heated to a temperature of over 10^7 K to trigger a fusion reaction. Then, the nuclei have enough kinetic energy on average for a significant fraction of them to fuse on collision.

$$^2_1H + ^3_1H \rightarrow ^4_2He + ^1_0n \text{ plus } 17.59 \text{ MeV}$$

Induction heating brings the gas to high temperatures: electric coils round the chamber act as the primary coils of a transformer and the plasma nuclei act as the secondary. Alternating current at high frequency in the primary coils induces a current of ions, which means the ions gain kinetic energy. The high temperature can also be reached by firing powerful lasers into the gas.

At these high temperatures, the ordinary solid matter of a container would melt or evaporate. So the plasma has to be held in a 'magnetic bottle': a strong field makes the high-speed nuclei move in circles or tight spirals in the shape of a hollow doughnut – a torus – well away from the walls of the chamber.

Fig 17.34 shows details of the equipment used, called a **tokamak**.

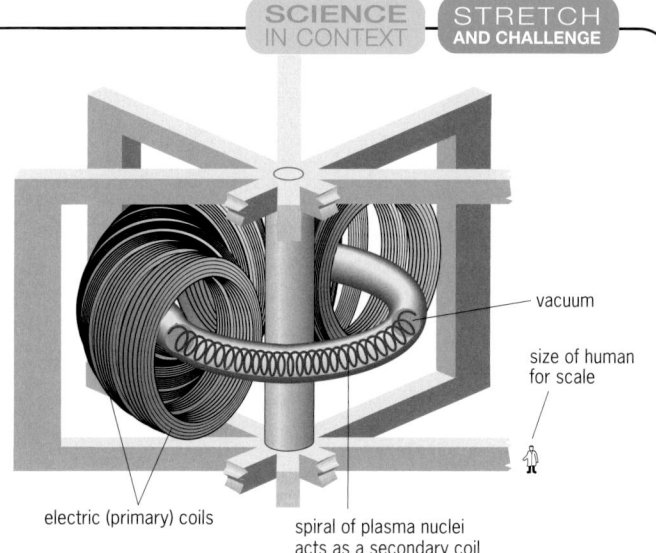

vacuum

size of human for scale

electric (primary) coils

spiral of plasma nuclei acts as a secondary coil

Fig 17.34 A tokamak nuclear fusion reactor

In 1997 the Joint European Torus (JET) tokamak produced 16 MW of power for 2 seconds – a world record. Even so, more energy was supplied to the machine to produce the result than was obtained from fusion.

The advantages of fusion as a source of energy are that the raw material is deuterium, which is easily extracted from the sea, and the end product is non-radioactive helium. However, highly radioactive tritium is formed during the reaction (Fig 17.35). Also, neutrons released during fusion are captured by the chamber walls, so making new, radioactive isotopes. It is therefore unlikely that controlled fusion will become a practical energy source until well into the twenty-first century.

A fusion plant could operate for a whole year, generating 7 billion kilowatt-hours of electricity, using just 100 kg of deuterium and 3 tonnes of lithium. A coal fired power station would generate 11 million tonnes of carbon dioxide to produce the same annual output.

In 2005 a group of countries containing half the world's population agreed to build a new tokamak – the International Thermonuclear Experimental Reactor (ITER) – at Cadarache in France. This will cost €5bn and should be operational by 2016.

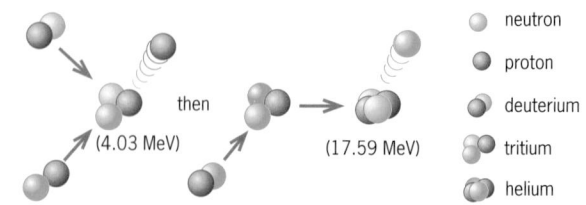

then

(4.03 MeV)   (17.59 MeV)

neutron
proton
deuterium
tritium
helium

Fig 17.35 A likely fusion reaction in a tokamak

Nuclear power station operators would like to store all wastes deep underground but it is difficult to get agreement on where to do this. The other problem is how to decommission a nuclear power station when it becomes obsolete and is no longer economical to run. A large, slightly radioactive mass of building material has to be made safe – and this could involve burying the whole site in concrete.

Dealing with waste is so costly that nuclear power may be no cheaper than power from conventional power stations using fossil fuels. But, of course, the true environmental cost of using fossil fuels is not yet paid. For example, the consequences of acid rain and the more distant and unknown effects of global warming are yet to be seen.

10 USES AND DANGERS OF RADIOACTIVITY

THE SMOKE DETECTOR

Most radioactive sources used in industrial and other applications are artificial radioactive isotopes. They are made from stable elements by using the stream of neutrons from a nuclear reactor. Being uncharged, neutrons can penetrate the atomic nucleus quite easily. When an ordinary stable nucleus gains extra neutrons, it becomes unstable with a probability of decaying by either negative or positive beta emission, as explained above.

Most applications of radioactivity are in industry or medicine, but the most common is found in almost every home – the smoke detector (Fig 17.36). It uses a small amount of the nuclide americium-241 ($^{241}_{95}$Am) with a half-life of 433 years. There are tiny amounts of it in mineral ores of uranium, but commercially it is produced by irradiating plutonium with neutrons in a nuclear reactor.

As a nuclide with a comparatively massive nucleus, americium-241 decays by the alpha process. In the smoke detector, alpha particles in a steady stream collide with molecules in the air and ionise them. The ions move towards the electrodes, maintaining a small continuous current. Smoke particles from a fire are much bigger than air molecules and are more likely to intercept the alpha particles, absorbing them and so decreasing the ionisation current. When the current drops, an alarm is triggered via an electronic amplification system.

THE DANGERS OF IONISING RADIATIONS

Living cells contain complex molecules which are easily damaged by ionising radiation. The key molecules likely to be damaged are DNA and RNA. They are involved in the production of proteins, which include the enzymes that control the synthesis of all the biochemicals needed for the growth and reproduction of cells.

Alpha radiation is heavily ionising and can be most damaging to cells, so alpha emitters are dangerous if they enter the body. But alpha radiation is easily absorbed: its range in air is only a few centimetres and a sheet of paper is enough to act as a shield (Fig 17.37, overleaf).

Beta particles are less ionising but have a longer range. So they can penetrate deeper into the body from external sources. Anyone working with beta emitters must wear protective clothing.

Gamma radiation is the least ionising but far more penetrating, so is considered the most dangerous.

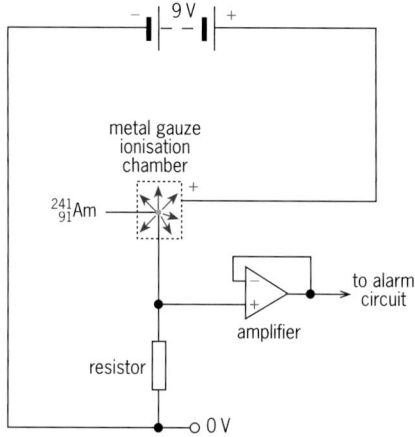

Fig 17.36 How a smoke detector works

Fig 17.37 Shielding from ionizing radiations

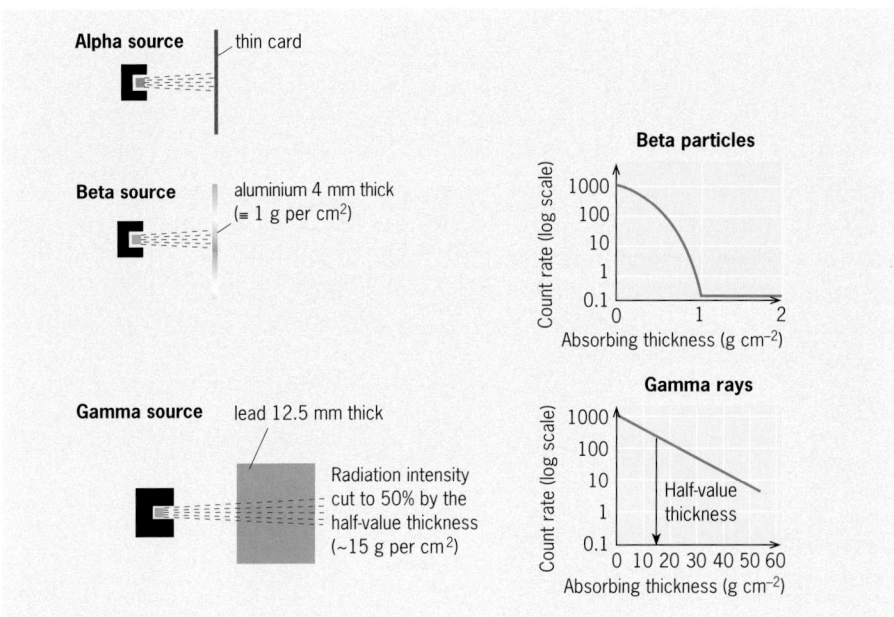

Table 17.6 Units related to radioactivity

Quantity	Unit	Definition
Activity	becquerel (Bq)	decay rate in decays per second
Dose	gray (Gy)	energy absorbed in tissue from radiation, in J kg⁻¹
Dose equivalent	sievert (Sv)	a measure of likely tissue damage, calculated as: dose × quality factor

? QUESTION 16

16 **a)** Why is gamma radiation less damaging to the human body than alpha radiation?

b) Why is more care is taken to shield workers from gamma sources than from alpha sources?

MEASURING THE BIOLOGICAL EFFECT

The variety of radiations and their differing penetration and ionising effects mean that simply measuring the activity of a source doesn't tell us much about the effect the emissions may have on the body. What matters is a combination of the energy released in the body by the ionising radiation and the relative ionising effect on living tissue.

The energy absorbed in the tissue is measured as the **dose**, in units of joules per kilogram, called the **gray** (Gy):

$$1 \text{ Gy} = 1 \text{ J kg}^{-1}$$

To allow for the different ionising abilities of the radiation, we multiply the energy absorbed per kg in grays by a **quality factor** which depends on the radiation: for X-rays, gamma rays and beta particles the factor is 1; for alpha particles it is 20. The result is a quantity called the **dose equivalent**, and this is measured in **sieverts** (Sv).

Table 17.6 summarises the units related to radioactivity.

Older units still in use:
curie = 3.7×10^7 Bq
rad = 0.001 Gy
rem = 0.001 Sv

Background radiation

The average dose equivalent of background radiation in the UK is 2.6 millisieverts per year. The sources of this background are shown in Fig 17.38.

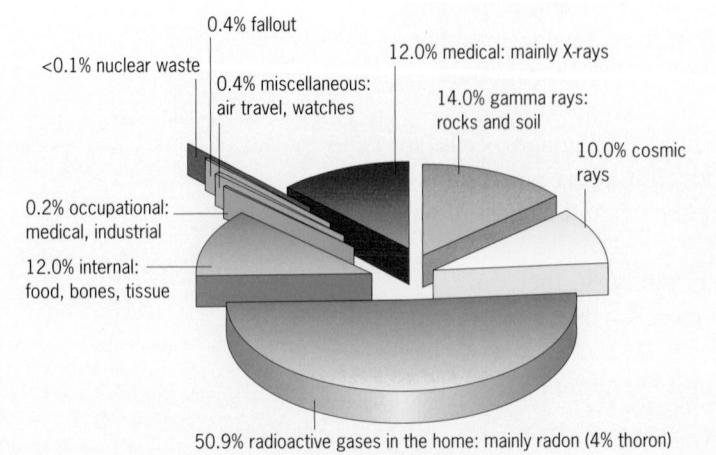

0.4% fallout

<0.1% nuclear waste

0.4% miscellaneous: air travel, watches

12.0% medical: mainly X-rays

14.0% gamma rays: rocks and soil

10.0% cosmic rays

0.2% occupational: medical, industrial

12.0% internal: food, bones, tissue

50.9% radioactive gases in the home: mainly radon (4% thoron)

Fig 17.38 Sources of background radiation as averages in the UK

SCIENCE IN CONTEXT | STRETCH AND CHALLENGE

Carbon dating

The carbon dioxide in the atmosphere is used by plants to build their main structures: roots, stems, trunks, branches, leaves and seeds. Atmospheric carbon is a mixture of the main isotope carbon-12 (98.89%), carbon-13 (1.11%); also tiny traces of carbon-14, which is radioactive with a half-life of 5730 years. It is being formed continuously as high-energy cosmic rays from space collide with atmospheric nuclei. They break up, producing neutrons and other fragments. The neutrons then enter nitrogen nuclei, which are disturbed enough to lose a proton and so form carbon-14. The process is:

$$^{14}_{7}N + ^{1}_{0}n \quad ^{14}_{6}C + ^{1}_{1}p$$

Carbon-14 eventually combines with oxygen to form carbon dioxide, CO_2. Both $^{12}CO_2$ and $^{14}CO_2$ in the atmosphere are taken up by plants. Therefore, carbohydrates in all plants contain radioactive carbon in the same ratio as carbon-14 to carbon-12 in the atmosphere at any time. So do carbohydrates in animals and other organisms whose tissues contain carbon derived from plants.

Fig 17.39 A carbon-containing sample is burnt and the amounts of carbon-12 and carbon-14 it produces are analysed, with the results displayed on screen

Fig 17.40 Examples of the bristlecone pine tree, famous worldwide for its use in setting the scale for radiocarbon dating

When a plant dies, its store of carbon-14 stops being recycled, so that as radioactive decay occurs the proportion of carbon-14 decreases. Thus the ratio of carbon-14 to carbon-12 in a piece of wood, say, many hundreds of years old, will give a measure of the time that has elapsed since that piece of wood died.

A modern piece of wood has an activity per kilogram (its specific activity) due to carbon-14 of 250 s^{-1}. Say the specific activity of wood from an old building is 125 s^{-1} kg^{-1}, then the wood must be one half-life old: 5730 years. More generally, if the zero age specimen has a specific activity A_0 and the specimen of age t has a specific activity A then $A = A_0e^{-kt}$ where k is the decay constant of carbon-14 (see pages 326–328.

As an example, suppose A was measured to be 50 s^{-1} kg^{-1}.

Then we can say:

$$50 = 250 \times e^{-kt} = \frac{250}{e^{kt}}$$

or: $$e^{k} = 5$$

giving:

$$kt = \ln 5 = 1.61$$

Now, as explained on page 327, $k \times$ half-life = ln 2

A half-life of 5730 years means a decay constant k of (ln 2)/5730 per year, so the age of the specimen is:

$$t = \frac{1.61}{k} = 5730 \times \frac{1.61}{0.693}$$

$$= 13\,300 \text{ years}$$

Carbon dating is not an exact method. The energy of the beta particles emitted is low and some would get absorbed inside the material, so small samples are vaporised to avoid this (Fig 17.39). But with such small samples, the error in counting these random events is significant, especially with older materials of low activity.

The method also assumes that cosmic ray activity has been constant over many thousands of years, though it has not. To correct for this, the radioactivity in the wood of tree rings of living trees (bristlecone pines in California) many thousands of years old has been used to calibrate radiocarbon dates much more accurately (Fig.17.40). Now, the accuracy of dating is about ±200 years in the range 600 to 10 000 years. More recently (2001) an Anglo-American team studied – of all things – a 50 cm long stalagmite that grew in a Bahaman cave during the last major ice age about 20 000 years ago. It has been preserved by being under water deep inside the cave system. Their investigations showed that the levels of carbon-14 fluctuated wildly during the time the stalagmite was growing. It suggests that we should add perhaps 8000 years to current accepted values for artefacts and fossils that are about 30 000 years old.

Carbon dating is the best-known dating technique. It has revolutionised the work of archaeologists, geologists and palaeontologists. At the same time, they are also using longer-lived radioactive nuclides to date materials over far greater time spans. For more, see Chapter 26.

SUMMARY

This chapter has dealt with radioactivity and the nature and basic structure of the atomic nucleus. Having studied it you should:

- Know the properties of the ionising radiation emitted by radioactive sources, including range, ionising ability and shielding.
- Know how the radiations are detected and monitored (Geiger counter, solid state detector, etc.).
- Know the sources of radiation (including background radiation) and understand the concepts of activity and decay.
- Know that activity decreases exponentially, giving rise to a half-life for the decay of a particular active nuclide.
- Know how to estimate a half-life from a graph of activity.
- Know that the decay is random, based upon a probability of a decay occurring.
- Be able to use the mathematics of decay and the decay constant.
- Know how the atomic nucleus was discovered and some details of the Geiger–Marsden experiment.
- Know that the nucleus consists of two kinds of nucleon – protons (positive charge) and neutrons (uncharged).
- Know that the number of protons in the nucleus decides its atomic number (proton number) Z and that the mass number (nucleon number) A is the sum of the numbers of protons and neutrons.
- Know that nuclei of the same element have the same number of protons but may have different numbers of neutrons (isotopes).
- Know that nucleons are held together in a nucleus by the strong nuclear force, whilst protons repel each other due to their electric charge.

- Know how the masses of nuclei may be measured.
- Know how a mass spectrograph works and that it provides the evidence for mass differences between nuclei.
- Know how the size of a nucleus is related to its nucleon number, and that all nuclei have much the same (very high) density.
- Know what happens in the nucleus when decay occurs and understand the concept of a radioactive decay series.
- Know that for a nucleus to be stable there must be a balance between the numbers of protons and neutrons.
- Understand that forces in the nucleus give rise to a negative potential energy (binding energy) which is observed as a loss in mass (mass defect).
- Understand the significance of the plot of binding energy per nucleon (BEPN) against nucleon number A, and use it to explain how nuclear fusion or fission may produce energy.
- Be able to describe some theories about the cause of radioactive decay, for the alpha, beta minus and beta plus, and gamma processes, and the discovery of the neutrino.
- Be able to explain nuclear fission, chain reaction and nuclear waste, and the simple workings of a nuclear reactor.
- Know the advantages and disadvantages of nuclear power.
- Know the uses and dangers of radioactive sources and their emissions.

 Practice questions for this chapter are available at www.collinseducation.co.uk/CAS

18

Imaging

18 IMAGING

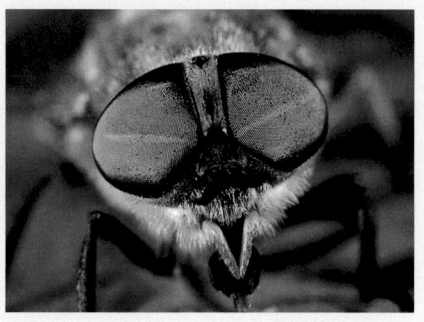

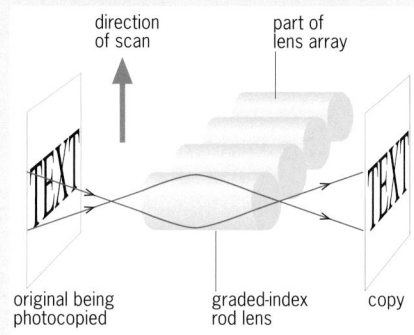

direction
of scan

part of
lens array

original being
photocopied

graded-index
rod lens

copy

An insect's eye and a photocopier both use an array of rod-shaped lenses to produce an image. Each rod provides part of the image, and all the parts contribute to a complete picture

Tailored eyes

Optical lenses, such as the lenses in a camera viewfinder, a telescope or a microscope, allow us to see the images of a wide range of objects. In these instruments, a lens (or several lenses) takes the image to the eye, which itself has a lens, too. But an image can be formed by many lenses packed side by side in a layer. The eyes of insects have this arrangement, with hundreds of small rod-shaped lenses, each directing part of the image to the creature's brain.

A photocopier has a similar imaging system. Up to several million cylindrical 'microlenses', each only a few micrometres across, form a flat array, which scans the item being copied a line at a time. The light from particular points on the copied item passes through the microlenses, and on to the detector, to build up a complete image. The refractive index of the microlenses is graded, which means the microlenses don't have to be 'lens-shaped'.

Microlenses are also used in producing the image on the liquid crystal display (LCD) screen of a portable laptop computer. The brightness and clarity of the image are steadily being improved and, at the same time, the energy required to power the equipment is being reduced.

The ideas in this chapter

In today's world, images have become as important as writing – or even speech – as a means of communicating ideas. Images are rich in information: we say that 'a picture says more than a thousand words'. Fig 18.1 shows some symbols that clearly convey ideas more rapidly and simply than words.

Every day we experience the communicating power of images, particularly through television and advertising. Also, current physics and technology convert complex data into images – from particle tracks in accelerator detectors (see Fig 24.31(c), page 496) to ozone concentrations measured by satellites. In this chapter, we will be looking at the basic science and the techniques used to produce images.

First, the chapter deals with the working of a simple thin lens, and how lenses work in imaging devices such as the human eye, cameras, telescopes and microscopes. Images are also produced by mirrors, both flat and curved. The chapter goes on to show how images are displayed and recorded. (The way images are transmitted is left till Chapter 21, Communications.) Finally, we look briefly at some modern methods of imaging which rely on advances in physics and involve complex technology.

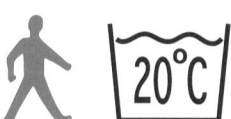
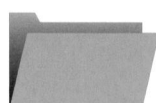

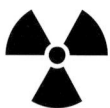

Fig 18.1 Symbols we see regularly and which instantly convey information more rapidly than words

1 HOW A CONVERGING LENS FORMS AN IMAGE

We are familiar with convex glass lenses. They have equal surfaces that we can think of as parts of a sphere, and are called **spherical** (or simple) **lenses**. Figs 18.2 and 18.3 show what happens to the wavefronts of light waves when they pass through a simple glass lens. A lens like this, which alters a plane wavefront to make the light waves pass through a point, or **focus**, is called a **converging** or **positive** lens.

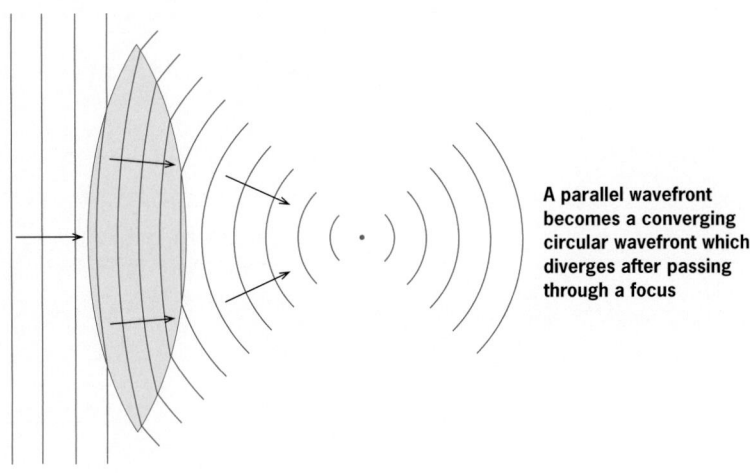

A parallel wavefront becomes a converging circular wavefront which diverges after passing through a focus

Fig 18.2(a) Plane light waves passing through a simple lens

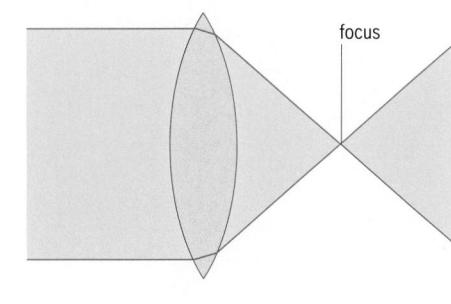

focus

Fig 18.2(b) Beam diagram

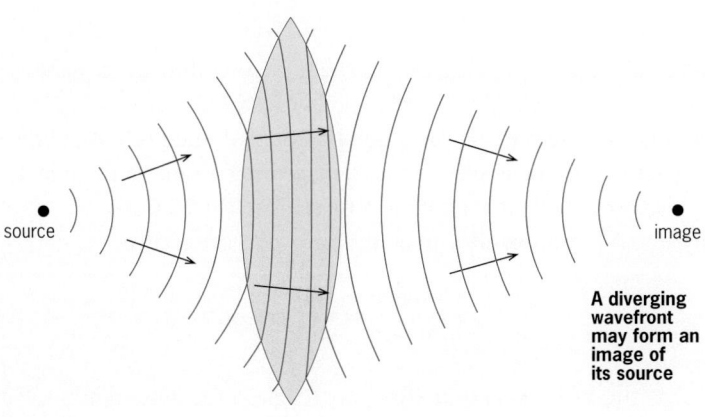

source

image

A diverging wavefront may form an image of its source

Fig 18.3(a) Diverging light waves passing through a simple lens

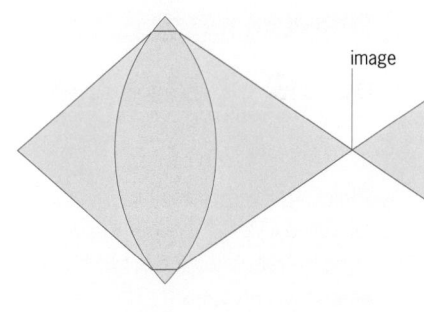

image

Fig 18.3(b) Beam diagram

In Figs 18.2 and 18.3 you can see that the wavelengths of the light are shorter after they pass across the air–glass boundary. This is because the speed of the waves is less in glass than in air, and the waves don't go as far in each period of the wave motion. This drop in speed causes **refraction**, meaning that the light changes direction wherever the wavefront is not parallel to the boundary. (See Chapter 15, pages 290–292, for more about refraction.)

Wave diagrams like Figs 18.2(a) and 18.3(a) are hard to draw, and they also hide some of the features of the light paths. Here, it makes sense to revert to an old but very useful model of light which assumes that light travels in straight lines. Figs 18.4 and 18.5 show **ray diagrams**. Where this ray model breaks down (as it will), we shall use the more advanced wave model.

Figs 18.4 and 18.5 show just some of the light rays we could draw. The rays show the *direction* of the waves, which means that the rays are at right angles to the wavefront. When a ray hits the glass surface, it is refracted as shown. Notice in Fig 18.5 that the light ray hitting the centre of the lens does so at 90° and that light rays increasingly far from the centre of the lens hit the surface at smaller and smaller angles. We will return to this soon.

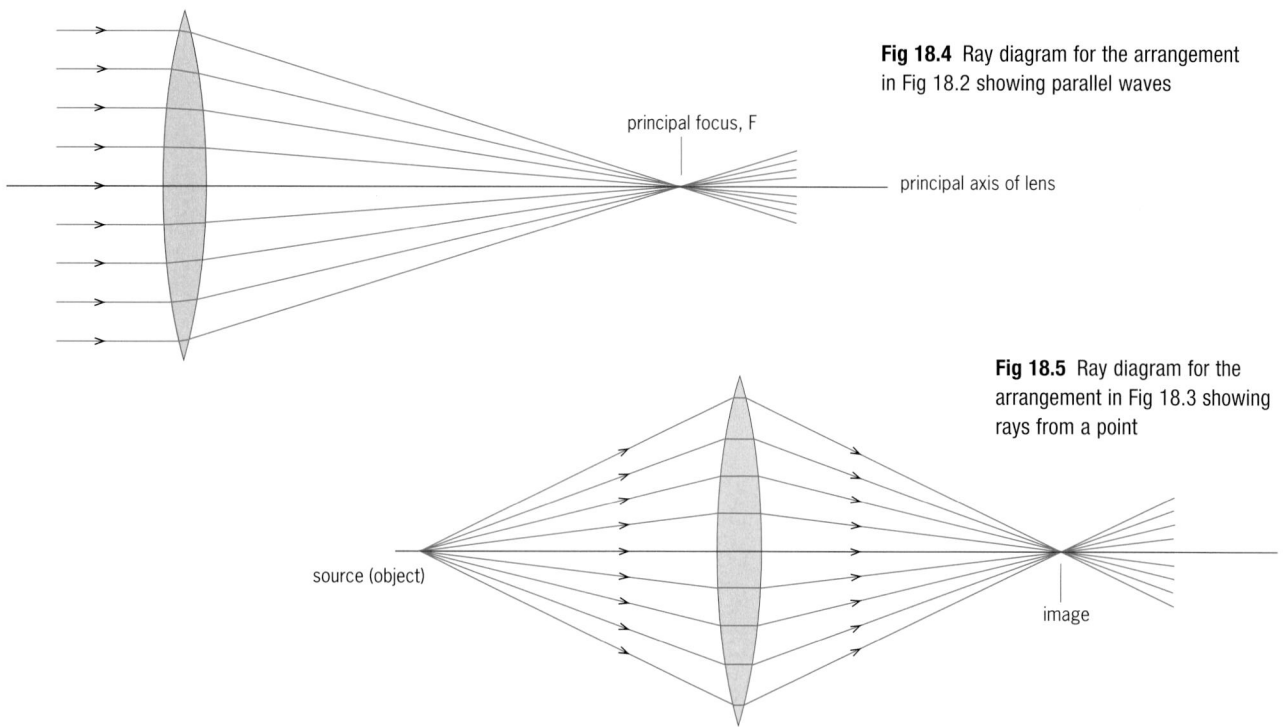

Fig 18.4 Ray diagram for the arrangement in Fig 18.2 showing parallel waves

Fig 18.5 Ray diagram for the arrangement in Fig 18.3 showing rays from a point

? **QUESTIONS 1–2**

1 Draw an accurate diagram showing the path of a ray of light going from air into water. The ray reaches the water surface at an angle of 45°. The refractive index of water is 1.33.

2 Light of frequency 5.0×10^{14} Hz enters some glass.
a) Light travels at 3.0×10^8 m s^{-1} in air. What is the wavelength of the light in air? (Remember the wave equation $v = f\lambda$.)
b) The frequency of the light stays the same in the glass, but the light slows down to a speed of 2.0×10^8 m s^{-1}. **i)** What is its wavelength in the glass? **ii)** What is the refractive index of the glass?

Let's now look at Fig 18.6(a), which shows light passing through a plane surface, such as the surface of a glass block. The line at right angles to the boundary is the **normal**, and we can see that the angle i made with the normal by the incident ray is greater than the angle r of the refracted ray. At the same time, as i increases, so r increases, while remaining less than i; see Fig 18.6(b).

The light rays are obeying **Snell's law**, the **law of refraction**:

$$\frac{\text{sine of angle of incidence}}{\text{sine of angle of refraction}} = \frac{\sin i}{\sin r} = \text{constant, } n$$

The constant n is the **refractive index** (air to glass for glass lenses).

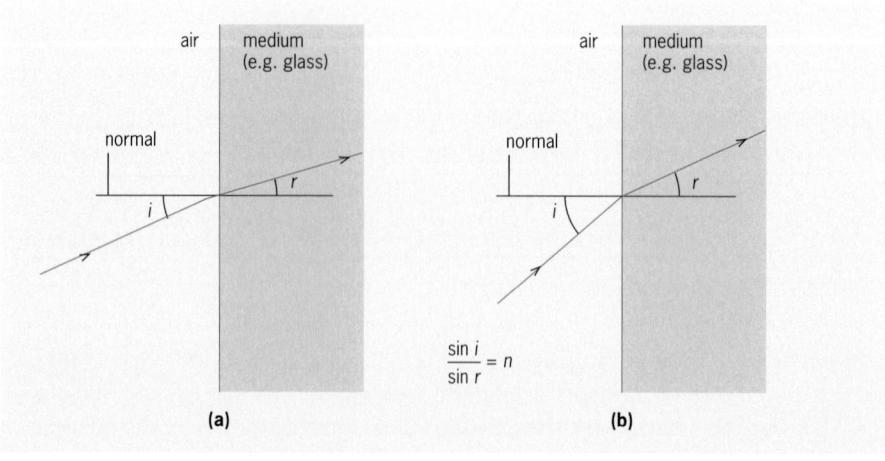

Fig 18.6 The angles which define the law of refraction. The angle of incidence is larger in **(b)** than in **(a)**

We can now look at Fig 18.7, which is part of Fig 18.5 in close-up, and shows rays from a point source passing through a lens. The radius lines of the curved surface are shown extended beyond the surface as normal lines. We can see again that the law of refraction applies to the rays as they cross the air–glass boundary.

The spherical geometry of the simple lens makes the rays converge (but not accurately) to one point or **focus**. For parallel rays (that form a plane wavefront), this point is called the **principal focus**, as in Fig 18.4. The distance of this point from the centre of the lens is called the **focal length** of the lens (CF in Fig 18.8 below). A lens has *two* principal focuses (or foci), one on each side of the lens, at equal distances from it (F and F′ in Fig 18.8).

In practice, the focus for simple spherical lenses is only at a point if the diameter of the lens is very small compared with the radius of curvature of its surfaces. Otherwise, the lens forms a partly blurred image. A lens defect like this, caused either by the shape or the material of the lens, is called an **aberration**. For a lens with spherical geometry, it is called **spherical aberration**. Removing aberrations is technically difficult, which explains why good optical instruments, such as camera lenses, are expensive.

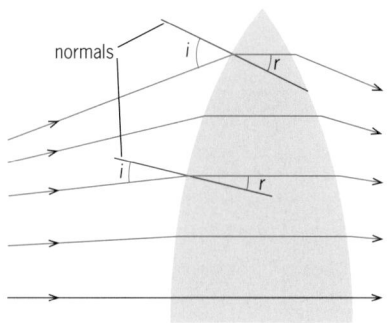

Fig 18.7 Refraction of light by a simple lens

PREDICTING THE IMAGE

Fig 18.8 shows how a simple lens forms an image of an object. We can *predict* the position and size of an image either by drawing or by using formulae.

Drawing to find the image

We can draw any number of rays to help us find the position and size of an image, but the three rays that are most helpful to draw are shown in Fig 18.8, with the usual labels we use when drawing ray diagrams.

Fig 18.8 shows an upright object OX close to a lens. The object could be anything, but by convention it is drawn simply as an arrow. As Fig 18.4 showed, any ray that is parallel to the **principal axis** of the lens is refracted to pass through the principal focus, F. In this way, we can predict the direction of the ray labelled 1 in Fig 18.8. Note that in ray diagrams such as this, the rays are assumed to change direction at a line that represents a plane in the centre of the lens.

We use the same idea for ray 2. Going through F′, it emerges from the lens parallel to the principal axis.

Fig 18.8 The image made by a converging lens, showing the main symbols and terms used, and the rays drawn in constructing a ray diagram. In conventional **ray diagrams** the rays are drawn as if everything happens in the middle of the lens or mirror at the axis perpendicular to the principal axis. This means that we can exaggerate the vertical scale for clarity and still get accurate results. The insert shows the **optical path** (what really happens)

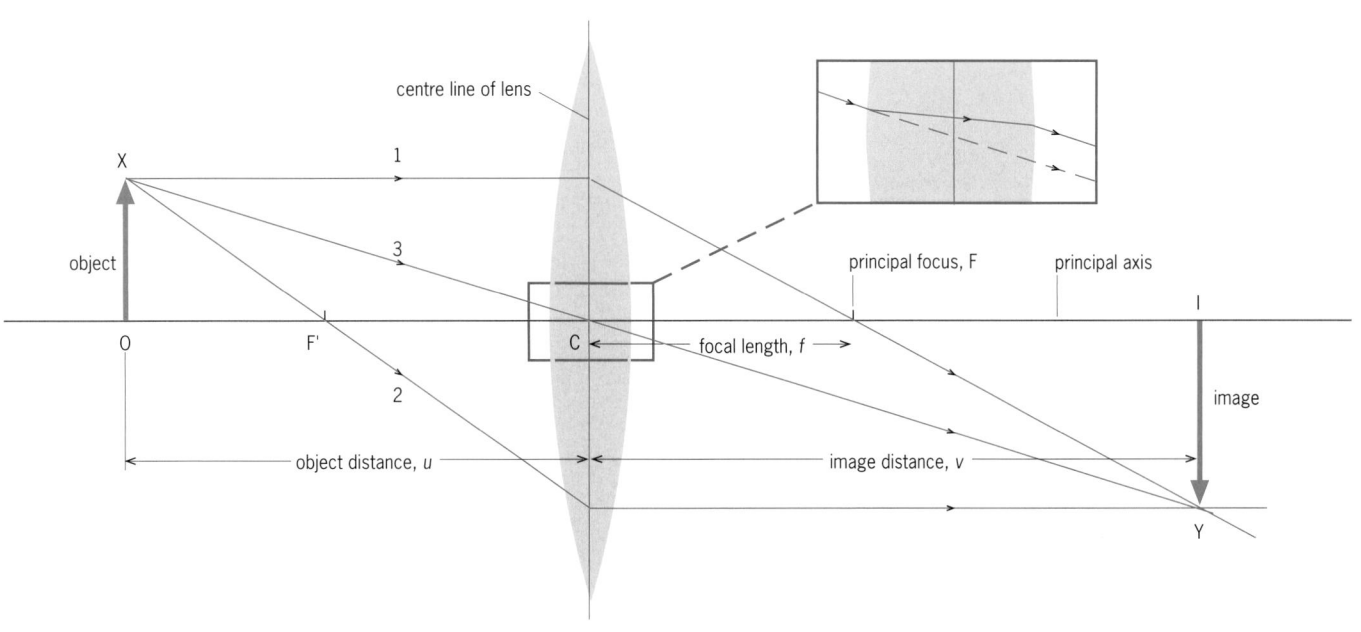

3 Check that you have understood
Fig 18.8 and followed the
description for constructing a ray
diagram. Show that an object, 5 cm
tall, placed 10 cm from a lens, of
focal length 6 cm, produces an
inverted image 15 cm from the lens.
The image should be 7.5 cm high.
By drawing on A4 graph paper, you
can use a scale of 1:1 for both
vertical and horizontal distances.

4 Use the lens formula to check the
results for image distance and size
that are given in question 3.

The third useful line, for ray 3, goes straight through the centre of the lens – it does not deviate. (But see the close-up drawing. At the centre of the lens, the two faces are parallel to each other. If the lens is thin compared with the distances of object and image, which we assume, the slight sideways displacement of the ray is not significant.)

All three rays pass through the same point, Y. They all started at X, and it is clear that a screen placed at Y would catch them all together again: Y is a *focused image* of X. Similarly, any point on OX would give a focused image of itself somewhere between I and Y. IY is a **real image**. A real image is one that can be caught on a screen: surprisingly some images can't and are called **virtual** images (see below).

These construction rays can be drawn to scale to find the position and relative size of the image of any object placed in front of the lens. Objects viewed through a lens, and their images, are usually much smaller than the distances they are from the lens. In such cases, it is best to make the vertical scale larger than the horizontal one.

Finding the image by formula

It is usually quicker and more accurate to find the position and size of an image by using the **lens formula**:

$$\frac{1}{u} + \frac{1}{v} = \frac{1}{f}$$

where u is the distance of the object from the lens centre, the *object distance*, v is the distance of the image from the lens centre, the *image distance*, and f is the *focal length* of the lens. To find the size of the image we can use the equation

Image size = object size × V/U.

You can now find the position and size of any image simply by inserting the other given values in the formula.

2 THE IMAGE IN A DIVERGING LENS

Fig 18.9 shows a lens with *concave* spherical surfaces and what happens to parallel light rays (that is, a plane wavefront coming from a distant object) when they pass through it. The rays are refracted so that they seem to diverge from a single point, F. This point is the principal focus of a diverging lens. As light doesn't actually come from the point, or pass through it, it is a virtual focus. (See the description of the plane mirror on page 361 for more about the word 'virtual'.)

Fig 18.10 shows how a diverging lens forms an image of an object. As for a converging lens, you would see the image by looking at the object through

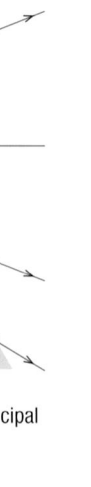

Fig 18.9 A diverging lens has a virtual principal focus and a negative focal length

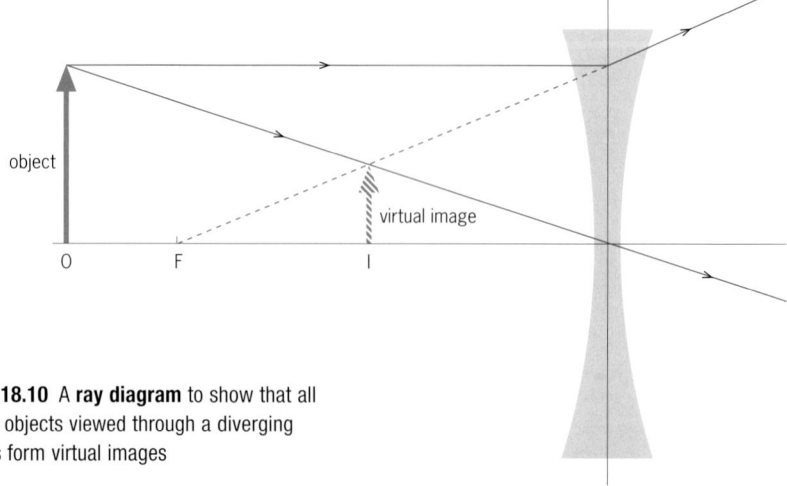

Fig 18.10 A **ray diagram** to show that all real objects viewed through a diverging lens form virtual images

the lens. But light doesn't actually pass back through the diverging lens to the image, so you cannot catch the image on a screen. It is therefore a virtual image.

The sign convention

The lens formula works for all simple optical devices (even mirrors, as explained on page 363). But we have to know whether the images, principal focuses – and even objects – are real or virtual. Where they are virtual, the convention is to give *negative* values to distances measured from them to the lens or mirror. For example, the principal focus of a diverging lens is virtual, so its focal length is given a negative sign.

Suppose we place a real object 20 cm from the diverging lens as shown in Fig 18.10. The principal focus of the lens is 10 cm from the lens, so its focal length is –10 cm. The lens formula gives:

$$\frac{1}{20} + \frac{1}{v} = -\frac{1}{10}$$

$$\text{So:} \quad \frac{1}{v} = -\frac{1}{10} - \frac{1}{20} = -\frac{3}{20}$$

$$\text{and:} \quad v = -\frac{20}{3} = -6.7 \text{ (cm)}$$

So the distance of the image from the lens centre is 6.7 cm, and the negative sign tells us that the image is also virtual.

> ✔ **REMEMBER THIS**
> Converging lenses have positive focal lengths and are often called *positive* lenses. By contrast, diverging lenses are called *negative* lenses.

3 THE POWER OF A LENS AND ITS IMAGE QUALITY

In optics, lenses are usually described in terms of their **power**. The more powerful the lens, the closer to the lens is the image that the lens forms of a distant object. The power of a lens is defined as the reciprocal of its focal length f measured in metres:

$$\textbf{power} = \frac{1}{f}$$

The unit of power is called the **dioptre**, symbol D, and so a lens of focal length +10 cm (0.1 m) has a power of +10 D. A diverging lens of focal length –5 cm (–0.05 m) has a power of –20 D. This way of describing lenses lets us work out what happens when two lenses are used together. The combined power of the lenses is simply the sum of the powers of each lens, bearing in mind their signs, as shown in Fig 18.11.

> **? QUESTION 5**
>
> 5   A camera lens is made of two components, a diverging (negative) lens of focal length 69 mm, and a converging (positive) lens of focal length 29 mm. What are:
> **a)** the powers of each component,
> **b)** the power of the combination,
> **c)** the focal length of the combination?

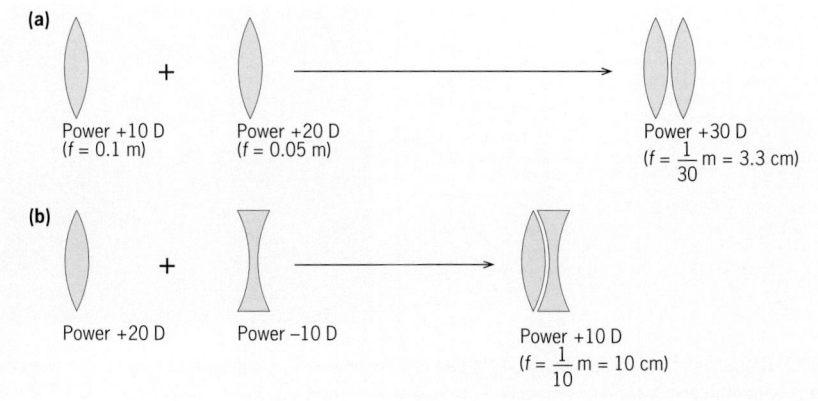

(a)
Power +10 D
(f = 0.1 m)   +   Power +20 D
(f = 0.05 m)   →   Power +30 D
(f = $\frac{1}{30}$ m = 3.3 cm)

(b)
Power +20 D   +   Power –10 D   →   Power +10 D
(f = $\frac{1}{10}$ m = 10 cm)

Fig 18.11 Lens combinations: **(a)** two positive, **(b)** positive plus negative. In combination, the powers of lenses are added

THE CAMERA LENS AS AN EXPENSIVE HOLE

We have seen that the quality of the image made by a lens depends on its shape (see spherical aberration, page 357). Image quality also depends on the aperture of the lens, that is, the part of the lens through which light is allowed to pass. (Though the lens diameter is fixed, the aperture can be varied.)

A lens of large diameter captures more light and produces a brighter image than a smaller diameter lens. However, it is difficult and expensive to correct for aberrations in large aperture lenses. So, for example, in ordinary cameras with a single lens, the lens is usually 'stopped down' to make the picture sharper. The light used to form the image passes through the central region only of the lens (see Fig 18.12), and this reduces spherical aberration.

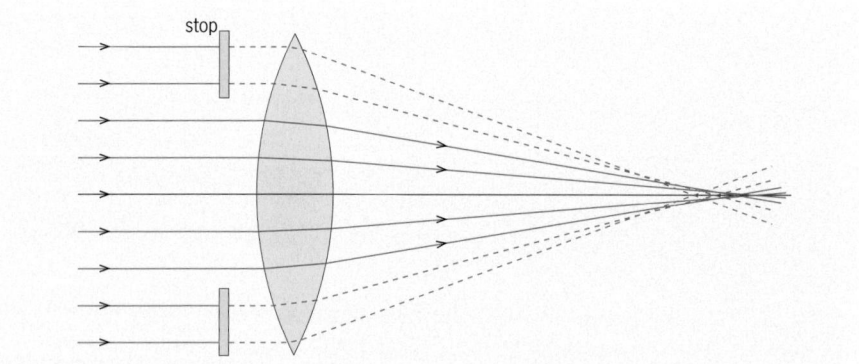

Fig 18.12 'Stopping down' to reduce lens aperture and so correct spherical aberration. A 'stop' excludes the outer rays which would have been brought to a focus closer to the lens than the inner rays

The quality of the image is also affected by **diffraction** (see Chapter 15, pages 298–299). The image is blurred as points on the object become circular diffraction patterns. Points on the image subtending an angle smaller than a certain value of θ (see Fig 18.13) are not seen as separate; their **resolution** is not possible. θ is determined by wavelength λ and aperture d in the **Rayleigh criterion**:

$$\theta \approx \frac{\lambda}{d}$$

Diffraction effects are reduced when the aperture is large, so accurate optical instruments have a design conflict. Large aperture means better resolution, as the Rayleigh criterion tells us, but more spherical aberration. Small aperture reduces aberration but worsens resolution.

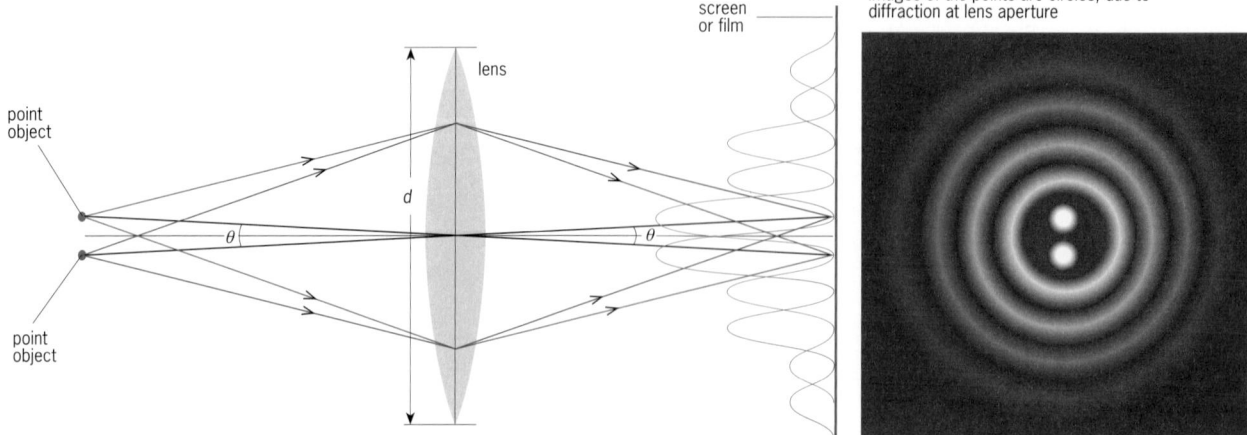

Fig 18.13 Diffraction: the images of two points can just be 'resolved', meaning that they can be seen as separate, when the points subtend an angle θ at the lens such that $\sin \theta \approx \theta > \lambda/d$

4 MIRRORS

Plane mirrors are the most common optical devices we come across. The ordinary household mirror is a sheet of flat glass, 'silvered' on the back with a layer of metal paint (the metal is usually aluminium), which is then protected by a coat of ordinary paint.

Light passes through the glass and is reflected by the silvering. A plane wavefront is reflected as a plane by a flat mirror, and the geometry results in the well-known rule:

the angle of incidence equals the angle of reflection.

The angles are shown in Fig 18.14, and are measured from the **normal** line drawn at right angles to the surface.

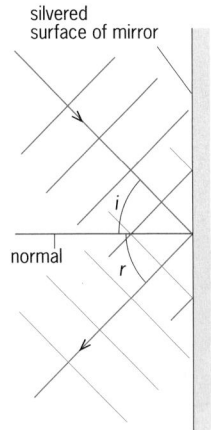

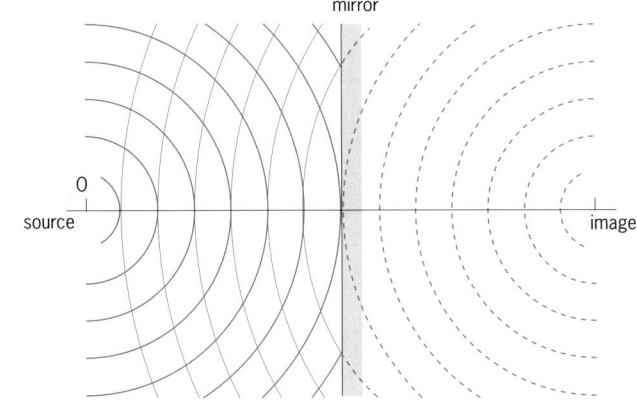

Fig 18.14 Plane waves reflected in a plane mirror. The angle of incidence *i* equals the angle of reflection *r*

Fig 18.15 Waves from a point source O reflected in a plane mirror. Circular waves are reflected so that they appear to come from the image, which is as far behind the mirror as O is in front

As shown in Fig 18.15, the image of an object reflected in a plane mirror is behind the mirror and as far from the mirror as the object is. Notice that light does not pass through the mirror, and the image is really an optical illusion. It isn't really 'there' – you couldn't, for example, catch it on a photographic film placed at the image position. The image is therefore a **virtual** image. Compare this image with the one produced by the lens in Fig 18.5 which is formed from rays of light and can be caught on a photographic film. Our brain perceives ('sees') virtual images by making them into 'real' ones using another optical device – our eyes.

An ordinary glass mirror produces a blurred image because of multiple reflections – see Fig 18.16. Such a mirror is not suitable for optical instruments which need to give sharp images. There are two main solutions to this problem.

Front-silvered mirrors

These have the metallic layer on the front surface. Very fine metal particles are deposited on glass either from solution or from metal vapour in a vacuum. The large mirrors used in reflecting telescopes (see page 368) are made in this way. The metal surface is easily damaged, by touching or corrosion, and has to be treated with care.

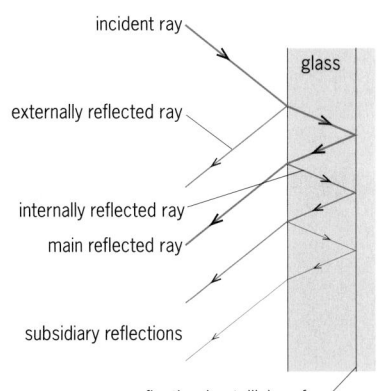

Fig 18.16 Ordinary 'silver'-backed mirrors produce blurred images because multiple reflection occurs

REMEMBER THIS

Total internal reflection occurs at angles of (internal) incidence greater than c, the critical angle. By Snell's law (page 356):

$$\frac{\sin 90°}{\sin c} = n \quad \text{or} \quad n = \frac{1}{\sin c}$$

See Fig 18.17.

REFLECTING PRISMS AND SNELL'S LAW

A glass (or clear plastic) **reflecting prism** provides a much cheaper and more practical plane mirror by using the effect of **total internal reflection**.

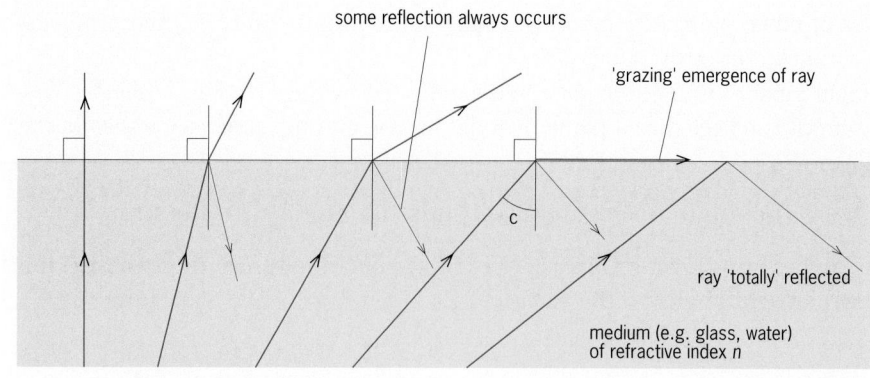

Fig 18.17 How total internal reflection occurs

For an explanation of how optical fibres use total internal reflection to carry information please see the How Science Works assignment for this chapter at www.collinseducation.co.uk/CAS

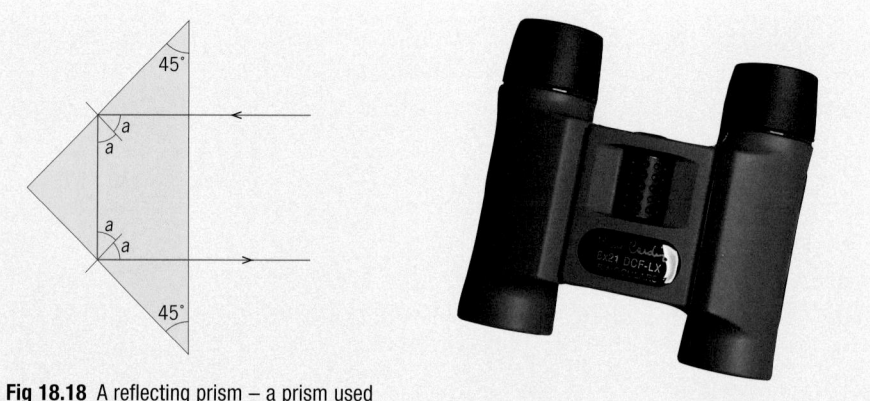

Fig 18.18 A reflecting prism – a prism used as a mirror. Angle a must be greater than the critical angle c for the material used

Fig 18.19 The use of prisms allows binoculars to be compact

Fig 18.16 showed light rays which were partly internally reflected. Fig 18.17 shows how total internal reflection occurs when the angle of incidence of a ray exceeds the **critical angle** c for the medium. When a ray reaches the inside of a plane boundary (say, between air and glass) at an angle of incidence greater than the critical angle, it cannot pass through the surface.

The relationship, given by **Snell's law**, between the refractive index of a medium and its critical angle, is $n = 1/\sin c$.

The action of a prismatic mirror is shown in Fig 18.18. Such mirrors are used in some cameras and binoculars, Fig 18.19.

5 OPTICAL INSTRUMENTS: SINGLE-COMPONENT DEVICES

THE MAGNIFYING GLASS

A single converging lens can be used as a magnifying glass – sometimes called a simple microscope. The object is placed closer to the lens than the principal focus. As shown in Fig 18.20, the lens produces a magnified virtual image which is upright. The eyepiece lens of a (compound) microscope or telescope may act as a magnifying glass in this way.

? QUESTION 6

6 An object is placed 4 cm from a converging (positive) lens of focal length 6 cm. Show (by calculation or by drawing) that the image produced is virtual, 12 cm from the lens and 3 times as large as the object.

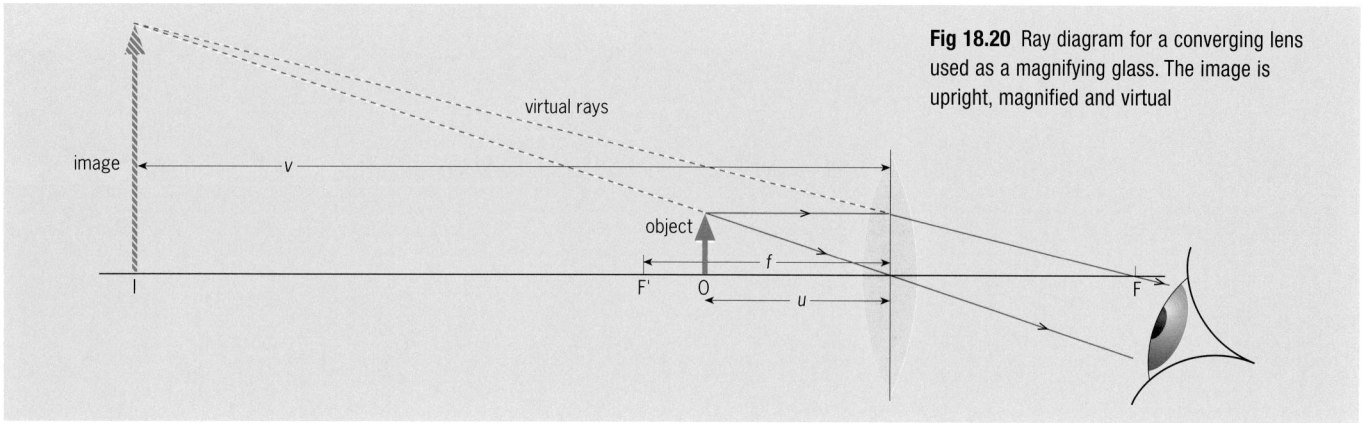

Fig 18.20 Ray diagram for a converging lens used as a magnifying glass. The image is upright, magnified and virtual

SPHERICAL MIRRORS

The concave mirror

A spherical mirror has much the same image-forming properties as a glass lens. As shown in Fig 18.21, the concave mirror focuses parallel rays to a point – its principal focus, F. To find the image of an object placed in front of a mirror, we can use the same kind of ray-drawing technique as for a lens (see Fig 18.22).

Similarly, we can use the same formula relating object distance, image distance and focal length as we use for the lens, namely: $1/u + 1/v = 1/f$.

A concave mirror can be compared with a positive (converging) lens, and can produce both real and virtual images. Concave mirrors are used as shaving and make-up mirrors in their virtual, magnifying mode. As with a lens used as a magnifying glass (see above), the object has to be nearer the mirror than the principal focus. Concave mirrors are also used as the *objectives* in large astronomical telescopes (see the description of the Newtonian telescope on pages 367–368).

The simple geometry of the circle in Fig 18.21 shows that the focal length f of the mirror is half the radius of curvature of the sphere of which the mirror is a section, so that PC = $2f$. This focal length applies only if the angle made between the edges of the mirror and its sphere's centre is very small, in other words, that the aperture of the mirror is small compared to its radius. Otherwise, we find that the image is blurred, a form of spherical aberration like that shown in Fig 18.12. Spherical aberration may be avoided for large mirrors by making the shape parabolic.

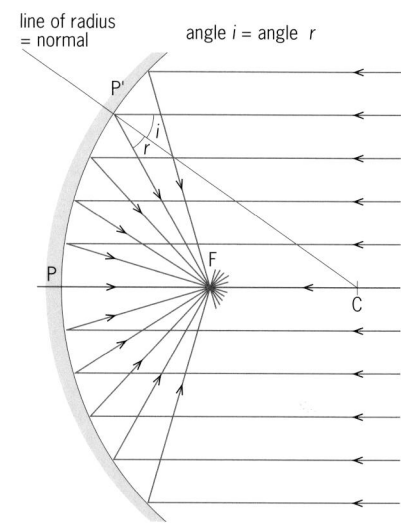

Fig 18.21 A concave spherical mirror. Parallel rays are focused at F. Distance PF = f, radius PC = $2f$ (spherical aberration not shown)

Fig 18.22 Finding an image for a concave mirror by a **ray diagram**. A line perpendicular to the principal axis defines the position of the reflecting surface

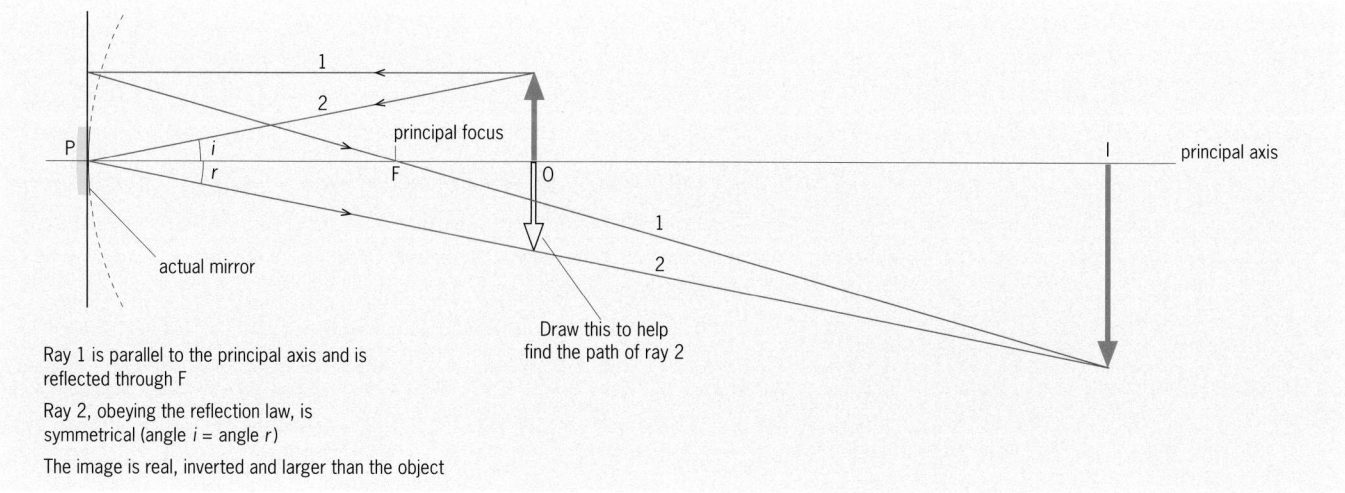

Ray 1 is parallel to the principal axis and is reflected through F

Ray 2, obeying the reflection law, is symmetrical (angle i = angle r)

The image is real, inverted and larger than the object

The convex mirror

Convex mirrors act like concave (diverging) lenses. Their focal lengths are negative and they form virtual images of real objects (Fig 18.23). They are used to give a wide field of view in car rear-view mirrors, in blind exits or entrances and as security mirrors in shops (Figs 18.24 and 18.25).

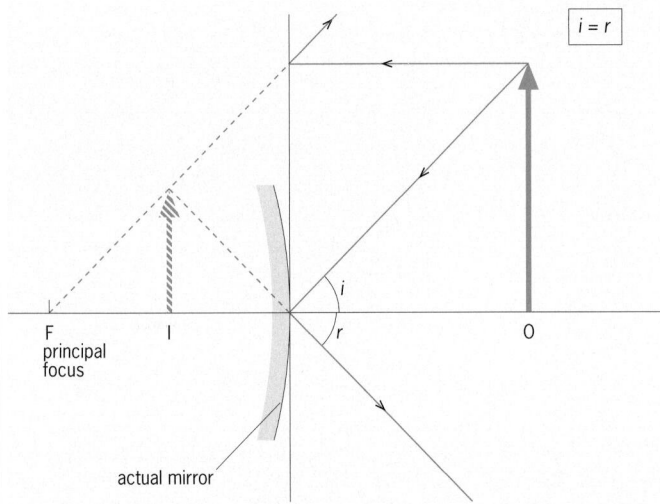

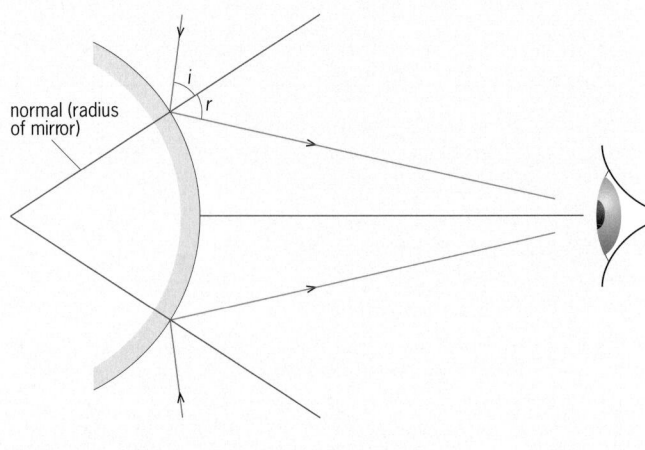

Fig 18.23 Ray diagram for the image formed by a convex mirror. The image is upright, virtual and smaller than the object

Fig 18.24 A convex mirror gives a wide field of view. It produces a diminished picture of a large area

? QUESTIONS 7–9

7 Find, by drawing or calculation, the position and size of the image of a child 1.4 m tall who stands 2 m from a convex (diverging) mirror of focal length 4 m. Where would such a mirror be useful?

8 **a)** Draw a scale diagram (use graph paper) to find the position and size of an image made in a concave mirror. Data: radius of curvature of mirror 80 cm; distance of object from mirror 20 cm; height of object 4 cm.
b) Check the results obtained in **a)** by calculation using the formula $1/u + 1/v = 1/f$.

9 Find, by drawing or by calculation, the position and size of the image produced when a slide 24 mm by 32 mm is placed 40 mm from a concave mirror of focal length 36 mm. Is the image real or virtual?

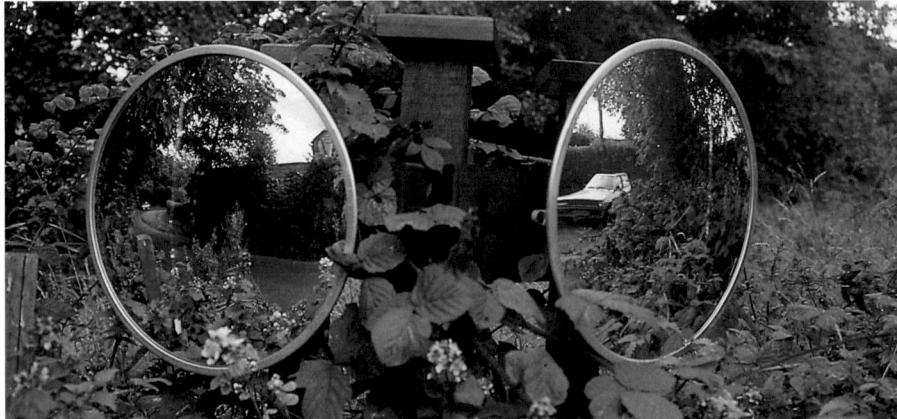

Fig 18.25 Convex mirrors are used as security mirrors in shops and on roads at sharp bends and concealed entrances

6 OPTICAL INSTRUMENTS WITH TWO COMPONENTS

THE ASTRONOMICAL REFRACTING TELESCOPE

An astronomical telescope is designed not only to *magnify* the apparent size of distant objects but also to *gather as much light* as possible. In the traditional **refracting telescope** which uses glass lenses, the light gathering task is done by a large-aperture lens at the front of the instrument called the **objective** lens. The objective and eyepiece lenses work together to produce the magnified image.

Fig 18.26(a) shows the light rays from distant objects forming a 'pencil' of light that passes through the telescope. In optics, a distant object producing almost perfectly parallel rays (a plane wavefront) is said to be at **infinity**.

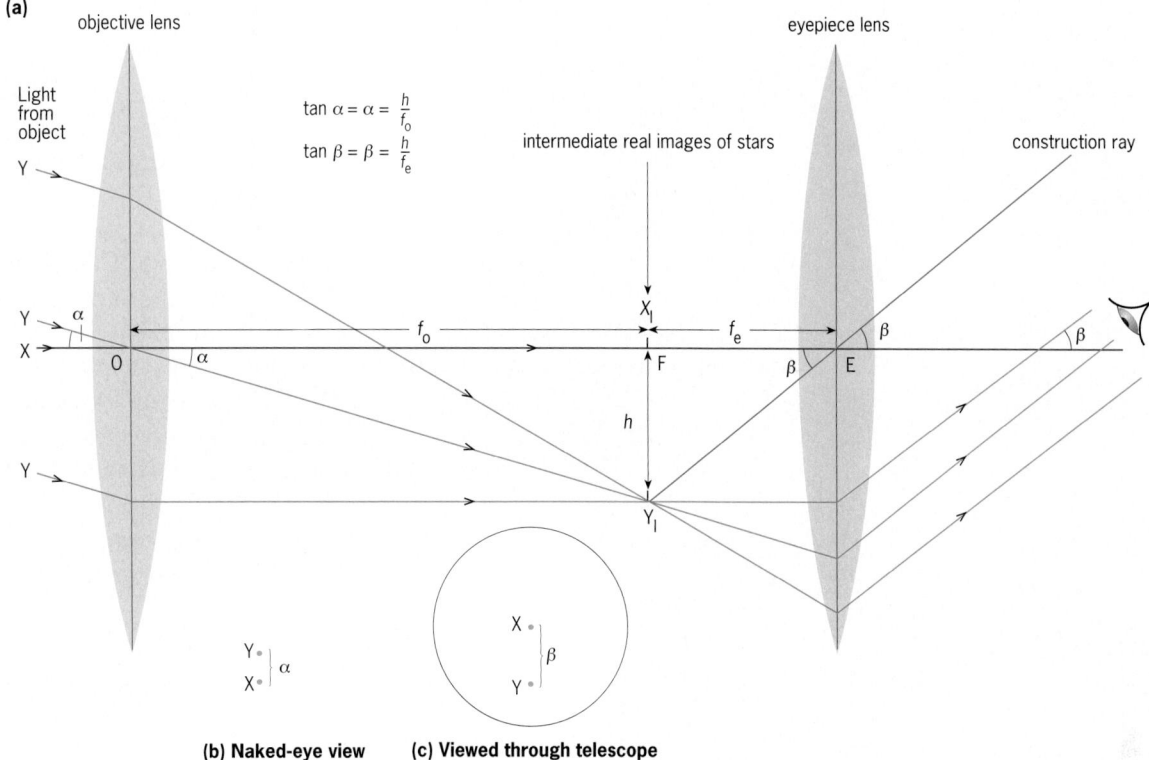

(b) Naked-eye view   (c) Viewed through telescope

In the diagram:

$$\tan \alpha = \alpha = \frac{h}{f_o}$$

$$\tan \beta = \beta = \frac{h}{f_e}$$

Follow the rays Y in Fig 18.26(a) from left to right. The objective lens forms a real image of the object in the plane of its principal focus, F. The eyepiece is placed so that F is also at the position of the plane of *its* principal focus. Accordingly, the final pencil of light leaving the eyepiece and entering the eye is composed of parallel rays. The image is virtual, upside down (inverted) and also at infinity. The telescope set up like this is in normal adjustment, the usual arrangement for viewing distant objects. The position of the eyepiece can be altered to produce a real image, on a photographic plate, for example.

Fig 18.26 A ray diagram showing how a telescope concentrates light so that images look brighter, and separates the light coming from distant objects – it magnifies. Angles α and β have been exaggerated for clarity

Magnifying power

Fig 18.26(a) shows that the emerging set of rays from the eyepiece makes a larger angle, β, with the central axis of the telescope than angle α made by the incoming rays. What this means is shown in Figs 18.26(b) and (c).

Imagine that we are studying a system of two stars, X and Y. Without the telescope, we would see the system as quite small, as in Fig 18.26(b). Suppose star X is at the centre of the picture. It sends light along the main axis of the telescope. Star Y is off-centre and sends light at angle α. When the light emerges from the telescope we see that Y appears to be further apart from X, as shown in Fig 18.26(c). In other words, the image of the system appears larger than with the naked eye. With a telescope, stars appear brighter and further apart, and we are able to see faint objects that were previously invisible.

The magnifying power of the telescope is simply the ratio of the image size seen with the telescope and the image size seen without it. The ratio is also the ratio ($\tan \beta / \tan \alpha$) which, when the telescope is in normal adjustment, is also the ratio:

$$\frac{\text{OF}}{\text{FE}} \quad \text{or} \quad \frac{f_o}{f_e}$$

where f_o is the focal length of the objective and f_e is the focal length of the eyepiece.

✔ REMEMBER THIS

For angles θ smaller than 5° or so, we have $\sin \theta = \tan \theta = \theta$ radians.

? QUESTION 10

10 An astronomical telescope has an objective lens of focal length 1.2 m. What should the focal length of the eyepiece be to produce a magnifying power of 150?

The angles α and β are usually very small, so we can write (using radians):

$$\text{magnifying power} = \frac{\beta}{\alpha}$$
$$= \frac{f_o}{f_e}$$

Where do you put your eye?

A simple telescope is designed for use with the human eye. This means that all the light gathered by the objective has, eventually, to form a beam that just fits the pupil of the eye – nominally taken to be 5 mm in diameter. Fig 18.27 shows the extent of a beam of light entering the objective that can reach the eyepiece and so be used to form the final image.

R is the position of the eye ring, the hole you look through in telescopes and binoculars. The eye is best placed at R because this is where the emerging beam is smallest, ensuring that:

● the light is most concentrated, so the image is **brightest**;
● all of the useful light entering the objective is seen, so we have **the greatest field of view**.

It can be shown that the position and size of the eye ring are the same as the *image of the objective lens made by the eyepiece*.

Fig 18.27 A **ray diagram** showing the eye ring of a telescope at position R

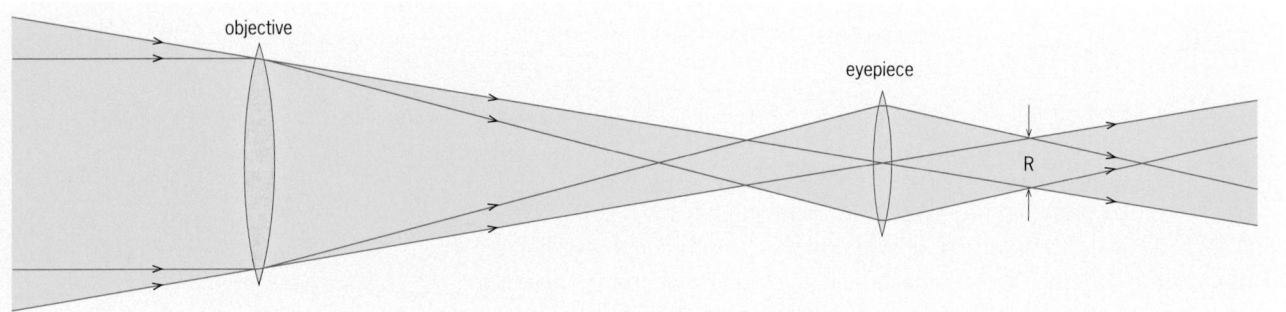

Defects of a refracting telescope

Refracting telescopes have their name because they use lenses, which refract light, to bring the light rays to a focus. It is hard to make large refracting astronomical telescopes because the large objective lens suffers from several kinds of aberrations. The most inconvenient of these is **chromatic aberration**, shown in Fig 18.28. Rays of different colours are focused at different distances from the objective. (See page 291 for more about this.) Also, as a lens has to be thick in the middle, a large aperture lens has a large mass, making it not only expensive but difficult to mount and control.

? QUESTION 11

11 A typical reflecting telescope used by amateur astronomers has a mirror of focal length 1.2 m. What is its magnifying power when used with an eyepiece of focal length 40 mm? It is possible to buy eyepieces of focal length 2.4 mm. Can you think of any disadvantages in using an eyepiece of such short focal length?

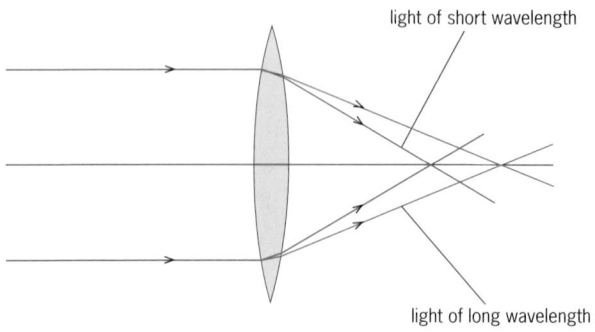

Fig 18.28 In chromatic aberration, shorter wavelengths are focused nearer to the lens than longer wavelengths

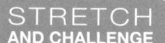

Galileo exploits the telescope's potential

At the great annual fair at Frankfurt-am-Main in Germany in 1608, a wandering trader was offering a novelty for sale – a tube with a lens at each end, one concave and the other convex. When you looked through the tube, it magnified distant objects seven times. In October, a Dutch spectacle maker applied for a licence to make and sell similar 'telescopes' (meaning 'far seers') but was refused because so many other people were already making them. By the following year, they were available for sale in London, Paris and in Italy.

Galileo Galilei was then one of the most famous 'natural philosophers' in Europe – the word 'scientist' was not yet in use. Galileo is still revered as one of the greatest physicists of all time, but unlike some physicists, he was also smart. In August 1609 he went to his employers, the Senate of Venice, and offered them a device – a telescope – which would enable their trading fleets to see enemy ships long before the enemy could see them. The grateful senators immediately doubled his salary, just a few days before the local spectacle makers learned about telescopes and started making them for sale.

This kind of commercial smartness made the senators of the great trading Republic of Venice quite proud. A professor of physics and mathematics who could outsmart *them* was worth keeping, and they gave him a contract for life.

In fact, Galileo was (as far as we know) the first person to explain how the telescope worked. His improved design is named after him (while the man at the Frankfurt Fair was never known). Fig 18.29 shows how it produces an image.

The Galilean telescope uses a negative lens for an eyepiece, which means that the telescope can be shorter than the later – and better – astronomical telescope, and it produces its image the right way up. The only place you are likely to see one is in theatres as the binoculars called 'opera glasses'.

Galileo used his telescope to look at the mountains on the Moon and the satellites of Jupiter. His observations convinced him that the old ideas of the nature of the Universe were wrong: the heavens were *not* 'perfect' – and the Sun *was* at the centre of a Copernican solar system of moving planets. It was these ideas that got him into trouble with the Catholic Church in Italy.

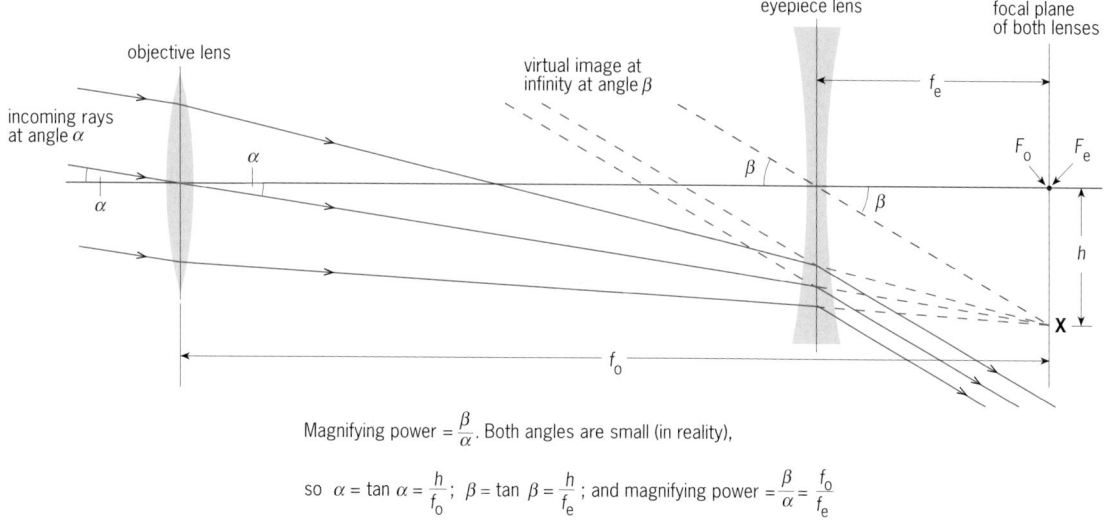

Magnifying power $= \dfrac{\beta}{\alpha}$. Both angles are small (in reality),

so $\alpha = \tan \alpha = \dfrac{h}{f_o}$; $\beta = \tan \beta = \dfrac{h}{f_e}$; and magnifying power $= \dfrac{\beta}{\alpha} = \dfrac{f_o}{f_e}$

Fig 18.29 Ray diagram: The Galilean telescope is shorter than an astronomical telescope of the same power and produces an upright image. The image would be formed at X, but the eyepiece straightens out the rays. The 'virtual object' for the eyepiece is at its principal focus, so rays are made parallel and the image is at infinity

REFLECTING TELESCOPES

Some of the defects of refracting telescopes can be avoided by using a curved mirror as the objective, as in the **Newtonian reflecting telescope**. The mirrors in such telescopes do not suffer from chromatic aberration, and spherical aberration may be removed by making the shape slightly parabolic rather than perfectly spherical. Remember that the larger the aperture, the more light can be collected and the better the resolution, as diffraction problems are reduced.

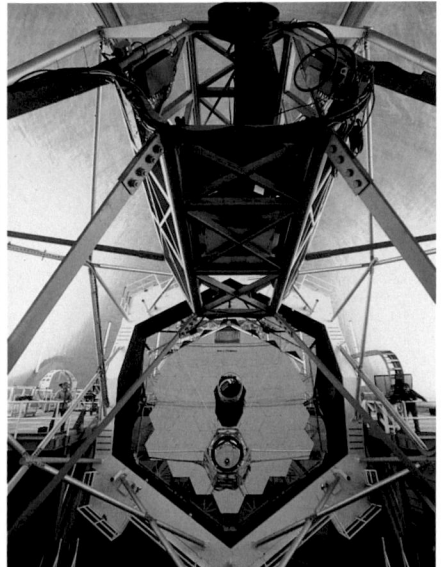

Fig 18.31 The world's largest reflecting telescope at Mauna Kea in Hawaii. Its mirror consists of 36 smaller hexagonal mirrors controlled by computer to work together in making an image

> ### ? QUESTION 12
>
> 12 Why doesn't a Newtonian telescope suffer from chromatic aberration?

The objective mirror in Fig 18.30 produces a real image of a distant object at its principal focus, F. This is usually offset by using a plane mirror so that the eyepiece can be mounted conveniently at the side, out of the way of incoming light. Apart from using a mirror as the prime focusing device, the reflecting telescope works just like a refracting type as far as size and magnification are concerned.

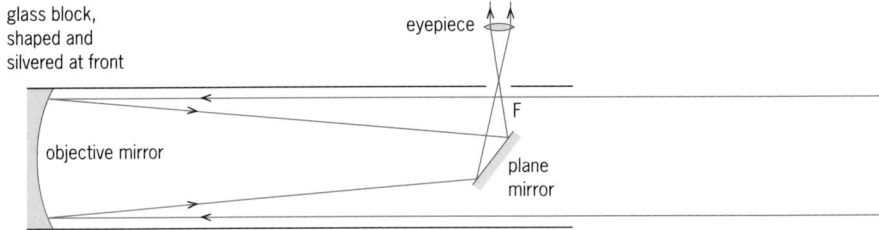

Fig 18.30 The Newtonian reflecting telescope uses a concave mirror instead of a lens as the objective, so avoids chromatic aberration

While the largest refracting telescope has an objective lens 1 m in diameter, the largest reflecting telescope, the Mauna Kea telescope in Hawaii, Fig 18.31, has an objective mirror with an aperture of 10 m diameter. It is not easy to make large mirrors, but with the aid of computers several smaller mirrors can be made to combine images so that the effective aperture is increased. (The largest single-mirror telescope, at Zelenchukskaya, Russia, is 6 m in diameter.) Even larger apertures are now obtained by using *adaptive optics* (see Chapter 25, section 5) and also by combining signals from widely spaced optical telescopes, with suitable time delays, to produce a higher-resolution signal. This technique has long been used with radio telescopes.

> STRETCH
> AND CHALLENGE
>
> # The Cassegrain telescope
>
> We have seen that large magnifications require a long focal length. This means that the tube of a Newtonian telescope is inconveniently long, especially for amateur users. A Cassegrain system reduces the length considerably, as shown in Fig 18.32. It uses a convex *secondary mirror* which extends the focal length, forming the image via a small hole in the main mirror. As it is technically much easier to make a spherical mirror than a parabolic one to the accuracy required, simple spherical mirrors are used with a glass *correction plate*. Its complex shape counteracts the defects of the mirrors.
>
>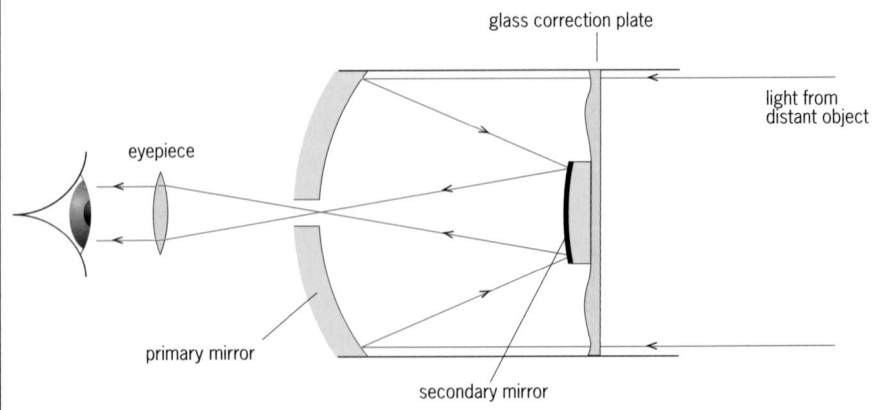
>
> **Fig 18.32** Arrangement in a Cassegrain telescope. The secondary mirror allows the tube to be short

THE COMPOUND MICROSCOPE

A compound microscope consists of two lenses, a lens combination which reduces aberration. It is designed to produce an enlarged virtual image of a small object. Light gathering is not as important as it is in a telescope, since the object can be brightly illuminated if necessary. Fig 18.33 shows how a microscope forms its image.

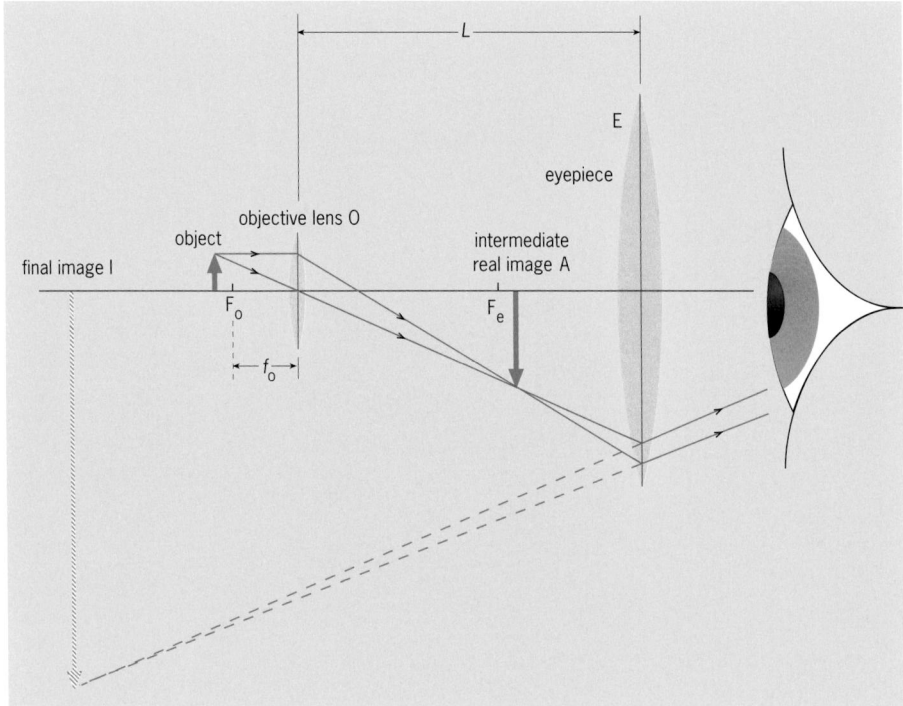

Fig 18.33 A **ray diagram** showing the formation of an image in a compound microscope. In practice, the final image is roughly 25 cm from the eye and eyepiece

The objective lens O forms a slightly magnified (intermediate) real image of the object at A. A is just inside the focal length of the eyepiece E, so that the final image I is virtual and highly magnified. It is usually arranged so that this final image is formed about 25 cm from the eye. This is the *near point* of the eye, where we normally place something that we want to see as large as possible (see below).

Magnification in a compound microscope

The magnification produced by the compound microscope depends on where the final image is actually formed. The microscope is focused by moving the object closer to or away from the objective lens, a high power lens (with a small focal length).

We can find an approximate value for its magnification, which is good enough for everyday purposes, as follows.

Assuming that the final image is 25 cm from the eyepiece, as in Fig 18.34, we can find an *approximate* value for the magnification M_e produced by this lens. We can assume that the intermediate, real image is formed close to the principal focus f_e of the eyepiece:

$$\text{magnification} = \frac{\text{image distance from eyepiece}}{\text{object distance from eyepiece}}$$

$$M_e = \frac{25}{f_e}$$

Fig 18.34 The magnifying power of a compound microscope

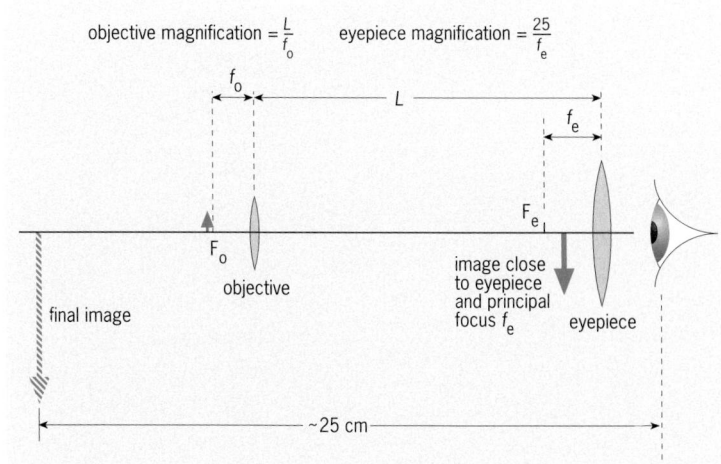

objective magnification $= \dfrac{L}{f_o}$ eyepiece magnification $= \dfrac{25}{f_e}$

? QUESTIONS 13–14

13 Telescopes are usually made so that different magnifying powers are produced by changing the eyepiece (see question 11). Microscopes are made so that it is easy to change the objective lens, for example by having three on a swivelling mount.
a) Suggest a reason for this difference between the instruments.
b) The three objective lenses of a laboratory microscope are labelled ×10, ×20, ×40. What does this tell you about the focal lengths (or powers) of the three lenses?

14 A compound microscope is often used to produce a real image on a screen. Explain how the position of the eyepiece lens has to be adjusted to do this.

The objective lens has a very small focal length. The object is placed close to the principal focus of the objective f_o and forms a real image close to the eyepiece, which also has a small focal length. So the image distance for the first image is almost the distance L between the lenses, and therefore roughly the length of the microscope tube. So, with measurements in centimetres, the magnification M_o produced by the objective is approximately:

$$M_o = \frac{L}{f_o}$$

The total magnification of the compound microscope is therefore:

$$M = M_o M_e = \frac{25L}{f_o f_e} \quad \text{(measurements in cm)}$$

BINOCULARS

Binoculars are a pair of telescopes, one for each eye. The magnifying optical principles are the same as in the astronomical telescope described above. The practical difference is that the tube is much shorter, and so the final image is upright.

Both these effects are produced by using reflecting prisms (see Fig 18.18). The light travels along the tube three times, so that the optical path is roughly three times the length of the binoculars. The prisms are arranged so that they invert the telescope image, which means it is finally the right way up.

7 CAPTURING IMAGES

The images formed by optical (and other imaging) devices can be 'caught' and stored in a variety of ways, ranging from the biochemical method using eyes and brain, through the traditional photochemical processes of film and plate cameras, to the newer systems, which include video cameras, charge-coupled devices (CCDs), magnetic discs and compact discs.

While the imaging process itself (using lenses and mirrors) depends on the *wave* aspect of light, image-capturing systems generally rely on the *particle* aspect of light. It is the energy of the photon that determines how the devices work and are designed.

THE HUMAN EYE

Focusing
Details of the eye are shown in Fig 18.35(a). Light entering it is focused by two lenses. First, the light meets the **cornea**, a curved layer which is transparent and fairly hard. It acts as a fixed focus lens and in fact does most of the refracting of the light entering the eye. Then the light reaches the **lens**. It refracts the light only slightly, mainly because it is surrounded by substances of almost the same refractive index as itself, and so the refraction (change in speed and direction) of light at the lens surfaces is quite small.

The job of the lens is to adjust the focal length of the cornea–lens combination, allowing for a range of object distances between about 25 cm at the **near point** and infinity at the **far point** for the normal eye.

The focal length of the eye lens is adjusted by changing its shape: the radii of curvature of its surfaces are changed by a ring of muscle round the lens called the **ciliary muscle**, and Fig 18.35(b) shows how it alters the shape of the lens.

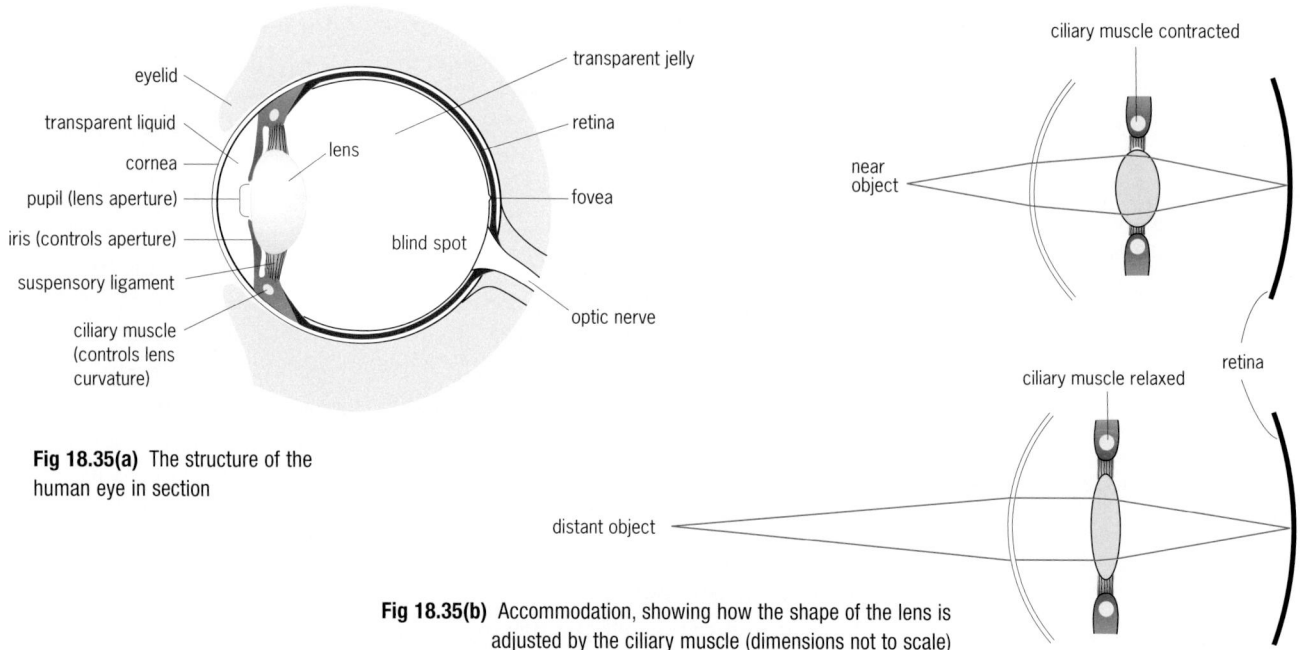

Fig 18.35(a) The structure of the human eye in section

Fig 18.35(b) Accommodation, showing how the shape of the lens is adjusted by the ciliary muscle (dimensions not to scale)

When the eye is relaxed, the radial suspensory ligament keeps the lens in tension. The eye forms clear images of objects at the far point (infinity, rays parallel), and the focal length of the cornea–lens combination is the length of the eye – about 17 mm. When the eye looks at a near object (rays diverging), the ciliary muscle contracts, the lens becomes fatter, and the focal length is shortened, in order to refract the rays to form a focused image on the retina. Rapid change in lens shape relies on swift feedback between brain and eye, and is called **accommodation**.

Sensing

The quantity of light entering the eye depends on the size of the **pupil**, the hole in the **iris**. Its size is controlled by the muscles of the iris. The light travels on to reach the **retina** which contains two types of light-sensitive cells, called **rods** and **cones** because of their shape. It is the functioning of these cells that enables us to 'see'. Briefly, this is the mechanism. The rods and cones contain light-sensitive pigment molecules. Photons of particular energies (frequencies) reach the pigment molecules. These molecules absorb energy and a reversible photochemical reaction is triggered. The molecules then rapidly lose energy in a process that generates an electrical potential, and a signal is transmitted to the brain via the **optic nerve**.

The **fovea** is the point on the retina directly in line with the lens. The fovea is where an image is resolved in the finest detail and is the part of the retina most crowded with cones. The rods are more numerous away from the fovea. The average human eye contains about 125 billion rods but only 7 billion cones.

Rods can 'distinguish' between different intensities of light, but not between light of different frequencies (photon energies). They are more sensitive at low light intensities, and are particularly effective for seeing in the dark. Since there are more of them away from the centre of the retina, at night, faint objects are most easily seen 'out of the corner of the eye'. If we suddenly move from bright light to darkness, or a light is switched off, it takes our eyes time to adjust to the dark and make out our surroundings. In this time, the photochemical pigment in the rods,

> **? QUESTION 15**
>
> 15 Why does the cornea produce more of a focusing effect than the eye lens?

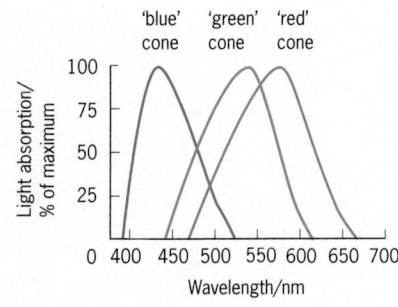

Fig 18.36 The absorption spectra for the three cone pigments in the retina. Each type of cone has a maximum sensitivity at a particular wavelength (at the peak) where light absorption is taken as 100 per cent for that type. (Cones for blue light are in fact much less sensitive than for green and red light)

which was broken down by bright light, is gradually resynthesised. When the retina is again sensitive to dim light, we say it is **dark-adapted**.

Cones allow us to see colour. Theories of colour vision vary, but it is generally accepted that there are three types of cone which are sensitive to overlapping regions of the spectrum, centring on the **red**, **blue** and **green** wavelengths, as shown in Fig 18.36.

It is thought that the enormous range of colours we can see around us is due to different combinations of the three types of cone being stimulated, and to the way the brain interprets the signals from them. Red, blue and green are the **primary colours** of optics, and any pair of these colours produces the secondary colours:

- red + green (or minus blue) produce the sensation of **yellow**,
- red + blue (or minus green) produce the sensation of **magenta**,
- green + blue (or minus red) produce the sensation of **cyan**.

When all three types are strongly stimulated by the energy range of photons found in daylight, the brain interprets the signals as 'white'. (In reality, colour vision is much more complicated than this simple description suggests.)

Defects of the eye

The near point is the closest distance at which we can see objects clearly, and this depends largely on the strength or weakness of the ciliary muscles – look back to Fig 18.35(b). The distance of the near point increases with age: at 10 years, it is about 18 cm; in a young adult, 25 cm; and by the age of 60, it may be as much as 5 metres.

This age-related defect is called **far sight** or **hypermetropia**. The eye lens is too weak, so that near objects are blurred because their images are formed behind the retina. Fig 18.37 illustrates these defects and how spectacles with positive lenses can correct them.

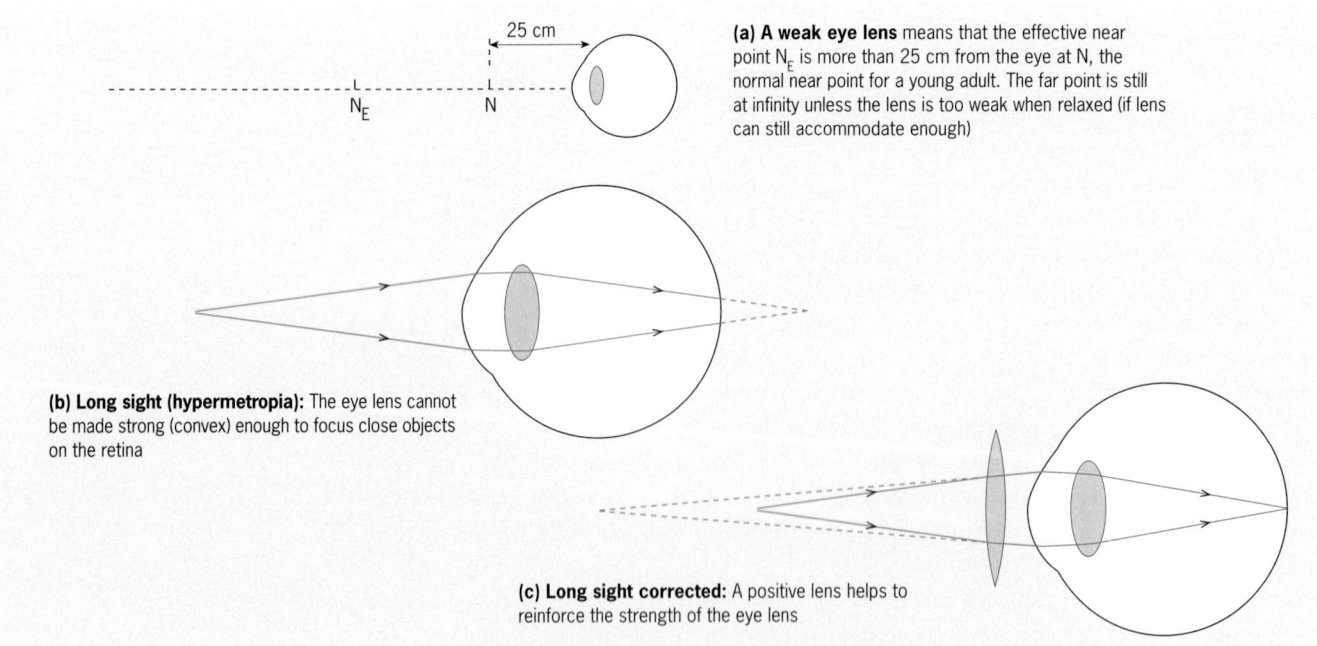

25 cm

N_E N

(a) A weak eye lens means that the effective near point N_E is more than 25 cm from the eye at N, the normal near point for a young adult. The far point is still at infinity unless the lens is too weak when relaxed (if lens can still accommodate enough)

(b) Long sight (hypermetropia): The eye lens cannot be made strong (convex) enough to focus close objects on the retina

(c) Long sight corrected: A positive lens helps to reinforce the strength of the eye lens

Fig 18.37 Long sight and its correction

Another common defect is **short sight** or **myopia**. In this case the eye's ciliary muscles are too strong and, even when relaxed, the lens is too powerful. This means that distant objects are focused in front of the retina. Negative lenses correct this defect, as shown in Fig 18.38.

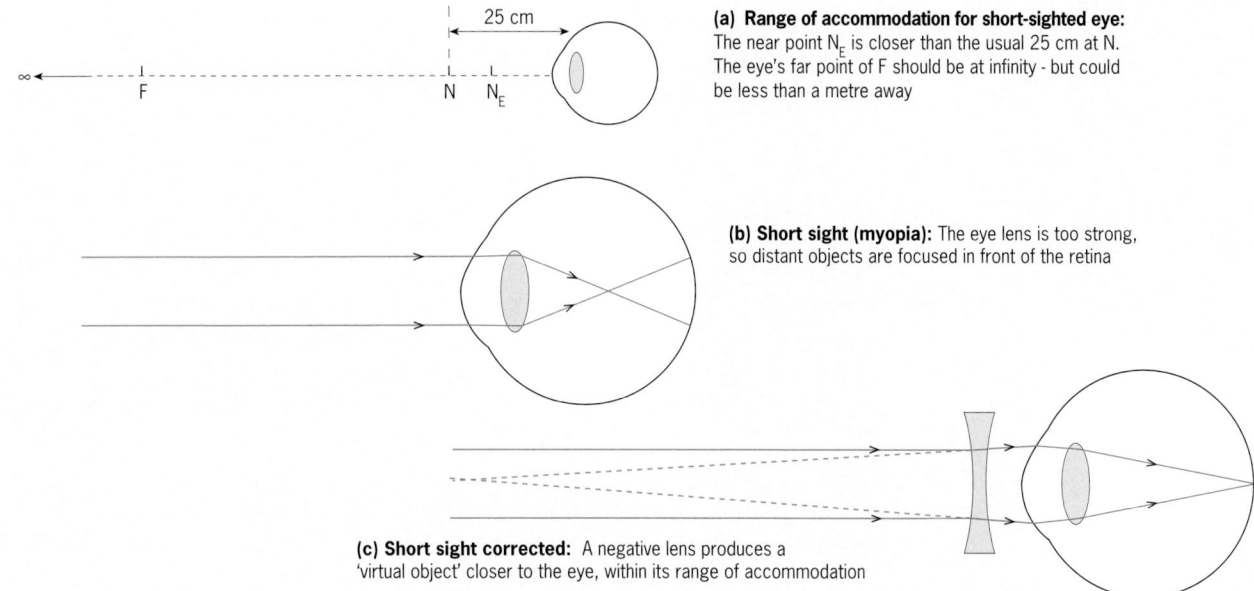

(a) **Range of accommodation for short-sighted eye:**
The near point N_E is closer than the usual 25 cm at N.
The eye's far point of F should be at infinity - but could be less than a metre away

(b) **Short sight (myopia):** The eye lens is too strong, so distant objects are focused in front of the retina

(c) **Short sight corrected:** A negative lens produces a 'virtual object' closer to the eye, within its range of accommodation

Fig 18.38 Short sight and its correction

The lens in the ageing eye tends to get less and less flexible, so that it becomes practically a 'fixed focus' device. Then, a person may need two pairs of spectacles – one for seeing close objects clearly ('reading glasses', with positive lenses) and one for seeing distant objects clearly (with negative lenses or weaker positive ones). Some people wear **bifocals**, spectacles with lenses that have a 'long distance' part and a 'reading' part, or **varifocals** with gradual variation from top to bottom.

At any age, the eye lens may have a condition called **astigmatism**. The eye cannot focus at the same time on vertical lines and horizontal ones, and a point source tends to be seen as a line. This is because the lens is not spherical and, for example, the radius of curvature in the horizontal direction is not equal to the radius in the vertical direction. Astigmatism is corrected by lenses with curvatures that counterbalance the eye lens curvatures.

DIGITAL CAMERAS

Digital cameras use **charge-coupled devices**, known as CCDs. CCDs are also used as the sensors which capture the images in astronomical telescopes (Fig 18.39). A CCD consists of a large number of very small picture element detectors, called **pixels**. A good digital camera will have a CCD with an array of perhaps 16 million pixels, each a tiny electrode built on to a thin layer of silicon.

When a photon hits the silicon layer, an electron–hole pair is created. A pixel electrode collects the charge produced, which depends upon the intensity of the light falling on the silicon. After a brief time, the electrodes are made to release the charge they have collected in a programmed sequence as the pixels are scanned electronically. The scan produces a digital signal consisting of a linear sequence of numbers, which can be stored in a small magnetic memory device. This is later transferred to a computer which can display the image on a screen and transfer it to a colour printer, or send it across the internet.

Digital 'movie films' can be taken similarly by camcorders and stored on tape or on disc, but larger memories are needed.

Colour pictures require three sets of sensitive areas with colour filters (red, green, blue) which produce a more complicated output signal containing colour as well as brightness information.

> **? QUESTION 16**
>
> 16 Estimate the focal length of your cornea–eye lens combination when you look at an object 25 cm from your eye (and see it clearly in focus).

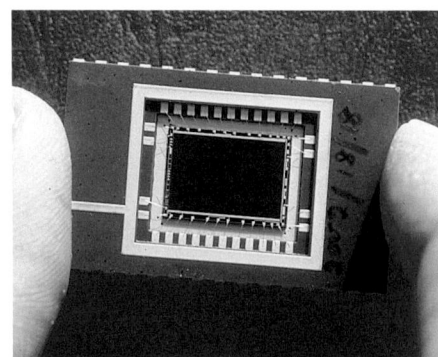

Fig 18.39 A CCD as used in an astronomical detector. Many millions of photon-sensitive pixels occupy the central rectangle

REMEMBER THIS
A nanometre, symbol nm, is 10^{-9} metres.

CCDs are sensitive to light of wavelengths from 400 nm (violet) to 1000 nm (infrared). Their main advantage in both scientific and everyday applications is their *efficiency*. Photographic film uses less than 4 per cent of the photons reaching it. The 'wasted' photons simply miss the sensitive grains in the film, or fail to trigger a chemical change. CCDs can make use of about 70 per cent of the incident photons, partly because they cover a larger area but mainly because the pixels are more sensitive than the chemicals in a film. (The eye is only about 1 per cent efficient at sensing photons.)

In astronomy, the collection time can be made very much longer than in a TV camera, allowing detail in a faint object to build up. Even so, the detection efficiency of CCDs means that the time of exposure is much less than is needed for a chemical photographic image. Also, the output current is proportional to the number of photons arriving, which means that the intensity of spectral lines and the brightness of stars can be measured more accurately than is possible with photographic methods.

Photographic plates do have the advantage that the light-sensitive grains are smaller than CCD pixels, so they can produce images with better resolution. But CCDs can be 'butted' together to make larger image areas. CCD technology is developing rapidly and may well take over from chemical photography as LCD display screens (see below) take over from cathode ray tube displays.

Scanners are now commonly used to convert a photograph into a stream of data for storage in a computer. They work by digitising the photograph's continuously varying light intensities and colour.

DISPLAY SCREENS

We already see a great deal of the world on our TV screens, and developments in information technology have made everyday communication through electronic mailing systems more common than the printed word. There are two main kinds of video screen used to display the information: the **cathode ray tube** (**CRT**), with a phosphor screen which is made to glow by high speed electrons, and the **liquid crystal display** (**LCD**), where the image is produced by a scanning process.

The cathode ray tube

Cathode ray tubes (CRTs) with phosphor screens are the oldest type: 'cathode rays' was the name given to streams of what were later discovered to be electrons. They were emitted from the negative electrode (cathode) of a high voltage discharge tube. Nowadays, electrons are produced by heating a metal oxide. Energy transferred from the electrons as they reach the screen makes the phosphor coating emit light.

CRTs are not only the most common tubes for TV receivers, radar devices and computer monitors but are also in such useful laboratory equipment as cathode ray oscilloscopes. CRTs waste energy by having to heat the electron emitter, and they need high voltages (over 2 kV) to accelerate the electrons to energies capable of exciting the phosphor. However, the technology is well established and CRTs are likely to be in use for some time.

Liquid crystal display screens

Many portable devices, such as calculators, watches and laptop computers, use liquid crystal displays (LCDs). The principle behind the image production is that the crystal is able to polarise light, and so can cut out light polarised in certain directions. This polarising effect in liquid crystals can be switched on and off by applying an electric field to it. In an LCD screen an array of small liquid crystal picture elements (pixels) is back-lit by a bright screen. A pixel can be changed from bright to dark electronically, and the array of pixels can be controlled by a data signal just like the screen of the cathode ray tube in a TV set.

Each pixel is connected individually to a **thin film transistor** (**TFT**), many thousands of these making up a large single block – a kind of microchip. This individual control of each pixel means that the pixels can be brighter, and the brightness can also be changed faster, so that the screen is 'refreshed' more often. As these types of screen (Fig 18.40) become cheaper and larger, they are already competitive with CRTs for computer monitors, and are taking over for television screens.

BEYOND THE VISIBLE SPECTRUM

An image is a record of *information*. Increasingly, the information is being coded digitally (see Chapter 21). The object used as the basis of an image need not be visible to the eye, that is, it need not be a source or reflector of visible light waves. The whole range of radiation in the electromagnetic spectrum may be used to make an image. For example, X-rays, ultraviolet and infrared have been used for a long time to make visible images on photographic film (see Fig 18.41). Images of soil and even the depths of the sea can be made using radar of different wavelengths, as described in Chapter 15.

Images are now also made using sound, electrons (as waves), and even changes in the tiny magnetic fields of spinning nuclei.

Ultrasound imaging

Ultrasound scanners are now commonly used in medicine to investigate and diagnose disorders. Ultrasound consists of sound waves of very high frequency and correspondingly small wavelength. Body tissues of different types absorb and reflect these sound waves to varying degrees, and images can be made of organs deep within the body.

You can read more about ultrasound imaging in the next chapter (page 381). Remember that sound is not part of the electromagnetic spectrum.

Magnetic resonance imaging

Hospitals commonly run appeals to raise funds for a 'scanner'. This is a device that can probe body systems in even more detail than ultrasound, using a technique that relies on the magnetic property of atomic nuclei and is known as magnetic resonance imaging, or MRI. The low intensity electromagnetic waves used (at radio frequency) do not affect biological tissues. (See page 389 for more about this.)

IMAGING THE ULTRA-SMALL

The transmission electron microscope

Quantum physics produced the greatest surprise of all when it suggested that, just as light waves have a particle aspect, so material particles should have a wave aspect (see page 316). The realisation that electrons – as waves – could be used to produce images in much the same way that light waves do, led to the development of the **electron microscope** (Fig 18.42 overleaf).

It is helpful to compare the diagram with that of Fig 18.33. An electron beam is projected through a series of electromagnets shaped in a ring which act as 'lenses' to change the direction of the beam. The first lens is a **condenser** lens. This lens may be used to make the beam parallel, or to focus on the target (the object being

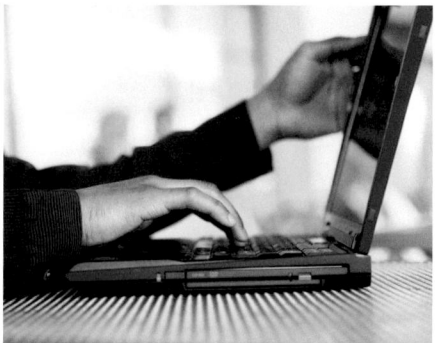

Fig 18.40 Modern laptop computers and, increasingly, desktops, use TFT technology to produce the image, with a large saving in energy and unwanted heating

? QUESTION 17

17 Compare the advantages and disadvantages of using liquid crystal screens and cathode ray screens for video display.

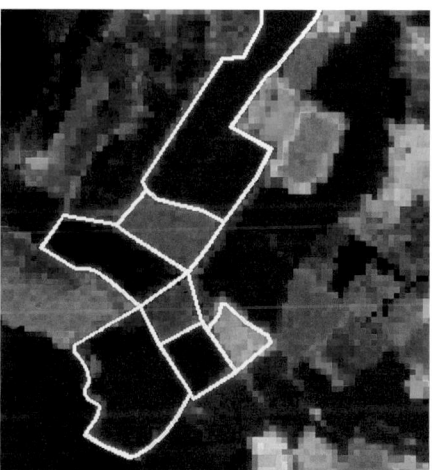

Fig 18.41 A satellite image of farmland. The red and infrared radiation reflected from the land varies according to the crops growing on it, and a computer converts these variations into different colours

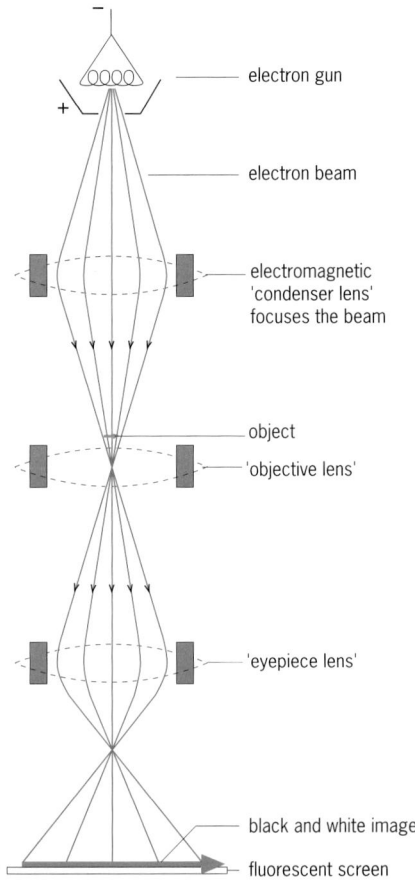

electron gun

electron beam

electromagnetic 'condenser lens' focuses the beam

object

'objective lens'

'eyepiece lens'

black and white image

fluorescent screen

Fig 18.42 The operation of the transmission electron microscope. The electron 'rays' are focused by powerful coil magnets, as in a TV tube. Their wave property allows detail in an object to be imaged

? QUESTION 18

18 The momentum p of an electron is related to its wavelength λ by the de Broglie formula $p = h/\lambda$, where h is the Planck constant.

a) Explain why this relationship means that in the electron microscope, shorter wavelengths require higher accelerating voltages than longer wavelengths.

b) Estimate **i)** the momentum and **ii)** the kinetic energy of the electrons in a typical electron microscope.

c) Hence calculate the accelerating voltage required for the microscope. Data: mass of electron 9.1×10^{-31} kg, $h = 6.6 \times 10^{-34}$ J s, elementary charge $e = 1.6 \times 10^{-19}$ C.

studied) to increase the 'illumination'. The second magnetic ring acts as the **objective** lens, and forms a magnified image of the target. The third electromagnet acts rather like the **eyepiece** on a light microscope, magnifying the image further and forming an image on a screen or on photographic film (Fig 18.43).

The problem with making images of any kind with waves is that of diffraction (see page 297). Diffraction affects the *resolution* of an image, that is, how far apart objects or details in an object must be before they can be seen as separate in an image. The limit of resolution for a microscope or telescope is defined by the Rayleigh criterion (see page 360).

The clarity of the image is determined by the wavelength – the shorter the better. Blue light has the shortest wavelength in the visible range, though ultraviolet may be used with photomicrography. The visible wavelengths are of the order of a few hundred nanometres – about 3 to 5×10^{-7} m.

In an electron microscope, electrons are accelerated to a high speed before hitting the object being studied. The higher the speed, the shorter the wavelength (see page 316), and so the better the resolution. The wavelength of an electron in an electron microscope is typically about 10^{-11} m – about 10 000 times shorter than the wavelength of light, and therefore the resolution is 10 000 times better. But as with light microscopes there are aberrations (distortions). The basic ones are:

- the magnetic field is not absolutely accurately defined (i.e. the lens has defects),
- electrons tend to repel each other and so their paths deviate to produce imperfections in the final image,
- as electrons pass through the target they slow down – and so are not focused to the right spot in the final image.

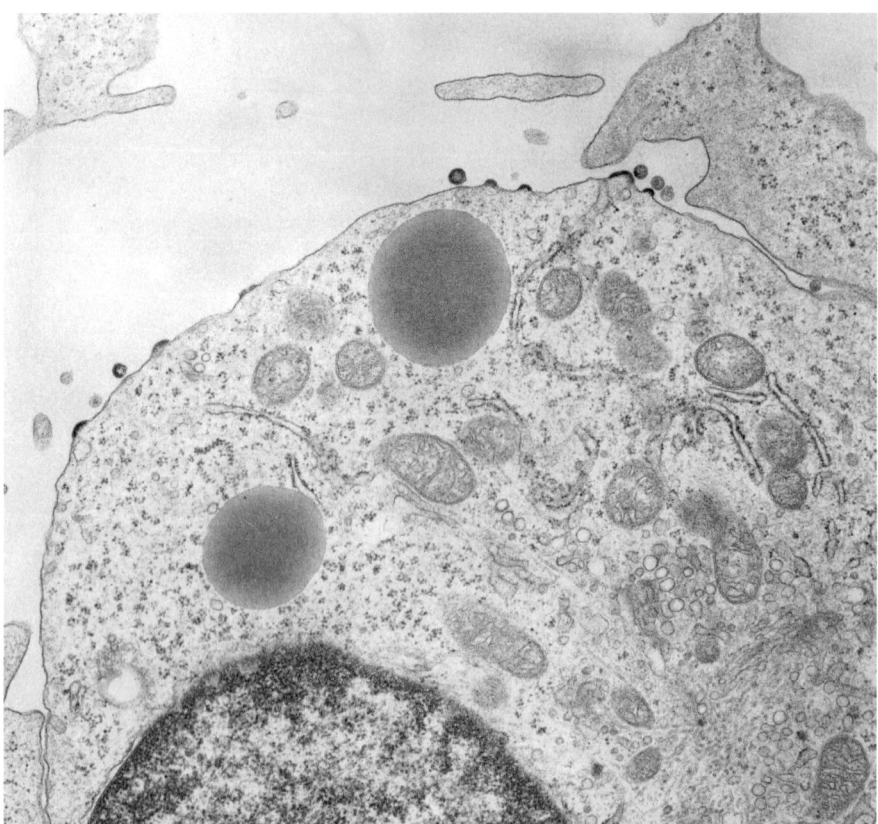

Fig 18.43 A transmission electron micrograph: part of a white blood cell known as a T-cell (its dark nucleus is bottom left). The cell's role is to combat infection, but it has itself been infected with HIV. The AIDS virus particles multiply inside it, and can be seen as small dark spheres budding off its outer surface at the top of the picture

The scanning tunnelling microscope

The image in Fig 18.44 was produced by a scanning tunnelling microscope. It shows the actual atoms at the surface of a crystal of silicon. The image was formed by exploiting a strange property of the electron, the fact that it can behave as if it is in several places at once: by quantum theory, an electron could be at any place defined by its wave equation (see Chapter 16, page 318).

In the scanning tunnelling microscope, a very fine needle passes at a constant tiny distance over the surface of an object, like the needle of a record player over the groove of a record, but not quite touching it. The needle has a probability of 'capturing' electrons on the surface, even though physics suggests that the electrons do not have enough energy to escape. The electrons are imagined as **tunnelling** through a potential energy barrier.

The greater the number of electrons there are at a position on the surface – at the outer boundaries of atoms – the more the electrons will 'tunnel'. The variation in current they produce can be used to build up an image at the atomic level of detail. All this is done with just a small positive voltage on the needle.

The scanning tunnelling microscope has the following advantages over the electron microscope: it is very useful indeed for studying surfaces that would be damaged by high-voltage electron bombardment, and it does not require a vacuum to produce the images.

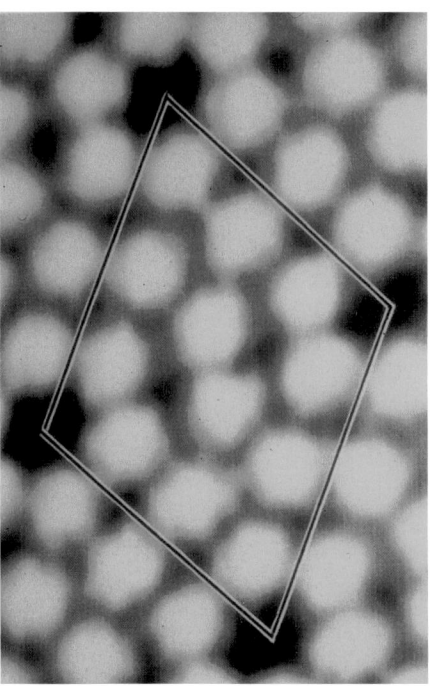

Fig 18.44 The scanning tunnelling microscope gives us images of individual atoms at surfaces. In this image of a silicon crystal magnified 45 million times, the orange spots are each a silicon atom, and the faint extensions between some atoms represent the electrons binding atoms together. The diamond indicates the repeating pattern in the crystal

SUMMARY

As a result of studying the topics in this chapter you should:

- Understand the importance of images and imaging in modern life.
- Understand how lenses form images, and be able to distinguish between real and virtual images.
- Know how to find the position and size of images in single lenses and mirrors both by drawing and by calculation, using the lens formulae:

$$\frac{1}{u} + \frac{1}{v} = \frac{1}{f} \quad \text{and} \quad M = \frac{v}{u}$$

- Understand the meaning of power in dioptres for a lens, as $1/f$ (in metres).
- Understand resolution and its calculation by the Rayleigh criterion:

$$\theta = \frac{\lambda}{d}$$

- Understand total internal reflection and the significance of the critical angle, given by $n = 1/\sin c$.

- Understand how a range of optical devices work (magnifying glass, refracting and reflecting astronomical telescopes, compound microscope), including the eye, its possible defects and their correction.
- Be able to calculate the magnifying powers of telescopes and microscopes, using the formula

$$m = \frac{f_o}{f_e}$$

- Understand the basic physical principles underlying some modern imaging systems such as CCDs, display screens, the ultrasound scanner, magnetic resonance imaging, the electron microscope and the scanning tunnelling microscope.

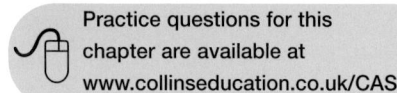

Practice questions for this chapter are available at www.collinseducation.co.uk/CAS

19

Medical physics

19 MEDICAL PHYSICS

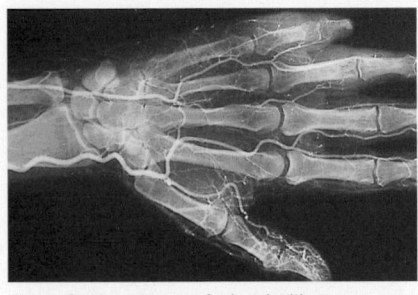

Above: An X-ray image of a hand with a contrasting dye used to highlight the vein structure

Below: An infrared image showing variation in haemoglobin density as yellow where it is at a low level, and red and blue at higher levels

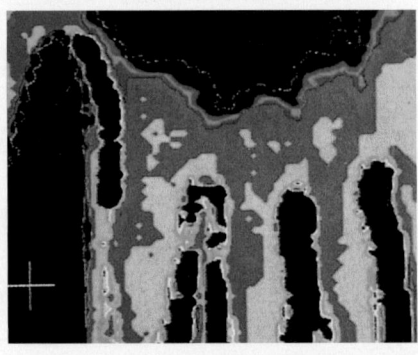

For more information on how electrical technology has advanced medical physics with the development of the electrocardiograph (ECG) please see the How Science Works assignment for this chapter at www.collinseducation.co.uk/CAS

An inside look

Most children playing with an electric torch have noticed the red glow that comes through their hand when they put it over the lens. Light passes through quite easily, but it doesn't give a clear picture of what is under the skin because the soft tissue scatters light.

An X-ray image of a hand is a fine-tuned version of the picture using torchlight. Blood vessels can be shown clearly when the blood is injected with a dye that strongly absorbs photons.

A different picture is obtained when a very short pulse of infrared light from a laser is used. The light that penetrates the hand and comes straight out the other side is detected in an equally short time, while scattered photons, which take longer to pass through the hand because they travel further, are not recorded. So the resulting image is sharp.

Images from infrared are not yet as clear as X-ray images because resolution with this technique is still poor. However, they can be useful because the colours indicate the quantity of haemoglobin (the oxygen-carrying compound) in blood. An advantage is that infrared radiation does not ionise atoms, so it is safer to use than X-rays.

With improvements such as computer enhancement giving better resolution (detail) of images, both infrared and visible light imaging could become very safe techniques for both patients and medical workers.

The ideas in this chapter

This chapter deals with the use of physics to **diagnose** (Part A) and **treat** (Part B) illnesses and other medical conditions that mar a person's life, happiness and comfort. Most of the techniques described use radiations of one kind or another, covering most of the electromagnetic spectrum. Even radio is used, to supply energy to the oscillating magnetic fields used in magnetic resonance imaging (MRI). Some techniques involve the use of particles such as beta particles and positrons, emitted by radioactive elements. To use all these radiations, specialist detecting instruments are needed, as well as highly technical means for producing and directing the beams.

Medical physicists need to be aware not only of the beneficial effects of radiations but also of the possible harmful effects that they might have on patients and on medical personnel.

Much of the basic physics involved here is dealt with in earlier chapters, particularly Chapter 15 Electromagnetic radiation and Chapter 17 The atomic nucleus.

PART A: PHYSICS IN MEDICAL DIAGNOSIS

A trained observer can find out a great deal about the state of health of the human body by looking at it, examining by touching it, studying substances from it, and listening to its internal noises. Usually, the patient can also describe the nature and site of any pain. But until the end of the nineteenth century, finding out more required **invasive techniques**, such as cutting an organ open in an exploratory operation. This carried the risk of trauma (damage and shock) and infection. But in 1895 Wilhelm Konrad Röntgen discovered X-rays. He saw that they cast a shadow of a hand on a luminous screen. One of his X-ray images revealed the bones and the ring on a finger of his wife's hand. Within weeks of the discovery, doctors were using home-made X-ray machines to look at broken bones and other internal structures. They did so with dangerous enthusiasm, not knowing that X-rays were ionising radiations that could harm living tissue.

X-rays are an example of a **non-invasive** method for probing deep into the body without cutting into it. Doctors now use a wide range of non-invasive (and often less risky) techniques, both as probes for diagnosis, and also to provide treatment. These involve not only X-rays but also high-frequency sound waves (ultrasound), high-frequency radio waves, light, infrared and ultraviolet radiation and subatomic particles.

1 IMAGING USING ULTRASOUND

Ultrasound waves are longitudinal pressure waves at a frequency well beyond the upper limit of human hearing (>20 kHz). Low intensity ultrasonic waves pass through tissue without causing harm, and are reflected at the *boundaries* between different biological structures. These *reflections* allow images (body scans) of internal organs to be created by an **ultrasound scanner**.

THE PIEZOELECTRIC TRANSDUCER

Typical diagnostic frequencies are in the range 1 to 5 MHz. Such high frequencies are produced by an electromechanical effect known as **piezoelectricity**. Certain crystals, such as quartz (SiO_2), produce an electric charge on their surfaces when compressed. The effect is used in the everyday piezoelectric gas igniter: squeezing the handle compresses a crystal and the charge produced makes a spark to ignite the gas.

The effect is used in reverse to produce ultrasound. A high-frequency alternating voltage applied to the crystal surface makes the crystal compress and expand at the same frequency, and the crystal's vibrations generate the ultrasound waves. Vibrations are best at one of the crystal's natural **resonant frequencies** – determined by its size and how it has been cut – and so the applied voltage is tuned to match one of the crystal's resonant frequencies.

Fig 19.1 shows a typical ultrasound emitter. It uses a piezo-crystal of lead zirconate–lead titanate, PZT. It is a more efficient energy converter than quartz,

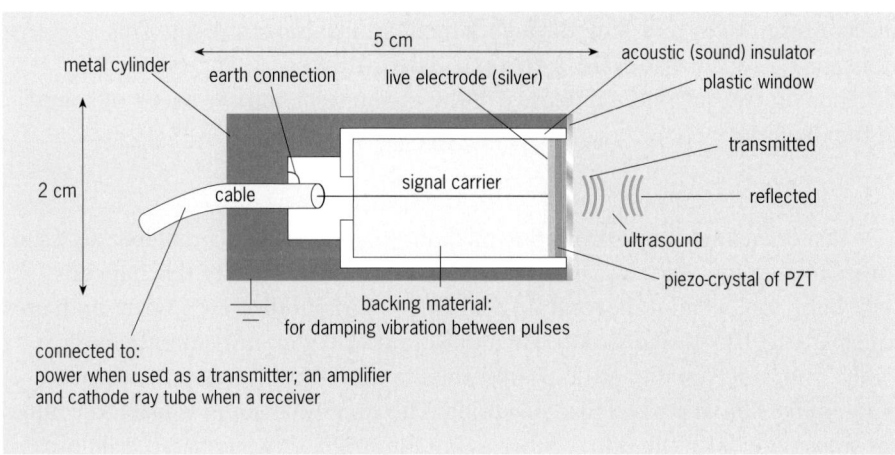

connected to:
power when used as a transmitter; an amplifier
and cathode ray tube when a receiver

Fig 19.1 A typical piezoelectric transducer for medical use

? QUESTION 1

1 Explain what resonance is, and give two examples of a resonating effect or system.

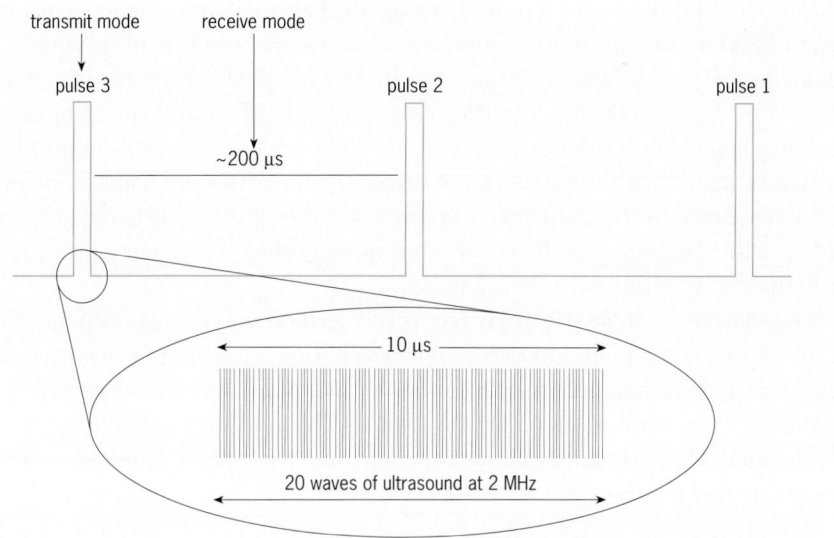

Fig 19.2 Ultrasound pulses used in diagnostic scans

and so can produce higher power output. The emitter also acts as a receiver: incoming waves alter the crystal's vibrations which, in turn, generate electrical signals. The piezoelectric element can be thought of as a **transducer**, a device that changes a signal from one energy form to another. As an emitter it converts electric potentials to mechanical vibrations, and as a receiver it converts the energy of mechanical vibrations into varying electric potentials.

The ultrasound is produced in short pulses, typically 10 µs long, with a gap of a few hundred microseconds between pulses (Fig 19.2). Typically, the beam has a mean power of 0.1 mW.

BUILDING AN ULTRASOUND IMAGE

With the transducer in the 'receive' mode, the reflections from different layers in the body return before the next pulse is transmitted. The result is displayed on the screen of a cathode ray oscilloscope as a set of line peaks as in Fig 19.3. Each peak shows the position of a reflecting surface and the height of the peak shows how reflective the surface is. This is called an **A-scan**.

A **B-scan** produces an image that is easier to interpret. The probe is scanned across the body in a series of lines, just as a TV screen works. The strength and position of the return signal are stored electronically, then transferred to produce an image on a TV screen. The signal strength now controls the brightness – and even the colour – of a spot on the screen, so building up a two-dimensional image, Fig 19.4.

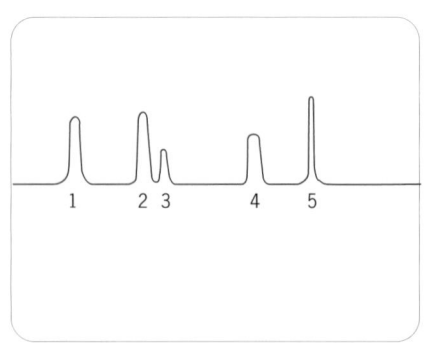

Fig 19.3 An A-scan: peaks identify surfaces 1 to 5 at increasing depths in the body

Just as electric currents experience resistance in a conductor, ultrasound also meets resistance in travelling through a medium like human tissue. This resistance is called **specific acoustic impedance**, Z. The value of Z depends on two factors: the density of the medium, ρ, and the speed of sound in the medium, c:

$$Z = c\rho$$

When the sound moves from one medium to another with a different acoustic impedance, some of the wave is reflected back. (Remember that this happens with light, too, when it moves from one medium to another, even when both are transparent.) This is one reason why ultrasound waves do not enter the body easily – not only are they strongly absorbed in air if there is a gap between emitter and skin, there will also be strong reflection. So a liquid is used to couple the transmitter with the skin – either a thin film of oil or water-based cellulose

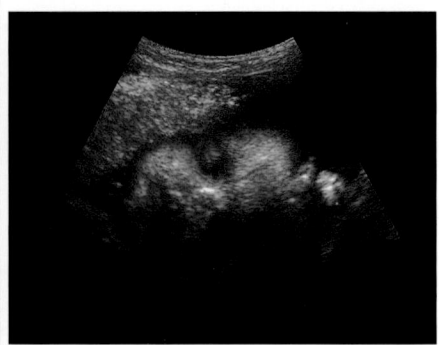

Fig 19.4 Ultrasound scan of the face of a full-term (9 month) fetus

jelly. But it is this very reflection property that ultrasound imaging relies on. It can be shown that the fraction a of energy that is reflected when ultrasound moves from a medium 1 to a medium 2 is given by the relationship:

$$\alpha = \frac{\text{energy reflected}}{\text{energy transmitted}} = \frac{(Z_2 - Z_1)^2}{(Z_2 + Z_1)^2}$$

where the Z values are for the two different media. Table 19.1 gives the values of Z for some biological tissues.

Table 19.1 *Z* values for biological tissues

Medium	Density/kg m^{-3}	Ultrasound speed/m s^{-1}	Z/kg m^{-2} s^{-1}
air	1.3	330	429
water	1000	1430	1.43×10^6
blood	1060	1570	1.59×10^6
brain	1025	1540	1.58×10^6
fat	952	1450	1.38×10^6
muscle (average)	1075	1590	1.70×10^6
bone (varies)	1400–1908	4080	5.8–7.8×10^6

ULTRASOUND IMAGE QUALITY

As we have seen, the ultrasound image is formed from a set of reflection pulses from material at different depths in the body section scanned. The sharpness of each reflection depends on the duration of the transmitted pulse: if the pulse is too long, then echoes will overlap. But if the pulse is too short, the energy carried is small and the reflections may be too weak to be detected above the background 'noise' of the detection system. Thus, the best pulse length is a balance between the two.

Another problem is multiple reflections: the reflected pulse from a boundary may be bounced back into the patient to be reflected once again. This gives multiple overlapping signals which reduce clarity. Also, since the image of an area of the body is built up over time using a scanning procedure, any movement of the patient or internal organ means that linear images taken at different times do not match, and the compound image will be blurred.

Resolution

The image of an object in the body is made up of reflections from small details. **Diffraction** will occur if the wavelength used is too large. Then, the image will lack clarity, making **resolution** poor. As a general rule, ultrasound will just resolve details of the same size as its wavelength. This means that if we need to resolve detail to a level of 1 mm, the ultrasound must have a wavelength equal to or smaller than 1 mm. Diagnostic ultrasound uses frequencies in the range 1 to 15 MHz, resolving details as small as 0.1 mm.

BLOOD FLOW MEASUREMENT

One useful application of ultrasound is the measurement of the rate at which blood flows in blood vessels. The method uses the **Doppler** principle. The ultrasound is reflected by blood particles (red blood cells) and, as the particles are moving, the reflected waves are shifted in frequency by an amount determined by the speed of the blood.

> **? QUESTION 2**
>
> 2 The speed of ultrasound in brain tissue is 1540 m s^{-1}. What frequency of ultrasound has a wavelength that can resolve detail to 0.1 mm?

Ultrasound frequencies of 5 to 10 MHz are used to make images. The beam enters the blood vessel at an angle θ (Fig 19.5). The frequency shift Δf is measured and related to blood speed v by the formula:

$$\Delta f = \frac{2fv\cos\theta}{c}$$

where c is the speed of the ultrasound.

Fig 19.6 shows a typical Doppler scan.

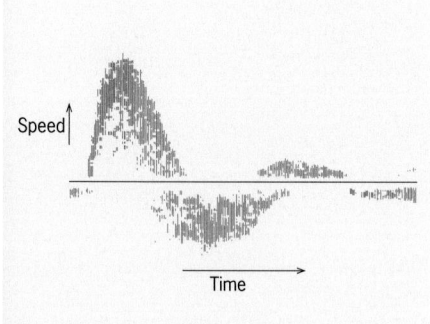

Fig 19.5 Using ultrasound to measure blood flow

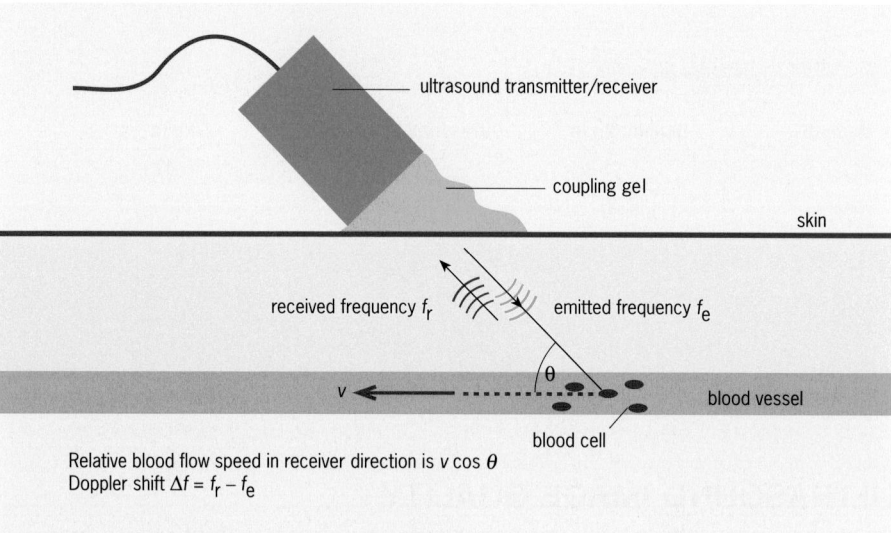

Relative blood flow speed in receiver direction is $v\cos\theta$
Doppler shift $\Delta f = f_r - f_e$

Fig 19.6 Typical Doppler scan for an artery using an ultrasound scanner. This shows how the speed of blood changes with heartbeat

DANGERS OF ULTRASOUND

Ultrasonic waves carry energy. Some of it is absorbed in tissue and causes heating. Bones are particularly energy absorbent. At some frequencies, small objects in the body could resonate and literally be shaken to pieces. So care is taken to keep a low combination of exposure time and intensity. Ultrasound can also cause **cavitation**, the production of small gas bubbles which absorb energy, expand and may damage surrounding tissue. Damage is unlikely at the frequencies and intensities used for diagnosis, but is useful in some kinds of treatment (see page 394).

2 IMAGING WITH X-RAYS

PRODUCTION OF X-RAYS

X-rays are ionising electromagnetic radiations (photons) with short wavelengths (of about 10^{-8} to 10^{-12} m) and correspondingly high photon energies (of about 100 eV to 1 MeV). Diagnostic X-rays give best results at energies of about 30 keV, and are produced by bombarding a tungsten anode with electrons accelerated through potential differences of 60 to 125 kV. Fig 19.7 shows the arrangement in a typical diagnostic X-ray machine.

X-rays are produced when electrons are rapidly decelerated as they strike the anode. It becomes very hot, so the usual material is tungsten which has a very high melting point. The electrons also disturb (excite) tungsten atoms which then emit more high-frequency photons at particular wavelengths. These photons add a line spectrum of **K** and **L lines** to the continuous spectrum produced by the decelerating electrons (see Fig 19.8(a)).

The spectra in Fig 19.8 show that the distribution of photon energies depends on the target anode and the tube voltage and current, as explained in the next sections.

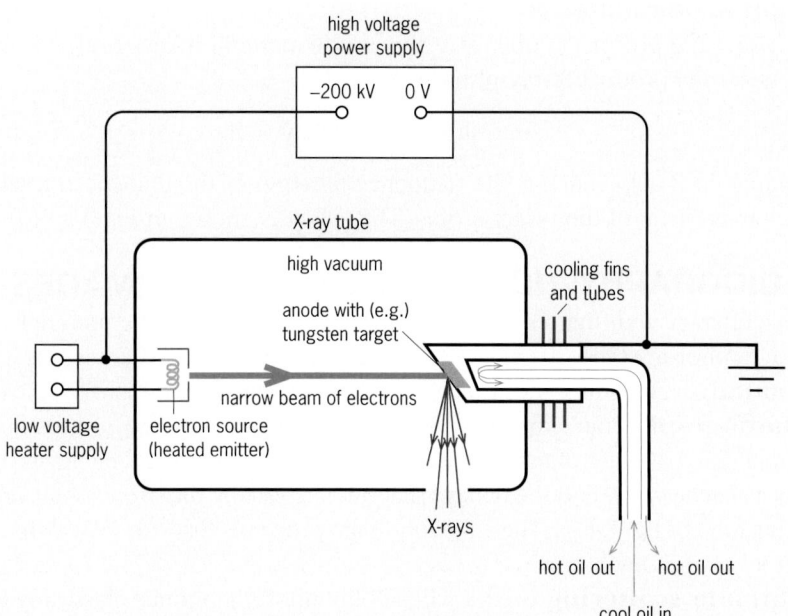

Fig 19.7 Plan of the X-ray machine. The anode is strongly heated by the electron impact. It must be cooled, and may also be rotated to reduce wear on the target metal

Fig 19.8 Continuous spectra showing typical energy distributions for an X-ray tube. Note that $E = hf$

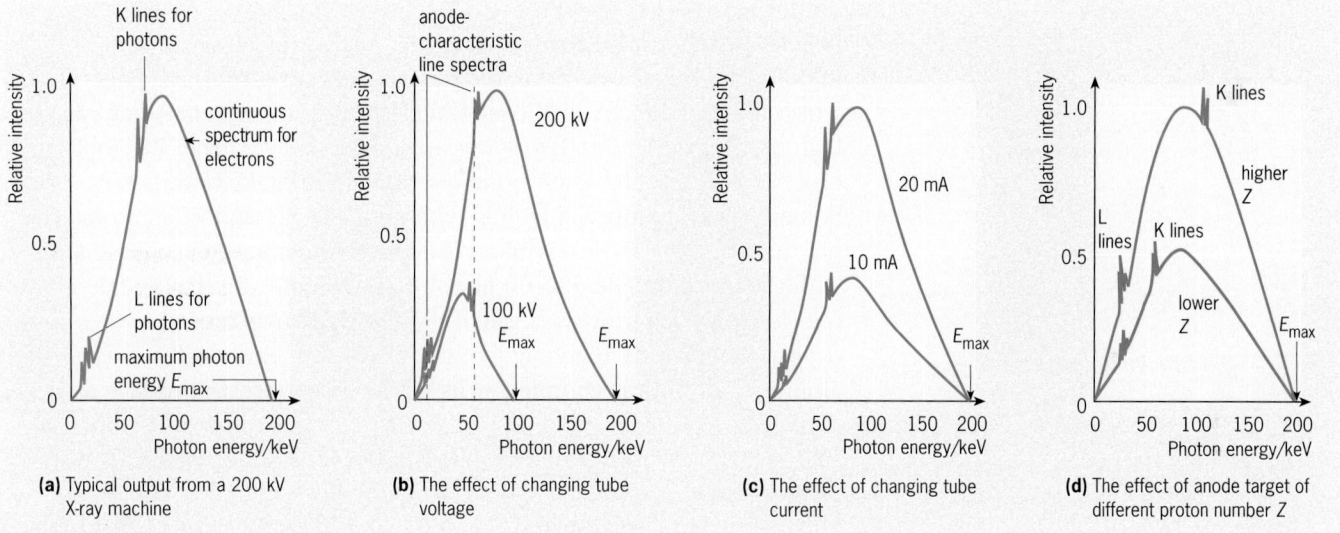

(a) Typical output from a 200 kV X-ray machine

(b) The effect of changing tube voltage

(c) The effect of changing tube current

(d) The effect of anode target of different proton number Z

Tube voltage

The higher the potential difference through which the electrons move, the more kinetic energy E_k they gain, and so the higher the frequency f of the X-ray photons produced:

$$\text{maximum energy of photon } hf = E_k = eV$$

where h is the Planck constant, e is the electronic charge and V is the accelerating voltage. Most electrons lose energy in heating the anode, and only a few have this maximum energy. Fig 19.8(b) shows the effect of increasing tube voltage.

Tube current

Increasing the tube current, which means increasing the number of electrons moving from cathode to anode, increases the number of X-ray photons produced:

$$\text{beam intensity} \propto \text{tube current}$$

This effect is shown in Fig 19.8(c).

> **? QUESTION 3**
>
> 3 **a)** Explain why high-energy X-rays have short wavelengths.
>   **b)** Explain why increasing the electron current produces more X-rays rather than X-rays with more photon energy.

Target anode material

Increasing the proton number Z of the anode material increases the likelihood that electrons produce X-ray photons:

$$\text{output beam intensity} \propto Z$$

A change in Z also changes the frequency (energy) of the line spectra, which are characteristic of the target atoms. This effect is shown in Fig 19.8(d).

RADIOGRAPHY: HOW X-RAYS PRODUCE IMAGES

X-rays interact with matter in various ways. In all of them, the material removes photons (absorbs energy) from the direct beam and so causes **attenuation**, meaning that the energy of the beam is diminished.

Radiography, the term given to producing images with X-rays, relies on the fact that different types of tissue cause differing attenuations. An X-ray image is really a *shadowgraph* and the darkest shadows are cast by the strongest absorbers (attenuators) of the X-rays. There are four main processes that can reduce the intensity of an X-ray beam:

- **Simple scattering** occurs when X-ray photons bounce elastically off the nuclei of atoms. They do not lose energy but change direction–so that they do not reach the detector.
- A photon may instead **ionise** an atom, transferring all or most of its energy in doing so. This is essentially the **photoelectric effect** (see page 310) in which the photon energy liberates an electron from an atom. X-rays have high energy and tend to knock out inner orbital electrons in this ionising process. (Ions usually result from loss of outer orbital electrons.)
- Sometimes a photon will collide with an *outer* electron in an atom. The photon acts as a particle with a particular momentum, which it shares with the electron. The photon goes off at an angle after losing energy to the electron. This process is called the **Compton effect**.
- A photon with very high energy that travels very close to the nucleus of an atom may disappear completely. Its energy is enough to produce a pair of particles – an electron and a positive electron (a positron). The photon's energy has been converted to matter in a process called **pair production** (see Chapter 24). The energy has to be high enough to satisfy Einstein's relationship $E = mc^2$, where m is the sum of the masses of the two particles produced.

Measuring the total attenuation

Each of the four processes produces attenuation which depends on the mass of matter interacted with, and this is measured in terms of the **mass attenuation coefficient** μ_m. Table 19.2 shows how μ_m for the four processes depends on the photon energy E and the nuclear charge, that is, the number of protons Z in the nucleus.

Table 19.2 Attenuation processes for X-rays in matter

Process	How μ_m depends on photon energy E	How μ_m depends on Z	Photon energy range in which the process is important in soft tissue
simple scatter	$\propto 1/E$	$\propto Z^2$	1–20 keV
photoelectric effect	$\propto 1/E^3$	$\propto Z^3$	1–30 keV
Compton scatter	falls very gradually as E increases	does not depend on Z	30 keV–20 MeV
pair production	increases slowly as E increases	$\propto Z^2$	above 20 MeV

As a general rule, attenuation gets less as photon energy increases, so the higher the X-ray energy, the more the photons penetrate matter. In diagnostic radiography, an optimum photon energy of about 30 keV produces the best contrast between different types of tissue. This is because at 30 keV energy the main attenuation process is the *photoelectric effect*, with absorption proportional to the cube of the proton number Z. This means that bones, which are mainly calcium with $Z = 20$, produce significantly more attenuation per unit mass than soft tissue (mostly water with hydrogen: $Z = 1$ and oxygen: $Z = 16$).

HOMOGENEOUS BEAMS

It is not easy to obtain an intense beam of X-rays containing photons of just one energy – a **homogeneous** or **monoenergetic** beam. A near-monoenergetic beam can be obtained by **filtering** it: the beam passes through a metal sheet which absorbs some X-ray photons, more of the low-energy photons than the high-energy ones – as you should be able to deduce from the second column of Table 19.2. This means that when an X-ray beam is filtered, the beam becomes more penetrating.

In the ideal case, a near-monoenergetic beam is attenuated in matter to give the percentage transmission curve shown in Fig 19.9. The shape of the graph should be familiar: it is an **exponential fall**. This is because each small distance Δx in the material produces a small attenuation $-\Delta I$, which is proportional both to Δx and to the beam intensity I:

$$-\Delta I = \mu I \Delta x \qquad [1]$$

μ is a constant for a given X-ray wavelength in a given attenuating material, and is called the **linear attenuation coefficient**.

In any situation where the *change* in a quantity is proportional to the (varying) quantity itself, the result is an exponential change. We can rewrite equation 1 as:

$$\frac{\Delta I}{I} = -\mu \Delta x$$

or, in calculus notation:

$$\frac{\mathrm{d}I}{I} = -\mu \mathrm{d}x \qquad [2]$$

Integrating equation 2 gives:

$$\ln I = -\mu x + C \qquad [3]$$

where I is the intensity at a depth of penetration x. C is a constant which we can identify by the fact that when x is zero, the beam has its starting unattenuated value I_0, so:

$$\ln I_0 = C$$

Putting this value for C in equation 3 gives:

$$\ln I - \ln I_0 = -\mu x$$

or

$$\ln \frac{I}{I_0} = -\mu x$$

which we can write as:

$$\frac{I}{I_0} = \mathrm{e}^{-\mu x} \qquad [4]$$

This is shown by BC in Fig 19.10; note that filtering the beam makes it **harder**, that is, more penetrating.

? **QUESTION 4**

4 The average values of Z for muscle and bone are 7.4 and 13.9 respectively. Estimate the ratio of attenuation due to the photoelectric effect between equal masses of bone and muscle.

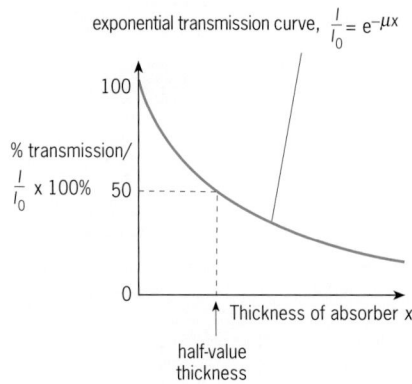

exponential transmission curve, $\frac{I}{I_0} = \mathrm{e}^{-\mu x}$

Fig 19.9 Ideal graph for attenuation of a near-monoenergetic X-ray beam

✔ **REMEMBER THIS**

As an example of exponential change, think of radioactive decay: the amount of a radioactive material that decays in a given time depends on the amount of material there is, and that amount varies with time.

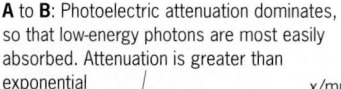

A to **B**: Photoelectric attenuation dominates, so that low-energy photons are most easily absorbed. Attenuation is greater than exponential

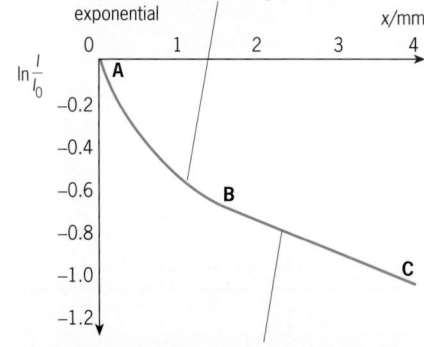

B to **C**: The beam is now 'hard', with attenuation obeying an exponential law: $I = I_0\, \mathrm{e}^{-\mu x}$

Fig 19.10 A logarithmic plot of attenuation in a typical X-ray beam after passing through a total thickness x (mm) of a metal. Filtering out low-energy photons makes the beam harder

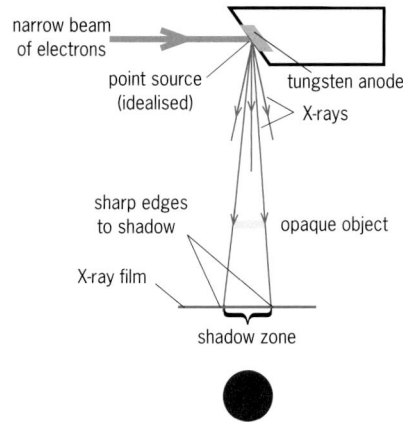

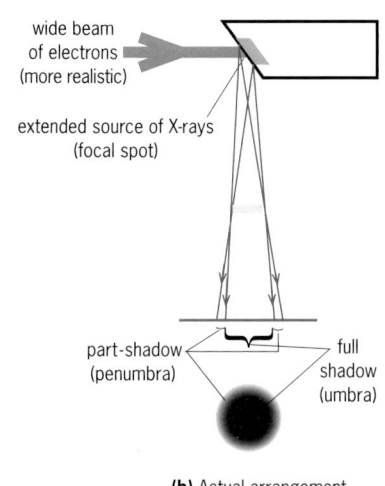

Fig 19.11 The sharpness of an X-ray image is affected by the size of the source

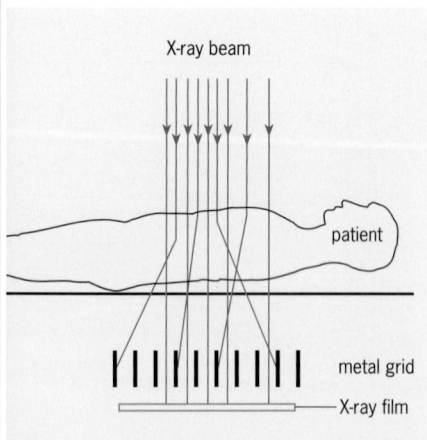

Fig 19.12 A metal grid is used to remove scattered X-rays. This improves contrast (the size of the grid spacing is exaggerated)

Fig 19.9 on the previous page shows that for a filtered, monoenergetic beam we can define a **half-value thickness** (compare *half-life* in radioactivity) which is the thickness of a material that cuts the X-ray intensity by a half. We can use equation 4 to state the half-value thickness $x_{\frac{1}{2}}$ in terms of the linear attenuation coefficient μ as follows:

$$I = \tfrac{1}{2} I_0$$

so:

$$e^{-\mu x_{\frac{1}{2}}} = \tfrac{1}{2}$$

or:

$$e^{\mu x_{\frac{1}{2}}} = 2$$

giving:

$$x_{\frac{1}{2}} = \frac{\ln 2}{\mu}$$

The inverse square law

As with light, in a vacuum the energy of X-rays spreads out from the source according to the inverse square law. This means that the intensity decreases as $1/r^2$ where r is the distance from the source.

X-RAY IMAGE QUALITY

The X-ray image or shadowgraph is usually produced on special photographic film. The sharpness of the image is affected by the *size of the X-ray source*, known as the **focal spot**, and the *scattering* effect as photons pass through the object.

A point source produces perfectly sharp shadows, see Fig 19.11(a). But X-rays originate in a small spot of finite size on the tungsten anode as in Fig 19.11(b), and so the shadow contains an edge effect – a **penumbra**. The penumbra can be reduced by placing the film as close to the object (part of the patient) as possible.

Photons scattered by nuclei in the object carry no information and merely blur the final image, reducing *contrast* between the darker and lighter areas. To minimise this effect, a filter grid is used as shown in Fig 19.12. Only unscattered photons can reach the film.

Clearer pictures would be produced if higher energy (harder) beams were used and the exposure time increased. But this would increase the risk of damage to the patient because atoms in living cells would be ionised, and that increases the risk of cancer.

Improvements in detection systems allow better images with quite low beam intensities. For example, a fluorescent (phosphor-coated) screen placed in front of and behind light-sensitive film will absorb X-rays and re-emit the energy as light in a pattern matching the X-ray image. Fig 19.13 shows how the phosphors and light-sensitive film are arranged. The film is much more sensitive than ordinary X-ray film, so images can be produced using low intensity X-ray beams.

When an X-ray image of the digestive system is required, the patient swallows a harmless suspension of barium sulphate (a 'barium meal'). This enhances image contrast, since barium atoms have a high Z value. Similarly, harmless high-Z dyes can be injected into blood (see the photo at the beginning of this chapter).

COMPUTERISED TOMOGRAPHY (CT)

This technique for X-ray imaging was developed in the 1970s, and is a great improvement on traditional X-ray imaging techniques. A narrow beam of X-rays is rotated around the patient and after passing through the body is detected electronically. The body is surrounded by several hundred photon detectors, whose outputs are fed to a computer. This analyses the data and forms an image of a narrow slice of the body on a monitor screen: a **CT scan** (Fig 19.14). This method produces images with good resolution and does so very quickly – so that changes in 'real time' can be observed. The technique is particularly useful for diagnosing damage (e.g. lesions) in the brain, where exploratory surgery is not usually possible. (See also PET scanning, page 394.)

3 MAGNETIC RESONANCE IMAGING (MRI)

This technique gives images of tissues deep in the body by using radio waves and a rather obscure property of nuclei, their **nuclear magnetic resonance**, or **NMR**. The process is now generally called **magnetic resonance imaging**, **MRI**, and targets the hydrogen nuclei which form such a large component of living tissue.

The nucleus of an atom spins. It is also charged, and a spinning charge generates a magnetic field. Just as one magnet becomes aligned in the presence of another (e.g. a compass needle in the Earth's magnetic field), so hydrogen atoms are aligned in a magnetic field. The field has to be very strong, and a hydrogen nucleus can align itself in one of two ways, which correspond to two different quantised energy states.

The magnetic field of the nucleus is along its axis of spin. When an external field is applied, the spin axis itself rotates in an effect known as **precession**. The Earth's axis, for example, precesses in a period of 23 000 years or so about a line perpendicular to the plane of its orbit. The rate of precession of the hydrogen nucleus, the **Larmor precession**, is a lot quicker; in a field of strength 1.5 tesla, the frequency is about 63.8 MHz, which is in the radio frequency (RF) range at 42.577 MHz. When an extra, weaker magnetic field is applied which is made to oscillate at this frequency, the direction of the nucleus' magnetic axis reverses. Most of the nuclei align in the direction of the field, but some align in the opposite direction, giving rise to two different quantised energy states. (see Fig. 19.15.)

The frequency of the applied RF signal is chosen to match the precession frequency of the hydrogen nuclei so that **resonance** can occur (Fig 19.16). The magnetic component of the electromagnetic wave supplies the energy to cause the reversal of the spin alignment of many nuclei. The energy taken from the radio wave depends on the number and distribution of the nuclei in the sample: molecules of biological tissue contain plenty of hydrogen nuclei in water and carbohydrates. In simple **absorption** MRI this loss is measured and used to build up the image.

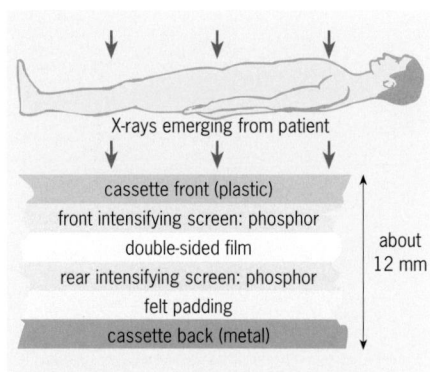

Fig 19.13 Arrangement of film and phosphors in an intensifying screen cassette (patient and cassette not to scale)

? QUESTION 5

5 **a)** Suggest why ordinary light-sensitive film is more sensitive to light than X-ray film is to X-rays.
b) Explain the advantage of using two layers of phosphor as shown in Fig 19.13.

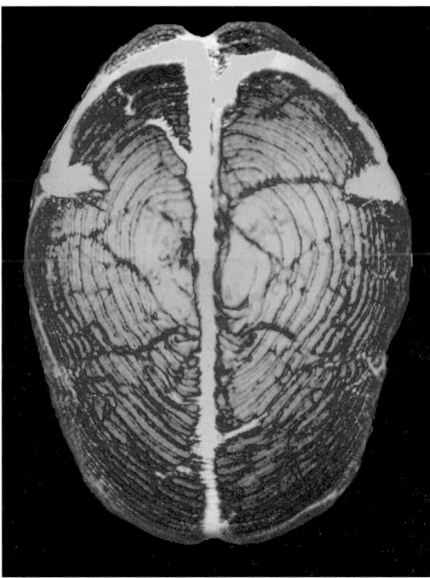

Fig 19.14 CT scan of the brain

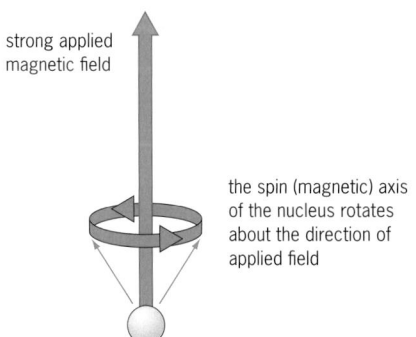

(a) The Larmor precession. The spin axis of the nucleus rotates about the main applied field at a very high frequency

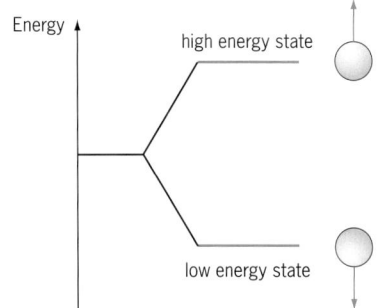

(b) When a further field is applied, oscillating at the right frequency (causing resonance), the direction of the nuclear spin axis reverses. This takes energy from the applied field

Fig 19.15 Nuclear magnetic resonance

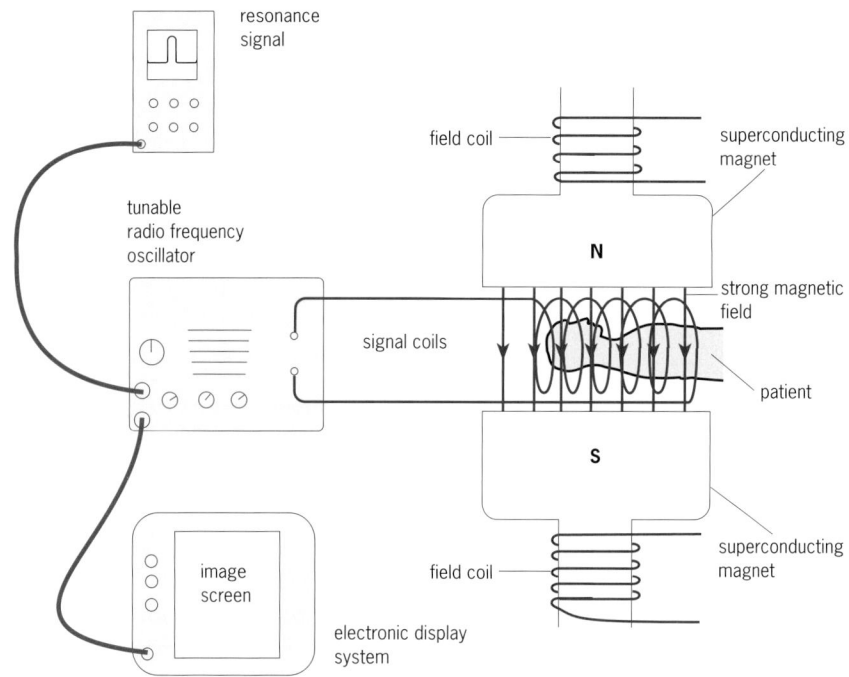

Fig 19.16 Schematic diagram of a magnetic resonance imaging system. At the correct radio frequency, the tiny hydrogen nucleus magnets oscillate (resonate), taking energy from the signal. The image is built up by scanning (not shown), using the variations in the detected signal strength

A better method is to send the RF signal as a short **pulse**. This realigns the nuclei as before, but after a time the nuclei return to the normal arrangements of their alignment in the steady magnetic field. The effect due to the pulse decays in a way similar to the decay of charge in a capacitor or of radioactive nuclei. This is characterised by a time constant called the **relaxation time**, typically about 1 second. As the precession rearrangements decay, the nuclei emit a radio signal at the same frequency as the original pulse. The character of the signal is decided by the number and distribution of the hydrogen nuclei in the tissue and is used to create the final image. The relaxation time depends on the molecule of which the hydrogen is a part – in water the relaxation time is longer than in more complex molecules, for example. This means that the decay signal is complex and carries information about the different molecules in the tissue – hence providing contrast. By changing the timing of the pulses, the signal can be better matched to the relaxation times of the different components of the tissue. In practice, the pulsing is repeated many times, and in more complex ways, so building more detail in the final image (Fig 19.17). Further improvement is produced by injecting chemicals with magnetic properties that enhance contrast.

MRI can produce images of slices of a tissue. This is done by making the steady magnetic field graded in strength from strong to weak. The strength of this field decides the resonance frequency of the precession of the nuclei, so by choosing the appropriate frequency the system can target a slice of the tissue that has that particular field strength.

Magnetic resonance imaging needs expensive equipment, but it is a particularly useful technology for probing delicate areas of the body such as the brain (Fig 19.17). This is because the energy carried by the radio signal is very small and at a frequency far from the frequencies at which molecules of the body vibrate, so it does no damage. Lower frequencies (such as those in microwave ovens) might provide information – but at the expense of cooked tissue!

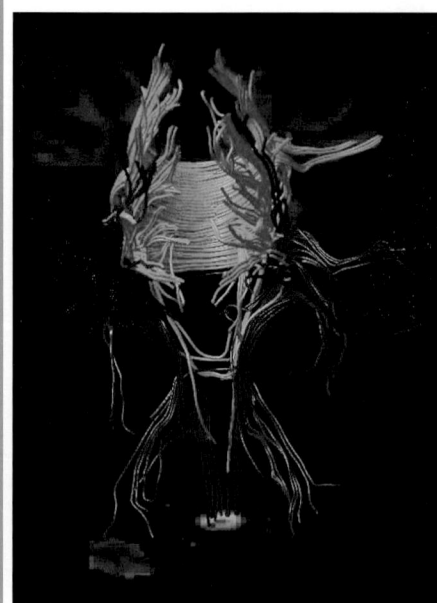

Fig 19.17 Using better computer programs MRI can even show individual brain cell paths in living tissue, and so monitor changes during ageing or illness

4 IMAGING USING LIGHT

Images can be made of the inside of hollow organs by sending a beam of light into them through optical fibres. This is the principle of the **endoscope** (Fig 19.18). There are two bundles of very narrow optical fibres. The illumination bundle carries light to the object being studied, and the image bundle carries back reflected light to provide the image (Fig 19.19). The image fibres are aligned *coherently* (Fig 19.20) so that the mosaic image formed best matches the object. This image is viewed or photographed through a magnifying eyepiece.

The bundle of fibres is in a flexible probe that is inserted into the body, for example at either end of the digestive system, or through blood vessels to view the heart. The tool aperture is used in treatment, for example, to introduce a powerful laser that can be focused on a small area of unhealthy tissue to burn it away.

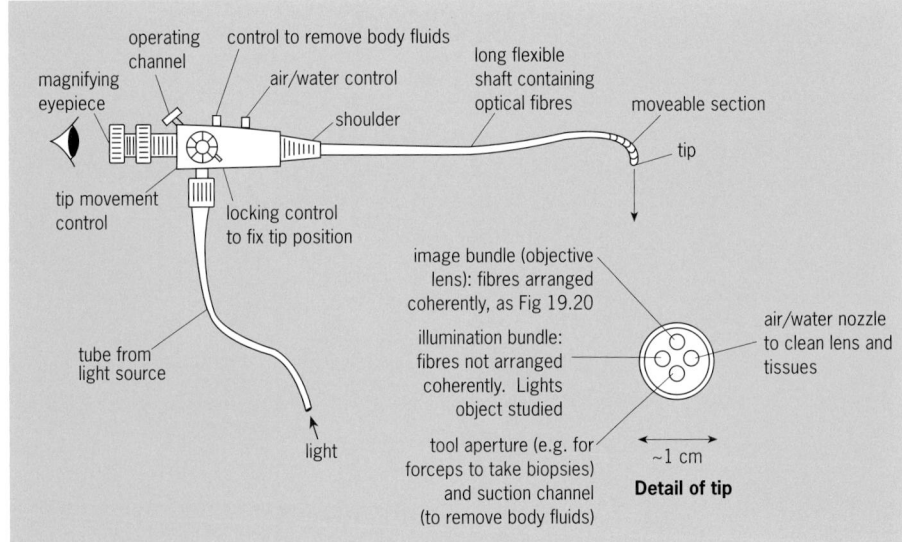

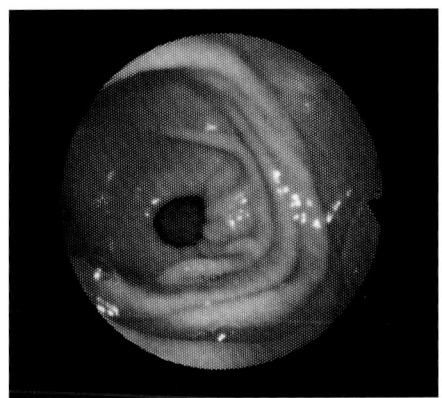

Fig 19.18 The main features of an endoscope

Fig 19.19 An image of the exit from the stomach into the duodenum, taken with an endoscope. Each tiny facet of the image corresponds to the end of an optical fibre

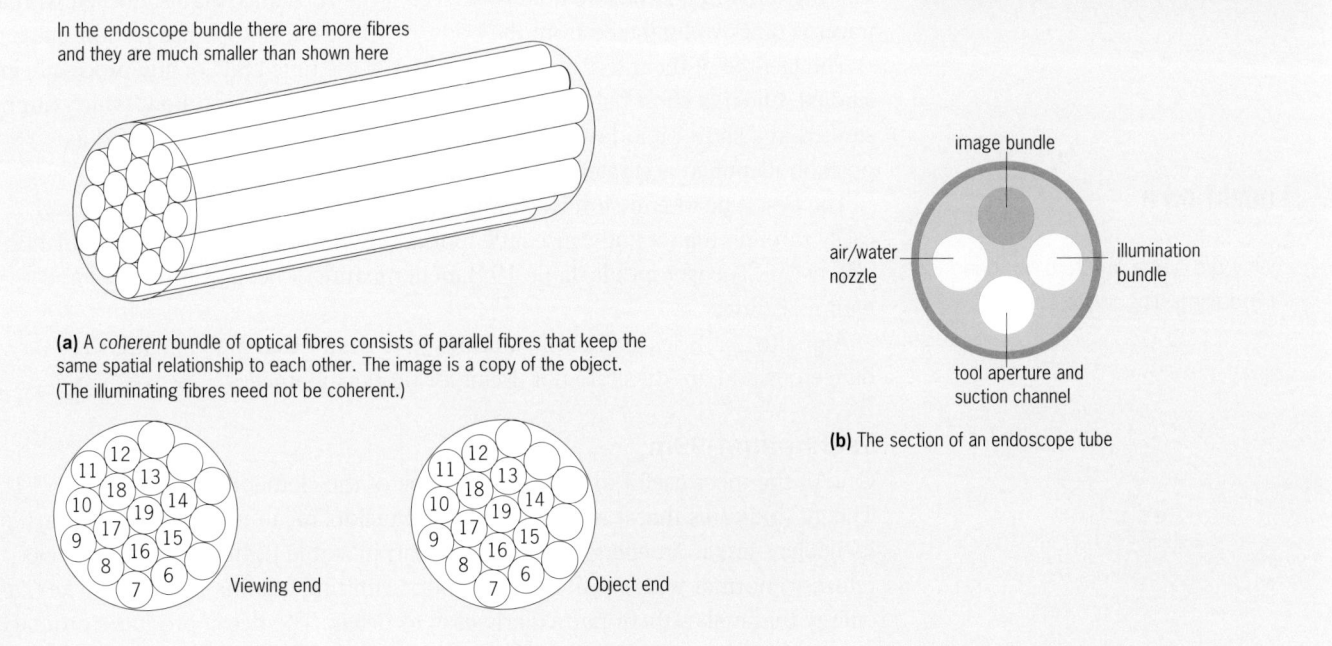

(a) A *coherent* bundle of optical fibres consists of parallel fibres that keep the same spatial relationship to each other. The image is a copy of the object. (The illuminating fibres need not be coherent.)

(b) The section of an endoscope tube

Fig 19.20 (a) Optical fibres in (b) an endoscope tube

5 IMAGING USING RADIOACTIVE TRACERS

Radioactive nuclides emit ionising radiation. This can be detected by film, by a Geiger counter or by a scintillation counter.

In diagnoses, radioactive nuclides are injected into the bloodstream and their passage through an organ is followed using one of various detection instruments.

Alternatively, specific areas can be **radiolabelled**. Biochemical processes involving a series of chemical reactions can be followed using a radioactive isotope of an element in a compound in the series. For example, the uptake of iodine in the thyroid gland is checked by using radioactive iodine.

Table 19.3 shows some of the medical uses for a range of radioactive tracers.

Table 19.3 Some radioactive tracers used in medicine

Organ/tissue	Tracers	Uses
General body composition	^{3}H, ^{24}Na, ^{42}K, ^{82}Br	Used to measure volumes of body fluids and estimate quantities of salts (e.g. of sodium, potassium, chlorine)
Blood	^{32}P, ^{51}Cr, ^{125}I, ^{131}I, ^{132}I	Used to measure volumes of blood and the different components of blood (plasma, red blood cells) and the volumes of blood in different organs. Also used to locate internal bleeding sites
Bone	^{45}Ca, ^{47}Ca, ^{85}Sr, ^{99m}Tc	Used to investigate absorption of calcium, location of bone disease and how bone metabolises minerals
Cancerous tumours	^{32}P, ^{60}Co, ^{99m}Tc, ^{131}I	Used to detect, locate and diagnose tumours; ^{60}Co is used to treat tumours
Heart and lungs	^{99m}Tc, ^{131}I, ^{133}Xe	Used to measure cardiac action: blood flow, volume and circulation. Labelled gases used in investigations of respiratory activity
Liver	^{32}P, ^{99m}Tc, ^{131}I, ^{198}Au	Used in diagnosing liver disease and disorders in hepatic circulation
Muscle	^{201}Tl	Diagnosis in organs; in particular, heart muscle
Therapy	^{32}P, ^{131}I	^{131}I used in treatment of cancerous thyroid; ^{32}P used in treatment of certain blood cancers
Thyroid	^{99m}Tc, ^{123}I, ^{125}I, ^{131}I, ^{132}I	Used to investigate thyroid function. ^{132}I is especially useful for pregnant women and for children
Brain	^{11}C, ^{13}N, ^{15}O	These emit positrons (beta$^+$) which interact with electrons to emit gamma rays in positron emission tomography (PET)

The quantity of tracer used must be as small as possible to minimise harmful ionising radiation. Exposure time is reduced if the substance that is labelled with a tracer is quickly eliminated from the body, or when the isotope has a short half-life.

The lifetime of the tracer must be matched to the time scale of any process being studied. Often, a short half-life is useful, as in monitoring blood flow, which can be studied in a short period of time. The tracer should be easy to detect and its position identified accurately.

The best type of emission is gamma (γ) radiation because gamma rays travel easily through matter and cause little ionisation. But low-energy beta (β) radiation is also useful. The isotopes in Table 19.3 are a mixture of beta, positron (β^+) and gamma emitters.

Alpha (α) particles are heavily ionising. This means that alpha emitters are very dangerous and are therefore not useful for producing images.

Technetium-99m

One of the most useful tracers is an isotope of the element **technetium**: $^{99m}_{43}$Tc. The 'm' indicates that it is a **metastable** nuclide, meaning that the nucleons in its nucleus are at an energy level higher than in stable technetium. Such nuclei return to normal with a half-life of 6 hours, emitting gamma rays of 140 keV, an energy that makes them particularly easy to detect. The decay produces ordinary technetium-99 which is a naturally occurring radioactive material but has a half-life of 216 000 years, and so it is practically stable, emitting very little radiation.

> **? QUESTION 6**
>
> 6 Why are alpha emitters not used for producing diagnostic images?

Radiation detectors in medicine

The basic methods of detecting ionising radiations are covered in Chapter 17, pages 323–324. Most have been adapted to medical diagnosis and for monitoring in radiotherapy.

A **Geiger counter** is used to measure beta radiation to detect contamination or spillage of radioactive materials. The counter is battery driven and is usually portable. It may include a warning buzzer to show when contamination has reached a dangerous level. Miniature Geiger counters are small enough (20 mm square by 2 mm) to be used inside the body.

An **ionisation chamber** is sometimes used to monitor exposure to radiation and is more accurate than the ordinary film badge described on page 398. The ionisation chamber measures the small current or charge collected when the gas inside the chamber is ionised.

Gamma radiation is of great use in medical diagnosis, since it produces very little damaging ionisation. For the same reason, it is difficult to detect with a Geiger counter or ionisation chamber. The preferred method is to use a series of **photomultiplier tubes** arranged to form a **gamma camera**.

A photomultiplier works in the following way. A gamma ray (emerging through a patient, say) reaches an ionic crystal substance, such as sodium iodide, which emits light when hit by the gamma ray: the crystal *scintillates*. Because of this effect, the gamma camera scan is called a **scintigram.** The number of light photons emitted depends upon the gamma ray's energy. The photons then hit a photocathode, a material that ejects electrons when bombarded by photons in the *photoelectric effect*. The number of electrons is multiplied using a sequence of charged metal plates called **dynodes** (see Fig 19.21). Electrons collide with the plates and have been accelerated enough to liberate secondary electrons from the plates. There may be ten dynodes, each producing four secondary electrons for each incident electron. The electron current is thus multiplied by a factor of 4^{10}, that is, by about 10^6. The whole system is called a photomultiplier tube.

The gamma camera consists of an array of photomultiplier tubes connected to a recording and display system (Fig 19.22(a)). An image is formed which matches the distribution of gamma emissions from the patient (Fig 19.22(b)).

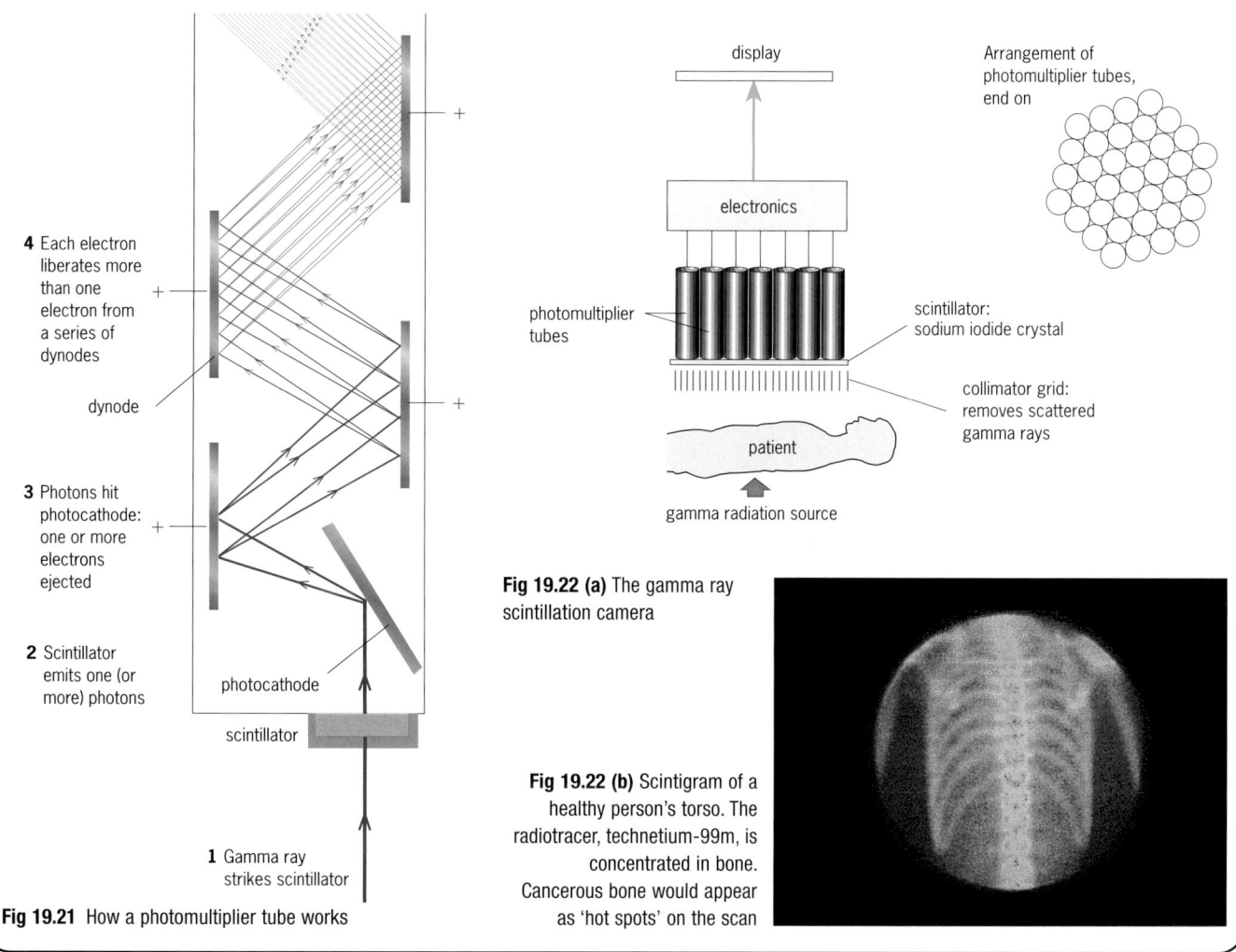

4 Each electron liberates more than one electron from a series of dynodes

dynode

3 Photons hit photocathode: one or more electrons ejected

2 Scintillator emits one (or more) photons

photocathode

scintillator

1 Gamma ray strikes scintillator

Fig 19.21 How a photomultiplier tube works

display

Arrangement of photomultiplier tubes, end on

electronics

photomultiplier tubes

scintillator: sodium iodide crystal

collimator grid: removes scattered gamma rays

patient

gamma radiation source

Fig 19.22 (a) The gamma ray scintillation camera

Fig 19.22 (b) Scintigram of a healthy person's torso. The radiotracer, technetium-99m, is concentrated in bone. Cancerous bone would appear as 'hot spots' on the scan

POSITRON EMISSION TOMOGRAPHY (PET)

Certain isotopes decay by emitting **positrons** (positive electrons), the antimatter twin of the electron – see Chapter 17, page 341. In diagnosis positron-emitting isotopes such as oxygen-15, carbon-11 and nitrogen-13 are used to label compounds that are injected into the body. The compounds chosen are those which tend to collect in specified parts of the body. Once there the emitted positrons immediately collide with electrons and they annihilate each other, emitting a pair of gamma rays. The patient is surrounded by **gamma photon detectors** (similar to the gamma camera described in the Science in Context box on the previous page). See Fig 19.23. The output from the gamma detectors is fed to a computer which uses the data to construct 'real-time' artificially coloured images on a monitor.

The technique is particularly useful for imaging such delicate structures as the brain. For example, when the brain is active the most active parts increase their use of glycogen, as a source of energy. Glycogen labelled with oxygen-15 can then show which parts of the brain are most active when doing different activities such as mathematics, reading, listening to music, etc. (Fig 19.24).

Fig 19.23 Arrangement of detectors for a PET scan. The scintillators and photomultipliers are arranged radially around the patient in a grid

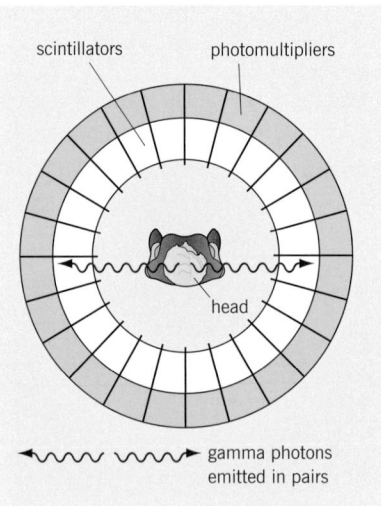

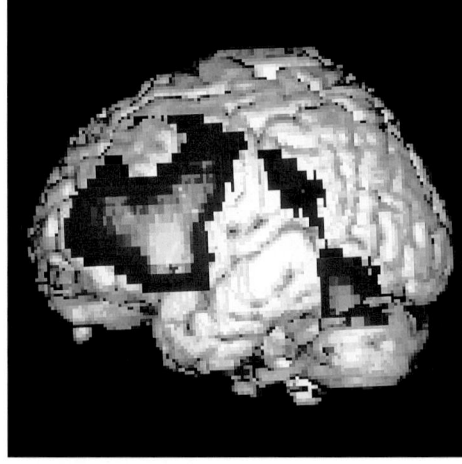

Fig 19.24 PET scan of the brain of a patient who is performing a language-generation exercise

PART B: PHYSICS IN MEDICAL TREATMENT

Many physical diagnostic processes can also be adapted to provide treatment, known as **therapy**.

6 THERAPY USING ULTRASOUND

Ultrasound is used to heat small volumes of tissue and destroy small tumours, malignant groups of (cancerous) cells. This requires more intense ultrasound beams than are used in diagnosis, but causes little or no harm to surrounding tissue when a wide beam is accurately focused, or when several beams meet at the point being treated.

Bladder stones can be shattered by the resonance effect when the ultrasound frequency matches their natural frequency of vibration. We have seen (page 384) that **cavitation**, produced when small air bubbles absorb energy and expand, can be harmful. But used carefully, cavitation also promotes wound healing and the repair of damaged bones.

7 THERAPY USING IONISING RADIATIONS

Ionising radiations can kill living cells and both **X-rays** and radiations from **radioactive nuclides** are used to treat malignant (cancerous) tumours in **radiotherapy**.

For treating tumours deep within the body, higher-energy X-ray photons are required. Lower-energy photons are more easily absorbed in soft tissue (see Table 19.2, page 386): they fail to reach deep into the body and may also cause damage to the tissues that absorb them.

High-energy X-rays are produced by using high voltages, of up to 2 MV compared with the 120 kV used to produce diagnostic X-rays. The output beam of high-voltage tubes contains a wide range of photon energies and the lower-energy photons are removed by metal filters (aluminium, tin, lead and gold). The X-rays are delivered by several beams which converge on the site of the malignant cells (Fig 19.25). This reduces the harm to surrounding tissue. Alternatively, a single beam can be used while the patient is rotated about the target point.

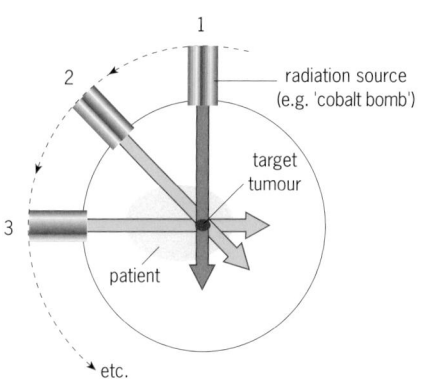

Fig 19.25 Multiple beam therapy. Short doses of radiation are given at each of a number of positions (1, 2, 3 etc.). Only the tumour receives the dose each time. The same effect can be obtained by rotating the patient about the axis of the tumour

The production of artificial isotopes

Most of the radioactive materials used in medicine do not occur naturally but are produced in nuclear fission reactors at nuclear power stations from natural, often stable, isotopes. Usually, a sample of the natural isotope is irradiated with neutrons obtained as a by-product in the reactors (see pages 344–347 for more about nuclear fission reactors).

One reaction involves the capture of a neutron by the nucleus, which then immediately emits a gamma ray and also becomes a radioactive isotope of the original nuclide. This is the n,γ reaction. For example: ordinary sodium-23 is converted to radioactive sodium-24:

$$^{23}_{11}Na + ^{1}_{0}n \rightarrow ^{24}_{11}Na + \gamma$$

In this process the element stays the same. Not all the nuclei will be changed. It is chemically impossible to separate the two isotopes, so that you cannot get a pure sample of the active isotope. Ordinary sodium is the **carrier** for radioactive sodium. Phosphorus-32 and potassium-42 are other examples of tracers that can be produced by neutron irradiation.

A pure sample of the radioactive isotope phosphorus-32 can be made using another reaction: ordinary (stable) sulphur is irradiated by neutrons and the irradiated nuclei emit protons in the n,p reaction:

$$^{32}_{16}S + ^{1}_{0}n \rightarrow ^{32}_{15}P + ^{1}_{1}p$$

The new nuclide is chemically different from the irradiated nuclide, and so it can be separated chemically. This process is also used to produce carbon-14 from nitrogen-14, and sulphur-35 from chlorine-35. These pure and entirely radioactive substances are called **carrier-free**.

Other processes include the n,α reaction, which also produces pure samples. Phosphorus-32 is an example:

$$^{35}_{17}Cl + ^{1}_{0}n \rightarrow ^{32}_{15}P + ^{4}_{2}\alpha$$

The phosphorus is then separated chemically from the chlorine. This process is also used to produce hydrogen-3 (tritium) from lithium-6.

The very useful tracer isotope metastable technetium-99m is produced when the radioactive isotope of molybdenum, $^{99}_{42}Mo$, decays by beta emission:

$$^{99}_{42}Mo \rightarrow ^{99m}_{43}Tc + ^{0}_{-1}e + \bar{v}$$

(Inside the nucleus, $n \rightarrow p + e^- + \bar{v}$.)

This process has a half-life of 67 hours, and the technetium can be produced using a 'molybdenum-cow', a column of alumina into which the molybdenum has been absorbed. When required, the technetium can be flushed out with a saline solution, leaving the insoluble molybdenum behind, although the solution must then be cleaned of aluminium and other impurities.

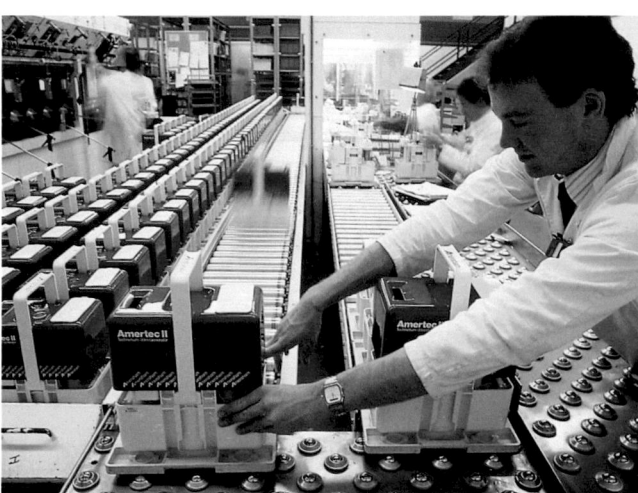

Fig 19.26 Production line for technetium-99m sources

Fig 19.27 The 'cobalt bomb' used in teletherapy. Gamma rays from the cobalt-60 source have an energy of 1 MeV (compared with X-rays which have energies of 8–10 MeV), often used to treat secondary cancers

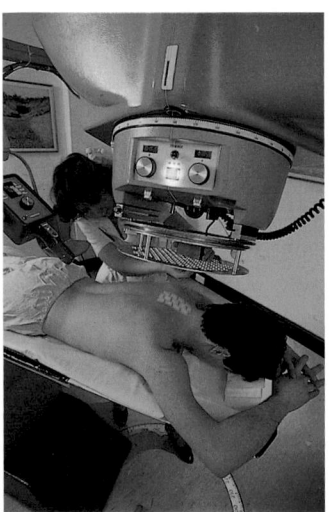

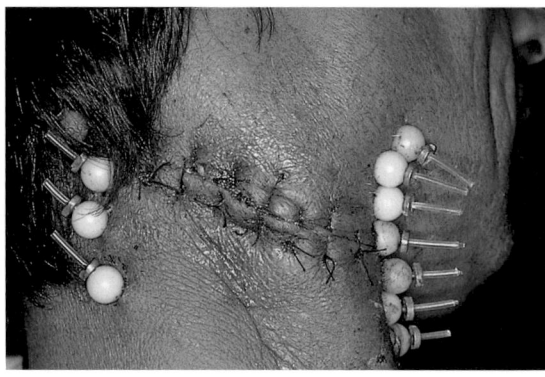

Fig 19.28 Implant needles, here containing radioactive iridium, being used to treat a lymphatic cancer. The needles may remain in place for 24 hours to one week

In some cases, the therapy requires even more energetic photons. These are actually 'artificial' gamma rays, produced in **supervoltage devices** – linear or circular electron accelerators (described in Chapter 24). These instruments accelerate electrons using potential differences between 4 MV and 42 MV, and the electrons give rise to the high-energy photons.

Teletherapy uses high-energy gamma rays from radioactive nuclides. ('Tele' means 'at a distance'.) These gamma rays bridge the gap between X-rays and photons from supervoltage devices. The nuclides commonly used are caesium-137 and cobalt-60 (Fig 19.27). Both have long enough half-lives for the output from the source to be roughly constant during a course of treatment. The source is placed in a lead-lined steel container which emits the gamma rays through a small aperture. The source has the advantage of being small, and simpler to use than X-ray machines. However, it cannot be turned off, and is a small but significant radiation hazard for the medical staff working with it.

Implanted radiation sources are also used to treat malignant tumours. These deliver a small but continuous dose of radiation at the site of the tumour, which kills the cells. 'Needles' (Fig 19.28) contain a radionuclide (such as radium-226 or gold-198). The use of small sources can produce very localised effects. This is especially important with radium which is an alpha emitter.

Unsealed sources can be injected or ingested (swallowed), and are used when they accumulate selectively in malignant tissue. For example, radioactive iodine accumulates in the thyroid gland and so is used to treat cancer of that gland. Colloidal suspensions of gold-198 target malignant cells carried in fluids lining the lungs and in the abdominal cavity.

PHYSICAL, BIOLOGICAL AND EFFECTIVE HALF-LIFE

The activity of a radioactive isotope decreases with time with an exponential decay signified by its **physical half-life** (see page 326). Here we will denote this by t_r. But when the isotope is in the body it effectively gets weaker because it is usually removed from the body by biological routes: the waste removal processes of respiration, urination and defaecation. By how much each of these processes decreases effective activity depends upon the chemistry of the isotope and the part of the body in which it is used. For example,

Dilution analysis

HOW MUCH PLASMA DOES THE PATIENT'S BLOOD CONTAIN?

Plasma is the colourless liquid in the blood that carries – amongst other things – the blood cells that make blood red. Plasma contains proteins which can be labelled with iodine isotopes such as I-131, at the rate of about one atom of the isotope per protein molecule in a sample of plasma. The most common method is to label the protein serum albumin with I-131, which has a half-life of 8 days and emits gamma rays. Labelled serum albumin in a volume v of distilled water is injected into the blood stream. A sample of *equal* activity is diluted with a known volume of distilled water and kept as a comparison standard. Fifteen minutes later a blood sample is taken and centrifuged to separate out the plasma.

The activity of this sample is compared with that of an *equal volume* (the comparison sample) in a **scintillation counter**. The gamma photons collide with atoms and energise them. As the electrons fall back to the lower state they emit light photons. These photons are few and are detected by using a **photomultiplier tube** (see the Science in Context box on page 393).

Calculating the result

Suppose the sample from the body has an activity p, and the standard sample an activity s. The value of p will be less than s because the injected sample has been diluted by the volume of plasma in the patient's body, whilst the standard sample has been diluted by a much smaller known volume of water.

A volume v of tracer is injected into a body with plasma volume V.

Suppose the original activity of the tracer was A. Then for the body sample, this is reduced by a factor v/V, so $P = A.v/V$.

For the reference sample the activity is reduced by a factor d. So $s = A/d$.

They both started off with the same activity and both have been reduced by an equal amount due to normal decay. Thus it is fair to compare the activities bearing in mind just the dilution effects. A just cancels so we have:

$$\frac{s}{p} = \frac{1}{d} \div \frac{v}{V}$$

and, as the original activities were the same:

$$\frac{s}{p} = \frac{V}{vd}$$

and:

$$V = \frac{vds}{p}$$

In practice, a number of corrections have to be made to allow for such things as background radiation. An average man of body mass 70 kg has a blood plasma volume of about 3 litres.

iodine-131 is used to label the human protein *serum albumin* (see the Science in Context passage above). I-131 has a physical half-life of 8 days, but it is removed from the body with a half-life of 21 days; this is its **biological half-life**, t_b. The **effective half-life**, t_e, is a combination of the two:

$$\frac{1}{t_e} = \frac{1}{t_r} + \frac{1}{t_b}$$

EXAMPLE

Q What is the effective half-life of technetium-99m in the body when its biological half-life is 15 hours? The half-life of Tc-99m is 6 hours.

A Inserting the data into the formula gives

$$\frac{1}{t_e} = \frac{1}{6} + \frac{1}{15}$$

$$= \frac{(5+2)}{30}$$

So $t_e = \frac{30}{7} = 4.3$ hours

8 THERAPY USING LASER TREATMENT

Laser light carries energy and can be focused into a small volume. This energy can destroy living tissue. Malignant tissue (for instance, a cancer tumour) absorbs laser radiation more strongly than healthy tissue: the output from lasers is usually pulsed and each pulse contains a definite quantity of energy. The wavelength of radiation, its intensity and the time of exposure are chosen to suit the absorption properties of the tumour.

In the eye, a detached retina can be spot-welded – *coagulated* – back on to the wall of the eyeball by laser light, as in Fig 19.29.

A laser can produce light with enough energy to cut through tissue. As it does so, it 'heat seals' blood vessels and so there is less bleeding than during scalpel surgery. With this technique, diseased parts of the liver can be removed, whereas using a knife might lead to a life-threatening loss of blood.

Darkly pigmented tissues absorb best and this is why lasers are also used to decolour skin blemishes, such as 'port wine' birth-marks, see Fig 19.30.

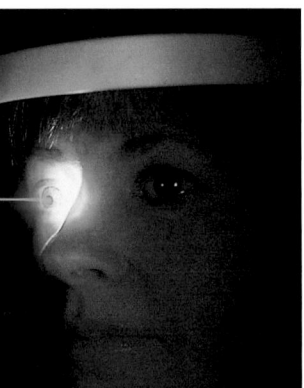

Fig 19.29 (left) Laser eye surgery

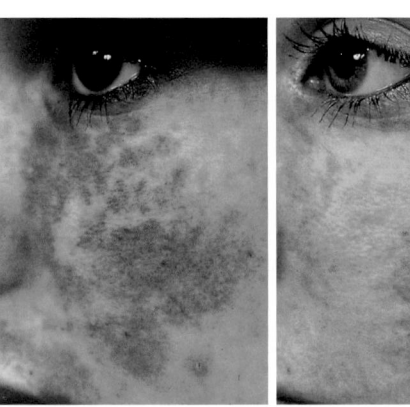

Fig 19.30 (right) A 'port wine' birth-mark: before and after laser treatment

9 MONITORING RADIATION DOSE OF HEALTH WORKERS

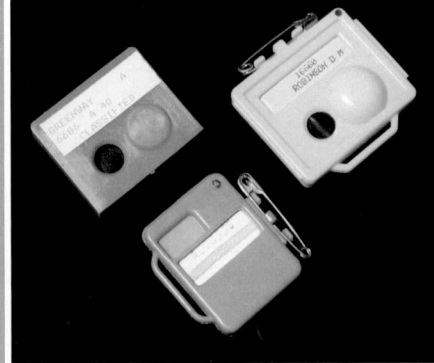

Fig 19.31 (a) Types of film badge worn by medical workers to monitor exposure to radiation

Medical workers and patients are protected as far as possible from unnecessary exposure to ionising radiation, by careful monitoring of the **radiation dose** they receive.

The most common monitoring device for medical workers is the **film badge**, see Figs 19.31(a) and (b).

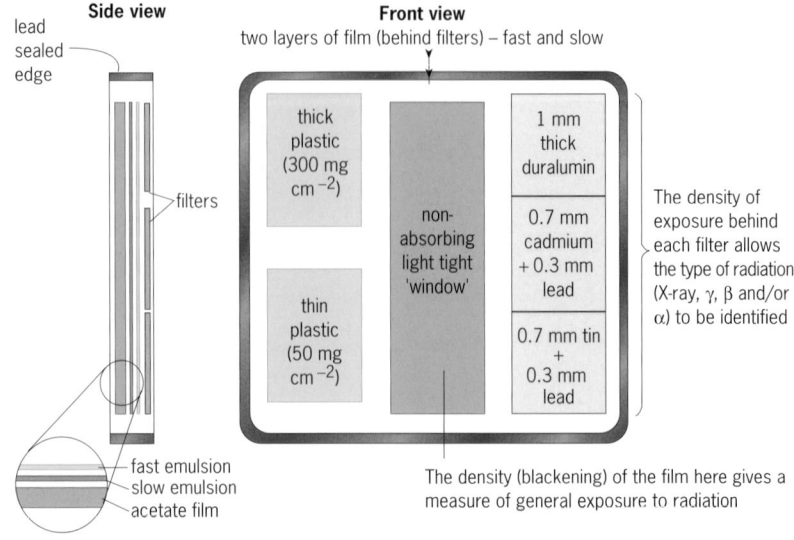

Fig 19.31 (b) A film badge dosimeter

The film badge contains two types of film: one is fast (sensitive), the other slow (less sensitive). The films are in a light-tight box and radiation enters through three windows. One is 'open': the light-tight cover does not include an absorber and lets all the radiation through. The other two areas are covered with several absorbing filters which have two functions: to indicate the *degree* (total exposure) of irradiation, and to identify the *type* of radiation:

- Irradiated film shows darkening when it is developed, and the **image density** depends on the total exposure to radiation.
- Low-energy radiation darkens the part of the film with no absorber or a low absorber in the way, but has little effect in other parts. The higher the energy of the photons and particles, the more likely they are to pass through the filters of increasing thickness or density, and so the more likely they are to reach and affect the underlying film. Blank areas show that no high-energy radiation has been received. In general, the contrast between the different areas of the film indicates the range of radiations the user has been exposed to.

The filters and film speeds are chosen to simplify analysis of the type and degree of exposure. The badges are cheap, reliable and sufficiently accurate for their monitoring task, measuring exposure dosage to about 20 per cent.

SUMMARY

After studying this chapter, you should understand and be able to describe the following main topics and techniques related to medical physics:

- How non-invasive techniques are important for diagnosis and treatment.
- That ultrasound is generated and detected by piezolectric crystals, and is used to produce images.
- How ultrasound is used for diagnosis, body scanning and blood flow measurements; there is a relationship between the frequency used and the resolution obtained.
- How X-ray beams of different types are generated and detected to produce images.
- That X-rays interact with matter: they become filtered and attenuated ($I = I_0 e^{-\mu x}$), and so may be controlled to produce images (shadowgraphs).
- That X-rays for treatment are generated by high voltages. X-rays reach the patient as multiple beams or as a single beam in rotational treatment.

- How magnetic resonance imaging is used as a non-hazardous imaging technique.
- How ingested and injected radioisotopes are used for body measurements, diagnosis and therapy.
- How medically useful radioisotopes are produced (e.g. technetium-99m) from naturally occurring isotopes.
- How the following instruments are used to detect and monitor ionising radiations and to make images: film, Geiger and scintillation counters and photomultiplier tubes.
- What safety aspects are involved in the use of ultrasound and ionising radiations.

 Practice questions for this chapter are available at www.collinseducation.co.uk/CAS

20

Condensed matter

20 CONDENSED MATTER

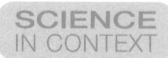

Transistors have transformed our lives

In 1948, William Shockley filed a patent for his new invention, the junction transistor. He had combined the theory of quantum mechanics from earlier in the century with the fast-growing knowledge of new materials and their uses. Ten years later, the electronic revolution began with the appearance of transistor radios and the first modern computers.

Since then, improved theory and technology have led to miniaturised devices of silicon, germanium and, more recently, gallium arsenide and other semiconductor compounds. Some devices have only a few layers of atoms, so that conduction is effectively within a two-dimensional surface. Electronic equipment containing these tiny devices fills our homes and workplaces. It is not often in history that a single technological breakthrough has had such far-reaching effects.

What development will have such an impact in the future? It could be a superconductor that operates at room temperature. With such a device, we could in theory transmit electrical power over any distance with practically no energy losses.

Physics will continue to have the potential for changing our world when applied with the right materials.

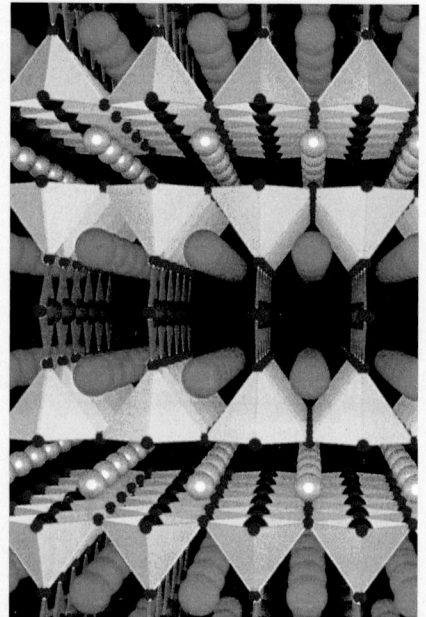

Computer-generated model of the high-temperature superconductor yttrium–barium–copper oxide, $YBa_2Cu_3O_{6.5}$. Yttrium atoms are marked in grey, barium in green, copper in blue and oxygen in red

The ideas in this chapter

You see that this chapter is titled 'Condensed matter', but it might have been called 'Solid state physics'. So why wasn't it? Partly because 'Condensed matter' is more fashionable. But, more importantly, 'solid' obscures the fact that atoms and electrons in all materials are in constant motion, and 'physics' hides the need for an input from chemistry and the Periodic Table.

In this chapter we shall look at the way quantum theory, as discussed in Chapter 16, has led to a better understanding of how materials behave and how this in its turn has led to new devices hardly imagined before the arrival of the theory. We shall look at semiconductors, semiconductor lasers, superconductors, and magnetic material.

1 ATOMS AND THEIR OUTER ELECTRONS

All atoms consist of a nucleus of protons and neutrons surrounded by electrons. A simple model of the atom has electrons moving round the nucleus in a series of orbits, like planets orbiting the Sun. But the theory of this simple model could not justify precise orbits with electrons having fixed energies. With the arrival of quantum theory, electrons could be treated as waves confined around a circular path or, more accurately, as three-dimensional waves filling the near space around the nucleus. Just as we can set up standing waves on a string attached at one end with the other end fixed (Fig 20.1), so the waves associated with the electrons can be thought of as standing waves set up as if confined within a spherical box.

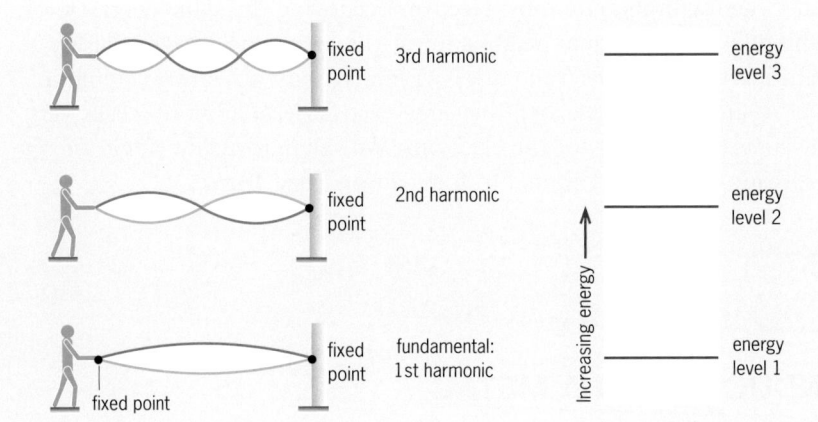

Fig 20.1 Standing waves on a string. Each mode has an associated energy which can be shown as an energy level

Many different modes of 'vibration' of the electron wave become possible, and each of these modes involves a different amount of energy. The different modes of vibration lead to a series of **energy levels**, which we can think of as like the energies associated with a series of planets moving around a central body.

The properties of an atom (excluding properties due to the nucleus) rely on the possible energy levels that the electrons can occupy in their wave-like form. So we represent the atom as a series of available electronic energy levels, see Fig 20.2(a). The number of electrons available to fill up the energy levels depends on the atomic number of the particular atom. If the atom is in its ground state, that is if it has not been excited, the electrons fill the levels one by one, starting from the bottom level. The bottom level corresponds to the level that, on average, is nearest to the nucleus. (If we go back to thinking of the electron as a particle, then it moves around very rapidly and we cannot be sure where it is at any one time, but we can say some on average are nearer to the nucleus than others.) Only two electrons can occupy each level; this comes from quantum theory. Even these two electrons themselves must have different properties. We can imagine them as spinning tops: the two electrons in any single energy level must spin in opposite directions. This is shown by tops spinning upright and upside-down in Fig 20.2(b). We show two tops representing two electrons filling the lowest level, one top representing an electron partially filling the second level, and then empty levels.

When atoms come together to form compounds, it is the outer **valence** electrons in the highest filled energy levels that interact. We can picture that above this are empty levels and below there are inner electrons which are more tightly bound (Fig 20.3). If two identical atoms are brought very close

REMEMBER THIS

It requires slightly different amounts of energy to set up the different modes of vibration of a string.

? QUESTION 1

1   Standing waves are set up in a string of length 4 m. Calculate the wavelengths of the first four harmonics. Show that they correspond to lengths of 8/n metres, where n is an integer.

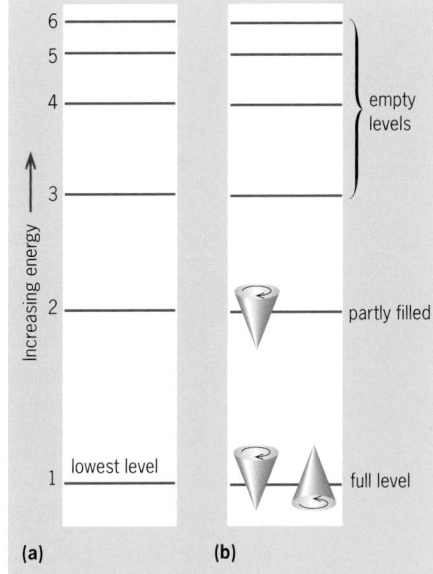

Fig 20.2 (a) Available electron energy levels in an atom
(b) Electrons with spin occupying two of the levels. Electrons are represented by tops spinning upright or upside-down

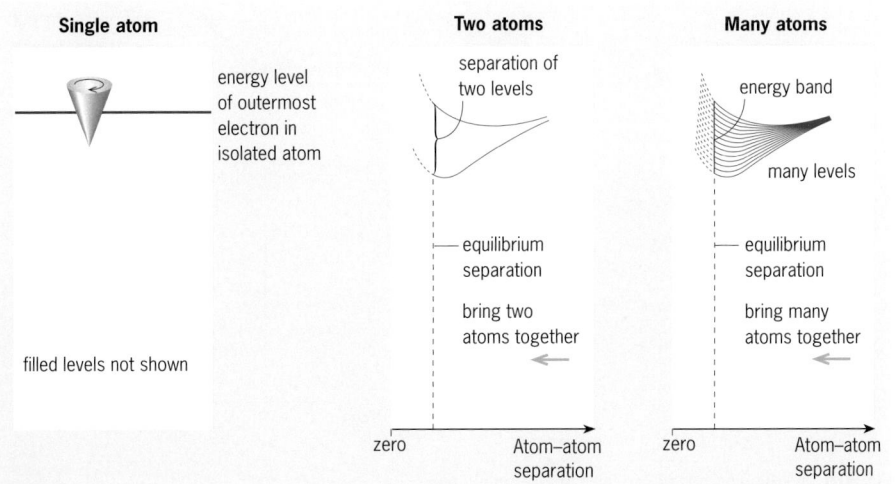

Fig 20.3 Creating electron energy bands by bringing atoms close together

together, each with its outermost electron occupying the same energy level, then the two levels of equal height split in value, producing very slightly different levels for the electrons to sit within. When we bring a very large number of atoms together, then the same very large number of levels, very closely spaced, will exist for the electrons. We say that such a single energy level spreads out (in magnitude) to form an **energy band**.

2 METALS, INSULATORS AND SEMICONDUCTORS

CONDUCTION IN A METAL

Conduction in a metal arises because free electrons can circulate among a lattice of ions (Fig 20.4). The ions are the original atoms minus their 'freed' outer electrons which belong to no particular atom. There may be more than one outer electron per atom; it would be two for an atom of an element from Group 2 of the **Periodic Table** (see page 331).

The electrons move very fast: their speed is about 10^5 m s^{-1}. But their velocities are in all different directions so the electrons make no net progress in one direction along a conductor. However, when an e.m.f. is applied to the ends of a metal conductor, the electrons *do* move slowly round the circuit, forming a current. We say *slowly* as they move with a **drift velocity** which is typically 10^{-5} m s^{-1} but can vary by orders of magnitude depending on the cross-sectional area of the conductor and the current carried.

This model fits our band model. The electrons in the current are moving within an energy band. Just as people in a crowd cannot move around unless there is an area to move into, so electrons cannot move around within the energy bands unless there is a vacant *energy* space in which to move. If all energy states are filled, the electrons cannot change their energy.

To move round a circuit easily, an electron needs to be able to move within the energy bands as well as spatially through the material. So for good conduction in the metal, it is best to have a large number of filled and a large number of unfilled energy states. This can easily happen if *filled* and *unfilled* levels in isolated atoms spread apart and start to overlap when the atoms are brought close together (Fig 20.5). Below these overlapping levels, there are likely to be other completely filled levels. The number of levels depends on where the atoms are in the Periodic Table.

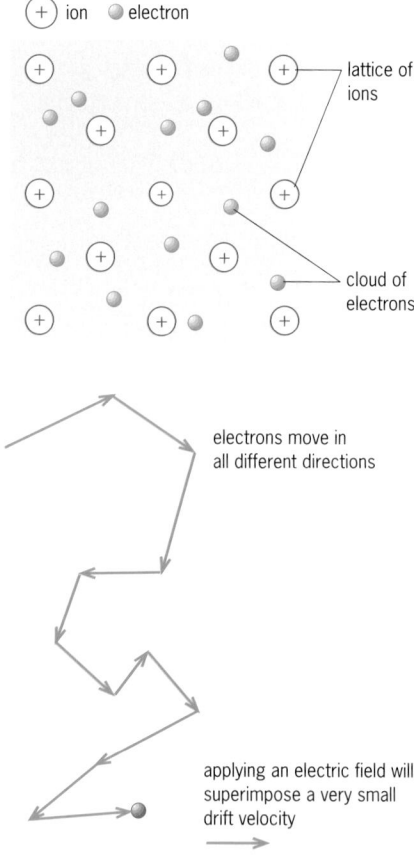

Fig 20.4 A metal consists of electrons dispersed and moving freely within a lattice of ions. If an e.m.f. is applied, the electrons drift slowly round the circuit

? **QUESTIONS 2–3**

2 Briefly, explain electronic differences between atoms from different columns of the Periodic Table.

3 Assume that there is an electrical circuit around your room and that it includes a light bulb. Estimate how long, on average, it will take for a particular electron to complete the circuit from the moment you switch on. Approximately what total distance will the electron have travelled during this time? Why does the light go on instantaneously?

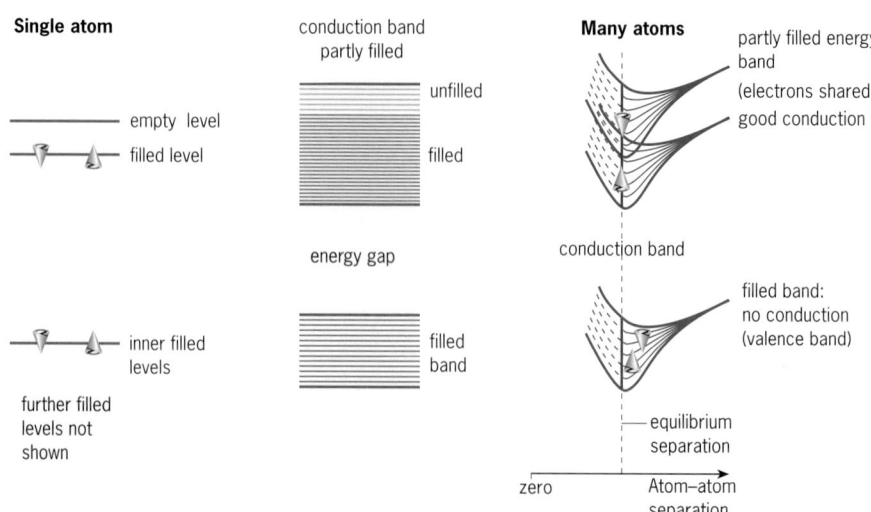

Fig 20.5 Overlapping bands can lead to incomplete filling

Now we have built up a model for the metal in which we have a lower filled band, a large energy gap where no electrons can exist, and the partially filled band in which the electrons can move around, independent of any particular atom.

When the metal is heated, the electrons go faster, but only by a very small fraction of their initial speed. Meanwhile, the ions also warm up and vibrate with larger and larger amplitude. The circulating electrons make more collisions with the ions (the lattice) and are slowed down. So the conductivity of a metal decreases as the temperature increases (Fig 20.6).

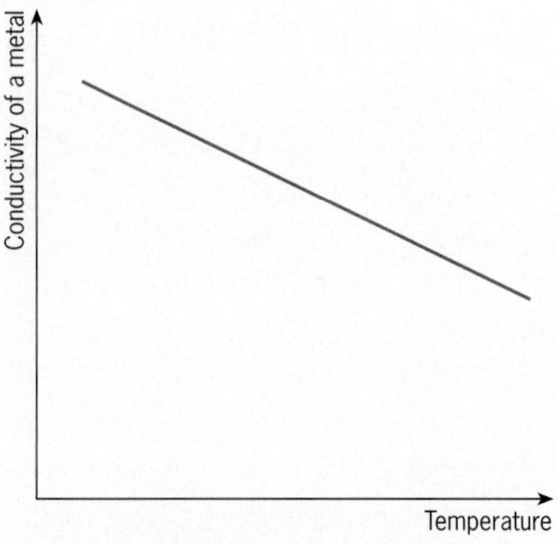

CONDUCTION IN AN INSULATOR

An **insulator** has a lower, *filled* electron band, a bandgap that is quite large, and then another band which is empty, as in Fig 20.7(a). The electrons cannot move around in the filled band because there are no vacant energy states to move to, nor can electrons jump the gap to the unfilled band. Consequently the insulator has a very low electrical conductivity. Even if we heat the insulator, we cannot excite electrons to move from the filled to the unfilled band because it requires too large an energy jump.

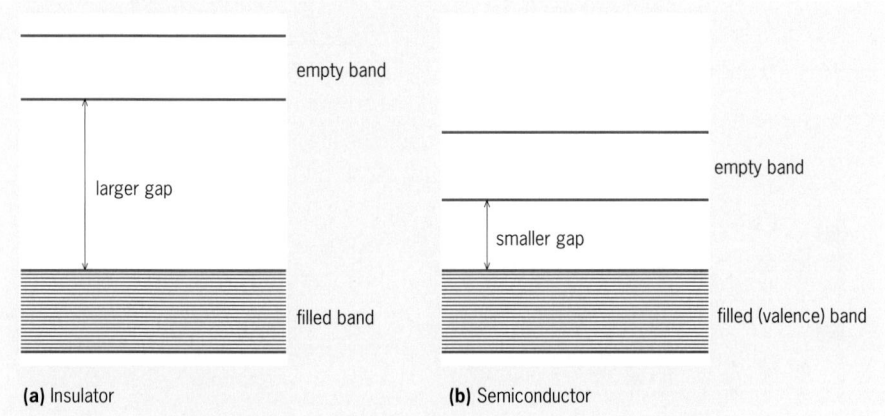

(a) Insulator **(b)** Semiconductor

Fig 20.6 Variation of conductivity of a metal with temperature

Fig 20.7 Band structure of
(a) an insulator,
(b) a semiconductor at 0 K

CONDUCTION IN A PURE SEMICONDUCTOR

Semiconductors have had a massive impact on the design and usefulness of electronic equipment. Computers are amongst the best known and most useful equipment that contain them. Computers are only of a manageable size and speed of operation because semiconductor devices can be made very small and so electrons have to move only tiny distances. As the name suggests, a semiconductor carries current less easily than a metal, but much better than an insulator. This is because it contains free charges which carry current, but fewer than in a metal.

At 0 K, the band structure of a semiconductor looks similar to that of an insulator; filled band, bandgap and unfilled band, as in Fig 20.7(b). The difference between the semiconductor and the insulator is that the semiconductor's bandgap is small. Electrons in the filled band require only a little energy to excite them into the higher band.

We can estimate whether electrons will be excited thermally by comparing the energy required to jump up through the energy gap with the magnitude of kT where k is Boltzmann's constant and T is the temperature of the semiconductor measured in kelvin. Typically, the bandgap energy is quite a lot larger than kT, but sufficiently small for the thermal energy to excite a significant number of electrons to make the jump (see the How Science Works passage overleaf). Once electrons are excited into the upper band, they can move freely and so the semiconductor can carry electricity. This upper band is called the **conduction band**.

Conduction electrons in an intrinsic semiconductor

Suppose an electron needs energy E to escape from its surroundings, and that this energy is supplied thermally. The temperature T (in kelvin) multiplied by the Boltzmann constant k indicates the amount of energy available to the electron. It can be shown that the number of electrons which acquire enough energy E to jump the energy gap is proportional to $e^{-E/kT}$.

In fact, for N atoms, each with an electron available to break free, the number of electrons n which actually do so is given by:

$$n = N\,e^{-E/kT}$$

The expression $e^{-E/kT}$, which gives the ratio of the number of electrons excited to the total number of existing electrons available for excitation, is called the **Boltzmann factor** and this same factor exists in other examples of thermal activation. Another common example of a process where this factor comes in is diffusion, where an atom or ion needs to be excited above an energy barrier before it can jump to an adjacent site.

The number n rises rapidly as the temperature T increases (Fig 20.8). It is these electrons which reach the conduction band and allow electrical conduction in a semiconductor. The resistance of a semiconductor decreases as the number of carriers increases: double the number of carriers, and the resistance halves, and so on. It is not difficult to see that the resistance will vary proportionally to $e^{E/kT}$.

Additionally, by escaping from the lower valence band, each electron leaves behind a gap called a 'hole'. We can liken this effect to a passenger moving from a bus queue on to the bus. In the queue, as a person leaves, the rest move up, one by one, to fill the gap left by the previous person. You will see a gap move down the queue in the opposite direction to the actual movement of the passengers (Fig 20.9). Similarly, in the valence band of the semiconductor, once a gap or hole is left, an adjacent electron can jump into it. Applying an e.m.f. to the semiconductor makes electrons jump like this. With repeated jumps of electrons, one after another, holes move through the semiconductor in the opposite direction to the electrons.

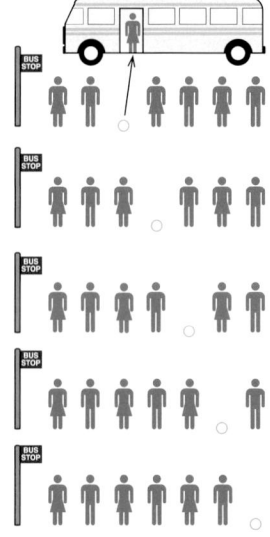

Fig 20.9 The movement of people to fill a space in a bus queue is similar to the movement of electrons to fill a hole in the valence band of a semiconductor

Electrons move under the influence of the e.m.f. towards the positive potential (corresponding to the bus-stop sign), while the holes in the valence band move the opposite way. It is as if the holes have a positive charge. So we say that such a semiconductor has electrons in the conduction band and holes in the valence band and that both act as

carriers of charge. The electrons move against the electric field as they have negative charge, the holes move with the field as they are of positive charge.

We get the overall conductivity by adding together the contributions from both types of charge. Their contributions must be added as, although they have opposite charge, they also move in opposite directions. When electrons that are excited into the conduction band leave behind an equal number of holes, we describe the semiconductor as intrinsic and the conduction as intrinsic conduction.

Because far fewer charges move in a semiconductor than in a metal, a semiconductor has a lower electrical conductivity. This lower conductivity is slightly offset by the 'mobility' of the electrons (their ability to move in an applied e.m.f.), which is much higher for a semiconductor than for a metal: the drift velocity of semiconductor electrons is usually many metres per second.

As the temperature of a semiconductor is increased, the mobility of the electrons (and the holes) decreases, just as it does in a metal. But the increased temperature enables more electrons to be excited from the valence to the conduction band. This effect happens rapidly as the temperature effect is exponential and it swamps any variation of the mobility. Overall, as temperature rises, the increased number of carriers increases the conductivity of the semiconductor (Fig 20.10).

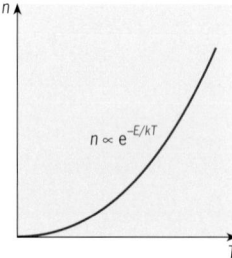

Fig 20.8 How the number of electrons moving into the conduction band varies with temperature

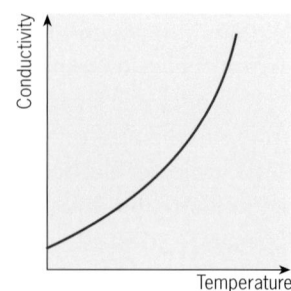

Fig 20.10 Variation of conductivity of an intrinsic semiconductor with temperature

EXAMPLES OF SEMICONDUCTOR MATERIALS

Typical semiconductor materials are the elements silicon (Fig 20.11(a)) and germanium, with atoms in a structure like that of diamond (page 151). The atoms are *covalently* bonded, meaning that adjacent atoms *share* outer electrons and come from Group 4 of the Periodic Table (see page 331).

For silicon the bandgap is 1.1 eV and for germanium it is 0.67 eV. kT measured in eV at room temperature is 0.026 eV, that is, $(8.6 \times 10^{-5} \times 300)$ eV.

Another commonly used semiconductor material is the compound gallium arsenide (Fig 20.11(b)), with a bandgap of 1.43 eV. Gallium is from Group 3 and arsenic from Group 5. The atoms take up alternate sites in the diamond structure and are also covalently bonded: adjacent atoms share electrons (unlike ions which lose or gain electrons).

Compound semiconductors are similar in behaviour to single-element conductors. For example, although gallium arsenide is a more complicated material to prepare and to use than single-element semiconductors, it is popular. The reason is that the electrons move through gallium arsenide very much faster than they do in silicon or germanium, so devices operate more rapidly. Other, less used, semiconductor materials contain atoms of three different elements.

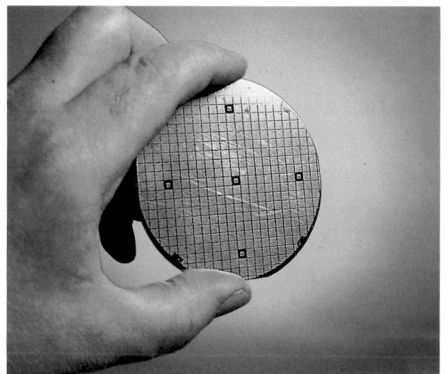

Fig 20.11(a) A silicon sheet: each square is doped (see page 408) and becomes an integrated circuit

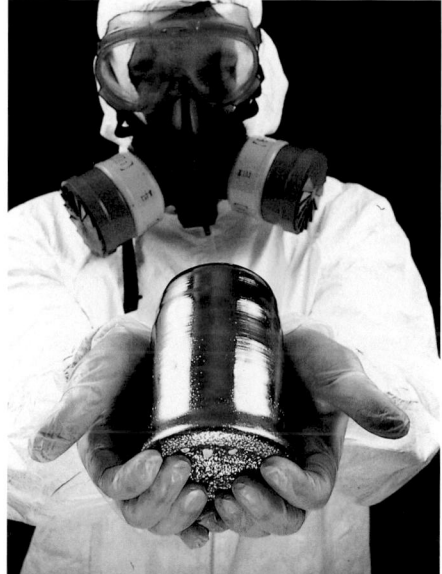

Fig 20.11(b) Gallium metal rods and arsenic nuggets are fused at high temperature to form this lump of gallium arsenide

By altering the proportions of elements and compounds, semiconductors can be made with the right bandgaps for their use. For example, semiconductors used in infrared cameras can be made to detect light of infrared frequency. The incoming photons of light each have an energy equal to the semiconductor bandgap energy and are absorbed as they excite electrons up across the gap. In reverse, light is emitted by semiconductor lasers that are designed to produce light of a particular frequency and colour. They are used in CD players and for optical communications.

THERMISTORS AND LIGHT-DEPENDENT RESISTORS

Thermistors detect variations in temperature and so are rather like thermometers, while LDRs, light-dependent resistors, detect variations in light level. Varying the temperature of thermistors changes the number of available electrons for conduction, while incoming light alters the number in LDRs.

A thermistor is made of a semiconductor material such as nickel oxide. Its resistance very rapidly decreases exponentially (not linearly) as its temperature rises because the number of free carriers increases exponentially. As we have

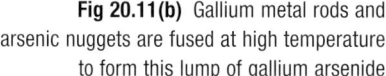

REMEMBER THIS

The energy required to excite electrons from the valence to the conduction band is always stated in eV rather than in J.

? QUESTIONS 4–5

4 What is 1 eV when measured in J?

5 Estimate the fraction of electrons which are excited from an energy band through an energy gap of 1.1 eV at a temperature of 300 K. What is the fraction at 600 K?

seen, increasing the temperature, and hence thermal energy, excites more electrons into the conduction band. Because of this rapid change of their resistance, thermistors are useful for measuring temperature (see page 257).

A typical variation of resistance for a thermistor is from 4.7 kΩ at room temperature to 270 Ω at 100 °C. So thermistors are used in electronic circuits where big changes of output signal are required for small variations in temperature. For example, a thermistor can be used with a computer to monitor a process that produces thermal energy, such as a chemical reaction. Being sensitive to a tiny energy change, the thermistor gives rise to a large input signal that is used to record and control the process.

LDRs are usually made of cadmium sulphide which has a bandgap of 2.6 eV – larger than the bandgap for a typical semiconductor. For LDRs, it is photons of light which provide the energy to excite the electrons from the valence into the conduction band. The dark resistance of an LDR is typically 1 MΩ, and this decreases with increasing light intensity to 1 kΩ or less, depending on the magnitude of intensity. LDRs are also easily incorporated into electronic circuits (page 183).

CONDUCTION IN A DOPED SEMICONDUCTOR

The precise conducting properties of semiconductors used for transistors (see page 409), thermistors and LDRs are controlled by adding very small amounts of 'impurity' which is a very tiny quantity of another element. The process of adding the impurity is called **doping** and the extra material is the **dopant**. Dopant atoms go into positions in the original semiconductor lattice to replace a few of the atoms of the pure material. Their size must be similar to the size of the atoms they are displacing. Assuming we start with a Group 4 semiconductor such as silicon, then we choose either a Group 3 element such as boron or a Group 5 element such as arsenic or phosphorus. Choosing to replace with a Group 3 or a Group 5 element leads to quite different changes.

Arsenic-doped silicon

Starting with a lattice of silicon atoms as in Fig 20.12(a), each atom shares its outer four electrons with four other atoms and shares a further four electrons from its neighbours to establish a filled shell of eight electrons. Conductivity occurs when some of the electrons are excited thermally into the conduction band. If we now replace a few silicon atoms with arsenic, each arsenic atom brings with it an *extra* electron, as in Fig 20.12(b). This extra electron in arsenic is easily excited into the conduction band. For the bulk material, the band structure diagram on the right of Fig 20.12(b) shows these extra arsenic electrons within the energy band diagram just below the conduction band.

? **QUESTION 6**

6 Sketch the variation of resistance of a thermistor with temperature.

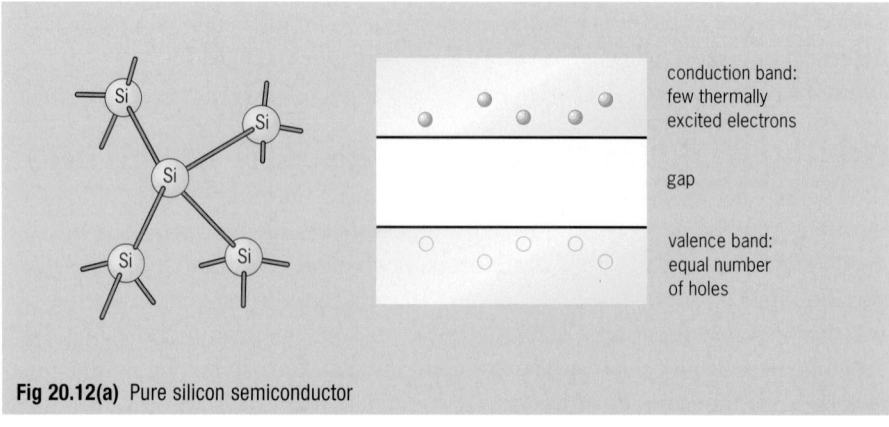

conduction band: few thermally excited electrons

gap

valence band: equal number of holes

Fig 20.12(a) Pure silicon semiconductor

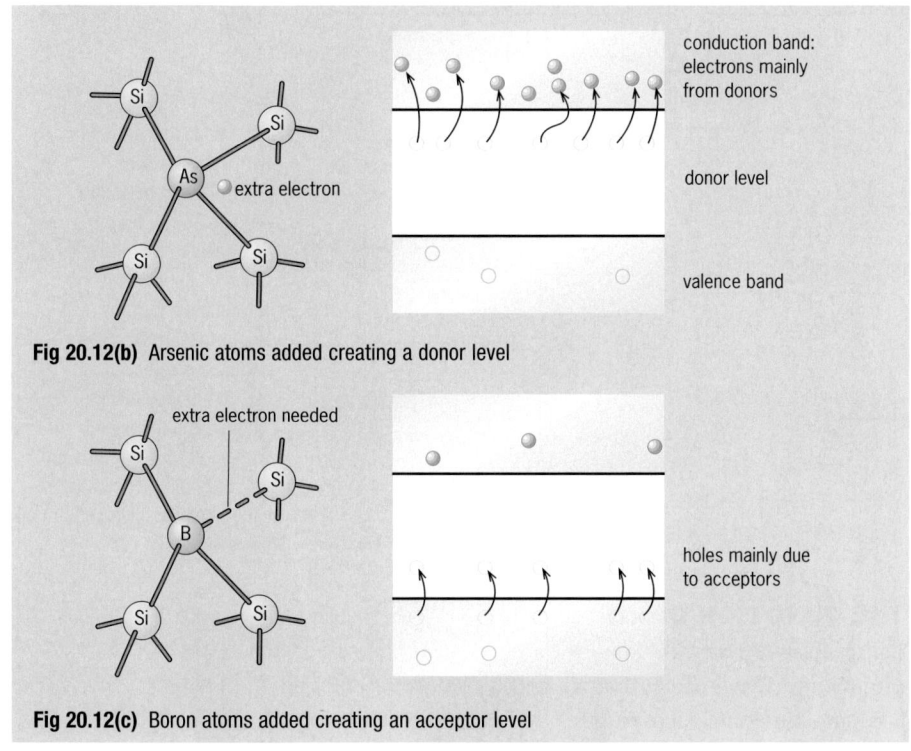

Fig 20.12(b) Arsenic atoms added creating a donor level

Fig 20.12(c) Boron atoms added creating an acceptor level

? QUESTION 7

7 How would you expect the conductivity to vary with temperature for an extrinsic n-type semiconductor in which the carrier concentration is due to donors? (Remember that the conductivity will depend on the carrier concentration and the carrier mobility.)

✔ REMEMBER THIS
The Hall effect

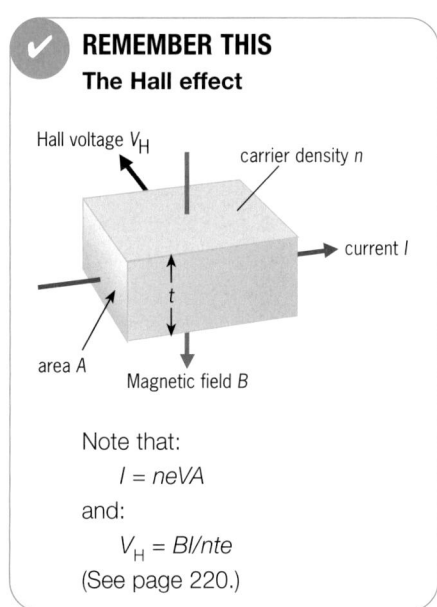

Note that:

$$I = neVA$$

and:

$$V_H = BI/nte$$

(See page 220.)

? QUESTION 8

8 Explain how the Hall voltage can tell us which type of carrier exists in an extrinsic semiconductor.

At room temperature they are thermally excited up into the conduction band. By controlling the number of dopant atoms we can control the number of current-carrying electrons and hence the conductivity. The dopant atoms are referred to as **donors** because they are giving up electrons and the semiconductor is called **n-type** because it has *negative*-type carriers.

Boron-doped silicon

We can instead add boron atoms as a dopant. They have one electron *less* than the silicon atoms and the lattice can easily take up electrons from the valence band. This leaves holes in the valence band to carry current. The boron atoms are called **acceptors** as they are taking up electrons and the semiconductor is called **p-type** (*positive* carriers). As in Fig 20.12(c), we represent the acceptors on the energy band diagram at a level just above the valence band.

A semiconductor in which the conduction is dominated either by electrons from donor atoms or by holes from acceptor atoms is called an **extrinsic** semiconductor.

We can either have an *n-type* semiconductor in which the carriers are predominantly electrons or a *p-type* semiconductor in which the carriers are holes. For either case, we can find out the number of carriers by measuring the Hall voltage (see page 219).

THE TRANSISTOR

The transistor was invented in 1951 by John Bardeen, Walter Brattain and William Shockley, at the Bell Research Laboratories in the USA; it is used very widely as a controllable switch.

The **pnp transistor** consists of a thin layer of n-type material sandwiched between two thicker regions of p-type material. The transistor turns on and controls a large current through one of a pair of **pn junctions** (see the Stretch and Challenge passage overleaf) by passing a small current through the other. Transistors are particularly suited for controlling the on–off binary logic used in computers. They are available as discrete circuit components or as parts of integrated circuits.

The pn junction

A pn junction consists of a piece of p-type semiconductor joined to a piece of n-type semiconductor. The lattice of atoms in which the p-type and n-type impurities are inserted is often the same material. Excess holes exist in the p-type material and extra electrons in the n-type material and it is these which can carry current.

Very close to the junction, the holes and electrons cancel each other out, so that there are very few free carriers here. This region is called the depletion layer (Fig 20.13). Because there is now a shortage of holes on the p side of the junction, it is as if there is a negative charge there relative to the rest of the material, and the shortage of electrons on the n side makes this a positively charged region. This gives rise to a contact potential (Fig 20.14) maintained by the distribution of holes and electrons; there are no charge carriers, so there is no current.

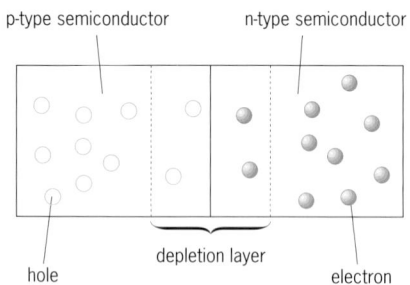

Fig 20.13 A pn junction showing the depletion layer

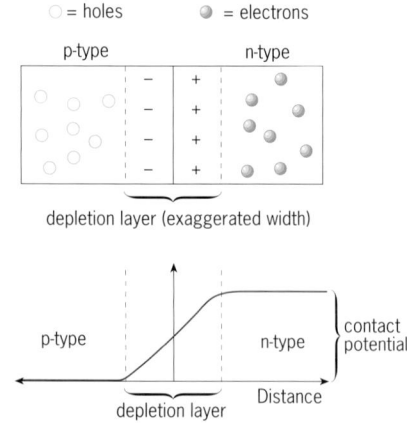

Fig 20.14 The contact potential across the depletion layer

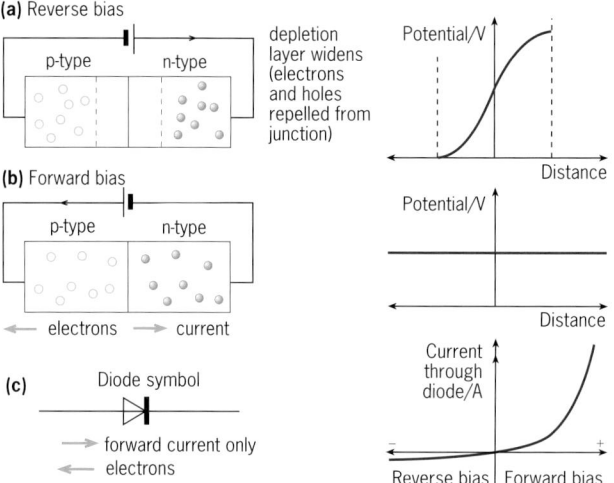

Fig 20.15 A pn junction in reverse and forward bias. **(a)** In reverse bias, electrons and holes are attracted away from the junction and there is a large potential to be overcome, preventing a current. **(b)** In forward bias, the potential is removed. **(c)** The junction diode symbol, and the overall variation of current through the diode as the potential is varied both positive and negative

THE JUNCTION DIODE

Let us apply a *reverse bias* to the pn junction. This means that we apply a voltage difference across the junction with a positive voltage going to the n-type side and a negative voltage to the p-type side. This increases the contact potential, see Fig 20.15(a), and attracts even more free carriers (both holes and electrons) away from the contact region.

If we apply the voltage difference the other way round, in *forward bias*, the applied potential difference will cancel the contact potential, see Fig 20.15(b). The depletion layer is narrowed and then removed and the pn junction conducts normally. Hence the junction passes current in forward bias but not reverse bias, see Fig 20.15(c), and can be used as a junction diode for rectification, meaning that current is allowed to pass in one direction only (as described on page 241).

THE LIGHT-EMITTING DIODE

A light-emitting diode (LED) is made from a junction of two semiconductors, gallium phosphide and gallium arsenide. A current passes one way only, as in an ordinary junction diode, but when current passes through the junction light is emitted as electrons drop between energy levels.

Red, yellow and green LEDs have been in use for some time, but more recently blue LEDs have become practicable. For blue light ($\lambda = 450$ nm), a forward voltage drop across the junction of 2.8 V is needed. Gallium nitride (GaN) LEDs have been developed with forward voltages of 3.4 eV ($\lambda = 360$ nm) and aluminium nitride (AlN) LEDs with ultraviolet outputs (6.2 eV).

LEDs can now be made as bright as a 500 W traffic light while using just one-tenth of the energy. They are taking over from battery-thirsty filament bulbs in, for example, bicycle lamps; and, because they respond (light up) more quickly, they are ideally suitable for car stoplights. Ultraviolet LEDs could also replace the gas discharge tubes used in fluorescent lighting.

? QUESTIONS 9–10

9 Show that for an LED to emit yellow light ($\lambda = 600$ nm), electrons of charge e must fall through a voltage difference of 2.0 V. (Remember, the energy of a photon is hf.)

10 A car stoplight becomes visible some time after the brakes have been put on. A bright red LED lights up 0.25 s faster than a filament lamp. Make a quantitative estimate of the effect this advantage has in traffic travelling at motorway speed.

3 SEMICONDUCTOR LASERS

We have discussed how semiconductor material can be produced by doping and how electrons can be excited into a higher energy level – into the conduction band. This usually happens because the bandgap is small and the electrons are thermally excited. A very extensive application of semiconductors is now to produce lasers – devices to produce coherent light (see page 296). For instance, semiconductor lasers are used in CD players and DVD readers to read off the digital data on the discs and are used for reading barcode labels in most supermarkets (see Fig 20.17). They have the advantages of being small, cheap, highly reliable and efficient. For these semiconductors to act as lasers, there has to be a method of controlling the electron populations in higher energy levels.

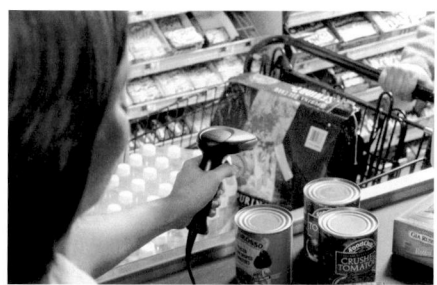

Fig 20.16 Use of a laser scanner in a supermarket

How a laser works

A laser requires electrons to fall in large numbers between an upper and a lower energy level such that a photon of a precise energy and frequency is emitted by each. In a semiconductor laser this occurs in a thin layer, and much of the emitted light is reflected back and forth between the two ends, where mirrors are positioned, as this light causes (stimulates) further electrons to drop spontaneously between the levels (Fig 20.18(a), overleaf). This sets up an intense beam of photons reflected back and forth. One of the mirrors is made to be a total mirror, but the other is made to be only partially reflecting so that some light gets through as a precise monochromatic beam in which the waves of light are in phase. This beam is the laser light.

Population inversion

It is easy to realise that it is necessary to have more electrons in the upper level (level 2) than in the lower level (level 1) or else the stimulation will not occur in the required direction. If the number of electrons in level 2 is N_2 and in level 1 is N_1, N_2 needs to be greater than N_1. This is called **population inversion**. However, the number of electrons in each level would normally be governed by the Boltzmann expression (page 406) and the higher level would be expected to contain fewer electrons than the lower level. Some way must therefore be found to increase the number in the higher level and, as this is analogous to filling a water reservoir at a higher level, this is referred to as **pumping**.

As rather a lot of electrons must be excited between the levels, when there are only two levels, it is best to keep up the population of the higher level at the required steady level by filling it from an even higher level. There will be a steady fall of electrons from this third level. Meanwhile, the population of the third level is kept up by the actual pumping, usually the application of a high electric potential difference – a voltage that can supply enough energy to take electrons from the lowest (ground) level up to the third level (Fig 20.18(b)). The principles are the same whether we are talking about levels in semiconductor lasers or in gas lasers but, in the case of semiconductor lasers, high potential difference means only about 3 V.

As electrons fall from our original level 2 to our level 1, the lower level 1 will be filling up. This is not satisfactory and we need to empty it steadily.

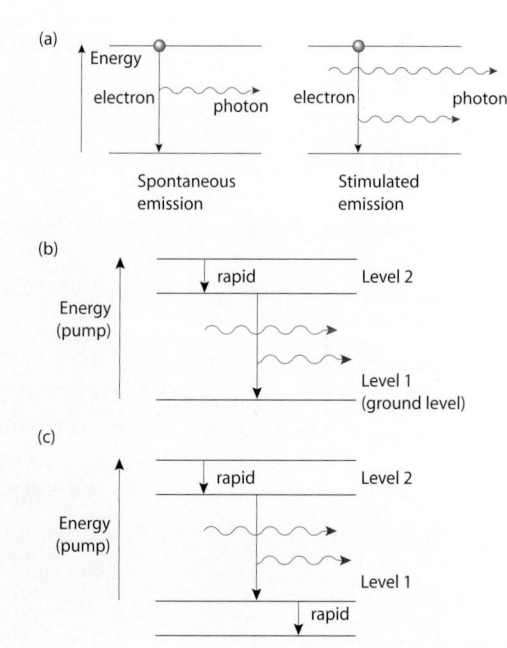

Fig 20.17 Types of emission between levels
(a) Spontaneous and stimulated emissions compared
(b) Stimulated emission in three-level laser
(c) Stimulated emission in four-level laser

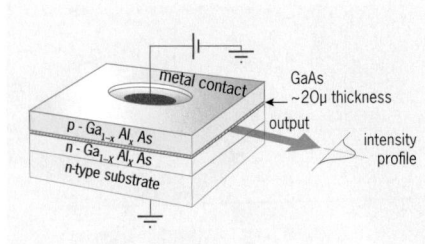

Fig 20.18 Semiconductor laser diode

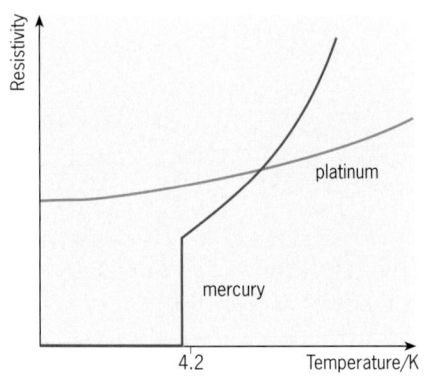

Fig 20.19 Resistivity of platinum and mercury at very low temperatures

? **QUESTION 11**

11   What would happen if the temperature suddenly went up or the current density increased significantly through the superconducting coils of the magnet in a magnetic resonance imager?

This is done by having a lower energy level, a fourth level, a bit below our original ground level (Fig 20.18(c)) and we excite from this level. We arrange for the filling of level 2 to be fast compared with the movement between levels 2 and level 1, and similarly the emptying of level 1, such that the population ratio N_2/N_1 (>1) is maintained. We now have a **four-level laser**.

Structure of a semiconductor laser

Fig 20.19 shows the basic structure of a semiconductor laser diode. For example, the active region, which may be of the order of 0.2 m thick, can be gallium arsenide. This is sandwiched with gallium aluminium arsenide, one side being doped p-type and the other side being doped n-type to provide the filling and the emptying. However, the precise processes rely on the principles of pn junctions (see the Stretch and Challenge box on page 410) and are beyond the scope of the present discussion. These layers are deposited on a cleaved substrate and metal contacts are added to both outer surfaces. In the case of gas lasers, pumping is liable to be very inefficient, but in the case of semiconductors there can be 70% efficiency.

4 SUPERCONDUCTIVITY

In 1911, a Dutch physicist, Heike Kammerlingh-Onnes, was investigating what happened to the electrical resistivity in metals as he reduced their temperature down to that of liquid helium, 4.2 K. He found that the resistivity of platinum levelled out to a constant low value. Impurities in the platinum, however small in number, scattered the electrons and added a finite resistance.

The great surprise came when he used high-purity mercury. Below 4.2 K it appeared to have no resistivity at all, yet on an increase in temperature, the resistivity shot up at 4.2 K (Fig 20.16). Some important change was happening at this temperature.

The critical temperature at which mercury becomes a superconductor is called the **transition temperature**. A metal which can 'go superconducting' has a transition temperature below which resistivity drops to zero and it becomes a superconductor. In addition, both the current density in the superconductor and any external magnetic field adjacent to it must be below critical values.

An important application of superconductivity is *superconducting magnets* which are held at low temperature using liquid helium. The current through the coils of the electromagnets keeps flowing indefinitely and there is no heating of the wire. The magnetic fields produced are exceptionally stable and in medicine are used in scanners for magnetic resonance imaging (MRI) of the human body (see page 389). Also, the fact that there is little electrical noise in superconductors means that they can be used in low-noise devices.

MAGNETIC LEVITATION AND THE MEISSNER EFFECT

A superconductor can keep a permanent magnet suspended above its surface – see Figs 20.20(a) and (b). As the magnet starts to fall it induces an e.m.f. and hence a current in the superconductor, obeying Faraday's law (see page 226): charge flows around at the surface of the superconductor totally unresisted. And, in agreement with Lenz's law (page 226), the effect of this current is to oppose the motion of the magnet, so it remains levitated.

To explain more fully, the current rises to the value that produces a magnetic field which exactly matches and opposes the magnet's field. The internal 'supercurrent' at the superconductor surface can flow continuously and so it behaves as another magnet. Its poles are in the opposite direction to those of the permanent magnet, and the magnets repel. The separation adjusts until the force of repulsion exactly balances the gravitational field.

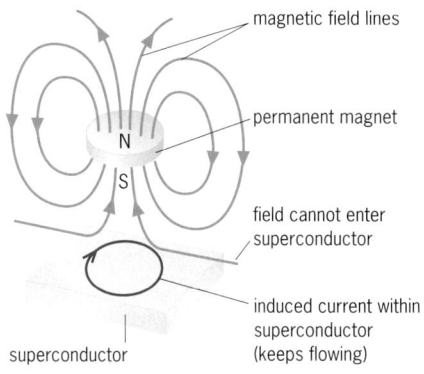

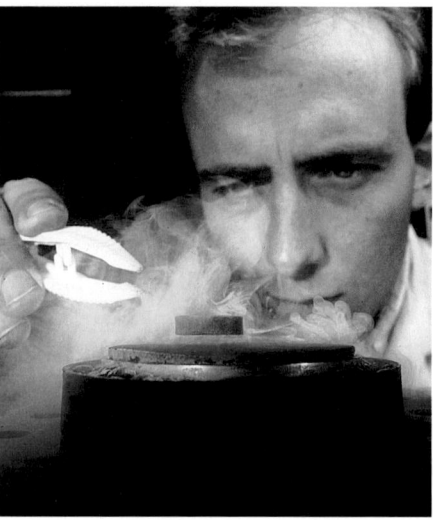

Fig 20.20(b) Magnetic levitation above liquid nitrogen-cooled yttrium–barium–copper oxide

For more on Ohm's Law, semiconductors and superconductors please see the How Science Works assignment for this chapter at www.collinseducation.co.uk/CAS

Fig 20.20(a) A magnet levitating above a superconductor

The field lines of the permanent magnet are excluded from entering the surface of the superconductor, and this is named the **Meissner effect**.

The Maglev train in Japan uses the levitation effect to reduce friction.

When a superconductor is placed in parallel lines of magnetic flux, the field lines are pushed out and bend round it (Fig 20.21). This is not the case for an ordinary metal, nor when the superconductor 'goes normal'.

Only advanced quantum mechanics can explain superconductivity, so we shall not attempt it here!

HIGH-TEMPERATURE SUPERCONDUCTORS

Interest in superconductors was reinforced in 1987 when a superconductor with a transition temperature as high as 92 K was discovered. This is the material illustrated at the start of the chapter; it has the approximate formula $YBa_2Cu_3O_{6.5}$ and is often called YBCO because it contains yttrium, barium, copper and oxygen.

Table 20.1 shows the transition temperature (without any magnetic field present) for YBCO compared with some other metals. Further materials with high transition temperatures have been discovered since then and, like YBCO, they are compounds with imprecise ratios of elements.

These 'high-temperature' superconductors are likely to be more useful than the low-temperature superconductors. In particular, their transition temperature is above that of liquid nitrogen, which is relatively cheap and can be used to cool the superconductor (see Fig 20.20(b), in which the vapour is that of liquid nitrogen). Unfortunately, it has so far proved difficult to make these high-temperature superconducting compounds in bulk form with tensile strength. It may be some years before useful superconductors at room temperature are made. Currently, transition temperatures up to 135 K have been achieved and even higher if pressure is applied to the superconductor.

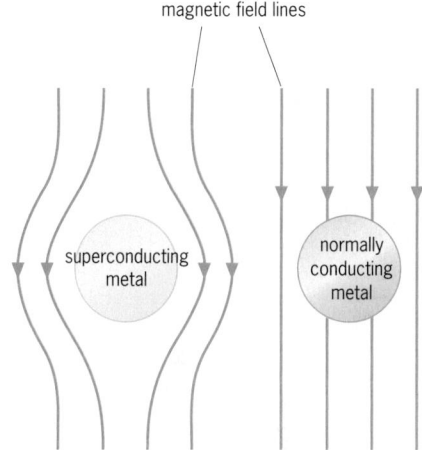

Fig 20.21 A superconductor excludes magnetic field lines, but a normally conducting metal does not

Table 20.1 Transition temperatures for some superconducting materials

Material	T_c/K
Al	1.20
Hg	4.15
Pb	7.19
Nb	9.26
Nb_3Ge	23.2
YBCO	93
$Tl_2Ba_2Ca_2Cu_3O_{16}$	125

5 MAGNETIC MATERIALS

We usually connect magnetic fields with moving charges (electrons) within a wire and, as a current passes through the wire, we detect the associated magnetic field round the wire (see page 213). But many atoms themselves

? QUESTION 12

12 List three possible applications for room-temperature superconductors (if and when they become available). Explain the advantage of a superconductor over a conventional conductor in each case.

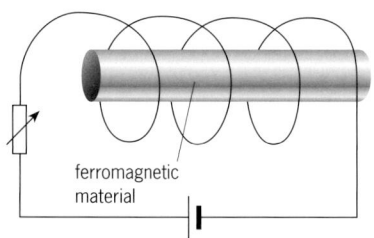

Fig 20.22 Magnetising a specimen in a solenoid

 REMEMBER THIS

Remember (from page 213):

$$B = \mu_0 nI$$

(where n is the number of turns per unit length of the solenoid), so the magnetising field is proportional to the magnetising current.

Fig 20.23 Magnetisation loops for **(a)** a soft magnetic material and **(b)** a hard magnetic material

have so-called **magnetic moments**. That is, they behave rather like very small bar magnets. As in a current-carrying wire, the magnetic field which we detect in a ferromagnetic material must arise from moving charges: in the material, the field arises from the motion of certain unpaired outer electrons in its atoms.

Whereas many atoms have magnetic moments, once these atoms are in combination as ions or molecules, the magnetic moments usually combine and cancel. It is only the atoms of certain elements, such as iron, nickel and cobalt (transition elements, see the Periodic Table, page 331), that have magnetic moments which align in such a way as to maintain the magnetism in the bulk material. These are called **ferromagnetic materials**.

To form a permanent magnet from ferromagnetic material, the magnetic moments of its atoms are lined up in the same direction by inserting the specimen into a solenoid (Fig 20.22). Current through the turns of the solenoid is gradually increased and the magnetic field along the axis of the solenoid increases in proportion.

The magnetisation of a specimen follows the magnetising current, but not always linearly. Look at Fig 20.23(a): starting from zero magnetisation, the magnetisation curve follows AB; when at B the specimen has reached magnetic **saturation**. At this stage, all the atoms with magnetic moments have become aligned with the magnetic field. If the current in the solenoid is now decreased, the magnetisation in the specimen also decreases, but lags, following curve BC. When the current through the solenoid is zero and the magnetising field is also zero, there remains a residual value of the magnetic induction at C called the **remanence**. This means that the material remains partly magnetised.

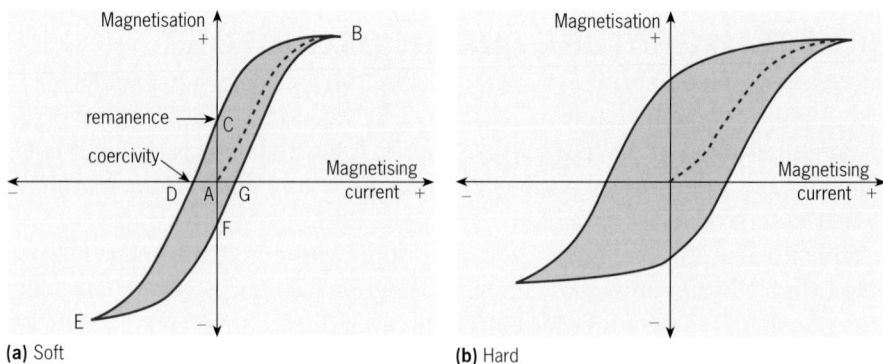

(a) Soft   **(b)** Hard

We now reverse the current in the solenoid. The reverse magnetic field from the solenoid must reach a particular value, the **coercivity**, at D before the field in the specimen has been eliminated. At this stage, the magnetic moments of the atoms in the material will be randomly aligned. Alternatively, the magnetic moments may be aligned *within* **domains**, but the domains will then be randomly aligned. Further increase in the reverse magnetic field now starts to produce a reverse magnetisation in the specimen that ultimately saturates at E.

As we continue to cycle the current, the field in the specimen follows the outside loop BDEGB. The area enclosed within the loop represents the energy lost (ultimately heating the magnet). If this area is small, then the specimen consists of a **soft** magnetic material. If the area within the loop is large and coercivity is large, then it is a **hard** magnetic material, as in Fig 20.23(b). This makes sense as it needs a large amount of reverse current to drive a hard material into its reverse magnetisation.

A good analogue model of what is happening can be demonstrated in two dimensions using a grid of magnetised needles. The model grid is placed between large magnetising loops (Helmholtz coils, see page 218). Initially the directions of all the little magnets average out and there is no preferred direction (Fig 20.24(a)). You may however notice that there are local regions where the magnets are lined up; these are analogous to the domains we have mentioned. There is a local internal magnetic field within each domain but the fields average out overall throughout the material. We now apply an external magnetising field (by passing a current through the Helmholtz coils) and the magnets start to line up. Domains switch gradually until there is the alignment shown in Fig 20.24(b). This means we have gone up the steep part of the loop starting from A in Fig 20.23(a). Notice that the magnets have aligned along a natural direction arising from the way the magnets have been arranged – in this case on a square grid. In single crystals a similar thing happens with the alignment of the magnetic moments of the atoms according to the structure. However, this preferred direction of magnetisation is slightly mis-oriented with respect to the external field. The field strength must be increased significantly to pull all the little magnets into line with it (Fig 20.24(c)). This corresponds to the flattening of the loop in Fig 20.23(a) as we come towards position B. If we then reduce the magnetising field, the little magnets gradually swing back to their preferred alignment. As the field is reduced to zero, magnets in some of the domains switch singly or in groups, but it needs a substantial reverse field to cause a large switching of the domains.

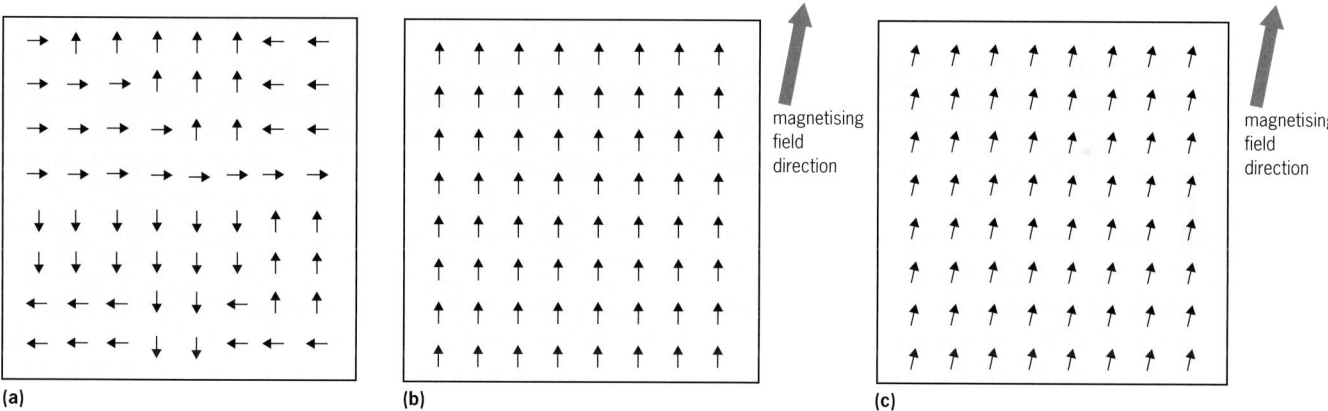

(a) (b) (c)

Fig 20.24 The grid of magnetised needles **(a)** before the external field is applied and **(b)** fully aligned with one another by the action of an external field but needing a further increase in applied field strength **(c)** to pull them into exact alignment with the field

A hard material is suitable for a permanent magnet where we want it to be difficult to reverse the direction of magnetisation. It is difficult to alter the magnetisation within the domains. A soft material, that gives little opposition to change of magnetisation so that energy loss is small, is suitable for a transformer core. Steel cannot be easily magnetised and is a *hard* magnetic material; iron can be easily magnetised and is *soft*.

Let us look again at the curves in Fig 20.23. Choose a particular magnetising current, and you will see that it has two possible maximum values of magnetisation for the specimen. (This is apart from high current in the solenoid, when the magnetisation has saturated.) Which value applies in practice depends on whether we are increasing or decreasing the current in the solenoid, since the value of the specimen's magnetisation depends on its previous magnetisation history, shown as the path taken on the magnetising current–magnetisation graph. And so we say that the value for the specimen is path dependent, a property we call **hysteresis**.

QUESTION 13

13 In a magnetic material the magnetic moments of atoms are aligned. If you used a solenoid to demagnetise a specimen would you use d.c. or a.c. current? Can you think of another way of demagnetising the specimen without using a solenoid?

✔ **REMEMBER THIS**
Remember Faraday's law of electromagnetic induction:
$$\varepsilon = -N \, d\Phi/dt$$
(see page 226).

When an electromagnet is used to make measurements or obtain data such as magnetic resonance in a varying magnetic field, the hysteresis is kept small. This is done by using a very soft magnetic material, when the solenoid current–magnetisation variation will be close to a single curve. Then, the energy loss within the magnetic material during the cycle is negligible.

Low energy loss is particularly necessary in transformer cores and so these are usually made from iron (with about 3 per cent silicon). However, iron has a low electrical resistivity so that it is necessary to make the core from laminated sheets to prevent eddy currents. The eddy currents arise from electromagnetic induction (see Chapter 11); the higher the frequency of operation of the transformer, the larger is the induced e.m.f. setting up the eddy currents. If one can use a soft magnetic material that is also insulating then lamination becomes unnecessary. Ceramics such as ferrite ceramics can be used but usually only when the transformers are small. Metallic glasses have been developed that are easy to magnetise in all directions.

If a magnetic material is heated sufficiently there is enough energy to overcome the interaction between the magnetic moments of the atoms so the material is no longer capable of magnetisation. The temperature at which this occurs is called the **Curie temperature**. In the model of magnetic needles, a similar effect can be produced by inserting energy through shaking.

SUMMARY

By studying this chapter you should have learned the following:

- When atoms come close together, electron energy levels split and spread out to form energy bands.
- Conduction in a metal occurs because electrons can move among partially occupied energy levels of the conduction band.
- Insulators cannot conduct electricity because they have a filled valence band and an empty conduction band separated by a large energy gap.
- A pure semiconductor has a small energy gap between valence and conduction bands, and so electrons can be thermally excited into the conduction band at finite temperature, leaving an equal number of holes in the valence band.
- Semiconductors can be doped with donor and acceptor impurities to produce n-type and p-type semiconductors respectively.
- The electrical conductivity of a metal decreases with temperature, whereas that of an intrinsic semiconductor increases with temperature.

- The Hall effect can be used to find the type and number of carriers in an extrinsic semiconductor.
- Semiconductor lasers are small and efficient.
- Lasers depend on population inversion achieved by pumping.
- Superconductors require the temperature to be below a critical value, in order to have negligible resistance.
- Superconductors exclude magnetic field; this is the Meissner effect.
- Soft and hard magnetic materials exhibit hysteresis loops, with small and large enclosed areas respectively.

 Practice questions for this chapter are available at www.collinseducation.co.uk/CAS

21

Communications

21 COMMUNICATIONS

Every second counts

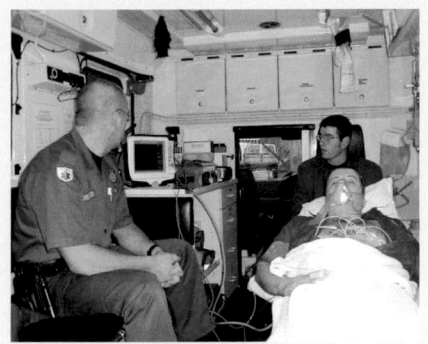

Modern computer and communications technology saves lives

Heart attacks are still one of the biggest killers in Britain. The first hour after the initial attack is crucial. If the correct treatment and drugs can be given in this time most sufferers will survive to lead full lives. This has been known for many years and has been one of the reasons why survival rates are much poorer for heart attack victims who live in more remote areas.

The paramedics shown in the photograph serve a rural area of west Wales which is a good hour from the nearest general hospital. They are now able to use the latest modern communications technology to save more lives. They use portable cardiac sensing and monitoring equipment to measure the patient's vital signs. These are transmitted instantly, sometimes using the mobile phone network, sometimes by satellite link, to a heart specialist at the hospital. The specialist can diagnose as accurately as if the patient were in the hospital, then give appropriate instructions to the paramedics. All this can be done while the patient is on the way to hospital so that drugs can be administered immediately on arrival, without wasting more time in doing further tests.

The ideas in this chapter

The example above is just part of a communications revolution that we are living through. The growth of the internet and the mobile phone network has been logarithmic in the last decade (see Fig 21.1).

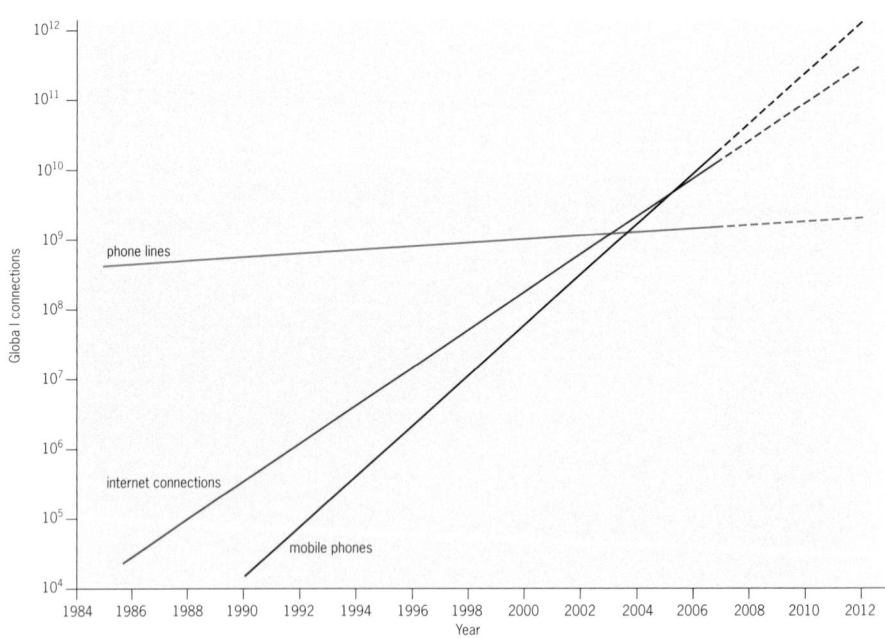

Fig 21.1 The recent increase in internet and mobile phone use shown graphically. Note the vertical scale is logarithmic

As the demand for communication capacity increases, the technology must strive to provide it. The radio spectrum is highly congested, but the use of light in optical fibres is making broadband (high capacity) systems possible. The future is very exciting.

In this chapter, we will be answering the question: 'How is it possible to transmit so much information so easily?' But first we need to understand some important aspects of radio and telephone communication.

1 RADIO COMMUNICATION

Sound offers a flexible means of communication between people. We come equipped with our own transmitter and receiver – our voice and our ears. It does have some disadvantages, though: sound does not carry far, and if several people 'transmit' at the same time, the 'receiver' finds it very difficult to sort the messages out.

Fig 21.2 Radio waves, shown in relation to other parts of the electromagnetic spectrum, with their frequencies and main uses in radio broadcasting, services, television and satellite

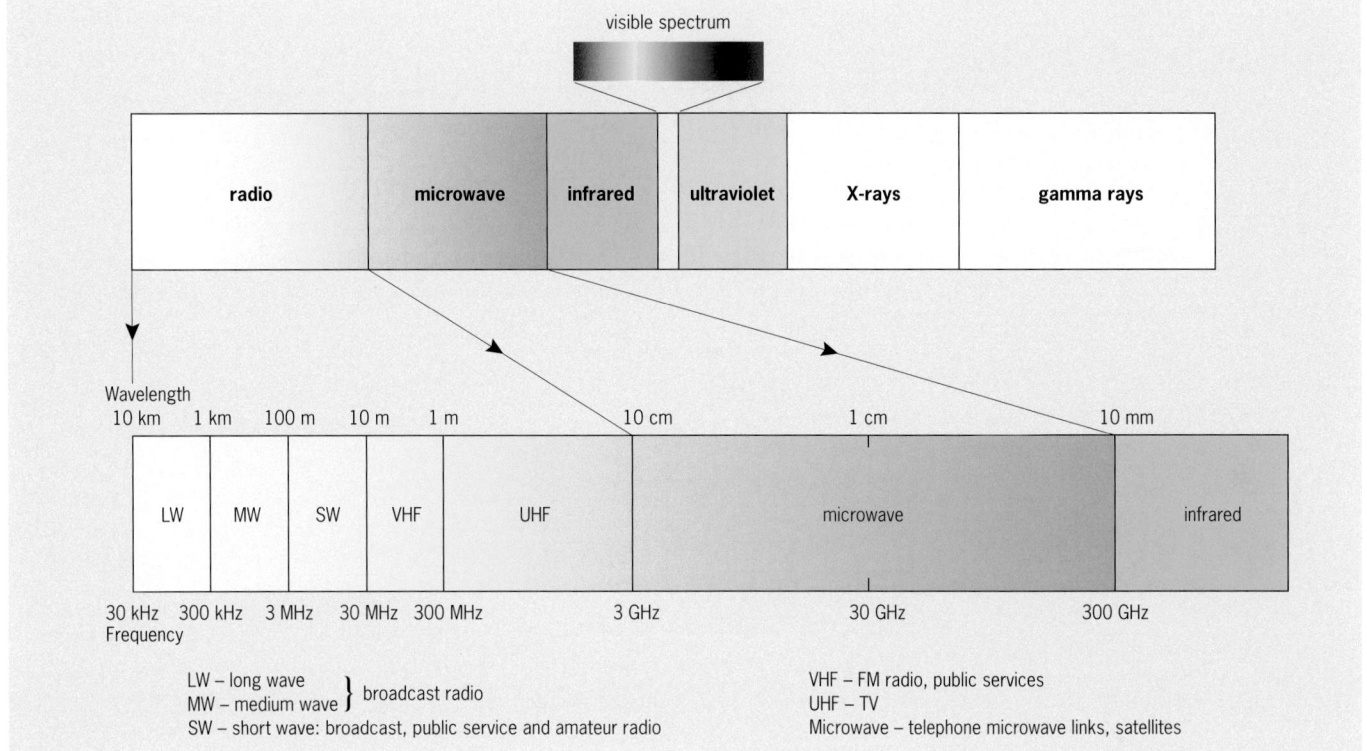

LW – long wave ⎫
MW – medium wave ⎬ broadcast radio
SW – short wave: broadcast, public service and amateur radio

VHF – FM radio, public services
UHF – TV
Microwave – telephone microwave links, satellites

Radio waves offer one answer because they 'carry' the sound (or any other information we send) much further – as electromagnetic waves, travelling at a speed of 3×10^8 metres per second in a vacuum. Fig 21.2 shows where radio waves fit into the electromagnetic spectrum, and some of the features of the **radio spectrum**.

Radio waves have frequencies ranging from tens of kilohertz to thousands of megahertz. The sound waves we hear on the radio and telephone are within the range of human hearing; that is, from about 20 Hz to 20 000 Hz. Generally, radio waves have frequencies far higher than the frequency of the sound information that they 'carry'.

THE TRANSMITTED SIGNAL

Communication systems using radio waves can transmit a variety of information which can be received at its destination as sound, video pictures or data of various types. But before we look at the signal that is received, let's see what a transmitted signal consists of.

There are two signals that go to make the signal being transmitted. First, there is a radio signal of constant **amplitude** and **frequency**, which is often called the **carrier wave**. This carries the information from the second signal, the **information signal**, which is combined with the carrier. The information signal fluctuates (varies), as the information changes. It can also be intermittent, meaning it may stop and start. The two signals – the carrier signal and the information signal – are combined in a process called **modulation**.

✔ REMEMBER THIS

kilohertz	=	10^3 Hz
megahertz	=	10^6 Hz
gigahertz	=	10^9 Hz

? QUESTION 1

1 Using the equation:
speed = frequency × wavelength,
a) calculate the wavelength of the radio signals with these frequencies: **i)** 200 kHz, **ii)** 1 MHz, **iii)** 100 MHz, **iv)** 500 MHz, **v)** 10 GHz;
b) calculate the frequency of radio signals with these wavelengths:
i) 200 m, **ii)** 80 m, **iii)** 2 m, **iv)** 20 cm, **v)** 10 mm.

Both sound and radio travel as waves (see Chapter 6).

When a microphone converts sound into a changing electrical voltage, we refer to it as a *signal*: the information carried by the sound wave is transferred to the signal.

Similarly, in a radio, the received radio *wave* is converted to a *signal* that is then processed by the radio: the signal is a fluctuating voltage which then causes a fluctuating current to flow along a wire.

THE MODULATION PROCESS

There are several different ways of achieving modulation. In the simplest type of modulation used to transmit simple codes such as Morse code, the radio wave is merely switched on and off.

More complex methods of modulation are needed to transmit sound information such as speech or music. The two methods, namely **amplitude modulation** (AM) and **frequency modulation** (FM), which are used by broadcasting stations (such as Radio 1, Virgin, Channel 4 television, and so on), are described below.

2 AMPLITUDE MODULATION (AM)

When the information signal is combined with the carrier wave, the amplitude of the carrier signal is altered. Fig 21.3 is a block diagram for a simple **amplitude modulated** radio transmitter designed to transmit sound signals. Read through the notes on the diagram to see how the signal is built up.

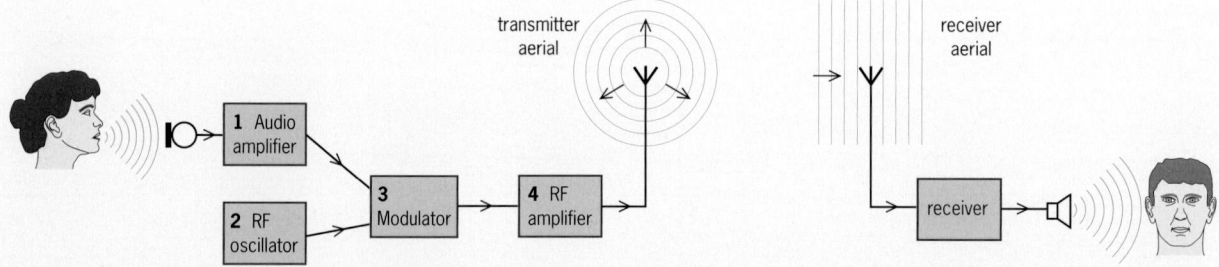

1. Audio amplifier: a microphone converts the sound into an electronic signal, which is usually very small, so an amplifier makes it larger.

2. Radio frequency oscillator: an oscillator is a circuit that generates an electronic 'carrier' signal, in this case, a radio frequency signal, of constant amplitude and frequency.

3. Mixer or modulator: the circuit in which the information signal, in this case the signal produced from the sound, and the carrier are combined.

4. Radio frequency (RF) amplifier: the signal produced by the modulator is a more complex radio frequency signal. A special amplifier makes this signal stronger before it is fed into the aerial which 'radiates' the signal.

Fig 21.3 Block diagram for an amplitude modulated radio transmitter

THE MODULATOR SIGNAL

The signal from the modulator is quite complex, as Fig. 21.4 shows. It is a mixture of signals fed into the modulator. It is easier to understand if we think about a transmitter sending a simple sound (audio) signal such as a pure tone – a note of single frequency. Let's call it f_0, as in Fig 21.4(a). The radio frequency carrier signal has a frequency of f_c. As in Fig 21.4(b), f_c would be a much higher frequency than f_0.

The mixer combines these two signals (Fig 21.4(c)) to produce two new frequencies as well as the two signals we started with. The two new signals are the sum and the difference of f_0 and f_c (see Fig 21.5):

$$(f_c + f_0) \text{ and } (f_c - f_0)$$

The output of the mixer contains all four frequencies:

$$f_0, f_c, (f_c + f_0) \text{ and } (f_c - f_0)$$

Three of the frequencies at the output of the modulator are roughly the same; they are all radio frequency signals. The odd one out is f_0. As an audio frequency signal, its frequency is much lower than the other three. The last stage in our simple

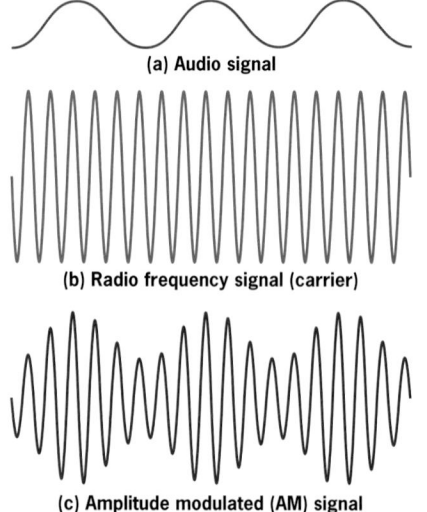

(a) Audio signal

(b) Radio frequency signal (carrier)

(c) Amplitude modulated (AM) signal
= (a) + (b), the signal at the output of the modulator

Fig 21.4 Graphical representation of audio, radio and amplitude modulated (AM) signals

transmitter is an amplifier. It is a radio frequency amplifier which only amplifies the three radio frequency signals. f_0 is effectively filtered out; it doesn't reach the aerial.

Fig 21.5 shows a useful way of displaying the three radio frequency signals that are transmitted. It is a **frequency spectrum** and shows the carrier and the two other frequencies either side of it.

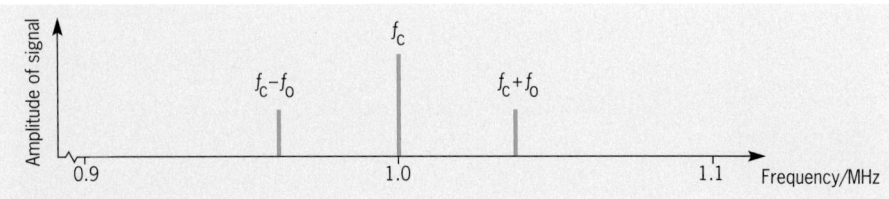

Fig 21.5 The three radio frequency signals transmitted by an amplitude modulated radio transmitter, shown as a **frequency spectrum**. (A device called a **spectrum analyser** is used to display the different frequencies present in a signal as a frequency spectrum)

BANDWIDTH

In most real radio transmissions, the sound signal will be more complex than the single tone mentioned earlier. Instead of a single pure frequency, it will be a range of audio frequencies representing, say, a person's voice or the music of a group. For telephone communication and most radio, the sound is transmitted in a **band of audio frequencies** ranging from 300 Hz to 4 kHz. We would say that this signal has a **signal bandwidth** of slightly less than 4 kHz. When this band of frequencies is used to **amplitude modulate** the **carrier**, the resulting output is the carrier, f_c, and two **sidebands**.

In amplitude modulation, the signal transmitted includes all the frequencies shown in Fig 21.6. The sidebands are the important part because they carry the information. (It would be pointless to just send the carrier signal.)

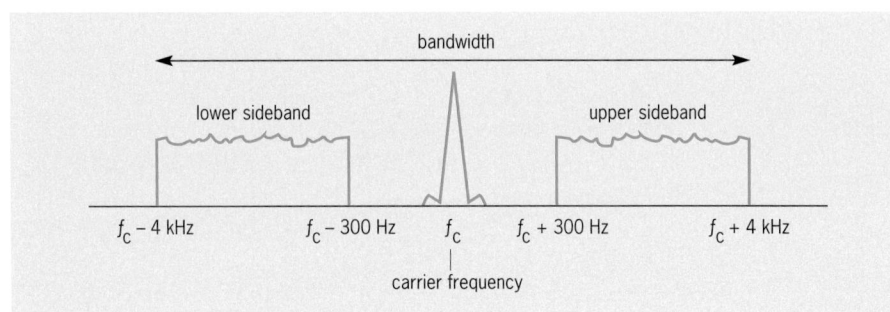

Fig 21.6 Frequency spectrum of a typical medium wave band station with an audio bandwidth of 300 Hz to 4 kHz. Notice the upper and lower sidebands

> **? QUESTION 2**
>
> 2 A carrier frequency signal of 1 MHz is modulated with an audio signal of 10 kHz. Calculate the 'sum and difference' frequencies produced by the modulator.

The signal transmitted covers a range of frequencies, and we say that the transmitted signal has a bandwidth. The bandwidth of the signal just described and shown in the diagram is 8 kHz. That means that this radio station occupies 8 kHz of frequency space. The space the station occupies is often described as a **channel** and in this case the **channel bandwidth** is 8 kHz. Notice also that:

$$\text{channel bandwidth} = 2 \times \text{maximum audio frequency}$$

Radio transmissions are organised into bands by international agreement. They are given names relating to their wavelengths, for example, the 'medium wave band' and the 'long wave band'. Each band itself covers a particular range of frequencies. The medium wave band covers a range from 500 kHz to about 1.6 MHz (Fig 21.9).

> **? QUESTION 3**
>
> 3 What is the channel bandwidth of the medium wave band described in the text?

Fig 21.7 The medium wave band showing the carrier frequency of some of the radio stations broadcast in the United Kingdom

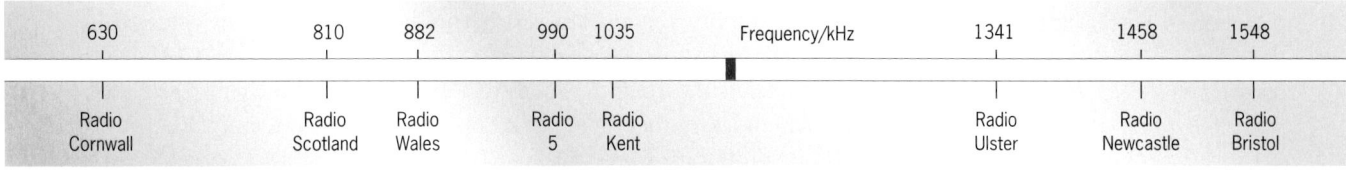

If radio stations on a band wanted to use amplitude modulation to transmit signals over a range similar to that in Fig 21.8, they could each be allowed 10 kHz of frequency space. This would avoid any overlap of adjacent stations, and they could operate without interfering with each other.

Depth of modulation

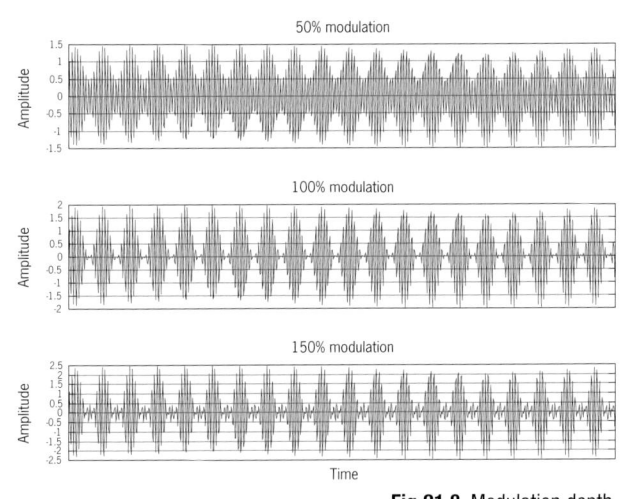

Fig 21.8 Modulation depth

When two signals are added together as in amplitude modulation, the relative amplitude of the two signals is also important. If the carrier amplitude is much larger than the signal, then the modulation will be weak and would be difficult to use effectively. On the other hand, if the signal amplitude is too large, then the result is 'over-modulation', which results in a distorted signal being received. The amount or 'depth' of modulation is usually expressed as a percentage. Fig 21.8 shows three examples of amplitude modulated carriers.

At 50% depth of modulation, the minimum amplitude of the modulated carrier is half of the maximum amplitude. At 100% the minimum is just zero. If the depth of modulation increases any more, then the signal received would be distorted.

Power distribution in amplitude modulation

Amplitude modulation is quite inefficient. The information to be transmitted is contained in the sidebands, yet most of the energy transmitted is contained in the carrier signal. Although this is a disadvantage, receivers for amplitude modulation signals are easy and cheap to make.

As the depth of modulation increases, more energy is carried by the sidebands and less by the carrier but, as explained in the "Depth of modulation" box (page 420), there is a limit at 100% modulation depth before the signal would be distorted. At this point, the efficiency reaches a maximum of 33%.

It should also be noticed that the information contained in each sideband is the same. It should only be necessary to actually transmit and receive one sideband to access the information. This leads to a far more efficient type of amplitude modulation called 'single sideband' or SSB. SSB is more efficient in terms of the energy transmitted and also uses a smaller portion of the frequency spectrum; it has a narrower bandwidth. This means that more SSB transmissions can be allowed in the same band space as ordinary amplitude modulated signals. However, SSB receivers are more complex and expensive.

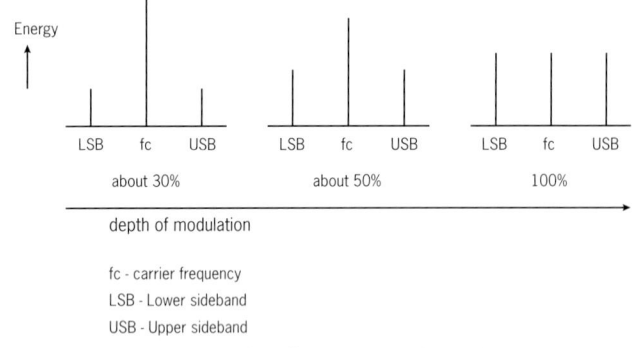

Fig 21.9 Frequency spectra for different depths of modulation

QUESTION 4

4 What is the maximum number of radio stations, each allowed a bandwidth of 10 kHz, that could operate on the medium wave band without interfering with each other?

3 FREQUENCY MODULATION (FM)

Frequency modulation is another very common form of modulation. FM gives a far better quality signal than AM because AM is very easily affected by 'noise' and FM is not.

Noise means the random signals that are present in all circuits, and the atmospheric noise in the signal picked up by the aerial in a radio. Electrical noise can also be produced by electrical machinery, such as drills or vacuum cleaners.

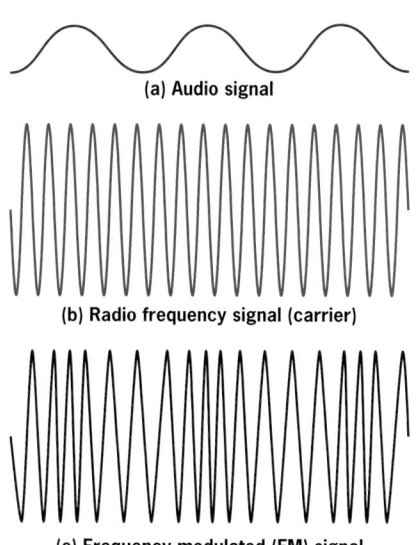

(a) Audio signal

(b) Radio frequency signal (carrier)

(c) Frequency modulated (FM) signal

Fig 21.10 Graphical representation of audio, radio and frequency modulated (FM) signals

Whatever the source, the noise is a signal which affects and interferes with the *amplitude* of the information signal being received, and so, in a radio, you will hear a signal distorted by crackles and hiss.

Since FM is a *frequency* variation, changes in amplitude do not affect it nearly as much. The mathematics of FM is more complicated and beyond the scope of this book, but the results are important.

As Fig 21.10 shows, in FM the audio signal which carries the information is used to modulate the *frequency* of the carrier signal (rather than the amplitude, as in AM). The spectrum of an FM signal is also more complicated than the AM signal spectrum. There are many more sidebands and the channel bandwidth is greater, as shown in Fig 21.11.

FM is used for stereo sound transmissions where high quality reproduction is important. For stereo quality the signal bandwidth is 20 kHz, which is sufficient to cover the range of human hearing (often quoted as 20 Hz to 20 kHz). Because FM requires a very big bandwidth, FM stations in Britain are allowed a channel bandwidth of 150 kHz. This means that the signals need to be transmitted on a frequency band which is much higher than for AM. The FM radio stations in Britain fit into a band from 88 MHz to 108 MHz.

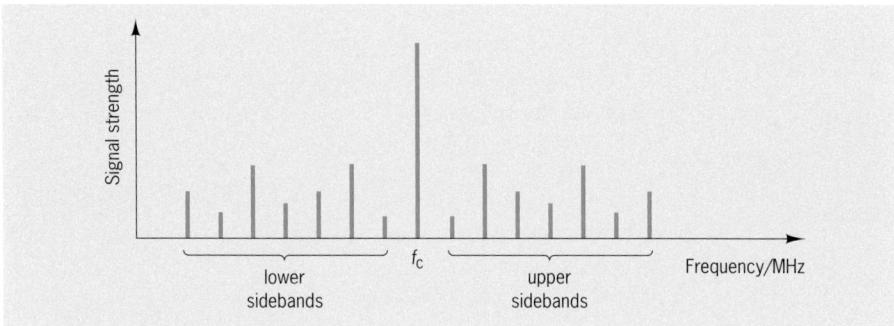

Fig 21.11 Frequency spectrum for an FM signal. Notice the larger number of sidebands than in AM

4 AM AND FM: ANALOGUE METHODS OF MODULATION

RADIO AND TELEPHONE SYSTEMS

So far, we have concentrated on radio signals. Telephone signals can also be amplitude modulated or frequency modulated. Many telephone signals can be sent down a cable – or, today, an optical fibre – in a band like a band of radio signals. We will look at optical fibres later, on page 434.

Amplitude modulation and frequency modulation are **analogue methods** of modulation. By 'analogue' we mean that there is a direct relationship between the information signal and the electronic signal that is transmitted. In the case of radio, the loudness and pitch of the sound are used to change the *amplitude* and *frequency* of the transmitted signal. Analogue signals change continuously, covering a range of possible values.

> **? QUESTION 5**
>
> 5 **a)** Why are stereo signals not transmitted on the medium wave band?
>
> **b)** What is the largest number of stereo stations that could use the British FM band?
>
> **c)** Capital Gold transmits on 1548 metres. Why would the station prefer to be FM?

STRETCH AND CHALLENGE

Noise

Noise is a very important characteristic of all communication systems. It is a nuisance but almost impossible to avoid. You will find that the main advantage of different communication techniques is their ability to overcome 'noise'.

Switch a television to a channel that has not been tuned in and you will see white speckles fill the screen. This is noise. Turn the volume of a CD player up high without a CD in it. The hiss you hear is noise due to the random motion of electrons in the system.

Engineers design systems so that the signal carrying the information is always stronger than the noise signal. This is measured as the **signal-to-noise ratio**.

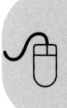 For more information about this please see the CAS website at www.collinseducation.co.uk/CAS

The way radio waves travel

Radio waves travel at the speed of light. The Voyager spacecraft sent messages straight back to Earth from the outer edge of the Solar System over 5000 million km away in just over four and a half hours. But the distance and paths followed by radio waves on Earth are affected by the Earth itself and on the state of the upper atmosphere which itself changes with time of day, season and the level of solar activity.

At low frequencies, radio communication depends on the wave travelling (being propagated) in contact with the surface of the Earth; this is called surface or ground wave propagation (Fig 21.12). During the daytime, broadcasts from medium waveband stations can travel nearly 200 km like this. Above 2 MHz, a surface wave weakens rapidly with distance (it is attenuated).

At frequencies between 2 MHz and about 20 MHz, radio waves are reflected off the ionosphere, a layer of ionised

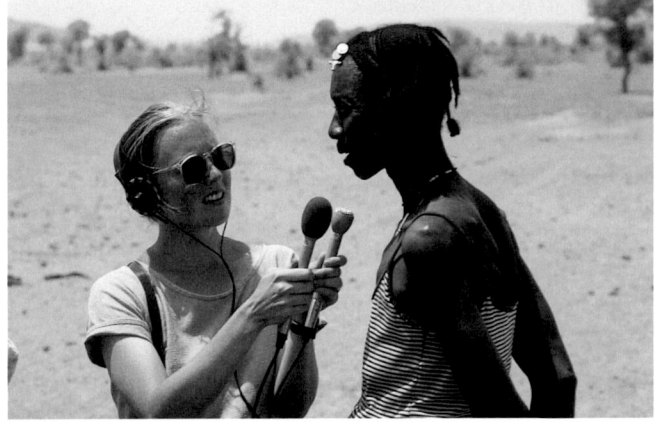

Fig 21.13 Radio brings us the voice of people from the most remote parts of the world

molecules which reaches from about 40 km to about 300 km above the Earth's surface. Using this mode of propagation, radio waves can travel 4000 km in one 'hop' and can easily travel round the Earth with several hops. When a radio wave travels like this, it 'skips' over large areas where the signal strength will be very weak.

The upper limit of ionospheric propagation varies with the sunspot cycle, which goes through eleven-year cycles of activity. At periods of high sunspot activity, the upper frequency can reach 30 MHz.

Above 30 MHz, radio waves travel mainly by space wave, which is a line-of-sight wave. Both Earth-bound and satellite TV use this mode of propagation. Range is then limited by the curvature of the Earth. At these frequencies, the ionosphere has little effect.

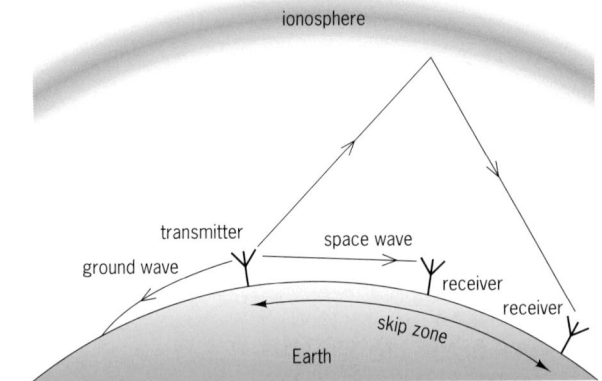

Fig 21.12 The three main modes of propagation of radio waves

As shown above, such signals take up a slice of frequency space, occupying a small part of the electromagnetic spectrum. Both AM and FM signals travel a limited distance, and beyond this they are so weak that they are difficult to detect.

Limitations of AM and FM

We have seen that AM and FM are widely used in radio and telephone communication. Some television systems use AM for picture information and FM for the sound. So AM and FM are certainly effective means of communication, but they cannot provide the flexibility and reliability required for some modern communications.

They are also very open: once a signal is transmitted, anyone with a suitable receiver can listen in. They are both 'real time' systems, which means that the signal can be received only at the time it is transmitted. As radio airwaves become more congested, this is a disadvantage.

5 DIGITAL COMMUNICATIONS

It is now possible to send a complete message over the radio that takes only milliseconds to transmit. Signals can also be coded so that only the person they are intended for can receive them. This system is called **packet radio** and has been used for about twenty years by radio amateurs and for longer by military and commercial users. In packet radio, the transmitted signal is converted to a series of very short pulses which are compressed together into a very short period of time, usually only milliseconds. These signals are computer messages, pages of text compiled and decoded by a computer at each end.

Personal computer-based videophones (Fig 21.14) allow us to communicate face to face. We can have video conferences with each person seen in their window on the monitor screen. In the time since we wrote the first edition of this book, communication from computer to computer over the **internet** has become a part of our everyday lives. The text you are now reading was first sent to the publisher by **email**. Many of us send *text* messages to our friends over our **mobile phones** (see page 435).

These are just some of the changes that have been made possible because of **digital systems**. In using them, communications technology has surprisingly reverted to the first effective electrical method used to transmit information, that is, Morse code, which consists of a series of short and long pulses.

A pulse is made by switching the signal 'on' for a short time. In Morse code, long pulses ('dashes') are three times as long as short ones ('dots'). Combinations of pulses are used to represent letters, and these are strung together to make words and sentences. Samuel Morse devised his code to take advantage of the new wire telegraph that he invented in 1837. Messages could be sent over very long distances – the first transatlantic cable carrying Morse came into use in 1858, while the first transatlantic telephone line wasn't laid until 1956. Digital transmissions are less affected by noise interference, they can travel further and still be detected, and they take up less frequency space, so that more stations can use the same band.

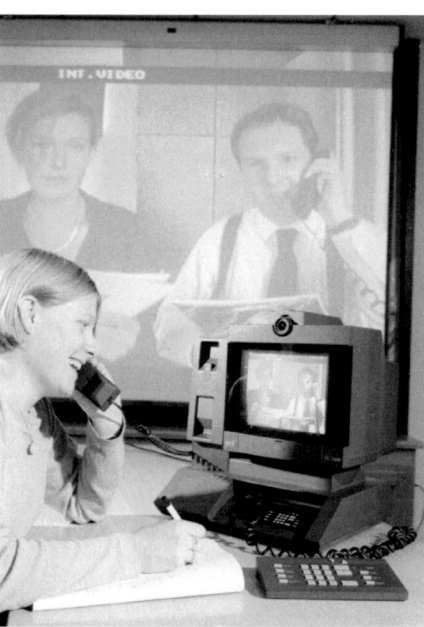

Fig 21.14 In a video-conference we can see the people we are talking to by telephone

Fig 21.15 Morse code for the letters A (· —) and B (— · · ·)

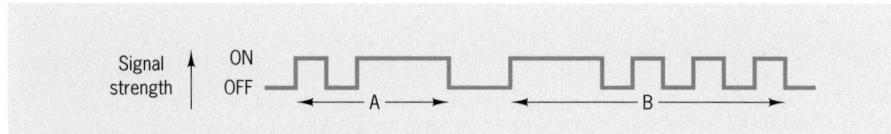

WHAT IS A DIGITAL CODE?

Morse code is a simple **digital code** (see Fig 21.15). Electronic digital codes and digital signals are also very simple: they have only two values. They are either 'on' or 'off'. A digital signal is made up from combinations of 'on' and 'off' pulses. 'Off' is given the code '0' and 'on' the code '1'.

The binary code

A simple code in common use is the **binary code**. The binary number system is based on just two digits, 0 and 1 (as compared to the ten used by the decimal system – 0 to 9). Table 21.1 shows what signals equivalent to the binary codes for decimal numbers 1 to 15 look like.

The third column of the table shows each binary number represented as a 'four-bit' binary word. Each digit of the binary number is called a **bit** (from **bi**nary digi**t**). Zeros are added as extra bits to the left of any number that is less than four bits. Digital signals are made up from four-bit words or multiples of them: 8 bit (called a **byte**), 16 bit, 32 bit, or even 64 bit.

DIGITAL SIGNALS

Images and sounds are changed into digital codes, and the codes are transmitted as pulses. Then the receiver equipment changes the pulses back into the original sounds or images. Let us look further at this process.

Table 21.1 Decimal and binary equivalents

Decimal	Binary	Four-bit binary
0	0	0000
1	1	0001
2	10	0010
3	11	0011
4	100	0100
5	101	0101
6	110	0110
7	111	0111
8	1000	1000
9	1001	1001
10	1010	1010
11	1011	1011
12	1100	1100
13	1101	1101
14	1110	1110
15	1111	1111

Fig 21.16 After travelling a long distance, a digital signal loses its original shape. This is because of dispersion, the same effect that causes different frequencies of light to be split up when they pass through a triangular prism. The 'square' digital pulse is made up of a large number of different frequency signals – see pages 430–431. The different frequencies travel at different speeds

Digital signals are easy to receive. All the receiver needs to do is to detect whether a pulse is high or low. Digital signals, transmitted either as a radio signal or down a telephone line, tend to change after they have travelled some distance. Fig 21.16 shows how a very regular pulse changes as it travels a long distance. But as long as the receiver can still distinguish between 'high' and 'low', the original signal can be reproduced accurately. Analogue signals do not have this abrupt 'high'–'low' pattern. They change continually and become corrupted over much shorter distances.

Older undersea telephone systems use special equipment that amplifies and reshapes the analogue signal. They are called *repeaters* and are required every 3 nautical miles. Modern digital systems which use optical fibres have repeaters every 30 nautical miles. The digital repeaters change the corrupted pulses, like that on the right in Fig 21.16, back into perfect pulses, as shown on the left.

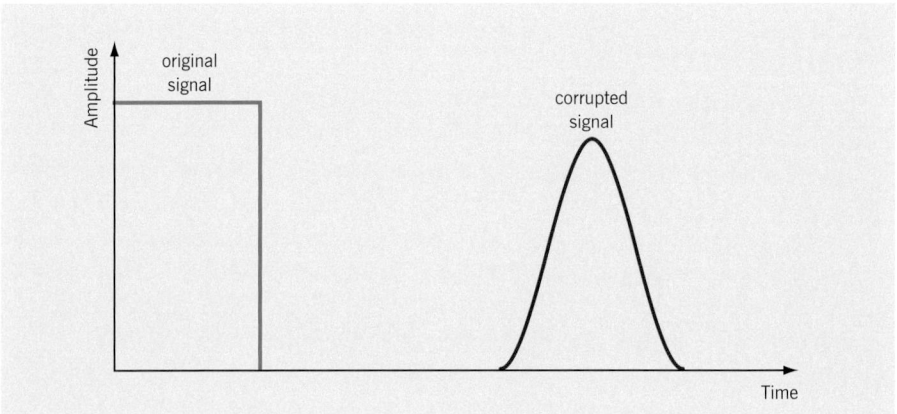

6 SIGNAL CONVERSION

Many signals that we wish to send start out as analogue signals. Examples are speech or music which change continually. To benefit from the advantages of a digital system, the analogue signal must first be changed into a digital signal. This process is called **analogue-to-digital conversion**. The digital signal is then transmitted, and at the receiver it is turned back into an analogue signal. This is called **digital-to-analogue conversion**. Ideally, the received signal should be a perfect reproduction of the analogue signal we began with.

PULSE CODE MODULATION (PCM)

There are several ways that signals can be converted into digital pulses. We will look at one of them, **pulse code modulation** or **PCM**, which is the method commonly used in communication systems.

In particular, let's see what happens inside a digital telephone line using PCM. Fig 21.17 shows the analogue–digital–analogue conversion system

Analogue-to-digital conversion

First, the microphone changes the sound of a voice into an electronic analogue signal which is an alternating voltage which varies over a range of voltages and frequencies. The signal travels in this form to a local telephone exchange where it is changed into a digital signal using PCM.

The voltage of the analogue signal is measured – it is **sampled** – several times during each cycle of the signal. The samples are very short pulses of varying amplitude and taken together they show the same shape as the original analogue signal, as in Fig 21.18. The number of pulses per second is called the **sampling rate**.

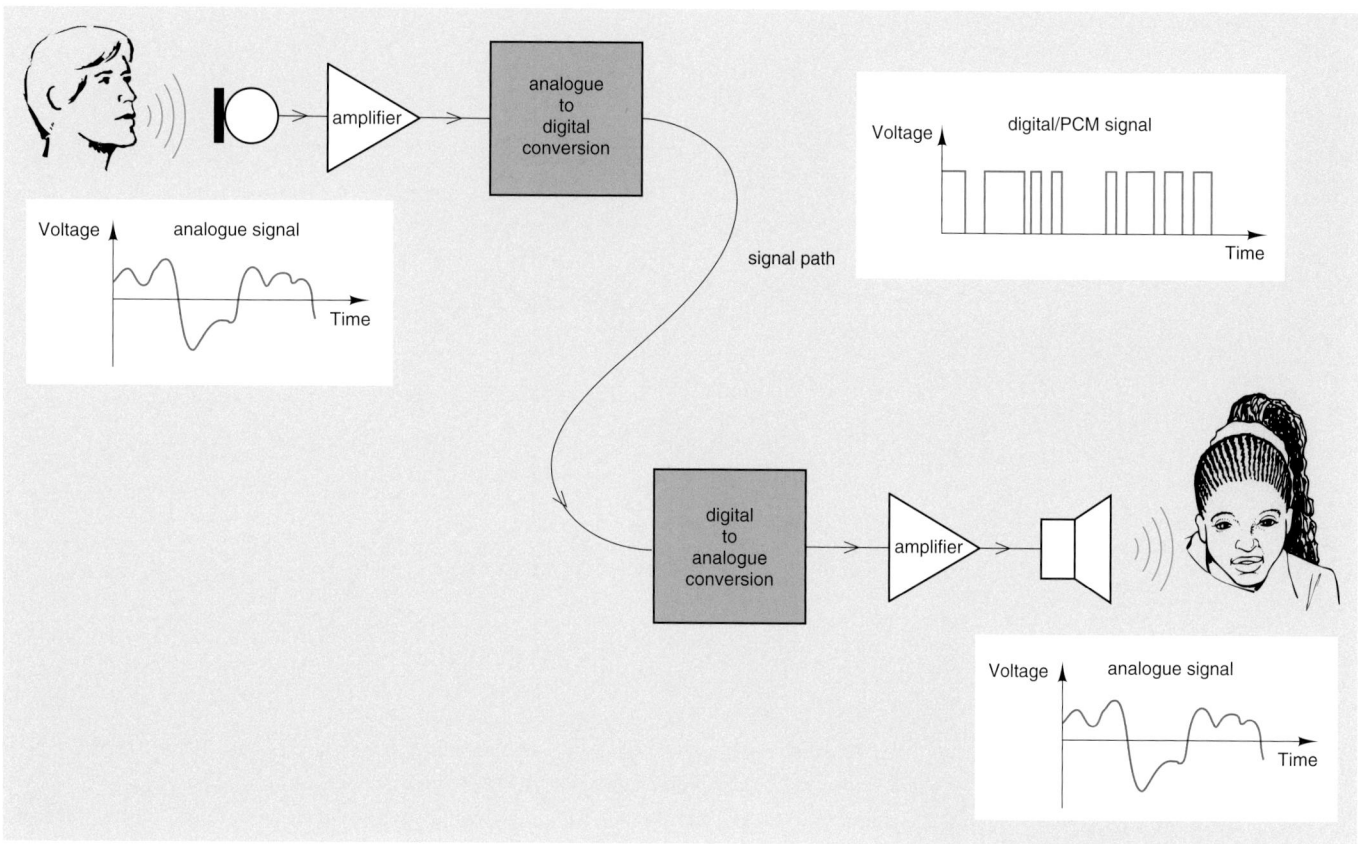

Fig 21.17 Block diagram showing the function of the main parts in an analogue–digital–analogue conversion system

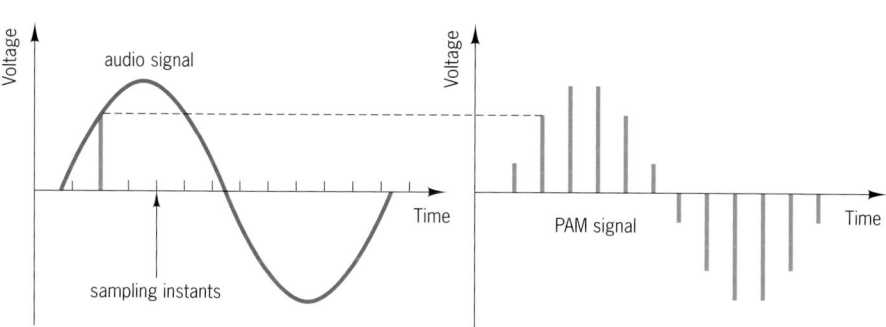

Fig 21.18 The sampling of an audio signal, and the resulting pulse amplitude modulated (PAM) signal

The sampling rate will depend on the highest frequency present in the signal to be sampled and is related to it by a simple formula:

$$\text{sampling rate} \geq 2 \times (\text{maximum frequency in signal})$$

Fig 21.19 (overleaf) shows how this works. Fig 21.19(a) shows two digital pulses. We look for the most obvious simple signal that could be represented by these samples. The simplest signal is a sine wave. Figs 21.19(b) and (c) show two possible signals. They have different amplitudes but they are of the same frequency.

When lower frequency signals are sampled at the same rate there will be more samples for each complete cycle of the signal. Reconstructing these signals will be far easier and more accurate.

When the signal has been sampled like this it is described as **pulse amplitude modulated (PAM)**.

The next step is to convert the varying amplitude pulses into a binary code. The maximum analogue voltage, which depends on the microphone and the amplifier used, is subdivided into a fixed number of levels. This process is called

> ## EXAMPLE
> Digital telephone systems use the same practical rules as for AM, with a maximum audio frequency signal of 4 kHz. A sampling rate of 8000 times per second is twice that maximum frequency.

Fig 21.19 Sampling at twice the signal frequency

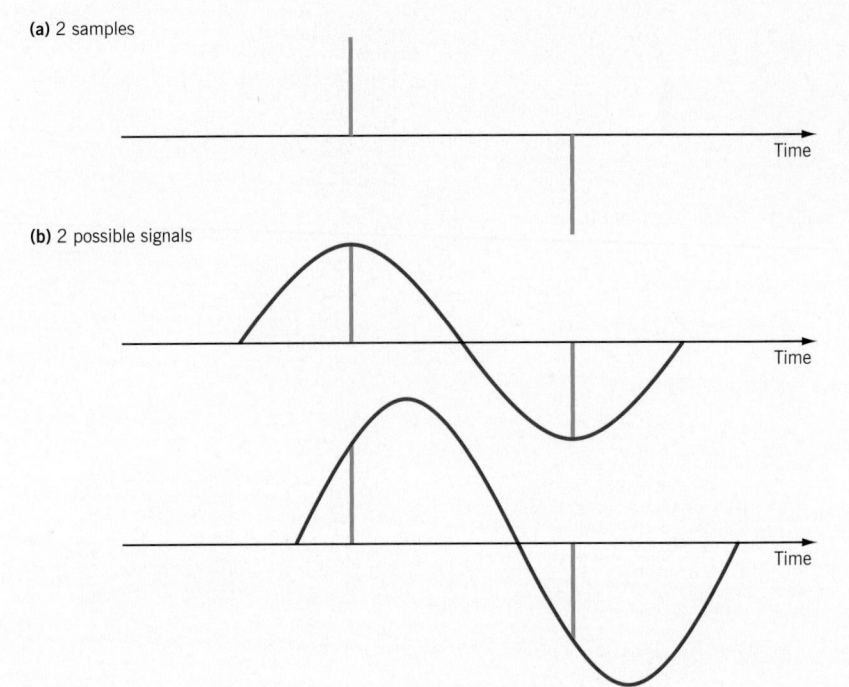

(a) 2 samples

(b) 2 possible signals

Table 21.2 The voltage and corresponding binary code of each successive sample taken of the signal shown in Fig 21.18

Sample	Level or voltage/V	Code
1	1	001
2	3	011
3	5	101
4	7	111
5	5	101
6	3	011
7	1	001

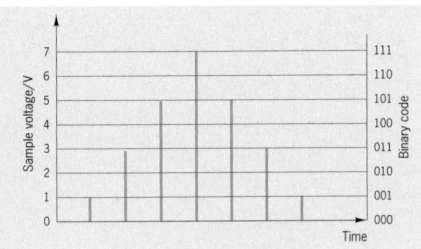

Fig 21.20 Amplitude pulses are converted into a binary code

quantisation and the levels are called **quantisation levels**. For example, if the maximum signal voltage is 1 volt, this would be the highest level. If sixteen quantisation levels were used, then the first level above zero would represent 1/16 volt. Each sampled pulse is then measured and matched to these levels and is given the value of the closest level. As shown in Fig 21.20, each amplitude pulse is given a digital code which is a binary number. The size of the number, that is, how many bits it has, depends on the number of quantisation levels. If there are eight levels (including zero), as in Fig 21.20, then a three-bit code will do. See Table 21.2.

Fig 21.21 The binary code and digital waveform for the example in Fig 21.20

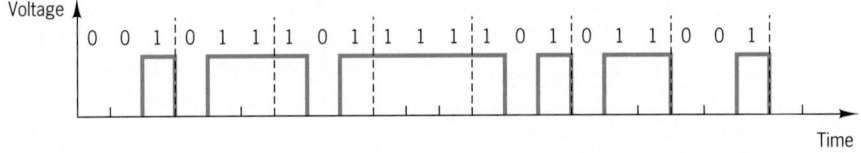

To summarise, the number of quantisation levels determines the number of bits in the code for each pulse. Each pulse is represented by a binary number with the same number of bits, no matter what its level, and each binary number is called a **word**. All samples with a value in a particular range are given the same binary code.

Each binary code is then transmitted in sequence, starting with the first sample. If the binary signal were displayed on an oscilloscope, it would look like a series of pulses, each having the same amplitude, but these pulses would now have different lengths. The digital signal for our example is shown in Fig 21.21.

Each binary digit is allocated a fixed period of time. The length of the pulse is the time for which it is high or low. Binary zeros (0) are represented by zero volts, and binary ones (1) by a fixed voltage (often, +5 V is used). A series of several consecutive 1's or 0's represents a longer pulse. The signal is now **pulse code modulated**.

In a telephone system, these digitised pulses are transmitted along a coaxial cable, or they are converted into pulses of infrared radiation and sent along an optical fibre. They may even be transmitted as pulses of radio waves at microwave frequencies. The information from the Voyager space probes was sent back to Earth as a PCM radio signal.

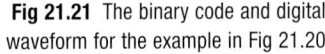

? QUESTIONS 7–9

7 Why would 16 quantisation levels need a four-bit number?

8 Why is it better to send pulses of the same amplitude rather than pulses of varying amplitude?

9 Pulse code modulation is also used for digital audio recording. Some compact discs use a 32-bit code. How many quantisation levels would this give?

Digital-to-analogue conversion

At the receiver, the process is reversed. As it arrives, each binary word is decoded by the receiver as the voltage equal to the *mean* of the relevant quantisation level.

As the samples are decoded, they are reassembled to make the original analogue signal. Fig 21.22 shows the digital signal changed back into a pulse amplitude modulated (PAM) signal. This is further processed to give the original analogue signal.

The quality of reproduction depends on the number of quantisation levels, that is, how close together they are within the range used. More levels means bigger binary codes. Larger binary codes can be sent within the same time by giving each binary digit a shorter time.

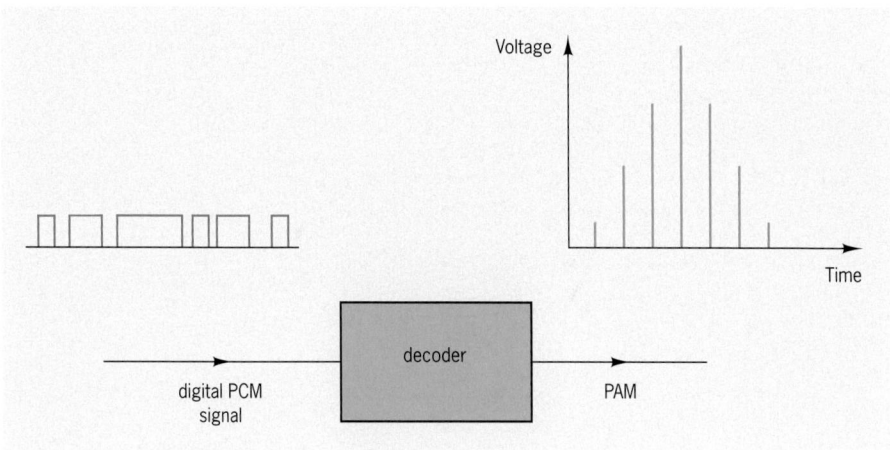

Fig 21.22 The digital signal arrives at the receiver, which decodes it to reproduce the original pulse amplitude modulated signal

QUANTISATION ERRORS

Reconstructed signals may be distorted if quantisation levels are too widely spaced. Several samples which may have been slightly different in the original signal could be given the same value when the signal is reconstructed. An example is shown in Fig 21.23. The difference between the original sample and the reconstructed sample has the same effect as noise in analogue signals – it affects the amplitude. The difference in amplitude between the two signals – the original and the reconstructed – is a measure of the 'noise'. Fig 21.23 shows that the signal-to-noise ratio is better as the samples get bigger. For small samples the ratio is very small.

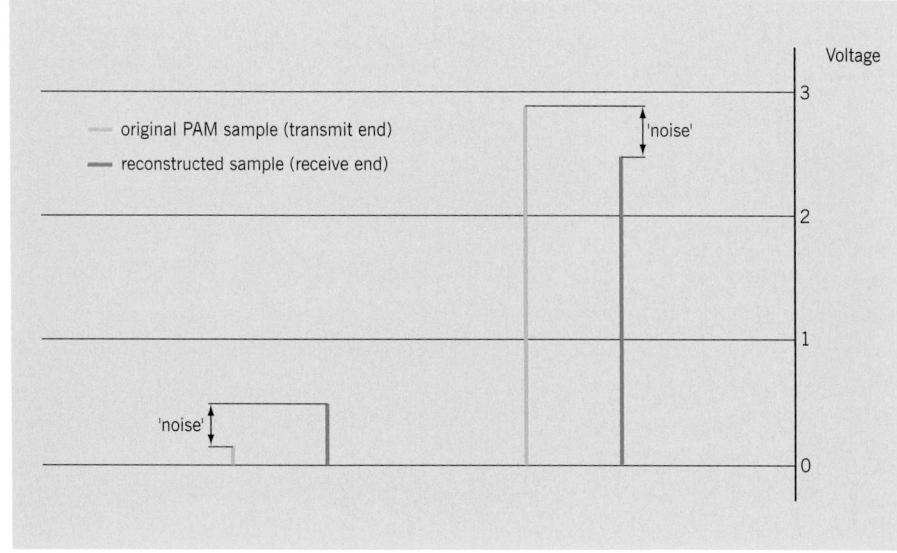

Fig 21.23 Quantisation distortion

429

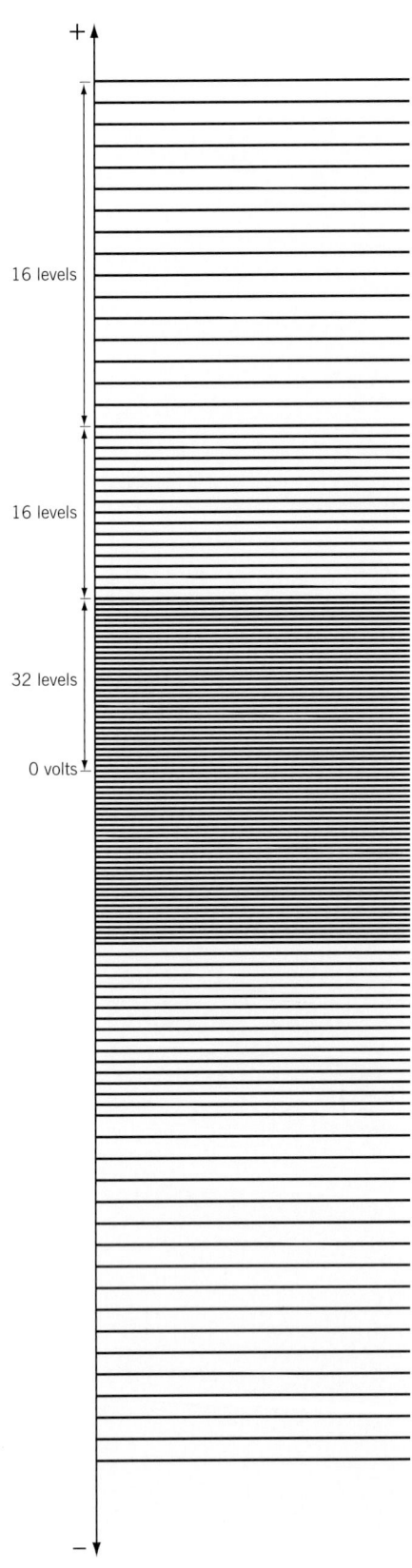

Fig 21.24 Companding quantisation levels

There is a very simple technique which overcomes this potential problem. Instead of all quantisation levels being equal, a non-linear scale is adopted. The process is called **companding**. Fig 21.24 shows an example of companding similar to that used in sound recording. The first 32 levels are equal but very close together; the next 16 are also equal but slightly further apart than the first 32. Above these there are 16 more equal levels which are slightly further apart again. This scheme continues for higher levels and is duplicated for negative samples, giving a total of 256 quantisation levels. Each sample could be encoded as an 8-bit word ($2^8 = 256$).

DIGITAL SIGNALS AND BIT RATES

An analogue signal would be described by its 'frequency range', such as that for a radio station. This term has no meaning for a digital signal. Instead, we describe a digital signal by the number of bits – binary digits – per second.

To calculate the **bit rate**, we need to know the sampling rate and the number of quantisation levels. The sampling rate is the number of samples every second. The levels determine the binary code and the number of 'bits per sample' required.

So the bit rate is given by:

$$\text{bit rate} = (\text{sampling rate}) \times (\text{number of bits per sample})$$

The **medium** through which a signal travels will place a limit on the maximum frequency and on the maximum bit rate. We will look at this in more detail on pages 433–435.

EXAMPLE

Q Calculate the bit rate for a signal which has a sampling rate of 8 kHz and where 16 quantisation levels have been used.

A The sampling rate is 8000 per second.
16 quantisation levels can be coded by a 4-bit binary number because $16 = 2^4$.
So :

$$\text{bit rate} = (\text{sampling rate}) \times (\text{number of bits/sample})$$
$$= 8000 \times 4$$

The bit rate for the signal = 32 000 bits per second

BANDWIDTH OF DIGITAL SIGNALS

The bandwidth of a digital signal depends on the 'mode' of transmission. Let's start thinking about what seems straightforward at first; that is, to send a series of 1's and 0's, rather like the signal in Fig 21.21. The 1's and 0's are a series of pulses, ideally 'square' pulses with very short transition times between 1 and 0.

Fig 21.25(a) shows a simple 'square wave' signal – a pattern of alternating 1's and 0's. This looks very simple but when we examine such a signal on a spectrum analyser (Fig 21.25(b)) we see that it is far from simple, especially when we compare it with a spectrum for a pure sine wave signal (Fig 21.25(c)).

The sine wave spectrum contains only one peak corresponding to the frequency of the signal. The square wave signal contains many peaks, each gradually getting smaller. If we look carefully we can see that the spectrum includes only odd harmonics (f, $3f$, $5f$, $7f$, etc.)

(The spectrum can be explained using a mathematical technique first developed by the French mathematician Baron Jean Baptiste Joseph Fourier (1768–1830), called **Fourier analysis**. Fourier showed that any periodic signal can be made up by adding together a simple pure sine wave signal and some of its harmonics.)

If a square wave is actually made up of all these different components then its bandwidth is theoretically huge. However, in practice we can get away with using a far narrower bandwidth.

The minimum bandwidth is calculated from the time period for a single bit. If this time is t seconds then the bandwidth has a lower limit given by:

frequency bandwidth $\Delta f \geq 1/t$

Use of the minimum bandwidth effectively filters out all the harmonics and only allows the fundamental frequency signal through. This means that the signal at the receiver looks like a pure sine wave, as shown in Fig 21.26.

This is not a problem because the original pattern of 1's and 0's is still preserved in the received signal. It is very simple to 'regenerate' the original signal electronically using a circuit called a **Schmitt trigger** (Fig 21.27). The bandwidth in practice is thus determined by the period of a single bit.

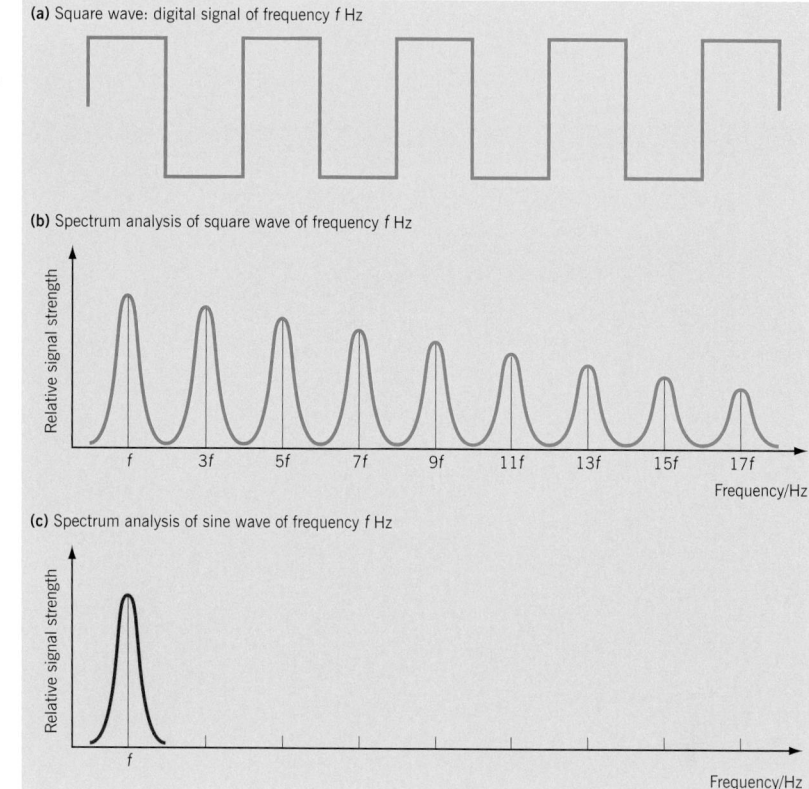

Fig 21.25 A square wave signal and its spectrum analysis compared with that for a pure sine wave signal

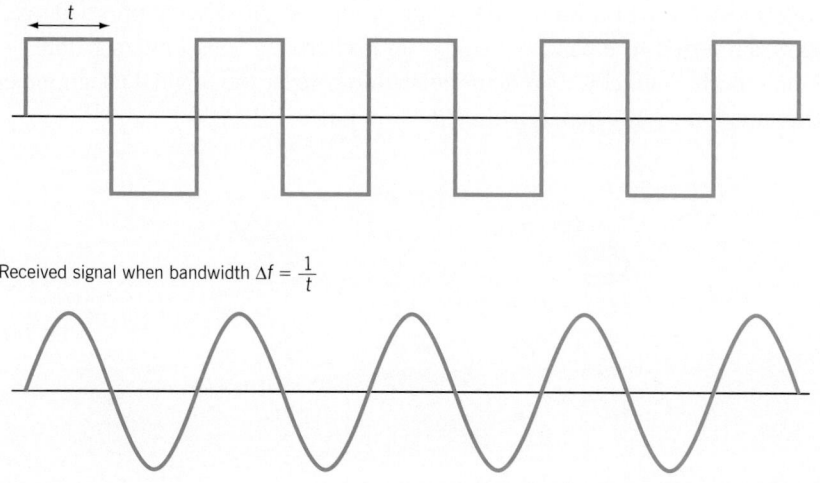

Fig 21.26 Transmitted and received signals using a bandwidth of $\Delta f = 1/t$

For example, telephone systems use a bit length of 2 to 3 µs. At 2 µs this means that the bandwidth necessary to transmit would be $1/2$ µs^{-1}, which is 500 kHz (0.5 MHz) or 500 kilobits per second.

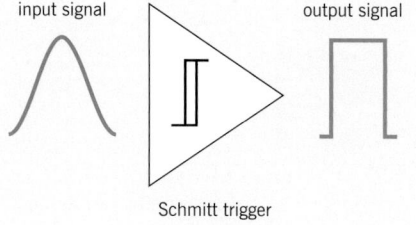

Schmitt trigger

Fig 21.27 Received signal before and after Schmitt trigger circuit

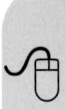

For more information on digital communications, modems and the internet please see the How Science Works assignment for this chapter at www.collinseducation.co.uk/CAS

This is quite a large bandwidth. It would not be possible to send such a signal down an ordinary telephone connection which is just a pair of copper wires. Modems manage to overcome this using a different way of sending a digital signal.

7 MULTIPLEXING

We have seen different ways of transmitting information. The next question is: How can we send more than one signal along a telephone cable at the same time? Alternatively, how do modern communication satellites handle thousands of telephone calls at a time? **Multiplexing** is the process that achieves this, by combining many individual signals and sending them together in one signal.

FREQUENCY DIVISION MULTIPLEXING

Analogue signals can be assembled to produce bands rather like a band of radio signals. A band containing several signals is called a **group**. This grouping together of analogue signals is called **frequency division multiplexing**.

Let's see how four telephone lines can be multiplexed together to form a small group. This is shown in Fig 21.28(a), with each telephone line representing a line with one telephone connected to it.

As each telephone call comes in, it is amplitude modulated with a carrier signal. The first carrier signal is at 1.01 MHz, the second at 1.02 MHz, the third at 1.03 MHz and the fourth at 1.04 MHz. The band is made up from four channels; each channel is allowed 10 kHz of bandwidth (Fig 21.28(b)). At the multiplexer, all the channels are combined to give a **multiplexed signal**.

The cable from the telephone exchange therefore carries a band of frequencies from 1.00 MHz to 1.05 MHz. This is our 'group'. At the destination exchange, the process is reversed. The band of frequencies is filtered to split it into separate channels. Each channel is then demodulated to recover the original telephone call. (Demodulation of AM signals is described on pages 449–450.)

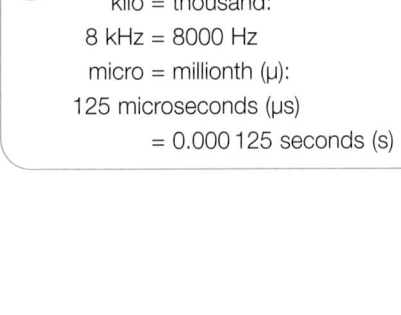

REMEMBER THIS

kilo = thousand:
8 kHz = 8000 Hz
micro = millionth (μ):
125 microseconds (μs)
   = 0.000 125 seconds (s)

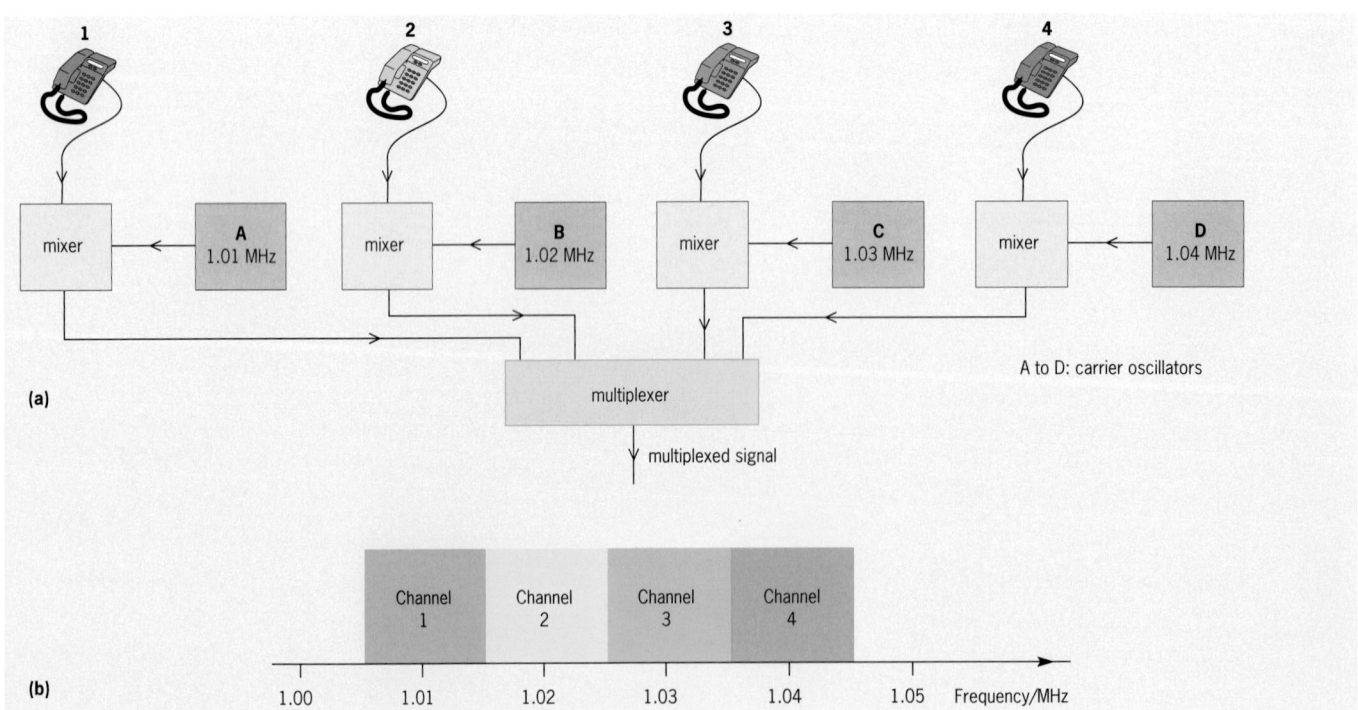

Fig 21.28 Block diagram and bandwidths for four multiplexed telephone lines

TIME DIVISION MULTIPLEXING

Digital signals are multiplexed using a different method, called **time division multiplexing**.

In the Example of pulse code modulation on page 427, the analogue signal is sampled at a rate of 8 kHz. That means that samples are taken every 125 μs (125 microseconds). But each sample lasts for only 2 or 3 μs, and that leaves over 120 μs free between samples – time in which the system would not be carrying any information. For the system, this is wasted time.

In time division multiplexing, this 'free' time is used to fit in other signals. In practical systems, at least 30 channels are multiplexed. Just three channels are shown in Fig 21.29.

Fig 21.29 Three channels which are time division multiplexed

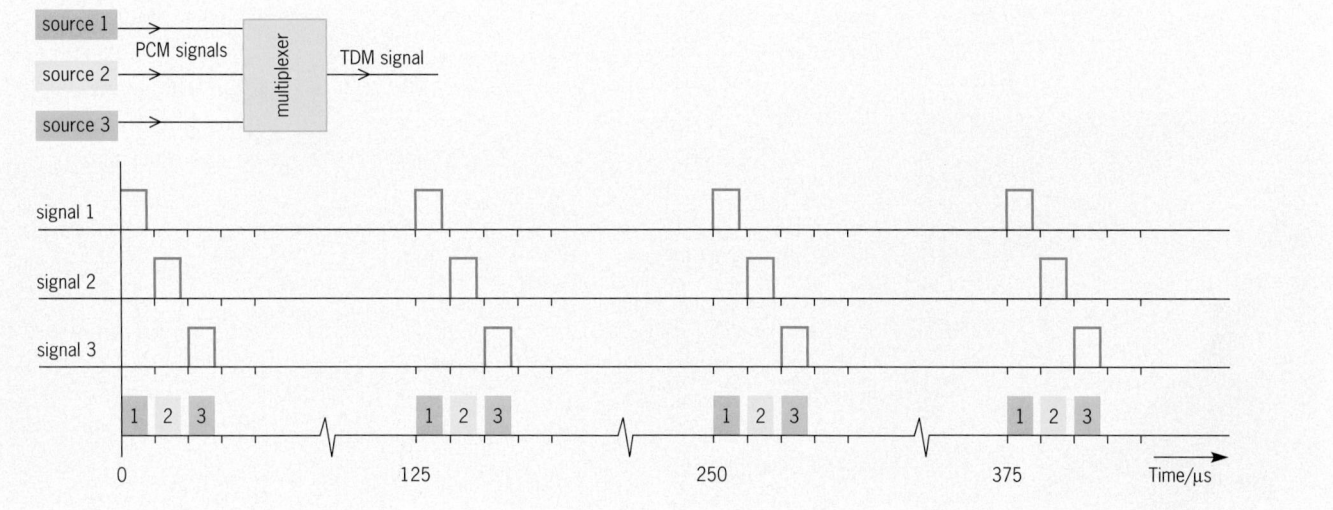

8 MEDIA: HOW SIGNALS TRAVEL

Radio waves can travel through free space or along a coaxial cable. Electrical signals can travel down a wire, and light pulses can be sent along an optical fibre. Free space, coaxial cable, wire, optical fibre – all these are referred to as **media** through which a signal can be sent. Each has its uses, and when you make a telephone call, it is possible that your message may be travelling through every one of these media. Let's follow a long-distance call from a caller in Britain via satellite to her uncle in California, as shown in Fig 21.30.

Fig 21.30 Simple block diagram for a transatlantic telephone call

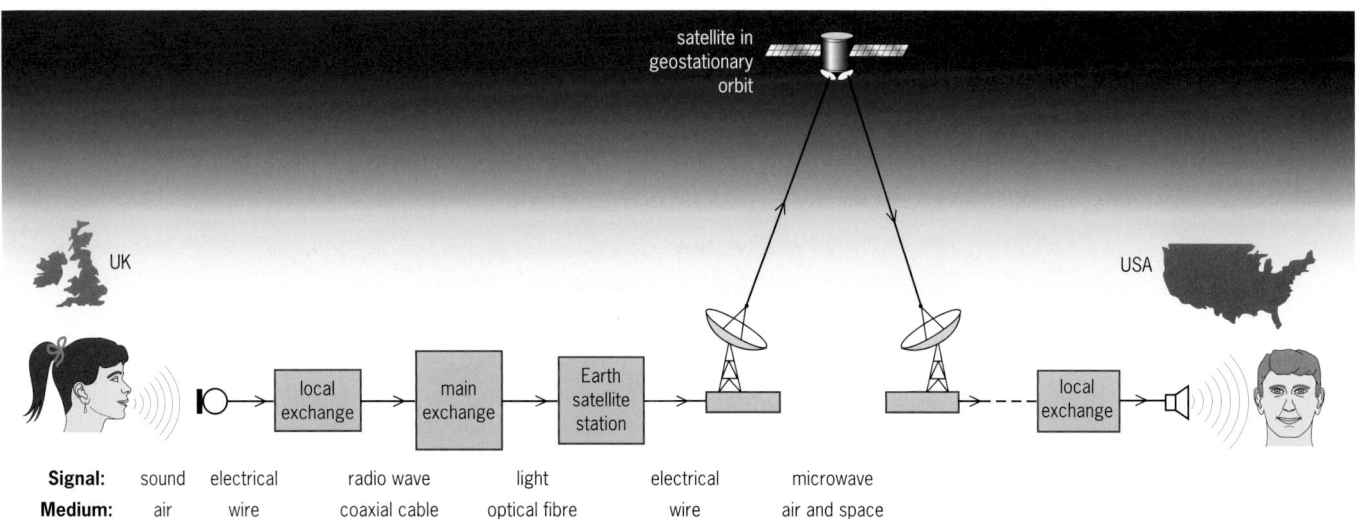

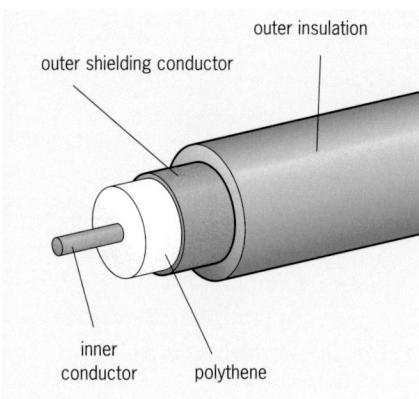

outer insulation

outer shielding conductor

inner conductor   polythene

Fig 21.31 The structure of a coaxial cable which carries radio waves

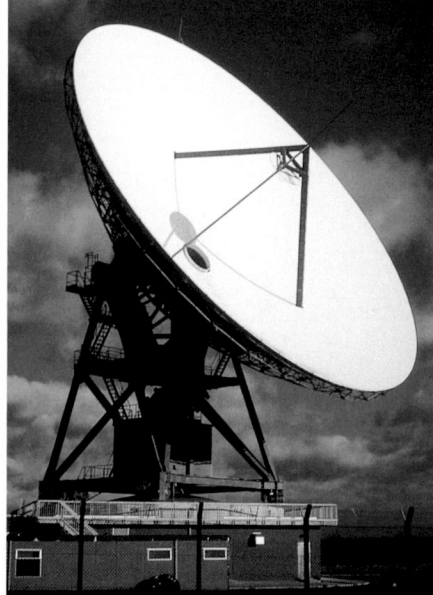

Fig 21.32 The satellite dish at British Telecom's ground station at Madley in Herefordshire, where international telephone calls are relayed

? QUESTION 10

10 What happens to the signal during the last lap of this call?

Our call would first travel as an electrical signal from the telephone to the local exchange along a **copper wire** (wires are in pairs for a complete circuit). These wires are likely to carry only one call at a time – but that's all right because that's all a single phone can handle.

At the local exchange, our call would be digitised and multiplexed with other calls from the area, and sent to a bigger exchange at the nearest large town. All the calls could travel along a coaxial cable as a radio wave.

A **coaxial cable** is a cylindrical wave guide: the radio wave is guided along the cable between the inner and outer conductors which are shown in Fig 21.31. The space between the conductors is filled with polythene or a similar dielectric material. Coaxial cables can carry radio signals with frequencies of tens of megahertz or tens of megabits per second.

Our long-distance call, and many other transatlantic calls like it, would then be directed from the large exchange to a satellite ground station (Fig 21.32). The link between the exchange and the ground station is by **optical fibre** and, to use it, the signal has to be converted from electrical pulses into pulses of light. Infrared is used in high-speed optical systems. The frequency of infrared is of the order of 10^{14} Hz, a million times higher than the upper frequency limit of coaxial cables. With bit rates approaching 10^{14} bits per second, we can see that an optical fibre is capable of handling vast amounts of information. Here, it means a vast number of phone calls all at the same time.

An optical fibre is made from a fine cylinder of glass about 5 μm in diameter. This is the **core**, and is enclosed by **cladding** which is made from a less dense glass. If light enters the core at a large enough angle, it will be trapped in the core because the beam is totally internally reflected at the boundary between the core and the cladding. The beam travels down the fibre after multiple reflections, as shown in Fig 21.33.

Signals travelling down a fibre are not affected by electrical interference, and they are very secure because they do not create a magnetic field which a current flowing down a wire would create.

At the satellite ground station (Fig 21.32), the signal is converted back into an electrical signal (it continues to be digitised). This is then transmitted up to a geostationary satellite, now as a **microwave** signal. The microwaves have frequencies of about 10 GHz (10 gigahertz or 10^{10} Hz). Microwaves don't have the signal-handling capacity of optical signals, yet they allow thousands of telephone calls and several television channels to be transmitted at the same time.

The satellite retransmits the signal down to another ground station in America. Our call may then be directed to its destination by optical fibre or coaxial cable, or both. Its last lap to the telephone in California will probably be by wire – unless our caller's uncle is using a mobile telephone.

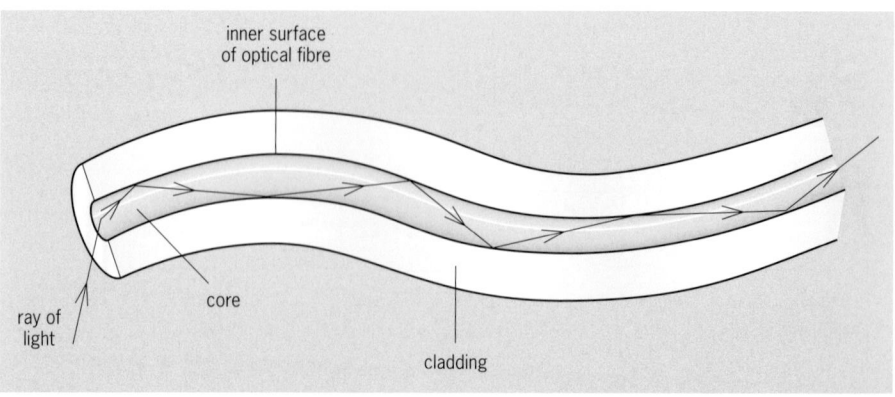

inner surface of optical fibre

ray of light

core

cladding

Fig 21.33 Light travelling along an optical fibre

In fact transatlantic telephone calls now travel by undersea optical fibre cables. It is the vast potential of optical fibre systems that makes the 'information superhighway' possible. The optical fibre systems being installed now are handling only a small fraction of what they are capable of carrying, and there is plenty of room for expansion over the next decade or two.

9 MOBILE PHONES

Mobile telephones are based on a technology that has been in use for many years. They are very low-powered radios with a range of no more than 10 km. The system works because the country is covered by a network of small 'cells', each centred on a **base station** (Fig 21.34). This is why mobile phones are sometimes called **cellphones**.

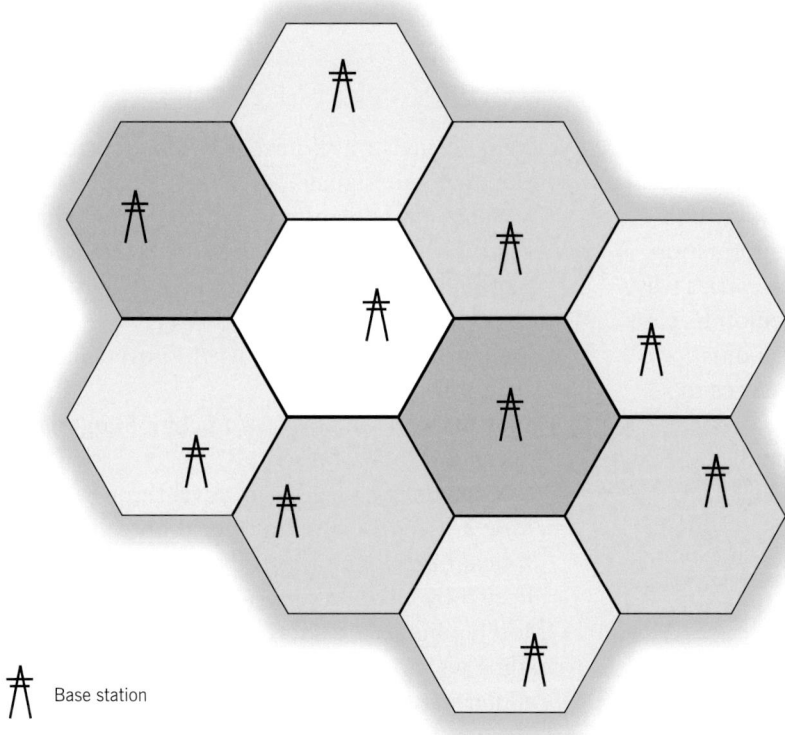

Fig 21.34 The cellular network

☥ Base station

The size of a cell varies around the country, depending upon:
geography and terrain – high-frequency radio signals travel by line of sight so hills, trees and buildings can get in the way,
the frequency used – cells using higher frequencies are smaller because the signal doesn't travel so far,
the number of users within the cell – there is a limit to the number of calls a base station can handle and so in urban areas cells are smaller.
The base station is in reach of any mobile phone within that cell. The mobile phone sends a radio signal to the base station at one frequency; the base station sends the return call back to the mobile at a slightly different frequency. This is an example of **duplex** communication – sending at one frequency and receiving at another.
The base station connects the mobile call to the rest of the telephone network, whether that is another part of the mobile cellular network or the network of

? QUESTIONS 11–12

11 For efficient transmission a simple radio transmitter should have an aerial which is about a quarter of a wavelength long. Estimate the size of the aerial in a mobile phone.

12 Find out more about modern digital systems and prepare a presentation on mobile telephones.

ordinary *land lines* (often referred to as the Public Switched Telephone Network or PSTN). These connections are either ordinary telephone lines, usually optical fibres, or microwave links. Each base station is connected to each of the other base stations by a central switching network. This makes sure that the mobile user is automatically transferred from one base station to another if a call is being made while moving from one cell to another. The cells overlap so that the mobile is always within range of a base station.

In the UK mobile phones use radio frequencies in the ranges 872–960 MHz, 1710–1875 MHz and 1920–2170 MHz.

Today's digital mobile phones use two different technologies. Currently most use the **GSM** or **G**lobal **S**ystem of **M**obile communication which uses the 900 MHz and 1800 MHz bands. GSM is recognised across the world and it enables mobile phones to be used in different countries.

In the future it is expected that more mobiles will use the **UMTS** or **U**niversal **M**obile **T**elecommunications **S**ystem. This uses the higher frequency, 2 GHz, band and offers video and multimedia options to mobile users.

SUMMARY

Having studied this chapter, you should be able to understand the following:

- Electromagnetic waves, in particular radio waves and light waves, can be used to carry information.
- The process of adding information to a carrier wave is called modulation. Two types in common use are amplitude modulation and frequency modulation.
- Signal bandwidth is the range of frequencies in a signal.
- For an amplitude modulated signal, channel bandwidth = 2 × audio signal bandwidth.
- The bandwidth for a frequency modulated signal is much greater.
- For a digital signal, bit rate = sampling rate × number of bits per sample.
- The bandwidth for a digital signal should be at least f Hz where $f = 1/t$ and t is the time for one bit.
- Noise is a random signal that is always present in circuits. Atmospheric noise and other interference from electrical machinery can also affect signals.
- Analogue and digital signals can be converted from one to the other.

- Digital signals travel further without corruption than analogue signals.
- Pulse code modulation is a digital modulation method used for communications and audio recording which enables very high quality reproduction.
- Companding is a method used to overcome quantisation distortion.
- Multiplexing is the process of combining many signals into one.
- Electromagnetic waves can travel through space, along a wire or along an optical fibre.
- Optical fibres offer a huge bandwidth and are not affected by electrical interference.
- Mobile phones are short-range low-powered radios which connect via base stations in the cellular network.

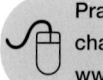 Practice questions for this chapter are available at www.collinseducation.co.uk/CAS

22

Physical electronics

22 PHYSICAL ELECTRONICS

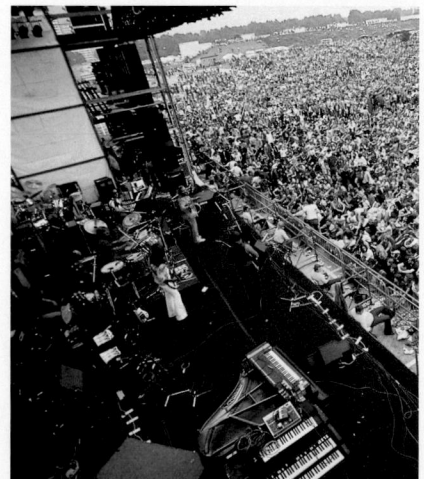

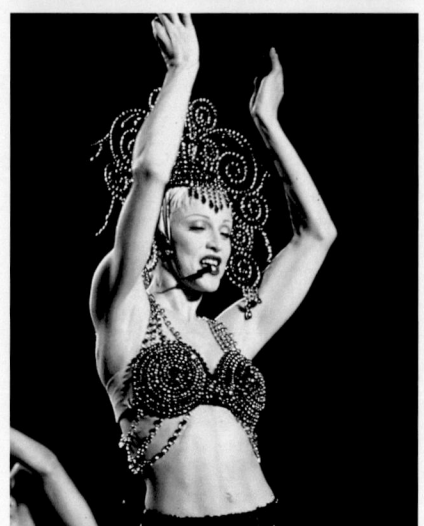

When pop groups perform on stage, they no longer have to put up with a clutter of wires and speakers because of the progress made in electronic sound engineering.

Singers and musicians cannot hear directly what other members of the band are playing. Up until recently, they have had to rely on monitor speakers on stage to play back the sound of the band, to get their own timing and sound levels correct (with other speakers directed at the audience).

Now, thanks to miniaturised electronic circuits, singers and players can wear a tiny earpiece instead of listening to the monitor speakers. Sound engineers mix the sound from all the instruments and voices and send it to a radio transmitter about 100 metres from the stage. Each musician carries a battery-powered receiver that picks up the signal from the transmitter and sends it along a wire to the earpiece. The receivers have volume controls, so each musician can adjust the sound to a comfortable level.

This system has several advantages. The stage is safer without stray speakers and wires and the musicians need not suffer from hearing damage because they can control their own sound level. The dreadful howling noise which used to come from sound feedback into amplifiers is a thing of the past. And the audience hears a better sound because it comes only from speakers directed at them.

Above: A stage cluttered with wiring restricts the musicians
Below: Madonna can move freely around the stage wearing a radio microphone and an earpiece

The ideas in this chapter

This chapter describes the behaviour of electronic circuits and systems. Electronics is a practical subject, so it will be best if you try the circuits out and check that they behave in the way described here. Only then will you fully understand the ideas in this chapter.

Electronic devices perform a vast range of tasks. For example, an electronic system in washing machines allows different types of material to be washed at the right temperature for the right length of time. The system controls water flow into and out of the machine, and heats the water if necessary. It also controls the rinsing and spinning.

As another example, some car radios tune themselves automatically to the strongest signal. Though the driver may not know it is happening, on a long journey, the radio retunes as the car travels between the range of one transmitter and the next. This ensures that the sound output remains as clear as possible.

In this chapter we will look at the principles of some of the most useful electronic circuits and systems.

1 ELECTRONIC SYSTEMS

INPUT, PROCESS AND OUTPUT

Any electronic system can be broken down into three parts as shown in Fig 22.1. Electronic systems respond to **input** signals. A signal is something that varies with time and carries information. For example, some of the signals we human beings respond to are changes in temperature or light intensity, changes in sound level or the weight of a bag of sugar. These signals could also apply to electronic systems.

The input block converts the input signal – the information – into an electronic signal. This will be a voltage which changes to reflect the changing information. The electronic signal is passed into the **process** block. For the time being, we will simply say that this block 'processes' the signal. The rest of this chapter describes some different types of process device.

The signal coming out of the process block is still an electronic signal but it has been changed, that is, it has been processed. The last block, the output block, responds to this processed electronic signal and changes it into some other form – such as a sound or light signal, or perhaps it turns a motor on or off.

The input and output blocks use devices that convert signals from one form to another. These are called **transducers**.

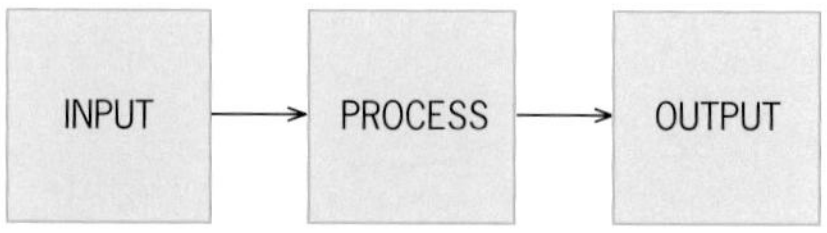

Fig 22.1 Block diagram of any electronic system

TRANSDUCERS

Transducers can be divided into **input transducers** and **output transducers**. Input transducers are devices that convert some physical quantity, such as temperature or light level, into a voltage or some other electrical quantity. Input transducers are sometimes referred to as **sensors**.

A microphone converts the changes in air pressure of sound into a changing voltage. A light-dependent resistor responds to changes in light intensity by changing its resistance. This change of resistance can be used in a simple circuit to produce a changing voltage (Fig 22.2).

> **? QUESTION 1**
>
> 1 What physical quantity could these input transducers change into electronic signals?
> **a)** a thermistor,
> **b)** a strain gauge,
> **c)** a photodiode.

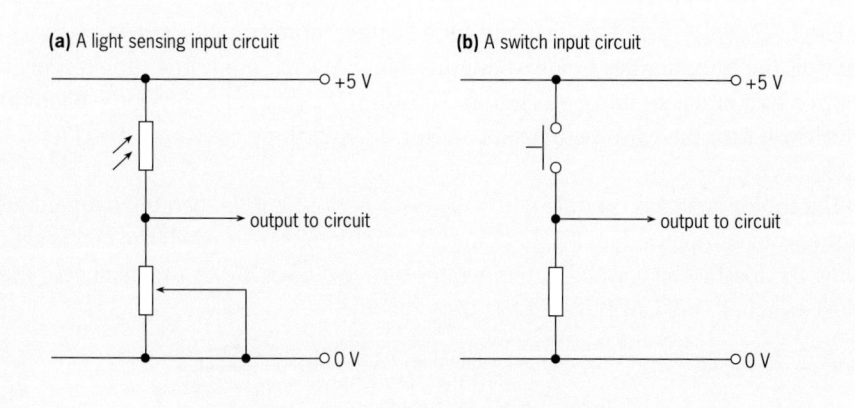

Fig 22.2 Examples of input circuits

Output transducers change electronic signals back into some physical quantity. For example, a loudspeaker converts an electronic signal into changes in air pressure – that is, sound.

Electronic systems can be divided into two kinds, although there are many examples where they are used together to make useful systems. These two parts are **digital** systems and **analogue** (or linear) systems.

> **? QUESTION 2**
>
> 2 What physical quantities do these output transducers change electronic signals into?
> **a)** a motor,
> **b)** a bulb,
> **c)** a heater.

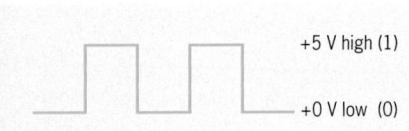

Fig 22.3 A 'square' wave with a 'peak' voltage of 5 V, typical for a digital signal

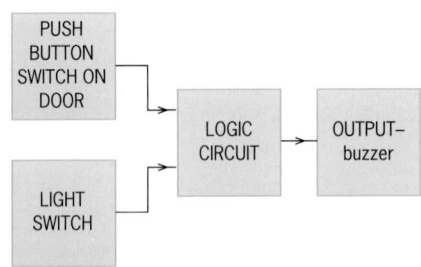

Fig 22.4 Block diagram of a lights-on alarm system in a car

Table 22.1 Combinations of switches for the lights-on alarm

Light switch	Door switch	Audible warning
off	open	off
off	closed	off
on	open	off
on	closed	on

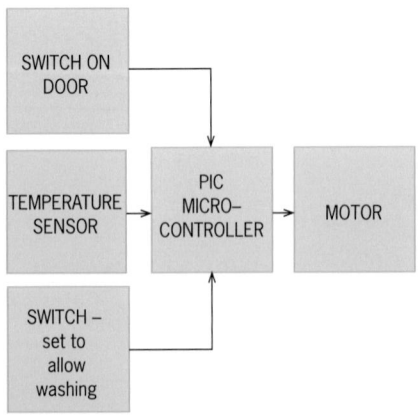

Fig 22.5 Block diagram of the control system for a washing machine

2 DIGITAL SYSTEMS

Digital systems process digital signals. A digital signal is one which has discrete values (that is, separate as opposed to continuous, possibly varying values). The switch in Fig 22.2(b) produces a digital signal. The switch is either open or closed, so the voltage output of the circuit will be either 0 V or 5 V, which is the usual voltage range of the power supply. In simple digital systems there are only two possible signal states. These two states are called **low** and **high**.

Some circuits are designed to make digital signals. An **astable** produces a square wave – it has a frequency and amplitude just like the sine wave more typical of alternating signals, but the signal alternates sharply between a high and low value (Fig 22.3).

The square wave is a digital signal that changes at a regular rate. If the period (time for one cycle) is constant, circuits like this can be used for timing.

DECISION CIRCUITS – LOGIC GATES AND PROGRAMMABLE MICROCHIPS

Most new cars have an audible alarm that warns the driver that the lights are on when the car door is opened. The electronic system that does this uses two inputs:

- A push-button switch which is *closed* when the door is opened.
- The light switch – off when the lights are off and on when the lights are on!

There is one output (Fig 22.4), which activates the buzzer that produces the audible warning. Table 22.1 shows the possible combinations in a **truth table**.

The design of a system that behaves as described in the truth table is quite simple if we use one of a group of very useful digital circuits called **logic gates**. These are simple electronic elements which make decisions about an output based on one or more inputs. The simplest logic gate, the **NOT gate** or **inverter**, has only one input; other logic gates have two or more inputs. See the Stretch and Challenge box opposite.

Fig 22.5 shows the block diagram for a slightly more complex system, which controls the programmes of a washing machine. At each point in a programme, the control system has to make a decision. For example, there are only some conditions which will turn the washing machine motor on, and these are summarised in Table 22.2.

The motor switches on only when the door is closed *and* when the temperature of the water is higher than 55 °C (2 and 3 in Table 22.2), *or* when the dial is set to allow the load to be washed at temperatures of less than 55 °C, in which case the wash switch is on (1 in Table 22.2).

Table 22.2 Combinations of conditions for the motor of a washing machine

Water temp. sensor	Wash switch	Door	Motor
<55 °C	off	open	OFF
<55 °C	off	closed	OFF
<55 °C	on	open	OFF
<55 °C	on	closed	ON [1]
>55 °C	off	open	OFF
>55 °C	off	closed	ON [2]
>55 °C	on	open	OFF
>55 °C	on	closed	ON [3]

Logic gates and truth tables

The inputs and outputs to and from logic gates will depend on the power supply, but are often 0 V or 5 V. An input or output at 0 V is described as 'low' and an input or output at or near 5 V is 'high'. The low and high voltages at inputs or outputs are given the binary codes 0 and 1. Truth tables using these digits summarise the behaviour of logic gates. Fig 22.6 shows the circuit symbols and the truth tables for several useful logic gates.

Fig 22.7 shows a simple circuit for testing a two-input logic gate. The two switches allow each input to be set at either low or high.

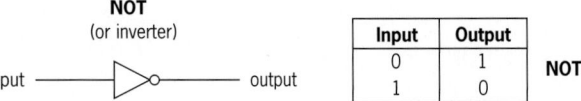

NOT
(or inverter)

Input	Output	
0	1	**NOT**
1	0	

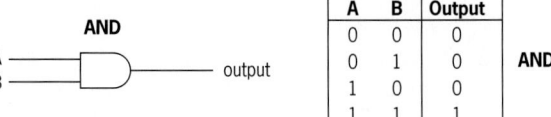

AND

A	B	Output	
0	0	0	
0	1	0	**AND**
1	0	0	
1	1	1	

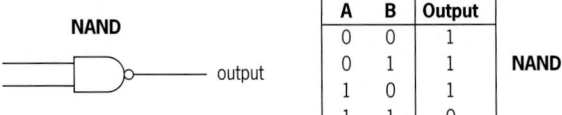

NAND

A	B	Output	
0	0	1	
0	1	1	**NAND**
1	0	1	
1	1	0	

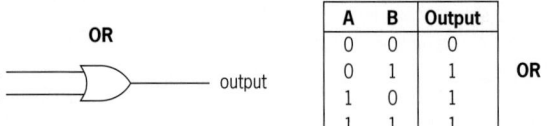

OR

A	B	Output	
0	0	0	
0	1	1	**OR**
1	0	1	
1	1	1	

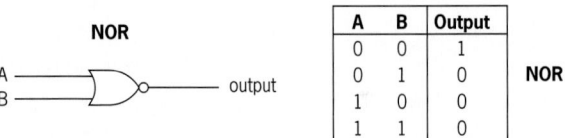

NOR

A	B	Output	
0	0	1	
0	1	0	**NOR**
1	0	0	
1	1	0	

Fig 22.6 Symbols and truth tables of common gates

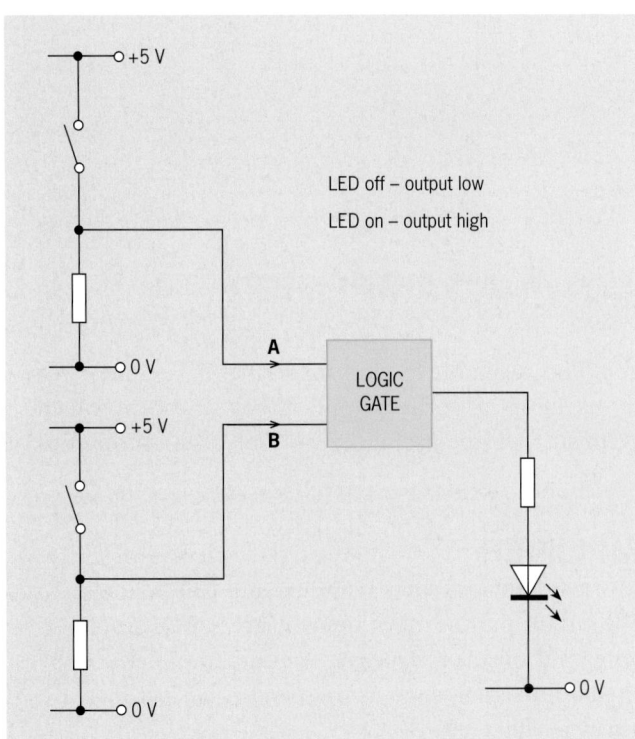

LED off – output low
LED on – output high

Fig 22.7 A simple circuit for testing a two-input logic gate. When the switch is open the input (A or B) into the gate is low. The switch is closed to make the input go high. The LED monitors the output

? QUESTION 3

3 Look at the truth tables above and compare them with Table 22.1. Which gate could be used to make the decisions necessary in the lights-on warning system in a car?

This design problem could also be solved using a combination of logic gates but today it is far more likely to be solved using **programmable microchips** or **PICs**. PIC stands for Peripheral Interface Controller. It is a simple computer equipped with inputs and outputs, memory and microprocessor, all contained on a single microchip. PICs are very adaptable – they will do what the program tells them to do. The inputs and outputs can be digital or analogue.

The advantage of using a PIC in a washing machine system is that it can be programmed to carry out a variety of different washing cycles, which can be simply selected by a switch.

3 ANALOGUE SYSTEMS

Many electronic circuits are designed to respond to signals that change over a wide range of values, like the varying temperature of the water in the washing machine. These are known as **analogue systems**.

A circuit very similar to those in Fig 22.2 can be used as a temperature-sensing input board (Fig 22.8). The thermistor is joined to a variable resistor to make up a potential divider. The voltage at the output of this circuit will change with temperature. The output voltage range can be adjusted by changing the variable resistor since the variable resistor changes the sensitivity of the circuit.

QUESTION 4

4 List four other physical quantities which change in a way similar to temperature.
Suggest a transducer or sensor which could convert each of those quantities into a changing electrical quantity.

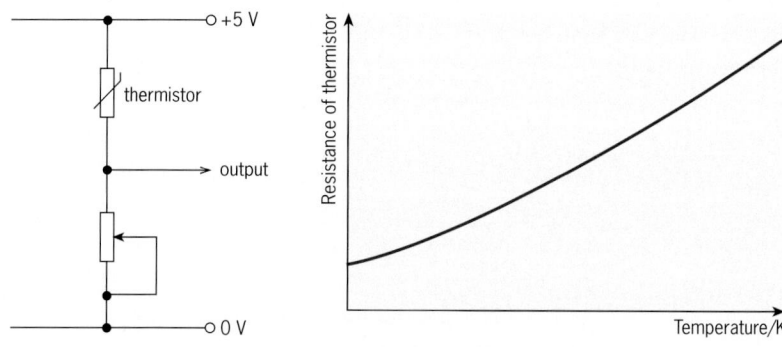

Fig 22.8 A 'temperature-sensing' input board, with a graph showing how the resistance of the thermistor varies with temperature

4 THE OPERATIONAL AMPLIFIER

There is a family of amplifiers available in chip form (that is, as integrated circuits), which are very useful in all sorts of applications. These are called **operational amplifiers**. It will be useful first to look at the properties of a simple amplifier.

THE SIMPLE AMPLIFIER

We are all familiar with audio devices such as radios and CD systems. An audio amplifier is an important part of all of these systems. The amplifier takes a small, weak signal and makes it stronger. A good amplifier preserves the characteristics of the audio signal, such as frequency, and just increases the amplitude of the signal, as in Fig 22.9.

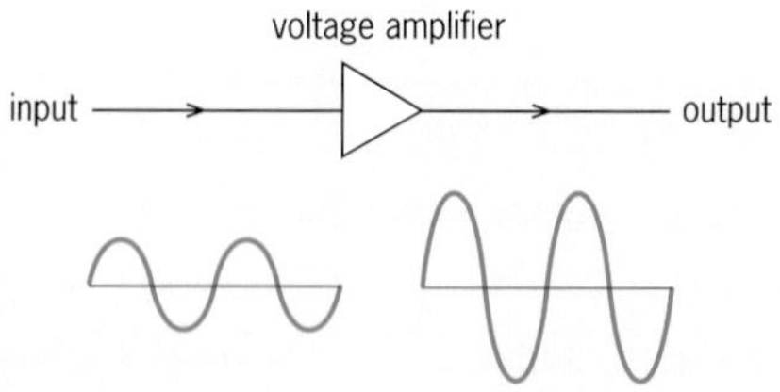

The amplitude of the signal going into and out of the amplifier could be measured in volts, and so the amplifier may be described as a **voltage amplifier**. The output voltage will be bigger than the input voltage: the ratio of the output to the input is called the **gain** of the amplifier. The gain may be expressed as a number (such as 10 times) or may be measured in **decibels** (**dB**).

Fig 22.9 A simple voltage amplifier showing input and output signals

The decibel

Very often in electronics we wish to compare the relative amplitude of two signals. The signals could be the input to and output from an amplifier, and the ratio could be very large, sometimes as big as millions. For this reason it is easier to use a logarithmic scale, as shown in Table 22.3.

Table 22.3

Linear scale, N	1	10	100	1000	10 000	100 000
Logarithmic scale, $\log_{10} N$	0	1	2	3	4	5

We use a unit called the **decibel**. By definition, the ratio of two signals in decibels is:

$$dB = 20 \log_{10}\left(\frac{V_2}{V_1}\right)$$

where V_1 and V_2 are the peak voltages of the two signals. (Although we could use the r.m.s. voltages – see Chapter 12.)

REMEMBER THIS

The decibel is defined as:

$$dB = 10 \log_{10}(P_2/P_1)$$

But remember that power, $P = V^2/R$, so that:

$$dB = 10 \log_{10}\left(\frac{V_2^2/R}{V_1^2/R}\right)$$

$$= 10 \log_{10}(V_2/V_1)^2$$

$$= 20 \log_{10}(V_2/V_1)$$

EXAMPLE

Q The input to an amplifier has a peak voltage of 0.2 mV. The output has a peak voltage of 2 V. What is the gain of the amplifier?

A

$$\text{Gain} = \frac{\text{output voltage}}{\text{input voltage}} = \frac{2\text{ V}}{0.2\text{ mV}} = 10\,000 \text{ times (or} \times 10\,000)$$

Or, in dB:

$$\text{Gain} = 20 \log_{10}\left(\frac{V_{\text{out}}}{V_{\text{in}}}\right) = 20 \log_{10} 10\,000 = 20 \times 4 = 80 \text{ dB}$$

Input and output impedance

When a signal passes into an amplifier, there is a current. The size of the current depends on the signal voltage at any instant, but it also depends on the **input impedance** of the amplifier. The impedance is measured in ohms.

The signal coming out of the amplifier is also a current and has a voltage (usually both are fluctuating) and is passed into another device or **load**. In the case of an audio amplifier, the load is usually a loudspeaker. The output of the amplifier behaves as a signal source. The current that this source drives through the load depends on the source voltage, the impedance of the load and the **output impedance** of the amplifier.

It helps to think of the output of the amplifier as a source of alternating e.m.f. with an internal resistance – rather as a battery is made up of a source of e.m.f. ε in series with its internal resistance r, as in Fig 22.10.

When the signal source is connected to a load, it operates most efficiently when the load impedance is the same as the output impedance of the amplifier. This is a result of the maximum power theorem.

Maximum power theorem

This is a useful idea from d.c. circuits that helps in the design of efficient electronic systems.

How does the energy transferred from a battery to a load depend on the resistance of the load? (See the circuit of Fig 22.10(a).)

Consider the two extremes of the load – that is, zero resistance and very high (infinite) resistance.

When the load has zero resistance ($R = 0$), the current I will be limited only by the internal resistance r of the battery and will therefore have a maximum value. However, the p.d. across zero resistance is zero. No energy is transferred in the load – but the battery will get very hot.

When the load resistance R is infinite, the current in the load will be very small. Again, the energy transferred in the load (IV) will be very small.

It is reasonable that for some value of load resistance in between, the energy transferred will be a maximum. That value can be found using calculus, as in the following Stretch and Challenge passage.

QUESTION 5

5   A signal of 5 mV is fed into an amplifier with a gain of 20 dB. Calculate the voltage of the output signal.

REMEMBER THIS

Impedance

We saw in Chapter 12 that capacitors and inductors have reactance in a.c. circuits. We treat electronic circuits as a.c. circuits, as the signals they process are often alternating. The combination of resistance and reactance is called impedance. Like resistance and reactance it is measured in ohms, and like reactance it depends on frequency. Impedance, Z, is given by:

$$Z = \sqrt{(R^2 + X^2)}$$

where R is resistance and X is reactance.

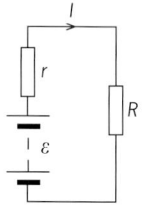

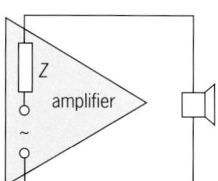

(a) A battery of e.m.f. ε with internal resistance r connected to a load resistor R

(b) The output of the amplifier – a source of alternating e.m.f. in series with the 'output impedance' of the amplifier connected to a load (a loudspeaker)

Fig 22.10 Analogy between a battery with internal resistance and a signal source

Derivation of the maximum power theorem

In the circuit of Fig 22.10(a) we have:

$$\varepsilon = Ir + IR$$

or:

$$I = \frac{\varepsilon}{r + R}$$

The power W in the load R is given by:

$$W = I^2R = \frac{\varepsilon^2 R}{(r + R)^2}$$

As R changes, so does W. W will be a maximum when dW/dR is zero:

$$\frac{dW}{dR} = \frac{d}{dR}\left(\frac{\varepsilon^2 R}{(r + R)^2}\right) = 0$$

That is:

the differential $= \dfrac{(r + R)^2\varepsilon^2 - 2\varepsilon^2 R(r + R)}{(r + R)^4} = 0 = 0$

Therefore: $\quad (r + R)^2\varepsilon^2 - 2\varepsilon^2 R(r + R) = 0$

This simplifies to: $\quad (r + R) - 2R = 0$

which gives the solution: $\quad r = R$

That is, the maximum energy transfer happens when the load resistance is the same as the internal resistance of the battery.

The same idea works in electronic systems except that we are dealing with alternating signals rather than d.c. Instead of resistance we consider impedance, but the result is the same:

Maximum power is transferred when the output impedance is equal to the load impedance.

PROPERTIES OF OPERATIONAL AMPLIFIERS

The operational amplifier or **op-amp** is nearly the perfect amplifier. Fig 22.11 shows the basic characteristics of an op-amp.

Op-amps have some important properties:

1 They are **differential** amplifiers. They have two inputs and the output of the amplifier depends on the difference between them:

output = gain × *difference* between the two inputs

One input is called the **non-inverting** input and the other is the **inverting** input (Fig 22.11).

$$V_{out} = A(\varepsilon_1 - \varepsilon_2)$$

For example, if $A = 10^6$, $\varepsilon_1 = 0$ V and $\varepsilon_2 = 2$ μV, then:

$$V_{out} = 10^6(0 - 2) \text{ μV}$$
$$= -2 \text{ V}$$

Notice that when $\varepsilon_1 = 0$, the output is negative – the amplifier is said to 'invert' the input.

2 They have a very high gain A, typically 10^5 to 10^6, with some having gains up to 10^9. This gain is called the **open loop gain**.

3 All inputs and outputs are measured relative to earth (0 V). Most op-amps use a 'split rail' power supply which means that earth is taken as the mid-point of the power supply. The supply voltage limits the output voltage of the amplifier. V_{out} cannot be bigger than $\pm V$ (Fig 22.12).

4 The inputs draw very tiny currents – so small that we can consider that they draw no current at all. That is, they have a very high input impedance. (A typical op-amp will draw a current much smaller than a

For more information on impedance and voltage matching please see the How Science Works assignment for this chapter at www.collinseducation.co.uk/CAS

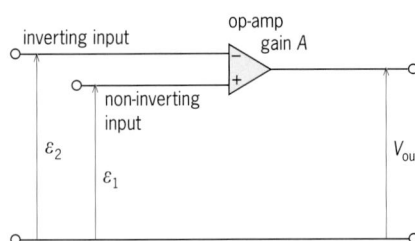

Fig 22.11 Symbol, inputs and output of an op-amp

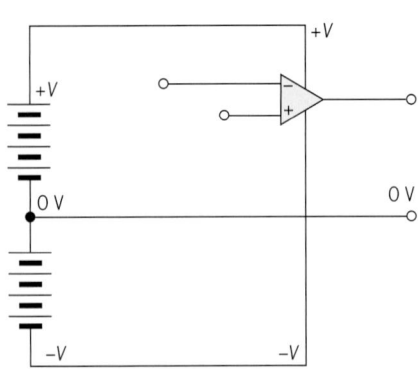

Fig 22.12 Op-amp using 'split rail' power supply

micro-amp, and often as low as nano-amps.) A voltage of 1 µV at the input will drive a current of 1 pA (1 pico-amp) into the op-amp (Fig 22.13).

5   The output impedance is very low. This means that the output can deliver quite a high current, up to 20 mA.

OP-AMPS IN USE

Op-amps are not used by themselves. The simplest circuits use resistors – in particular, one between the input and the output. This provides **feedback** between the output and the input and makes some very useful circuits possible. In the examples described, the feedback is **negative feedback**. This means that a fraction of the output is 'fed back' to the *inverting* input.

The inverting amplifier

In Fig 22.14, R_f is the value of the feedback resistor between the output and the inverting input. R_{in} is the input resistor value. The non-inverting input is earthed, that is, at 0 V.

You will find it easier to understand this circuit if you try it out. If the values of the two resistors R_f and R_{in} are equal, the output voltage will be the same size as the input but it will also be inverted. That is, an input voltage of +1 V will give an output of –1 V. To analyse how this circuit behaves, we must start at the output.

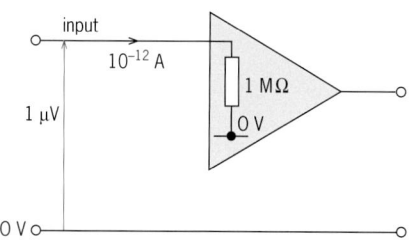

Fig 22.13 Op-amps usually draw little current

? QUESTION 6

6   How many times bigger than a pico-amp is a milliamp?

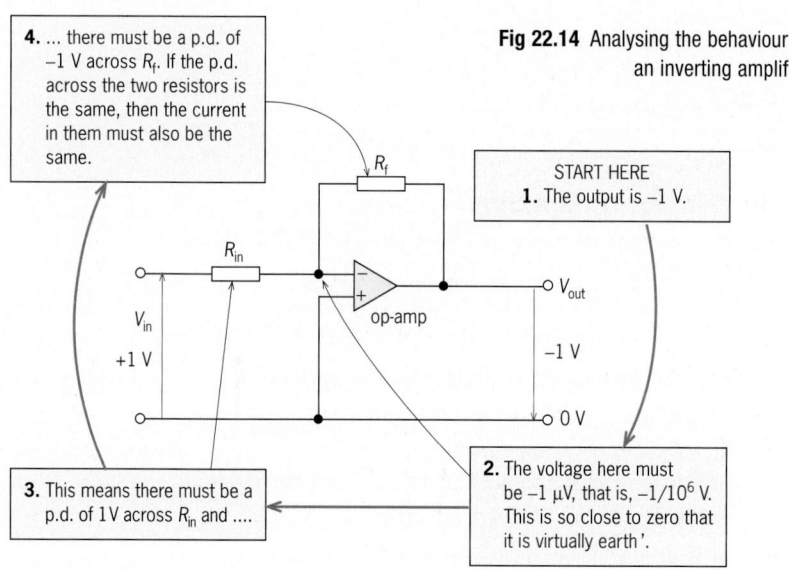

Fig 22.14 Analysing the behaviour of an inverting amplifier

4. ... there must be a p.d. of –1 V across R_f. If the p.d. across the two resistors is the same, then the current in them must also be the same.

START HERE
1. The output is –1 V.

3. This means there must be a p.d. of 1 V across R_{in} and ....

2. The voltage here must be –1 µV, that is, –1/10^6 V. This is so close to zero that it is virtually earth '.

R_f

R_{in}

V_{in}

+1 V

op-amp

V_{out}

–1 V

0 V

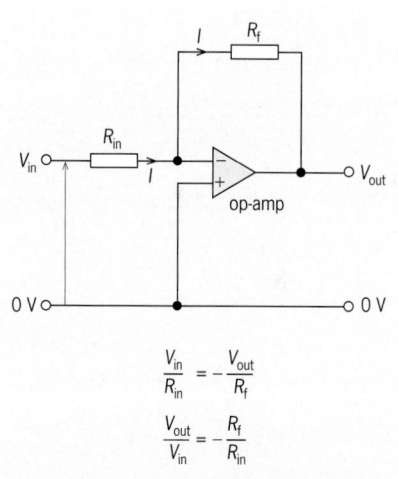

$$\frac{V_{in}}{R_{in}} = -\frac{V_{out}}{R_f}$$

$$\frac{V_{out}}{V_{in}} = -\frac{R_f}{R_{in}}$$

Fig 22.15 The inverting amplifier with its associated equations

The two resistors are effectively in series. The current drawn by the inverting input of the op-amp is very small compared with the current through the two resistors. This will still happen when the two resistors are not the same size since resistors in series have the same current in them. So the mathematics of this circuit is fairly simple (Fig 22.15).

The output voltage can be a precise multiple or fraction of the input – it depends only on the two resistors. Notice that the output voltage does not depend on any of the characteristics of the op-amp, yet the circuit would not work without it.

The circuit carries out a precise mathematical operation, in this case multiplication by a constant, the gain of this circuit (V_{out}/V_{in}), which is called the **closed loop gain**.

One way of looking at the circuit is to say that the output will become whatever value is necessary to make the difference between the two inputs equal zero. In this case, the output goes to a value that makes the inverting input zero. (The other input has been fixed at zero.)

The voltage of the power supply limits the maximum output voltage from the amplifier. No matter what the theoretical gain of a circuit, it is impossible for the output to be bigger than the supply voltage. Real op-amps saturate at one or two volts short of the power supply voltage.

For example, if an op-amp is operating from a ±15 V supply (Fig 22.16(a)), then the output will never be bigger than ±13 V, and so ±13 V is called the **saturation voltage**. This can be measured by plotting the transfer characteristic of the op-amp (Fig 22.16(b)).

The slope of the central part of the graph is the gain of the inverting amplifier, R_f/R_{in}.

Fig 22.16 (a) Op-amp circuit and **(b)** transfer characteristic

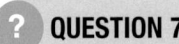

? QUESTION 7

7 What will be the overall gain of the circuit shown below?

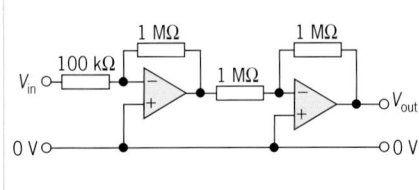

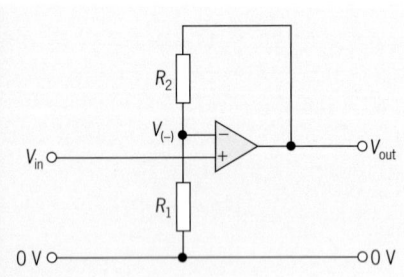

Fig 22.17 The non-inverting amplifier

? QUESTION 8

8 If in Fig 22.17 R_1 is 10 k$\,\Omega$, what value of R_2 would give a gain of 10?

The non-inverting amplifier

The op-amp can be used to make an amplifier that does not invert the input signal. The circuit is shown in Fig 22.17. This circuit also operates so that the difference between the two inputs is so close to zero that it can be taken as zero.

This time, neither input is connected to earth (0 V). If the input to the non-inverting input is V_{in}, then we assume that the voltage at the inverting input is also V_{in}.

R_1 and R_2 form a **potential divider** (see page 184). The voltage at the inverting input $V_{(-)}$ of Fig 22.17 is given by:

$$V_{(-)} = \frac{R_1}{R_1 + R_2} \times V_{out}$$

This is equal to the input voltage, V_{in}, so that:

$$V_{in} = \frac{R_1}{R_1 + R_2} \times V_{out}$$

The gain is thus:

$$\frac{V_{out}}{V_{in}} = \frac{R_1 + R_2}{R_1} = 1 + \frac{R_2}{R_1}$$

Again, this is the closed loop gain and it depends only on the two resistors.

There is one version of the non-inverting amplifier that is particularly useful. This is the **voltage follower**.

The voltage follower

Fig 22.18 shows a simple version of the non-inverting amplifier. The output is connected directly to the inverting input, which means that R_2 is zero. The other resistor in Fig 22.17, R_1, is removed. This is equivalent to making its size infinite. Therefore:

$$\text{gain} = 1 + 0/° = 1 + 0 = 1$$

So what good is an amplifier with a gain of 1?

The advantage of this circuit lies in the basic properties of the op-amp. The input draws a very small current and the output can provide a much larger current. The technical explanation is: 'It has a very high input impedance and a very low output impedance.' The following example illustrates the use of the voltage follower.

Fig 22.19 shows a voltmeter connected to measure the p.d. of 1 V across a 1 MΩ resistor. A typical moving-coil voltmeter might have a resistance of about 100 kΩ (please see the How Science Works assignments for Chapter 8 at www.collinseducation.co.uk/CAS), so this is not a very good way of measuring the p.d. since the voltmeter will draw most of the current and give an incorrect reading.

Fig 22.20 shows a better way of measuring the p.d. using a voltage follower. The op-amp input draws far less current than the voltmeter, but the output can provide enough current for the voltmeter. A typical op-amp will draw about 1 pA with a voltage of 1 V at the input, but will provide several milliamps at the output.

The voltage follower is a very useful little circuit and has some very interesting applications in physics. The examples in Fig 22.21, for instance, both require a measuring device that draws very little current.

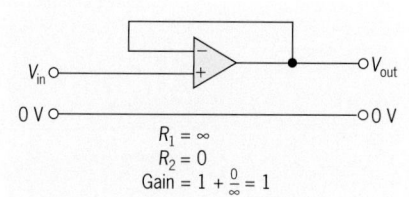

Fig 22.18 The voltage follower (compare this circuit with Fig 22.17)

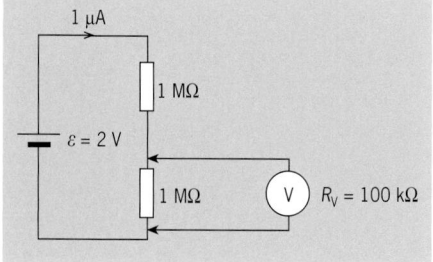

Fig 22.19 A voltmeter connected to measure the p.d. of 1 V across a 1 MΩ resistor (1 μA × 1 MΩ = 1 V). But what happens when the voltmeter is added?

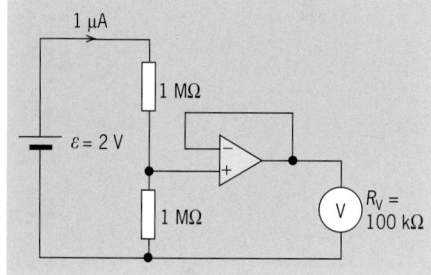

Fig 22.20 The voltage follower allows the use of the same voltmeter without the effect on the current

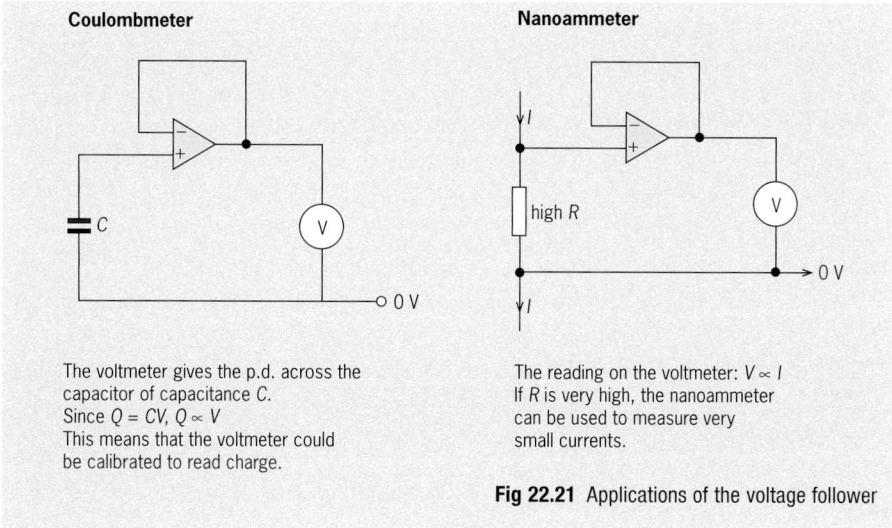

Coulombmeter

The voltmeter gives the p.d. across the capacitor of capacitance C.
Since $Q = CV$, $Q \propto V$.
This means that the voltmeter could be calibrated to read charge.

Nanoammeter

The reading on the voltmeter: $V \propto I$.
If R is very high, the nanoammeter can be used to measure very small currents.

Fig 22.21 Applications of the voltage follower

? QUESTIONS 9–10

9   How much current would the voltmeter in Fig 22.19 draw with a p.d. of 1 V across it? Estimate the reading on the voltmeter.

10   In the circuit of Fig 22.20, where does the 'extra' current come from?

The comparator

The op-amp can be used as a switch. There is no feedback, so the two inputs do not have to be the same. The output depends on the difference between the two inputs. In Fig 22.22, an op-amp with an open loop gain of 10^6 has a voltage of 13 μV at the non-inverting input. (The inverting input is held at 0 V.) The output will be at +13 V, the saturation voltage.

If the input is reduced by 13 μV to zero, the output also becomes zero. If the input is further reduced to –13 μV, the output shoots down to –13 V. A change of 26 μV (0.000 026 V) is enough to switch the output of the op-amp from positive saturation to negative saturation.

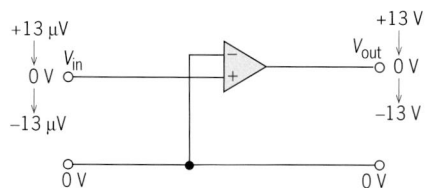

Fig 22.22 A basic comparator – the op-amp as a switch

Fig 22.23 A temperature-sensitive comparator

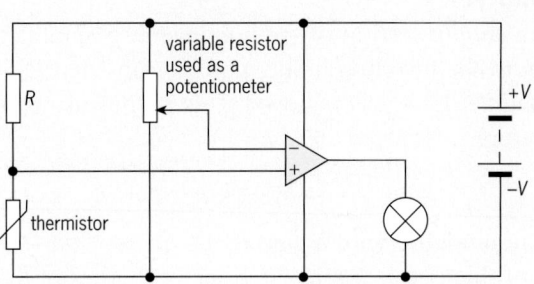

The op-amp can also be used as a voltage **comparator**. Fig 22.23 shows a typical application of this.

The thermistor and the fixed resistor, *R*, form a potential divider, which fixes the voltage at the non-inverting input of the op-amp. As the temperature rises, this voltage increases as the resistance of the thermistor increases. (If the temperature falls, the voltage will decrease.) The voltage at the inverting input is set by the variable resistor which is used as a potentiometer.

The potentiometer is set so that the voltage at the inverting input is the same as the voltage at the non-inverting input. The difference between the two voltages will then be zero and the lamp at the output will be off. As soon as the temperature increases, the voltage difference will be greater than zero and the lamp will light.

Comparators are very sensitive switches. The temperature need only change by a very small amount before the voltage difference exceeds 26 μV.

5 RADIO RECEPTION

We shall finish this chapter by looking at a simple radio designed to receive amplitude modulated signals. (See Fig 21.3, page 420, for a block diagram of an AM transmitter.)

A transmitter adds an audio frequency signal to a radio frequency carrier to produce the amplitude modulated signal which is transmitted.

A radio receiver receives this signal and carries out the reverse process, eventually 'un-mixing' the radio signal to produce the original audio frequency signal. Fig 22.24 is a block diagram showing the important parts of an AM receiver.

The radio signal is transmitted as an electromagnetic wave and the signal is 'picked up' by an aerial. A length of wire makes a very effective simple aerial; many radios use a telescopic metal rod.

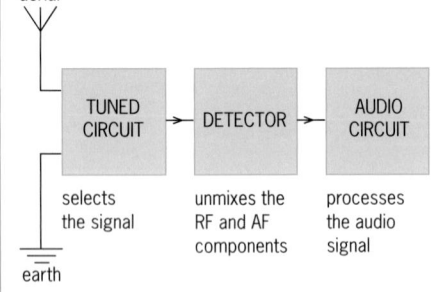

Fig 22.24 AM receiver block diagram

ELECTROMAGNETIC WAVES AND AERIALS

Electromagnetic waves have an electric field component and a magnetic field component. Different kinds of aerial respond to one or other of these components (Fig 22.25).

In the presence of a radio signal, free electrons in a wire or telescopic aerial oscillate to produce an alternating current at the same frequency as the radio signal. The oscillation of the electrons in the wire aerial is induced by the *electric field* component of the radio wave. (See Fig 15.3, page 285.)

Most radios designed to receive medium and long wave signals use a ferrite rod aerial, which consists of a coil of wire wound on a ferrite rod. This aerial responds to the *magnetic field* component of the radio wave. The changing magnetic field induces a current in the coil. The ferrite rod concentrates the local field, making it stronger inside the coil.

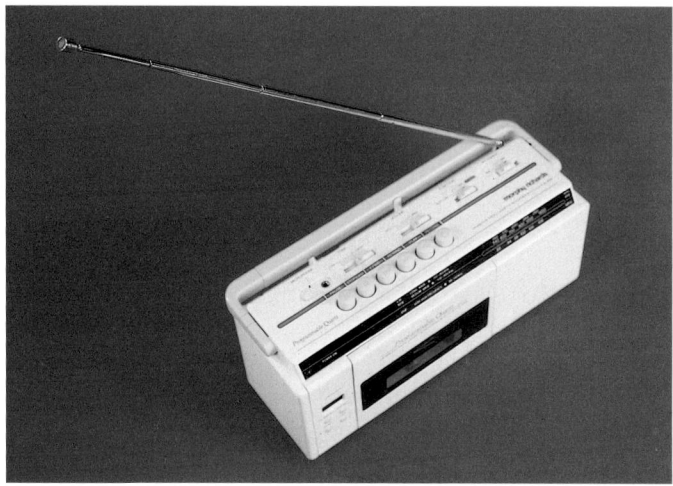
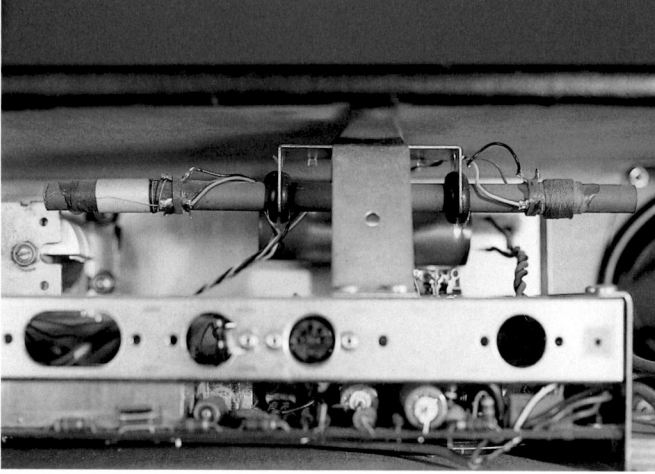

Fig 22.25 Left: A radio with a telescopic aerial responds to the electric field component of the radio wave
Right: A radio with a ferrite rod aerial responds to the magnetic field component

The problem is that there are many radio signals, each with a different frequency and each inducing a current of the same frequency as the radio wave. The aerial carries all these alternating currents into the radio. The **tuned circuit** selects one signal out of the many present in the aerial (Fig 22.26).

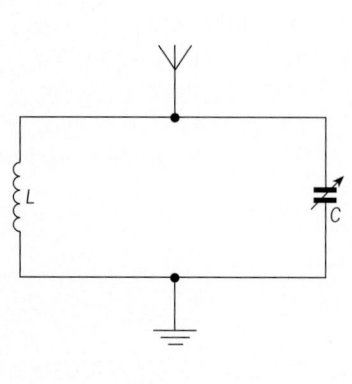

Fig 22.26 The tuned circuit

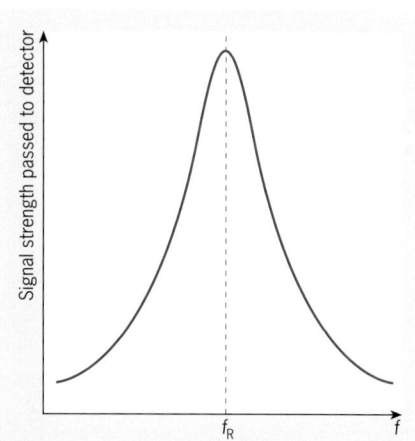

Fig 22.27 Resonance curve for parallel LC circuit

The tuned circuit is a parallel LC circuit. That is, it is a capacitor in parallel with an inductor (see page 246). Most tuned circuits use a variable capacitor so that the circuit can be 'tuned' to cover a range of frequencies. The parallel LC circuit has a resonant frequency.

If the resonant frequency matches a signal from the aerial, this signal will be passed on. The tuned circuit behaves like a filter, blocking some signals and allowing a narrow range of frequencies through (Fig 22.27).

The 'ideal' tuned circuit allows only one signal to pass through, so that the signal produced by the radio is free from interference from other signals. However, the tuned circuit must allow a band of frequencies through that is equal to the bandwidth of the AM signal (see page 422).

Simple radios also need a good earth wire in contact with the ground to allow unwanted signals to be carried away. Note that this literally means the earth, not the mains power supply earth.

The next stage is the 'un-mixing' or **demodulation** of the selected signal. A very simple and effective demodulator can be made using a single diode and a capacitor. The diode actually rectifies the signal, that is, it allows current in only one direction. The rectified signal still contains the lower frequency signal and the radio frequency carrier.

 QUESTION 11

11   A variable capacitor can be varied between 200 pF and 500 pF. It is used in a tuned circuit intended to cover the medium wave band, that is, from 0.5 to 1.5 MHz. Calculate the size of a suitable inductor to be used with the capacitor to make a tuned circuit.

✔ **REMEMBER THIS**
Remember from Chapter 12 that the resonant frequency of a parallel LC circuit is:

$$f = \frac{1}{2\pi}\sqrt{\frac{1}{LC}}$$

Fig 22.28 Demodulation

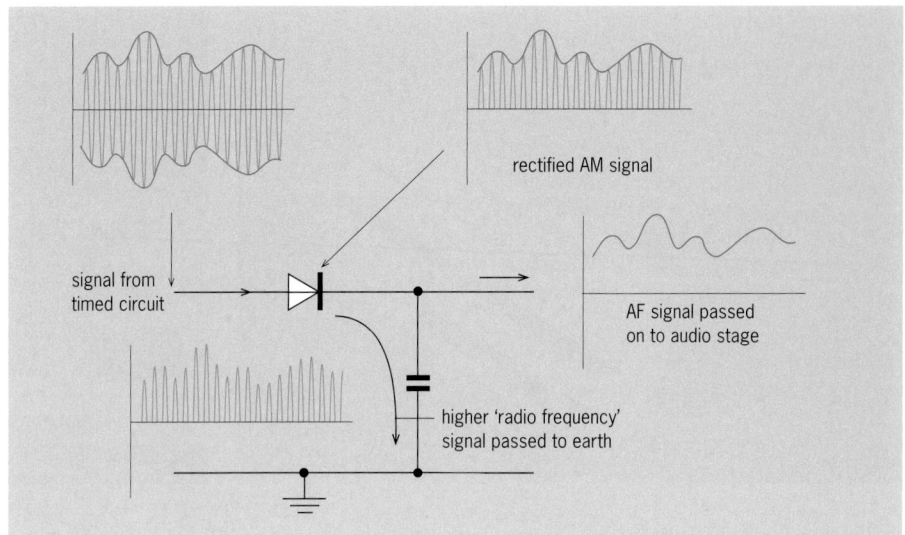

The capacitor is chosen so that its reactance is low at the frequency of the radio signal. The radio frequency part of the rectified signal then passes through the capacitor to earth (Fig 22.28).

The lower, audio frequency part of the rectified signal is not strong enough to drive a loudspeaker, but it can be amplified by an audio amplifier.

As its name suggests, the audio amplifier is designed to amplify audio frequency signals. A good amplifier should amplify equally over the whole of the audio frequency range (20 Hz to 20 kHz), although for most simple radios a much narrower range still gives acceptable results. Fig 22.29 shows a simple 'crystal set' radio.

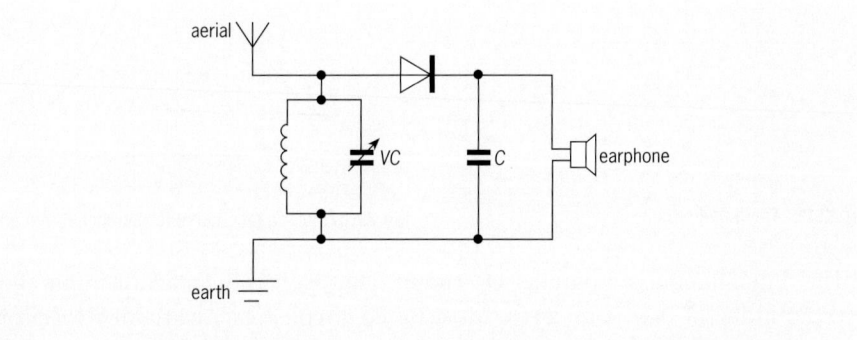

Fig 22.29 The simple crystal set will drive a high impedance earphone when tuned to a strong signal. A good aerial and earth are very important to this simple radio. Note that there is no power supply!

SUMMARY

After studying this chapter you should:
- Know that any electronic system can be broken down into three parts: input, process and output.
- Understand the terms transducer and sensor.
- Know that there are two kinds of electronic system: digital and analogue.
- Understand the terms op-amp, inverting amplifier and non-inverting amplifier.
- Understand the principles of radio reception.

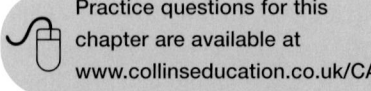
Practice questions for this chapter are available at www.collinseducation.co.uk/CAS

23

Spacetime physics

23 SPACETIME PHYSICS

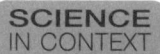

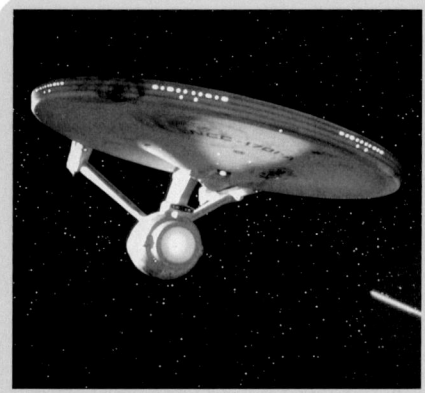

'TO BOLDLY GO…'

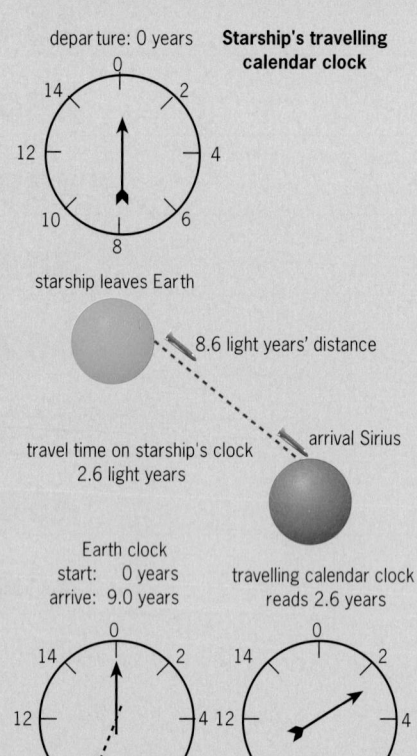

Starship's travelling calendar clock

departure: 0 years

starship leaves Earth

8.6 light years' distance

travel time on starship's clock
2.6 light years

arrival Sirius

Earth clock
start: 0 years
arrive: 9.0 years

travelling calendar clock
reads 2.6 years

The trip to Sirius: traveller's elapsed time is 2.7 years; stay-at-home's elapsed time is 9 years. Another example: light measured on Earth takes 120 000 years to cross the diameter of our Galaxy. A starship travelling at almost the speed of light could cross it in a few days – as measured by its own clock. As it did so, the Earth would get more than 120 000 years older

Time flies

The Voyager 2 spacecraft was launched by NASA in 1977. Its mission was to visit each of the outer planets and take close-up photographs and other measurements. It took 12 years to reach Neptune, its final port of call in the Solar System. It is now travelling in the direction of the star Sirius, leaving the Solar System at a speed of about 10 km per second. Sirius is a comparatively near star, 8.6 light years away, and Voyager 2 should be near it after a journey lasting 300 000 years or so.

The laws of relativity forbid any object that has mass from travelling faster than c, the speed of light, which is about 3×10^8 metres per second. But the laws also tell us that a starship could get to Sirius in a shorter time than you would calculate in the usual way.

If we could break the laws of physics and travel at the speed of light we could reach Sirius and get back in 17.2 years. Then, relativity theory shows that our starship clock would record a time interval of zero!

But how quickly could we do it, at a speed *close* to the speed of light, say? The answer depends not only on how *fast* the starship goes, but also on where the clock is that measures the time. The maths is very simple – although the ideas are very strange. Suppose NASA wants a starship to get to Sirius 8.6 light years away in just 9 years. To do this it would have to travel at a speed of $0.96c$, that is, $8.6c/9.0$. Relativity treats distance and time as almost interchangeable, and a version of Pythagoras' theorem is used to calculate the time:

(time elapsed on ship's clock)^2 =
    (time elapsed on NASA clock)^2 − (Sirius distance in light units)^2

Putting in the values, we get:

(time elapsed on ship's clock)^2 = $(9)^2 − (8.6)^2$

This gives a ship's time interval of 2.7 years. Mission control back at Houston will have aged 9 years. For a round trip, the astronauts would be 5.3 years older, the NASA ground team 18 years older.

This is the famous 'twin paradox': a twin in the spacecraft would come back younger than her brother back at NASA. It is a paradox because it is hard to explain why the effect is not symmetrical, that is, why each twin isn't younger than the other!

The ideas in this chapter

This chapter deals with the early twentieth-century revolution in our understanding of space, time and movement caused by that obscure young patents clerk Albert Einstein. Using just two simple ideas he worked out that time and distance are inextricably linked. This led to straightforward conclusions that seemed to be unbelievable paradoxes. No massive object can travel faster than light. Time for a moving object passes more slowly than for one at rest. And it is impossible to tell which one *is* at rest. Moving objects appear shorter. Energy and mass are equivalent: $E = mc^2$. Light rays are bent by gravity. Time passes more slowly near a gravitational mass than in emptier space.

You will have to think hard to cope with all this. You will meet the idea of a 'thought experiment'. You will learn about the key experiments that support this still strange view of the Universe: the Michelson–Morley experiment, and the extra life of muons.

1 SPACE AND TIME

Chapter 1 brought out the close relationship that exists in modern physics between distance and time, and we saw that the main link is the *speed of light*. Distance is measured in the unit of the metre, itself based upon the *distance light travels in a unit of time* (Fig 23.1). This chapter extends this basic and simple relationship more fully.

THE TWO BASIC IDEAS

Einstein built his special theory of relativity using two basic ideas or *postulates*:

- the constancy of the speed of light,
- the laws of physics are the same for any two systems (e.g. laboratories, atoms, spacecraft) that move relative to one another with a steady speed.

The first postulate is hard to accept but easy to understand and use. The second is more subtle – there is more about this later.

Light speed

The idea that the speed of light (in empty space) is a constant for all observers seems absurd. It says that however fast you travel, light still shoots away from you – or towards you – at the same speed of $2.997\,924\,58 \times 10^8$ m s^{-1}. If you drive a *car* faster, you can catch up with the one in front. But however fast your spacecraft goes you can never even *gain* on the light wave in front. Light doesn't obey the ordinary laws of *relative* motion. This led Einstein to call his theory a **principle of relativity**.

The consequence of the principle is that *distances, time intervals* and the *time at which an event occurs* will be different for observers who move at a *steady velocity* with respect to each other. This chapter covers such simple situations, with objects moving at constant velocities.

In time dilation we observe that processes take longer to happen in objects that are moving relative to us. The effect is most dramatic at relative speeds close to the speed of light. Time dilation leads to other effects: objects *shrink* in the direction of travel – the **Lorentz contraction** – and their *mass increases*.

We begin by considering the idea of time.

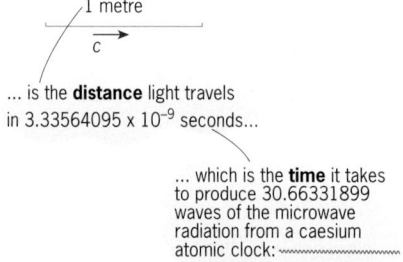

... is the **distance** light travels in 3.33564095 x 10^{-9} seconds...

... which is the **time** it takes to produce 30.66331899 waves of the microwave radiation from a caesium atomic clock: ～～～～～～～～～

Fig 23.1 Light in the form of microwave radiation from caesium defines both time and distance

2 A (VERY) BRIEF HISTORY OF TIME

The idea of time turns out to be fundamental to (Einsteinian) relativity. So we begin by recalling some aspects of time and its measurement that you probably take for granted.

TIME AND CLOCKS

Clocks do two things. They tell us the *time of day*, and they can be used to define a *time interval*. As mechanical clocks were improved and became more widely available in the early seventeenth century, the idea grew that they measured something that flowed steadily, as described by Isaac Newton:

absolute, true and mathematical time, of itself, and from its own nature, flows equably without relation to anything external.

Newton had defined a kind of clockless time. But it doesn't work.

Whose time is it?

A **muon** is a short-lived small particle of matter created when there is an energetic collision, for example a collision in a particle accelerator or caused by cosmic rays. The muon is highly unstable and very fast, with a half-life of about a millionth of a second. But when particle physicists study muons, their lifetime is seen to be many times longer (see page 461). So the external observer and the high-speed muon seem to experience time at different rates.

SETTING A CLOCK

A clock is anything that can be used to measure time. Ordinary clocks tend to use oscillating systems such as a pendulum or a vibrating quartz crystal. But very long times, such as the age of the Earth, can be measured using the half-lives of radioactive materials. The half-life of a beam of muons can also 'tell the time'. The radioactive material and the beam of muons are sorts of clocks. *But how do we actually compare clocks?*

Imagine that watches and clocks could easily be set to microsecond accuracy. Suppose you check your watch by looking across the town square at the town clock (Fig 23.2). If it says one o'clock exactly and your watch agrees exactly, you are happy. But the town clock is 120 metres away; when you *see* the town clock at one o'clock it is already one o'clock + $(120/c)$ seconds, where c is the speed of light. Your wristwatch will be slow by 0.4 microseconds.

If you set your watch by the radio time signal beeps, it might be slower by far more. The national master clock is at Rugby, Warwickshire. Its signal for one o'clock has to travel to the radio station, then to you – say 400 km altogether. Timed exactly according to this signal, your watch would be slow by 1.3 milliseconds. This is a very long time by the standard, for example, of the clock in a computer running at 100 MHz which easily measures time to an accuracy of 10^{-8} s.

But it's no problem to a person seeking maximum accuracy. If you know how far you are from the master clock, you can easily work out the correction to ensure that your watch tells the same time of day. Also, however fast or slow the 'time carrier' (the signal or process that 'carries' the time), your watch could still be an accurate measurer of *time intervals*.

The problems occur when clocks start moving, *relative to each other*.

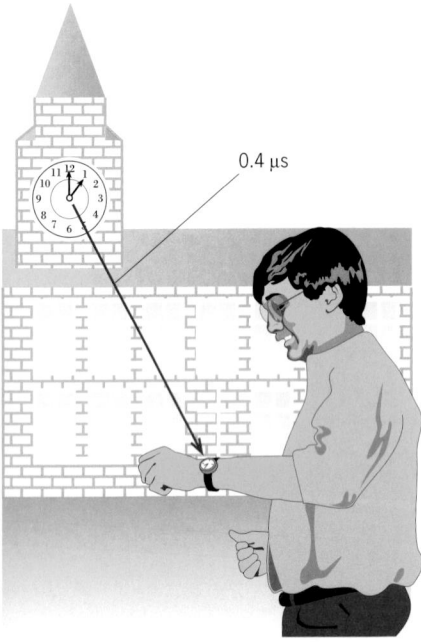

0.4 µs

Fig 23.2 Comparing the time on a stationary clock and watch

3 MOVING CLOCKS AND THE LAWS OF PHYSICS IN MOVING REFERENCE FRAMES

A REMINDER ABOUT EVERYDAY RELATIVITY

Chapter 1 explained *frames of reference* and 'everyday' relativity. A reference frame can be simply you, your laboratory and your measuring instruments.

Four hundred years ago, Galileo realised that he could not prove that the Earth moved – or stayed still – simply by making measurements of objects moving about on Earth. His example was a goldfish bowl in a ship's cabin. The fish move about the bowl in exactly the same way whether the ship is moving or not (as long as the ship is sailing at a steady speed on a calm sea). Movement of the goldfish or water in the bowl gives you no clue about the movement of the ship. For that you would have to look out through the porthole at the shore – and then you would have to assume that it is the ship and not the shore that is actually moving.

Imagine you are sitting at a desk and drop your pen on to it from a height of a few centimetres. It should fall directly below where you let it go. Exactly the same would happen if you were sitting in an aircraft travelling at a steady speed where you and the cabin are the reference frame (look back at Fig 1.15, page 14). But from a frame of reference outside yours, dropping the pen would be seen as moving sideways as well as falling down (Fig 23.3).

The motion of the aircraft is adding a sideways motion to the pen. This is simply in accordance with the laws of mechanics: speeds add up.

LIGHT DOESN'T BEHAVE LIKE PENS – OR ANY FORM OF MATTER

The strange fact that emerged towards the end of the nineteenth century was that light doesn't behave like falling pens, with an observed movement that differs according to the reference frame. Nor does light behave like bullets fired from a moving gun. For example, if a gun is fired while moving towards a fixed target, the bullets move faster to the target than if both gun and target are stationary. This agrees with the ideas of Galileo and Newton, that any object in a moving frame of reference has the speed of the reference frame (the gun, in the case of the bullets) as well as any extra speed of its own. Experimenters thought that light would behave like objects and gain *extra* speed when the light source and the observer were moving towards each other relatively. But in spite of very careful measurements, the experiments all failed to show that this happens.

Albert Michelson and Edward Morley carried out the experiments described in the following Stretch and Challenge passage on the behaviour of light. The implication of the null result (a result that disproves the starting assumption) is as follows. If you are travelling in a rocket at half the speed of light and send out a light beam ahead of you, you would measure the speed of the light as *c*, as you would expect. But *c* would also be the speed measured *by any other observer moving at any other steady speed relative to your rocket.* Compare this with throwing a pen forwards in a train.

For pens: pen speed, v_p, plus train speed, v_t, equals $(v_p + v_t)$
For light: light speed, c, plus rocket speed, $0.5c$, equals c

This is shown in Fig 23.4. The meaning of this null result was profound: its explanation was one of the great turning points in physics.

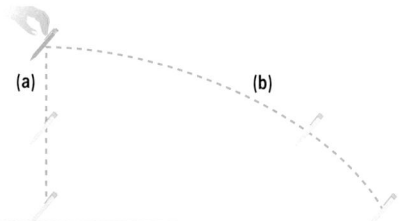

Fig 23.3 Dropping a pen in two frames of reference: **(a)** the passenger's and **(b)** someone hovering outside as the plane passes – a stationary observer

 REMEMBER THIS
Look back to pages 13 to 15 in Chapter 1 to remind yourself about frames of reference.

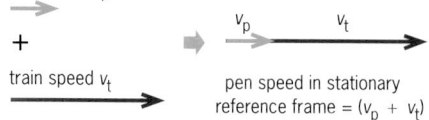

(a) Throwing a pen forward in a moving train
pen speed v_p
+
train speed v_t
pen speed in stationary reference frame = $(v_p + v_t)$

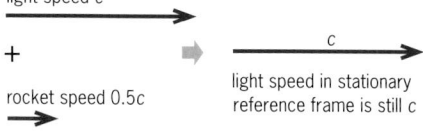

(b) 'Throwing' a light beam forward in a moving rocket
light speed c
+
rocket speed $0.5c$
light speed in stationary reference frame is still c

Fig 23.4 (a) Objects obey Galileo's ideas and Newton's laws: speeds add up. **(b)** Light doesn't go any faster or slower, however hard you 'throw' it

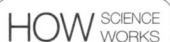

The Michelson–Morley experiment

It seemed obvious in the late nineteenth century that, if light is a wave, there must be a medium to carry it: scientists thought that, since light travelled through the vacuum of space, a vacuum should have at least some of the properties of a material. Just as sound waves are carried by air, so light waves were imagined as disturbances in what was called a luminiferous (or light-carrying) aether (pronounced ether) occupying all space (and all matter too) in the Universe. Light and all bodies were thought to travel through it.

Starting in 1880, the American physicist and naval officer Albert Michelson (Fig 23.5) carried out experiments to measure the speed of the Earth through the aether. He found it a harder task that he had expected. When he moved to the University of Cleveland, Ohio, he was joined by chemistry professor Edward Morley.

The two scientists assumed that light travels at a constant speed c in the aether. Their aim was to measure the speed of the Earth as it moved through the aether, relative to the speed of light. If, for example, the Earth was moving through the aether in the same direction as the light beam of their experiment, then (they thought) the light should appear to be travelling slower than c because of a sort of Doppler effect. Think of a road (the aether) with a cyclist (the Earth) moving along it. A car (light) travelling at constant speed comes up from behind the cyclist and overtakes. The car will approach and move away from the cyclist at a speed that is slower than its actual speed.

So when the Earth moves at speed v in the same direction as a beam of light, Michelson and Morley expected a light speed of less than c, namely (c − v). And a light beam moving in the opposite direction should have a speed of (c + v).

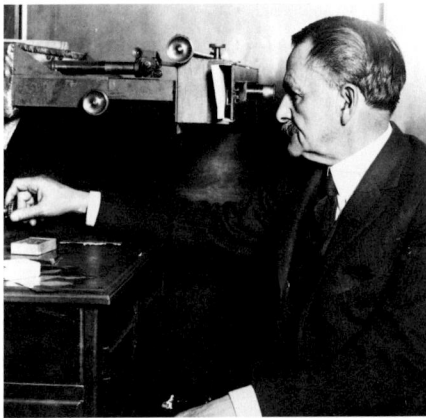

Fig 23.5 Albert Michelson was born in Strelno, Poland, but emigrated to the USA and became a physicist serving in the US navy. He was an instructor at the US Naval Academy when he began his research, but then left to become a professor of physics at Cleveland, Ohio. There, he was joined by the chemistry professor Edward Morley. The famous experiments that they carried out produced null results, providing the first crack in the well-built structure of nineteenth-century physics

Not knowing in which direction the Earth was travelling through the aether, Michelson and Morley arranged their apparatus to measure light speeds coming from different directions. Since every 6 months the Earth's direction changes by 180°, they also hoped that any change of the Earth's direction relative to this aether would affect their light-speed measurements, too. The interferometer they used is shown in Fig 23.6.

Simply, Michelson and Morley measured the time taken for light to travel along a pair of equal-length arms placed at right angles to each other. If at one time the Earth was stationary relative to the aether, beam 1 and beam 2 would take the same time to cover the equal distances. But if the Earth in its orbit then moved through the aether in the direction of one of the arms – so the experimenters thought – the time taken would be different for the two light beams.

Michelson and Morley measured time in a very modern way for over a hundred years ago – in terms of the number of complete waves made by the light along each arm and observed as an interference pattern at the screen. The light was monochromatic and therefore of constant frequency and wavelength. So, when the apparatus was rotated through 90°, if light took longer to travel along one arm than before rotation, the number of waves would be greater in that direction. The apparatus was sensitive enough to detect a time difference equivalent to a hundredth of the time period t of one wavelength. They expected to see a difference of up to four hundredths of t, estimated from the known speed of the Earth in its orbit. A simple account of the mathematics they used is given below Fig 23.6.

But after many experiments there was never any difference between sets of results: there was always a null result. Compared with the aether, the Earth appeared to be at rest – even when it swung to the other side of the Sun and was travelling in the opposite direction!

This null result – finally confirmed in 1887 – led first to the theory that electrical forces (i.e. connected with the electromagnetic waves of light) will shrink any object when it moves through the aether. This was the Lorentz–FitzGerald contraction theory: it explained the result – but otherwise led nowhere!

Then in 1905, Einstein, who probably didn't even know about Michelson and Morley's experiment, produced a much more radical theory based on two simple assumptions about the nature of physics and of light. Not only did it explain the null result; it also predicted the other 'relativistic' effects that had not then been observed.

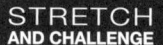 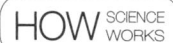

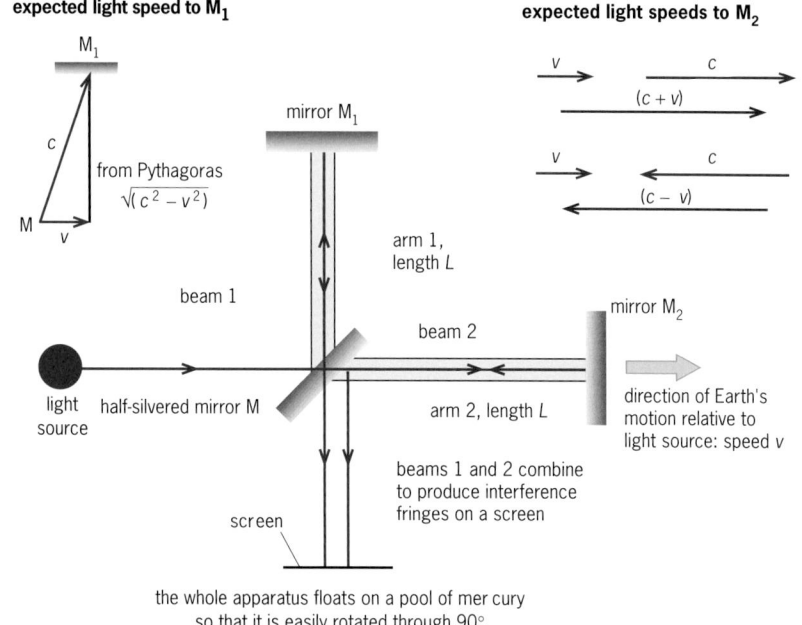

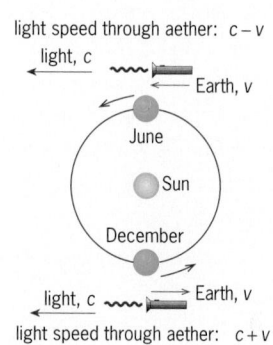

Fig 23.6 (a) The interferometer that Michelson and Morley used to measure the velocity of the Earth through the aether (space), and the mathematical explanation of their results

(b) What Michelson and Morley expected to find

The beam is split by the half-silvered mirror M. Beam 1 goes along arm 1, length L, and beam 2 along same-length arm 2. For beam 2, relative to Earth, the light speed to the right is $(c - v)$. But when it travels left after reflection at M_2, it is $(c + v)$.

So it takes a total time T_2 to travel from the half-silvered mirror to M_2 and back of:

$$T_2 = \frac{L}{c - v} + \frac{L}{c + v} = \frac{2Lc}{c^2 - v^2} = \frac{2Lc}{c^2\left(1 - \frac{v^2}{c^2}\right)} = \frac{2L}{c}\left(1 - \frac{v^2}{c^2}\right)^{-1}$$

Beam 1 travels to and from mirror M_1 at the same speed of $(c^2 - v^2)^{1/2}$, so that it takes a time of

$$T_1 = \frac{2L}{(c^2 - v^2)^{\frac{1}{2}}}$$

to do the double journey.

This can be rearranged as:

$$T_1 = \frac{2L}{c}\left(1 - \frac{v^2}{c^2}\right)^{-\frac{1}{2}}$$

Thus the time difference is:

$$T_2 - T_1 = \Delta T = \frac{2L}{c}\left[\left(1 - \frac{v^2}{c^2}\right)^{-1} - \left(1 - \frac{v^2}{c^2}\right)^{-\frac{1}{2}}\right]$$

Now, v^2/c^2 is very small, so that we can expand the brackets according to the binomial theorem:

$$(1 - x)^n = 1 - nx \text{ (for } x \ll 1)$$

You can do this to show that the expression for ΔT simplifies to Lv^2/c^3.

Michelson and Morley determined the value of ΔT by swinging the whole apparatus through $90°$, so swapping one arm for the other. They expected this to cause the interference pattern to change by moving the fringes sideways by an amount equal to a path difference due to a time difference *twice* ΔT:

$$\text{path difference} = c \times 2\Delta T$$

which corresponds to a shift of n fringes such that:

$$\text{path difference} = n\lambda = 2c\Delta T$$

so that:

$$n = \frac{2c\Delta T}{\lambda} = \frac{2Lv^2}{\lambda c^2}$$

? QUESTION 1

1 In the apparatus of Fig 23.6, L was 10 m and the light had a wavelength of 5×10^{-7} m. Show that this corresponds to a fringe shift of about 0.4 × fringe width if the Earth moves at a speed of 30 km s^{-1}.

4 EINSTEIN'S THEORY

Albert Einstein produced the theory that explained the null results of the Michelson–Morley experiment. The Lorentz–FitzGerald theory was seriously flawed since it was invented to explain just one effect (see the previous Stretch and Challenge passage). Einstein produced a formula for contraction with a simpler (if at first unbelievable) assumption about the constancy of the speed of light.

EINSTEIN'S TWO ASSUMPTIONS

Einstein took account of the nature of light and the fact that it was an electromagnetic effect. His theory was based on two simple assumptions (or 'postulates'):

- Physical laws – mechanical, optical and electromagnetic – are the same in all uniformly moving frames of reference.
- The speed of light in a vacuum is the same for all observers, in all uniformly moving frames of reference.

To recap: your frame of reference is the set of objects like tables, chairs, clocks or metre rules that happen to be at rest relative to you. You, and these things, could well be moving with respect to other objects – think of doing experiments in a train or an aircraft. An experimenter in another train travelling past you would be in a different frame of reference. If the relative motion of your frames are at a constant velocity, they are called **inertial** frames – frames in which things that are moving keep moving at the same velocity, things at rest stay at rest, so showing **inertia** (see page 27).

> ### ✔ REMEMBER THIS
> Frames of reference are called **inertial frames** when they are not accelerating in a straight line or rotating. In these frames, Newtonian relationships like $F = ma$ apply simply, whereas in rotating frames we experience imaginary forces like centrifugal and Coriolis forces.

5 STRETCHING TIME – TIME DILATION

The first and very surprising consequence of Einstein's principle of relativity is called **time dilation**. This means that:

> **a process that takes a certain time to occur in a moving system is observed to take a _longer_ time by someone outside that system than by someone moving _with_ the system.**

For example, in Fig 23.7, the observer outside the system could see a clock in a moving spacecraft move its second hand, say, 10 seconds, and also see that this took 11 seconds measured by her own watch. Meanwhile, an observer in the moving system would also see that while his watch counted 11 seconds, the outsider's watch changed by 10 seconds. Both would say that the other person's watch counted seconds too slowly. The situation is _symmetrical_: either could say that the other is moving; neither has the right to declare that they are at rest relative to the Universe at large.

A mathematical proof of time dilation is very simple and needs no more than an understanding that distance = speed × time, and a knowledge of Pythagoras' theorem. Other proofs use even less mathematics.

There are two difficulties: one is believing the final result, the other is in setting up a scenario in which time dilation is important. In his popular explanations, Einstein used the situation of a moving train being struck by lightning, with

Fig 23.7 Time measured from inside and outside systems

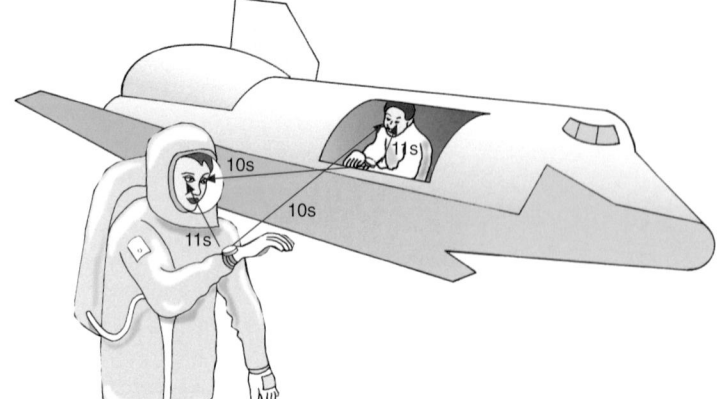

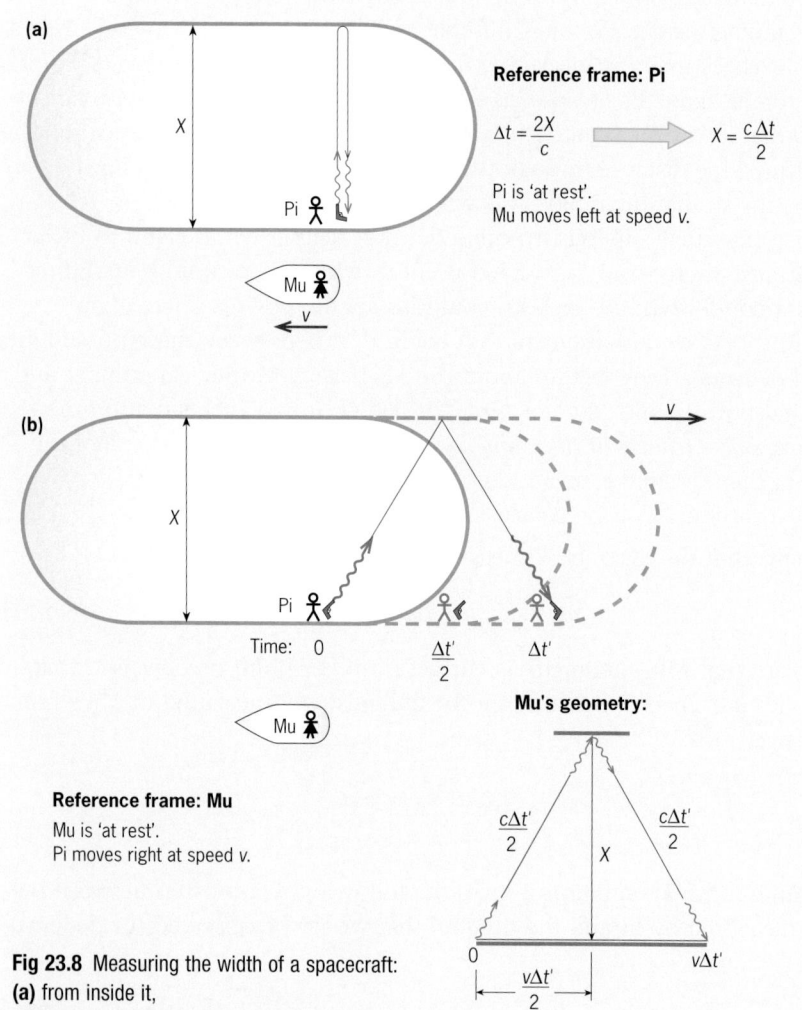

Fig 23.8 Measuring the width of a spacecraft:
(a) from inside it,
(b) from a spacecraft moving past it

$$X^2 = \left(\frac{c\Delta t'}{2}\right)^2 - \left(\frac{v\Delta t'}{2}\right)^2$$

But:
$$X = \frac{c\Delta t}{2}$$

so:
$$\left(\frac{c\Delta t}{2}\right)^2 = \left(\frac{c\Delta t'}{2}\right)^2 - \left(\frac{v\Delta t'}{2}\right)^2$$

which simplifies to
$$c^2(\Delta t)^2 = c^2(\Delta t')^2 - v^2(\Delta t')^2$$

Dividing by c^2:
$$(\Delta t)^2 = (\Delta t')^2 - \left(\frac{v^2}{c^2}\right)(\Delta t')^2$$

$$(\Delta t)^2 = (\Delta t')^2\left(1 - \frac{v^2}{c^2}\right)$$

Changing the subject of the formula gives:
$$(\Delta t')^2 = \frac{(\Delta t)^2}{\left(1 - \dfrac{v^2}{c^2}\right)}$$

so that:
$$\Delta t' = \frac{\Delta t}{\sqrt{1 - \dfrac{v^2}{c^2}}} = \gamma\,\Delta t$$

γ is the **Lorentz factor**.

the guard on the train and the station master some distance away arguing about exactly when the strike occurred – hardly the first thing either would worry about under the circumstances!

We shall imagine a scenario – a thought experiment – that would be more common nowadays: a measurement made by astronauts in 'deep space'. The mistake to avoid here is to think that relativity works only in outer space, and is only of significance to astronauts. Instead, bear in mind that one of the consequences of relativity and time dilation is the equivalence of mass and energy, according to the well-known formula $E = mc^2$. This relationship describes the source of the energy that powers stars – and so makes life possible on Earth.

Back to our scenario: a large, strange, deserted spacecraft is found in space, and is boarded by an astronaut, Pi, who is given the task of measuring its internal dimensions. He does this using an infrared gun, which measures distance X in terms of the time taken for an infrared pulse to go to and from an internal wall, as shown in Fig 23.8(a).

As Pi does this, his twin, Mu, sees him through the window of a scout vehicle from the space station where they both work. She decides to check the measurements which he has radioed in. Mu is doubtful: measuring with the same kind of infrared gun, she does not agree that the pulse travelled through space as shown in (a).

When Pi and Mu return to the space station, Mu tells Pi that, as the spacecraft was moving, the pulse actually travelled a greater distance than $2X$, along two sides of a triangle, as in Fig 23.8(b). She suspects that there is something wrong with Pi's timing system. Pi points out that his infrared gun is exactly the same as Mu's. They check them by measuring the same distance inside the space station, and the results agree. Pi also asserts that the deserted spacecraft was actually at rest, and that it was the scout vehicle that was doing the moving. Therefore, when Mu measured the distance through the window, her infrared pulse followed the longer path – so that her timing was wrong. They argue inconclusively.

At this stage their supervisor points out that neither could claim to be at rest – because there is no third fixed point to which they could refer. Either viewpoint could be true – or both could in fact be moving. There is no physical process or measurement that could decide between these possibilities. He then delivers a long lecture about the Michelson–Morley experiment and shows that both Pi and Mu can agree, provided that in each situation the measuring pulse *travels at the same speed through space*, irrespective of the motion of the transmitter or another observer.

This leads to the following conclusions (refer to Fig 23.8).

Mu accepts that the distance X measured by Pi is given by:

$$2X = c\Delta t, \text{ i.e. that } X = \frac{c\Delta t}{2} \qquad [1]$$

> ? **QUESTION 2**
>
> 2 Calculate the value of the Lorentz factor for a speed of 2×10^8 m s^{-1}.

Both accept that Mu's geometry is correct from her point of view, and that this implies a *different* time of flight for the pulse $\Delta t'$, measured in Mu's frame of reference, so that:

$$X^2 = \left(\frac{c\Delta t'}{2}\right)^2 - \left(\frac{v\Delta t'}{2}\right)^2 \qquad [2]$$

Substituting for X in equation 2 gives the following relationship between the time Δt measured by Pi and the time $\Delta t'$ that would be observed (or deduced) by Mu:

$$\Delta t' = \frac{\Delta t}{\sqrt{1 - \dfrac{v^2}{c^2}}} = \Delta t\left(1 - \frac{v^2}{c^2}\right)^{-\frac{1}{2}} \qquad [3]$$

This result is worked out in detail beside Fig 23.8, and is the effect known as **time dilation**. It is a consequence of the fixed and unvarying speed of light, and the result applies to any time interval $\Delta t'$ that we measure, using *our* clocks, for a process taking a time Δt in a body moving at speed v relative to us. The process could be a pendulum swinging, a body ageing, a muon decaying or a light wave oscillating.

The quantity:

$$\frac{1}{\sqrt{1 - \dfrac{v^2}{c^2}}} \qquad \text{or} \qquad \left(1 - \frac{v^2}{c^2}\right)^{-\frac{1}{2}}$$

is called the **Lorentz factor**. It is awkward to write but it keeps turning up in relativistic expressions, so it is often written as γ, so that the time dilation effect becomes $\Delta t' = \gamma\Delta t$, as shown in Fig 23.8.

TIME DILATION IS SYMMETRICAL

We could work out that time dilation is symmetrical by looking at it from Pi's point of view, which would assume that Mu was doing the moving. This would produce an identical result, except that Pi would deduce that it

> **REMEMBER THIS**
>
> **The meaning of time**
>
> Time is not an abstract 'out there' entity – as Newton seemed to assume. Time is measured by change and so needs *things* changing for it to make sense. Time is a property of a set of objects that exist together in their own **frame of reference**. They carry their *own* time – often called **proper time** (compare French *propre* – own, not as in *proper*ly dressed!). This is also called *wristwatch time* – you carry it around with you. If you are moving relative to me you have your own proper time. And so do I because I am moving relative to you. At relative speeds near the speed of light – and for places in gravitational fields of different strengths (see page 468) – proper times differ.

was Mu's time that was going slow. As we saw in Fig 23.7, the (Einsteinian) relativistic situation is fundamentally symmetrical.

SOME EVIDENCE FOR TIME DILATION: DETECTING MUONS

Early experiments investigating new subatomic particles of matter used the debris formed when high-speed particles called cosmic rays collided with the nuclei of atoms high in the atmosphere. In these debris were to be found particles called muons (see Chapter 24). Muons are unstable and decay with a half-life of 2.2 microseconds. They were detected by balloon flight experiments at a height of about 2 km above a high-mountain observatory. But 80 per cent were still detected at the observatory. The muons are travelling at a speed of $0.996c$ and would take 6.7 μs to travel 2 km, which is about 3 half-lives. This means that we would expect the muon flux to have decreased by one-eighth to 12 per cent. The explanation for the 'extra' muons observed is time dilation, which means that the half-life is increased by the factor γ. At this speed $\gamma = 11.2$, so the muons' half-life in the observatory's frame of reference becomes 24 μs. Therefore the time of flight from balloon to observatory is about one-third of a half-life and only about 20 per cent of the muons decay in this time.

TIME DILATION LEADS TO LENGTH CONTRACTION

A cosmic physicist travelling with the muons as in the last subsection could measure their progress by using the same kind of calculation. Her measurement of the time from balloon to observatory would be 'our time' divided by γ, i.e. 6.7/11.2 μs = 0.6 μs. At a speed of $0.996c$ the distance travelled is 0.6 μs $\times$ $0.996c$ = 180 m. So for the moving object the distance in our atmosphere looks much shorter than we see it to be. In another scenario, if a 2000 m long spaceship approached us at this kind of speed it would look to us to be 180 m long.

We know that it is all relative. These results reinforce the fact that time and space (distance) are interdependent.

More formally, in this example we can extend the relationship $\Delta t' = \gamma \Delta t$:

$$\text{time measured by us} = \gamma \times \text{muon time}$$

to relate the distances involved. Within a reference frame distance travelled is proportional to time, so that we can write:

$$\frac{x_0}{x} = \frac{\Delta t'}{\Delta t} = \gamma$$

Here x_0 is the distance between the balloon and the observatory in our frame and x is the distance as measured by the physicist travelling with the muons.

In general, a length x in one frame (e.g. the length of a moving object such as a spaceship as seen by us on Earth) measured from another frame, the length being in the same direction as the relative velocity v, is given by:

$$x = \frac{x_0}{\gamma} \qquad \text{or} \qquad x = x_0 \left(1 - \frac{v^2}{c^2} \right)^{\frac{1}{2}}$$

where x_0 is the length as measured in the object's own frame (e.g. the length of the spaceship as the occupants would measure it). Note that when the object is moving with respect to us we see it to be shorter, so to get our observed value x we *divide* by γ, which is always greater than 1. This always means a **length contraction**, known as the **Lorentz–FitzGerald contraction**.

? QUESTION 3

3 A muon is created in the upper atmosphere by a collision between a cosmic ray and an oxygen nucleus. The muon moves Earthwards at a speed of $0.998c$. In its own reference frame, the muon has an expected lifetime of 2×10^{-6} s.

a) Show that its expected lifetime in a laboratory on Earth is about 30 microseconds.

b) How far will it travel before decay, **i)** in its own reference frame, **ii)** as observed in the laboratory?

? QUESTION 4

4 Centaurian spacecraft are spherical. What shape would a Centaurian spacecraft appear to have as it passes you at a relative speed of $0.5c$?

A CLOSER LOOK AT THE LORENTZ FACTOR γ

At the heart of the Lorentz factor is the quantity $(1 - v^2/c^2)$. As the size of v gets closer and closer to that of c, v/c and therefore v^2/c^2 get closer and closer to 1. Thus the quantity in the brackets gets closer and closer to zero, and so does its square root.

The Lorentz factor γ is the inverse of this square root, so as the square root gets smaller and smaller, γ gets larger and larger. The result of *multiplying* by γ, as in $t' = \gamma t$ and $m = \gamma m_0$ (see below), is therefore a very large value as v approaches c. When v equals c, γ becomes an infinite number.

When we *divide* a quantity by the Lorentz factor, the result approaches zero for high values of v. This is equivalent to *multiplying* the quantity by

$$\sqrt{1 - \frac{v^2}{c^2}}$$

It will help you to look now at Fig 23.9, which shows how the Lorentz factor γ varies with v up to values close to the speed of light. Nothing changes very much until $v = 0.6c$ or thereabouts. Then, for $v > 0.995c$, the Lorentz factor increases very rapidly indeed for small fractional increments of speed.

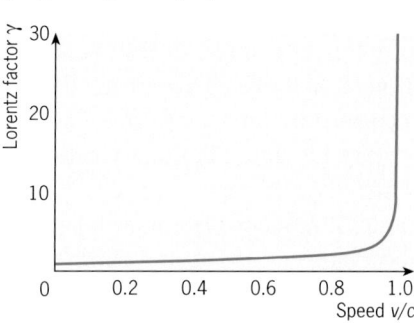

Fig 23.9 The graph shows that the Lorentz factor γ increases very rapidly to an infinite number at speeds over 95 per cent of the speed of light

? **QUESTION 5**

5   State some ways in which everyday life would be different if light travelled at 13 m s^{-1} (that is, at about 30 miles an hour).

6 MASS AND SPEED

One of the more surprising and significant consequences of Einstein's theory of relativity is that the *mass* of a moving body increases with speed. The mass of the object will be m, compared with the mass m_0 that it has at rest in our reference frame. So:

$$m = \gamma m_0$$

The **rest mass** m_0 of the body is especially significant in particle physics. The 'mass' of an object such as a proton or electron quoted in tables is its rest mass. At speeds up to about $0.2c$ the actual mass of a particle is very close to its rest mass (Fig 23.10). The particle's observed mass increases very rapidly at speeds close to that of light as it is multiplied by the Lorentz factor.

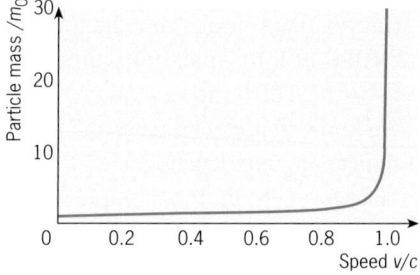

Fig 23.10 The mass of a moving particle increases as the Lorentz factor increases. At speeds over 95 per cent of light speed, there is a rapid mass increase to an infinite value

The mass acquired by a moving particle due to its motion is just as 'real' as what we call its 'ordinary' mass. The gravitational force on it increases in accordance with Newton's gravity law, and it becomes harder for a force to accelerate it, exactly in accordance with Newton's laws of motion.

The relativistic mass formula given above explains why no object that has mass can travel faster than the speed of light in a vacuum. An accelerating force does work which appears as the kinetic energy of the object. As the speed approaches c, the mass increases and so does kinetic energy. If it could reach the speed c, it would have infinite mass and so infinite kinetic energy, and to get this result the force would have to be either infinite or act for an infinite time, so no object with *rest mass* can travel at the speed of light.

? **QUESTION 6**

6   Estimate the mass your body would have if you travelled at $0.999c$. Bearing in mind that you are actually travelling at this speed relative to some distant galaxy, explain why you don't in fact feel this extra massiveness.

7 MASS AND ENERGY

The best known equation (and one of the shortest) in all physics is:

$$E = mc^2$$

Don't make the mistake of thinking that the Einstein mass–energy relationship applies only to high-speed particles and nuclear reactions. We can justify it in words by considering what happens when you heat a gas. Most of the energy put in to make the gas 'hotter' goes to make its molecules move faster. As they move faster they gain more mass as shown by the equation:

$$m = \gamma m_0$$

When a cup of coffee cools down, it loses energy – and also loses the mass-equivalent of that energy. *Any gain in energy is a gain in mass.*

THE MASS–ENERGY OF AN ATOM

The mass of an atom is made up of the rest masses of its particles (nucleons and electrons), together with mass due to both their kinetic and their potential energies. As the nucleons move around in the region of the nucleus and the electrons move around outside the nucleus, kinetic energy is continually being interchanged with potential energy.

Since we are concerned with changes of energy relating to changes of mass, the formula is often written:

$$\Delta E = c^2 \Delta m$$

This relation applies to such things as the burning of a fuel, where the final mass of the chemical products is always less than the initial masses of the reactants.

The mass change in a normal chemical reaction is tiny. It is far too small to worry about when doing ordinary chemical calculations. More mass gets converted to energy in nuclear reactions like fission and fusion; but even so, there are practical physical reasons that make it impossible for all the energy equivalent of the rest mass of the nuclei to be converted to, say, kinetic energy. Ultimately, any process would end with everything in a stable form of matter: protons, electrons and neutrinos (see Chapter 24).

The mass of a massless particle

A photon of light has zero *rest* mass. But it has energy E and so, from the Einstein mass–energy relationship, it must have an equivalent relativistic mass given by:

$$m = E/c^2$$

Photon momentum

This means that a photon also has momentum p:

$$p = mc = E/c$$

de Broglie again

The energy of a photon is given by the Planck–Einstein relation

$$E = hf$$

where h is the Planck constant and f is the frequency of the radiation. We can write this in terms of light speed and wavelength λ:

$$E = hf = hc/\lambda$$

Now, as the momentum p of a photon is E/c, we can also see that:

$$p = \frac{E}{c} = \frac{hc}{c\lambda} = \frac{h}{\lambda}$$

which is the de Broglie relationship, which you first met for electrons on page 316.

> **? QUESTION 7**
>
> 7 Which would have a greater force exerted on it in a gravitational field, a photon of red light or a photon of blue light? Would their motion be different in the field? Explain your answer.

Relativity explains electromagnetism

The magnetic effect of a current (of moving charges) appears as a force. The force is always caused by the *relative* motion of charged particles – the electrons drifting along in a wire, say, and the electrons in a detector such as a Hall probe. Magnetic forces are a consequence of *relativistic time dilation*.

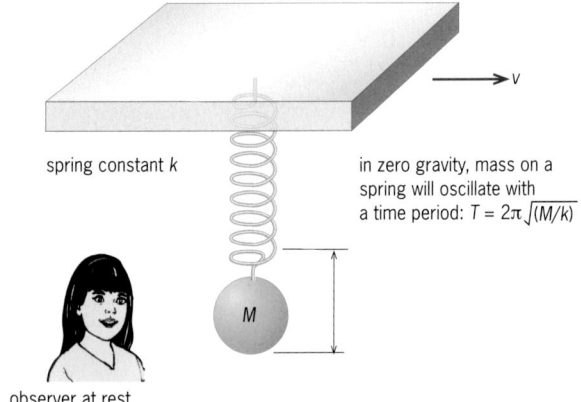

Fig 23.11 An oscillating system viewed sideways. *T* increases when the system moves at speed *v*. *M* gets larger and *k* gets smaller

Consider a mass *M* on a spring (Fig 23.11). It will oscillate if disturbed with a time period *T*:

$$T = 2\pi\sqrt{\frac{M}{k}}$$

where *k* is the spring constant (force per unit extension).

When such an oscillating system moves relative to us *sideways* at a speed *v*, *T* changes by the usual dilation factor γ. In effect, this appears to us as either *M* getting larger or *k* getting smaller. Some advanced mathematics shows that it is a combination of both effects: the mass increases, and the force decreases by a factor of order v^2/c^2.

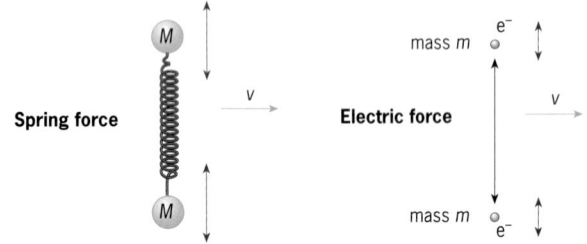

Fig 23.12 A pair of electrons can oscillate like two masses on a spring. If they move relative to a stationary observer, the period of oscillation increases: again, *M* increases and the force decreases. The force (electric) decreases in all directions

We have imagined a force due to a spring, but any force will be affected in this way when the masses move relative to us, as in Fig 23.12.

Now consider two wires with electrons free to move among fixed positive ions, as in Fig 23.13. When there is no current in the wires there is no net force between them. The forces exist but balance out, as Fig 23.13 shows:

$$\frac{\text{attraction between}}{\text{opposite charges}} = \frac{\text{repulsion between}}{\text{like charges}}$$

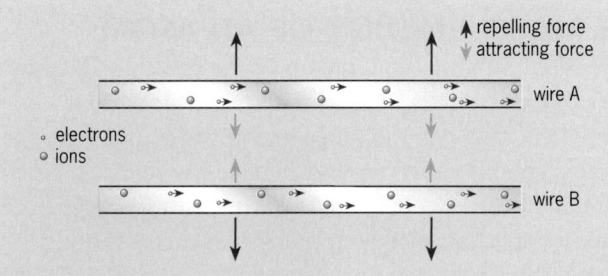

There are two pairs of attracting forces and two pairs of repelling forces:

Attracting: 1. electrons in A and ions in B
                    2. electrons in B and ions in A

Repelling: 3. ions in A and ions in B
                 4. electrons in A and electrons in B

With no current, all forces are equal and cancel out. With a current of moving electrons, force 4 gets less. There is a net attraction between the wires: this is electromagnetism.

Fig 23.13 Magnetism is a consequence of relativity

But when the wires carry a current, electrons are moving with a mean speed *v* relative to us (and the fixed positive ions). We have seen that as *v* increases, *M* increases, and so the force decreases. So the force of repulsion between the electrons gets less. The net force of attraction is now greater than the net repulsion force. As a result, the wires are pulled together. This is the effect we call **electromagnetism**.

8 OTHER EFFECTS DUE TO RELATIVITY

RELATIVISTIC MOMENTUM, ENERGY AND 'MOMENERGY'

Momentum
The momentum of a moving body is given by $p = mv$. If v is very large then the increase in mass means we have to write:

$$\text{momentum } p = \gamma m_0 v$$

The total energy of a moving mass
The work done in accelerating a body is transferred to its kinetic energy. At speeds very much smaller than c, the kinetic energy E_k is given by the formula $E_k = \frac{1}{2}mv^2$. However, for higher speeds we need to use the relativistic form of the equation, which allows for the relativistic increase in mass. The formula becomes:

$$E_k = \gamma m_0 c^2 - m_0 c^2$$

where m_0 is the rest mass of the body. Rearranging gives:

$$\gamma m_0 c^2 = E_k + m_0 c^2$$

The quantity $\gamma m_0 c^2$ is the **total energy** E of the moving body, consisting of its kinetic energy E_k plus its rest-mass energy $m_0 c^2$:

$$E = E_k + m_0 c^2$$

The 'momenergy' formula
In many cases, such as in particle physics, the momentum of the particle is better known than its speed, so this relationship is often written in terms of momentum p:

$$E^2 = p^2 c^2 + (m_0 c^2)^2$$

See the Stretch and Challenge passage below for a proof of this relationship and Chapter 24 for examples of its use.

At very high speeds, say at $0.999c$, the rest-mass energy is negligible compared with the body's kinetic energy, so that the energy formula reduces simply to:

$$E = pc$$

This is the same formula as that for a photon given on page 463.

STRETCH
AND CHALLENGE

Derivation of the 'momenergy' formula

The aim is to get rid of the speed term v in favour of momentum p.

Start with the relationships $p = \gamma m_0 v$ and $E = \gamma m_0 c^2$. Square both to get

$$p^2 = \gamma^2 m_0^2 v^2 \quad \text{and} \quad E^2 = \gamma^2 m_0^2 c^4$$

Use these to get a relationship for $E^2 - p^2 c^2$, converting γ^2 to get it in terms of v and c:

$$\gamma^2 = \frac{1}{\left(1 - \dfrac{v^2}{c^2}\right)}$$

so:

$$E^2 - p^2 c^2 = \frac{m_0^2 c^4 - m_0^2 v^2 c^2}{\left(1 - \dfrac{v^2}{c^2}\right)}$$

The right-hand side simplifies (try it!) to just $m_0^2 c^4$, so we have:

$$E^2 - p^2 c^2 = m_0^2 c^4$$

which is simply rearranged for the momenergy formula:

$$E^2 = p^2 c^2 + m_0^2 c^4$$

9 GENERAL RELATIVITY

Spacetime grips mass, telling it how to move:
mass grips spacetime, telling it how to curve.

This single sentence carries the seeds of general relativity. It began with Einstein doing one of his famous **thought experiments**.

Imagine standing in a closed box, like a lift. You can't see outside the box, but feel a force at your feet. When you drop a pen it falls to the floor with a constant acceleration. What can you deduce about where you are, without having any contact with the outside world?

Two possible situations could cause these effects:

● the closed box is on a planet like Earth, i.e. in a *gravitational field*,

● the box is somewhere in space, perhaps part of a spaceship being accelerated 'upwards' so that there is a force on your feet – you have to accelerate with the box.

But were these effects caused by a downward all-pervading force (gravity), or by the fact that the box was being accelerated upwards? In each case you would feel the force on your feet, i.e. you experience what we call your 'weight'. When the pen was let go it was either 'attracted by gravity' or failed to be given the acceleration that the spaceship engines were giving to the box and you.

Einstein drew one of his simple but world-shattering conclusions from this 'experiment': *inside such a closed box there is no experiment that can be performed that would allow you to tell which situation you are in.* He stated a **principle of equivalence**: inertial forces (those that cause acceleration) are completely indistinguishable from gravitational forces: i.e. they are **equivalent**.

He then applied his *theory of special relativity* to this situation and borrowed some advanced geometry (from his teacher, Hermann Minkowski) to extend it to the Universe at large. This extended theory is called the **general theory of relativity**.

First, Einstein abolished gravity as a 'force that acts through space'. He replaced it with geometry – a simple consequence of the *curvature of spacetime*. Fig 23.14 provides an analogy. Imagine two people flying aeroplanes due north at a steady speed from two points on the Equator. They both travel in straight lines – but will inevitably find themselves getting closer and closer together – ultimately colliding at the North Pole. Is there some mysterious force pulling them together? No. It is all because the Earth is a sphere: its surface is curved.

Fig 23.14
Q: What mysterious force draws A and B together?
A: No force – it's just geometry

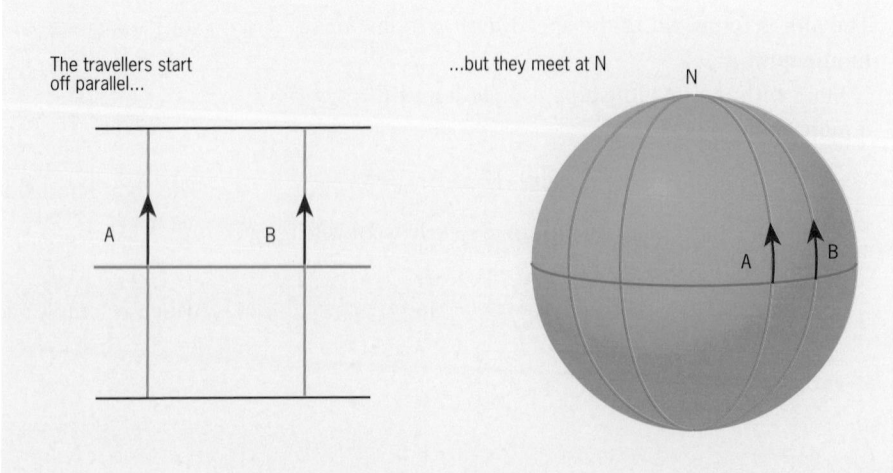

The travellers start off parallel...   ...but they meet at N

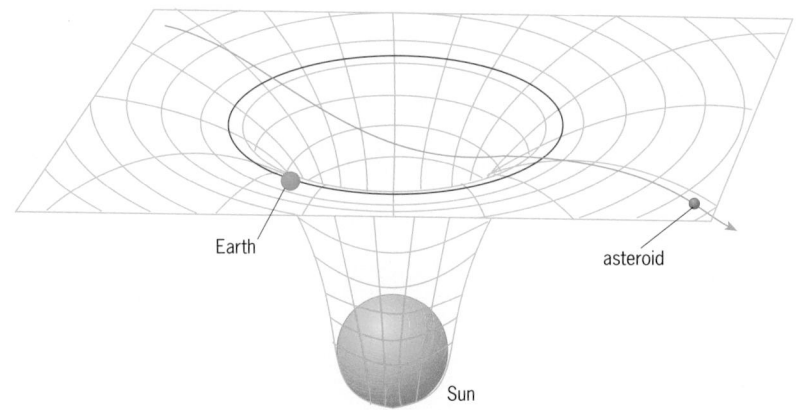

Fig 23.15 Spacetime is curved
Q: What mysterious force draws the asteroid towards the Sun?
A (Newton): Gravity – but I can't explain it.
A (Einstein): No force needed. It's just geometry and I can explain it – even if you can't understand it!

Einstein showed that a lump of matter caused the spacetime around it to be curved. Two masses travelling near each other, such as the Earth and the Moon, will move in 'straight lines through spacetime' – *but we see them as moving in curved paths*. The Earth has more mass, so its spacetime-curving effect is greater. Both bodies orbit around the same point, but the Moon orbits in a larger, less curved path. An asteroid may fall into the Sun and the Earth orbits around it because they follow paths in curved space (Fig 23.15).

DOES THE GENERAL THEORY WORK?

Anybody (who's clever enough) can come up with ingenious theories about the Universe. The success of a theory lies in its **explanatory power** and its **predictive ability**.

Explaining the behaviour of the planet Mercury

Einstein was able to explain a fact that Newton's laws couldn't, to do with the orbit of the planet Mercury. Like the orbits of all the planets, that of Mercury is an ellipse. The ellipse is also 'in orbit': it rotates around the Sun such that its point of furthest distance (the perihelion) swings around the Sun at a rate of about 1.56° (or 5600 seconds of arc) per century (Fig 23.16). This effect is caused mostly by effects due to the gravitational forces from other planets, as calculated using Newton's laws. But there was a discrepancy of 40" (40 seconds) of arc. Einstein's new theory explained this difference.

Predicting the 'bending of light'

Einstein produced another thought experiment. Fig 23.17 overleaf shows what he said would happen to a ray of light in an accelerating spaceship. As it crosses from one side to another the point B has moved on so that the light – travelling in a straight line – hits the wall below it (a). But the spacemen wouldn't *see* that. For them, in their reference frame of the spaceship, point B hasn't moved at all but the light has bent downwards (b). But are they accelerating in space – or just standing still in a gravitational field? If they couldn't look outside they wouldn't know. So according to the principle of equivalence, light would also appear to bend in a gravitational field.

Light travels in straight lines – even in Einstein's model. But he predicted that it would seem to bend in gravitational fields. The stronger the field, the more that light would be seen to curve. But as he pointed out, it wasn't light that was bending, it was space itself (see Fig. 23.15). A light ray passing close to the Sun would follow a *straight* line in *curved* space, called a geodesic.

Fig 23.16 The orbit of Mercury swings ('precesses') around the Sun. Newton's theory predicted this but at the wrong rate. General relativity gets it right

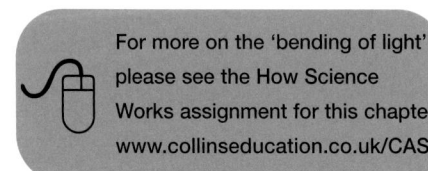

For more on the 'bending of light' please see the How Science Works assignment for this chapter www.collinseducation.co.uk/CAS

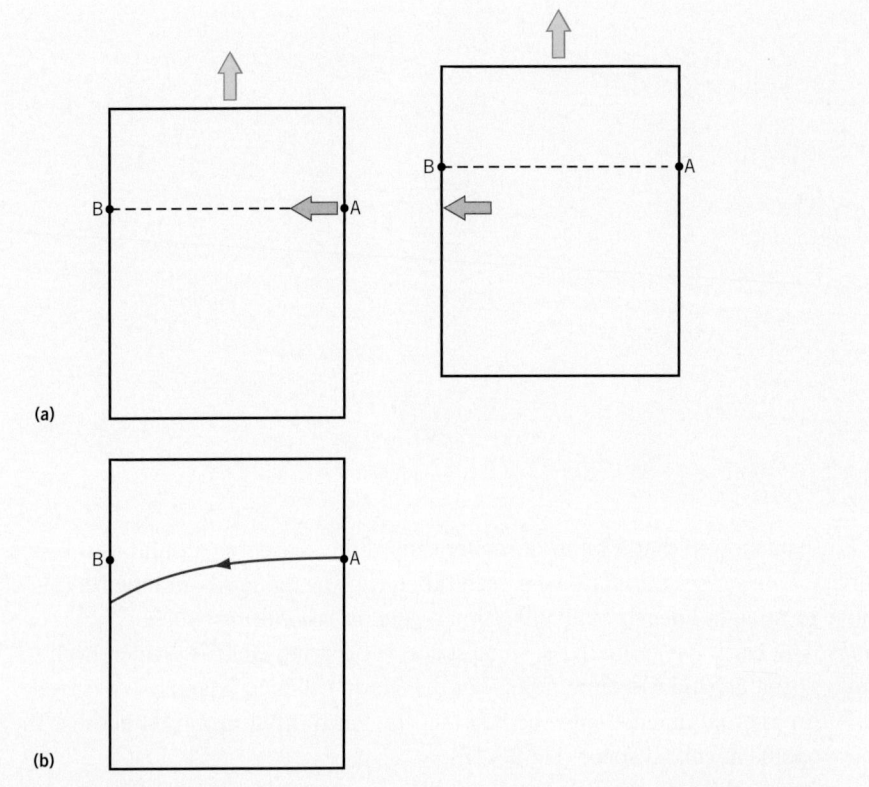

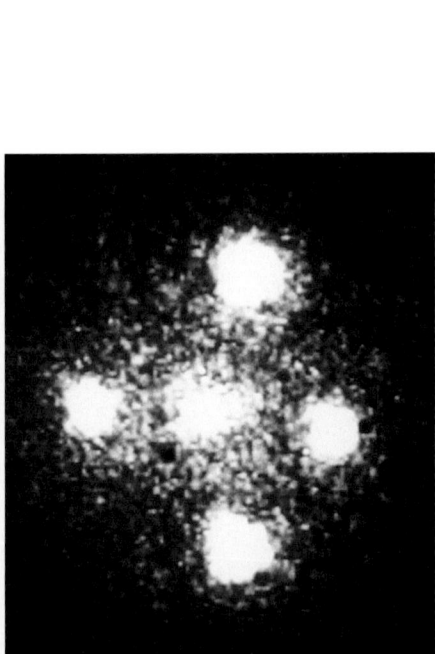

Fig 23.18 The Einstein cross, or Huchra's cross after its discoverer. The central spot is a relatively nearby galaxy; the four outer spots are images of a distant quasar, formed by the gravitational lensing effect of the intervening galaxy

Fig 23.17 (a) A photon leaves A towards B. But by the time it crosses the spaceship B has moved on. This is a view from an (imaginary) external reference frame. Light has travelled in a straight line. **(b)** Inside the spaceship the travellers see the light hit the wall at a point below B and assume or observe that it curved to get there. But in a gravitational field light has travelled in a straight line in curved space

Einstein calculated that a light ray that just 'grazed' the Sun would be deflected by 1.75" of arc. But it would be too close to the Sun to be seen except in a solar eclipse. There was a solar eclipse on the 29th May 1919 and two expeditions set out to test Einstein's prediction. The deflections they measured were:

Sobral (Brazil)	1.98" ± 0.12"
Principe (West Africa)	1.61" ± 0.30"

This gravitational bending of light is now seen on a regular basis by astronomers. Very massive objects such as galaxies produce a lensing effect: objects further away from the galaxy can form several images as light is bent around the massive object (Fig 23.18). The lenses have severe aberration!

Gravity and time

Another prediction of the general theory of relativity is that clocks slow down in a gravitational field: the stronger the field, the slower they go. A light wave is a sort of clock (it is the basis of our standard of time, after all – see page 454). Imagine an excited atom emitting a photon on the surface of a planet – and another doing the same well away from the planet. The first photon will have a lower frequency (longer wavelength) than the second: its clock is ticking (oscillating) more slowly. This is the **gravitational red shift**. It also means that the photon has less energy. The more massive the object, the less energy a photon emitted at its surface will have. For a black-hole-sized gravity field it will have no energy at all. This is the fundamental reason why black holes are black. But this effect has been detected in gamma rays emitted from different atoms just a few metres apart in the Earth's field.

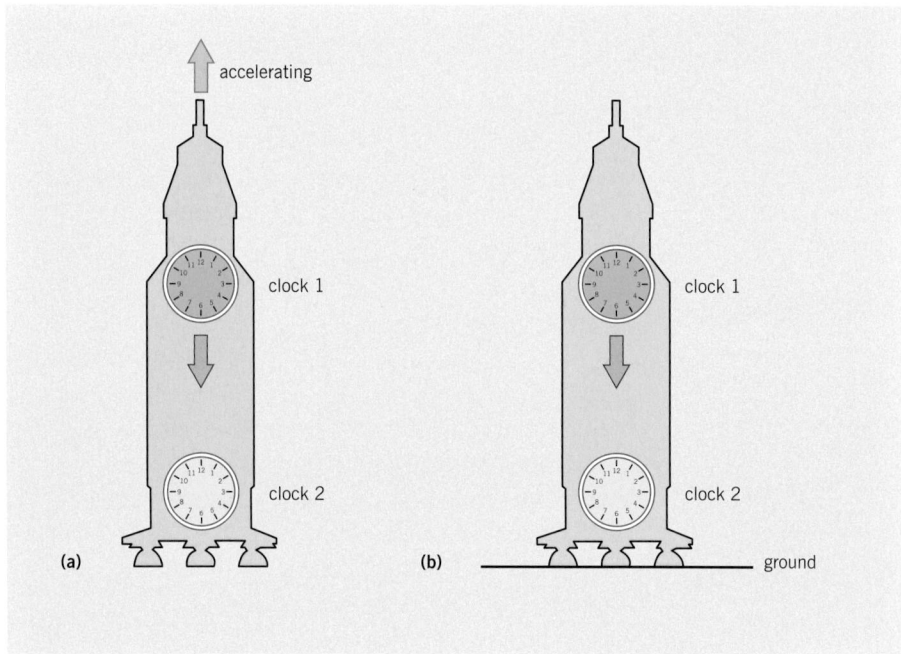

Fig 23.19 (a) Rocket accelerating in space **(b)** Rocket at rest on surface of a planet

A simple explanation of the effect uses the principle of equivalence. Look at Fig 23.19. In (a), clock 1 is at the front end of a rocket accelerating through space and clock 2 is at the back end. In (b) the rocket is at rest on a planet. Clock 1 is higher above ground than clock 2.

Both clocks are very accurate atomic clocks, configured as emitters and detectors of radiation that measure time using the frequency of photons (e.g. a caesium clock, see page 453). In the accelerating rocket, clock 2 sends out its standard signal of accurately known frequency (a photon) to clock 1. At the time of emission both clocks, as part of the rocket, are travelling at the same speed. Clock 1 observes the photon emitted from clock 2 and compares it with its own 'photon clock'. Now clock 1 will be moving faster by the time the photon reaches it than clock 2 was when it sent it out, because light has taken time to travel between the clocks. So the light from clock 2 will appear *Doppler shifted* to clock 1, with a lower frequency compared to its own standard photon. (Imagine the same number of waves having to be stretched out over the extra distance that clock 1 has travelled in the time the photon takes to reach it.)

An observer at clock 1 comparing this clock with clock 2 will deduce that clock 2 is 'running slow', i.e. that the time signal it produces is 'dilated'. This effect is nothing to do with the principle of relativity, it is just the simple Doppler effect. But now consider the second rocket stationary on a planet. According to the principle of equivalence, the rocket need not be accelerating in empty space to produce the same effect – it could be just sitting on the ground at rest in a gravitational field. An observer locked inside the rocket at the level of clock 1 can't tell the difference between acceleration and gravity, remember, so clock 2 still appears to be 'going slower'. Clock 2 is now experiencing a *gravitational time dilation*, and as the frequency appears reduced and wavelength increased, it is called a *gravitational red shift*.

The general theory of relativity is now the basis of large-scale cosmological theory. But a major problem still exists: there is no acceptable 'theory of everything' that includes both gravity and quantum physics.

SUMMARY

In this chapter you have learned how a simple principle – the constancy of the speed of light in a vacuum for all observers moving at a steady speed – leads to some remarkable consequences about the nature of time, space (distance), mass and energy. You have learned how the extension of this special (restricted) theory of relativity was extended to a general theory of relativity using the principle of equivalence.

In particular you should now:

- Understand the principle of the Michelson–Morley experiment and the significance of its null result.
- Know the two hypotheses of Einstein's theory of special relativity which explained the null result in the Michelson–Morley experiment.
- Understand the concept of a frame of reference.
- Be able to explain what is meant by a *thought experiment* and be able to describe examples, e.g. time signals in moving vehicles leading to the effects of special relativity, light passing through an accelerating spacecraft illustrating the principle of equivalence.
- Understand how Einstein's hypotheses lead to the Lorentz factor γ in time dilation.
- Understand and be able to use the formulae relating the Lorentz factor to time, distance and mass:
  $$t' = \gamma t \qquad x' = \gamma x \qquad m = \gamma m_0$$
- Appreciate that mass increases with speed, thus setting a maximum limit (c) to the speed a body can attain.

- Understand the equivalence of mass and energy and $E = mc^2$ (or $\Delta E = c^2 \Delta m$).
- Know about relativistic energy, and that momentum is linked by the energy and momentum–energy equations:
  $$E = \gamma m_0 c^2 = E_k + m_0 c^2$$
  $$E^2 = p^2 c^2 + (m_0 c^2)^2$$
- Appreciate the significance of the principle of equivalence of inertial and gravitational forces.
- Explain the effect of gravity on time in terms of a thought experiment based on the principle of equivalence, and how this also explains gravitational red shift.
- Remember how the general theory of relativity was supported by its ability to explain the anomalous values for the precession of the orbit of Mercury and to predict the bending of light passing close to the Sun.

The derivations of formulae are not usually required for A-level examinations.

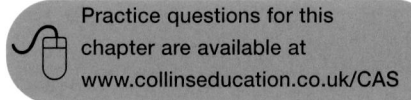

Practice questions for this chapter are available at www.collinseducation.co.uk/CAS

24

Deep matter

24 DEEP MATTER

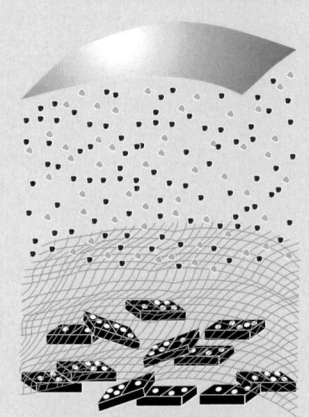

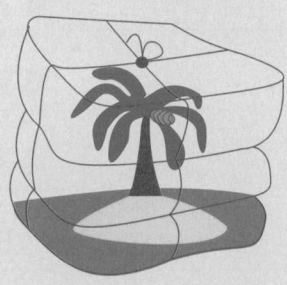

Warning to children

Children, if you dare to think of the greatness, rareness, muchness, fewness of this precious only endless world in which you say you live, you think of things like this:
Blocks of slate enclosing dappled red and green, enclosing tawny yellow nets, enclosing white and black acres of dominoes, where a neat brown paper parcel tempts you to untie the string. In the parcel a small island, on the island a large tree, on the tree a husky fruit. Strip the husk and pare the rind off: In the kernel you will see blocks of slate enclosed by dappled red and green, enclosed by tawny yellow nets, enclosed by white and black acres of dominoes, where the same brown paper parcel – Children,

leave the string untied! For who dares undo the parcel finds himself at once inside it, on the island, in the fruit, blocks of slate about his head, finds himself enclosed by dappled green and red, enclosed by yellow tawny nets, enclosed by black and white acres of dominoes, with the same brown paper parcel still untied upon his knee.

And if he then should dare to think of the fewness, muchness, rareness, greatness of this endless only precious world in which he says he lives – he then unties the string.

Robert Graves (1895–1985)

Scientists once thought that atoms were indivisible – the word 'atom' means 'cannot be cut'. They looked more closely, and found electrons, protons and neutrons. Again, they thought these were the smallest particles. Then physicists found they were not, but were divisible into a whole array of even smaller particles.

Where does this subdivision end, and will we ever know we have found truly fundamental particles? These are questions to which there is so far no definite answer.

The ideas in this chapter

In a study of the world of subatomic particles we are entering a very strange world indeed. What we see about us in everyday life is, on the whole, *stable* matter.

The theory of how the world of stable matter came about is called the **standard model**. This model says that about 15 billion years ago there was a 'singularity', a highly unstable point which was the entire Universe. Then, time and space began in the **Big Bang**. Chapter 26 deals in more detail with this stage in the development of the material of the Universe.

Today, researchers into the fundamental particles of matter use very large **particle accelerators** at international laboratories such as CERN (Centre Européen de Recherche Nucléaire) and other large international and national laboratories.

However, the most highly energetic particles come free: they are the **cosmic rays** that arrive from outer space – particles (most of them protons) which have been accelerated in the magnetic fields of exploding stars to speeds approaching the speed of light. See Figs 24.1(a), (b), (c).

The practical application of particle physics is not as remote from everyday life as you might imagine. For instance, particle accelerators and detectors are routinely used in hospitals to diagnose and treat diseases (see Chapter 19). Archaeologists and art researchers do detection work with these expensive pieces of equipment. They have also been used to discover and improve new materials for industry and the home, such as superconducting materials, semiconductors and video screen surfaces.

This chapter deals with how particles were discovered and are detected and manufactured in experiments with very large machines – the particle accelerators. It describes how physicists explain and predict the events of the subatomic world, which will involve quantum physics and relativity theory, the existence of both matter and antimatter, deep inelastic scattering and how events can be summarised in **Feynman diagrams**. You will learn about the types of particles that exist or are postulated to exist (hadrons, baryons, quarks, leptons, bosons) and the **conservation rules** that determine the reactions and relationships between them.

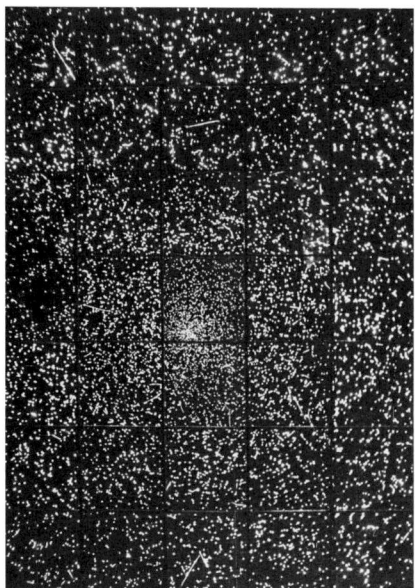

Fig 24.1(b) One particle from space travelling close to the speed of light collides with an atomic nucleus in the atmosphere. The kinetic energy is converted to new particles. More collisions create more particles, giving the 'cosmic ray shower' of about 2×10^5 particles. The shower core is seen as a 5 m $\times$ 7 m area by a discharge chamber array

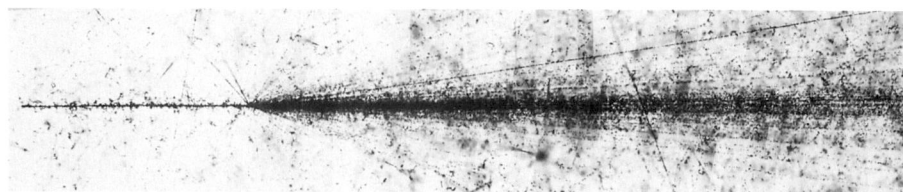

Fig 24.1(a) A very high-energy iron nucleus from a cosmic ray collides with a silver or bromine nucleus in photographic emulsion, producing a jet of particles (about 850 mesons)

What you should know before tackling this chapter

The basis of atomic and nuclear physics is covered in Chapters 16 and 17. You should know the following things about the size and nature of a typical atom:

- An atom is about 10^{-10} m across and consists of a small central nucleus just 10^{-14} m across surrounded by a 'cloud of wavy particles', the electrons.
- The nucleus contains practically all the mass of an atom and (except for hydrogen) is made up of two types of nucleon: protons and neutrons. Protons are stable, but free neutrons (not in an atom) decay as shown in Fig 24.2 (and see page 491). This can also happen inside a nucleus which has too many neutrons.
- An electromagnetic force binds electrons to the nucleus.
- A strong nuclear force binds nucleons together inside the nucleus.
- There is also a rather more mysterious weak nuclear force that is (for example) involved in beta decay (see box on page 494).

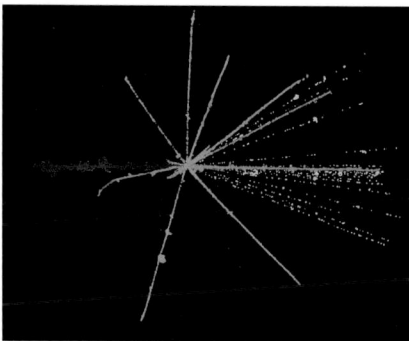

Fig 24.1(c) A cosmic ray sulphur nucleus (red) collides with a nucleus in photographic emulsion. (Green: fluorine nucleus; blue: other nuclear fragments; yellow: 16 pions.)

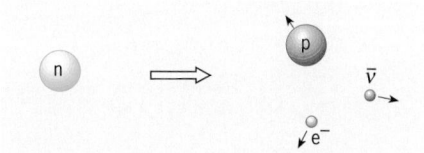

Fig 24.2 A neutron is stable only inside a nucleus. Free neutrons decay with a half-life of 900 s. Charge, momentum and mass–energy are conserved

This chapter has many terms and ideas that may be unfamiliar to you. Take it step by step and check your understanding before moving on. It may help you to refer now and then to Table 24.16 on page 493: it lists all the particles mentioned and their properties, and you can gradually build up a picture of them all.

> **? QUESTION 1**
>
> 1 Outline the arguments to support the ideas that:
> **a)** the electromagnetic force is stronger than the gravitational force,
> **b)** the strong nuclear force is stronger than the electromagnetic force.

1 THE SIMPLE ATOM GETS COMPLICATED

The simple Rutherford–Bohr model of an atom had three particles: neutron, proton and electron. But the observed energy spectrum of beta particles emitted in radioactive decay showed the need for another particle, the **neutrino**, which carries off both energy and momentum. This is a very small, uncharged particle, with a mass of zero or close to zero (see page 343).

Then the British theoretical physicist Paul Dirac said in 1930 that, mathematically, each charged particle had to have a matching antiparticle, of identical mass but of opposite charge. So there had to be an electron with a positive charge. This anti-electron or **positron** was first observed experimentally in 1932.

Again because theory suggested it, the Japanese physicist Hideki Yukawa proposed in 1935 that another particle ought to exist, with a mass between that of an electron and a nucleon. This was called a **meson** (the Greek word for 'middleweight'). In fact, Yukawa and his colleagues found *two* 'mesons'. One had the properties predicted by Yukawa and is now called a **pion** or **pi meson**. This is a genuine meson, as the name is now used. The other turned out to be a kind of giant electron now called a **muon**.

TOO MANY PARTICLES?

More and more 'mesons' – middleweight particles – were discovered in the next thirty years, together with other particles which were more massive than the nucleons. This was all very confusing, and rather like the state chemistry was in before the idea of a Periodic Table (Table 17.4) and the theory of electron shells. The equivalent theory in particle physics is the 'standard model', involving the particles discussed in this chapter.

The first new particles discovered were thought to be the building blocks of ordinary matter and were called *fundamental* particles. But by the 1960s there were even more of these 'fundamental' particles than there were elements in the Periodic Table! Most existed only for extremely short periods of time. To understand and categorise them, physicists needed to identify their properties and compare them. We will look at this shortly, and describe what are now seen as fundamental particles. But first we look at how particles are discovered.

2 DISCOVERING PARTICLES

The electron was the first subatomic particle to be discovered, in 1897. The cathode ray tube technique used then (see page 218) is used in **particle accelerators** today (see Fig 24.3). In the cyclotron, for example, charged particles are accelerated in a magnetic field at right angles to their direction of motion, which makes them move in the arc of a circle. In a given magnetic field, the radius of the circle depends on the charge, mass and speed of the particle.

These accelerated particles are then used in collisions to produce other subatomic particles, rather like the formation of particles by cosmic rays (Fig 24.1). **Particle detectors** enable the newly formed particles to be located and identified. It is not these particles that are seen, but their tracks formed as ionised particles of the material they pass through. As we shall see, neutral particles leave no tracks themselves, but other clues of their presence can be detected.

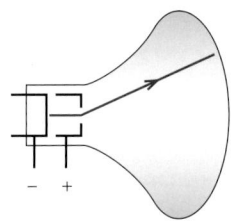

name	cathode ray tube
particles	electrons
energy	1 keV (1×10^3 V)
discoveries	mass and charge of electron

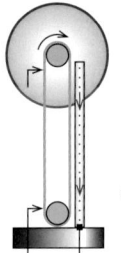

name	van de Graaff generator
particles	protons/small ions
energy	10 MeV (10×10^6 V)
discoveries	structure of nuclei

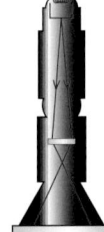

name	electron microscope
particles	electrons
energy	25 keV (25×10^3 V)
discoveries	structure of crystals, viruses and cells

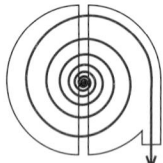

name	cyclotron
particles	protons/small ions
energy	25 MeV (25×10^6 V)
discoveries	structure of nuclei and transmutation of elements

name	linear accelerator
particles	electrons/positrons/protons
energy	50 GeV (50×10^9 V)
discoveries	evidence for quarks, tau lepton

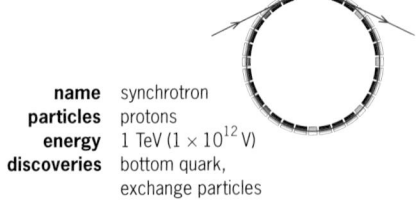

name	synchrotron
particles	protons
energy	1 TeV (1×10^{12} V)
discoveries	bottom quark, exchange particles

Fig 24.3 Particle accelerators have been used to produce the range of particles described in this chapter

ENERGY AND MATTER

Accelerated (highly energetic) particles are useful for the investigation of new particles because of a consequence of the **special theory of relativity** – that energy and mass are interconvertible (see page 463).

Fig 24.4(a) shows a **bubble chamber**, a type of detector of charged particles important historically but now obsolete. An incoming proton travels at a speed very close to the speed of light. It has very high kinetic energy. As it collides with a stationary proton (a hydrogen nucleus), this energy creates all the new particles and provides them with the kinetic energy to move away. Following the Einstein relation $E = mc^2$:

mass–energy of incoming proton → masses plus kinetic energies of
new particles produced

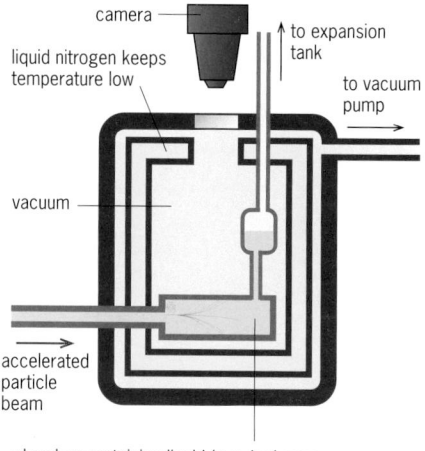

Fig 24.4(a) A bubble chamber. The beam enters the chamber, and the liquid pressure is momentarily reduced at the expansion tank. This allows liquid in the chamber to boil only at points where ions are present. So tracks of bubbles appear where there are charged particles at that moment

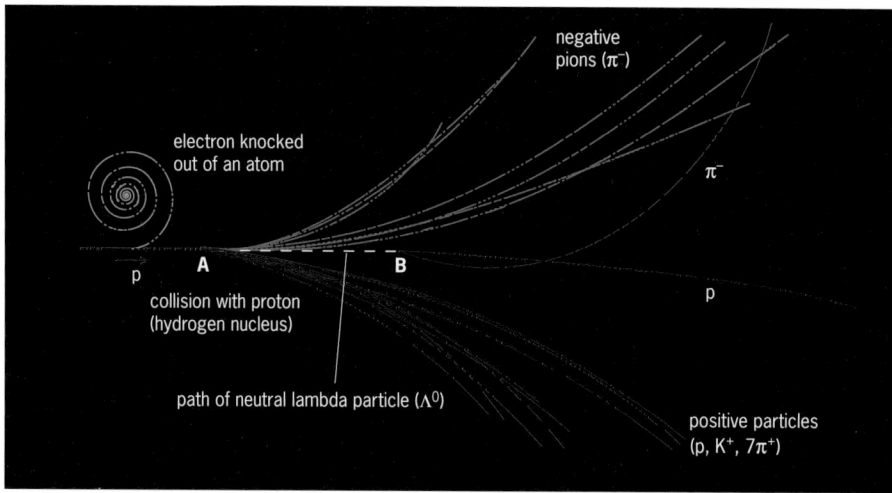

Fig 24.4(b) A high-energy proton collides with a stationary proton, producing 18 new particles

Fig 24.4(b) shows an example of such a collision (at A). The bubble tracks of some particles arc downwards, and others arc upwards. The small tightly curved spiral is from an electron knocked violently out of an atom by the incoming proton, showing that particles curving upwards are negatively charged, while those curving downwards are positively charged. At B, two particles appear as if from nothing. They are a newly created proton and a negative meson known as a **pion**, symbol π^-. We have to guess that these two particles were formed at B by a decay or a collision involving a neutral particle that left no track as it travelled from the first collision at A to the start of the two new tracks at B.

SOME COLLISIONS AND DECAYS

Particles that are observed in a detector, such as a bubble or cloud chamber, tend to do one of two things:

- In simple collisions, they collide with a nucleus already there, and then may possibly break up the nucleus and/or create new particles.
- They self-destruct by 'decaying' into other particles or by colliding with an antiparticle.

We now look at both kinds of events in more detail.

Simple collisions

Look at Fig 24.5(a) overleaf, showing the structure of a cloud chamber, and Fig 24.5(b) which shows collisions between alpha particles and the nuclei of hydrogen, helium and nitrogen as observed in the cloud chamber. The tracks in this and similar diagrams have been (redrawn and) artificially coloured to make things clearer.

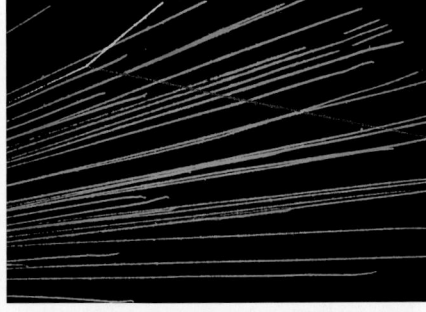

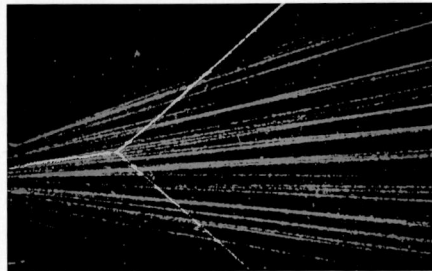

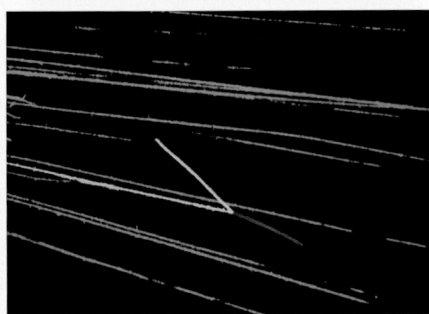

Fig 24.5(b) Three cloud chamber pictures of alpha particle collisions.
Top: An alpha particle (yellow) in hydrogen; the heavier alpha particle is deflected only slightly as it hits the hydrogen nucleus. (The green alpha particles are not involved in collisions.)
Centre: An alpha particle colliding with a helium nucleus. An alpha particle is a helium nucleus, so both have the same mass and their paths diverge at right angles.
Bottom: An alpha particle in air, hitting a nitrogen nucleus. The nitrogen nucleus is 3.5 times heavier, and the alpha particle bounces back from it at a sharp angle

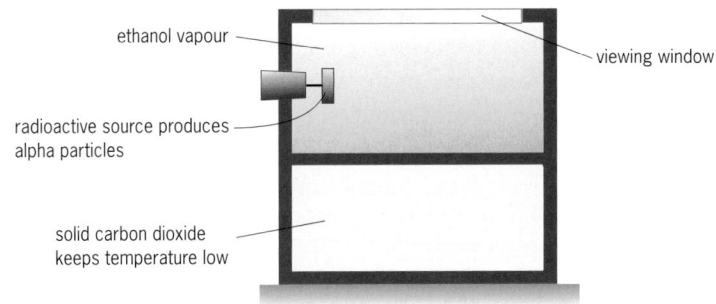

Fig 24.5(a) A cloud chamber. Ethanol condenses round charged particles in the chamber, and so forms tracks of moving particles made of tiny droplets

The pictures show that the angle between the tracks of the alpha particle and the nucleus after collision is decided simply by the ratio of the mass of the alpha particle to that of the nucleus it hits.

For another simple collision that indicates different masses, look back at Fig 24.1(c) in which a heavy cosmic ray particle, in this case a sulphur nucleus (red track), collides with a nucleus in the photographic emulsion. The heavy blue tracks are nuclei, the thin yellow ones are the tracks of smaller, less ionising particles identified as pions.

Particles that decay

Unstable particles are like unstable (radioactive) nuclei: for a particular particle we can predict *what* will happen, but not *when*. The newly created particles will decay, eventually, into the **stable particles of matter**, which are protons, electrons and neutrinos. Occasionally, the electromagnetic particle the **photon** is emitted, or the decay is completely to photons, leaving no matter behind. As with radioactive nuclei, we can be certain that half the number of any type of unstable particle will decay in a particular time, so we use the idea of the *half-life* of the particle.

We now know that every known particle has its antiparticle, equal and opposite in its properties. For example, the positron is an antiparticle, exactly the same as an electron but opposite in charge. Particles and antiparticles make up what we call **matter** and **antimatter**.

When an antiparticle collides with its ordinary-matter particle twin, they annihilate each other. Their mass–energies are converted to new particles, namely photons and massive particles, that appear in the detector.

3 THE SEARCH FOR ORDER: CLASSIFYING PARTICLES

The problem facing researchers was how to put all these new particles into some sort of order, and perhaps find out *why* they existed. Researchers started off by naming them with Greek letters, more or less randomly as they turned up. These are a few examples:

μ	mu 'mesons' or muons	Ξ	xi particles
π	pi mesons or pions	Σ	sigma particles
K	kappa mesons or kaons	Ω	omega particles
Λ	lambda particles		

You don't need to remember the details of these particles for examinations, but should recognise them when you meet them in questions.

Matter and antimatter

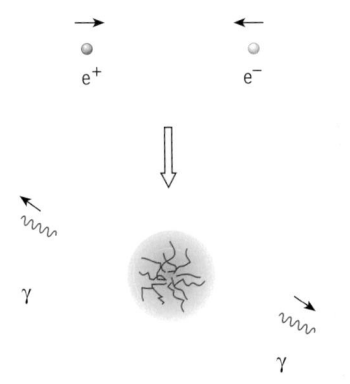

Fig 24.6 Annihilation of an electron–positron pair converts their mass–energy into photons. Momentum is conserved by the photons of equal mass–energy moving away in exactly opposite directions. Note also that charge is conserved

When a particle meets its antiparticle there is instant annihilation of mass. The mass–energy of the pair appears as new particles (supplying both mass and kinetic energy) and/or radiation. The most commonly observed matter–antimatter collision is that for electrons:

electron + positron → 2 photons
$$e^- + e^+ \rightarrow 2\gamma$$

Why *two* photons? This is because photons carry not only energy but momentum, as explained below. Momentum has to be conserved. If we think of the two particles meeting head on with the same speed, the original momentum adds to zero. If the result was a single photon, the momentum would not be zero. The momentum can only be the same before and after the collision with two photons carrying *equal quantities* of momentum travelling in *opposite* directions, as in Fig 24.6.

Pair production

Just as an electron–positron pair can annihilate to produce photons, so photons with enough energy can 'decay' into these and even more massive particles. Fig 24.7 shows such an event seen in a bubble chamber; it is called **pair production**. The event occurs only in a strong electric field – near a charged nucleus for example.

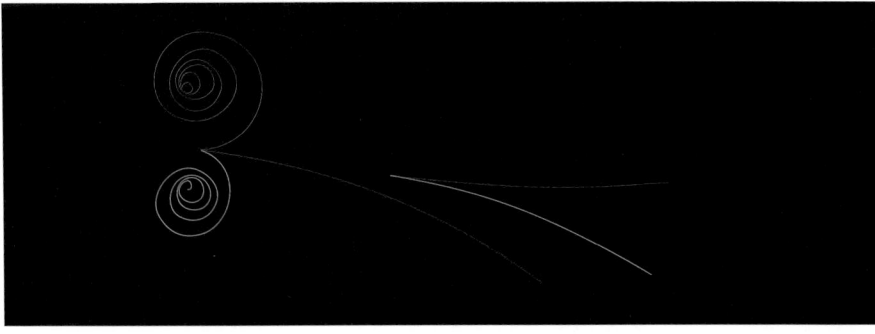

Fig 24.7 Gamma ray photons (not detected) enter the bubble chamber from the left. One photon decays to an electron–positron pair, with the electron spiralling down and the positron up. (The straighter track is for an electron displaced by the same photon from an atom in the chamber.) On the right is the decay of a second photon to an electron–positron pair

? QUESTION 2

2 Read the text above and the caption for Fig 24.7. Which electron– positron pair has the greater energy? Explain your answer.

The basic properties of matter were well known to these researchers, but more properties had to be discovered before a clear system of classification was produced. These basic properties are *charge* and *mass*.

CHARGE

Charge is either positive or negative. It is also 'quantised': both positive and negative charge on ordinary particles come in simple multiples of the elementary charge, $-1e$ or $+1e$, of value $\pm 1.6 \times 10^{-19}$ C (but see page 483 for the peculiarities of quarks). However charge is no great help in solving the problem of *classifying* so many particles.

MASS

Mass seemed a good basis for classification, and particles discovered in the 1940s and 1950s were put into three groups mainly by mass, as in Table 24.1. There were problems with this grouping: a muon is nearly as massive as a pion, for example, although as we shall see they belong to completely different families of particle. Also, new particles were

Table 24.1 An attempt to classify particles on the basis of mass

Name	Mass	Examples
mesons	medium	pions, kaons
baryons	heavy	protons, neutrons, lambda, sigma, xi
leptons	light	electrons, muons, neutrinos

discovered, such as some new mesons (middleweights) which were heavier than the proton. But, as we shall see next, the groups had properties other than mass that made them fundamentally different.

NEW FUNDAMENTAL PROPERTIES

Charge and mass were not enough to make the distinctions between all the particles found, so workers identified other common properties. These properties are just as fundamental and mysterious as charge and mass, and physicists have given them weird names including *charm, bottomness, baryon number* and *strangeness*. Using these properties, physicists have been able to simplify what has been called the *particle zoo*, as we shall see later. One such property is whether the particle responds to different kinds of force.

MATTER AND FORCES: HADRONS AND LEPTONS

We are familiar with the fact that charge is acted upon by electromagnetic forces, and that mass is acted upon by gravity. A key to identifying the differences between particles was the way they were affected by these and other forces.

Protons in a nucleus are affected by electromagnetic forces and by gravity. But they stay inside the nucleus, in spite of the strong electric force of repulsion due to their positive charges, because there is another, stronger force holding them together. This is the **strong nuclear force**.

All particles that 'feel' the strong nuclear force are called **hadrons**, subdivided into **mesons** and **baryons**. Most particles that do not 'feel' the strong force are called **leptons**. This distinction neatly separated most particles into two significant groups, as in Table 24.2: pions are hadrons, and 'feel' the strong nuclear force, while electrons and muons are leptons and are unaffected by the strong force. (This broad classification could be developed further, whereas the grouping of Table 24.1 could not.)

Table 24.2 Examples of hadrons which feel the strong nuclear force, and leptons which do not. Note that gravitons (if they exist) and photons are non-hadrons

Hadrons	Non-hadrons
mesons, e.g. pions, kaons, eta mesons	**leptons**, including electrons, muons, neutrinos
baryons, e.g. protons, neutrons, omega, sigma and lambda particles	photons, gravitons (if they exist)

The lepton family is described in more detail opposite.

Another important difference between hadrons and leptons is that *leptons have no substructure* – they are (as far as we know) genuinely *fundamental* particles – while hadrons are built from even smaller (fundamental) particles called **quarks** (see page 483).

Most hadrons and leptons are *unstable*: they very quickly decay into other particles, and finally end up as the only stable particles in the Universe – protons, electrons and neutrinos. Even the neutron is unstable, since outside a nucleus it decays with a half-life of about 11 minutes to a proton, an electron and an antineutrino:

$$\text{n} \rightarrow \text{p} + \text{e}^- + \bar{\text{v}}$$

PARTICLES AND ANTIPARTICLES

Each hadron has its *antiparticle*, for example:

proton and antiproton	p$^+$ and p$^-$
neutron and antineutron	n and $\bar{\text{n}}$
kappa meson (or kaon)	K$^+$ and K$^-$

Antiparticles are often represented by using a bar over the symbol, as for the antineutron, especially when they have no opposite charge.

THE WEAK NUCLEAR FORCE

As well as being affected by the electromagnetic force, charged hadrons are affected by a force called the **weak nuclear force** and, since they all have mass, they are affected by *gravity*.

The weak force seems the most mysterious of all the forces. Like the strong force, it acts over a very short range. However, modern theory shows that when particles have a high enough energy, the weak force and the electric force become the same **electroweak** force. We will see on page 492 that the weak force seems to work as one quark changes into another.

LEPTONS

Leptons are generally much less massive than hadrons (Greek: hadron = heavy, lepton = small). Leptons are affected by three of the four fundamental interactions (forces): the electromagnetic (if charged), the weak and gravity.

There are three kinds of lepton: **electrons e**, **muons μ**, and **tauons τ**. Each of these is associated with its own kind of **neutrino ν**.

Electrons and neutrinos are stable particles, but both muons and tauons decay. Their decay is due to the weak force, so lifetimes are much longer than for the unstable hadrons. The tauon is much more massive than the other leptons and has enough mass–energy to decay into hadrons. Each property of a particle is in general associated with a number, which helps to explain the reactions in which they are involved. For example, charge is either +1 or −1. The number associated with 'lepton-ness' is the **lepton number** (+1 for leptons, −1 for antileptons). Table 24.3 shows the main leptons and their neutrinos.

Table 24.3 Leptons and their neutrinos. Each associated neutrino is subtly different from the others

	Leptons			Antileptons		
	Electron	Muon	Tauon	Positron	Muon plus	Tauon plus
Symbol	e^-	μ^-	τ^-	e^+	μ^+	τ^+
Neutrinos	ν_e	ν_μ	ν_τ	$\bar{\nu}_e$	$\bar{\nu}_\mu$	$\bar{\nu}_\tau$
Lepton no.	+1	+1	+1	−1	−1	−1

4 LOOKING FOR PATTERNS OF BEHAVIOUR

So far, we have seen how particles are classified in terms of well-known properties, like mass and charge, and their response to forces. But the key to the fundamental nature of particles was in investigating what happens *and what does not happen* when particles interact or otherwise change, either naturally by spontaneous decay or when they interact at high energies.

THE RULES OF BEHAVIOUR

Fundamental particles must obey the basic ground rules of physics, which should be well known to you. These are:

- **Momentum conservation**. In any interaction between particles in a system, the total momentum must stay constant.
- **Mass–energy conservation**. In any interaction between particles in a system, mass–energy must neither be created nor destroyed.
- **Charge conservation**. In any interaction between particles in a system, the total electrical charge in the system must not change.

The following examples illustrate these rules.

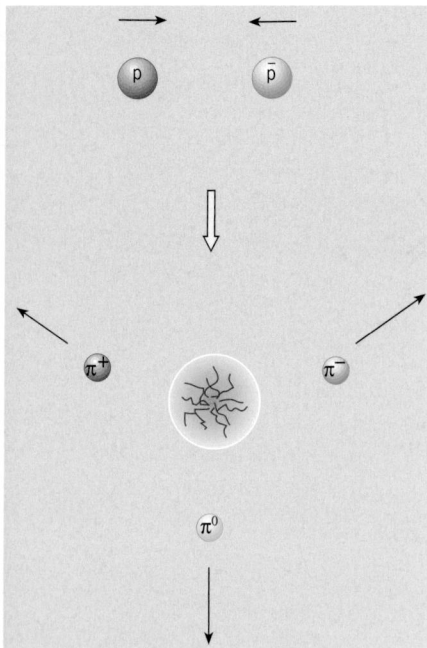

Fig 24.8 Proton–antiproton annihilation

Example 1. Neutron decay

$$n \rightarrow p + e^- + \bar{\nu}_e$$

The neutron has mass–energy of 939.6 MeV, the proton has 938.3 MeV and the electron 0.5 MeV. The neutron can thus change into the particles on the right with an energy of about 0.8 MeV left over to be shared by the kinetic energy of the products and the creation of the antineutrino. The neutron has zero charge and so the sum of the charges on the products is also zero.

Example 2. Proton–antiproton annihilation

$$p + \bar{p} \rightarrow \pi^+ + \pi^- + \pi^0$$

This reaction clearly conserves charge. The combined mass–energy of the protons is 1876 MeV. The mass–energy of each charged pion is 140 MeV, with 135 MeV for the neutral pion. Since the mass–energy of the protons is more than enough to produce the total mass of the pions (415 MeV), they fly off at very high speeds, in the directions that conserve momentum (Fig 24.8).

Example 3. When the expected doesn't happen

Particle physicists soon realised that there were some possible changes that did obey the three basic conservation laws but which never actually occurred, even when enough energy was supplied. For example, a proton did not spontaneously decay into a positron and a neutral pion, even though charge, energy and momentum could all be conserved.

$$p \nrightarrow e^+ + \pi^0$$

This is just as well, otherwise all protons would eventually decay and the atomic nucleus – hence atoms, chemistry, life, stars – could not exist!

WHY SOME CHANGES COULD NOT HAPPEN: THE DISCOVERY OF BARYON NUMBER

Many other proposed changes were never observed in practice. So physicists decided that there must be some sort of 'charge' that would not be conserved by these changes – the equations would not balance. A theory was proposed that particles possess (or lack) another property that must be conserved. It was a quality that, for example, a proton possessed but that neither electrons nor pions did.

Evidence built up that this new kind of charge was possessed only by the heavier particles, the baryons. Unlike electric charge, there was no *force* associated with it. But like electric charge it came in same-size 'chunks'. It is called **baryon number**, B.

The proton and neutron were given baryon number +1, and electrons, neutrinos, positrons and pions had baryon number 0.

Thus, proton decay could not occur because baryon number would not be conserved, the two sides in Example 3 did not balance:

$$\text{baryon equation:} \quad +1 \neq 0$$

But when a neutron decays into a proton (Example 1 above), baryon number *is* conserved because the neutron also has a baryon number of +1.

Now look back at the reaction in Example 2, in which two baryons (proton and antiproton) are converted to pions. Here the right side is entirely of pions, and so has *zero* baryon number. Thus the left side must also have zero baryon number. This can be true only if the antiproton has a *negative* baryon number ($B = -1$); see Table 24.4.

Now in Table 24.2 (page 478) mesons and baryons are grouped together as hadrons. But note that mesons have a baryon number of 0. Leptons also have baryon number 0 but have their own conserved property, **lepton number** L: as Table 24.3 (page 479) shows, leptons must have lepton number number +1 or −1. To conserve lepton number, when leptons are made out of non-leptons they are made in pairs:

$$\pi^- \rightarrow \mu^- + \bar{\nu}_\mu$$

Pions are not leptons (Table 24.2), so the left side of the equation has a lepton number 0. On the right side is a muon of lepton number +1 and a muon antineutrino with a lepton number −1.

MORE NON-EVENTS LEAD TO MORE NEW PROPERTIES

Identifying reactions that seemed never to happen became an important tool in classifying particles. This approach led to **strange particles** – particles with a conserved property called **strangeness**. This was to be explained by the theory of quarks (see page 483), which dramatically simplified the task of classifying particles.

STRANGENESS AND TIME

Reactions that involve the strong nuclear force seemed to happen on a very short time scale, typically 10^{-23} s. This is the time it takes for the fastest possible effect – the strong interaction – to cross a nucleus at the speed of light.

A typical reaction involving strongly interacting particles takes this very short time. For example:

$$p + \pi^- \rightarrow K^0 + \Lambda \qquad time = 10^{-23}\ s$$

The Λ (lambda) particle is unstable and breaks up – but oddly, it does so in a time of about 3×10^{-10} s.

Let us put this into an everyday time scale. When you drop a china cup on to a hard floor, it breaks up in less than a millisecond. (For a rough estimate, consider how long it takes a shock wave travelling at the speed of sound to cross a cup. The cup usually breaks into several pieces, all produced at much the same time, all of random sizes.)

Both of the times for the particle reactions are very short, but one is 10^{13} times longer than the other. On the cup scale of time, it was as if you dropped a cup, which immediately (at least, in 10^{-4} s) broke into two large pieces. Then, *three years later*, these two pieces broke up into lots of smaller pieces.

The new exceptionally long-lived particles were not clearly identified by mass, charge and baryon number, so they were simply called **strange particles** and labelled as K (kappa – a kaon), Λ (lambda), Σ (sigma), Ξ (xi) and Ω (omega); see Table 24.5.

Table 24.4 Some particles and their baryon numbers

Particle	Baryon no. B
baryons, e.g. proton, neutron, sigma	1
baryon antiparticles, e.g. antiproton	−1
mesons, e.g. pion, kaon; leptons, e.g. electron, positron	0

✔ **REMEMBER THIS**

As shown in Table 24.3, there are three pairs of leptons and each pair is associated with its own lepton number. This complicates things but does allow useful predictions about those ghostly leptons, the neutrinos.

? **QUESTION 4**

4 Look at Table 24.4 for the baryon numbers of the particles to check which of the following reactions would not occur because baryon number is not conserved. (All equations conserve charge.)
a) $\pi^+ + n \rightarrow K^0 + \Sigma^+$
b) $\pi^+ + p \rightarrow K^+ + \Sigma^+$
c) $K^+ + n \rightarrow \pi^0 + \pi^+$

Fig 24.9 A cup cannot break up faster than it takes for the shock wave to pass through it

? **QUESTIONS 5–6**

5 Calculate how long it takes for a disturbance to travel across a nucleus (10^{-14} m) at light speed (3×10^8 m s^{-1}).

6 Show that a cup takes less than a millisecond to break. (First estimate the size of a cup. The speed of sound in a ceramic is about 5000 m s^{-1}.)

Table 24.5 Some strange particles and their strangeness values

Particle	Strangeness S	Particle	Strangeness S
K$^+$, K^0 (mesons)	+1	Σ (baryon)	−1
K$^-$, $\bar{K}^0$ (mesons)	−1	Ξ (baryon)	−2
Λ (baryon)	−1	W (baryon)	−3

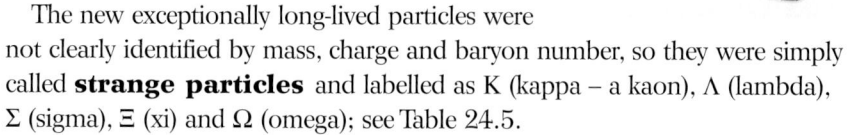

7 Test the following reactions for conservation of strangeness:
a) $\pi^- + p \rightarrow K^+ + \Sigma^-$
b) $K^- + p \rightarrow K^+ + \Xi^-$
c) $\pi^- + p \rightarrow K^- + \Sigma^+$
d) $\pi^+ + n \rightarrow \pi^+ + \Lambda$
Table 24.16 on page 493 may be useful.

The fundamental 'charge' or property called **strangeness**, symbol S, was needed to explain this behaviour. Particles can have strangeness numbers from +3 to −3. This introduces the idea of 'threeness', which we return to soon.

The strangeness of interactions is conserved only for reactions in which the strong force is important (see the Stretch and Challenge passage below). For example, we can produce the larger baryons, called **hyperons**, by colliding an electron and a positron at very high speeds. The collision has enough energy to make a large number of particles (Fig 24.10). When this happens, if hyperons are produced, they have to be as *pairs* with equal but opposite strangeness:

$$e^- + e^+ + a\ lot\ of\ mass\text{–}energy$$
$$\rightarrow \Lambda^0 + \bar{\Lambda}^0\ plus\ other\ particles$$

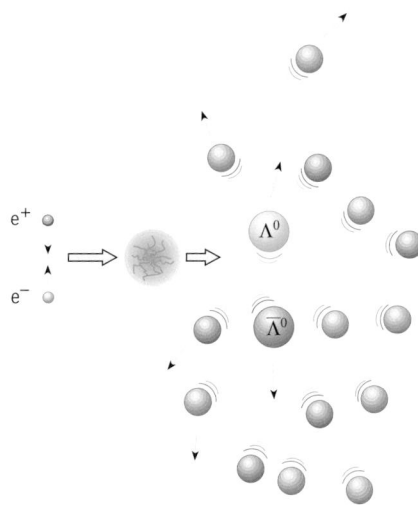

Fig 24.10 Electrons and positrons collide at high energies to produce a lambda and an antilambda particle (both strange) plus lots of other particles, mostly mesons

The ordinary baryons (protons and neutrons) have zero strangeness. Strange particles Λ and Σ have *negative* strangeness, and their antiparticles have *positive* strangeness.

Breaking the law of strangeness conservation

Some conservation rules work only when the strong force is involved, others only for the weak force. One rule is the conservation rule for strangeness. It has been found that strangeness-carrying particles can decay into particles with zero strangeness, *thus breaking the conservation law.* But they can only do this via the weak interaction, and when they do, they can only change the total strangeness number by just one step at a time.

For example, a **xi hyperon** (also called a cascade hyperon) first decays into a lambda hyperon in a weak interaction, gaining strangeness of +1. Then the lambda hyperon changes into hadrons (particles responding to the strong force but here interacting via the weak force) of strangeness 0, again with a strangeness change of unity.

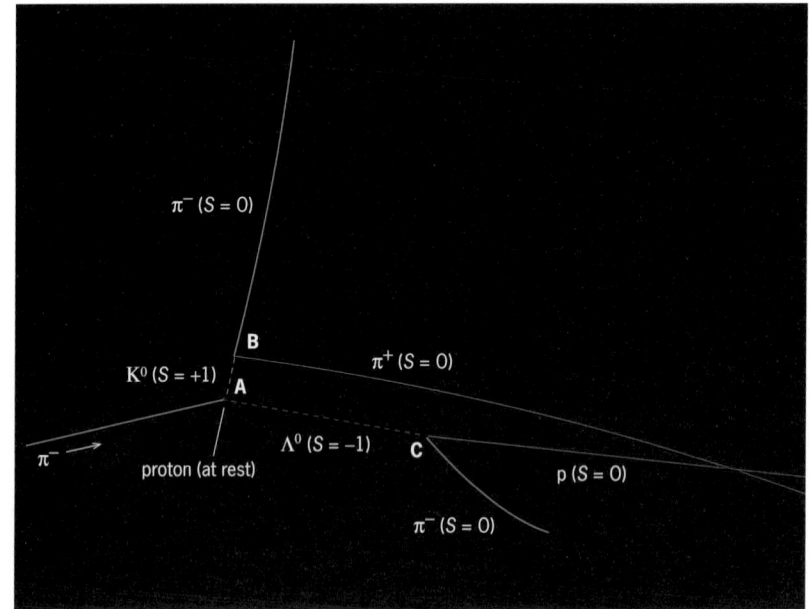

Fig 24.11 Another example of non-conservation of strangeness is shown by these tracks. A pion interacts with a proton to produce two strange particles (K^0, Λ^0), which leave no tracks. These then decay as shown. Strangeness is conserved at A (strong interaction), but changes by ±1 at B and C

Step 1:
$$\Xi^- \rightarrow \Lambda^0 + \pi^-$$
$$S = -2 \qquad S = -1 \qquad S = 0 \qquad \Delta S = +1$$

Step 2:
$$\Lambda^0 \rightarrow \pi^- + p^+$$
$$S = -1 \qquad S = 0 \qquad S = 0 \qquad \Delta S = +1$$

5 QUARKS BRING ORDER OUT OF CONFUSION

The ways described above for classifying particles were immensely helpful – interactions could be predicted. But like the Periodic Table in Mendeleev's day, there was no underpinning *theory* or *model* of particles which explained *why* the patterns existed.

Then a revolutionary new theory was suggested to explain the 'threeness' referred to opposite: the heavy particles (baryons) might in fact be simple combinations of *three smaller particles*. This theory required a startling idea, that *electric charge has to be subdivided into thirds*: the new particles could have charges of 1/3 or 2/3 of the electronic charge.

At the time, very few physicists believed in the *real* existence of these hypothetical particles, at first not even the American physicist Murray Gell-Mann (born 1929), who suggested the new particles and named them **quarks**.

This theory was later supported by experiments in which individual protons were bombarded by very energetic electrons. Just as the Geiger–Marsden alpha particle bombardment experiment showed that the atom has a small central mass, so these experiments showed that the density of a proton was not uniform, suggesting that it *was* made up of even smaller masses. These turned out to be the quarks. See pages 500–501 for more about the technique used – deep inelastic scattering.

The quark model of hadrons

The original simple quark model said that there were three quarks. These are now called the **up**, **down** and **strange** quarks. They are summarised in Table 24.6. As well as having fractional charge, quarks also have fractional baryon number.

Table 24.6 The first quarks

Quark	Symbol	Charge/e	Baryon no.	Strangeness
Up	u	+2/3	+1/3	0
Down	d	−1/3	+1/3	0
Strange	s	−1/3	+1/3	−1

Table 24.7 and Fig 24.12 show how these basic quarks are arranged in the most common baryons: protons and neutrons. The combination of fractional charges on the quarks explains why protons are positive and neutrons have no net charge.

Table 24.7 Quarks in protons and neutrons

	Proton	u	u	d	Neutron	u	d	d
Charge	+1	+2/3	+2/3	−1/3	0	+2/3	−1/3	−1/3
Baryon no.	+1	+1/3	+1/3	+1/3	+1	+1/3	+1/3	+1/3
Strangeness	0	0	0	0	0	0	0	0

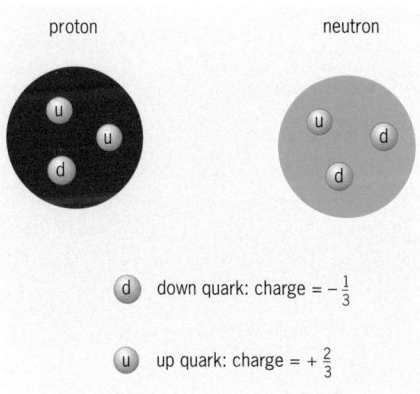

d down quark: charge = $-\frac{1}{3}$

u up quark: charge = $+\frac{2}{3}$

Fig 24.12 The quark structure of the proton and the neutron

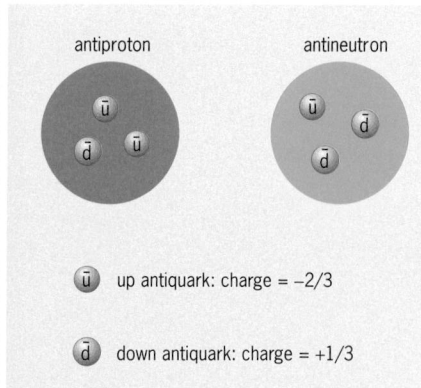

up antiquark: charge = –2/3

down antiquark: charge = +1/3

Fig 24.13 The quark structure of the antiproton and the antineutron

8 Use Table 24.9 to explain why:
a) the antiproton has negative charge and zero strangeness,
b) the lambda has zero charge and unit negative strangeness.

ANTIQUARKS

But of course, quarks must have **antiquarks**, and these were needed to explain the existence of mesons (the middleweight hadrons). Table 24.8 lists the three original antiquarks. In antiquarks, charge and strangeness have swapped over compared with the corresponding quarks. Fig 24.13 shows how antiquarks combine to produce the antiproton and the antineutron – and shows how a neutral particle can have an antiparticle version.

Table 24.8 The three basic antiquarks

Antiquark	Symbol	Charge/e	Baryon no.	Strangeness
Up	$\bar{u}$	–2/3	–1/3	0
Down	$\bar{d}$	+1/3	–1/3	0
Strange	$\bar{s}$	+1/3	–1/3	+1

QUARKS IN BARYONS

Table 24.9 lists the quark content of some baryons. Note that all baryons are made of quarks and all antibaryons are made of antiquarks. The baryon number of a quark is +1/3 and of the antiquark –1/3, which explains why the baryon numbers are either +1 or –1 for these particles.

Table 24.9 Quarks in some baryons

Particle	Proton	Antiproton	Neutron	Antineutron	Lambda	Antilambda
Quarks	uud	$\bar{u}\bar{u}\bar{d}$	udd	$\bar{u}\bar{d}\bar{d}$	uds	$\bar{u}\bar{d}\bar{s}$
Charge	+1	–1	0	0	0	0
Strangeness	0	0	0	0	–1	+1

QUARKS AND ANTIQUARKS MAKE MESONS

The significant difference between mesons and baryons (both are types of hadrons) is that mesons have baryon number 0. This is because mesons are made up of a quark and an antiquark, whose baryon contribution always cancels out. Table 24.10 lists the quark content of some mesons and their antiparticles.

Table 24.10 The quarks in some mesons

Meson	π^+	π^-	π^0	K^+	K^-	K^0	$\overline{K^0}$ antikaon	φ phi
Quarks	$u\bar{d}$	$\bar{u}d$	$u\bar{u}$	$u\bar{s}$	$\bar{u}s$	$d\bar{s}$	$\bar{d}s$	$s\bar{s}$

Table 24.10 clearly shows that the π^- is the antiparticle of the π^+: what was a quark in the particle has become an antiquark in the antiparticle, and vice versa. It also shows that some particles are their own antiparticles – changing an *up quark* for the *up antiquark* and vice versa makes no difference to the π^0.

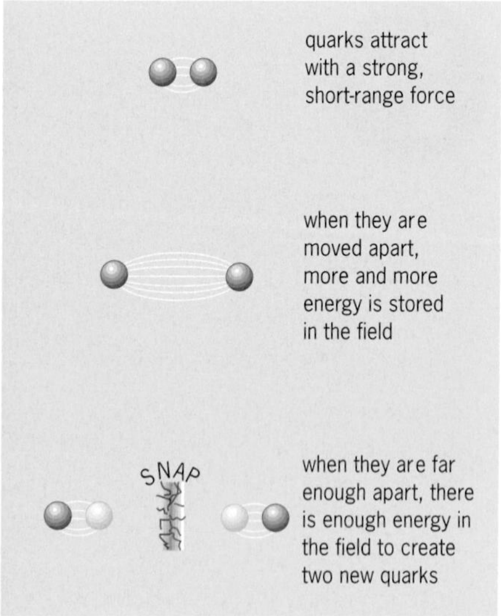

WHY SINGLE QUARKS DON'T EXIST

Quarks are 'invisible': they never appear on their own. Whenever there is enough energy to pull apart a pair of quarks in a pion, the energy is always enough to *create two more quarks*, which combine to form another pion (Fig 24.14). So all we see – and all we get – are pions.

quarks attract with a strong, short-range force

when they are moved apart, more and more energy is stored in the field

SNAP

when they are far enough apart, there is enough energy in the field to create two new quarks

Fig 24.14 Why single quarks never actually appear

AND ANOTHER THING ... *COLOUR*

Some combinations of quarks might seem possible – but have never been found to exist. To explain this yet another property has been given to the hard-working quark: **colour** (or **colour charge**). The rule is that only colourless (or white) combinations can exist. Just as white light can be created by mixing red, green and blue (the primary colours) so baryons can be made with only a combination of three quarks that produce a colourless result. So a proton has a *blue up*, a *red up* and a *green down* quark. A quark can carry any colour, so that an up quark can be red, blue or green. Fig 24.15(a) shows quark colour combinations for the proton and the neutron.

But how can a two-quark object like a meson manage to become colourless? Think about white light combinations: these can be made using secondary colours, e.g. yellow. Yellow is red plus green (or white minus blue). Yellow is often called 'minus blue'. So antiquarks are needed – each carrying a 'secondary' colour, here called antiblue, antired or antigreen. Mesons are made from a quark and an antiquark, so that for example a π^0 meson can exist with a *blue up* quark and an *antiblue up* antiquark (Fig 24.16).

Antibaryons contain only antiquarks with anticolours, see Fig 24.15(b).

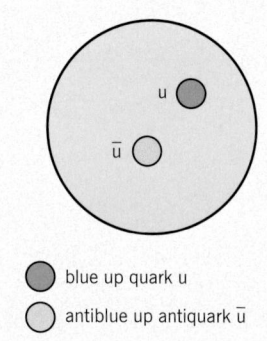

Fig 24.16 A π^0 meson has two quarks, shown here as blue and antiblue (yellow)

MORE QUARKS

The three quark–antiquark pairs listed in Tables 24.6 and 24.8 are insufficient to describe the structure of all the known hadrons. Table 24.11 is an up-to-date list of quarks and the 'flavours' that they have. How they were predicted and discovered is explained next.

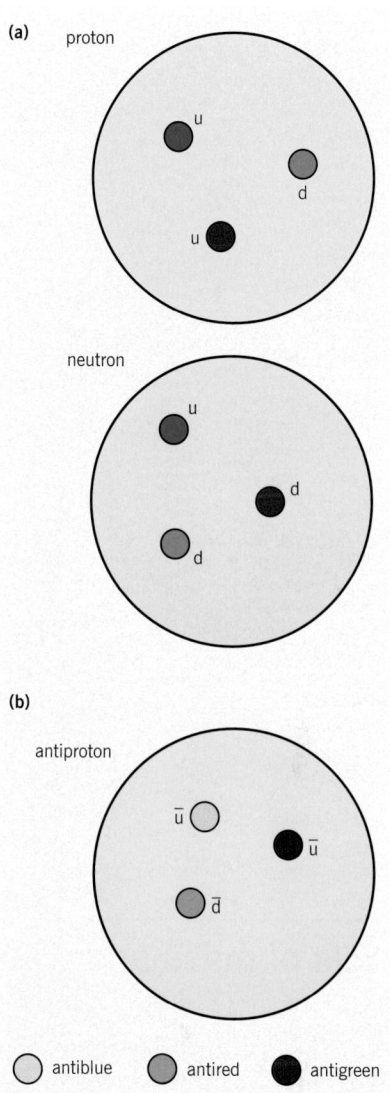

Fig 24.15(a) Colourless baryons: blue + red + green = white; and **(b)** a colourless antibaryon: antiblue + antired + antigreen = white

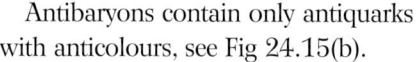

Table 24.11 All the quarks and their numbers

Name	Symbol	Charge	Baryon no.	Flavour			
				Strangeness	Charm	Topness	Bottomness
Quarks							
up	u	+2/3	+1/3	0	0	0	0
down	d	−1/3	+1/3	0	0	0	0
strange	s	−1/3	+1/3	−1	0	0	0
top	t	+2/3	+1/3	0	0	+1	0
bottom	b	−1/3	+1/3	0	0	0	+1
charm	c	+2/3	+1/3	0	+1	0	0
Antiquarks							
up	$\bar{u}$	−2/3	−1/3	0	0	0	0
down	$\bar{d}$	+1/3	−1/3	0	0	0	0
strange	$\bar{s}$	+1/3	−1/3	+1	0	0	0
top	$\bar{t}$	−2/3	−1/3	0	0	−1	0
bottom	$\bar{b}$	+1/3	−1/3	0	0	0	−1
charm	$\bar{c}$	−2/3	−1/3	0	−1	0	0

? QUESTION 9

9 Find the quark structure of the following hadrons, using Table 24.11 and the following data for the particles:

Particle	Charge	Baryon no.	Strangeness
Antiproton	−1	−1	0
Sigma minus	−1	+1	−1
Xi minus	−1	+1	−2
Kaon minus	−1	0	−1

6 THE REALLY FUNDAMENTAL PATTERN (POSSIBLY)

After accepting the quark model in the late 1960s, physicists noticed a new kind of symmetry – this time between *leptons* and quarks. Leptons contain no quarks (they are indivisible), and everything else does, so it makes sense to think of leptons and quarks as the basic, *really* fundamental building blocks of matter. Table 24.12 shows the pattern of leptons and quarks known by 1974 (omitting antiparticles).

Table 24.12 Lepton and quark families known about in 1974

Leptons			Quarks		
$Q = -1$	e^-	μ^-	u	?	$Q = +2/3$
$Q = 0$	ν_e	ν_μ	d	s	$Q = -1/3$

The pattern suggested that a quark should exist in the gap above the strange (s) quark. It was expected to have a charge of +2/3, and theory predicted that hadrons containing this quark should have masses of about 3 GeV/c^2. (See the Stretch and Challenge passage below for how mass and energy are interchangeable in particle physics.) Late in 1974, two laboratories announced the discovery of two new heavy hadrons, the J and psi (Ψ) particles. They turned out to be the *same* particle, with a mass of 3.1 GeV/c^2. Confusingly but appropriately, it is called the J/Ψ.

STRETCH AND CHALLENGE

Units of mass and energy in particle physics

Obeying the laws of relativity, the mass of a particle varies with its speed. This means that we have to use the value of its mass when it is not moving, its **rest mass** (see page 462). The principle of relativity also requires that mass and energy are equivalent, linked by the Einstein formula $E = mc^2$. In fact, particle physicists *measure mass in energy units*.

Investigations usually involve charged particles which are accelerated by high voltages and gain mass–energy as they accelerate. It is convenient for particle physicists to *measure energy and therefore mass in terms of an electrical unit*, namely the **electronvolt**, eV.

One electronvolt, 1 eV, is the energy gained by a particle carrying the electronic charge $e = 1.6 \times 10^{-19}$ C when it moves through a potential difference of 1 V.

$$1 \text{ eV} = 1.6 \times 10^{-19} \text{ C} \times 1 \text{ J C}^{-1}$$
$$= 1.6 \times 10^{-19} \text{ J}$$
and: $$1 \text{ J} = 6.25 \times 10^{18} \text{ eV}$$

The mass of a proton is 1.6726×10^{-27} kg. In energy units, this is equivalent to:

$$E_p = m_p c^2 = 1.6726 \times 10^{-27} \times (3 \times 10^8)^2 \text{ J}$$
$$= 1.5053 \times 10^{-10} \text{ J}$$

REST MASS IN GeV/c^2

The mass–energy of a proton is about 10^9 eV, or 1 GeV, a nice easy number to work with.

We need to be careful with this unfamiliar set of units. For example, from the Einstein formula we have:

$$m = E/c^2$$

so we can put

$$m = \frac{\text{energy in eV}}{(\text{light speed})^2} = \frac{\text{GeV}}{c^2}$$

Thus the rest mass of a proton m_p is written as 1, with units GeV/c^2, or:

$$m_p = 1 \text{ GeV}/c^2 = 1 \text{ GeV } c^{-2}$$

The masses listed in the tables in this chapter are given in units of GeV/c^2. Examples of calculations based on this unit are given on pages 503 and 504.

? QUESTION 10

10 Show that the energy equivalent of the mass of a proton is about 1 GeV.

CHARM ENTERS PHYSICS

Physicists then realised that the new particle was a heavy meson containing the predicted missing quark, carrying yet another conserved quantity called **charm**. The J/Ψ consists of two *charmed quarks*, one the antiquark of the other (c$\overline{c}$).

The new J/Ψ particle was predicted, but in the search for it, evidence was found for a particle that was not predicted at all. This was a *new lepton* – but an amazingly massive one, twice as heavy as a proton. This *third* kind of lepton was named the **tau**, τ.

This discovery ruined the existing pattern between leptons and quarks and if the lepton–quark pattern was to be preserved it meant that yet another pair of quarks should exist (see Table 24.13).

Quarks are never found alone, they have to be found indirectly – by finding particles with properties and interactions that could only exist if they carry the properties of their component quarks. Physicists named the new quarks **top** and **bottom** from their positions in the table, and had to invent two new conserved quantities, **topness** and **bottomness**.

Top and bottom quarks were predicted to be much more massive than other quarks (Fig 24.17), and so should produce equally massive combinations. Such particles need a great deal of energy to be created, and the new proton synchrotron opened in 1975 at Columbia University (New York State) with an energy of 30 GeV very soon found a new massive particle that was a combination of a bottom quark and an antibottom quark. This b meson was named the **upsilon**, Y. It has a mass of 9.5 GeV/c^2.

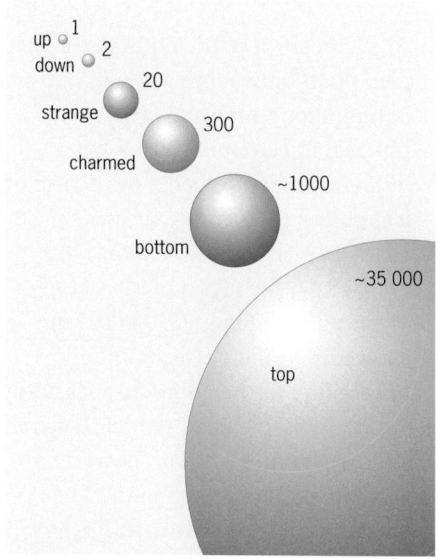

Fig 24.17 Quarks come in different sizes. The top quark is 35 000 times as massive as the up quark. Top quarks are hard to make

Table 24.13 Lepton and quark families known about in 1975

Leptons				Quarks			
$Q = -1$	e$^-$	μ$^-$	τ	u	c	top?	$Q = +2/3$
$Q = 0$	ν$_e$	ν$_\mu$	ν$_\tau$	d	s	bottom?	$Q = -1/3$

THE SEARCH FOR THE TOP QUARK

The missing piece of the jigsaw was the top quark. It was predicted to have a mass of more than 90 GeV/c^2, twenty times as massive as a bottom quark. A particle containing a top quark would have a mass greater than this.

The energy needed to produce such a massive particle is available when *protons* are made to collide with *antiprotons* in powerful synchrotrons. This was possible in the newly built 1800 GeV Tevatron collider at Fermilab (Chicago, USA), and in April 1994 evidence for the existence of the top quark was announced. Experiments in March 1995 matched a mass of about 175 GeV/c^2 for the top quark.

7 THE AMAZING IMPLICATIONS OF UNCERTAINTY

The uncertainty principle (see Stretch and Challenge box overleaf) has some amazing consequences for particle physics. It implies that a quantum of energy can exist for a very short time, *provided that the product of energy and time is less than the value of the Planck constant*, that is, if $\Delta E \Delta t < h/4\pi$.

This also applies to matter, since energy and matter are equivalent. So particles could also exist for very small times. These particles, called **virtual particles**, can be produced without breaking the law of conservation of mass–energy.

The significance of this feature of the uncertainty principle is seen as fundamental to a description of the nature of matter, as it exists now and in the early stages of the Universe. See the Stretch and Challenge box for more about this.

> ### ? QUESTION 11
>
> 11 An electron has a mass–energy of 8.2×10^{-14} J. For how long, in principle, could such a particle exist without the Universe noticing? ($h = 6.6 \times 10^{-34}$ J s)

The uncertainty principle

At the heart of particle physics is the idea of an uncertainty throughout nature, though not the everyday physical uncertainty caused by imprecise measurements or the use of techniques that cannot measure every factor in a complex situation.

In 1927, the German physicist Werner Heisenberg (1901–1976) showed that there was an inbuilt uncertainty in the ability to measure the state of any small particle, such as an electron or a photon, however accurate the instrumentation. His **uncertainty principle** has since been developed beyond the simple problem of measurement into a statement about the fundamental nature of the Universe.

Heisenberg imagined an experiment to measure the momentum and position of, say, an electron (Fig 24.18). One way of doing this would be to use an 'imaginary microscope' that could see the electron. This could only happen if a photon hit the electron and bounced back into the eyepiece. But the photon carries momentum and by its interaction with the electron would exchange some (unknown) fraction of its momentum, so that the electron would no longer have its original momentum.

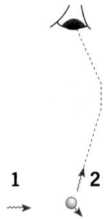

Fig 24.18 Heisenberg's imaginary experiment. You try to 'see' an electron using a photon microscope. But the photon has momentum and the collision moves the electron, changing its position and momentum. Thus, we cannot be certain of its 'observed' velocity or position

You could try to make this uncertainty in the momentum very small by using a photon of very small momentum. But a photon is also a wave that extends over space, having a characteristic wavelength λ. The position of the electron would not be determined to an accuracy better than the value of λ, and the smaller its momentum the larger is the wavelength of the photon. This means that by using a low-momentum (low-energy) photon we improve our knowledge of the electron's *momentum*, but lose accuracy in determining its *position* (Fig 24.19).

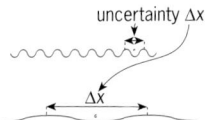

uncertainty Δx — high-momentum photon has high energy and small wavelength

Δx — low-momentum photon has large wavelength

Fig 24.19 Momentum–position and wavelength

The incoming photon has momentum h/λ, where λ is its wavelength and h is the Planck constant, value 6.6×10^{-34} J s (see page 309). The photon *could* transfer all this momentum to the electron. Thus the collision has produced an uncertainty in the electron's *momentum* of:

$$\Delta p = h/\lambda$$

As explained above, the uncertainty Δx in the *position* of the electron is of the order of the light wavelength, so we can put $\Delta x = \lambda$.

Multiplying both these uncertainties gives:

$$\Delta p \Delta x = \left(\frac{h}{\lambda}\right)\lambda = h$$

This represents the best possible accuracy. In practice, we must accept that the uncertainty is always greater, so we write:

$$\Delta p \Delta x \geq h \qquad [1]$$

The momentum–position formula

This is Heisenberg's simple treatment of the uncertainty principle. A fuller derivation gives

$$\Delta p \Delta x \geq h/4\pi$$

The uncertainty is *not* due to any method of measurement, but is in the nature of the moving object, whether a photon, an electron, a spaceship or anything else.

Uncertainty in energy and time

There is also an uncertainty in the *energy* of a photon or an electron; both have a wave and a particle aspect. The energy E of a photon of frequency f, for example, is given by $E = hf$.

Now think about trying to measure this energy by measuring the frequency. Suppose our frequency measurer is able to identify one wave (as above) and so measure to an accuracy of 1 Hz, and we try to measure the frequency of a 1000 Hz wave.

In 1 second we can say
$$f = (1000 \pm 1) \text{ Hz}$$
The uncertainty in the result is $\Delta f = 1$.

We can do better by taking a reading for a longer time, say 20 s, so that we measure 20 000 wavelengths.

Then the result could be put as
$$(20\,000 \pm 1)/20$$
This gives an uncertainty $\Delta f = 1/20$.

So for $\Delta t = 1$, $\Delta f = 1$.
For $\Delta t = 20$, $\Delta f = 1/20$.

In both cases: $\Delta f \Delta t = 1$ [2]

This is true, however accurate the measurement.

Now, both photons and particles are wavelike, with energy and frequency linked by $E = hf$. So we can write:

$$\Delta f = \Delta E/h$$

and from equation 2:

$$\Delta f \Delta t = \Delta E \Delta t/h = 1$$

giving: $\Delta E \Delta t = h$

Again, this is the best possible result, so in general we have an *uncertainty principle* involving energy and time that says:

$$\Delta E \Delta t \geq h \qquad [3]$$

The energy–time formula

Again, a more accurate relationship is

$$\Delta E \Delta t \geq h/4\pi$$

This means that if we wish to measure energy accurately we must take a long time to do the measuring.

8 WHAT HOLDS IT ALL TOGETHER? – FORCES AND EXCHANGE PARTICLES

Newton was worried by his theory of gravity. He thought it unscientific because the force of gravity was having to act through *empty* space, so there was nothing to transmit the force. This worry was ignored for centuries, but it is just as valid for the electric forces that travel through a vacuum as for gravity. Even on the small scale of the nucleus there seemed to be 'nothing' in between the nucleons that could carry the strong nuclear force. Modern physics recognises Newton's problem, and solves it by saying that the forces between particles are carried by *other particles*.

These are the **exchange particles** or **bosons**. Table 24.14 below lists the bosons needed to explain the four fundamental interactions.

FORCES AND INTERACTIONS

Forces always exist as pairs: when two particles exert any kind of force on each other, the force on one is the same as the force on the other, each acting in the opposite direction. This effect is called interaction between the particles. We commonly refer to the four *fundamental* interactions: electromagnetic, weak, strong and gravitational. As we shall see, when particles interact, there is always another particle that 'carries the force' – it 'mediates the interaction'. The mediating force-carrying particles known as exchange particles are in a group called **gauge bosons** – see Table 24.14. It is the possibility of virtual particles (see page 487) that underlies the idea of gauge bosons as particles that 'mediate the interaction' between particles.

Modern theory suggests that at very high energies all these forces merge into just one. There is experimental evidence that at very high energies the electromagnetic and weak forces are unified – they become the electroweak force.

Table 24.14 Gauge bosons

Interaction	Particle	Relative strength
Strong	gluon (g)	1
Electromagnetic	photon (γ)	10^{-2}
Weak	W, Z bosons	10^{-7}
Gravity	graviton (not yet found)	10^{-36}

TIME SCALES OF INTERACTIONS

Each interaction has a characteristic time scale (which is quoted as a half-life, see page 476). The stronger the force, the quicker things happen, so when two hadrons interact due to the strong force, events happen on a time scale shorter than about 10^{-10} s. This also applies to a hadron's internal change (an 'interaction' involving one particle), which we observe as a spontaneous decay.

In the weak interaction, things happen slowly. Normal weak interactions produce decays in about a millionth of a second – very slow by particle interaction standards. For example, a pi meson might decay in about 10^{-8} s by converting its two quarks into a muon and a neutrino (see Fig 24.27, page 492) via the weak interaction (mediated by a W boson).

The time scale of an interaction or change can be measured in detectors. The time gives valuable clues about the event involved, and hence the type of particle produced, even though it is not 'seen' by the detector.

PHOTONS

The most familiar boson is the **photon**, which carries the electromagnetic force (interaction) between charged particles.

Fig 24.24 in the Stretch and Challenge box is a diagram of an electron repelling another electron via the exchange of a **virtual photon**. This diagram is not realistic: it is a **Feynman diagram**, summarising a continuous and complicated process. Read the text in the box for help in interpreting the diagram.

In the gauge boson model of charged particles interacting, each particle is surrounded by a cloud of virtual photons. When one particle nears another, they exchange virtual photons. Since photons carry momentum there is an associated momentum exchange that we observe as a force causing a change in the velocity of both particles. The force mediated by photons can pull as well as push. At this level the concept of force is not very useful in fact; it is better to work purely in terms of momentum changes.

Imagine two electrons approaching each other. They exert a repulsive force on each other and do this by exchanging carriers of the electromagnetic force – photons. The closer they get to each other the more particles are exchanged, like eighteenth-century warships exchanging cannon balls. The photons are of course **virtual particles** which are never actually observed, something perfectly acceptable according to the uncertainty principle. Despite this, they carry momentum between the electrons which are both turned from their paths, conserving momentum in an elastic 'collision'.

W AND Z PARTICLES

The *weak* interaction can be mediated by one of two sorts of W particle, or a Z particle. W particles carry either positive or negative charge but Z particles carry no charge. A W particle changes either a quark or a lepton – see the Stretch and Challenge box for more details.

The carriers of the weak force have been detected outside a nucleus. Unlike photons, they have mass, of about 90 GeV/c^2.

GLUONS

When **quarks** interact inside a proton the force carrier is the **gluon**. The force is a short-range force of attraction – the strong nuclear force. Imagine the quarks moving around inside the small space – which has no 'boundary wall' – like angry ferrets in a sack kept together by mutual aggression! The gluon exchanges 'colour force' (see page 485) just as the photon exchanges electromagnetic force. The interaction changes the colours of the quarks as illustrated in the Feynman diagram of Fig 24.23. Gluons do not carry electric charge and are massless. They can change the colour of a quark but not its flavour (i.e. upness, downness, strangeness, etc.). The forces holding nucleons inside a nucleus are the result of gluons leaking temporarily, for quantum reasons, between one quark system (a proton, say) and another.

Bear in mind that gluons always *pull*, whilst photons can both pull and push.

STRETCH
AND CHALLENGE

Spin

An important property of photons, bosons, nuclei and nuclear particles is a characteristic called **spin**, an abbreviation for spin angular momentum. We imagine the particle rotating about its axis, as the Earth spins about the line joining its poles. But in quantum physics spin is quantised, and must have values such as 0, $\frac{1}{2}$, 1, $\frac{3}{2}$ etc, in units of $\hbar$.

The spin of a photon is linked with polarisation in the wave model. A photon has unit spin. The spinning of electrons and atomic nuclei gives rise to their magnetism. Electrons have spin $\frac{1}{2}$. For hadrons (baryons like protons, and mesons), the spin is the sum of the spins of the particles of which they are made: quarks. All quarks have half-integer spin: $\frac{1}{2}$. This means that ordinary baryons with three quarks have spin $\frac{3}{2}$, while mesons with two quarks have spin 1.

Interactions, decays and Feynman diagrams

Feynman diagrams model what is believed to happen when particles interact with each other and/or decay. They are named after Richard Feynman, who devised the diagrams to help illustrate such exchange processes. The diagram is not a picture of what happens; it just reminds us of the particles involved, and is used to keep track of particles and changes in complex interactions. It needs a very complex wave-quantum calculation to describe an interaction between particles completely.

READING A FEYNMAN DIAGRAM

The vertex

The vertex is where things happen. In Fig 24.20(a) a down quark changes into an up quark and emits an exchange particle. This has to carry away negative charge and is a W⁻ boson. Time goes from left to right. Particles are shown as straight lines with *time arrows* which meet at the vertex, and the particle symbol is at the free end of the line. The electromagnetic and weak bosons (photons, W and Z) are shown by a wavy line. There is no need for an arrow as they slope to show them moving forward in time.

Next the exchange particle creates a vertex. The virtual (W⁻) particle materialises into a pair of leptons: a **particle** (e⁻) and an **antiparticle** (an electron neutrino). See Fig 24.20(b). But the neutrino

has an arrow pointing back against the direction of time! This is because of the lepton conservation rule. A single lepton can't come from nowhere. The change at the vertex has to maintain a lepton number of zero. What comes out must go in. The convention therefore is that an antiparticle is always shown entering a vertex *against* the direction of time. It is thought of as a *particle going forward in time*. It really does work!

Combining vertices into Feynman diagrams

The full beta decay of a neutron is shown in Fig 24.21.

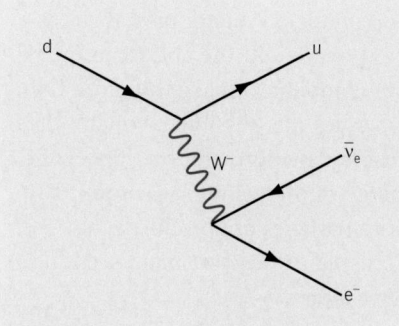

Fig 24.21 Beta decay of a neutron. A neutron becomes a proton when one of its d quarks becomes a u quark. The exchange particle W⁻ becomes a lepton pair. The neutron has turned into a proton. Compare with Figs 24.20(a) and (b)

Fig 24.22 shows the two vertices for positive muon decay. Positive muons are antiparticles of the ordinary negative muon. A positron and two neutrinos are emitted, with a W⁺ as the exchange particle.

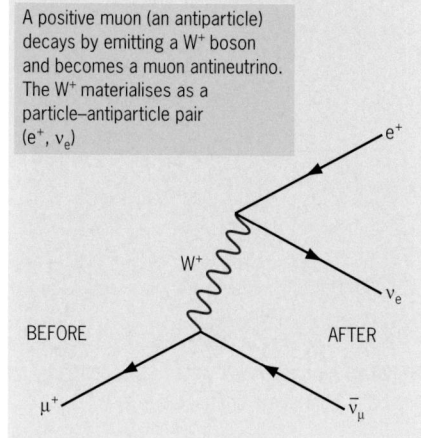

Fig 24.22 The decay of an antilepton. A positive muon decays via the W⁺ boson

Figs 24.23 and 24.24 show, respectively, exchange particles keeping quarks together and electrons apart. Gluons and photons are both massless, chargeless particles, and here simply exchange forces.

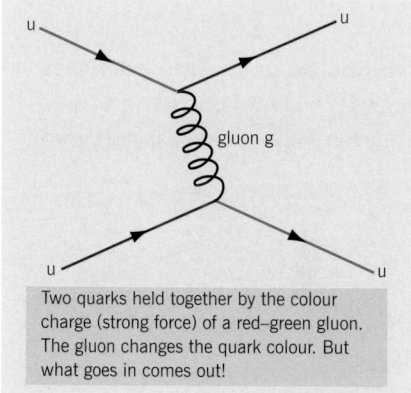

Fig 24.23 (Virtual) gluons keep quarks together. They do this by changing quark colour via the 'colour force'

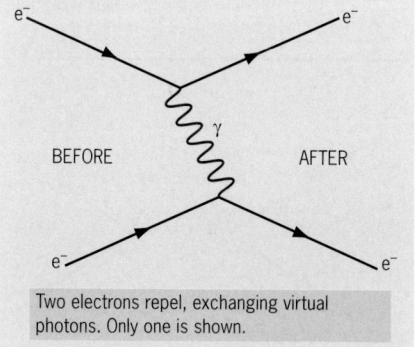

Fig 24.24 (Virtual) photons repel electrons when they get close

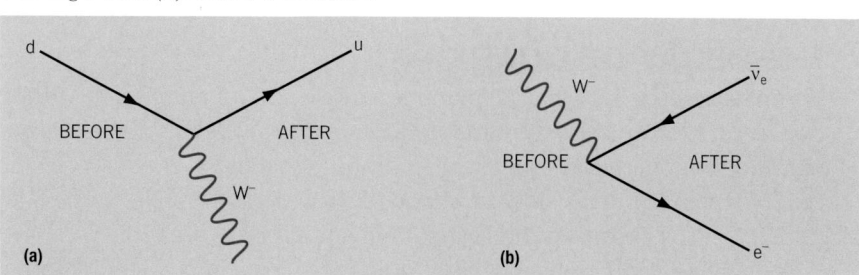

Fig 24.20 (a) A d quark changes to a u quark. This is what happens in neutron (or beta) decay **(b)** The W⁻ particle of (a) becomes a lepton–antilepton pair, conserving charge and lepton number – if the antineutrino is allowed to go backwards in time. This is what happens next in beta decay

491

Interactions, decays and Feynman diagrams (Cont.)

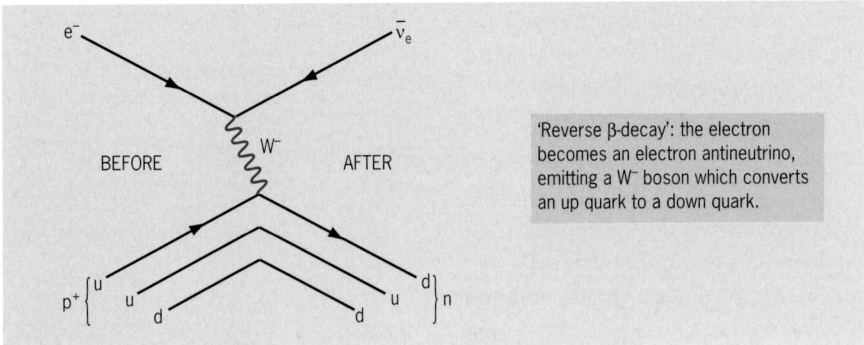

'Reverse β-decay': the electron becomes an electron antineutrino, emitting a W⁻ boson which converts an up quark to a down quark.

Fig 24.25 A proton is converted to a neutron by a change at the quark level (u → d). The other quarks are unaffected

In high-energy collisions between particles an electron can collide with a proton and 'reverse beta decay' to form a neutron. This is shown in Fig 24.25. An up quark in the proton changes to a down quark accepting the negative charge brought by the electron, mediated by the W⁻ boson. The antineutrino is there to balance the lepton books.

Gluons as exchange particles

Fig 24.26 shows one result of a collision between high-speed protons

producing a positive pion. There is enough energy to tear a gluon from a quark, which in turn carries enough energy to produce two more quarks. These have the same flavour but must be a quark–antiquark pair. But it is the u quark and the antidown quark that combine to make the pion. Other outcomes are possible involving the weak interaction, and the higher the energy of the colliding protons the more particles are produced, as discussed in the next main section of this chapter.

Virtual particles are unseen

Many new particles are produced by the collision of high-energy electrons and positrons in ring accelerators. Their production always involves the production of one or more virtual particles whose temporary and unseen existence can be inferred from the results, using Feynman diagrams which tend to be pretty complex!

To summarise

- Feynman diagrams are combinations of vertices at which things happen.
- They are to be read from left to right – the direction of time.
- Particles are shown by straight lines.
- Exchange particles (bosons) link vertices, and are shown by wiggly lines, without arrows.
- W particles are lepton-changing or quark-changing particles.
- Arrows show movement in time.
- Antiparticles are represented by arrows going backwards in time.

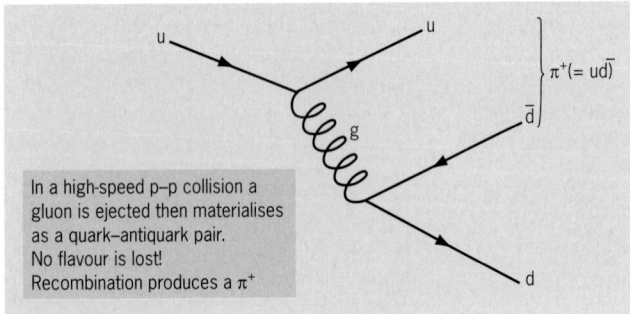

In a high-speed p–p collision a gluon is ejected then materialises as a quark–antiquark pair. No flavour is lost! Recombination produces a π⁺

Fig 24.26 One outcome of a high-energy proton–proton collision

? QUESTION 12

12 A positron–electron pair can interact to produce a pair of muons.
  a) Write down a particle equation, bearing in mind that charge must be conserved. (There are two possible answers.)
  b) Draw a Feynman diagram for the reaction, assuming that the reaction is mediated by a virtual Z boson.

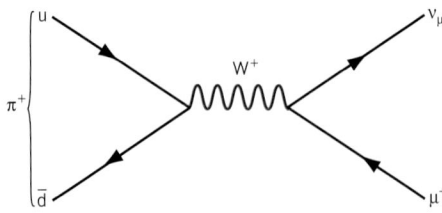

Fig 24.27 Pion decay. The quark–antiquark pair in the pion annihilate to form a W⁺ boson. This then changes to a lepton–antilepton pair. Is baryon number conserved?

THE DECAY OF QUARKS

Mesons are short lived: they contain a particle and an antiparticle. When a pion decays it forms a muon and a muon neutrino. Neither muons nor neutrinos contain quarks – they are leptons. 'Quarkness' is conserved, since a pion contains a quark and an antiquark. The decay is mediated by a W⁺ particle. This is shown in the Feynman diagram of Fig 24.27.

As explained in the previous Stretch and Challenge box, neutron decay (ordinary radioactive beta decay) is also the consequence of a quark decay. This is through the weak interaction, so needs the mediation of a W particle, in this case a W⁻. This is shown in Fig 24.21. A down quark has changed to an up quark. Again 'quarkness' is conserved, and so is baryon number.

QUARKS AND LEPTONS IN THE STANDARD MODEL

Matter is made up of just two kinds of particle: quarks and leptons. Table 24.15 shows the particles forming a pattern, displayed in three generations. Antiparticles have been omitted. It summarises currently accepted ideas and discoveries, although there is no accepted theory that can explain *why* the particles exist or predict their characteristics in detail.

Table 24.15 The three generations of the Standard Model

	Charge in units of electron charge	First generation	Second generation	Third generation
Quarks	+2/3	up (u)	charm (c)	top (t)
	−1/3	down (d)	strange (s)	bottom (b)
Leptons	0	electron neutrino (v_e)	muon neutrino (v_μ)	tau neutrino (v_τ)
	−1	electron (e^-)	negative muon (μ^-)	negative tau (τ^-)

A SUMMARY OF THE PARTICLES

This is given in Table 24.16.

Table 24.16 A summary of the particles

CLASS	Name and symbol		Particles Q	B	S	Quark content	Antiparticles Q	B	S	Quark content	Mass (GeV/c^2)	Half-life/s	Discovered, source
HADRONS — Baryons	proton	p	+1	+1	0	uud	−1	−1	0	$\bar{u}\bar{u}\bar{d}$	0.983	stable	1911–19 alpha scattering
	neutron	n	0	+1	0	udd	0	−1	0	$\bar{u}\bar{d}\bar{d}$	0.940	900	1932 alpha bombardment of beryllium
	lambda	Λ	0	+1	−1	uds	0	−1	+1	$\bar{u}\bar{d}\bar{s}$	1.115	2.6×10^{-10}	1951 cosmic rays
	sigma plus	Σ^+	+1	+1	−1	uus	−1	−1	+1	$\bar{u}\bar{u}\bar{s}$	1.189	0.8×10^{-10}	1953 cosmic rays
	sigma minus	Σ^-	−1	+1	−1	dds	+1	−1	+1	$\bar{d}\bar{d}\bar{s}$	1.197	1.5×10^{-10}	1953 accelerator
	sigma zero	Σ^0	0	+1	−1	uds	0	−1	+1	$\bar{u}\bar{d}\bar{s}$	1.192	6×10^{-20}	1956 accelerator
	xi minus	Ξ^-	−1	+1	−2	dss	+1	−1	+2	$\bar{d}\bar{s}\bar{s}$	1.321	1.6×10^{-10}	1952 cosmic rays
	xi zero	Ξ^0	0	+1	−2	uss	0	−1	+2	$\bar{u}\bar{s}\bar{s}$	1.315	3×10^{-10}	1959 accelerator
	omega minus	Ω^-	−1	+1	−3	sss	+1	−1	+3	$\bar{s}\bar{s}\bar{s}$	1.672	0.8×10^{-10}	1964 accelerator
	charmed lambda	Λ_c	1	+1	0	udc	−1	−1	0	$\bar{u}\bar{d}\bar{c}$	2.28	2×10^{-13}	1975 accelerator
Mesons	pi zero	π^0	0	0	0	u$\bar{u}$ or d$\bar{d}$	0	0	0	$\bar{u}$u or d$\bar{d}$	0.135	0.8×10^{-16}	1949 accelerator
	pion	π^+, π^-	+1	0	0	u$\bar{d}$	−1	0	0	$\bar{u}$d	0.140	2.8×10^{-8}	1947 cosmic rays
	K zero	K^0	0	0	+1	d$\bar{s}$	0	0	−1	$\bar{d}$s	0.498	$5 \times 10^{-8}, 1 \times 10^{-10}$	1947 cosmic rays
	kaon	K^+, K^-	+1	0	+1	u$\bar{s}$	−1	0	−1	$\bar{u}$s	0.494	1.2×10^{-8}	1947 cosmic rays
	J/psi	J/Ψ	0	0	0	c$\bar{c}$	0	0	0	$\bar{c}$c	3.1	10^{-20}	1974 accelerator
	D zero	D^0	0	0	0	c$\bar{u}$	0	0	0	$\bar{c}$u	1.87	10^{-17}	1976 accelerator
	D plus	D^+	+1	0	0	c$\bar{d}$	0	0	0	$\bar{c}$d	1.87	4×10^{-13}	1976 accelerator
	upsilon	Y	0	0	0	b$\bar{b}$	0	0	0	$\bar{b}$b	9.46	10^{-20}	1977 accelerator
LEPTONS	electron, positron	e^-, e^+	−1	0	0	—	+1	0	0	—	0.00051	stable	e^-1897 cathode rays, e^+1932 cosmic rays
	muon	μ	−1	0	0	—	+1	0	0	—	0.1056	2×10^{-6}	1937 cosmic rays
	tauon	τ	−1	0	0	—	+1	0	0	—	1.784	3×10^{-13}	1975 accelerator
	electron neutrino	v_e	0	0	0	—	0	0	0	—	<50 eV?	stable ?	1956 nuclear reactor
	muon neutrino	v_μ	0	0	0	—	0	0	0	—	<0.5 MeV?	stable ?	1962 accelerator
	tau neutrino	v_τ	0	0	0	—	0	0	0	—	<70 MeV?	stable ?	not yet observed
GAUGE BOSONS	photon	γ	**Charge** 0								0	stable	1923 X-rays scattered from electrons in atoms
	W	W^+, W^-	+1, −1								83	10^{-25}	1983 proton–antiproton annihilation (CERN)
	Z	Z	0								93	10^{-25}	1983 proton–antiproton annihilation (CERN)
	gluon	g	0								0	stable	1979 electron–positron annihilation (DESY)
QUARKS	up	u	**Charge** +2/3				**Baryon number** +1/3				~0.005		1964 (theory). Observed 1968–72 electron scattering (Stanford), neutrino scattering (CERN)
	down	d	−1/3				+1/3				~0.01		
	strange	s	−1/3				+1/3				~0.1		
	charmed	c	+2/3				+1/3				~1.5		1974 inferred from existence of J/psi particle etc.
	bottom	b	−1/3				+1/3				~4.7		1977 inferred from discovery of upsilon particle
	top	t	+2/3				+1/3				~175		1994/95

Quarks and the weak interaction

To follow this section, you need to refer back to the quark content of particles given in Table 24.16.

When a reaction is mediated by the weak interaction, one type of quark is *always* changed into another. The weak interaction is the only interaction that can do this. In all other cases, new quarks may be formed, but are formed in quark–antiquark pairs so that the total quantity of 'quarkness' remains constant. This is another way of saying that baryon number is conserved: a quark has baryon number $+1/3$ and its antiquark baryon number is $-1/3$.

For example, in the following *strong* reaction:

$$p^- + p \rightarrow n + \pi^+ + \pi^- + \pi^0$$

the quarks on the left side are $(\bar{u}\bar{u}d)$ and (uud). On the right we have (udd), $(u\bar{d})$, $(\bar{u}d)$ and $(u\bar{u})$. The extra quarks on the right side are a $(u\bar{u})$ pair and a $(d\bar{d})$ pair. In other words, if we count a quark as $+1$ and an antiquark as -1, the total quarkness on the left (3) equals the sum on the right.

The best known *weak* reaction is neutron decay:

$$n \rightarrow p + e^- + \bar{\nu}_e$$

On the left the quarks are (udd). On the right only the proton contains quarks (uud). Quarkness (baryon number) is conserved, but a down quark has turned into an up quark. This seems a minor result, but consider the reaction:

$$K^+ \rightarrow \pi^0 + \pi^+$$

On the left, the K^+ has quarks $(u\bar{s})$. On the right, the π^0 can be either a $(u\bar{u})$ or a $(d\bar{d})$ and the π^+ is $(u\bar{d})$. Quarkwise, the π^0 is self-cancelling. But to make the π^+, a *strange* antiquark has become a *down* antiquark. *This is the reason why strangeness is conserved in strong reactions, but may not be conserved in weak reactions.*

Whenever a quark changes type in a reaction, we can point to the weak interaction as its cause. Check that the following decays are due to weak interactions:

$$\Omega^- \rightarrow \Xi^0 + \pi^-$$
$$\Omega^- \rightarrow \Lambda + K^-$$

? QUESTION 13

13 Check that the quark total in the following reaction is the same on both sides:
$$K^- + p \rightarrow \Sigma^- + \pi^+$$
Is strangeness conserved in this reaction?

? QUESTIONS 14–15

14 Sketch the directions of magnetic field, electron velocity and the resulting force on the electron, which together make it move in a circle in the magnetic field.

15 Give the basic physical reasons why
a) more massive particles,
b) less highly charged particles
move in curves of larger radii in a magnetic field.

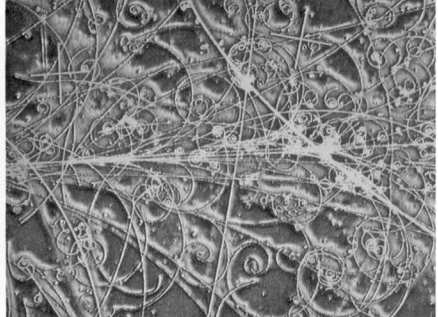

9 DETECTING SYSTEMS AND TECHNIQUES FOR FINDING SUBATOMIC PARTICLES

The most common techniques for finding the mass and charge of a particle of matter are based on the following: a charged particle moving at right angles to the direction of a magnetic field B experiences a force which acts perpendicularly to its direction of motion and the direction of the magnetic field. Remember that a force that acts at right angles to the direction of motion of a body makes it move in a circular path.

The radius r of the circle can be used to calculate the charge to mass ratio Q/m of the particle – provided its speed v is known:

$$Q/m = v/Br$$

Or

$r = p/BQ$, where p is the momentum of the particle.

Fig 24.28 shows the paths made by many particles as they move through a detecting device, in this case a **bubble chamber** (see opposite). The paths are curved, and particles carrying opposite charge curve in opposite directions – one clockwise, the other anticlockwise.

Nowadays, in large physics laboratories, interpreting the images is done by computers. The tracks of the particles are detected electrically and the data fed directly into the computer. No human eye actually sees the particle tracks, let alone the particles.

Fig 24.28 Bubble chamber photo with tracks of numerous particles, curving when the particles are charged

EARLY PARTICLE DETECTORS

The cloud chamber was one of the earliest detectors. You may have one at school or college. Another cheap detector is the simple **photographic plate**. These were used a great deal in the 1940s and 1950s to investigate the cheapest source of unusual or fast-moving particles – cosmic rays.

The **Geiger–Müller detector** is described on page 324. An array of GM detectors can track the path of a particle in three dimensions, and the same principle is used in the most modern detector system, the **multiwire array** described below.

MODERN PARTICLE DETECTORS

The bubble chamber

A bubble chamber (look at Fig 24.4(a) on page 475), the main tool for particle studies in the 1950s and 1960s, is a tank filled with 'superheated' liquid hydrogen. The liquid hydrogen is under pressure to keep it just on the point of boiling without actually doing so. When the pressure is slightly reduced, bubbles may form – think of opening a can of fizzy drink.

But the bubbles need something to trigger them, just like the water drops in a cloud chamber. Any particle moving through the liquid creates ions, around which tiny bubbles form and show the particle's path. The tank is in a strong magnetic field, so the charged particles follow curved paths. Fig 24.28 shows some paths of particles in a bubble chamber.

The drawback of the bubble chamber is that it only produces a bubble track when the pressure on the liquid is slightly reduced. This has to be timed just *before* the particle enters it – and as its arrival is unpredictable, it is easy to miss a particle of interest. Then, the pressure has to be increased to restore the bubble chamber to a bubble-free state. The cycle takes about a second, which is a slow process by modern standards.

The spark chamber

Spark detectors were designed to avoid the problem of the random picture-taking and long recycling time of bubble chambers. The detectors are arranged as a set of thin metal plates spaced closely together in an inert gas, forming a **spark chamber**, as in Fig 24.29. When a charged particle passes through, the gas along its track is ionised.

On each side are separate Geiger–Müller tubes which check that a particle of interest has passed into the spark chamber. If so, they immediately trigger a high voltage between the plates. The ions of the particle track are still there and they 'cascade' to produce a spark. At the same time, a camera shutter opens to photograph the spark track. The sparking clears the ions away very quickly when the voltage is switched off, so that the chamber is ready again in a fraction of a second.

Multiwire chambers

Multiwire chambers and **drift chambers** are a development of the spark chamber in which the plates are replaced by an array of many thin wires. A particle's trail is revealed by a pulse of the ions it produces moving on to the nearest charged wire. The wires are very close together and are connected separately to a computer recording system. They act like very many Geiger–Müller detectors in one large tube. In a drift chamber (Fig 24.30) the ions drift onto them under the action of an electric field produced by the other wires in the array. The drift speed of the ions is known, and a computer calculates the origin of the ions from the time they take to drift to the sensor.

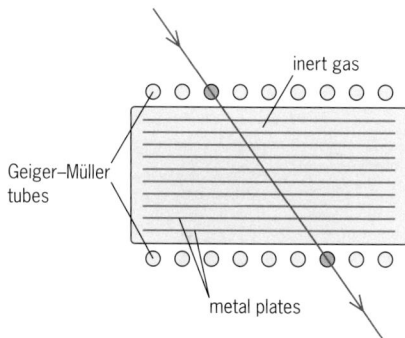

Fig 24.29 A spark chamber. The GM tubes act as 'coincidence' detectors. A particle has to pass through one in each row to trigger the operation of the spark chamber

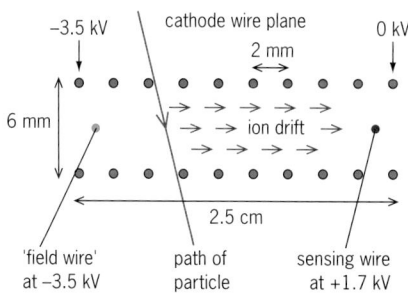

Fig 24.30 One of the many sensing elements in a drift chamber. The varying voltages on the cathode wires cause ions to drift towards the sensing wire at a steady speed. The arrival of a particle triggers a timing circuit and the times taken for ions to arrive at the sensing wires are used to calculate its track

Total detection systems

Total detection systems were developed and used in the **Large Electron–Positron (LEP)** collider, which was running at CERN (European Centre for Nuclear Research, Geneva) from 1989 until November 2000. It is being replaced by the **Large Hadron Collider (LHC),** which is due to begin work in 2008. This much larger system investigates collisions between more massive particles, and works on the same principles as the LEP, but instead of using electrons, a stream of protons moving in one direction collides with another stream moving in the opposite direction.

A series of detectors (Fig 24.31) is arranged around the chamber where particle collisions take place, and the signals produced by a very large number of collision events are processed by very sophisticated computer programming to yield information about the particles made in the collisions. The system produces a picture of the paths that the particles take and measures the energy they carry. It also compares the results with data from known particles held in memory and so can quickly identify novel events and products. It is expected that there will be one event of interest for every 10 million background events. See below for more detail about the LHC and its work.

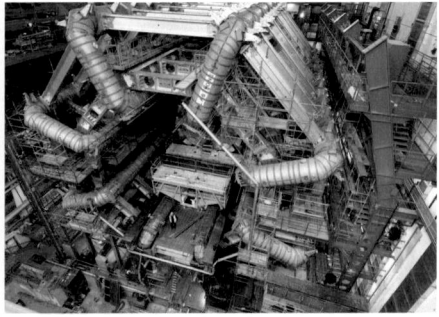

Fig 24.31(a) The new ATLAS detector system for the LHC

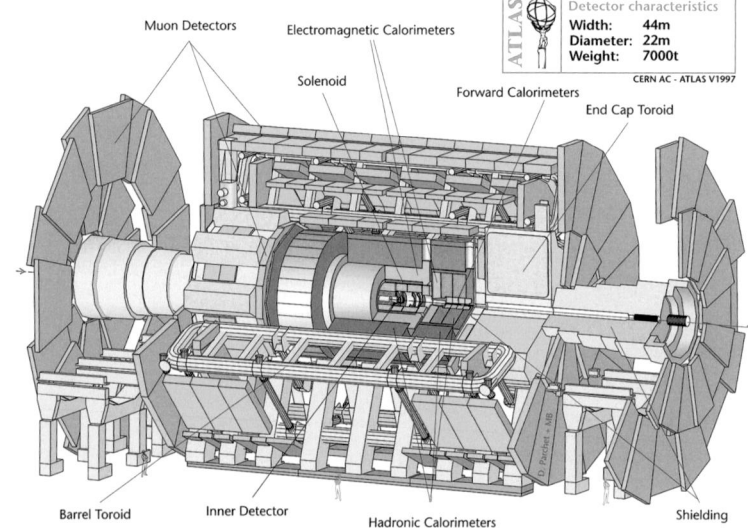

Fig 24.31(b) Cutaway diagram of the detector system. Collisions between protons and antiprotons take place in the yellow section. New particles spread out sideways and go through a series of detectors which measure their paths and energies. The sequence is shown in Fig 24.31(c)

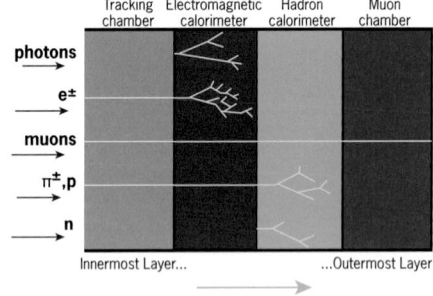

Fig 24.31(c) The particles are detected at different layers in the system, as shown here

10 MODERN PARTICLE ACCELERATORS

Modern particle accelerators are of three main kinds: linear accelerators (linacs), cyclotrons and synchrotrons.

LINEAR ACCELERATORS

In a linear accelerator, charged particles are accelerated along a straight evacuated tunnel by a set of switched anodes which produce a moving accelerating field, as in Figs 24.32(a) and (b). They are cheaper than accelerators with circular tracks because they don't need bending magnets, and cost depends mostly on that of the coils and the special steel required for the magnets.

The most powerful linear accelerator (linac) is at Stanford Linear Accelerator Center (SLAC) in California, USA (Fig 24.33). It is 3 km long and originally fired electrons with energies of 50 GeV at fixed targets. It provided the first experimental evidence for the existence of quarks. It has been upgraded to allow opposing

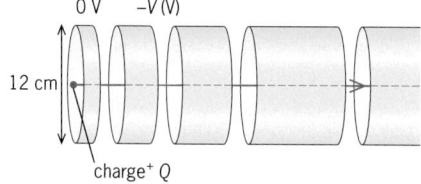

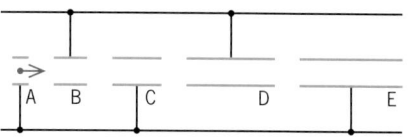

Fig 24.32(a) Part of a linear accelerator, like that at Stanford Linear Accelerator Center. The charged particle is accelerated by the field between the electrodes. It gains kinetic energy equal to the electrical potential energy transferred, QV

Fig 24.32(b) The particle moves from one electrode to the next in the linear accelerator: the same voltage difference is switched from A to B, B to C, and so on, so that the particle is always being accelerated. Why must each electrode be longer than the preceding one?

streams of electrons and positrons to collide at a combined energy of 10 GeV. The electrons come from a heated filament, just as in a TV set. Then they pass through a chain of 100 000 electrodes. The electrons leave one cylinder and are pulled towards the next by a comparatively small difference in voltage set up between the pair of electrodes at just the right time. The electrons are made to move close to the speed of light by very rapid voltage switching. This is done by feeding a high frequency radio signal to each electrode at just the right (but always changing) frequency to make the electrode more positive than the one before it. In effect, the electrons are surfing along this radio wave.

Linear accelerators (linacs) are both cheaper than circular accelerators, and much more efficient at feeding energy to electrons. This is because when charged particles are accelerated they emit radio waves and so lose energy, and when the particles move in a circular path they are always being accelerated towards the centre of the circle, even if they move at a constant speed round it.

The radiation emitted by accelerating particles is called *synchrotron radiation*. Since electrons have such a large charge compared to their mass, they lose a large fraction of their kinetic energy moving at high speeds in a circle. The effect is less for more massive particles such as protons.

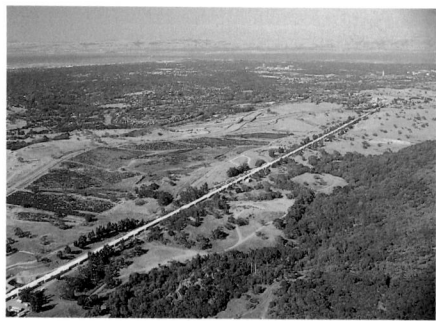

Fig 24.33 The 3 km building housing the accelerator at Stanford Linear Accelerator Center, California

CIRCULAR ACCELERATORS – CYCLOTRONS

In cyclotrons, a magnetic field forces charged particles to move in a circular path (Fig 24.34). The voltage on the D-shaped parts alternates so that the particles accelerate from one D to the other. The particles gain speed, so the path is actually an outward spiral. The maximum energy depends on how many times they can spiral before leaving the machine. Cyclotrons provide energetic particles for medical treatment and for the testing of advanced industrial materials.

Fig 24.34 The cyclotron. The potential of each D-shaped part alternates, so the positive particle is attracted from one part to the other, accelerating and spiralling out from the centre

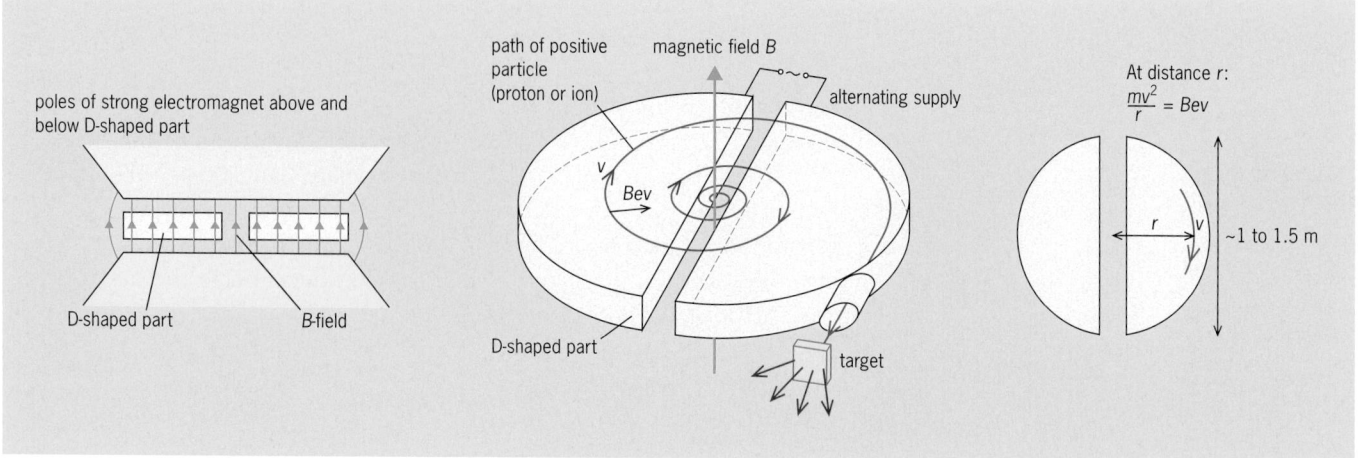

SYNCHROTRONS

At very high energies, particles become more massive because of relativistic effects near light speed. So in a cyclotron they take longer to complete a circuit and then the alternating voltage that accelerates them fails to synchronise with them.

Synchrotrons (Fig 24.35) overcome this problem: the frequency of the alternating voltage changes to match the increasing flight time of the particles. But at high energies the particles are moving at speeds so close to that of light that they actually make a circuit in a constant time: instead of getting faster, they just gain more momentum via an increase in mass. This effect underlies the design of synchrotrons.

They are very large machines. Particles are accelerated by passing through hollow anodes as in linear accelerators, but the track is circular. With a curved track, the particles can keep being accelerated without running out of track (as they eventually do in a linear accelerator) and in modern synchrotrons they keep moving in the circular path indefinitely, in *storage rings*.

Particles are first accelerated by smaller linacs or cyclotrons, then enter the synchrotron already travelling very close to light speed. They are held in a path of constant radius by strong magnetic fields, which are made even stronger as the particles gain more kinetic energy.

Most modern discoveries about fundamental particles come from **supersynchrotrons**. Their radius is very large, and superconducting coils are used to activate the electromagnets. Very large currents in superconducting coils avoid the heating effects that ordinary conductors would produce.

Fig 24.35 A synchrotron. A small group of particles is accelerated from one C-shaped hollow electrode to the other. The accelerating voltage switches from one electrode to the other as needed. The particles travel at a constant speed inside the electrodes

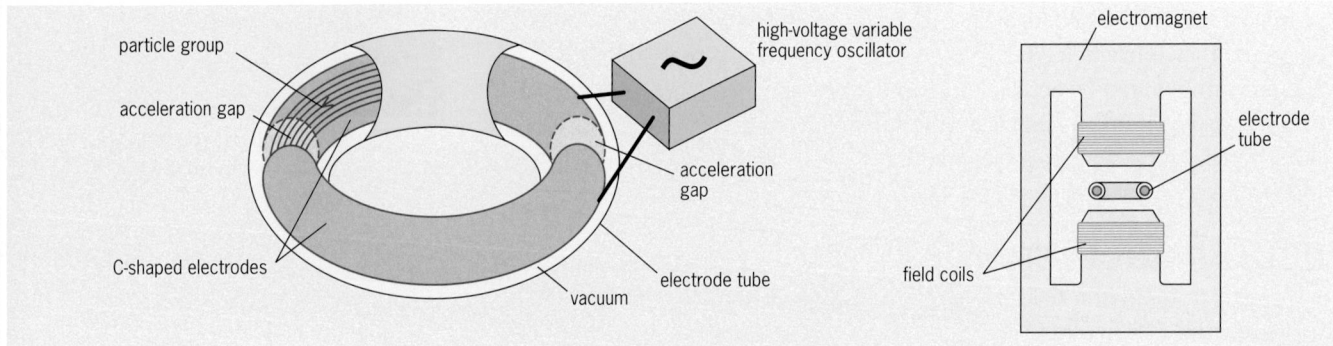

11 TARGETS AND COLLISIONS

FIXED AND MOVING TARGETS

High energies are required to investigate subatomic particles. In a collision, the 'spare' energy appears as a flux of particles. The larger the mass of a newly created particle, the greater the energy needed, which depends on the total accelerating voltage available.

In the late 1970s, the physicists at CERN came up with a brilliant idea. If you could fire two particles in opposite directions and make them collide, you would double the available energy at a stroke, without increasing the maximum kinetic energies of the particles. This was the principle used in the now obsolete **LEP** (Large Electron–Positron collider) and in the new **Large Hadron Collider (LHC)**; see Fig 24.36.

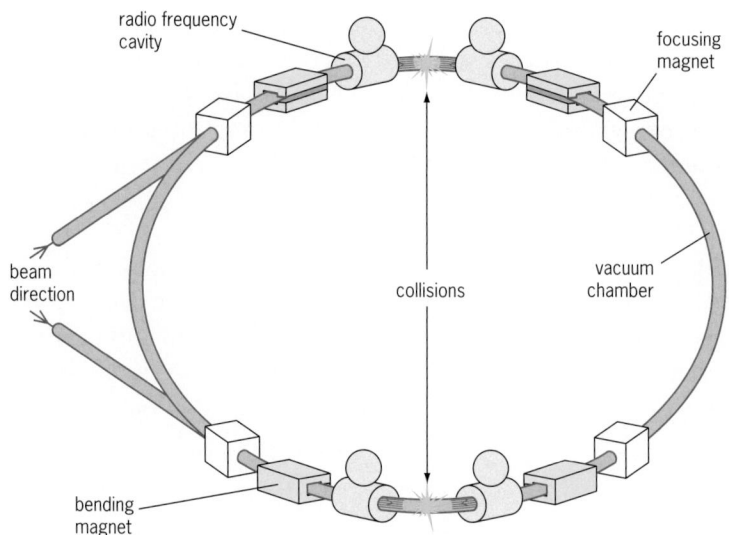

The LHC is designed to accelerate protons in opposite directions around the circular tunnel 27 km long in circumference. Each proton has an energy of 7 TeV (7×10^{12} eV), which means that it travels at 0.999 999 991 times the speed of light. The combined collision energy is thus 14 TeV, compared with 2 TeV obtained in the current highest energy system, Fermilab in Chicago, USA.

Only a small fraction of the protons in the beams actually collide when the beams cross, but with such a large number of particles ten billion collisions per second are expected during the course of an experiment. Hence the need for rapid data capture and analysis.

WHAT CAN HAPPEN IN COLLISIONS AT HIGH ENERGIES

Proton–proton collisions

Hit an atom hard enough and it emits photons as the excited atom goes back to its ground state. Hit a proton (a lot harder!): it also becomes excited, and a *very* short time later emits pions. Unlike photons, a pion is unstable and decays very quickly, in 10^{-8} s, into a muon and a neutrino. The muon (a kind of giant electron) decays more slowly, in 2×10^{-6} s, into an electron and a neutrino. The Universe is surprisingly full of neutrinos – which don't decay: about a thousand billion (10^{12}) pass through your body every second, at the speed of light.

Fig 24.37 shows a complex event in which a collision produces a starburst of tracks, including the production of pairs of pions. Fig 24.38 illustrates a relatively simple and fairly low-energy collision between two protons.

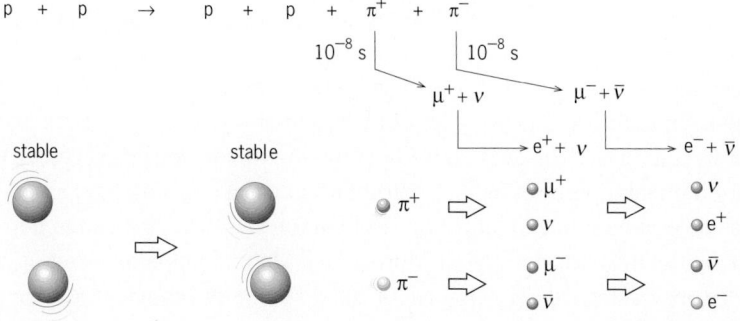

Fig 24.36(a) The arrangement of magnets, accelerators and experiments in the LHC collider at the European Particle Physics Laboratory at CERN, Geneva

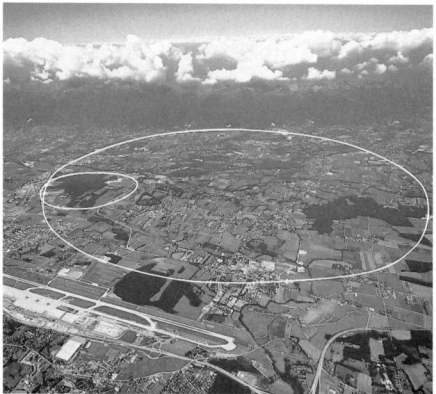

Fig 24.36(b) Aerial view showing where the CERN rings run underground. The LEP collider (large circle) is 27 km in circumference. The Large Hadron Collider (LHC) will occupy the same tunnel. The smaller circle marks the route of the super proton synchrotron

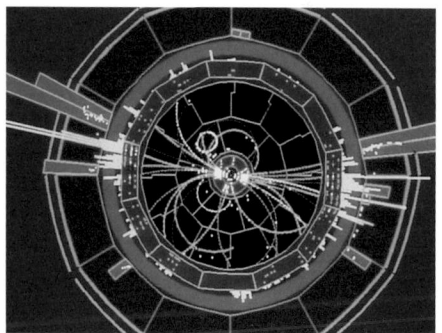

Fig 24.37 An image produced by the ALEPH detector computer, generated from the data reaching the detector systems: the decay of a Z^0 boson (a carrier of the electroweak force), via a quark–antiquark pair

? QUESTION 16

16 Use the data in the table in Fig 24.38 to check that:
a) charge is conserved,
b) baryon number is conserved.

Particle	Q	B	Particle	Q	B
proton	1	1	μ^-	−1	0
π^+	1	0	e^+	1	0
π^-	−1	0	e^-	−1	0
μ^+	1	0	ν	0	0

Fig 24.38 A simple collision with just enough spare energy to create two new particles, which then decay

Proton–antiproton collisions

When protons and antiprotons collide, they *annihilate* each other. The energy available is therefore not just their acquired kinetic energy but also the energy due to their rest masses. The rest-mass energy is small, however, compared with the kinetic energy for particles travelling close to the speed of light – and is usually ignored (see below).

Decays

The only **stable particles** we meet in particle physics are the proton, electron and neutrino (and their antiparticles). When a particle decays it must obey the conservation laws. Charge, mass–energy, momentum and baryon number are always strictly conserved. Strangeness can be 'lost' if the weak interaction is involved.

Mass–energy

In any decay, the new particles must always have less total rest mass than the original particle that decays. Any mass–energy left over will appear as kinetic energy in the new particles.

Momentum

In simple decays, we assume that the original particle is at rest and so has zero momentum. This means that the particles must move off in the particular directions and at the particular speeds which combine to produce zero momentum.

WHY STABLE PARTICLES ARE STABLE

The stable particles are stable because there is no particle with smaller mass that they can decay into without breaking a conservation law. *There is no baryon with less mass than a proton*, so it is stable. It could decay into pions and still conserve energy, charge and momentum – but this would not conserve baryon number. Pions are mesons with zero baryon number and so the decay is forbidden. Similarly, electrons could decay into neutrinos but for the fact that charge has to be conserved. (Refer back to Table 24.16 for categories of particles.)

12 DEEP INELASTIC SCATTERING

Deep inelastic scattering (DIS) is an extension of the scattering experiments like that of Geiger and Marsden that led to the discovery of the atomic nucleus. If the alpha particles used had had more energy they could have broken up the target nucleus, with results that might have been too confusing to evaluate at that time. The scattering would have been **inelastic** as the alpha particles lost energy in breaking up the nucleus, rather than the **elastic** scattering that Rutherford was able to assume.

But in 1968 high-speed electrons were used to probe the proton (hydrogen nucleus), contained in a tank of liquid hydrogen at the Stanford Linear Accelerator Center in California. This was about the time that theory was predicting that even such fundamental particles as the proton had internal structure, and should contain smaller objects with fractional charge and baryon number. These were named as quarks by the theoretical physicist Murray Gell-Mann. The pattern of scattering of the electrons confirmed the existence of small scattering centres inside the proton. These were identified as quarks.

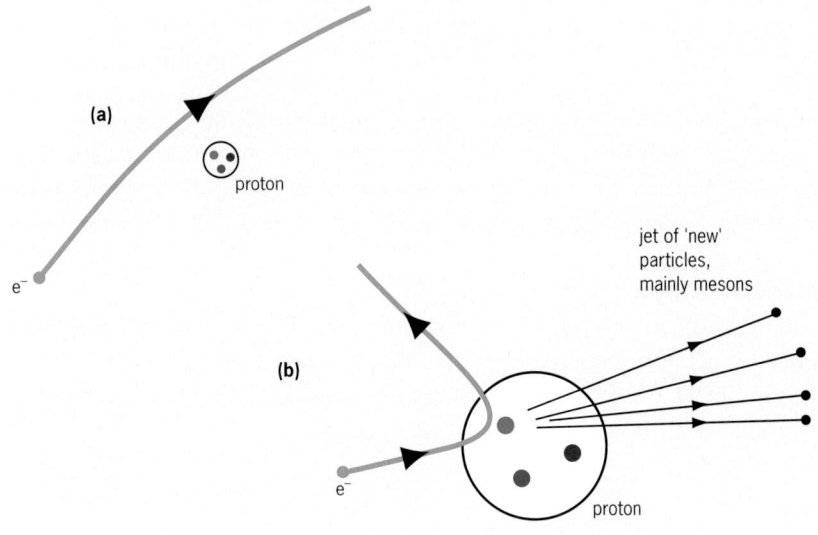

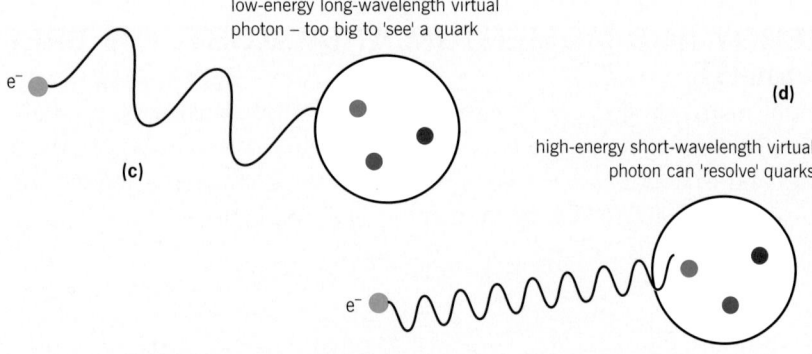

Fig 24.39 Low-energy and high-energy electron scattering
(a) Low-energy elastic scattering of an electron by a proton
(b) Deep inelastic scattering of an electron by a quark inside a proton. Energy is lost as new particles are created. The electron is scattered through a large angle
(c) Mediation by a low-energy virtual photon
(d) Mediation by a high-energy virtual photon

The interaction between particles is mediated by exchange particles, in this case by virtual photons between the incoming electron and the proton. When the electron kinetic energy is low these photons also have low energy, meaning an associated wavelength too large to 'see' the quarks. The electrons are scattered elastically through small angles. To resolve quarks, high-energy, short-wavelength photons are needed. When such a photon is emitted by a high-speed electron the electron recoils at a large angle. The photon also has enough energy to knock a quark out of the proton. But (see page 484) when quarks separate, new quarks are formed and the proton remains a three-quark object. The ejected quark breaks up into one or more quark–antiquark pairs observed as a jet of mesons. Fig 24.39 illustrates these processes.

This process of **deep inelastic scattering** is now one of the main tools of investigation in particle physics, with ever more massive and higher energy particles colliding with each other. The overall aim now is to find new more massive particles that can only be created with the 'spare' energy from inelastic collisions. We deal with such collisions next.

13 MASS, ENERGY AND TIME AT RELATIVISTIC SPEEDS

When particles approach the speed of light, their effective (inertial) mass increases. Thus both their kinetic energy and momentum can increase without much change in their speeds. This fact is a consequence of the **special theory of relativity**, discussed in Chapter 23. Here we will simply apply the results.

Relativistic mass

The mass of a particle at rest is its rest mass, m_0. This is the value quoted in reference books. For instance, the mass of an electron is 9.11×10^{-31} kg. The inertial mass of the particle moving at a speed v is however given by the formula:

$$m = \frac{m_0}{\sqrt{1 - \dfrac{v^2}{c^2}}} = m_0\left(1 - \frac{v^2}{c^2}\right)^{-\frac{1}{2}} = \gamma m_0$$

γ is the Lorentz factor (see page 460).

ENERGY AND MOMENTUM AT (ALMOST) THE SPEED OF LIGHT

In high-energy physics, energy calculations are simplest when we use the particle's momentum, p. The total energy of the particle, in relativity theory, is always and exactly $E = mc^2$ where m is the relativistic mass: $m = E/c^2$. For a particle moving at speed v, its momentum p is mv, hence:

$$p = mv = Ev/c^2$$

or: $$E = pc^2/v \qquad [1]$$

Now, for particles with very high energies, $v \approx c$, so:

$$E = pc \quad \text{and} \quad p = E/c \qquad [2]$$

Momentum units

Equation 2 means that:

$$\text{momentum units} = \text{energy units}/c$$

Just as particle physicists measure *mass* in units of GeV/c^2, so they measure *momentum* in terms of units GeV/c (see page 486).

Equation 2 ignores the rest-mass energy m_0c^2 of the particle. This means it also applies to photons, which have a rest mass of zero.

? **QUESTION 17**

17 Use the mass–speed relationship and a calculator to find how many times more massive a particle becomes when it is moving at 0.99c.

STRETCH AND CHALLENGE

EXAMPLE

Q In the electron–positron collider at CERN, the particles were accelerated to energies of 50 GeV. What percentage error is introduced into calculations by assuming that the rest masses are zero?

A The rest-mass energy of an electron is:

mass of electron × (speed of light)^2
= 9.1×10^{-31} kg × $(3 \times 10^8)^2$ m^2 s^{-2}
= 8.2×10^{-14} J

An electronvolt is 1.6×10^{-19} J, so the rest-mass energy:
= $(8.2 \times 10^{-14})/(1.6 \times 10^{-19})$
= 5.1×10^5 eV = 0.51 MeV
= 0.000 51 GeV

Thus: percentage error =
0.000 51/50 × 100 = 0.001%

MASSIVE PARTICLES AT SPEEDS CLOSE TO THE SPEED OF LIGHT: THE MOMENTUM–ENERGY FORMULA

For particles large enough for their rest mass to be significant, we need to use a more complete expression relating the conservation of total energy E and momentum p. This is derived on page 465 as:

$$E^2 = p^2c^2 + m_0^2c^4 \qquad [3]$$

Decays

Equation 3 is needed to calculate the mechanical outcome of particle decays. An example of this is shown below.

STRETCH AND CHALLENGE

EXAMPLE

Kaon decay

Q A positive kaon decays in about 10^{-8} s as follows:

$$K^+ \rightarrow \pi^+ + \pi^0$$

With what energy and at what speed do the pions move away?

A Suppose the kaon was at rest when the decay occurred. The rest mass of the kaon is 0.497 GeV/c^2. The total energy of the kaon has to supply the total energy of the pions, that is, both rest mass (of 0.140 GeV/c^2) and kinetic energy.

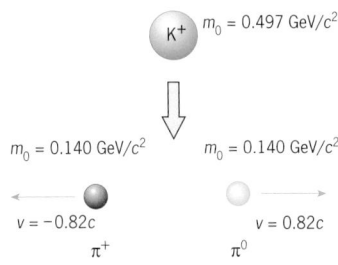

$m_0 = 0.497$ GeV/c^2

$m_0 = 0.140$ GeV/c^2 $m_0 = 0.140$ GeV/c^2

$v = -0.82c$ $v = 0.82c$

π^+ π^0

Fig 24.40 A kaon decaying into two pions. Charge, energy and momentum must be conserved

The pions have equal mass and share the kaon energy between them. Momentum is conserved, so the combined momentum of the pions must be zero: the momentum of the pions must be equal and opposite, and they must move apart with the same speed and the same kinetic energy.

Total energy for each pion
= 0.497/2 = 0.249 GeV.

We now use the momentum–energy formula to calculate the momentum p of a pion:

$$E^2 = p^2c^2 + m_0^2c^4$$

Rearranging:

$$p^2c^2 = E^2 - m_0^2c^4$$

So: $\quad p^2 = E^2/c^2 - m_0^2c^2$

The rest mass m_0 of each pion is 0.140 GeV/c^2.

So: $\quad p^2 = [(0.249 \text{ GeV})^2/c^2]$
$\qquad\qquad - [(0.140 \text{ GeV}/c^2)^2 c^2]$
$\qquad\quad = (0.249^2)(\text{GeV}^2/c^2)$
$\qquad\qquad - (0.140^2)(\text{GeV}^2/c^4)c^2$

and: $\quad p^2 = 0.0422 \ (\text{GeV}/c)^2$

giving: $\quad p = 0.205 \text{ GeV}/c$

TIP! Note that care needs to be taken with units – it is best to 'work them out' fully, as shown in the Example, using quantity algebra. If you find yourself multiplying or dividing by 9×10^{16} you are probably getting it wrong!

We can see how useful the chosen units are by finding the speed of each pion using equation 1 on page 502:

$$E = \frac{pc^2}{v}$$

that is:

$$v = \frac{pc^2}{E}$$

$$= 0.205 \times \frac{\text{GeV}}{c} \times c^2 \times \frac{1}{0.249 \text{ GeV}}$$

$$= \frac{0.205c}{0.249} = 0.82c$$

as shown in Fig 24.40.

Quarks and the weak interaction

In a collision, any new particles carry away kinetic energy *and* their rest mass energy. Both energies are provided by the total energy of the colliding particles.

We shall consider two situations involving a proton and an antiproton. In the first, the moving antiproton hits the proton which is a stationary target. In the second, both particles collide while moving with equal energies towards each other (as in a collider). The total energy of each moving particle is 2 GeV. Suppose that in each case a single particle is produced as a result of the collision. What total energy will this particle have?

A COLLISION WITH A STATIONARY TARGET

The total energy is 2 GeV for the moving antiproton plus the rest-mass energy of 1 GeV of the target proton, total 3 GeV (see Fig 24.41).

The total momentum is due to the incoming particle only, and is calculated (as on page 503) from:

$$p^2 = \frac{E^2}{c^2} - m_0^2 c^2$$

which gives:

$$p^2 = 3\left(\frac{\text{GeV}}{c}\right)^2$$

and:

$$p = 1.7 \text{ GeV}/c$$

The new particle must carry away exactly this quantity of momentum. To agree with equation 3 on page 503, its rest mass m_{new} must be given by:

$$m_{\text{new}}^2 = \frac{E^2}{c^4} - \frac{p^2}{c^2}$$

$$= 3^2\left(\frac{\text{GeV}}{c^2}\right) - 1.7^2\left(\frac{\text{GeV}}{c^2}\right)$$

so that: $\quad m_{\text{new}} = 2.5 \text{ GeV}/c^2$

This is in fact a Z particle.

COLLISIONS IN A COLLIDER

As in Fig 24.42, the energy for each colliding particle is 2 GeV, totalling 4 GeV. The total momentum before collision is zero, since each particle is moving with the same speed but in opposite directions. The momentum of the new particle must also be zero. This means that its *kinetic energy is zero*, so all the energy must appear as the rest mass of the new particle: which is thus 4 GeV/c^2.

This shows that the collider system is able to create particles of greater rest mass than the stationary target system is able to.

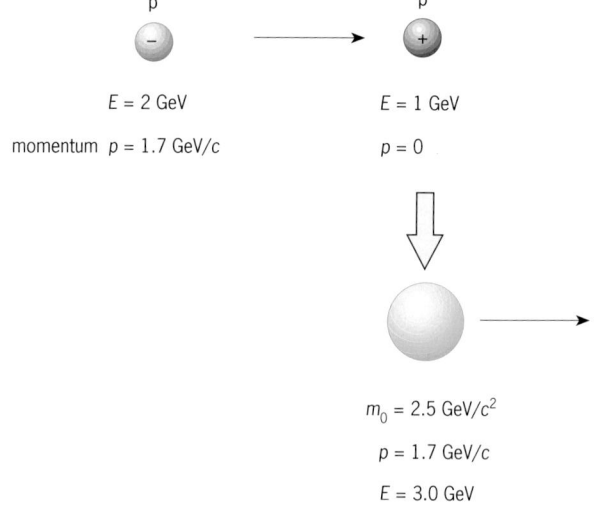

Fig 24.41 A moving antiproton colliding with a stationary proton: values before and after

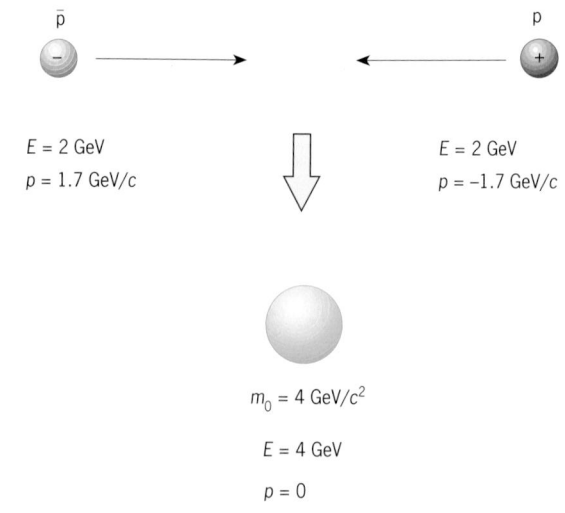

Fig 24.42 A moving antiproton colliding with a moving proton: values before and after

TIME DILATION: PARTICLES LIVE LONGER AT SPEED

Many of the new particles produced in accelerators decay with very short half-lives, and even at high speeds they would have decayed before reaching a detector except for the relativistic effect of **time dilation**. This effect is explained in Chapter 23, page 461, in connection with the detection of muons produced in the upper atmosphere by cosmic ray collisions. A particle that would decay in 10^{-8} seconds should travel just 3 m in this time at speeds close to light speed. In fact they travel 66 m and can be observed in detectors that are so large that they have to be several metres from the collision point where the particle was created. This is because to a stationary observer the particle's lifetime increases as a consequence of the special theory of relativity. To a fixed observer, the observed time $\Delta t'$ of a process occurring in a time Δt in a moving system is longer:

$$\Delta t' = \frac{\Delta t}{\sqrt{1 - \frac{v^2}{c^2}}} = \gamma t$$

A particle travelling at $0.999c$ would actually have a mean lifetime as observed increased from 10^{-8} s to 2.2×10^{-7} s, over 20 times longer, so that it can travel that much further on average (Fig 24.43).

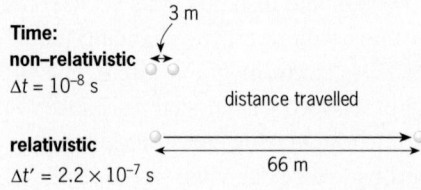

 REMEMBER THIS
Key formulae for relativistic motion
Lorentz factor

$$\gamma = \left(1 - \frac{v^2}{c^2}\right)^{-\frac{1}{2}}$$

Relativistic mass $m = \gamma m_0$

Total energy = kinetic energy + rest energy

$$E = E_k + E_0$$

Momentum $p = mv = Ev/c^2$

Total energy $E = mc^2$

Energy–momentum formula:
$E^2 = p^2c^2 + m_0^2c^4$

Time dilation: $\Delta t' = \gamma \Delta t$

? QUESTION 18

18 Check the value of 2.2×10^{-7} s for the relativistic mean lifetime for the particle in Fig. 24.43.

Fig 24.43 The effect of time dilation at $0.999c$. A particle with a lifetime of 10^{-8} s should travel 3 m at about the speed of light. Relativistic time dilation increases the observed lifetime to 2.2×10^{-7} s when the particle is travelling at $0.999c$. Thus the distance actually travelled is 66 m

MATTER AS WE KNOW IT

Fig 24.44 shows the two families, the quarks and the leptons, and their three generations. Each particle has its antiparticle. They make up all the matter and antimatter that has so far been discovered. But most of the Universe may consist of dark matter, which has not yet been identified.

Fig 24.44 The quarks and the leptons

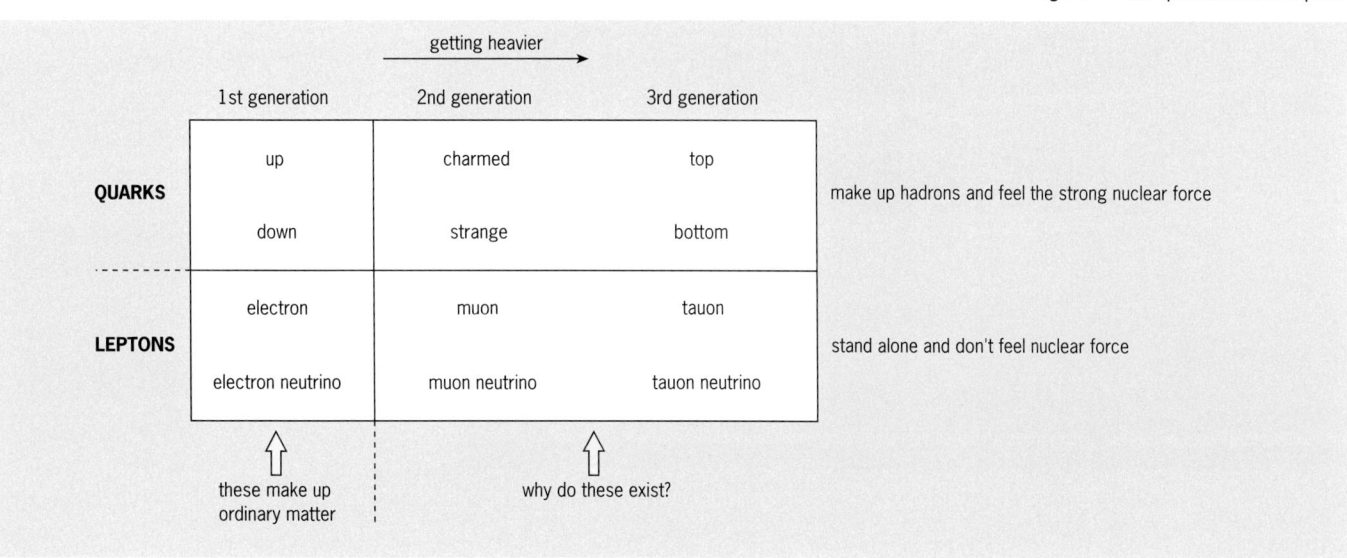

AND FINALLY...

Atoms and nuclei exist because they are made of particles *which cannot have the same set of quantum numbers while part of the same system.* The reason why is outside the scope of A-level physics.

This chapter has shown that the rules which define the behaviour of particles are due to the fundamental properties of quarks. *But no one knows why quarks have these properties.*

The rich variety of particles exists – and just for very short times – only in conditions of high energy such as during collisions in accelerators, in the interiors of stars and also at the time of the Big Bang. Most of the Universe makes do with protons, neutrons and electrons.

The next main goal of particle physicists is to find a particle called the **Higgs boson** which is important because its interaction with other particles is believed to be the source of their mass. Like all bosons, it is a 'field particle', which means that it carries a force of some kind.

We observe mass as something that makes it hard to accelerate something. The harder it is to accelerate, the greater the mass of the object. But imagine trying to push a sheet of aluminium in a strong magnetic field (see page 228). You feel a force opposing your efforts, which we explain as being due to eddy currents excited in the aluminium by its motion through the magnetic field. If you didn't know about magnetism and electricity, you might confuse this effect with the 'inertial force' that seems to stop you giving instantaneous velocity to a mass. In a similar way, the **Higgs field** opposes motion by exchanging virtual bosons – just as the exchange of photons mediates electromagnetic forces. The effect is to produce an interaction of some kind that appears as inertial resistance to motion. You can think of the Higgs boson as somehow making space 'sticky'.

The theory put forward by Peter Higgs (Fig 24.45) of Edinburgh University as long ago as 1964 is now seen to be very useful, as it links with the 'theories of everything' – superstring theory, supersymmetry and supergravity – now being explored by the 'super'-theorists. The mass of the Higgs boson is predicted to be between 0.1 and 1 TeV, so should be within the scope of the ATLAS experiment in the Large Hadron Collider at CERN.

Physics would quite like to know what causes mass – and be able to link quantum physics with Einstein's gravity theories.

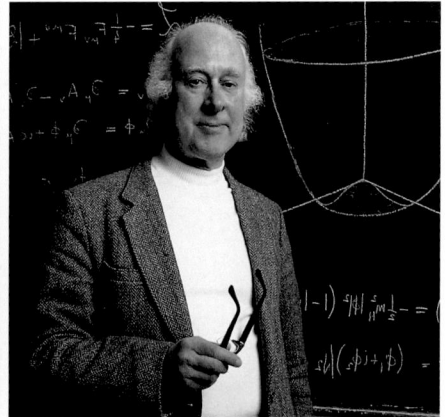

Fig 24.45 Peter Higgs, whose theory aims to unify electromagnetism, the weak and strong nuclear forces

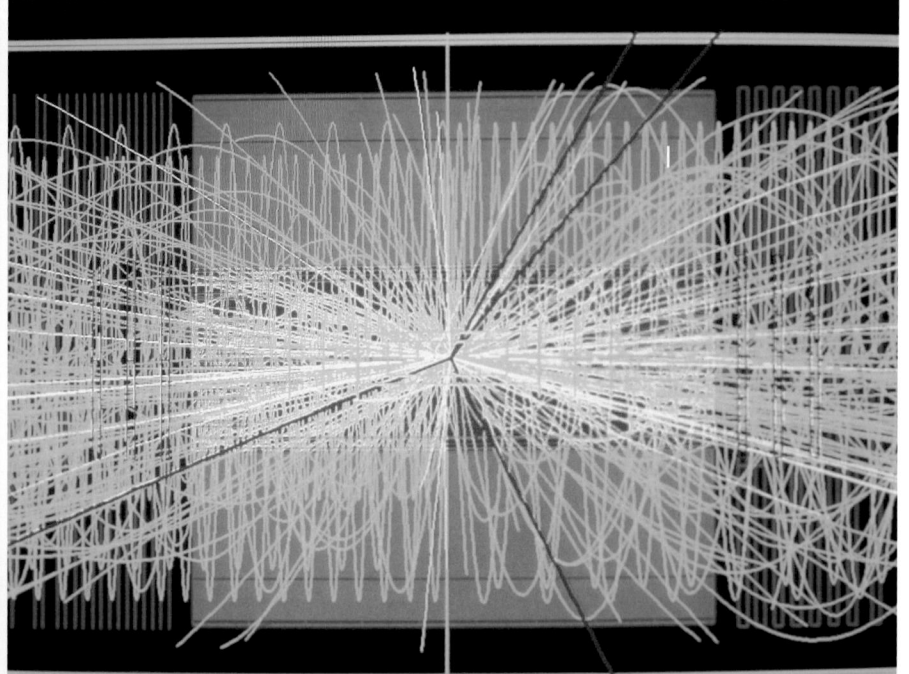

Fig 24.46 A computer simulation of an event expected by the Higgs theory. After a proton–proton collision, a Higgs boson decays to produce four muons – straight red tracks – and many other particles

For more information on the search for the Higgs boson please see the How Science Works assignment for this chapter at www.collinseducation.co.uk/CAS

SUMMARY

After studying this chapter, you should know and understand the following:

- Three particles – the neutron, proton and electron – are able to explain the main behaviours of stable atoms.
- The four types of interaction between particles require additional exchange particles – bosons – which mediate the interactions (they 'carry the forces').
- Many new particles have been discovered, initially from the collisions of cosmic rays (high-speed protons, electrons and atomic nuclei) and later from accelerator experiments.
- Each particle has an antiparticle, described as matter and antimatter.
- Particles and their antiparticles – hadrons (baryons, mesons) and leptons – are classified by rest mass and by other properties (baryon number, strangeness) and their response to forces.
- These properties were discovered by applying conservation rules in reactions.
- The behaviour, interactions and nature of hadrons may be explained more simply using the quark model.

- There are three lepton families and three quark families, arranged in successive generations.
- There are several types of accelerator, each based on a physical principle. Accelerators give particles high energies at which they interact.
- Many investigations involve deep inelastic scattering.
- There are several types of particle detector, each design based on a particular underlying physical principle but usually relying on the ability of a particle to cause ionisation.
- For simple reactions there are calculations and decays involving the masses, energies and momenta of high-speed, relativistic particles.
- Conservation rules enable particle interactions to be analysed.
- Feynman diagrams can be used to illustrate what happens in interactions and decays involving particles.

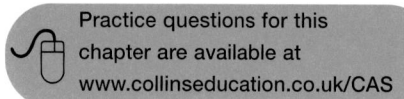

Practice questions for this chapter are available at www.collinseducation.co.uk/CAS

25

Astrophysics

Twinkle, twinkle little star

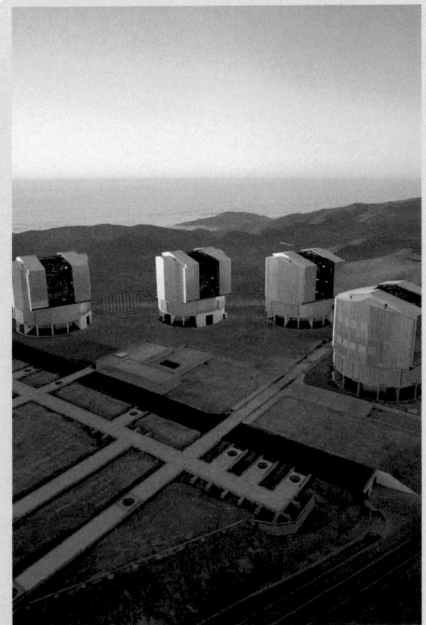

The four telescopes at the European Southern Observatory at Pinara Mountain, Chile

The Laser Guide Star in action

…and that's the trouble. Stars twinkle because of disturbances in the atmosphere, which alter the refractive index of pockets of air. This makes the image on the retina wander about slightly. Even with large telescopes the image on the CCD sensor will, over the time of viewing, blur over a small region instead of the small almost point-like image the star would make in perfect conditions. This 'seeing', as astronomers call it, will vary with the weather and the state of the atmosphere. Most modern Earth-based observatories are sited on high mountains, where the atmosphere above the telescopes is thin, and preferably in regions where cloud is rare or too low to affect the viewing. If you like sunshine in tropical climates, become an astronomer!

Another solution is to put the telescope well above the atmosphere in Earth orbit: like the Hubble Space Telescope and such temporary telescopes as the Hipparcos satellite (High Precision Parallax Collecting Satellite – see the Stretch and Challenge box on page 530).

The Hubble telescope has a small aperture (2.4 m) compared with ground-based telescopes such as the new Very Large Telescope system at the La Silla Pinara Mountain Observatory in Chile with four 8.2 m telescopes whose outputs can be combined. But these large telescopes would still have 'seeing' problems without the aid of an artificial star – **the Laser Guide Star (LGS)**.

At 90 km above the Earth, the atmosphere has a layer of sodium atoms. A tuned laser with well-defined wavelength is fired in the direction of any object the astronomers want to study. Sodium atoms are ionised over a small area and glow brightly enough for a small ancillary telescope to observe. The expected signal is well known and any deviations from the norm caused by atmospheric conditions are measured. Rapid, automatic computer work enables signals to be sent to a series of pistons underneath the mirror of the large telescope being used. This flexes to return the light from the star or galaxy, received after atmospheric disturbance as a distorted wavefront, to be sent to the detector in its pristine shape. This is known as **adaptive optics**.

Adaptive optics is also used at the world's largest single telescope, the Keck telescope at Mauna Kea in Hawaii (look back to Fig.18.31).

The ideas in this chapter

In this chapter, we look first at the main features of the Solar System (the Sun and its planets, asteroids and comets) and how they were formed. We then study the Sun as a typical star, the only star close enough to study in detail.

Our knowledge and understanding of the nearby Universe is based largely on the information of different forms of electromagnetic radiation. Though the nearest stars are mostly much larger and brighter than the Sun, they are so far away that they appear as tiny pinpoints of light, even in a large telescope. Yet we are able to gain a surprising amount of information from the tiny amount of electromagnetic radiation reaching us. Astronomers have fitted the different kinds of star into a pattern that links their sizes, brightness and ages. This pattern is the **Hertzsprung–Russell diagram**.

The brightest stars we see are relatively close and lie in our own branch of our own galaxy, which is called the **Milky Way Galaxy** and contains 100 billion stars. Galaxies in general will be dealt with in the next chapter.

The physics of stars is mostly to do with their sources of internal energy, and how they reach equilibrium by matching energy emission with the rate of energy production from nuclear and gravitational processes.

Finally, we consider what happens when a star's supply of energy is running out, and its steady state turns into the dramatic processes that produce red giants, white dwarfs, supernovas, neutron stars and black holes.

1 THE SOLAR SYSTEM

The planets move round the Sun in elliptical orbits, held in their paths by the gravitational force between them and the Sun. The Solar System also includes many smaller rocky objects called **asteroids** (see page 43) which form a belt between the orbits of Mars and Jupiter.

The total mass of the Solar System is about 2.0×10^{30} kg. Some 99.9 per cent of this is concentrated in the Sun. The largest planet, Jupiter, for example, has a mass of 1.899×10^{27} kg – less than 0.1 per cent of the Solar System's mass.

THE NUMBERS ARE ASTRONOMICAL

Astronomy requires very large numbers when distances are measured in standard SI units like metres and kilometres, so astronomers also use two other units of distance – the astronomical unit and the parsec. Popular astronomy also uses the light year; see Fig 25.1.

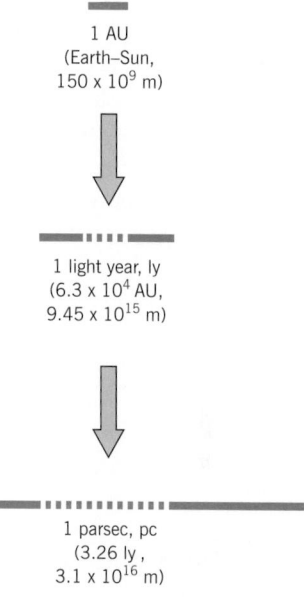

1 AU
(Earth–Sun,
150×10^9 m)

1 light year, ly
(6.3×10^4 AU,
9.45×10^{15} m)

1 parsec, pc
(3.26 ly,
3.1×10^{16} m)

Fig 25.1 Astronomical distance units

Fig 25.2 The Solar System planets: Mercury, Venus, Earth, Mars, Jupiter, Saturn, Uranus and Neptune

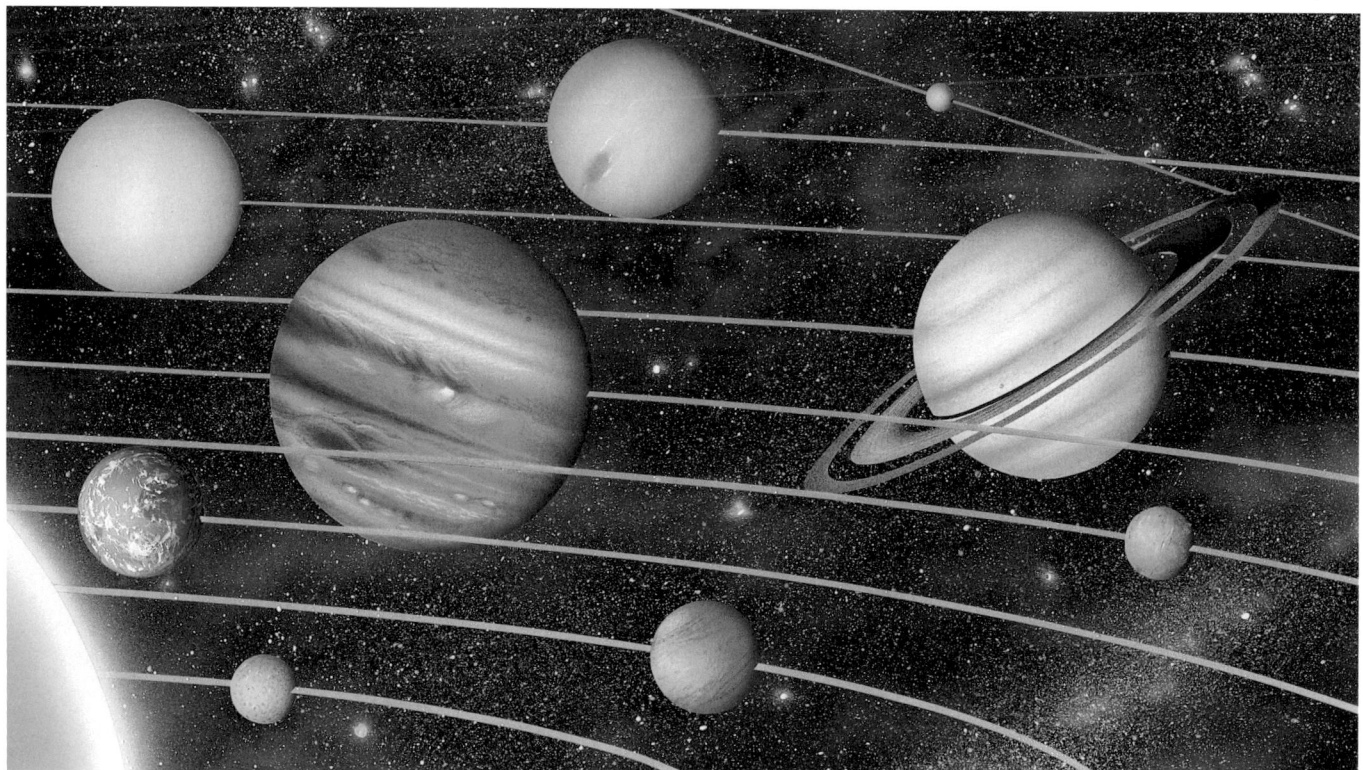

? QUESTIONS 1–3

1 An astronomy book states: the orbital distance of the planets from the Sun follows a regular spacing: roughly, each planet lies twice as far out as the preceding one. Use Table 25.1 to check this statement.

2 Put the numerical data in Table 25.1 into a spreadsheet. Use the data to investigate how such things as temperature, orbital period and rotational period vary with distance from the Sun for all the planets. Comment on any patterns you find.

3 Give two main chemical properties and two main physical properties of a) the inner planets, b) the outer planets.

The **astronomical unit**, AU, is the mean distance of the Earth from the Sun, 150×10^9 m. On this scale, Jupiter is just over 5 AU from the Sun and Pluto about 40 AU. The AU is a convenient unit for astronomers as it is the basis of a method for *measuring* astronomical distances using parallax, described on page 6–7. The AU gives rise to the second unit, the **parsec**, pc. Parsec is short for 'parallax second' and is the distance of a star which appears to shift its position in the sky by 1 second of arc as the Earth moves from the end of one diameter of its orbit to the other (see pages 529–530). It has a value of 2.06×10^5 AU (3.1×10^{16} m).

The **light year**, ly, is the distance travelled by light in 1 standard year, 9.5×10^{15} m. 1 pc is about 3.3 ly.

To get an idea of the scales measured by these units: the *nearest* star to Earth is Proxima Centauri, a very faint companion star of the brightest star in the constellation of the Centaur. It is at a distance of 4×10^{16} m, which is the same as 4.2 ly or 1.3 pc.

THE MAIN FEATURES OF THE SOLAR SYSTEM

Table 25.1 gives the main physical data of the Sun and planets. The planets form two groups, the **inner planets** and the **outer planets**. It is not easy to show them all to the same scale on a diagram, but with some artistic licence Fig 25.2 on the previous page illustrates their size. Space probes and satellites are providing remarkable pictures of the planets and information about their composition and appearance, revealing hitherto unsuspected rings and small satellites.

Table 25.1 Data on the planets

Planet	Mean distance from Sun (10^9 m)	Mean distance in AU (Earth = 1)	Period (Earth years)	Rotation period (hours)	Inclination of equator to orbital plane (degrees)	Surface temperature (°C)	Density (kg m^{-3})	Mass (Earth = 1)	Surface g-field (N kg^{-1})	Number of satellites	Name of largest satellite	Mass of largest satellite (kg)	Mean density of satellites (kg m^{-3})
Mercury	58	0.4	0.24	1416	0	350	5400	0.056	3.7	0			
Venus	108	0.7	0.61	5832	117	460	5300	0.815	8.9	0			
Earth	150	1.0	1	24	23	15	5500	1	9.8	1	Moon	7.2×10^{22}	3340
Mars	228	1.5	2	25	25	−20	4000	0.11	3.8	2	Phobos	9.6×10^{15}	2200
Jupiter	778	5.2	12	10	3	−73	1300	317.9	24.9	16	Ganymede	1.5×10^{23}	2000
Saturn	1427	9.5	29	10	27	−120	700	95.1	10.5	17	Titan	1.3×10^{23}	1800
Uranus	2870	19.1	84	11	98	−213	1600	14.56	8.8	15	Oberon	6.0×10^{21}	1600
Neptune	4497	30.0	165	16	30	−213	2300	17.24	11.2	8	Triton	2.2×10^{22}	2000

Earth data: Mass = 5.97×10^{24} kg   Radius = 6.38×10^6 m

THE INNER PLANETS

The four inner planets are Mercury, Venus, Earth and Mars, which all lie within 1.5 AU of the Sun. Then there is a belt of 'minor planets' and asteroids (see Fig 3.2, page 43) at an average distance of 2.8 AU, containing an estimated 50 000 objects. The inner planets and the asteroids are *rocky bodies* made of materials similar to the material on and in the Earth. Their cores are iron and nickel and they have lighter elements (mainly in compounds) such as oxygen, silicon, aluminium, magnesium with smaller quantities of potassium, sodium and calcium.

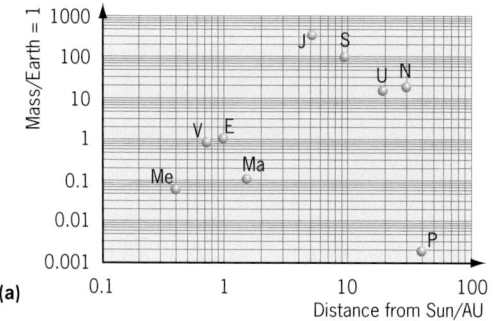

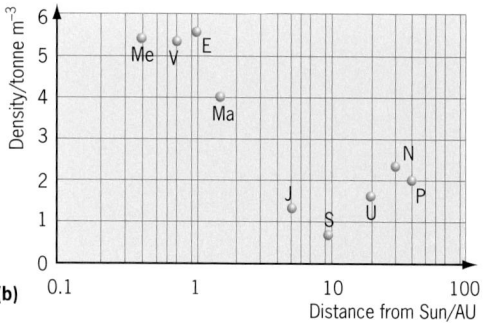

Fig 25.3 Plots for the planets:
(a) masses (log–log),
(b) densities (lin–log), against distance from the Sun

THE OUTER PLANETS

The outer planets, called the Jupiter group, are Jupiter, Saturn, Uranus and Neptune, plus an oddity, the 'double planet' Pluto–Charon. These planets are much further away from the Sun than the inner planets and are much larger, both in size and in mass. They are also much less dense, suggesting that their composition is different from the inner planets' composition. Their bulk must be mostly the light elements hydrogen and helium, which are gases at the planets' surfaces, but liquid or even solid at depth.

Pluto was discovered only in 1930: it is very small and is likely to be a rocky planet. Pluto is no longer classified as a planet. The International Astronomical Union decided in 2006 to restrict the use of the word planet to bodies orbiting a star which are massive enough for their own gravity to form them into a spherical shape. Pluto is now a **dwarf planet**.

Fig 25.3 shows mass and density data for the planets, plotted against distance from the Sun.

There are also **periodic comets** such as Halley's comet.

PERIODIC COMETS

Periodic comets move in very large orbits (Fig 25.4) which extend far beyond the orbit of Pluto, the furthest planet. Comets are much smaller than planets and are made of dust and the 'ice' of water and other gaseous elements (Fig 25.5).

Comets may have their origin in a region filled with a large number of objects (estimated to be 10^{12}) called the Oort Cloud (see Fig 3.1, page 42). The Oort Cloud is more than a thousand times more distant than Pluto, at the outer limit of the Solar System.

PLANETARY MOTION

All the planets are in orbit round the Sun and move in the same direction – anticlockwise when viewed from above our North Pole. Their paths all lie close to the same plane.

The orbits are elliptical, which means that sometimes they are further from the Sun than at other times. Books of data tend to give the *mean* distance of the planet from the Sun. For most planets this distance is usually quite close to the actual distance at any time, but Mercury and Pluto have more elliptical orbits. In fact, Pluto sometimes gets closer to the Sun than the next inner planet, Neptune.

The Sun is at one **focus** of the planet's ellipse (Fig 25.6, overleaf). Accurate prediction of a planet's motion requires very careful

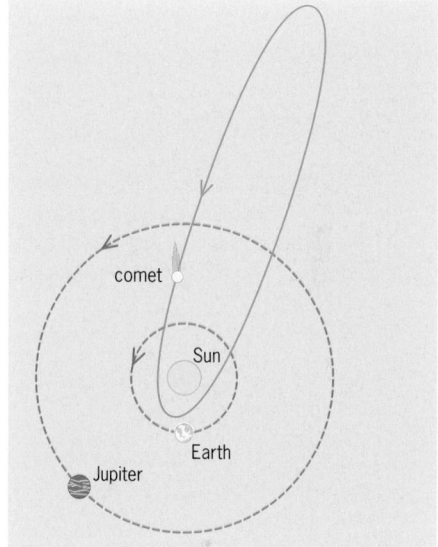

Fig 25.4 A typical orbit of a comet is a highly eccentric ellipse

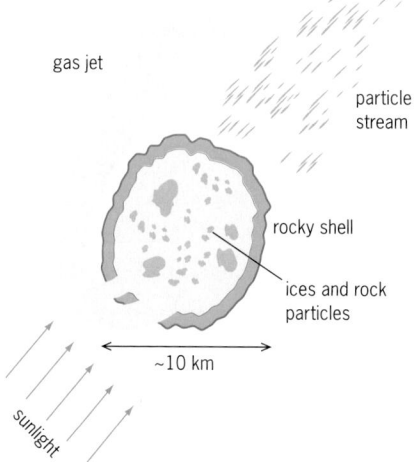

Fig 25.5 The structure of a comet head and the effect of sunlight

mathematics – not only is the mathematics of elliptical motion more complicated than that of circular motion, but each planet is affected by the gravitational forces between itself and other planets. However, the orbits of most planets are so nearly circular that we can assume circular motion and get good enough results for our purposes.

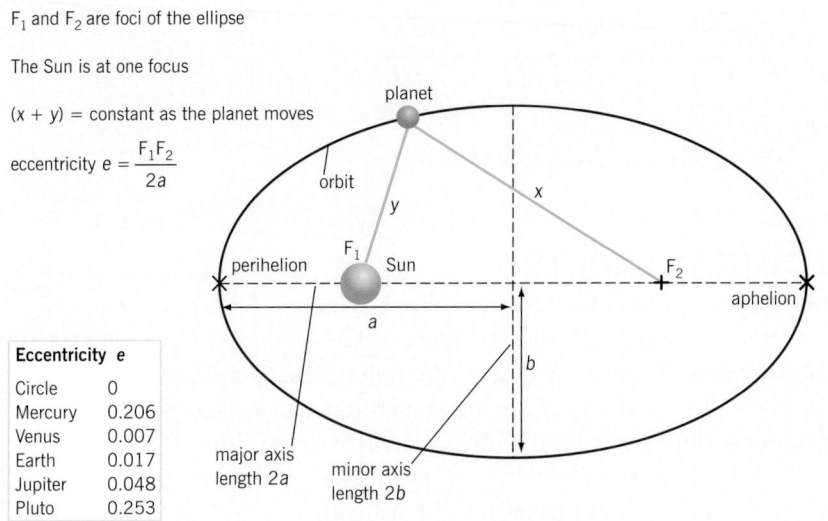

F_1 and F_2 are foci of the ellipse

The Sun is at one focus

$(x + y)$ = constant as the planet moves

eccentricity $e = \dfrac{F_1 F_2}{2a}$

Eccentricity e	
Circle	0
Mercury	0.206
Venus	0.007
Earth	0.017
Jupiter	0.048
Pluto	0.253

Fig 25.6 Planetary orbits are ellipses. In this diagram the eccentricity (a measure of the 'squashedness') of the orbit is exaggerated

THE LAWS OF PLANETARY MOTION

The gravitational force acting on the planet produces an inward acceleration v^2/r where v is the orbital speed of the planet at a distance r from the Sun. Newton's law of gravitation (see page 38) tells us the size of the force:

$$G\frac{Mm}{r^2}$$

where G is the universal gravitational constant, M the mass of the Sun and m the mass of the planet. So, by applying Newton's second law of motion, force = mass × acceleration, we have:

$$G\frac{Mm}{r^2} = m\frac{v^2}{r}$$

Making speed v the subject of the equation:

$$v = \sqrt{\frac{GM}{r}} \qquad [1]$$

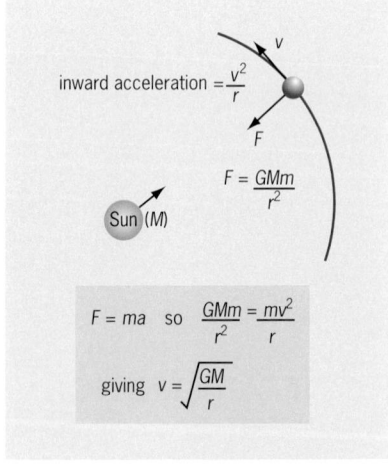

inward acceleration $= \dfrac{v^2}{r}$

$F = \dfrac{GMm}{r^2}$

Sun (M)

$F = ma$ so $\dfrac{GMm}{r^2} = \dfrac{mv^2}{r}$

giving $v = \sqrt{\dfrac{GM}{r}}$

Fig 25.7 Speed in orbit

which tells us that the speed of a planet in its orbit does not depend on its mass but only on its distance from the Sun. See Fig 25.7.

This is a very powerful result. For example, it allows us to calculate the mass of the Sun from the orbital speed of any planet. We also have to know the value of the gravitational constant G, a value which was not known in Newton's day and remains one of the most difficult of fundamental physical constants to measure accurately (see page 39).

Kepler's laws of planetary motion, and Newton's explanations

Newton produced his famous laws of motion in order to explain the motion of the planets. He used these, and the idea of gravity as a force, to deduce some laws of planetary motion already discovered by years of patient observation, particularly by the astronomer Johannes Kepler (Austria/Bohemia, 1571–1630) on the orbit of Mars. Three of Kepler's laws proved to be the most useful:

1 **The law of ellipses**. The orbit of each planet is an ellipse, with the Sun at one focus.

2 **The law of equal areas**. A line drawn from a planet to the Sun sweeps out equal areas in equal times, as in Fig 25.8.

3 **The harmonic law**. The *square* of the orbital period T of a planet is directly proportional to the *cube* of its average distance R from the Sun. This is usually written as:

$$\frac{T^2}{R^3} = \text{constant}$$

Newton gave a physical explanation and proof of Kepler's laws, using his laws of motion and the idea of gravity as a force obeying an inverse square law.

KEPLER'S LAW 1

Newton used his laws of motion and gravity to prove that a body moving in a gravitational field such as that produced by the Sun must move in a circle, an ellipse or a hyperbola. A hyperbola, unlike the other two, is an open-ended path; a comet, for example, may follow a hyperbola, and then it will never return.

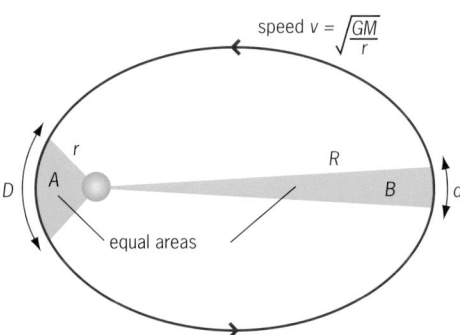

speed $v = \sqrt{\dfrac{GM}{r}}$

Fig 25.8 Kepler's second law of planetary motion says that the areas 'swept out' by the radius line in equal times are equal: area A = area B. This means that a planet covers the distances D and d in equal times so that it travels faster when close to the Sun

KEPLER'S LAW 2

Equation 1 on page 514 gives us a qualitative idea of Kepler's second law. As r decreases (as in Fig 25.8), the planet moves faster (v increases). In a given time, the line joining it to the Sun will sweep out an area such as A. When it is further from the Sun the planet will move more

slowly, so that the radius line will sweep out an area such as B. Areas A and B are equal if r increases enough to compensate for the decrease in v.

The simplest mathematical proof of Kepler's second law uses the fact that when a planet moves in its orbit its angular momentum is conserved (Fig 25.9):

$$\text{angular momentum } p = mvr = \text{constant} \qquad [2]$$

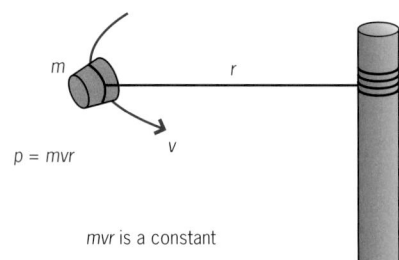

$p = mvr$

mvr is a constant

Fig 25.9 Conservation of angular momentum. When you spin an object (here a rubber bung) round a rod, as the string winds up r gets less but v increases to compensate

Look at Fig 25.10.

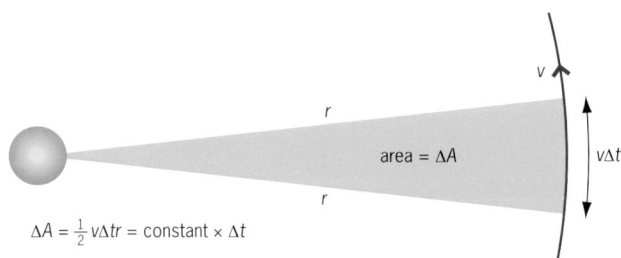

area = ΔA

$\Delta A = \frac{1}{2} v\Delta t r = \text{constant} \times \Delta t$

Fig 25.10 Diagram to illustrate proof of Kepler's second law

When the planet moves for a very short time Δt its radius line of length r sweeps out a small area ΔA. ΔA is (approximately) the area of a triangle of base $v\Delta t$ and height r. So:

$$\Delta A = \frac{1}{2} v\Delta t r = vr \times \frac{1}{2} \Delta t$$

But since m is a constant for any planet, from equation 2, vr is a constant. Thus the area ΔA is the same for any value of r when the planet moves for equal times Δt.

KEPLER'S LAW 3

Consider a planet moving at a speed v in a circle of radius r. The orbital period T is the time taken to complete one orbit, a circumference distance $2\pi r$ (Fig 25.11 overleaf). So:

$$T = \frac{\text{distance}}{\text{speed}} = \frac{2\pi r}{v}$$

Kepler's laws of planetary motion, and Newton's explanations (Cont.)

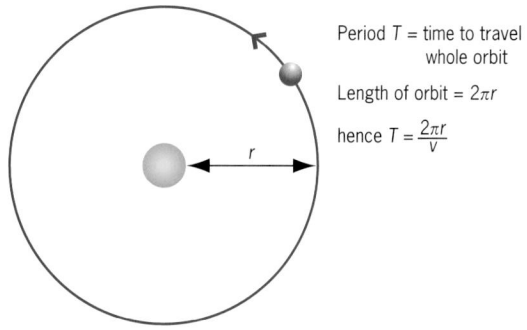

Period T = time to travel whole orbit

Length of orbit = $2\pi r$

hence $T = \frac{2\pi r}{v}$

Fig 25.11 Obtaining the period of orbit from speed and radius

From equation 1 on page 514:

$$v = \sqrt{\frac{GM}{r}}$$

and substituting for v gives:

$$T = 2\pi r\sqrt{\frac{r}{GM}}$$

When we square both sides we get:

$$T^2 = 4\pi^2 r^2\,\frac{r}{GM}$$

which we can simplify to:

$$T^2 = \frac{4\pi^2}{GM} \times r^3$$

That is, the square of the orbital period is directly proportional to the cube of the average distance between Sun and planet. This is normally given as Kepler's third law, in the form:

$$\frac{T^2}{r^3} = \frac{4\pi^2}{GM} = \text{constant}$$

This is a constant for all planets. It applies to all bodies orbiting in gravitational fields, but with different values of the constant, and may be used to help measure the masses of stars (see page 531).

? QUESTION 5

5   Use the data in Table 25.1 to check that Kepler's third law is true for the planets Venus and Mars. (You could use a spreadsheet for this calculation and tackle all the planets.)

2 THE FORMATION AND EVOLUTION OF THE SOLAR SYSTEM

A DUSTY, GRITTY UNIVERSE

The Milky Way contains a great deal of material that absorbs light and is often hard to detect. But it may be lit up by nearby stars, as in Fig 25.12. This shows a region of dark material in the constellation of Orion, an example of a **nebula** made of gas and dust, lit up by stars hidden behind it with others in front. The *gas* is identified from both its visible spectrum and radio spectrum as being mostly hydrogen. The interaction of the *interstellar dust* with light suggests that it is made of small grains of 'dirty ice', as shown in Fig 25.13.

Fig 25.12 An image in the visible spectrum of the nebula in Orion, 1500 light years from Earth. The bright central region of hydrogen gas hides a cluster of very hot stars called Trapezium which ionise the hydrogen with their ultraviolet radiation

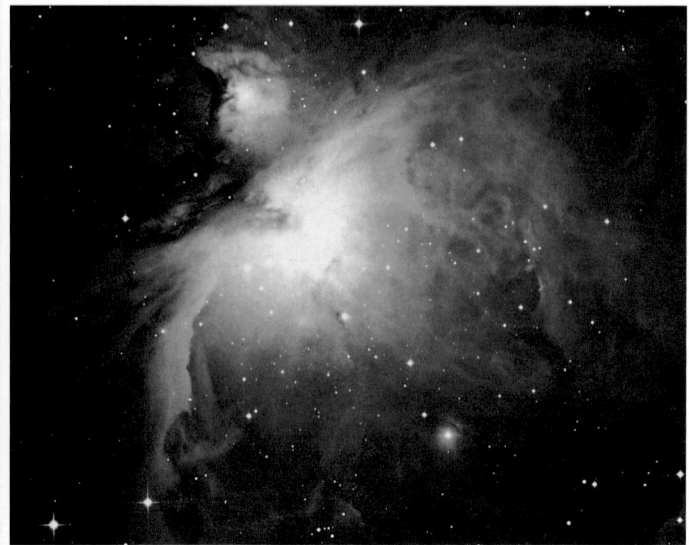

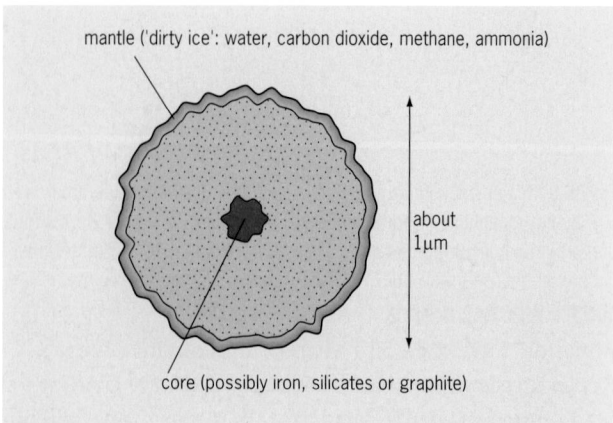

mantle ('dirty ice': water, carbon dioxide, methane, ammonia)

about 1μm

core (possibly iron, silicates or graphite)

Fig 25.13 A grain of interstellar dust. The core is thought to be of the same solids we find in meteorites. Like the mantle, the heads of comets are made of 'dirty ice', and the gases stream off to form the comet tails

Notice the two bright blue stars in the centre and below the centre on the right. Their colour indicates that they are very new stars, as are many others in this nebula.

The account that follows is thought to be broadly the way that the Sun and the planets of the Solar System were formed from both gas (mostly hydrogen with some helium) and dust, as well as the way in which other planetary systems now being found in our galaxy were formed.

THE FORMATION OF A STAR

To produce a star the size of the Sun would require a (roughly spherical) cloud of dust and gas a few light years in diameter. In the star's formation, much of the material is lost and doesn't end up in the star. The cloud may be stable for billions of years. During this time, the gravitational forces that tend to make it clump together are offset by the random thermal motion of the particles. Then the cloud starts a **gravitational collapse**. This may be triggered by a disturbance which makes a part of the cloud more dense than the rest.

Phase 1: gravitational contraction of the gas cloud

When the cloud starts to contract under gravity, gas and dust fall towards the centre of mass, gaining speed as potential energy is converted to kinetic energy. Collisions make the extra motion random. The gas gets hotter. Most energy remains trapped, but the cloud begins to lose energy as infrared radiation. At this point, we could detect the cloud from Earth as an infrared source (Fig 25.14).

Eventually, the core in the contracting cloud becomes white hot, but we cannot see it because the cooler outer layers absorb the radiation. Because infrared radiation is less easily absorbed, we observe the large dark cloud as a strong source of radiation, an infrared 'hot spot'. You can see several hot spots in Fig 25.14.

Phase 2: a protostar is born

From the start of collapse, it takes about a million years for a mass of gas to reach the stage of being a **protostar**. The core is several times larger than the star it will eventually become, and its heat generates an outflow of particles which blows away the gas and dust in the cloud that still surrounds it.

The hot core is now visible as a pre-main sequence star (see page 535). It continues to gain energy by a slow gravitational contraction. The material in the core is now a plasma, with all the atoms (mostly protons from hydrogen) stripped of their electrons.

Phase 3: a real star at last

After another 50 million years or so, the core is suddenly at a high enough density and temperature – about 10 million kelvin – to tap a new source of energy: nuclear fusion. Some protons now fuse together, eventually forming helium, in the proton–proton chain, a process called 'hydrogen burning' (see page 522). Vast quantities of energy are suddenly released as the core becomes a nuclear fusion reactor. The energy increases the temperature even further and hydrogen burning extends to more of the core.

The star reaches equilibrium

The cloud stops collapsing when the kinetic energy of the particles at all levels is great enough to balance the inward pull of gravity. Compare this with what happens in the Earth's atmosphere: the thermal energy of the air molecules makes them move fast enough not to be pulled to the surface by the Earth's gravity field.

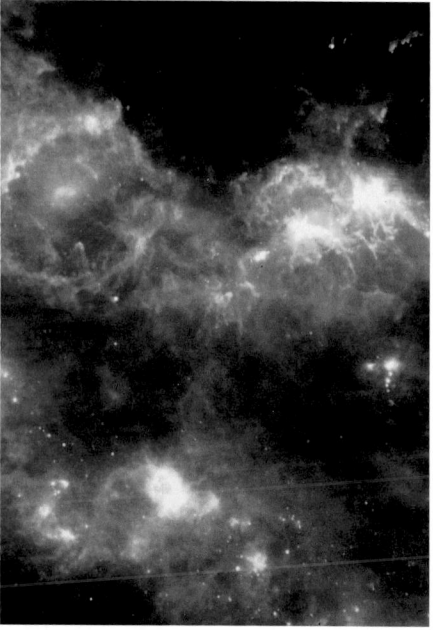

Fig 25.14 As shown by this infrared image of the Orion and Monoceros constellations, there are areas which are strong emitters of infrared radiation, possibly from heated dust grains. One region is the nebula in Orion shown in Fig 25.12, the bright patch seen here at top right

> **? QUESTIONS 6–7**
>
> 6 **a)** Suggest why hot gas clouds are less likely to collapse than cold ones.
>
> **b)** How could a 'chance disturbance' trigger a collapse in a cloud too hot to collapse of its own accord?
>
> 7 Explain why high temperatures are needed before nuclear fusion can begin.

THE FORMATION OF PLANETS AND THE INEVITABILITY OF SPIN

But while these dramatic events are going on in the core, the gas cloud itself is also changing.

Making a disc

All objects in the Milky Way – indeed in all galaxies – rotate about the centre of mass of the galaxy. Think about our original dusty nebula, such as the one in Fig 25.12. It gradually changes from a large mass to one with an axis. The outer edge moves faster than the inner edge, so the nebula spins very slowly on its axis: it has its own *angular momentum* about this axis (see page 72).

Now think of a mass of atoms, molecules and dust at a distance r from the centre of the nebula: it is rotating about the centre of the nebula at a very low speed v, and has angular momentum mvr. As the nebula contracts, this angular momentum is conserved, that is, mvr stays constant. Its mass m stays the same, but the mean value of r gets less, so *speed v* must increase. The result is that the shrinking cloud spins faster and faster.

Some of the gravitational force pulling the material inwards provides the centripetal force for the spinning mass. Less force is available to pull the particles inwards, so the rate of contraction is less than it would be if the cloud were not spinning. But this effect applies only to the direction at *right angles* to the axis of spin. There is no spinning *along* the spin axis, so the cloud condenses more rapidly in this direction, as shown in Fig 25.15. In **condensation**, small dust particles form when atoms and molecules clump together. The cloud eventually flattens into a pre-planetary disc.

We now have another possible equilibrium, when the rotational speed of dust and gas particles is just large enough to keep them in orbit. The gravitational pull of the new central star at the distance of the particles matches the centripetal force needed at that speed.

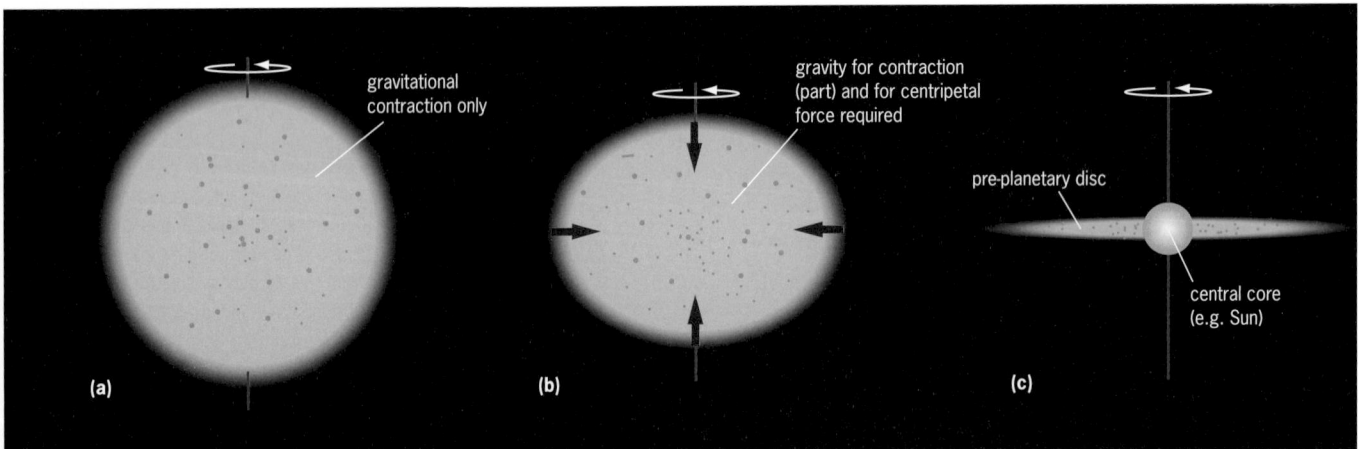

Fig 25.15 Why spherical spinning clouds go flat when they contract

Making planets

The dust grains are not moving in neatly ordered orbits. They have a large random motion and collisions still happen. The particles stick together to form clumps, a process called **accretion**. As the clumps get larger they are more likely to bump into others, so they get even larger. At a particular size a clump is large enough for its gravitational attraction to become significant – it has become a **planetesimal**, able to attract smaller particles to make an even bigger object.

As time goes on, the larger planetesimals grow even larger by accretion of smaller ones, eventually undergoing contraction and reaching the size of a **planet**. This process is shown in Fig 25.16.

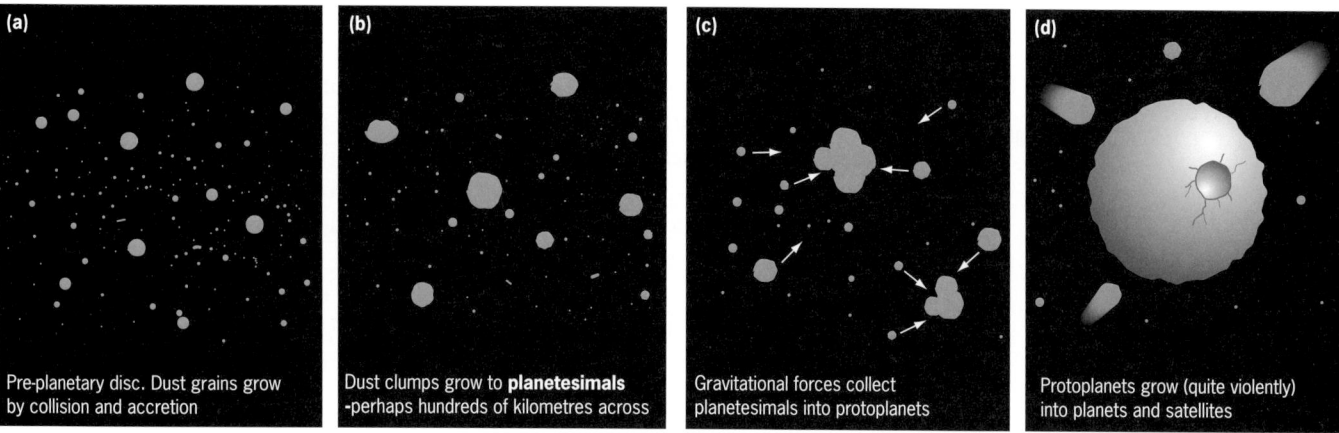

(a)	(b)	(c)	(d)
Pre-planetary disc. Dust grains grow by collision and accretion	Dust clumps grow to **planetesimals** -perhaps hundreds of kilometres across	Gravitational forces collect planetesimals into protoplanets	Protoplanets grow (quite violently) into planets and satellites

With the formation of new planets, there is intense heating when bodies make inelastic collisions with each other, and their kinetic energy becomes the internal energy of random motion of their particles. In the Solar System it is likely that at least the rocky planets became hot enough for their cores to be molten. This caused the separation of the planetary material into layers of different chemical structure and density.

The Sun and the planets were formed roughly at the same time. The Sun is estimated to be about 5 billion years old (5×10^9 y). Radioactive dating shows that the oldest rocks of the Earth and Moon are about 4.6 billion years old. Fig 25.17 summarises the standard model for the formation of the Sun and its planets.

Not everyone agrees with this model as the origin of the 'hot Earth'. It is likely that the main reason that the Earth was hot soon after its formation is the existence of radioactive isotopes. Remember that the half-life of uranium-238 is about equal to the age of the Earth. This means that at its formation the Earth had twice as much U-238 as it does now. It also contained much more of the shorter-lived radioactive isotopes, such as potassium-40, U-235, etc. What remains of these isotopes is the main source of geothermal energy today, even when their abundance is so much less.

Fig 25.16 The planetesimal theory

Evidence for the accretion model

There is not much evidence for the model of planetary formation just described, but all the rocky planets and many satellites have large impact craters which were made after the surface had cooled down and solidified (Fig 25.18). Such craters are harder to find on Earth because of its active geology (plate tectonics), its eroding atmosphere and the fact that two-thirds of its surface is covered by water. But there is still evidence of impacts on Earth (see page 43).

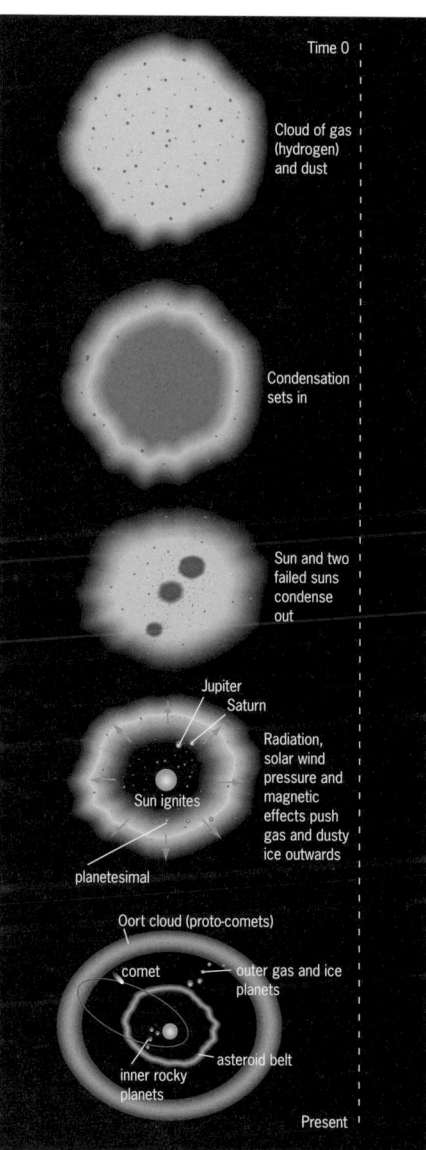

Fig 25.17 The standard model of the formation of the Solar System from a gas and dust cloud

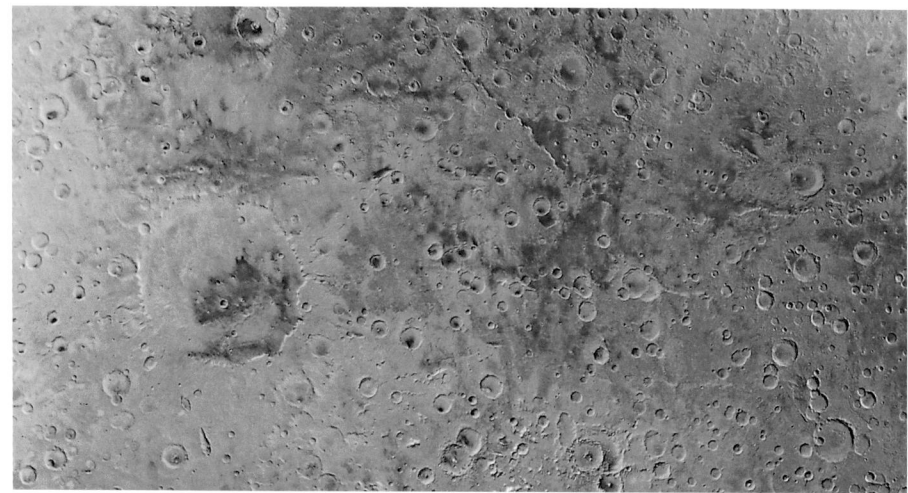

Fig 25.18 Craters on Mars, from images taken by Viking I and II space probes. The Huygens crater, centre left, is about 500 km in diameter

? **QUESTION 8**

8   Outline the evidence for the formation of planets and planetary satellites by accretion.

Why there are two main groups of planets in the solar system

Now think about the early stage of condensation, accretion and contraction. The new Sun created a large temperature gradient in the nearby surrounding cloud. Near the Sun, only those materials with a high melting point would solidify, such as rocks and metals with melting points above 400 or 500 K. Further out it would be cold enough for water ice to form – and even further out it would be cold enough to freeze compounds like methane and elements like hydrogen, oxygen and argon.

Gas particles are light and easy to move. The Sun emits not only radiation but also a stream of particles called the **solar wind**, containing protons and electrons. Both the radiation and the solar wind exert forces on particles near the Sun, and tend to push the lighter ones furthest.

It is assumed that this process began while the Sun was a protostar. The more massive particles of rock and metal were separated from the gases as rocks and metals formed planetesimals close to the Sun, whilst gases were forced further out and became 'icy' planetesimals made of frozen gases. It was these that formed the huge 'gas planets' of Jupiter and beyond.

3 THE SUN AS A STAR

The Sun is an average kind of star and its main physical characteristics are shown in Table 25.2.

We can measure the Sun's surface temperature in two ways:

●   Its spectrum can be plotted and fitted to the *black body curve* (see page 359).
●   The value of its energy output can be fitted into the Stefan–Boltzmann equation for radiation (see page 360).

The Sun's surface temperature of 5780 K provides a black body (temperature) radiation which is mostly in the infrared, but peaks at a wavelength of 500 nm which we see as a yellowish-green (Fig 25.19).

As mentioned on page 599, the *mass* of an astronomical object can be calculated from the period of any object that is in orbit round it. The *diameter* of the Sun can be measured from its angular diameter and the value of the astronomical unit (AU). This measurement gives us a solar radius of the visible sphere, the **photosphere**, of 7.0×10^8 m.

Table 25.2 Data about the Sun

Radius	6.966×10^8 m
Mass	1.989×10^{30} kg
Luminosity	3.863×10^{26} W
Surface temperature	5780 K
Core temperature (estimate)	$8{-}16 \times 10^6$ K
Average density	1410 kg m^{-3}
Age	$4.5{-}5 \times 10^9$ years
Composition at surface by mass	hydrogen 72%, helium 26%, other elements 2%

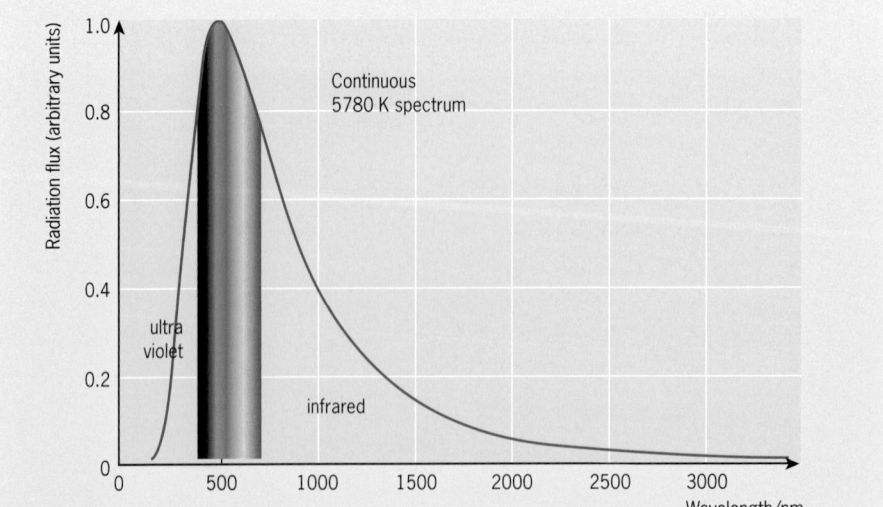

Fig 25.19 The continuous spectrum of the Sun

? **QUESTION 9**

9   Use the data in Table 25.2 to calculate the surface area of the Sun.

EXAMPLE

Q Find the average density of the Sun.

A The Sun has an average radius of 7.0×10^8 m, so its volume is:

$$v = (4/3)\pi r^3 = (4/3) \times \pi \times (7.0 \times 10^8)^3 = 1.4 \times 10^{27} \text{ m}^3$$

Its mass is 2.0×10^{30} kg, so its density is:

$$\rho = \text{mass/volume} = 1.4 \times 10^3 \text{ kg m}^{-3}$$

This is a little greater than the density of water.

THE LUMINOSITY OF THE SUN AND THE SOLAR CONSTANT

Luminosity L is a measure of the total radiation energy emitted by a star. At the distance of Earth's orbit, we measure the incident solar radiation energy to be 1.370 kJ per square metre per second (or W m^{-2}). This quantity is called the **solar constant** S. Some energy is absorbed in the atmosphere, so less than this quantity actually reaches the Earth's surface.

The Sun radiates evenly in all directions and so the radiation obeys an inverse square law. Its intensity I is:

$$I \propto \frac{1}{r^2}$$

The total radiation energy emitted by the Sun passes through a sphere of radius R at the distance of the Earth (1 AU) at the rate of 1.370×10^3 W m^{-2}. See Fig 25.20. We can therefore calculate the total radiation energy emitted by the Sun as $4\pi R^2 S$ where R is 1 AU (1.496×10^{11} m).

This value of luminosity may be used to calculate the Sun's surface temperature T, assuming that it obeys the Stefan–Boltzmann radiation law:

$$L = \sigma A T^4 = 4\pi R_s^2 \sigma T^4$$

where R_s is the radius of the Sun, A is its surface area and σ is the Stefan–Boltzmann constant, 5.57×10^{-8} W m^{-2} K^{-4}.

4 THE SUN IN MORE DETAIL

THE COMPOSITION OF THE SUN

The emission spectrum of the Sun has a number of dark lines in it (see Fig 16.13, page 315). The dark lines are due to absorption by cooler gases just above the hot visible surface that we see. The lines are called **Fraunhofer lines** after Josef von Fraunhofer (Bavaria, 1787–1826) who developed the spectroscope and discovered the dark lines. They indicate the elements that are present at the Sun's surface.

The *intensity* of the absorption lines for an element (Fig 25.21) can tell us how much of the element is present: the more of the element that is at the surface, the more absorption takes place and the darker the line. Such measurements show that the Sun's atmosphere consists of 72 per cent hydrogen,

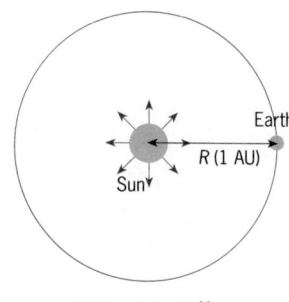
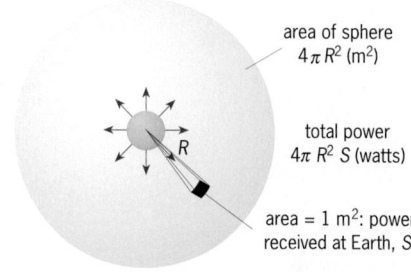

1 AU = 1.5 x 10^{11} m

area of sphere $4\pi R^2$ (m^2)

total power $4\pi R^2 S$ (watts)

area = 1 m^2: power received at Earth, S

Fig 25.20 Measuring the Sun's luminosity

? QUESTIONS 10–11

10 Use the data in the text to show that the luminosity of the Sun is 3.90×10^{26} W.

11 Use the data in the text to estimate the surface temperature of the Sun.

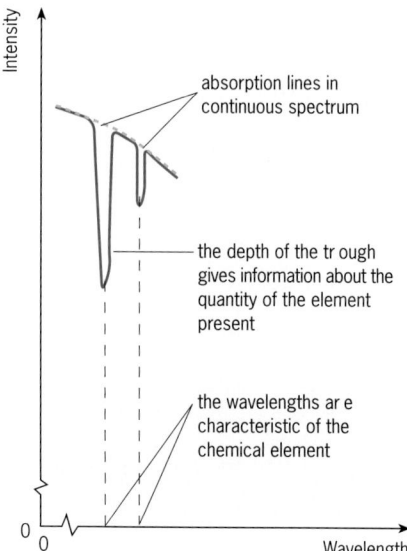

absorption lines in continuous spectrum

the depth of the trough gives information about the quantity of the element present

the wavelengths are characteristic of the chemical element

Fig 25.21 Fraunhofer lines are caused by the selective absorption of light wavelengths by cooler elements in the Sun's atmosphere

> ? **QUESTION 12**
>
> **12 a)** What are the two main features of the spectrum of radiation emitted by the Sun?
> **b)** Which feature **i)** allows a measurement of its surface temperature, **ii)** can be used to deduce the chemical composition of the solar atmosphere?

26 per cent helium and 2 per cent of what astronomers call *heavy* elements, those with more than two protons in the nucleus!

THE SUN AS AN ENERGY SOURCE

The Sun obtains its energy from **nuclear fusion**. In this process, positively charged nuclei collide with each other with enough kinetic energy to overcome the energy barrier produced by the electric *repulsion* forces between them. For this to happen, the particles have to be travelling at very high speeds, which are reached by a tiny fraction of the particles at any moment only when the temperature is more than about 10^7 K. The Sun's core is estimated to have temperatures in the range 0.8 to 1.6×10^7 K.

Nuclei are very small, and fusion reactions will be a continuous source of energy only when a plasma is at a density that is high enough for a sufficiently high rate of collisions. The plasma in the active core of the Sun is at high pressure and has a density 160 times that of water, 1.6×10^5 kg m^{-3}. This is high enough to maintain the reactions.

THE SOLAR FUSION REACTIONS

The fusion process that converts hydrogen to helium in the Sun is the **proton–proton chain**. This is the basic energy producing process in most stars. It is called '**hydrogen burning**', but is not the ordinary kind of burning (oxidation). The key reaction is the most difficult to 'arrange': two protons collide and stick together long enough for one of them to convert to a neutron. It does this by emitting a positron and a neutrino. The positron soon collides with a passing electron and they annihilate each other to form a pair of photons. The neutrino escapes in seconds as it has a very low probability of absorption by matter. The proton–neutron duo is deuterium, a fairly stable isotope of hydrogen. It lasts long enough for further collisions to take place.

The simplest process (but less likely to occur than the one described in the Stretch and Challenge passage opposite) is shown in Fig 25.22. Two deuterium nuclei merge. The net result is that 4 protons become 2 protons and 2 neutrons, and 2 new positrons annihilate 2 electrons.

Fig 25.22 The simplest version of the proton–proton chain

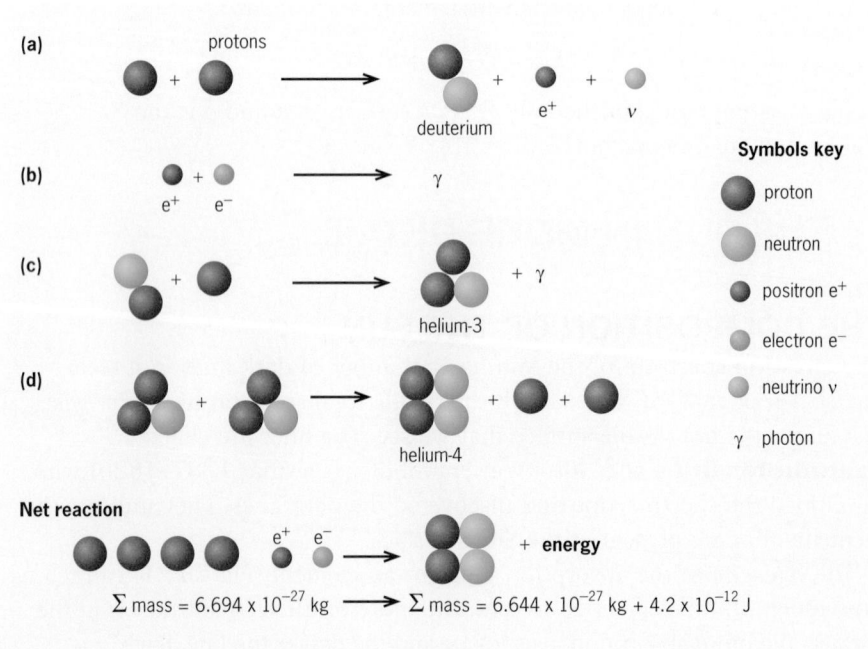

The most likely proton–proton reaction

This starts with deuterium as described in the main text. What happens next depends on the precise conditions in the core. The most likely is a collision between deuterium and another proton to form helium-3. This then collides with a helium-4 nucleus, resulting in the formation of beryllium-7, which in turn picks up a proton to form boron-8. Boron-8 is unstable and emits a positron and a neutrino to make beryllium again, now as Be-8. This too is unstable but undergoes fission to make two helium-4 nuclei.

$$^1p + {}^1p \rightarrow {}^2H + e^+ + \nu \qquad \text{(2 protons used)}$$
$$^2H + {}^1p \rightarrow {}^3He + \gamma \qquad \text{(1 proton used)}$$
$$^3He + {}^4He \rightarrow {}^7Be + \gamma$$
$$^7Be + {}^1p \rightarrow {}^8B \qquad \text{(1 proton used)}$$
$$^8B \rightarrow {}^8Be + e^+ + \nu$$
$$^8Be \rightarrow {}^4He + {}^4He$$

As in the simple process four protons combine to make *one* helium nucleus (check), and two positrons are created for swift annihilation.

The Sun in equilibrium

The Sun is in equilibrium, balancing its internal gas pressure against the force of gravity, and any changes are self-correcting. If the fusion reaction slowed down for some reason, the core would cool slightly and its particles would exert a smaller pressure. The force of gravity would cause a small collapse, and this would increase the temperature as gravitational potential energy becomes random kinetic energy. In turn, the rate of energy production by nuclear reactions would increase, the pressure of the hotter plasma would also increase, and so the balance would be restored.

THE INTERNAL STRUCTURE OF THE SUN

We can only observe the visible surface of the Sun (its photosphere) and have to deduce its internal structure by computer modelling using observations and calculations. The model in Fig 25.23 matches what we actually observe at the surface.

There are three main regions in the Sun: the energy-generating **core**, an **energy-transmitting zone** and an outer **atmosphere**.

? QUESTION 13

13 Use the Einstein relation $E = mc^2$ to show that to provide its luminosity of 3.9×10^{26} W, the Sun must lose mass at the rate of more than 4 billion kilograms per second.

Fig 25.23 The structure of the Sun

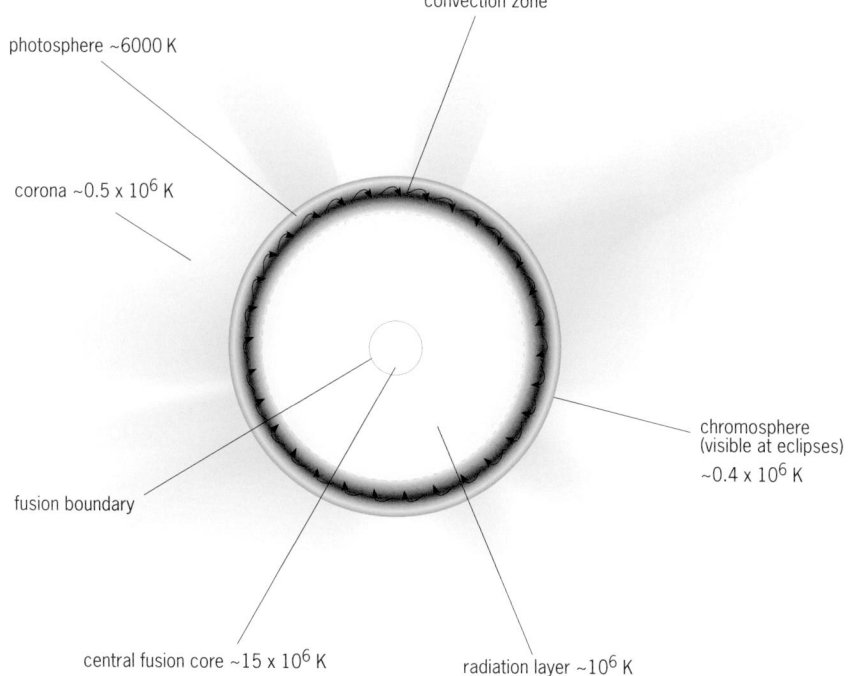

photosphere ~6000 K

convection zone

corona ~0.5 x 10^6 K

chromosphere (visible at eclipses) ~0.4 x 10^6 K

fusion boundary

central fusion core ~15 x 10^6 K

radiation layer ~10^6 K

? QUESTION 14

14 The region above the Sun's core is opaque to radiation, and efficient energy flow can only occur via convection. Explain why this is so. Relate your answer to what happens when heating water in a microwave oven.

The **core** is the site of the nuclear fusion reactions which provide the energy of the Sun. This energy travels to the surface first as **radiation** and then as **convection currents** in the cooler gases of the outer layers.

High-energy photons emerging from the core first supply energy to the gas of the **radiation layer**, making it hotter, but losing energy themselves as they do so. The heated gas expands and rises to form convection currents, just like water in a pan on a hot stove, in the **convection zone**.

This zone has a temperature which is low enough for hydrogen and helium *atoms* to form. Photons are still there as carriers of energy, but energy can be transported more quickly by convection than by photons. This is because the photons leaving the core are easily absorbed, by exciting or ionising the atoms. The convection zone is therefore opaque.

Convection ceases where the Sun's atmosphere becomes too thin. Energy now leaves the Sun as radiation, which means that it is the top of the convection zone that we actually see from Earth – the **photosphere**. Fig 25.24 shows what it looks like: it has a granular structure of light and dark areas when photographed using a filter which passes only the light from very hot hydrogen.

The Sun has two regions outside the photosphere, which can be seen only during an eclipse of the Sun. Next to the photosphere is the **chromosphere**, a very thin region of low density. It is seen as a flash of bright pink hydrogen light at the start of a solar eclipse. At total eclipse, we can see yet another zone of light-emitting gas, the **corona** (Fig 25.25). It is at a temperature of 500 000 K or so, and emits bright lines from highly ionised atoms – neon, calcium, iron and nickel, in addition to hydrogen. The shape of the corona suggests that magnetic fields are involved.

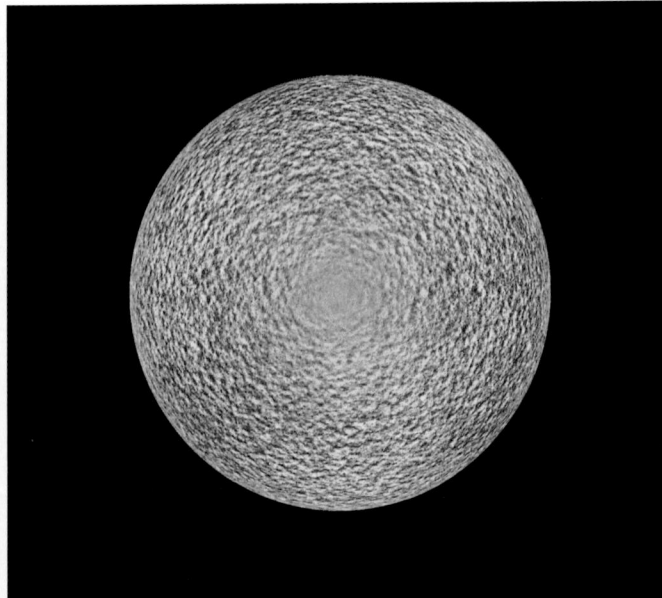

Fig 25.24 The convection cells at the outer limit of the Sun's convection zone. The image was taken by the SOHO spacecraft using the Doppler effect: areas of dark colour are hot gases welling up towards the observer and those of lighter colour are cooler gases moving down

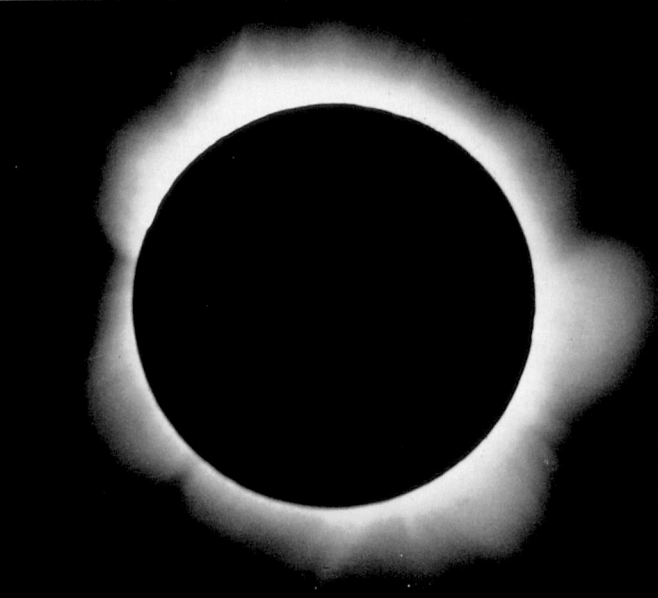

Fig 25.25 The Sun's corona during an eclipse

HOW LONG WILL THE SUN LAST?

The core of the Sun is believed to consist of helium and hydrogen in the ratio 60 per cent helium to 40 per cent hydrogen. Only about 10 per cent of the Sun's total mass of hydrogen is in the core. These are computer estimates as it is impossible to *measure* the amounts of hydrogen and helium at different levels in the Sun's interior. When the available hydrogen of the core is converted into helium, the proton–proton reaction will stop. The Sun as we know it will cease to exist – but see page 538 for what may happen next.

Computer models estimate that about 1×10^{29} kg of hydrogen is present in the core for conversion to helium. But only 0.7 per cent of the hydrogen's mass can be converted to *radiation energy* by way of the fusion reaction; the rest remains as helium. This means that the mass actually available for energy to keep the Sun going is reduced to 7×10^{26} kg.

We know that the Sun emits energy at the rate of 3.9×10^{26} W, or 1.2×10^{34} J per year. This is equivalent to a mass loss of:

$$\Delta m = \frac{E}{c^2} = \frac{1.2 \times 10^{34}}{9 \times 10^{16}} = 1.33 \times 10^{17} \text{ kg per year}$$

Thus, at a rough estimate, the Sun will use up its core hydrogen in $(7 \times 10^{26})/(1.33 \times 10^{17}) = 5 \times 10^{9}$ years.

5 THE EVIDENCE: TELESCOPES IN MODERN ASTRONOMY

We gain evidence about the nature of the Solar System and the wider Universe of stars, nebulas and galaxies by collecting information from the electromagnetic spectrum that reaches us from space. Until recently, all our telescopes have been ground-based, so this information has been filtered by the Earth's atmosphere. The atmosphere is transparent only to certain parts of the spectrum, absorbing almost all infrared, as well as X- and ultraviolet radiation. It also adds unwanted signals called 'noise' to other parts of the spectrum.

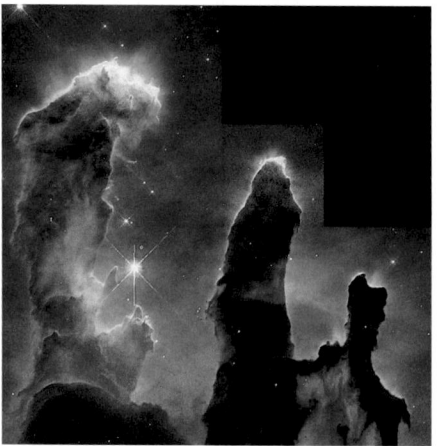

Fig 25.26 Gas clouds in the Eagle nebula, taken by the Hubble Space Telescope

TURBULENCE, TWINKLING AND 'SEEING'

Turbulence in pockets of air in the upper atmosphere affects light from stars, so that they seem to 'twinkle' (see page 510).

Seeing problems can be best (but expensively) avoided by using Earth satellites as platforms for instruments capable of detecting radiations at all frequencies. The most powerful instrument of this kind is the Hubble Space Telescope, launched in 1990, which has added greatly to our knowledge of stars and understanding of the Universe at large (Fig 25.26).

OPTICAL TELESCOPES

The basic physics of telescopes has been explained and discussed in Chapter 18.

The simple Newtonian reflector is the most commonly used optical telescope (look back to Fig 18.30, page 368). The image is formed on a photographic plate or (more often nowadays) by an electronic detector. The image is never perfect. There are three main problems:

- **Diffraction** produces a circular pattern rather than a point image of a star (or other object).
- **'Seeing'** gives loss of detail when air currents in the atmosphere cause random motion of the image that reaches the detector.

● '**Grain**' results because the detecting device has a lower limit to the size of object it can detect. This can be because of the size of the grains of light-sensitive chemical in a photographic plate, or the pixel size in a charge-coupled detector.

RADIO TELESCOPES

There are two main types of *radio* telescope, those with **dish** aerials and those with arrays of **linear** aerials.

Dish telescopes work in much the same way as reflecting telescopes, in that they gather as much of the signal as possible at as great a resolution as possible. They work at wavelengths which are very much longer than light, and the detector is a tuned circuit, as opposed to the photographic plate of an optical telescope.

As Fig 25.27 shows, the largest dish aerial is in a natural hollow in the ground at Arecibo in Puerto Rico. It has a diameter of 305 m. This telescope can only detect signals that enter it from overhead, so can only record whatever is above it as the Earth rotates. Steerable telescopes can point to any object above their horizon but have to be smaller. The largest is a 100 m diameter dish at the Max Planck Institute near Bonn in Germany.

REMEMBER THIS

Images are always diffraction patterns, and the larger the wavelength of a signal, the larger is the diffraction pattern produced. The critical value is the angular radius θ of the circular central peak of the diffraction pattern, as shown below.

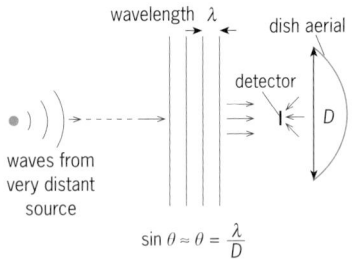

$$\sin \theta \approx \theta = \frac{\lambda}{D}$$

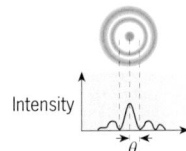

Diffracted image of a point source

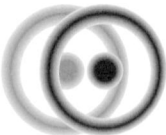

Two sources can be seen as separate if the central intensity maximum of one is on the first minimum of the other

? QUESTION 15

15 a) Estimate the diameter of a radio telescope operating at a wavelength of 0.21 m that could resolve as separate objects two radio sources with an angular separation of 0.5 arcseconds.
(1 second of arc = 1/3600 of a degree, or 4.85×10^{-6} radians.)
b) Suggest **i)** two possible sources of unwanted signals ('noise') in a radio telescope, and **ii)** two ways of reducing these signals.

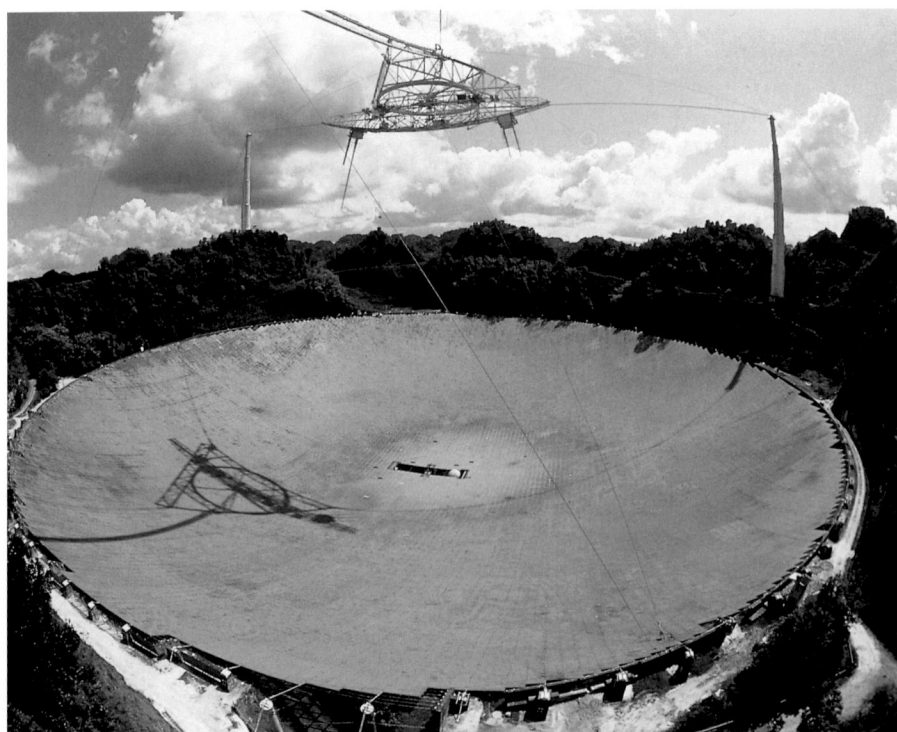

Fig 25.27 The Arecibo radio observatory in Puerto Rico. The dish reflects radio waves up to the receiving antenna suspended 130 m above the dish

Diffraction

Diffraction limits the accuracy with which any telescope can determine the position of an object. A dish of 100 wavelengths diameter can position an object within a region 1 degree wide, which is very much larger than the angular size of a star. Radio astronomy often uses the radio signal from molecular hydrogen at a wavelength of 0.21 m. This means that the early radio telescopes with dishes about 25 m or even 50 m wide could not pinpoint the positions of radio stars – stars emitting radio waves – accurately enough to match them with likely visible sources. A group of stars may be as close as 0.5 seconds of arc, and to separate their images would require a dish 50 000 wavelengths in diameter.

Receiving power

The larger the dish, the more energy the telescope can receive per second. This receiving power is simply proportional to the area of the dish:

$$\text{receiving power} \propto (\text{dish diameter})^2$$

Arrays of dish aerials

Small dishes give much better resolution when they are linked in arrays. This also increases the area of the receiving system and hence the receiving power.

Reflector smoothness

The dish of a radio telescope is made of metal which reflects radio signals in much the same way that a silvered surface reflects light. The surface need not be solid: in fact, it is usually a wire mesh, which is as good as a continuous metal surface provided that the gaps between the wires are less than one-twentieth of the shortest wavelength detected.

Line aerials

A simple aerial is a metal wire in which a signal voltage is induced when electromagnetic waves pass it, due to the electric component of the wave (look back at Fig 15.3, page 335). The signal is strongest when the length of the aerial is matched to the length of the electromagnetic wave. Then, there is resonance between the signal voltage and the wave that is being received. Such an aerial is 'tuned'. Everyday examples are the dipole aerials used for VHF radio and UHF TV reception.

Modern computer programs improve the radio image by adding up signals obtained at different times, enhancing the true signal and cancelling out noise.

Thousands of simple dipole line aerials can be connected together to give a non-steerable array, which makes a cheap but very sensitive system with good resolution (see Figs 25.28 and 25.29). It was an array like this at Cambridge that detected the first pulsar to be discovered (see page 542).

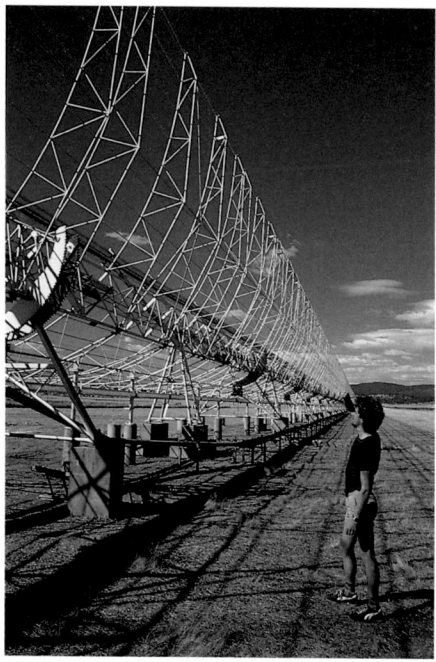

Fig 25.28 The array of line aerials at the Mills Cross radio telescope at Molongo in Canberra, Australia

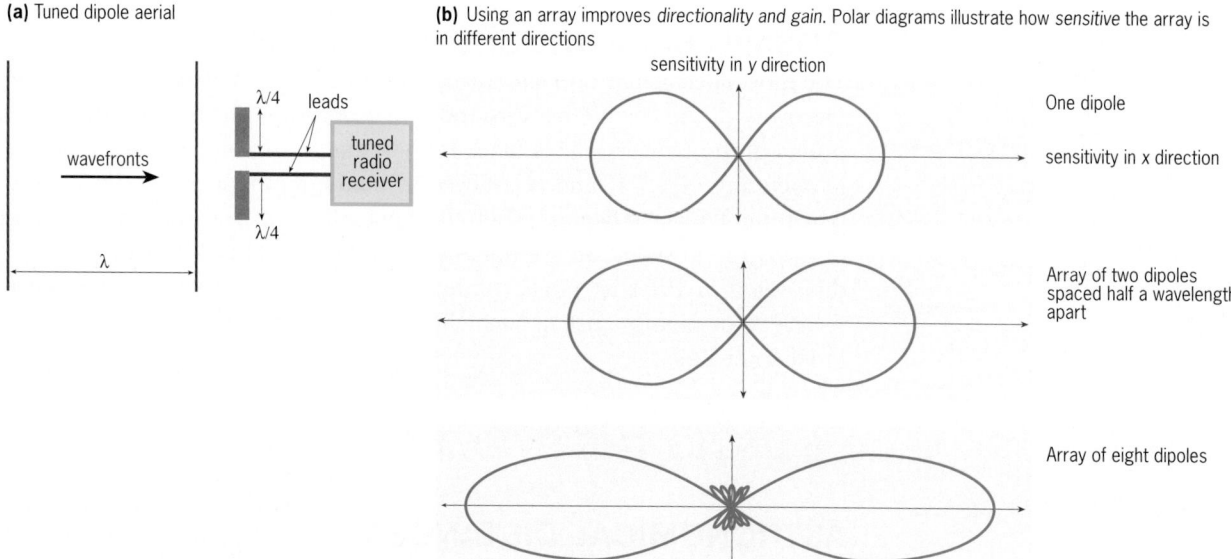

(a) Tuned dipole aerial

(b) Using an array improves *directionality and gain*. Polar diagrams illustrate how *sensitive* the array is in different directions

Fig 25.29 Line aerials. A single dipole aerial, see **(a)**, is directional. The response to an incoming signal is shown by polar diagrams, see **(b)**. The directionality and the efficiency of the aerial can be improved by using more than one dipole in an array

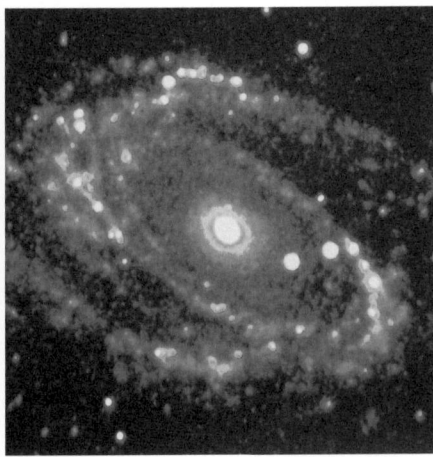

Fig 25.30 Taken by the Ultraviolet Imaging Telescope launched in 1990, this picture is the ultraviolet image of spiral galaxy Messier 81 in the Great Bear constellation. It is about 9 million light years away. The bright spots show where new stars are being formed

? QUESTION 16

16 a) What are the two main factors which determine the clarity of an image made by an astronomical telescope? Suggest two ways for improving images.
b) i) Do image detectors or recorders rely on the wave or particle nature of light? **ii)** What regions of the electromagnetic spectrum are observed by telescopes whose image detectors rely on wave aspects?
c) Why are large telescopes placed either on high, remote mountain peaks or in space?

SPECIALIST TELESCOPES: GAMMA RAY, X-RAY, ULTRAVIOLET AND INFRARED

Atmospheric absorption severely limits the use of ultraviolet, X-rays and infrared for observation, so balloons, high-flying aircraft, space laboratories and satellites have been used to collect data in these regions of the spectrum.

X-ray telescopes have been carried in the Uhuru satellite (launched in 1970, the first to carry an X-ray telescope), the ROSAT satellite in 1990, and several others. It is difficult to focus X-rays as they tend to go straight through materials or get absorbed in them. An ordinary mirror reflector is as useless as a lens would be. Instead, they are focused to a detector by a set of slightly angled cylindrical surfaces which they reach at grazing angles. As explained on page 544, X-ray sources are closely linked with detecting the existence of **black holes**.

Gamma rays are more penetrating than X-rays and reach ground level. There is a gamma ray telescope 10 m in diameter at the Whipple Observatory in Arizona, and NASA used the Space Shuttle to launch the Gamma Ray Observatory in 1991.

Hot stars – those with surface temperatures greater than 10 000 K – emit most of their energy as **ultraviolet radiation**. This region gives the most useful spectral lines for studying the composition of very hot stars and regions of space where new stars are being formed (Fig 25.30). Ultraviolet is strongly absorbed in the atmosphere, so most research uses satellite-borne telescopes. The Hubble Space Telescope also contains an ultraviolet instrument.

Ground-based infrared astronomy uses the narrow bands of wavelengths not absorbed by the atmosphere's carbon dioxide and water vapour. The electronic devices used to detect infrared have to be cooled close to absolute zero (about 2.5 K).

In 1983, IRAS, the Infrared Astronomical Satellite, mapped the whole sky at wavelengths between 12 and 57 μm. It detected some 250 000 infrared sources, identified as stars, galaxies and gas clouds. Five comets were also discovered. Some strong infrared sources are believed to be regions of space rich in gas and dust in which young stars are forming. The gravitational collapse of the cloud causes it to heat up (see page 517).

COSMIC BACKGROUND RADIATION

The most spectacular and significant event of infrared astronomy was the discovery of the cosmic background radiation, found to be uniform from all points of the Universe. This black body radiation is characteristic of a temperature of 2.7 K and is believed to be the remnant of the Big Bang with which the Universe began. (Though often called 'microwave', the wavelengths of background radiation are millimetres rather than micrometres.) It was discovered in 1964 as 'noise' while investigators were testing communications receivers for possible use at such short wavelengths. There is more about this in Chapter 26.

6 USING THE EVIDENCE

ASTRONOMICAL DISTANCES

Astronomical distances are large and very difficult to imagine. Yet the grand theories of cosmology (see Chapter 26) depend on knowing as accurately as possible the distances to the furthest parts of the Universe. Measurement started with the distance of the Sun from the Earth.

Measuring the astronomical unit (AU)

Distances are now measured scientifically in *light seconds*, but converted for everyday use to familiar units like metres (As described in Chapter 1). Astronomical distances are measured in terms of the Earth–Sun distance or astronomical unit (AU) and the parsec (pc), a unit derived from the AU (look back at Fig 25.1).

Kepler's third law can give us an accurate measurement of the ratios of distances in the Solar System. It states that for any planet, the ratio T^2/R^3 = constant, where T is the orbital period of the planet and R is its mean distance from the Sun. This is a consequence of Newton's laws (see pages 515–516). So, for the Earth and Venus we can write:

$$\frac{T_E^2}{R_E^3} = \frac{T_V^2}{R_V^3}$$

or, rearranging:

$$R_E^3 = \left(\frac{T_E}{T_V}\right)^2 \times R_V^3 \quad \text{where } R_E = 1 \text{ AU}$$

The orbital periods of the planets are known very accurately, and we can find the value of 1 AU in metres by measuring the distance of Venus from the Sun. This used to be very difficult, relying on very careful optical measurements. The distance from Earth to Venus has now been measured very accurately by radar. The rest is simple geometry, as shown in Fig 25.31.

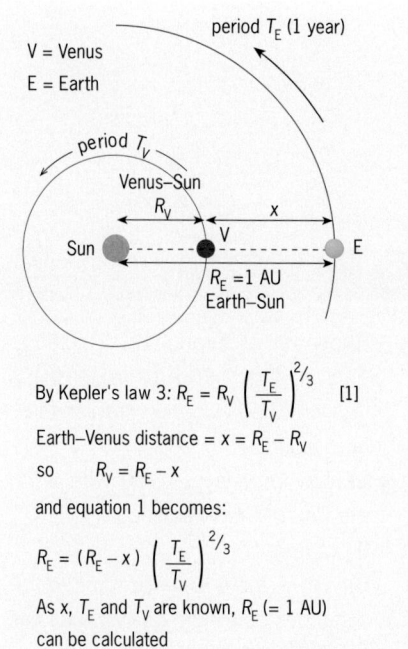

By Kepler's law 3: $R_E = R_V \left(\dfrac{T_E}{T_V}\right)^{2/3}$ [1]

Earth–Venus distance = $x = R_E - R_V$

so $\quad R_V = R_E - x$

and equation 1 becomes:

$R_E = (R_E - x)\left(\dfrac{T_E}{T_V}\right)^{2/3}$

As x, T_E and T_V are known, R_E ($= 1$ AU) can be calculated

Fig 25.31 Measuring the astronomical unit

MEASURING THE DISTANCE TO A STAR

Distances to the nearer stars are measured using **parallax**, as described on pages 6 to 7. What is measured is the apparent change in the angle of the 'line of sight' to a star, measured against the background of very distant stars, as the Earth moves from one end of the diameter of its orbit to the other. This gives a baseline 2 AU long, as Fig 25.32 shows. The Universe is so large that this method can only be used for stars that are relatively near to Earth. The measurement of distances to very distant objects is dealt with in Chapter 26.

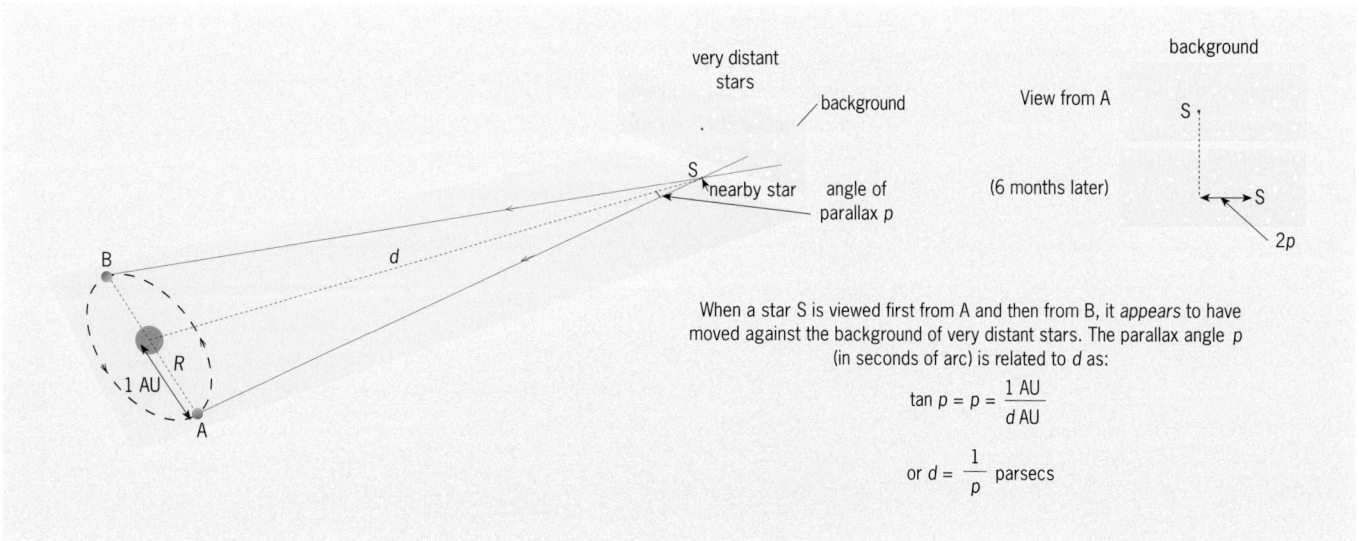

When a star S is viewed first from A and then from B, it appears to have moved against the background of very distant stars. The parallax angle p (in seconds of arc) is related to d as:

$$\tan p = p = \frac{1 \text{ AU}}{d \text{ AU}}$$

or $d = \dfrac{1}{p}$ parsecs

Fig 25.32 Parallax and the parsec

The parallax angle p is very small: the nearest star to Earth has a parallax angle of only 0.772 seconds of arc, or **arcseconds**. This is about 0.2 thousandths of a degree. If p is measured in radians, then we can write:

p radians $= R/d = 1/d$ AU $\qquad$ since $R = 1$ AU

So:

$$\text{distance } d \text{ of a star} = 1/p \text{ AU} \quad \text{when } p \text{ is in radians}$$

But astronomers always measure parallax in degrees rather than radians, in fractions of a degree called *arcseconds*: an arcsecond is a sixtieth of a minute of arc, which is in turn a sixtieth of a degree. Thus they use the distance unit called the **parsec**, pc, in a more convenient formulation:

$$d = 1/p \text{ parsecs} \quad \text{when } p \text{ is measured in } arcseconds$$

A parsec is more convenient because it comes directly from the measurement. It is also so much bigger than an AU that it is more appropriate for astronomical distances.

$$1 \text{ parsec} = 3.09 \times 10^{16} \text{ m} = 2.06 \times 10^5 \text{ AU} = 3.26 \text{ light years}$$

Measuring parallax requires very accurate instruments. Sirius is considered a very close star at a distance of 0.38 pc. Measuring the parallax angle of 0.38 arcseconds is like measuring the diameter of a 10p piece at a distance of five kilometres! The smallest angle that can be measured with suitable accuracy using a telescope is about 0.001 arcsecond. This allows measurement only of stars quite close to us.

The Sun is a member of the Milky Way Galaxy. This has a diameter of 25 000 pc, so most of the stars we can see are too far away to measure using parallax.

? QUESTIONS 17–18

17 Show that a distance of 1 parsec is equivalent to 2.06×10^5 AU. (Hint: you will need to convert radians to arcseconds.)

18 a) How far away is a star with a parallax of 0.001 arcsec in
i) pc, **ii)** AU?
b) Why is there an upper limit to the distances astronomers can measure using the parallax technique?

STRETCH AND CHALLENGE

Spectroscopic parallax

This is the method for finding the distances of stars that are too far away for trigonometrical parallax to be accurate. The name is completely misleading, as it has nothing to do with parallax at all! The method uses spectroscopic data for a star to find its surface temperature (i.e. spectral class), which gives its place along the horizontal axis of the Hertzsprung–Russell diagram (page 535). Then, by using the curve on the diagram, the absolute magnitude (M) is found – although not with great precision as the curve is so broad. The apparent magnitude (m) is measured and the distance D to the star calculated using the relationship (see page 534)

$$M = m + 5 - 5 \log D$$

Distances up to 10 Mpc have been measured using this method – with decreasing accuracy for the most distant. Trigonometric parallax is usable up to 100 pc for Earth-based measurements, but the Hipparcos satellite (active 1989–1993) surveyed 120 000 stars up to a distance of 650 pc.

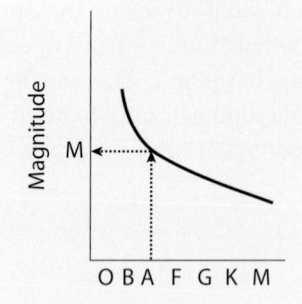

Fig 25.33 Finding *M* from spectral data

EXAMPLE

The star Spica, brightest star in the Virgo constellation, has an apparent magnitude of 1.0 and is classified as spectral class B on the Hertzsprung–Russell diagram (page 535), with a surface temperature of 150 000 K. Using the curve, the data allows us to say that its absolute magnitude lies between –3.2 and –5.0.
Inserting the data:

For $M = -3.2$: $\quad -3.2 = 1.0 + 5 - 5 \log D$

$$\log D = 1.8, \text{ and } D = 63 \text{ pc}$$

Check that, for the upper end of the range, the calculated distance is 158 pc.

The Hipparcos result based on trigonometrical parallax gave D as 80.38 pc.
(Note: spectrographic parallax is not completely accurate so values for close stars can be variable.)

THE TEMPERATURE OF A STAR

The temperature of a star is its *surface temperature*, the temperature of its photosphere. Most types of star produce a continuous spectrum of radiation that follows Planck's rule for *black body radiation* (see pages 308 and 520), although some cooler stars have more complex spectra which makes estimating temperature difficult.

Astronomers produce the spectrum of a star and measure the intensity over a range of wavelengths using a spectrometer (in the past, photographs were produced, but now recording is electronic). The observed spectrum is then matched to the black-body (Planck) curve to estimate the surface temperature T of the star (look back to Fig 16.1, page 307). The simplest method is to measure the wavelength of the maximum intensity in the spectrum, λ_{max}, and then use Wien's displacement law (see page 307):

$$\lambda_{max} T = 2.898 \times 10^{-3} \text{ m K}$$

Astronomical objects range in temperature from just above absolute zero to 10^5 K. This means that the maximum wavelengths in their spectra range from radio to X-rays.

MEASURING LUMINOSITY, THE ENERGY OUTPUT OF A STAR

The **luminosity** L of a star is a measure of the *total* radiant energy it emits per second. Thus L is measured in watts. The radiation follows an *inverse square law* so that the energy received per square metre per second, the **flux density** F at the Earth, is:

$$F = \frac{L}{4\pi d^2}$$

where d is the distance of the star in metres. F is a very small quantity and is the sum of radiation at all frequencies. This is difficult to measure on Earth, since most stars emit most of their radiation in the ultraviolet, which is absorbed in the Earth's atmosphere. Of course, a star's energy may also be absorbed by interstellar clouds as well, making measurement even more difficult.

MEASURING THE MASSES OF STARS

It is surprising enough that astronomers can measure the masses of stars many light years away. It is even more surprising that they can measure the masses of stars that they know are there but cannot see! The methods start with measurements of double or **binary stars**, pairs of stars close enough to orbit round each other.

Eclipsing binary star systems

The brightness of the star Algol in the Perseus constellation varies on a very short time scale: it goes from maximum to minimum brightness and back again in just a few hours (see Fig 25.34). This variation is because Algol is a pair of stars, one brighter than the other, that orbit around each other. So, seen from Earth, they pass in front of each other. We see them at maximum brightness when both stars are visible. When dim star K passes in front of bright star B, it 'eclipses' it and we get minimum brightness – P on the graph. There is a smaller dip in brightness at Q when star B cuts out some light from star K as it eclipses it.

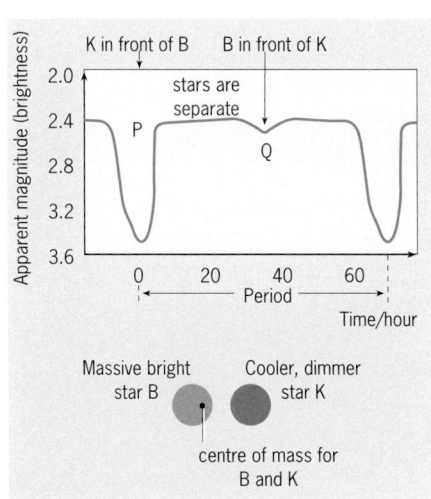

Fig 25.34 Graph for the variations in brightness of Algol, a binary star system

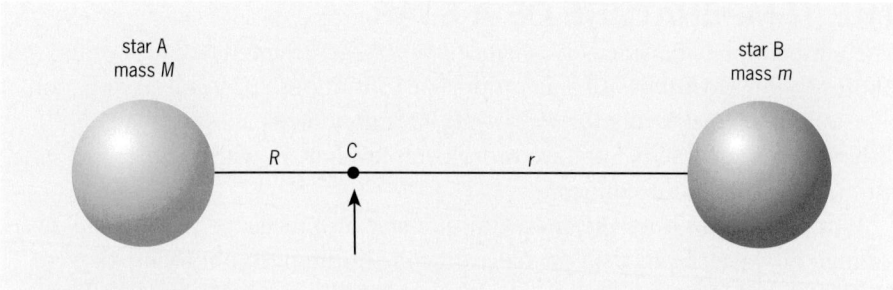

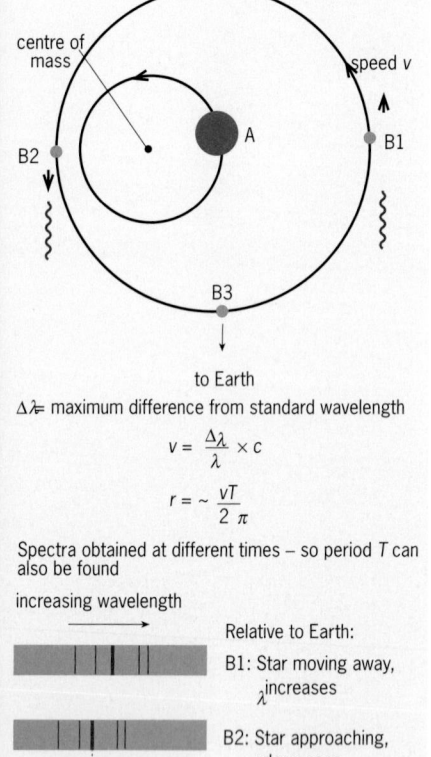

Fig 25.35 C is the centre of mass of the binary star system. Imagine two weights balancing on a lever: $MR = mr$

$$\Delta\lambda = \text{maximum difference from standard wavelength}$$

$$v = \frac{\Delta\lambda}{\lambda} \times c$$

$$r = \sim \frac{vT}{2\pi}$$

Spectra obtained at different times – so period T can also be found

increasing wavelength

Relative to Earth:
B1: Star moving away, λ increases

B2: Star approaching, λ decreases

B3: No relative line of light motion, no change in λ

Fig 25.36 Using the Doppler shift to find the speed of a component of a spectroscopic binary

? **QUESTIONS 19–20**

19 Why are stars more likely to form as binary or multiple star systems than as single stars, like the Sun? Why don't we notice this when we look into the night sky?

20 What is the difference between an eclipsing and a spectroscopic binary system? What main astronomical measurement can data from such systems provide?

Most stars are found in small groups, and often contain pairs of stars close enough together to orbit around their common centre of mass. Fig 25.35 shows the principle of a common centre of mass.

If both stars are visible, we can observe their motions and measure the period of each star. The smaller star is further away from the centre of mass and so moves more slowly with a longer orbital period. However, many binary stars are close enough for the period to be measured in hours rather than days or years.

The period of rotation is determined by the distance between the stars and their masses, and these are related by Kepler's third law (page 515–516), the law of moments (for centre of mass) and Newton's laws of motion.

When the stars are near enough to Earth to be seen separately in our telescopes, we can measure both the radii of their orbits and their orbital periods separately.

From this data the masses of the stars can be determined. The mathematics is not given here.

Spectroscopic binary star systems

Many binary star systems are either so close together or so far away from Earth that telescopes cannot separate them as two distinct objects. But when we study the spectrum of light from the stars we can detect *two sets of absorption lines*, one for each star. The absorption lines arise because elements in the outer, cooler atmosphere of a star absorb light from the star at particular wavelengths (see page 521).

We can also detect a Doppler shift for each set of lines from a binary star system (Fig 25.36). When one of the stars is moving towards us, the frequency of the light it emits increases (wavelength decreases). When it moves away from us, frequency decreases (wavelength increases). With c the speed of light, the change in wavelength $\Delta\lambda$ compared with the unaltered wavelength λ of a spectral line is proportional to the speed v of the star:

$$\frac{\Delta\lambda}{\lambda} = \frac{v}{c}$$

This allows us to measure the speed of each star in a binary system and also their orbital periods (see Fig 25.36). This data can be used to measure their separation and hence the masses of each star.

The simple treatment given here assumes that the stars' orbits are circles and that their planes are neatly edge-on to Earth. In fact, this is unlikely, and more complex calculations are required.

7 STAR TYPES

The Sun is a typical star since it emits both visible and invisible radiation as a result of *thermonuclear processes* in its core. Thermonuclear processes begin only when the density and temperature at the core are high enough, and this happens only when the mass of the gas cloud that forms the star is large enough for a big enough energy gain from its gravitational collapse. If the mass is too small, the body will be a *warm* star with a core temperature less than 10^7 K which emits mostly infrared radiation. Such stars are called **brown dwarf** stars.

Using the most powerful telescopes, the only differences we can see between stars is in their *colour* and *brightness*. These characteristics are the basis of what is still the most useful way of classifying stars.

COLOUR

The colour of a star is due to the spectrum of the visible light it emits. As explained on page 531, the emission spectrum can be used to measure *surface temperature*. The total energy that a star emits is called its *luminosity* (page 531), and this depends not only on its temperature but also on its size.

BRIGHTNESS: APPARENT AND ABSOLUTE MAGNITUDE

In 102 BC, the Greek astronomer Hipparchus made the first *measurement* of star characteristics, classifying them into six levels of *brightness*, which came to be called **magnitude**. Stars of the *first magnitude* were the brightest, and stars of the *sixth magnitude* were the dimmest, just visible to the eye on a very clear night.

Astronomers still use this idea of stellar magnitude, but they distinguish between **apparent magnitude** and **absolute magnitude** (see the Stretch and Challenge box below). A star may look bright because, though quite dim, it is very close to Earth; or it may be a more luminous object much further away.

The light emitted from a star obeys the inverse square law of radiation, so the quantity of energy received per unit area at a particular position is inversely proportional to its distance from the star. To find the star's 'real' brightness, we have to allow for this distance effect, as follows. We calculate how bright the star would look at a **standard distance of 10 parsecs** (32.6 ly). At this distance, the Sun would be classified as a rather faint star of magnitude 4.9.

> **? QUESTION 21**
>
> **21** What is the difference between apparent and absolute visual magnitude? Explain the reason for having an absolute magnitude.

STRETCH AND CHALLENGE

Apparent and absolute magnitude

The modern definition of apparent visual magnitude is now precisely logarithmic and is based on instrumental measurements of energy received in the visible part of the spectrum. The magnitude numbers have been chosen to fit as closely as possible to the historical naked eye observations. The brightness of a star (intensity of the starlight received on Earth) is measured using photographic plates or photoelectric sensors. This gives the **apparent magnitude** m of a star.

The eye perceives the brightest visible star to be roughly 100 times brighter than the faintest star. The scale of magnitude m is chosen so that stars *increase* in measured brightness by equal amounts as we go from $m = 6$ to $m = 1$. So the lower the number the brighter the star, and for the brightest we can see, $m = 1$. The scale chosen means that a star of magnitude 2 is 2.51 times as bright as a star of magnitude 3. There are 5 steps between 6 (faintest) and 1 (brightest), so

a star of magnitude 1 is brighter than a star of magnitude 6 by the ratio given by five steps:

$$2.51 \times 2.51 \times 2.51 \times 2.51 \times 2.51 = (2.51)^5 = 100$$

Instruments now allow astronomers to detect stars as faint as $m = 23$ or so. Table 25.3 shows the numbers of stars in the sky brighter than selected apparent visual magnitudes.

In Britain it is quite difficult to see stars as faint as magnitude 5.

Apparent and absolute magnitude (Cont.)

Table 25.3

Apparent magnitude	Number of stars brighter than the magnitude listed
5	1620
10	324 000
15	32 000 000
20	1 000 000 000 (10^9)

ABSOLUTE MAGNITUDE

The brightness a star would have if placed 10 parsecs from Earth is its absolute magnitude. The brightest star we see, of apparent magnitude 1, is more than 10 parsecs away and would appear much brighter if brought to this standard distance. If it appeared to be, say, 2.51 times brighter (i.e. *one magnitude brighter*), its apparent magnitude would become *zero*. Remember that brighter stars have smaller numbers. If it became 4 magnitudes brighter it would move from a magnitude of 1 to a magnitude of −3. All this works mathematically since we use a logarithmic scale.

We can't actually move stars around like this, but we can calculate how bright they would be 10 parsecs away. The **absolute magnitude** M of a star whose actual distance from Earth is D parsecs (Fig 25.37) is related to its apparent magnitude m by the formula:

$$M = m + 5 - 5 \log D$$

This relationship is sometimes quoted as

$$m - M = 5 \log\left(\frac{D}{10}\right)$$

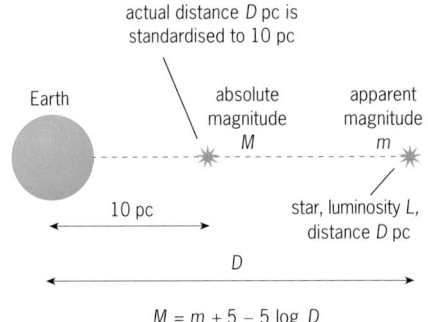

Fig 25.37 Apparent and absolute magnitude

? QUESTION 22

22 For the star Spica, D = 67 pc, m = 1.0. Use the formula in the text above to show that the absolute magnitude of Spica is −3.1.

? QUESTION 23

23 a) Why do we suppose that blue stars are hotter than red stars?
b) How is it possible for some red stars to be as bright (even absolutely) as blue stars?

8 THE HERTZSPRUNG–RUSSELL DIAGRAM

In 1913, Henry Norris Russell (USA, 1877–1957) had the ingenious idea of plotting stars according to two properties: their absolute magnitude M and their **spectral class** (or spectral type). Hot blue stars are labelled spectral class O, less hot and less blue stars are B type, yellowish-white stars like the Sun are labelled G, and so on (see Table 25.4 opposite).

Russell's plot looked like Fig 25.38(a). Note that he plotted the stars with the bluer stars on the left. As explained above, colour is related closely to the temperature of the star. This was realised by Ejnar Hertzsprung (Denmark, 1873–1967) and the plot is now called a **Hertzsprung–Russell diagram**, abbreviated to H–R diagram.

Modern astronomers use *luminosities* instead of the absolute magnitude values, and temperatures instead of spectral class, as shown in Fig 25.38(b). Being pretty independent in their ways, astronomers break the convention of labelling axes by scaling the x-axis with temperature *decreasing* as it goes from left to right.

You might expect that the hotter the star, the brighter it will be, and in general this is true. But Hertzsprung found that some stars were exceptions to this rule. Some were very bright but reddish in colour, so must be quite cool. He reasoned that they were bright because they were very large: they emitted radiation at a fairly low intensity per unit area but looked bright because they have a very large surface area.

A typical star of this kind is the red star in the constellation of Orion, called Betelgeuse. This star has a surface temperature of only 3100 K but is 20,000 times brighter than the Sun. It is so large that if it was in the Solar System its radius would extend to the orbit of Mars. Such a star is called a **red giant**.

There are also blue-white stars with a low luminosity: this means they must be small hot stars, and are named **white dwarf** stars.

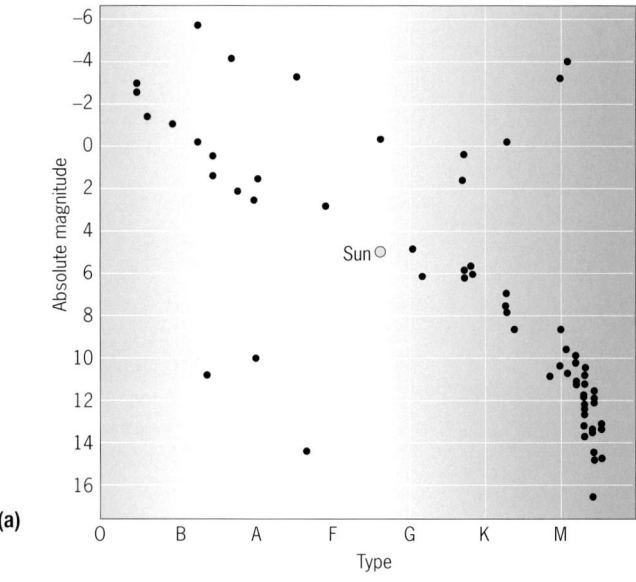

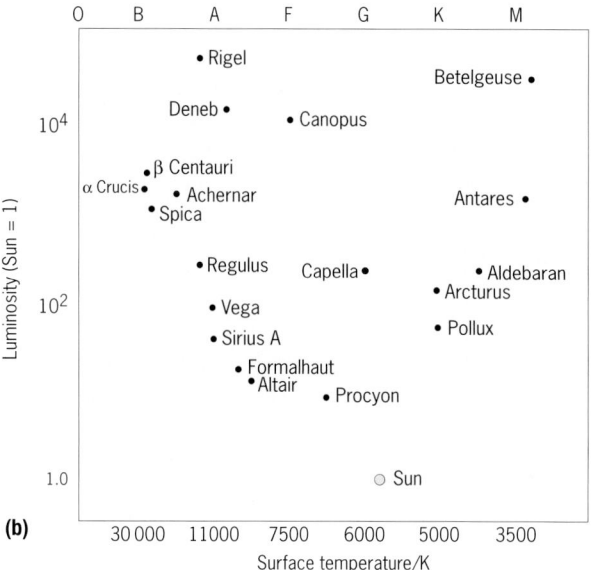

Fig 25.38(a) The absolute magnitude of the brightest and nearest stars according to their spectral class
(b) The Hertzsprung–Russell diagram for the brightest stars in the sky

Table 25.4 Relating spectral class to the surface temperatures of stars						
Colour	blue-white	blue-white	blue-white	bluish-white to white	white to yellowish-white	yellow-orange	reddish-orange
Spectral class	O	B	A	F	G	K	M
Surface temperature	30 000	11 000–30 000	7500–11 000	6000–7500	5000–6000	3500–5000	about 3500

STAR GROUPS IN THE H–R DIAGRAM

The stars on the H–R diagram of Fig 25.39 (overleaf) fall into three main groups. At the top of the diagram we have bright but rather cool stars. They are bright because they are large, as explained above, and are the **supergiant** and **giant** groups. At the very bottom of the diagram are the **white dwarf** stars, which are much fainter, but they range in temperature from about 6000 K to 20 000 K. Many stars plot on to a curving line, going from very bright and so very hot stars (blue-white) to small faint cool stars (reddish-white). These stars form the **main sequence** stars, and are, technically, also dwarf stars. The Sun is a typical main sequence star.

All the main sequence stars are small compared with the giants, but their masses vary from about a fifth of the Sun's mass to about 40 solar masses. A star's position on the main sequence is almost entirely decided by its mass and its age, as will be explained soon. Table 25.5 (overleaf) shows the main properties of some typical main sequence stars.

Fig 25.39 Star groups on the Hertzsprung–Russell diagram

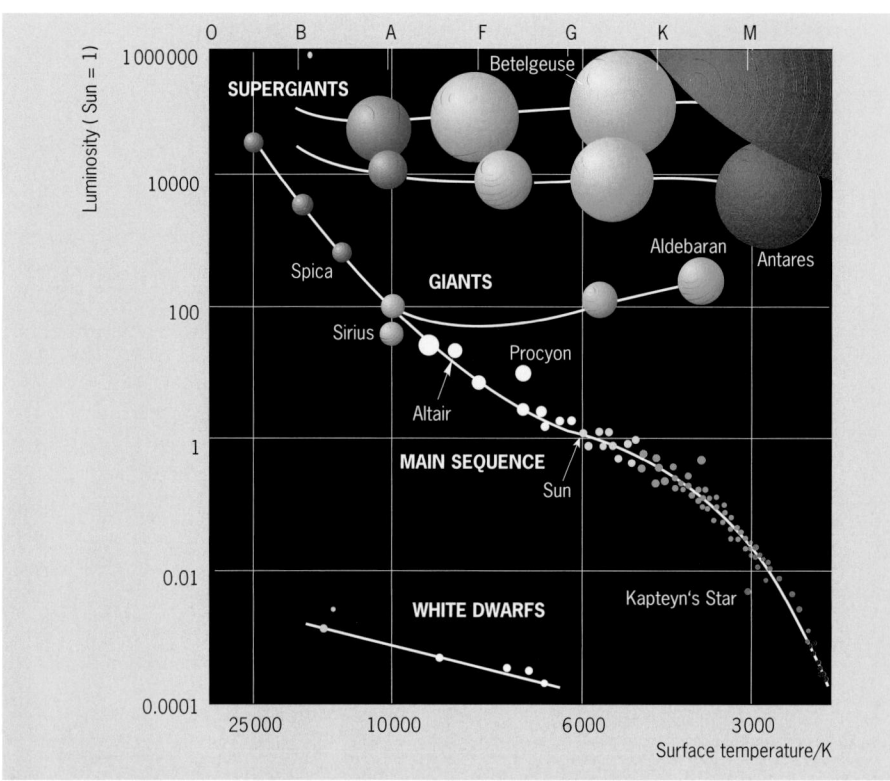

Table 25.5 Properties of some main sequence stars

Spectral class	Example	Surface temperature /K	Mass (Sun = 1)	Luminosity (Sun = 1)	Radius (Sun = 1)	Expected lifetime /10⁶ years
O	Naos	40 000	40	500 000	20	1
B	Spica	15 000	7	800	4	80
A	Sirius	11 000	2	26	2	2 500
F	Procyon	6 600	1.3	2.5	1.2	5 000
G	Sun	5 800	1	1	1	10 000
K	Alpha Centauri B	4 200	0.74	0.3	0.9	20 000
M	few named	3 300	0.21	0.01	0.3	50 000

WHY LARGE HOT STARS ARE RARE

Star catalogues contain data on many thousands of stars. Most are dwarf stars that occupy the cooler regions of the main sequence, and all are comparatively close to Earth. Large hot stars are rare. This is because the hotter the star, the shorter its lifetime (see Table 25.5).

Any very hot stars that formed in our neighbourhood at the same time as the Sun (about 5 billion years ago) have stopped being very luminous. The reason is that increasing the mass of a star increases the density and temperature of its core. In fact, doubling a star's mass increases its energy production by nuclear fusion by more than ten times. So it uses up its nuclear fuel ten times as quickly. To explain this fully, we need to think about how a star is formed and what happens to it as time goes on. So in the next section we look at **star formation** and **stellar evolution**.

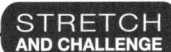
STRETCH
AND CHALLENGE

Identifying star types by their absorption line spectra

Light from hotter stars tends to be bluer than light from cooler stars. But more detail is needed to identify the main star types by their temperatures. This is done by using the line spectra of atoms in the outer atmosphere of stars that absorb photons on their way out of the star.

The key atom in this is hydrogen, and in particular the Balmer series of lines that occur for electron transfers between hydrogen's second energy level and any level above it (see page 286). These lines are in the visible light spectrum, and are labelled as:

line	alpha	beta	gamma	delta
wavelength/10^{-7} m	6.562	4.861	4.340	4.101

Most types of star emit these lines, but the strength of their absorption in the atmosphere depends on its temperature, and this is how stellar surface temperatures are measured. Stars are put into spectral classes based on temperature as explained in the text (page 534).

The Sun has fairly weak absorption of these lines, and cooler stars absorb even more weakly. Stars hotter than the Sun absorb the Balmer lines more strongly until they get very hot, when the absorption decreases again. Very hot stars can produce absorption by helium; cool stars absorb lines of metal ions (e.g. the Sun) and the coolest star type (M type) shows absorption by molecules that can exist in their cool atmospheres. Detailed study of spectra combined with data from laboratory experiments can give quite accurate measurements of star temperatures. Table 25.6 shows the main features of such absorption spectra.

Table 25.6 Features of absorption spectra by spectral class

Spectral class	Typical star	Surface temperature /K	Main features
O	Naos	30 000	few absorption lines and H lines weak. He lines and lines from highly ionised atoms present
B	Rigel, Spica	11–30 000	H lines stronger than for O, lines from non-ionised He
A	Sirius, Vega	7500–11 000	H lines strong; lines from singly ionised metals (e.g. Mg, Fe, Ca) and (weakly) some non-ionised metals
F	Canopus, Procyon	6000–7500	H lines get weaker; lines from singly ionised metals (e.g. Mg, Fe, Ca) and (more strongly than for A) some non-ionised metals
G	Sun, Capella	5000–6000	lines from ionised Ca are most obvious feature; lots of metal lines (ionised and neutral). H lines even weaker
K	Arcturus, Aldebaran	3500–5000	mostly neutral metal lines
M	Betelgeuse	3500	red giant stars; strong lines of neutral metals and molecules

9 THE LIFE AND DEATH OF STARS

STAR FORMATION – THE CLOUD CONDENSATION MODEL REVISITED

It is believed that all stars form in the way described for the Sun, that is, by the gravitational collapse of a large, very massive cloud of gas with a very tiny fraction of 'dust' (small solid particles). Large clouds may be a few light years in diameter with enough mass to produce stars much more massive than the Sun.

Large clouds tend to produce several stars rather than just one. Binary (double) stars are very common in the Milky Way; for example, Sirius, Algol, Capella, Alpha Centauri and Castor (Alpha Geminorum) are double stars, orbiting about a common centre of mass.

We also find many quite large groups of stars that are about the same age and probably formed from the same very large gas cloud at the same time. A typical example is the small constellation the **Pleiades** (Fig 25.40) which contains six very bright, young stars that can be seen with the naked eye. A telescope shows that Pleiades has about a hundred stars. Such groups are called **open clusters**, and some are close enough to Earth to make a

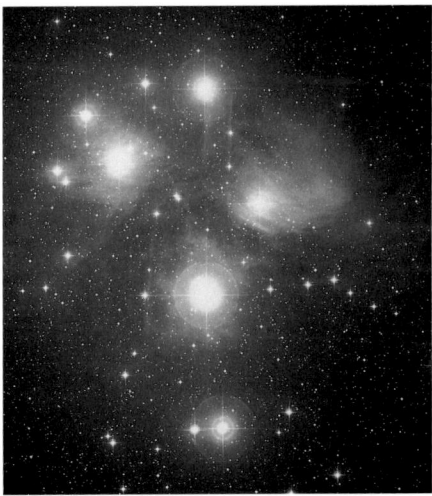

Fig 25.40 The main stars in the Pleiades, an open cluster in the constellation of Taurus. They are relatively young – about 50 million years old – and surrounding them is the cloud of cold gas and interstellar dust left over from the cluster formation. Light is seen reflected by the cloud

splendid sight through good binoculars. (Look back also to Fig 25.14, the infrared image of a star-forming gas cloud.)

REACHING THE MAIN SEQUENCE

A new hot *protostar* gets its energy from gravitational collapse. When nuclear fusion begins, it joins the main sequence at a position that depends on its luminosity and temperature – it is now a *zero-age main sequence star*. Stars on the main sequence have reached a stable balance between their rate of energy production and energy emission, and are no longer collapsing under gravity forces. But how long does a star remain stable and so remain on the main sequence?

THE MASS–LUMINOSITY CONNECTION

Compared with the Sun, a bright A-type star like Sirius has twice the mass and so twice the available hydrogen as a source of energy. But Sirius has a shorter expectation of life than the Sun because it emits radiation at much more than twice the rate of the Sun. This is because the increase in the rate of energy production means that the surface is much hotter – remember that the rate of emission depends on T^4 (Stefan–Boltzmann law).

In general, for stars on the main sequence, the luminosity L is approximately proportional to the third power of its mass (see Fig 25.41):

$$L \propto M^3$$

Roughly, the lifetime t of a star is inversely proportional to the square of its mass M:

$$t \propto 1/M^2$$

Thus, a star of double the Sun's mass should have a quarter of its lifetime. The most massive stars may have 50 solar masses, with a life expectation of 1/2500th that of the Sun. On the other hand, a star of 0.1 solar mass will have a lifetime 100 times greater.

As a result, it is not surprising that the Milky Way has more old, small, dull stars than large, hot, bright ones.

THE DEATHS OF STARS

When main sequence stars eventually run out of their main nuclear fuel, hydrogen, what happens next depends on the pressure and temperature in the core. This in turn depends on the star's mass. First let us consider the fate of a star the size of the Sun. Then we conside more and very massive stars.

THE DEATH OF A SMALL, SUN-SIZED STAR

Hydrogen fusion stops first in the central core, which then starts to cool down. But round the core is a spherical shell quite rich in hydrogen where fusion still occurs. As the inner core cools, its pressure decreases and gravity wins the long battle to make everything collapse. The hot hydrogen-fusing shell falls inwards and heats up even more as gravitational potential energy is lost.

The birth of a red giant

The rate of fusion in the collapsing shell increases, emitting more strong radiation, so that the next layer out in the star actually becomes hotter. This is the *convection zone* (see page 523), and it expands as it gets hotter. In fact, it expands so much that its outer surface, the *photosphere*, gets *cooler*. At this point, a star like the Sun would expand to reach as far as the orbit of the Earth.

The photosphere is now at about 3000 K instead of the 6000 K it was during the main hydrogen-burning period. But the increased surface area

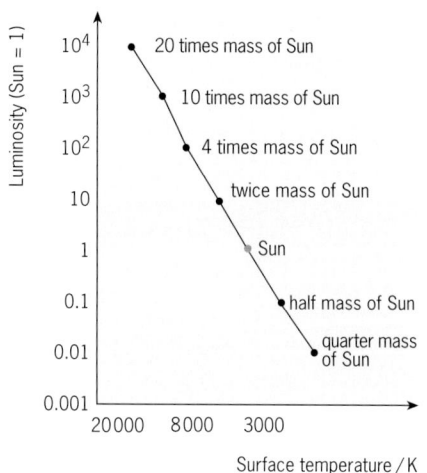

Fig 25.41 How mass, luminosity and temperature are linked for stars on the main sequence

means that more energy is emitted and the star becomes much brighter – its luminosity has increased by a thousand times. The star is now a **red giant**. Looking at the H–R diagram of Fig 25.42, note that by now the star has moved away from the main sequence and up towards the top right.

Even red giants don't last for ever

The story doesn't end there. The core is still collapsing gravitationally, and still getting hotter. It is now also very dense with all its particles very close together. Most of the hydrogen is used up and now there is helium and electrons.

When the core is hot enough, another nuclear fusion process begins: helium is converted to carbon by the **triple alpha process**. Two helium-4 nuclei first combine to form beryllium-8; then this combines with another helium-4 nucleus to form carbon-12.

This new energy-producing process in the superdense core starts up very quickly – in only a few minutes – and may generate enough energy to heat up the adjacent layer which is now also rich in helium. This may then trigger explosive reactions, and matter in the next outer layer of the red giant may be blasted away – in a 'superwind' lasting for some tens of years. Then, as it cools, the star settles down again. Every few thousand years this 'helium burning flash' occurs again. A star like this seems to be pulsating, its size and luminosity varying over a long time scale.

Old red giants may become planetary nebulas

This time scale is too long to have been observed. The theory has been developed to account for objects we *can* see, called planetary nebulas. They are falsely called 'planetary' because early observers with small telescopes thought that they were planets. A planetary nebula is formed when the red giant has ejected enough material to leave the hot superdense core bare and in view. It illuminates the expanding shell of gas which now surrounds it. We can see many objects like this: one is shown in Fig 25.43.

White dwarf stars

The dense carbon core is not hot enough for any more fusion reactions and is now a **white dwarf**. As time goes on, it cools and becomes invisible as a **black dwarf** star.

THE FATE OF A STAR MORE MASSIVE THAN THE SUN

In an ordinary smallish star like the Sun, the triple alpha reaction would be the end of the story. When all the helium is converted to carbon, the star's temperature is too low to trigger further fusion reactions and there is not enough gravitational potential energy available to raise the temperature by further collapse.

But stars more massive than the Sun can continue to create heavier nuclei *and* gain energy (see Chapter 17). For example, a carbon-12 nucleus can combine with a proton to make an isotope of nitrogen starting a sequence that goes via oxygen-15 back to carbon-12 again and a helium nucleus. Again four hydrogen nuclei are involved, ending up as two neutrons and two protons in He-4. This is the **CNO cycle**, the main energy source for hotter stars than the Sun. Further energy-producing reactions are possible as the star ages, causing the build-up of nuclei as large as iron. Making nuclei heavier

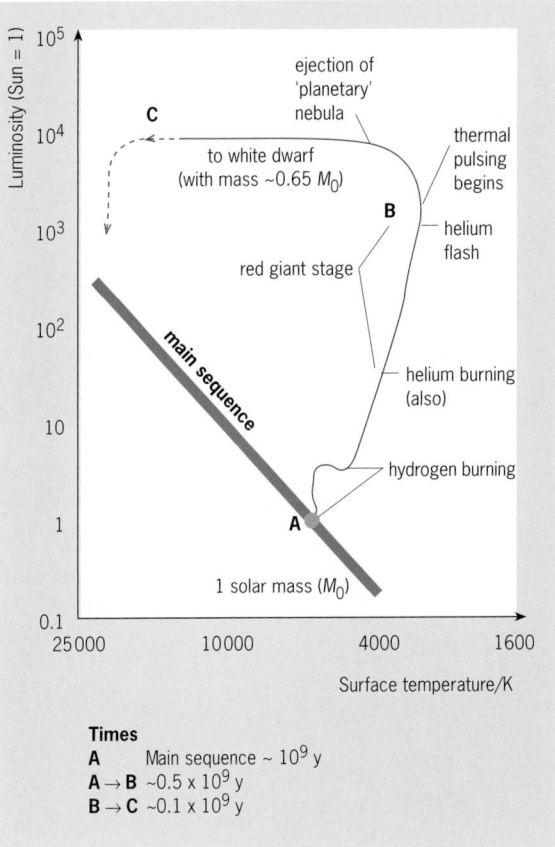

Times
A   Main sequence ~ 10^9 y
A → B ~0.5×10^9 y
B → C ~0.1×10^9 y

Fig 25.42 Final stages in the evolution of a Sun-sized main sequence star

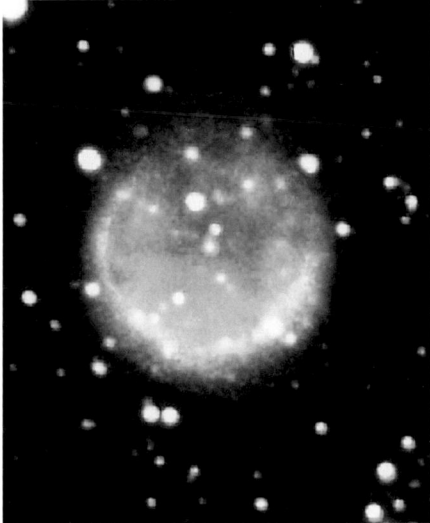

Fig 25.43 A planetary nebula in the constellation of Aquila. You can see the shell of gas emitted from the blue-ringed dying star in the centre

than iron absorbs energy; the heavier nuclei have been created in supernova explosions.

The theory supporting all this is backed up by laboratory experiments on Earth, and the theory predicts quite accurately the proportions of elements detected in the atmospheres of stars.

A five solar mass star

A main sequence star of five solar masses is a bright star, not only larger than the Sun but with a surface temperature of over 20 000 K. It gains its energy by converting its hydrogen to helium, but by a faster process than the simple proton–proton chain (page 522). The temperature in its core is more than double that in the Sun – about 3.4×10^7 K. Such a star emits 500 times as much energy per second as the Sun and, as explained above, it will spend less time on the main sequence. Its lifetime in this phase is only 400 million years, compared to 10 billion years for the Sun.

Once the core has been converted to helium it contracts and hydrogen falls inward to form a hydrogen-burning shell around the now quiescent core. This produces a great deal of energy, but the outer envelope of the star expands so that the emitted energy is spread over a much larger area. Therefore the surface temperature actually decreases and instead of getting brighter the star gets dimmer than it was before, becoming a **red giant** (see Fig 25.44).

The core continues to contract under gravity, so getting hotter, and helium is converted to carbon by the triple alpha process:

$$^4\text{He} + {}^4\text{He} + {}^4\text{He} \rightarrow {}^{12}\text{C}$$

This extra energy stops the star being a red giant and its surface temperature increases. This process then provides its energy for about 10 million years.

When the helium in the core is all converted to carbon, it ceases to produce energy. But burning may continue in a shell around the core and once again it becomes a red giant. The shell burning may provide enough energy to blow away the cooler envelope and the star will appear to get brighter. There are two possibilities for what happens next.

Fig 25.44 The evolution of a star of five solar masses. Stars larger than five solar masses follow a similar track but they may become supernovas that explode and end up as neutron stars

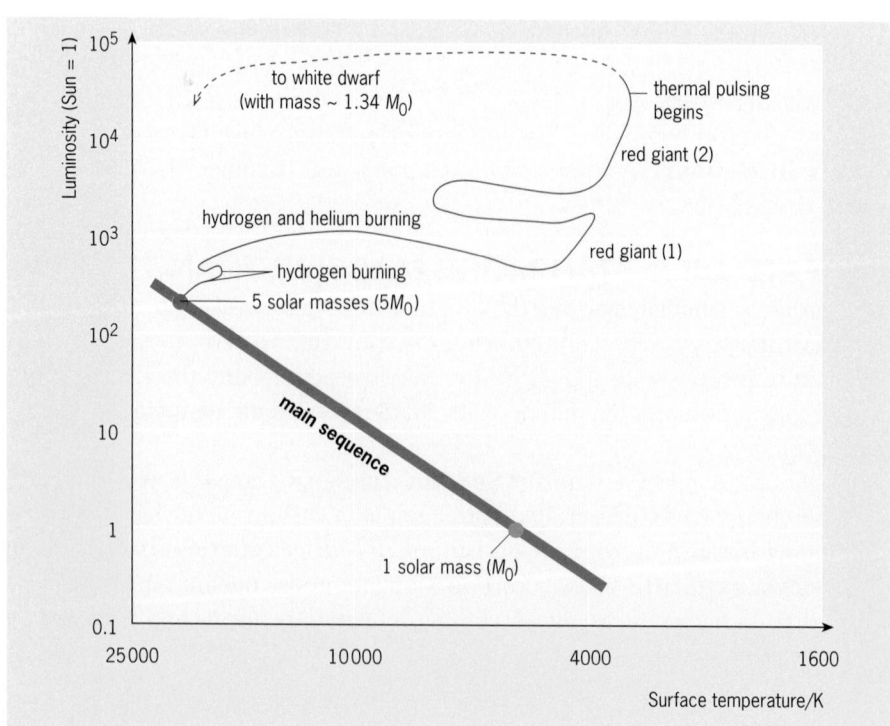

A degenerate black dwarf...

One is that the star continues to lose mass by its stellar wind and quietly becomes a white dwarf star, entirely of carbon and about 1.3 to 1.5 times the Sun's mass. With this mass the particles in the core becomes so packed together that gravitational forces cannot make the star any smaller. In this state, the matter is said to be *degenerate*. There is no energy to be had from gravitational contraction. The core gradually cools down and the end point is a **black dwarf** star.

...or a supernova?

Alternatively, the star might still be massive enough for its outer layers *not* to be degenerate. The star can still gain energy from gravitational contraction and so the carbon core can become hot enough for carbon burning to take place. The core is practically solid carbon, with nuclei and electrons very close together. Carbon nuclei convert to larger nuclei almost instantaneously across the entire core of perhaps 1.4 solar masses. The energy released in a few milliseconds is immense: *the rate of energy emission is equivalent to the power emitted by a whole galaxy of ten billion stars.* What we observe is a new *very* bright star appearing in the sky, a **supernova**. This a **type I** supernova. This is only likely to happen for a fairly low mass star if it is in a binary system, where it can gain extra explodable mass by accretion.

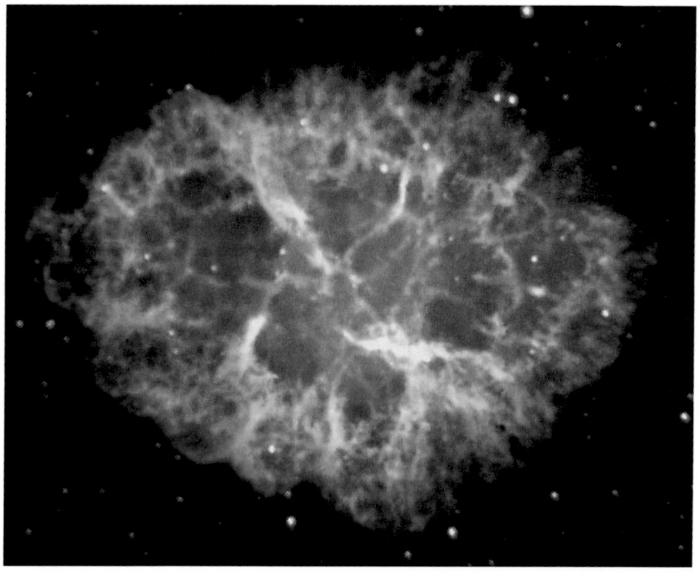

All the outer layers of the star are ejected at very high speeds – up to 10^7 m s^{-1}. The supernova reaches its peak of visibility after about 40 days when the hot material has expanded to the size of the Solar System.

In a typical galaxy, supernovas occur about once every 50 years. This hasn't happened nearby recently, so we haven't been able to study this spectacular astronomical sight at close quarters with modern techniques. The best known supernova remnant is the **Crab Nebula** (Fig 25.45). The supernova explosion happened in 1054 and Chinese astronomers observed it, courteously calling it a 'guest star'.

Fig 25.45 The Crab Nebula. The gas blown away from the star is green, yellow and red, and the blue glow is of energetic electrons spiralling through a magnetic field round the star's remnant, which is a **pulsar** – a rotating neutron star. (The nebula is 10 light years across, and about 7000 light years from Earth)

THE FATE OF VERY MASSIVE STARS

Stars with masses greater than about 8 solar masses develop central cores hot enough to trigger carbon burning in a steady non-explosive way. Nuclear fusion reactions gradually make successively larger nuclei until the central core is made entirely of iron nuclei – the largest nucleus which can be made with a net *release* of energy. Outside this iron-building core are layers of gradually decreasing temperature in which other reactions take place, each producing as heavy a nucleus as it can for the ambient temperature, see Fig 25.46.

Eventually, iron-building stops and, as we have seen before, the core stops producing energy and begins to contract under its own huge gravitational forces. The inner core gets hotter and hotter until at a temperature of 5 billion kelvin (5×10^9 K) the laws of physics produce the unexpected.

The outer layers of the star, and even the core itself, are partly supported by the *radiation pressure* of the photons in hot plasma. At a temperature over 5 billion kelvin, the photons have enough energy to break down the iron nuclei into helium nuclei. But in doing this, the photons lose a great deal of energy, so their radiation pressure suddenly drops and there is a rapid gravitational collapse.

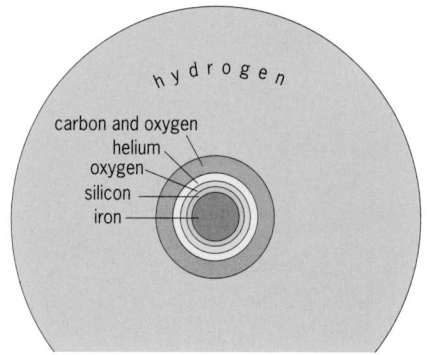

Fig 25.46 Late in the life of a very massive star, there are different types of nuclear fusion in the layers. When the iron core reaches a critically high temperature, its nuclei disintegrate into helium. The core then cools, collapses and triggers a supernova explosion

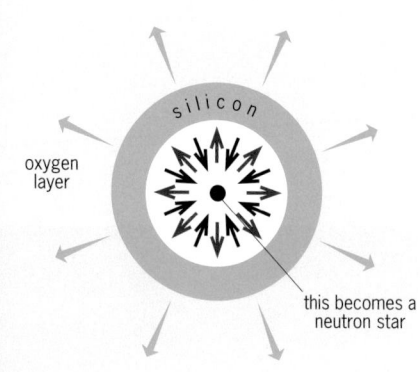

outward rebound blast ➤ infalling material ◄
flux of neutrinos due to disintegration of iron nuclei ➤

Fig 25.47 The massive star's core of neutrons collapses, and the surrounding material (in which reactions continue) falls into it and bounces off

atmosphere (5 cm thick) of iron nuclei vapour

solid outer crust (nuclei and electrons)

mantle (neutron-rich nuclei and neutrons)

central core (hadrons?)

superfluid core (neutrons, protons, electrons)

20 km

Point	Distance from centre/km	Density /kg m^{-3}
A	1	7×10^{17}
B	7	2.4×10^{17}
C	9	4×10^{14}
D	10	7×10^{9}

Mass ≲ 3 solar masses

Fig 25.48 The structure of a neutron star, based on theories of gravitational attraction and nuclear particles

Fig 25.50 Left: The magnetic field and radio emission of a pulsar, a rotating neutron star. The lighthouse effect makes neutron stars seem to pulse. With its strong magnetic field and high spin, the neutron star is a dynamo. The dynamo effect produces a strong electric field which pulls electrons from the surface and accelerates them. Accelerated electrons emit electromagnetic radiation, in this case at radio frequency. The effect is strongest where the magnetic field is strongest – at the poles

The outer layers fall catastrophically onto the core, which is still mostly iron. The core, originally about the size of the Earth, is compressed to a small sphere with a radius of just 50 km. This produces a concentration of matter which is denser than an atomic nucleus, a density at which electrons and the helium protons are forced together to become neutrons and neutrinos.

Meanwhile, the much greater mass of stellar material round the small core is collapsing inwards while undergoing different kinds of nuclear fusion. The temperature of this mass increases tremendously as its potential energy is lost, making the rate of the nuclear reactions increase explosively. The exploding matter falls onto the neutron core (Fig 25.47), bounces off it and creates a shock wave which blows all the outer material into space at very high speed. What we observe is another supernova explosion, called a **type II supernova**. This leaves behind the hot superdense core, a **neutron star** (Fig 25.48), which has a very strong magnetic field.

Pulsars

A pulsar is a rotating neutron star that emits short bursts (pulses) of radiation at radio wavelengths and at very regular intervals. (See Figs 25.45 and 25.49.)

The first pulsar was discovered in 1967 by 22-year-old research student Jocelyn Bell (now Burnell) and Professor Anthony Hewish whose team worked at the Mullard Radio Astronomy Observatory in Cambridge, England.

Jocelyn Bell noticed that one of the many radio sources detected by a very simple radio telescope produced sharp pulses at a very steady rate of just under one a second. The team wondered whether this could be a signal from some kind of extra-terrestrial civilisation. But more observations revealed similar signals from different parts of the sky. It was clear that this was a new type of astronomical object – a pulsating radio star or **pulsar**. Professor Hewish was awarded the Nobel Prize for the discovery in 1974.

The nature of pulsars was worked out by Thomas Gold (Austria and USA). In 1968 he suggested that they were in fact rotating neutron stars. A neutron star, with its strong magnetic field, has condensed from a much larger star which was rotating. So it will still have much the same angular momentum and, being very small, it should rotate very rapidly. A rotating magnetic field will emit radio waves continually, and it will do so along the line defined by the strongest concentration of lines of force (Fig 25.50).

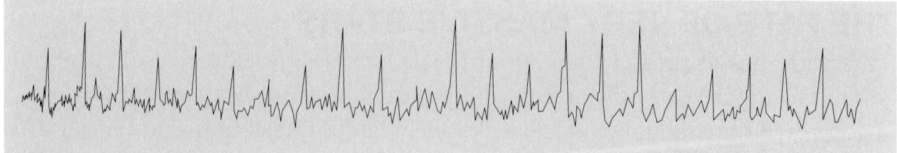

Fig 25.49 The signals from pulsar CPO 328, recorded with the radio telescope at Nançay in France. The pulses last 7 milliseconds and occur at intervals of precisely 0.714 518 603 seconds

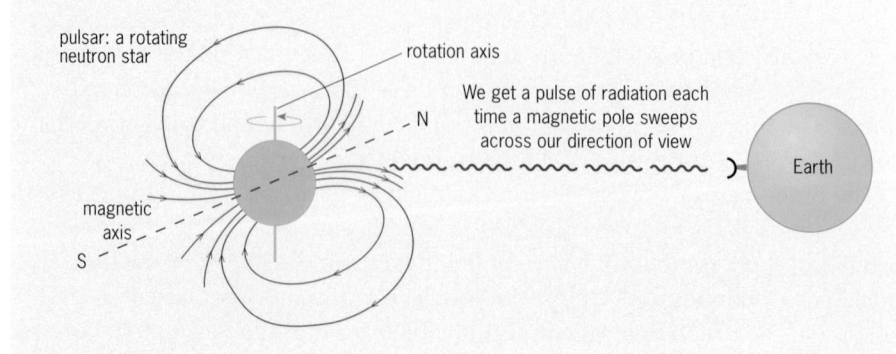

pulsar: a rotating neutron star

rotation axis

We get a pulse of radiation each time a magnetic pole sweeps across our direction of view

Earth

magnetic axis

As the neutron star rotates, its radio signal is detected by a radio telescope on Earth every time the magnetic poles face Earth. This is the *lighthouse model* of pulsars: the radio signal is seen at intervals, just as we see a flash when the rotating shield moves away from the light in a lighthouse.

The signal from the Crab pulsar (Fig 25.45) reaches Earth every 0.033 s, which means it rotates 30 times a second. It emits radiation at all wavelengths from radio to X-radiation, and its total pulse radiation loss is 10^{28} W. This is 100 times the total radiation emitted by the Sun. Earth also receives non-pulsed radiation from it, and its total luminosity, of 10^{31} W, is 10 000 times greater than the Sun's.

Supernovas and nucleosynthesis

The elements nickel, copper, gold, tin, platinum, lead, uranium, thorium – in fact, all elements with nuclei more massive than the iron nucleus – were formed in a type II supernova explosion. When the core collapses to form neutrons, many are ejected into the surrounding gas cloud that contains a range of nuclei. The neutrons penetrate nuclei freely and convert them to heavier and heavier nuclei. These then undergo radioactive decay (beta decay) to form stable elements.

The ejected gas cloud from a supernova explosion is later recycled to form other stars and planets. Apart from hydrogen, all the elements in your body were made in the core or atmosphere of an exploding star.

Black holes

It has been calculated that when a supernova remnant has a mass greater than about 2.5 solar masses, the neutron star formed is so dense and massive that no radiation can possibly escape from it. Then, the neutron star is a **black hole**.

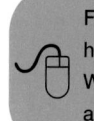

For more information on black holes please see the How Science Works assignment for this chapter at www.collinseducation.co.uk/CAS

Electromagnetic radiation is a form of energy, and according to relativity theory, the energy has an associated mass given by the Einstein formula $E = mc^2$. A photon of energy E (i.e. hf) has a mass:

$$m = E/c^2 = hf/c^2$$

The gravitational field of the neutron star acts on this effective mass. Its effect is not to *slow down* light leaving the star since this is forbidden by the laws of relativity. But just as a mass loses kinetic energy as it climbs in a gravitational field the photons lose their energy until it becomes zero, that is, until the photons cease to exist. Frequency f decreases due to the gravitational red shift (see page 468). Another way of looking at it is to consider the idea of *escape speed* (see page 53). An object is a black hole if the escape speed from its surface is greater than the speed of light.

A black hole must have a large mass in a very small sphere. This means that matter is crushed to a density much greater than that of a neutron star. The theory of black holes was first worked out by Karl Schwarzschild (Germany, 1873–1916), who calculated the largest radius a mass could have and still behave as a black hole: the **Schwarzschild radius**.

How big would the Sun be if it became a black hole?

The escape speed from a spherical mass is given by the formula:

$$v = \sqrt{\frac{2GM}{r}}$$

where M is the mass and r is its radius. G is the universal gravitational constant, 6.67×10^{-11} N m^2 kg^{-2} (or m^3 kg^{-1} s^{-2}) (see page 38). We can rearrange the relationship for escape speed c to give the Schwarzschild radius as $R_S = 2GM/c^2$; thus for light speed (3×10^8 m s^{-1}) and the Sun's mass (2×10^{30} kg) we can calculate the Schwarzschild radius R_S for the Sun as:

$$R_S = \frac{2 \times 6.67 \times 10^{-11} \times 2 \times 10^{30}}{9 \times 10^{16}} \text{ m}$$
$$= 3000 \text{ m}$$

The Schwarzschild radius is simply proportional to mass M. So, to be a black hole, the Earth, which has a mass about a three hundred thousandths of the Sun's mass, would have a Schwarzschild radius of just 1 cm!

On the edge of the event horizon

In general, matter is so dense in a black hole that its actual radius is smaller than its Schwarzschild radius (Fig 25.51). Then, the Schwarzschild radius defines a sphere called the event horizon. Nothing can escape from any point inside the event horizon.

? **QUESTION 24**

24 The escape speed from a black hole is greater than the speed of light. Describe what happens to a photon emitted from inside the hole along a radius, bearing in mind that light cannot slow down.

Fig 25.51 Light and the black hole

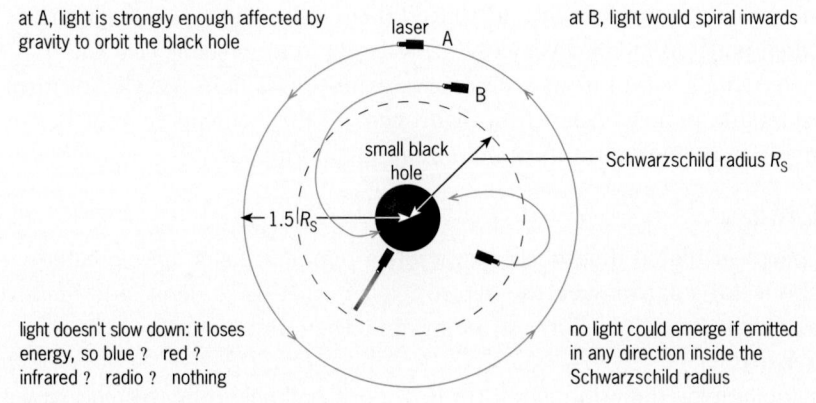

at A, light is strongly enough affected by gravity to orbit the black hole

laser A

at B, light would spiral inwards

B

small black hole

Schwarzschild radius R_S

1.5R_S

light doesn't slow down: it loses energy, so blue ? red ? infrared ? radio ? nothing

no light could emerge if emitted in any direction inside the Schwarzschild radius

Detecting black holes

As neither radiation nor matter can leave a black hole, how do astronomers ever find one?

Imagine a situation in which some material, such as gas or dust particles, is falling into a black hole. As it gets closer and closer, the material moves faster and faster. Collisions cause ionisation and the accelerated ions emit electromagnetic radiation in a very intense, directional polarised beam called *synchrotron radiation*.

The acceleration of particles close to (but outside) the event horizon of a black hole will be so great that the radiation is extremely energetic and will consist of X-ray photons. This suggests that where astronomers detect X-rays, they might find black holes.

Many stars are binary stars. Such stars orbit round a common centre of mass. Quite often, one star is large, massive and bright, whilst its companion is too faint to see. There is a star in the constellation Cygnus named Cygnus X-1 which orbits an invisible companion once every 5.6 days. We know this because its light has a Doppler shift with this period. The star has a high luminosity: it must be a very hot supergiant with a mass at least 15 times that of the Sun and a surface temperature of over 30 000 K. For a star of this mass to move at such a high speed of rotation, its invisible companion must also be very massive. It could, of course, be just a very large dead star, but theory suggests that very large dead stars should turn into black holes.

Another clue is that, as well as having the ordinary radiation expected from a large bright star, Cygnus X-1 also emits vast quantities of X-radiation – in fact at a rate of about 4×10^{30} W, which is 10 000 times the total power radiated by the Sun.

To explain these facts, astronomers have suggested the arrangement shown in Fig 25.52. The supergiant star is close enough to a black hole for its matter to be pulled away to form a disc round the black hole. Some of the material spirals into the black hole and some is propelled away by the gravitational slingshot effect. The accelerated matter moves fast enough to be ionised and so become the source of very intense X-ray photons.

10 THE WIDER UNIVERSE

This chapter has dealt with the basic physics of stars, and of the only planetary system we know about – our own Solar System. In 1996 evidence was found for the existence of large planets round nearby stars, and since then many more have been found.

Astronomers can study in detail only the nearest stars. These are relatively *very* near, being our closest neighbours amongst the estimated 100 billion stars in the Milky Way, which is 100 000 light years wide. And there are billions of galaxies in the observed Universe.

What exactly a galaxy is, and what other objects exist even further away than this is the topic of the next chapter, where we move on to even larger scales of time, energy and distance.

Fig 25.52 The black hole binary model for X-ray stars. Matter from the supergiant star is pulled away by the intense gravity field of the black hole. By the time it reaches the accretion disc, it is at a temperature of 10^6 K – hot enough to emit X-rays

SUMMARY

Having studied this chapter, you should:
- Know about the main features of the Solar System.
- Know that the motion of planets is described by Kepler's three laws, and how they are related to Newton's laws of motion and gravitation.
- Know the current model of the Sun, its source of energy and the formation of the Sun and planets by the gravitational collapse of a large cloud of gas and dust.
- Understand the nature and formation of the inner and outer groups of planets and know the differences between the two groups.
- Understand the origin and nature of comets and meteorites.
- Know how we obtain information about the Sun from a spectroscopic study of its radiation.
- Know the distance units used in astronomy (astronomical unit, parsec and light year).
- Know how it is possible to measure the mass, temperature and energy output (luminosity) of a star from measurements of its distance and a study of its spectrum.
- Know how stars are classified according to their spectra, and how this classification is related to

surface temperature and luminosity, as illustrated by the Hertzsprung–Russell (H–R) diagram.
- Know that stars are also classified according to their brightness, measured as apparent magnitude and absolute magnitude.
- Understand the meaning of apparent and absolute magnitude and be able to use the relationship between them and the star's distance: $M = m + 5 - 5 \log D$
- Know how stars of different masses form and evolve, leading to such objects and events as red giant stars, white dwarf stars, planetary nebulas, supernova explosions, neutron stars, pulsars and black holes.
- Be able to describe how stars similar to the Sun follow a path on the H–R diagram as they evolve to a final state.
- Be able to calculate the radius of the event horizon for a black hole from the Schwarzschild relation: $R_S = 2GM/c^2$

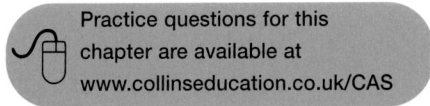
Practice questions for this chapter are available at www.collinseducation.co.uk/CAS

26

Cosmology

26 COSMOLOGY

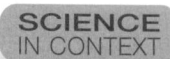
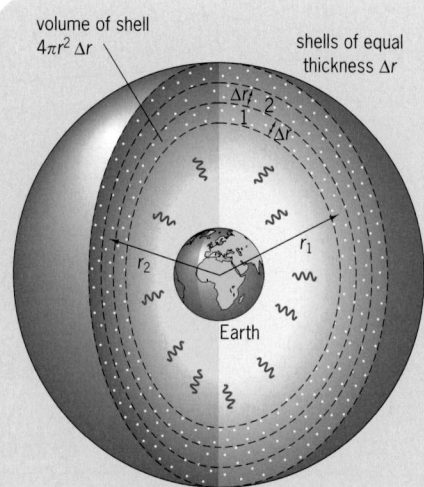

volume of shell
$4\pi r^2 \Delta r$

shells of equal
thickness Δr

Δr - 2
Δr

r_2 r_1

Earth

constant number of stars per unit volume N

Number of stars per unit volume of space = N

Volume of a spherical shell centred on Earth = $4\pi r^2 \Delta r$

So number of stars in each shell is proportional to r^2

Assume a constant mix of star types, on average; then light emitted from a shell is also proportional to r^2

But light obeys the inverse square law, getting weaker with distance, in proportion to $1/r^2$

So each shell produces the same intensity of light at the Earth. If there are an infinite number of shells, the night sky should be infinitely bright!

A strange darkness

With so many stars in the sky, why is it dark at night? This question puzzled astronomers in the seventeenth century and came to be known as Olbers' paradox, after Heinrich Olbers (Germany, 1758–1840) who posed it.

'The Newtonian Universe is infinite in size and contains an infinite number of stars', astronomers thought. 'So everywhere you look, your line of sight should end on the surface of a star, and the whole night sky should be as bright as the surface of an average star.' This is clearly not the case. Even the greatest astronomers could find no flaw with the argument, which is why it is called a paradox. The margin gives the argument mathematically.

But Olbers' paradox is no longer a puzzle. The Universe is still infinite and may well contain an infinite number of stars, but it is no longer a static Newtonian universe. Because of the way it is expanding, light from the very distant stars will never reach us: they are receding so rapidly that the energy of the light they emit is effectively reduced to zero. This conveniently leaves us with darkness at night.

Olbers' paradox. The intensity of light from each shell of stars decreases as r increases. But the number of stars in each shell increases as r increases – just enough to compensate

The ideas in this chapter

Cosmology is the study of the Universe as a whole. The Universe contains not only the very large – such as the huge groups of stars called **galaxies**. It also contains the very small – the particles of matter dealt with in Chapter 24. You will come across both in this chapter, which deals with the main features of the Universe, its age and size, and links the current theory of the Universe in the **hot Big Bang model**.

1 THE MAIN FEATURES OF THE UNIVERSE

 REMEMBER THIS
1 parsec (1 pc) = 3.26 light years

BEYOND THE SOLAR SYSTEM

The stars we see with the unaided eye (Fig 26.1) are the nearest stars to Earth, at distances ranging from just over 1 parsec (the star Alpha Centauri) to 500 or so parsecs.

We see the Milky Way as a broad, dispersed band of light in the night sky (Fig 26.2). A pair of binoculars shows that it is composed of a host of faint stars, all very close together in the field of view.

There are an estimated hundred billion stars in the Milky Way system. A collection of stars this size is called a **galaxy**. Plotted in the three dimensions, the stars form the patterns shown in Fig 26.3.

Most of the stars lie in a narrow **disc** with a central globular **nucleus**, now thought to contain a massive **black hole**. Surrounding the disc is a

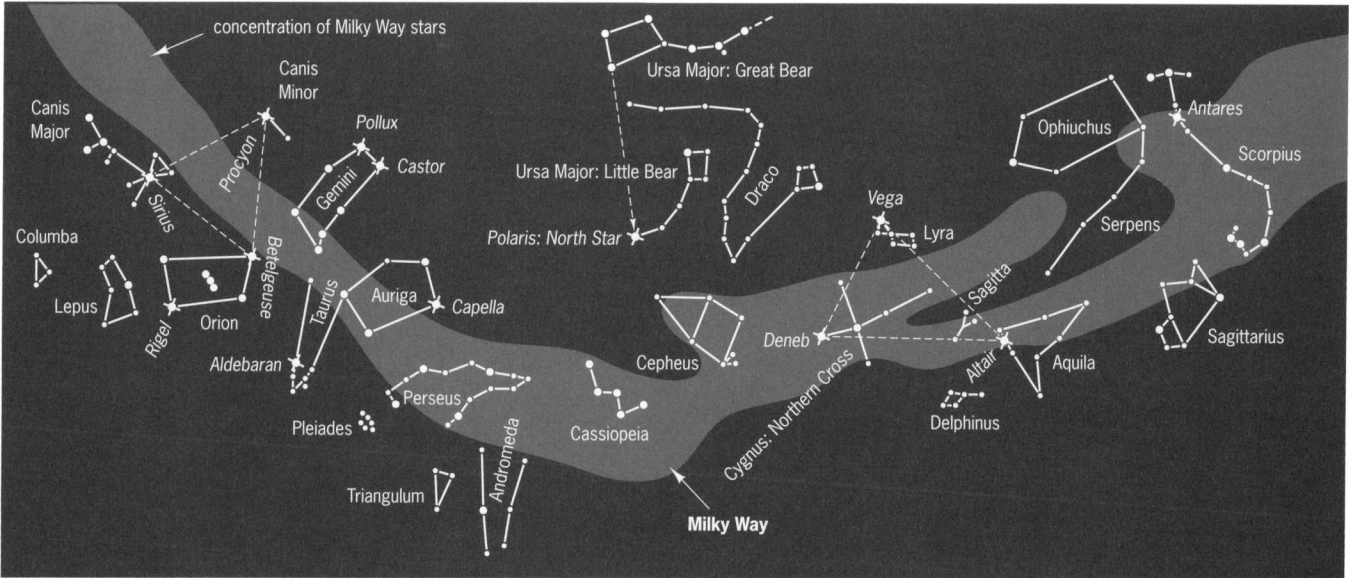

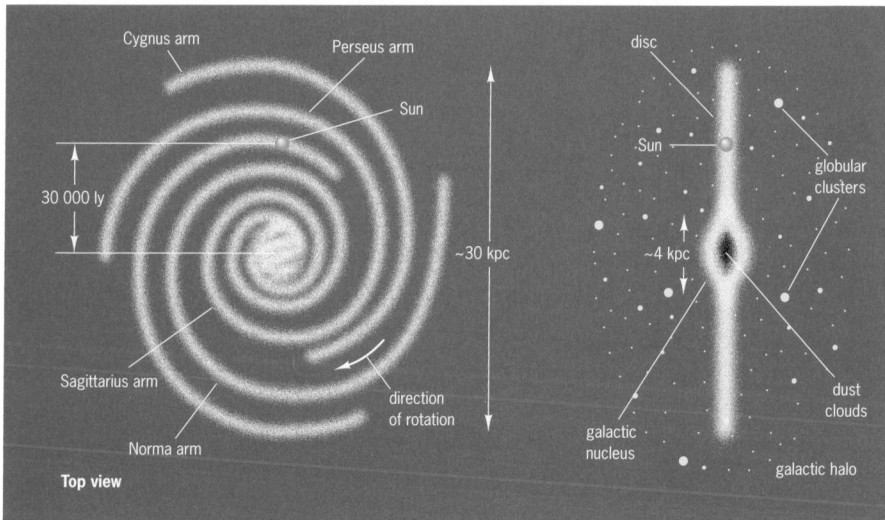

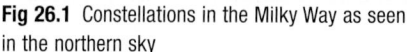

Fig 26.1 Constellations in the Milky Way as seen in the northern sky

Fig 26.3 Left: top view of the Milky Way Galaxy. The spiral arms of our galaxy have been mapped using radio waves emitted by the gas clouds they contain

Right: schematic model of the Milky Way Galaxy. The Sun is at the edge of a spiral arm, about 9 kpc from the galactic centre

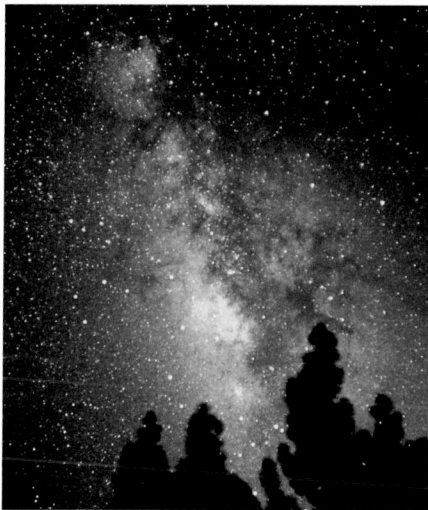

Fig 26.2 The Milky Way in the northern summer sky, seen as a band of stars and illuminated gas nebulae. Dust clouds block out the light of some stars

larger elliptical region, the **galactic halo**, which contains lone stars at a lower density, and a number of **globular star clusters**. Each cluster is 2 to 100 pc across, containing about a thousand to a million Sun-sized stars of roughly the same age, packed closely together.

As Fig 26.3 shows, the stars are arranged in long arms that spiral out from the nucleus, forming a disc 30 kpc in diameter. The Sun is a star of slightly below average size on the edge of a spiral arm, about two-thirds of the way out from the galactic centre.

Constellations are the patterns of stars we see in the sky with the unaided eye. These stars are usually far apart, some being much further away than others, the line of sight giving an illusion that they are somehow connected together. But most stars are in fact quite close together: in pairs, small groups (like the 'Seven Sisters' or Pleiades) or large **stellar clusters**. Stars in the more open galaxies like the Milky Way are about 5 light years (15 kpc) apart, on average. Galaxies are of course much further apart: in our local cluster they range from a few hundred kiloparsecs to a megaparsec or so.

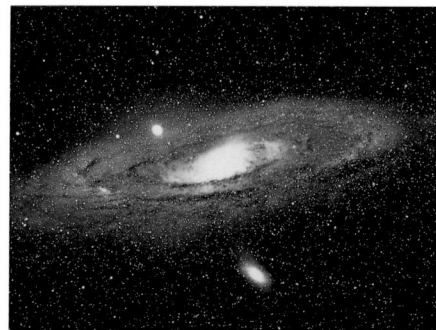

Fig 26.4 The Andromeda Galaxy, the only spiral galaxy we can see without a telescope. It is about twice as large as our own galaxy and is 770 kpc distant. (The two other bright objects are also galaxies)

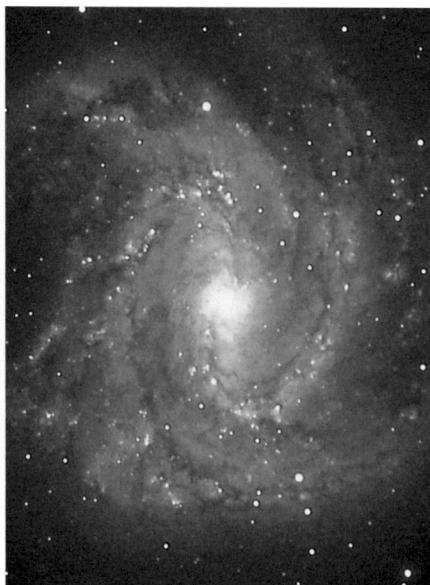

Fig 26.5 The Southern Pinwheel spiral galaxy M83, 10 kpc in diameter and some 10 million ly distant in the constellation of Hydra

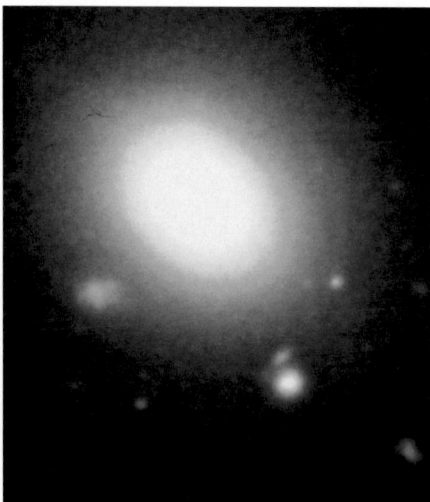

Fig 26.6 The elliptical galaxy NGC 1199

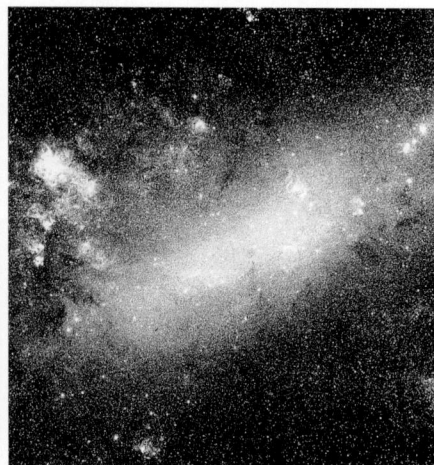

Fig 26.7 The Large Magellanic Cloud, an irregular galaxy

BEYOND THE MILKY WAY

Early astronomers discovered many bright objects larger than stars and looking like clouds of bright gas and dust, so they were called **nebulae** after the Latin for 'clouds'.

Charles Messier (France, 1730–1817) first drew up a list of nebulae, stellar clusters and galaxies, which was published as the *Messier Catalogue*. Most of the bright nebulae in the northern half of the sky are still labelled by Messier numbers. For example, the Andromeda Galaxy (Fig 26.4) is Messier 31, or M31 for short. In another system, the *New General Catalogue* of nebulae, galaxies and clusters, the letters NGC prefix the number.

Later, astronomers found that many of these nebulae were not clouds of gas but collections of very many billions of stars, very much further away than the ordinary stars in the Milky Way. They were called **extra-galactic** objects.

2 CLASSES OF GALAXIES

Galaxies fall into three main classes (see Figs 26.5 to 26.7):
- spiral galaxies, rather like the Milky Way
- elliptical galaxies, with no apparent structure
- irregular galaxies, with no definite shape or structure.

SPIRAL GALAXIES

A spiral galaxy is typically 30 kpc in diameter. Typically, it is a bright object in the sky, with many young hot stars in the arms, and with about 10^{11} stars producing a total luminosity 10^{10} times that of the Sun. It spins about its centre of mass, as shown in Fig 26.3.

The spectra of the stars in the arms show that they contain heavy elements (metals) which can only have been made in a supernova explosion (see page 541), so these stars are recycling material that has formed at least one star already. A spiral galaxy also contains a lot of hydrogen as **interstellar gas** at a density of about six atoms per cubic metre of space between stars.

We detect the gas from the radio waves it emits at a wavelength of 21 cm. Astronomers have worked out the positions of the spiral arms in our galaxy by plotting the Doppler change to this wavelength caused by their rotation.

The separate arms of a spiral galaxy are assumed to have been caused by huge compressive waves passing through the cloud of gas and dust from which the galaxy was formed. These waves compress the cloud and trigger the gravitational collapse that eventually leads to star formation.

ELLIPTICAL GALAXIES

Elliptical galaxies contain mostly old stars. They are not very bright and rarely contain traces of heavy elements (metals). On average, they are smaller than spiral galaxies, at 10 kpc or so, and much less luminous, at about 108 solar luminosity. Elliptical galaxies have little gas and dust, so it is likely that star formation has ceased.

IRREGULAR GALAXIES

Irregular galaxies are smaller than the first two classes, at an average size of 7 kpc. They have a mass of about 10^8 solar masses but at 10^9 solar luminosities they are quite bright for their mass. They contain young, metal-poor stars but are rich in gas and dust, so they have regions of active star formation.

ACTIVE GALAXIES AND QUASARS

Amongst these various types of galaxy are **active galaxies**. Active galaxies have compact energetic *nuclei*, small (by comparison) regions, which emit radiation strongly, with an intensity at least as great as that from a whole ordinary galaxy. The most likely explanation is that the nuclei contain a **supermassive black hole**, with masses 10^6 to 10^{10} solar masses. The black hole draws in surrounding material whose destruction gives rise to the energy output. It is now thought that, in general, galactic nuclei, of the kind we have at the centre of our Milky Way, also contain a smaller but still massive black hole.

Radio galaxies are also active galaxies, and cover huge areas of the sky, centred on a smaller galaxy (usually an elliptic one). The radio waves come from jets of ionised material ejected at high speed from the galactic nucleus: again, the energy seems to come from gravitational collapse, with a supermassive black hole the likely culprit.

Quasars are small, compact extremely bright objects, which emit as much as a 1000 times the energy as comes from a galaxy such as the Milky Way. Quasar stands for 'quasi-stellar' object, because they are nearer in size to stars than to galaxies: they are considered now to be 'naked' galactic nuclei. They were first discovered as intense radio 'stars'. The most likely energy source is the same as that for active galaxies, but they produce much more energy. Because they are so bright, they are the furthest objects we can see and obtain red shifts for.

3 MEASURING THE DISTANCES TO GALAXIES

The distances to the nearest stars can be found by triangulation – the method of **parallax** described on page 529. But extra-galactic objects such as galaxies are too far away to show parallax. Table 26.1 lists distances to some of the objects in the Universe, and the various methods that need to be used to measure the distances. These methods are also shown in Fig 26.8 and some of them are discussed in the following sections.

Table 26.1 Astronomical distances

Object	Comment	Distance	Measurement method(s)
Sirius	a nearby star	2.6 pc	parallax (trigonometry)
various	distant stars in our galaxy	up to 5 pc	parallax from satellite star colour – linked to luminosity
Large Magellanic Cloud	small irregular galaxy close to Milky Way Galaxy	50 kpc	cepheid variables
Andromeda Galaxy M31	largest galaxy (spiral) in our Local Cluster	770 kpc	cepheid variables
Virgo Cluster	nearest large cluster of galaxies in our Local Supercluster	20 Mpc	variables, novas (exploding stars), blue supergiant stars
Hercules Supercluster	nearest supercluster to ours	200–300 Mpc	supernovas, brightest galaxies in a cluster
Hydra Cluster	a large cluster of galaxies	1200 Mpc	brightest galaxies in a cluster
3C-324	furthest galaxy so far measured (radio)	2500 Mpc	red shift
Q0000-263	furthest quasar so far measured	3600 Mpc	red shift

Fig 26.8 Measuring the distances of astronomical objects

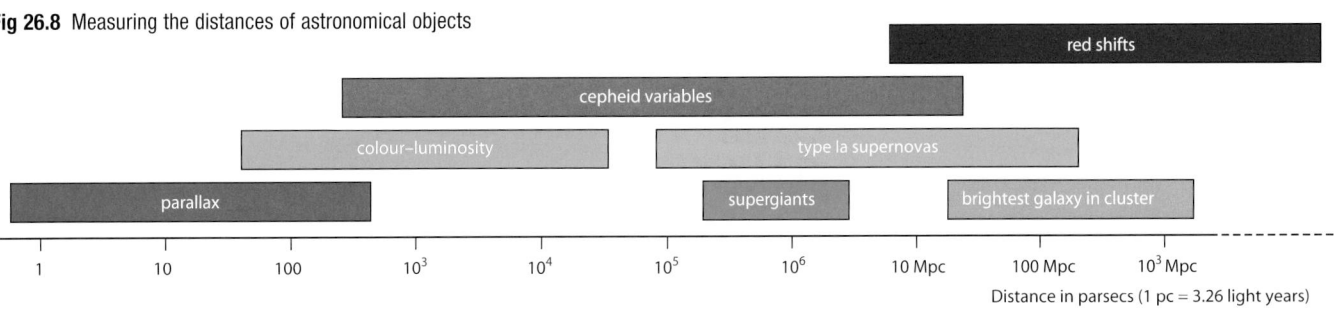

Distance in parsecs (1 pc = 3.26 light years)

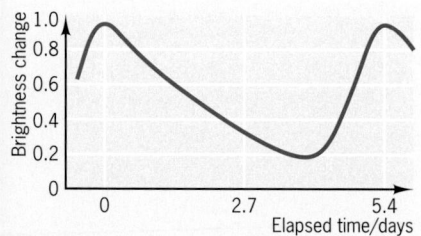

Fig 26.9(a) Brightness curve for the cepheid variable star Delta Cephei. The period of the variation in brightness is regular, with a peak-to-peak time of about 5.4 days

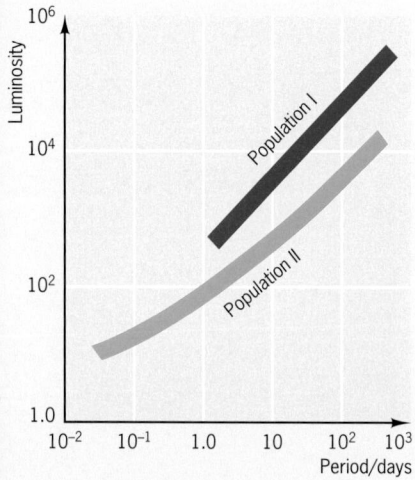

Fig 26.9(b) Simplified period–luminosity relation for cepheids, showing the linear relationship for absolute magnitude and the log of the period

? QUESTION 1

1 A cepheid variable of known absolute magnitude −2.5 is measured from Earth to have an apparent magnitude of 14.5. Show that the star is about 25 kpc away.

DISTANCE, BRIGHTNESS AND CEPHEID VARIABLES

Edwin Hubble (USA, 1889–1953) was the first astronomer to study galaxies and their distances in detail. This work, begun in 1924, used the 2.5 m diameter Newtonian reflector at Mount Wilson in California – the largest telescope in the world at the time.

He also used a very good method for measuring the distances to galaxies based on an odd kind of star called a **cepheid variable**, or cepheid for short, named after Delta Cephei in the constellation Cepheus, the first such star discovered.

These stars vary in their brightness very regularly over time, as shown in Fig 26.9(a). The astronomer Henrietta Leavitt (USA, 1868–1921) had found many cepheids in the irregular galaxies called the Magellanic Clouds (Fig 26.7) and was able to show that the period of the variation is related to the star's intrinsic brightness – its absolute magnitude, see Fig 26.9(b). Once the distance of a typical nearby cepheid had been found it was possible to calibrate the variation graphs. This allowed a simple calculation of a star's absolute brightness and hence its distance using the relationship between absolute (M) and apparent magnitude (m) and distance (D) in parsecs:

$$M = m + 5 - 5 \log D$$

(see Chapter 25, page 534).

Hubble used data about cepheids found in the Andromeda Galaxy M31 (Fig 26.4) to calculate its distance and confirmed that this was an extra-galactic object. (In 1923 it had been the first galaxy to have its distance estimated, at 450 kpc, using an assumption about its luminosity.) Unfortunately for Hubble, there are two kinds of cepheid star, and not knowing this at the time he used data for the wrong kind, so his measured distances for galaxies containing cepheids were all too low. For example, for M31 he obtained a distance of 330 kpc. It was later found to be 770 kpc.

Cepheids are brighter than the Sun, but even so, when they are too far away they get too faint to be useful for calculating differences. Recently the Hubble Space Telescope has extended the range from about 6 Mpc to about 17 Mpc.

USING VERY BRIGHT OBJECTS

The same magnitude–distance formula can be used to measure distances further out, using very bright stars of known luminosity, such as **supergiant** stars to 10 Mpc, and even **supernovas** (to 200 Mpc). The same method can be used to 1200 Mpc by assuming that the brightest galaxies all have much the same size and so have similar luminosity.

RED SHIFT

As the Universe is expanding (see page 554) light from distant objects shows a Doppler effect (see page 141) causing a shift of spectral lines to the red (long wavelength) end of the electromagnetic spectrum, and this can be used to measure very large distances. See page 555.

4 CLUSTERS AND SUPERCLUSTERS OF GALAXIES

Galaxies are clustered into groups, made of galaxies quite close together compared with distances to neighbouring groups. The Milky Way and the

Andromeda Galaxy are in fact the two largest galaxies in a **cluster** of 30 galaxies – the Local Group (Fig 26.10) – occupying a region of space about 1 Mpc across and affecting each other gravitationally. The largest two, the Milky Way and the Andromeda Galaxy, orbit each other and have the greatest gravitational effect on the whole group.

The **Virgo Cluster** is our nearest-neighbour cluster, about 18 Mpc away in the direction of the constellation Virgo. A small part is shown in Fig 26.11. It is a huge cluster, about 3 Mpc across, spanning a region of the sky 14 times as large as the Moon but too faint to be seen with the naked eye. It contains several thousand galaxies and its gravitational field is large enough to affect the movement of our own Local Group.

Distance measurements show that nearly all galaxies are grouped in such clusters. Clusters range in size from the very small with just an isolated pair of galaxies, to the very large. Large clusters may have galaxies widely spread out, or close enough to be tightly bound by a common gravitational field in which individual galaxies orbit.

Clusters of galaxies are themselves in larger groupings called **superclusters**. Our Local Supercluster is a roughly disc-shaped collection of 382 galaxy clusters about 700 Mpc across (Fig 26.12(a)), with the Local Group at the centre, and the Virgo Cluster at the edge.

There is then a 100 Mpc region of empty space before we reach the next supercluster (in the constellation of Hercules), as in Fig 26.12(b). This pattern of superclusters and voids continues on an even larger scale, as shown in Fig 26.12(c). This may resemble the way that matter arranged itself in the first moments of the early Universe.

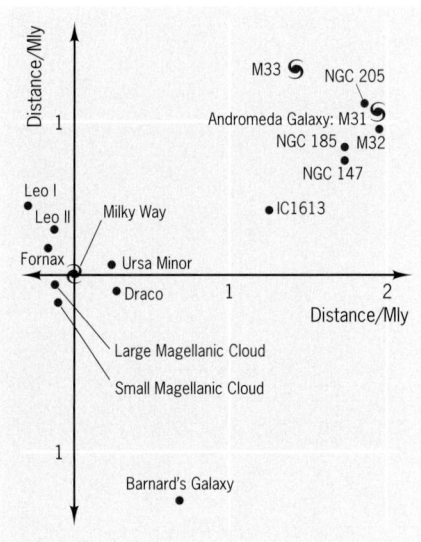

Fig 26.10 Some of the main galaxies in the Local Group, from a view above the Milky Way. Most of these galaxies are elliptical or irregular, M31 and the Milky Way being the largest. The Local Group occupies about a cubic megaparsec of space (Fig 26.12(a), centre)

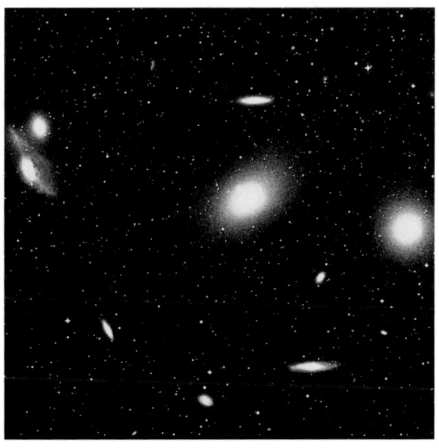

Fig 26.11 Elliptical and spiral galaxies in the Virgo Cluster which contains several thousand galaxies. At a distance of 19 Mpc, it is the nearest main cluster to the Local Group

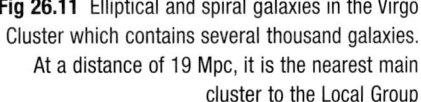
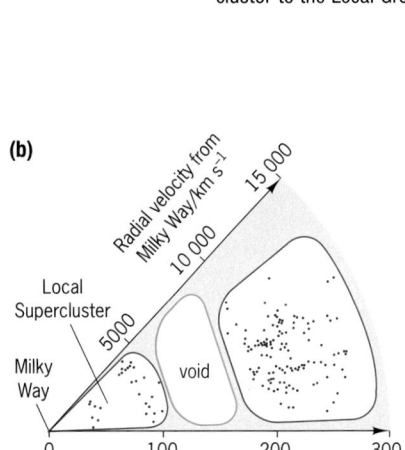
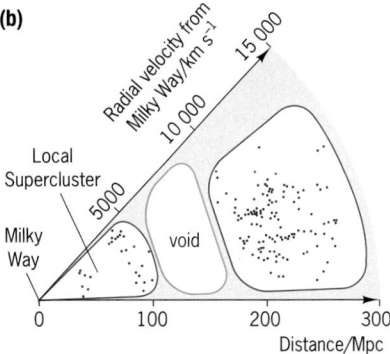

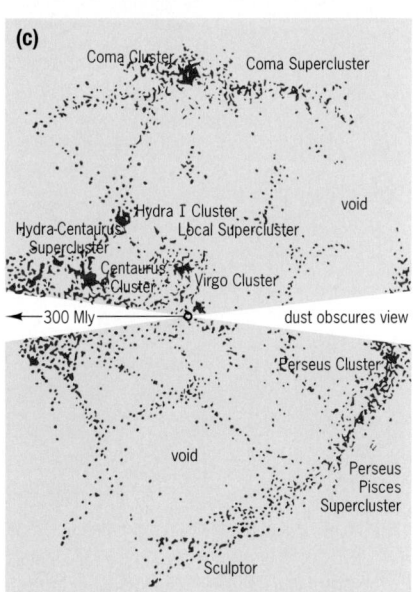

Fig 26.12 (a) The Local Supercluster with the Local Group at the centre. Each sphere represents a cluster of galaxies, and its size is proportional to the number of galaxies in it. Above disc: red; below disc: yellow
(b) Between the Local Supercluster and a neighbouring one, the Hercules Supercluster, there is a void with very few galaxies in it

(c) With the Milky Way at the centre, this is a two-dimensional picture of nearby clusters and superclusters, showing the voids between. In three dimensions, the clusters and superclusters look like fragmented bubbles, with the voids being the cavities in the bubbles. Each dot represents one or more galaxies

5 THE EXPANDING UNIVERSE

RED SHIFT

In 1929, Hubble used the Doppler effect to measure the speeds of 24 bright galaxies at different distances from Earth. He found that all of them were moving away from us, and the further away the galaxy was, the faster it was moving. He found a simple relation, called **Hubble's law**, between the distance D and the speed of recession v:

$$v = HD$$

where H is the **Hubble constant** (see page 556). The speed of recession v is obtained by measuring the red shift of a known spectral line due to the Doppler effect. Red shifts for galaxies in five comparatively close clusters are seen in Fig 26.13. Fig 26.14 shows these shifts plotted on a graph to calculate v.

The Doppler effect is a shift in frequency due to the relative motion between source and observer. In astronomy it is usually quantified in terms of a wavelength change $\Delta\lambda$. For a relative speed v, much smaller than the speed of light, we have a good approximation:

$$\frac{\Delta\lambda}{\lambda_e} = \frac{v}{c} \quad \text{or} \quad \frac{(\lambda_o - \lambda_e)}{\lambda_e} = \frac{\lambda_o}{\lambda_e} - 1 = \frac{v}{c}$$

Fig 26.13 Below: for each of the named galaxies, the H and K lines in the spectrum of ionised calcium shift towards the longer wavelength (red) end compared with a laboratory reference spectrum. The speed of recession is then calculated using the Doppler formula

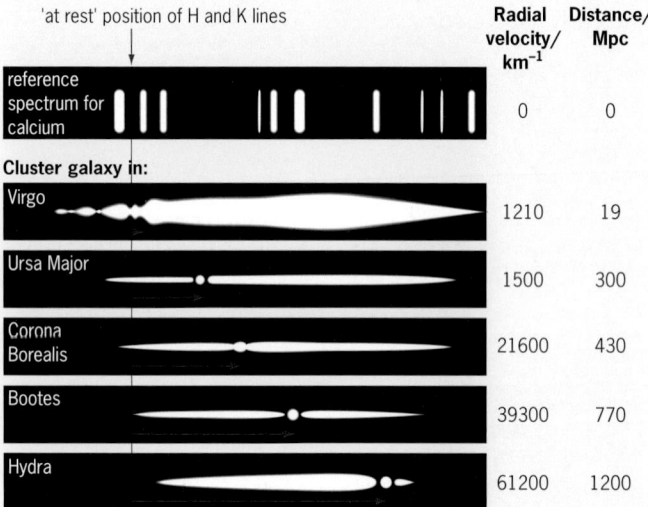

Fig 26.14 The data obtained from the spectra in Fig 26.13 is plotted here, showing a simple relationship between speed of recession and distance

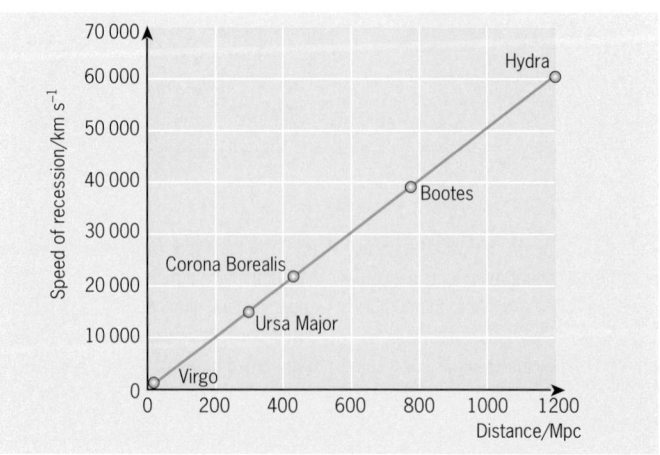

where λ_e is the wavelength of the radiation when *emitted*, λ_o is the wavelength *observed* on Earth, and c is the speed of light. In cosmology we are usually interested in light from objects moving away from us, so that λ_o is greater than λ_e, that is, the wavelength has 'shifted to the red' end of the spectrum.

The z factor

Astronomers define a quantity z as the red shift for small recession speeds v and hence small values of z:

$$z = \frac{\Delta\lambda}{\lambda_e} = \frac{v}{c}$$

or, incorporating Hubble's law:

$$z = \frac{H_0 D}{c}$$

These relations are modified to incorporate relativity theory for large values of v and z.

STRETCH AND CHALLENGE

The cosmological red shift

We observe a line spectrum emitted from a distant galaxy, a billion light years away, and find that the wavelengths of the lines have increased. A cosmological explanation of this effect is as follows. First we must remember that the light was emitted a billion years ago. Since then the space between us and that galaxy has increased due to the expansion of the Universe. This means that the space occupied by the wavelength of the light has increased *by the same factor*.

Fig 26.15 gives the simple mathematics of this effect, linking the expansion ratio to the z factor.

The red shift can also be explained using the Doppler effect, which links the speed of recession with the change in light frequency: see Chapter 6 for mathematical details of this.

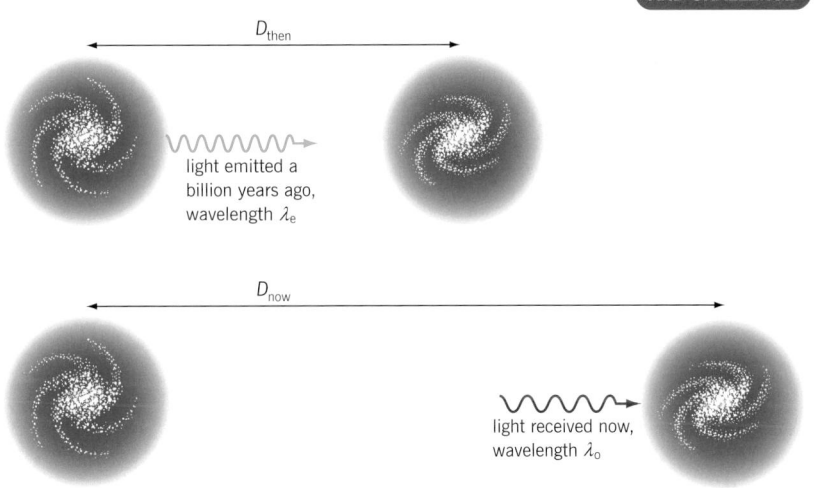

Fig 26.15 The cosmological red shift, z, time and the expansion of space

In Fig 26.15 space – and the photon's wavelength – have expanded by the same ratio:

$$\frac{D_{now}}{D_{then}} = \frac{\lambda_o}{\lambda_e} = \frac{(\lambda_e + \Delta\lambda)}{\lambda_e} = 1 + \frac{\Delta\lambda}{\lambda_e}$$

that is:

$$\frac{D_{now}}{D_{then}} = 1 + z$$

where z is now explained as a **cosmological** red shift.

EVERYTHING IS MOVING AWAY FROM EVERYTHING ELSE

It may seem that somehow the Earth is at the centre of a Universe that is doing its best to recede as far from it as possible. But this is an illusion. *Every large-scale feature* of the Universe is moving away from every other one. This is explained by general relativity theory as an expansion of space itself, carrying with it the matter it creates and is created by.

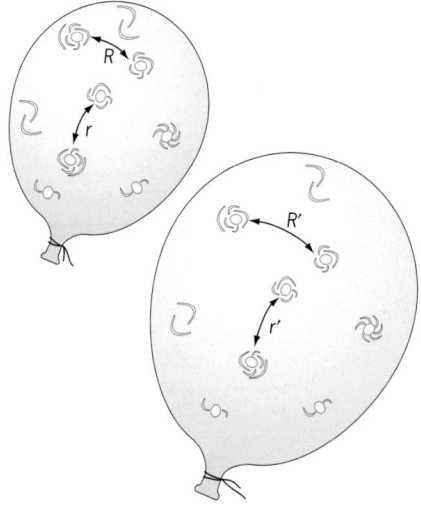

Fig 26.16 A model for Hubble expansion. When a balloon is blown up, every mark on it moves further away from every other mark. (One mark could be the Milky Way.) Each pair of marks moves apart at a rate proportional to their 'original' separation

Fig 26.16 shows a simple two-dimensional analogy. When a marked balloon is blown up, all the markings move apart. The rate of separation is the speed of recession and depends upon the separation, exactly as in Hubble's law.

THE HUBBLE CONSTANT *H*

The Hubble constant H is hard to measure accurately because distance measurements are so inexact for the furthest galaxies. The units of the constant are usually given as:

$$\frac{\text{speed in km s}^{-1}}{\text{distance in Mpc}}$$

The currently (2007) accepted value for H is 70.4 ± 1.5 km s^{-1} Mpc^{-1}. Fig 26.17 shows how the value as measured by astronomers has changed since Hubble's day. This is not because H is changing physically but because it is very hard to measure it accurately.

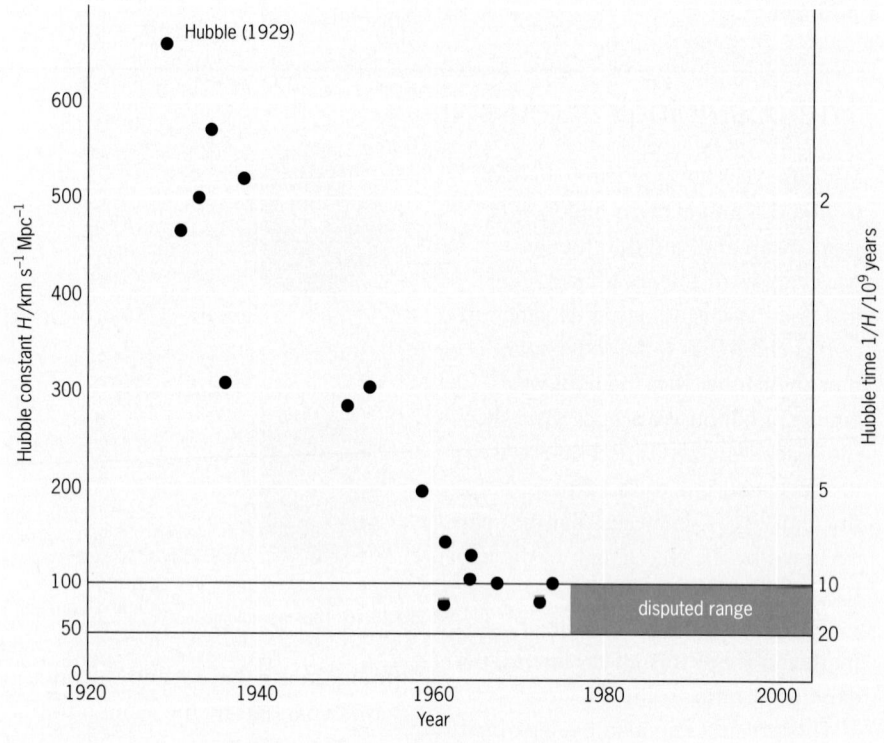

Fig 26.17 The calculated value of *H* has gradually become more reliable, and smaller. The data doesn't prove that *H* has changed, but the techniques for measuring distance have improved since Hubble's day. Over 300 measurements have been made in the last ten years or so

The Hubble constant and the age of the Universe

The Hubble constant gives us a rough measure of the age of the Universe. First assume that H has actually been constant since the Universe formed, a time T_H ago. In that time, any two points have moved apart by a distance in Mpc of D, at a steady speed v, so:

$$v = \frac{D}{T_H}$$

But also:

$$v = HD$$

So we have:

$$H = \frac{1}{T_H}$$

This gives the age of the Universe as:

$$T_H = \frac{1}{H} = \frac{1 \text{ Mpc}}{70.4 \text{ km s}^{-1}}$$

A megaparsec is 3.1×10^{19} km, so T_H comes to about 1.4×10^{10} years – 14 billion years (14 Gy or 14 *aeons*).

Hubble's own value for H was ten times larger than the currently accepted value above because he got his distances wrong. Hubble's estimate was 800 km s^{-1} Mpc^{-1}, making the Universe ten times younger, at 1.2 Gy, less than the age of the oldest rocks on Earth!

The discovery that the expansion of the universe is *accelerating* (see "Dark Energy" page 562) means that the Hubble constant varies with time. The final story is yet to emerge. Figure 26. 18 illustrates the possibility that the early universe expanded more quickly than the current rate, so giving a different value for its age.

> **? QUESTION 2**
>
> 2 Check the three quoted values for the age of the Universe in years using the three values of H given.

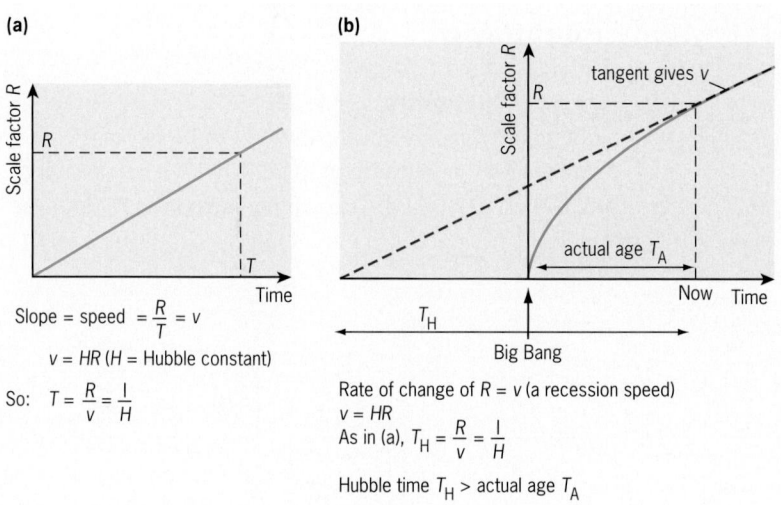

Fig 26.18 The Hubble constant gives a correct age for the Universe only if the Universe has expanded uniformly as in **(a)**, i.e. if H is constant over time. But if the expansion is as in **(b)**, with the rate decreasing, then the Universe is younger than we calculate from H. Here, labelling the vertical axis, the scale factor is a measure of the change in the size of the large distances in the universe caused by its expansion. See also page 561

> **✔ REMEMBER THIS**
> The four fundamental interactions are gravitation, the weak, the electromagnetic and the strong forces.

THE FIRST 3 BILLION YEARS: A PUZZLE

On the whole, we are more certain of what happened in the first three minutes of the Universe than in the first 3 billion years. Modern particle theory strongly supports the story given in the Stretch and Challenge box on pages 558–560. But according to the simple Big Bang model, the Universe should be full of galaxies spaced roughly equal distances apart, since originally the particles should have been spaced evenly apart. It would not be too difficult to model some instabilities which started the process of condensation into stars and galaxies. But we don't know how matter could have arranged itself into the galactic superclusters we observe and that give the structure of matter in the Universe the bubble-like *non-homogeneous* (uneven) appearance seen in Fig 26.12(c).

GUT and Guth

A way out of this problem was proposed in 1980 by the American theoretical physicist Alan Guth. He developed the supergravity theory, that at high enough energies, the fundamental interactions (forces) in nature become one. This is the grand unification theory or GUT, which predicts the very rapid inflation described on page 559. Any small random inhomogeneities (unevennesses) in the Universe just before the inflation are magnified as small bubbles of slightly differing density. Then, as time goes on, the Universe grows too fast to smooth itself out again, and the inhomogeneities remain as superclusters and clusters of galaxies (Fig 26.19).

Fig 26.19 It is thought that during and after expansion any inhomogeneities had no time to smooth themselves out because they were 'frozen' into the Universe by rapid inflation

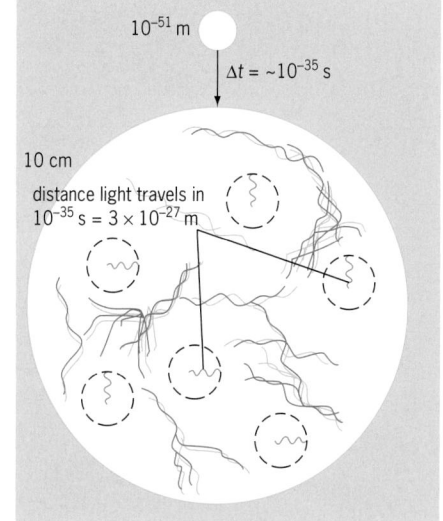

The Big Bang model of the Universe

The current model for the origin and nature of the Universe begins with a seeming impossibility and ends in uncertainty. The impossibility is that at the beginning everything must have been a single point – a **singularity**. This is not only difficult to imagine but it also means that no known laws of physics could apply.

The success of the model is that once we are past that first impossible moment, the laws of physics are able to explain most of the Universe's observable features. Of course, there are still many gaps in the theories and many observations that don't fit very well. There are also missing observations: no one has detected gravitational waves, let alone gravitons, the particles that theory predicts carry the gravitational force. There is also the puzzle that most of the mass that must be in the Universe to explain gravitational effects seems to be undetectable.

There follows a summary of the evolution of the Universe as described by the standard **Big Bang** model, shown in Fig

26.20, together with some of the main evidence in favour of the model. As you read, you may find it helpful to refer back to Chapter 24 for descriptions of subatomic particles.

DURING THE FIRST THREE MINUTES

If we run the film of the expanding Universe backwards, we reach a point where everything – spacetime, radiation and matter – is compressed into dimensions incredibly smaller than the size of a proton. At this very earliest stage, the four fundamental forces (interactions) of nature formed one single unified force, often called **supergravity**.

At 10^{-43} seconds

The micro-Universe has expanded to be about 10^{-35} m across at a temperature of 10^{32} K, with a mass–energy density of 10^{97} kg m^{-3}. Nothing surrounds it, not even a *space* or 'vacuum' since the Universe is all there is. At this

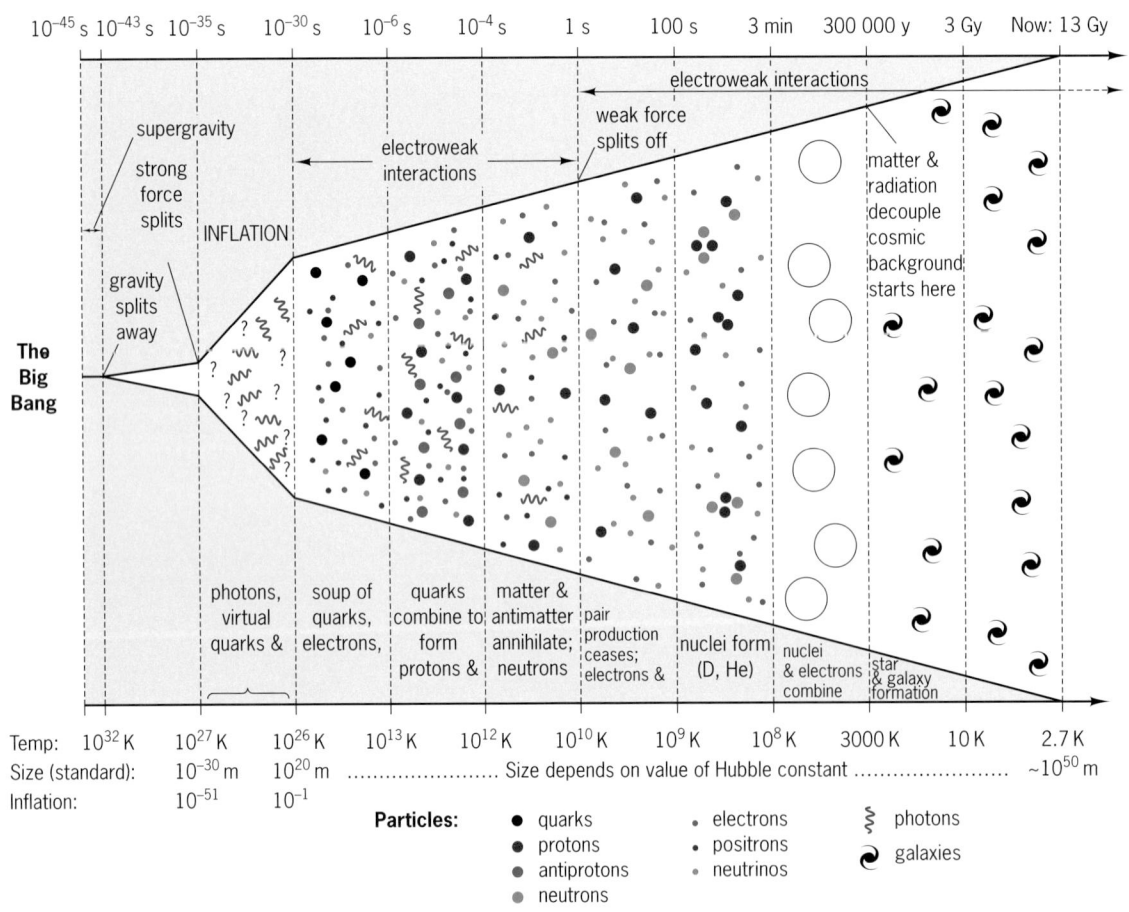

Fig 26.20 The standard Big Bang model for the development of the Universe

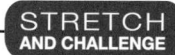

time, ordinary gravity splits away (decouples) from the original single force.

Expansion continues, and the tightly packed highly energetic photons convert some of their energy into a sea of *virtual quarks* which combine to form larger virtual particles and antiparticles. Virtual particles of matter exist for only a very short time. This is allowed by the Heisenberg uncertainty principle, provided that their mass–energy and lifetimes multiply to a smaller value than the Planck constant h.

After 10^{-35} seconds: a sudden rapid inflation

The Universe has been expanding steadily, while cooling. But at about 10^{-35} s, the *strong* force separates out, leaving the *electromagnetic* and the *weak* forces coupled together as the *electroweak* force. With the separation of the strong forces, there is a sudden increase in the rate of expansion, an **inflation**, which lasts until 10^{-30} s have elapsed. In this time, the Universe has expanded by a factor of 10^{50}, to become about the size of an orange.

By the end of this period of inflation, the Universe has cooled from 10^{32} K to about 10^{26} K. *Real* particles can now be formed from photons which have enough energy to produce particle–antiparticle pairs: *quarks* and *antiquarks*, *electrons* and *positrons*. So photons become fewer and less energetic. As expansion and cooling continue, the quarks combine to form very massive but short-lived particles (hyperons), and eventually the stable *protons* and *antiprotons*.

At one microsecond

A microsecond is a very long time in the early Universe. At this time it has reached the size of the Solar System and its temperature has dropped to 10^{13} K, too low for the creation of any more heavy particles from photons. In fact, the quantity of matter is now decreasing rapidly as protons combine with antiprotons, annihilating each other.

If protons and antiprotons had been created in exactly equal quantities, the Universe would now consist entirely of radiation, all at too low an energy to create more particles. Fortunately, there was an excess of protons over antiprotons in the ratio 10 000 000 001 to 10 000 000 000. This left enough protons over to make all the stars and galaxies that now exist.

At one second

The temperature has fallen to 10^{10} K, at which photons no longer have enough energy to create electron–positron pairs. There is a second great matter–antimatter annihilation as those that existed meet. This creates more

photons. But again, there is an excess of matter (electrons) over antimatter (positrons) which is just enough to match the protons' charge – so that the total electric charge in the Universe is zero.

At this stage the Universe is a hot plasma consisting of photons, electrons and protons in equal proportions. There is also a very large but unknown number of neutrinos.

Neutrons are produced by collisions between protons and electrons. But neutrons are unstable, and another equilibrium develops between creation and decay which eventually produces two neutrons for every 14 protons.

Later, at a slightly lower temperature, protons and neutrons can combine on collision to form the nuclei of deuterium (hydrogen with 1 proton, 1 neutron) and then helium. (The ratio of neutrons to protons, predicted by nuclear and particle theory, should have produced a hydrogen–helium ratio of 75 per cent to 25 per cent by mass. This ratio is confirmed by present-day observation.) Any larger nuclei are broken up by collision until the plasma cools down further.

At three minutes

Eventually, during the next three minutes, the stable isotopes of the light nuclei lithium (^{7}Li) and beryllium (^{9}Be) are formed – but in very tiny amounts. By this time, the average distance between particles is so large that they are extremely unlikely to meet and form larger nuclei. This process has to wait until nucleosynthesis in stars begins (see Chapter 25).

DURING THE NEXT 300 000 YEARS

In its first 300 000 years, the Universe is first a plasma consisting of electrons, protons and helium nuclei. All atoms are ionised. Photons are scattered by the charged particles and cannot travel without losing energy by collisions. We say the Universe at this stage is 'opaque' to radiation.

Eventually, the temperature drops to about 3000 K and nuclei rapidly capture electrons to form neutral atoms which photon energies are too low to break up. The Universe becomes transparent to its own radiation.

When the temperature falls a lot more, the maximum wavelength of the radiation is about 1 mm, in the near infrared. It is from this stage of the Universe's evolution that a relic of radiation at that time, **cosmic background radiation**, is still detectable. This radiation is roughly the same from all directions and shows a pattern of intensity at a range of wavelengths characteristic of black body radiation (pages 255 and 307) of a Universe which has cooled to about 3 K as it expanded.

The cosmic background radiation

The existence of a low-temperature radiation that fills all space was discovered by accident in 1965. It had been predicted as early as 1948 by George Gamow, Ralph Alpher and Robert Hermann, but later forgotten.

Arno Penzias and Robert Wilson, physicists working for the Bell Telephone Company, were testing a small, very sensitive radio telescope they had designed and built to detect radiation of 7 cm wavelength. They found a high level of 'noise' in the system which they couldn't eliminate. They also found that, unlike most noise in radio telescopes, it didn't vary with time of day or with the direction the telescope pointed. Eventually, they accepted that the signal wasn't noise in the machine but *radiation of cosmological origin*.

At a nearby university, physicists were reinventing the theories of Gamow, Alpher and Hermann, and the report of Penzias' and Wilson's discovery seemed convincing evidence in favour of the Big Bang model, which at the time had little evidence to support it.

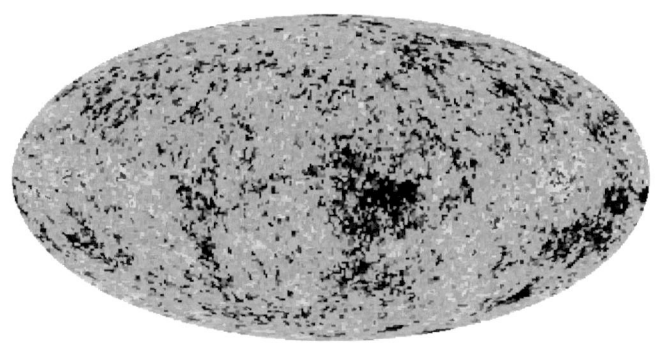

Fig 26.22 WMAP result: the Universe 14 billion years ago

Since then, many very accurate measurements have been made on the background radiation and have confirmed it as a relic of the primal universal radiation (Fig 26.21).

One problem with the radiation was that it was too uniform to be true! The variation and clustering of mass in the Universe was expected to be matched by a similar – if not so dramatic – variation in radiation density: whatever had caused matter not to be distributed uniformly should also have affected the radiation. The 'lumpiness' of the radiation was first measured by the Cosmic Background Explorer (COBE) satellite experiment in 1992. A much more detailed measurement was made by the Wilkinson Microwave Anisotropy Probe (WMAP) in 2006. In Fig. 26.22 darker shades show regions of lower radiation intensity coming from regions where, about 14 billion years ago, there was more matter. Its gravitational effect reduced the intensity of the radiation (see 'Black holes' page 543). The difference in intensity is tiny: a few parts in 100 000. Detailed study of the data supports the theory of early cosmic inflation (see page 559).

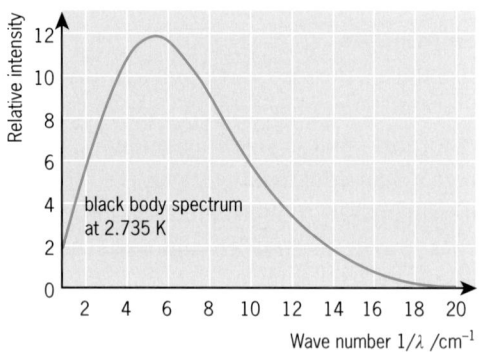

Fig 26.21 The spectrum of background radiation measured by the Cosmic Background Explorer (COBE) satellite

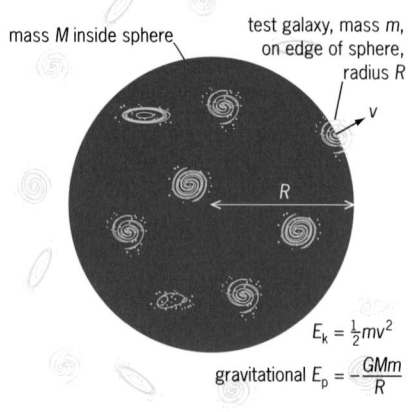

mass *M* inside sphere

test galaxy, mass *m*, on edge of sphere, radius *R*

$$E_k = \tfrac{1}{2}mv^2$$

gravitational $E_p = -\dfrac{GMm}{R}$

Fig 26.23 Gravity and the expanding Universe

6 CRITICAL DENSITY AND THE FUTURE OF THE UNIVERSE

We need Einstein's theory of general relativity for a full explanation of an expanding Universe. But the Newtonian model is good enough for us to construct some possible scenarios. Think of a galaxy at the edge of a large spherical volume of space inside the Universe, as in Fig 26.23. It contains clusters of galaxies, all moving apart from each other. Newtonian theory says that only galaxies *inside* the spherical volume will affect the motion of the galaxy. The effects of galaxies outside the sphere cancel each other out. Our chosen galaxy (and all others, because we can choose any sphere as long as it is large enough) will have a force on it tending to slow down its outward movement.

What eventually happens to the galaxy depends on much the same factors that decide whether an object thrown upwards from Earth will fall back or go off the planet having been given the escape velocity. This is essentially a battle between the kinetic energy of the galaxy and its gravitational potential energy, as explained on page 54.

Think about a galaxy of mass m at distance R from us (Fig 26.23). The sphere centred on us with a surface at the galaxy contains a mass M. According to Newton's law of gravity the force pulling inwards on the galaxy is

$$F = GMm/R^2 \qquad [1]$$

and the mass M in terms of the mean density ρ of the space inside the sphere

$$M = (4/3)\pi R^3 \rho \qquad [2]$$

By Hubble's law ($v = HD$, page 556) the galaxy is separating from us with a speed v such that

$$v = HR \qquad [3]$$

Does the galaxy have enough speed to 'escape'? If it does then the Universe will keep expanding forever following one of the paths shown in Fig 26.24. **Escape velocity** is a well-known idea (see page 53–54) and is given by the relationship

$$v^2 = 2GM/R \qquad [4]$$

with the quantities now referring to the sphere and the movement of the galaxy.

Using equations 2 and 4 we can put the possible escape velocity in terms of the density of the space inside the sphere:

$$v^2 = 2G(4/3)\pi R^2 \rho$$

The escape velocity will be just reached when the density has **critical** value ρ_c such that

$$\rho_c = v^2/[(8/3)G\pi R^2]$$

But we know that $v = HR$, so substituting for v we have

$$\rho_c = H^2 R^2/[(8/3)G\pi R^2]$$

which simplifies to

$$\rho_c = 3H^2/8G\pi$$

The large uncertain quantity here is H, the Hubble constant. Accepting the value favoured in this book the critical density is about 5×10^{-27} kg m^{-3} (about 1 hydrogen atom per cubic metre). Check this value for yourself.

The density of the Universe is not easy to measure. One way is to add up all the matter we can see in stars and galaxies, make some corrections for the clouds of invisible hydrogen gas and other small particles – and hope for the best. Cosmologists discuss the future of the Universe using the *density parameter* Ω which is the ratio of the measured density of the Universe to the critical density: $\Omega = \rho/\rho_c$. There are three possible fates for the universe.

1. $\Omega = 1$: the Universe will keep expanding but more and more slowly and eventually, at some time in the infinite future, come to a stop. It is a **flat** Universe.
2. $\Omega < 1$: the Universe expands for ever and ends up with a finite velocity at infinity. It is an **open** Universe.
3. $\Omega > 1$: the Universe will eventually stop expanding and its gravity will start pulling it backwards. It ends up in a hot dense phase – quite possibly as it started – in a Big Crunch. This is a **closed** Universe.

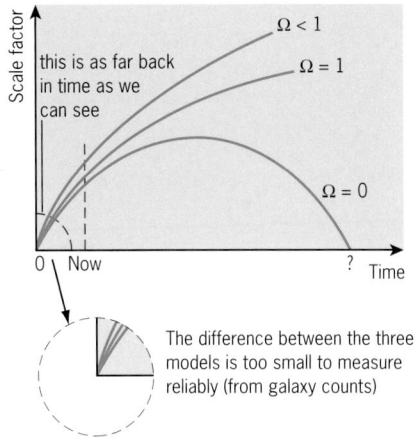

The difference between the three models is too small to measure reliably (from galaxy counts)

Fig 26.24 Three possible fates of the Universe, on a simple gravitational model. The scale factor of the *y* axis is any very large distance, undistorted by local gravitation

For more on missing matter and dark energy please see the How Science Works assignments for this chapter at www.collinseducation.co.uk/CAS

Table 26.2 The Universe

Radius today	13×10^9 ly
	1.2×10^{23} m
	4×10^9 Mpc
Hubble constant H_0	75 km s^{-1} Mpc^{-1}
Hubble time (age) $1/H_0$	13 Gy
Mass	5.7×10^{53} kg
Density	1.5×10^{-26} kg m^{-3}
Number of stars (Sun-sized)	2.9×10^{23}
Number of galaxies	1.6×10^{12}

The terms flat, open and closed are linked to the various **geometries** of space that fit Einstein's general theory of relativity.

To summarise: if there is too little matter we have scenarios 1 and 2, if enough scenario 3 will occur. Fig 26.24 illustrates these three possible futures. If ordinary matter were responsible for the fate of the Universe, scenario 2 occurs. But read on.

NINETY PER CENT OF THE UNIVERSE IS MISSING

Estimates of the density of matter in the Universe that are based on the matter we can actually see give very low values – about 4×10^{-28} kg m^{-3}, or one hydrogen atom to every 10 m^3. To keep the Universe expanding steadily, as in scenario 1 above, we need about 70 atoms in this volume of space. However, when astronomers measure the gravitational pull of the material in a galaxy, or even a supercluster of galaxies, they find that the visible material contributes only about 10 per cent of the gravitational mass.

The invisible material does not affect the light output, so is unlikely to be clouds of dust. (Even gas clouds form only 5 to 15 per cent of the mass of a galaxy.) The search is now on for the missing material. It could exist as unknown forms of matter such as *weakly interacting particles* (WIMPs), dead dark stars and planets (MACHOs) or *heavy neutrinos*. There could also be black holes, just small enough.

AND ANOTHER THING … *DARK ENERGY*

One of the most valuable indicators of cosmological distance is a very bright type of object called a **type Ia supernova**. They are valuable because not only are they very bright (and so can be detected even when they are very far away) but they all have almost exactly the same well-known maximum brightness. This allows distances to be measured for a range of galaxies in which they appear. Research teams working with these objects discovered (and announced in 1998) a quite unexpected result, linking the distances of the host galaxies with their rate of recession (*z* value).

Light takes time to travel. When we observe a distant galaxy we are looking at a stage of the Universe up to 10 billion years old. The surprising discovery was that the Universe is not expanding at a steady rate: H_0 is not constant with time. The Universe is expanding faster now than it was a billion years ago; it is **accelerating**. The theoretical implication of this discovery is that Einstein was right: his first model of the Universe contained a quantity called a cosmological constant which predicted the acceleration that has now been discovered. But back in the 1920s Hubble's work contradicted the existence of the cosmological constant and Einstein came to refer to it as his 'greatest mistake'. An accelerating Universe is not a constant energy system as considered in the scenarios above, rather the quantity of energy it contains must increase with time. This has been called **dark energy**, or **quintessence**, and has the effect of counteracting gravity. This energy causes *space* itself to expand faster and faster.

Had the effect been strongly in existence in the early Universe it would have stopped the gravitational collapse that has produced stars and galaxies, suggesting again that the dark energy is increasing with time. It is estimated to be now about two-thirds of the total energy in the Universe. The increase from a very small value over time can be explained by saying that the energy is proportional to the volume of space, and so increases naturally as space expands. It may be composed of particles and the search is now on for evidence of this.

Table 26.2 summarises data about the Universe.

SUMMARY

After studying this chapter, you should:

- Understand why Olbers' paradox suggests that a static, infinite Universe is an impossibility.
- Know that the Universe consists of stars and interstellar material grouped in units: galaxies, clusters of galaxies and superclusters.
- Know how the distances to stars and distant objects can be measured.
- Understand how the Doppler effect is used to measure the velocities of galaxies.
- Know about the observed expansion of the Universe on a large scale, red shift, Hubble's law and the Hubble constant.

- Know the standard Big Bang model of the Universe, the importance of particle physics in describing the first minutes of its evolution and be able to give evidence in support of the model (cosmic background radiation, cosmic abundance of elements).
- Know the age and possible fates of the Universe, linked to its density and the value of the Hubble constant.

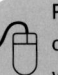 Practice questions for this chapter are available at www.collinseducation.co.uk/CAS

27

Energy consumption and climate change

27 ENERGY CONSUMPTION AND CLIMATE CHANGE

Are we changing the climate?

There is now little doubt that the average global surface temperature is on the increase. What is less certain is how much of the increase is caused by human profligacy, as we consume increasing amounts of energy and generate large amounts of carbon dioxide that passes into the atmosphere. How much does changing temperature change the world's climate? Were the UK floods of 2007 or the large-scale damage produced to New Orleans in 2005 as a result of a serious hurricane caused in any way by changing temperature and indirectly by human effects on the climate. However, temperature fluctuations have occurred naturally in the past. The UK has had hotter periods when wine-growing was prevalent and colder periods when the Thames froze and was used by skaters. Certainly, as the global temperature rises today, map-makers need to redraw the extent of many lakes and coastlines. The potential consequences for the human race are huge.

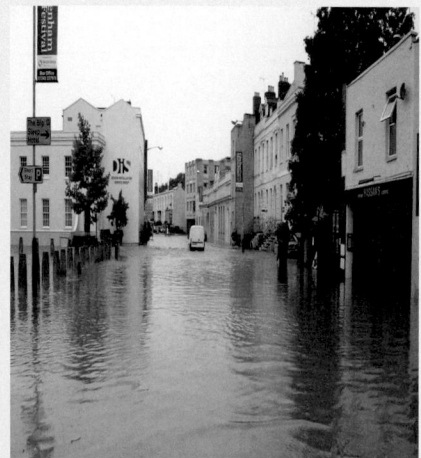

The effects of summer flooding in Cheltenham, 2007

The ideas in this chapter

We have seen how physics has helped us to explore and understand the very small and the very large, from nanoscale electronics to the Universe. But one of the biggest issues facing us today is the changing climate. This is a system of intermediate size but of incredible complexity. Understanding how temperature and climate are influenced is an inter-disciplinary topic in which physics plays an important role. In particular, we need to know just how much we are affecting the climate and how we might reduce the effects despite an ever-increasing population. In this final chapter we compare the Earth's energy sources. We explain the greenhouse effect and why it is important. We also compare ways in which we obtain our energy for power and heating and refer back to many topics in earlier chapters.

1 ENERGY FROM THE SUN

There are three main factors that determine the surface temperature of any planet in the Solar System:

- The radiation received from the Sun.
- The energy released internally in the planet (mostly due to radioactivity).
- The energy radiated away from the planet into space.

By far the biggest contribution to global energy comes from the Sun. The energy radiated from the Sun peaks in the visible part of the spectrum, and its total quantity is 3.8×10^{26} W. Of this, the Earth receives a tiny fraction, 1.353 kW m^{-2}, a quantity called the **solar constant**, S. But the Earth is not a perfect absorber: about 30% of the visible radiation is reflected – by clouds, ice, the sea and land. This reflected proportion is called the **albedo**, a, of the Earth: $a = 0.30$.

The radiation energy reaching the Earth heats the ground, the sea and the atmosphere. It evaporates water and powers the water cycle. However, the atmosphere is too 'transparent' to solar energy to be significantly warmed directly by solar radiation; it is warmed by contact with the ground. The heated, moving atmosphere then shares out the absorbed energy more evenly across the Earth: air heated near the ground in the tropics moves in convection currents towards latitudes near the poles. Convection in the oceans also helps to redistribute energy over the Earth. The Gulf Stream, for instance, brings warm water from the Caribbean area to western Europe.

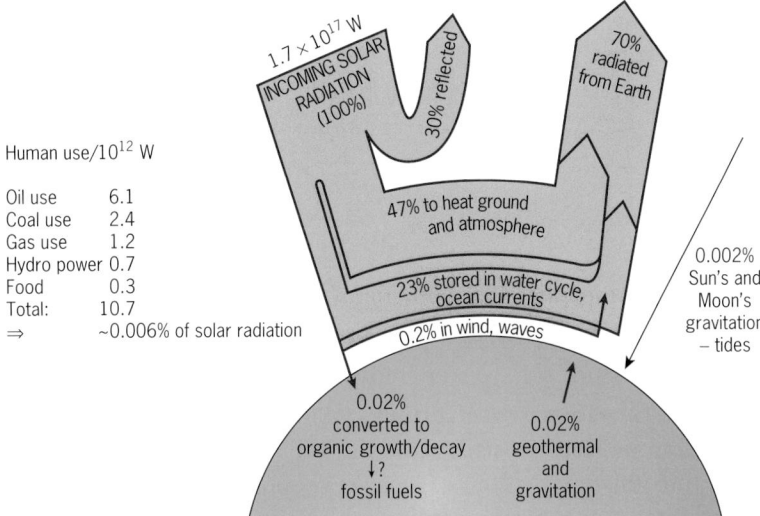

Fig 27.1 The energy balance of the Earth

Fig 27.1 shows what happens to the incoming energy on Earth. The warm Earth also radiates energy into space. The energy flows are represented by arrows and the figure is an example of a Sankey diagram. The widths of the arrows are proportional to the flow quantities. Such diagrams are used in other examples of flow. An equilibrium is established of a steady mean surface temperature because the power radiated equals the power delivered by the Sun's radiation:

$$P_{\text{absorbed}} = P_{\text{reradiated}}$$

We can estimate the effect of the atmosphere on the temperature of the Earth's surface in a calculation in which we assume that the Earth is 'bare', acting as a 'black body' (page 307), without an atmosphere, as in Fig 27.2.

Energy absorbed per second (in watts)
= solar constant S × (1 − albedo, a) × area of Earth disc

so: $P_{\text{absorbed}} = 1.353 \times 10^3 \times (1-0.3) \times \pi R^2 = 947\pi R^2$

where R is the mean radius of the Earth.

The radiation emitted is calculated using Stefan's law:

The radiation energy emitted per second per unit area by a black body at temperature T is σT^4

where σ is the **Stefan constant**, 5.57×10^{-8} W m^{-2} T^{-4}.

Total power radiated by Earth = $A\ T^4$

where A is the area of the whole Earth, that is, a *sphere* of radius R.
So the power radiated is:

$$P_{\text{radiated}} = 4\pi R^2 \times 5.67 \times 10^{-8} \times T^4$$

Equating absorption and radiation gives:

$$4 \times 5.67 \times 10^{-8} \times T^4 = 947$$

> **? QUESTION 2**
>
> 2   Explain why the continuous supply of radiant energy from the Sun does not produce a continuous rise in the temperature of the Earth.

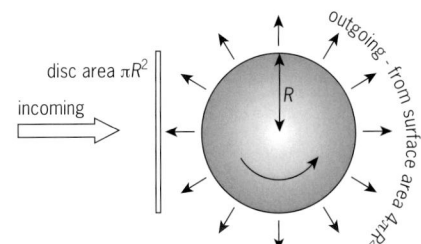

Fig 27.2 Energy exchange for a bare Earth

? **QUESTION 3**

3 Check the calculated value of −19 °C for the mean surface temperature of a bare Earth.

From this, the temperature of the bare Earth's surface is:

$$T = 254 \text{ K or } -19 \text{ °C}.$$

But the Earth is not bare, and the actual mean surface temperature is 288 K or +15 °C. A small part of the extra 34 degrees is due to an outflow of energy from the interior of the Earth, *but most of it is a result of the Earth having an atmosphere.*

The emissivity of the Earth's surface is important and can vary widely. In the most extreme desert regions, for instance Chile at 315 K, the emissivity is 550 W m^{-2}, whereas in a certain part of Indonesia where there are deep convection systems and the temperature can fall to 180 K, the emissivity can be as low as 60 W m^{-2}. The surface heat capacity C_s is defined as the energy required to raise the planet's surface by one degree and has units of J m^{-2} K^{-1}.

2 THE ATMOSPHERIC BLANKET

Molecules in the atmosphere contain energy in various ways.

- They have **translational kinetic energy**, as they move through space.
- They may spin and so have some **rotational kinetic energy**.
- They also have **vibrational energy**, alternately potential and kinetic as the atoms in molecules oscillate to and fro.

As a rough rule, the temperature of a gas is proportional to the mean translational kinetic energy of its molecules.

However, the energy that is important in making the atmosphere a 'blanket' for radiation from the Earth is the *vibrational* energy of molecules. Molecules can increase their vibrational energy by absorbing photons carrying exactly the right amount of energy to increase the vibrational energy by one quantum (Fig 27.3).

The energy required by a carbon dioxide molecule to jump up a quantum level happens to have a frequency that is close to the peak of the radiation emitted by the warm Earth, at 2×10^{13} Hz (infrared, at $\lambda = 15$ μm). Other gases can absorb energy in much the same way: ozone (O_3) requires energy at a photon frequency of 3×10^{13} Hz ($\lambda = 10$ μm), and water at 4 to 5×10^{13} Hz ($\lambda = 5$ μm).

THE GREENHOUSE EFFECT

The energy absorbed by a carbon dioxide molecule is re-emitted almost immediately as an infrared photon. Now, all the photons absorbed by carbon dioxide were travelling *outwards* from the Earth. But roughly half of the re-emitted photons (Fig 27.3(b)) are moving *back to Earth*.

✔ **REMEMBER THIS**

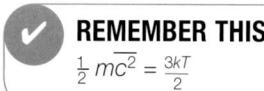

✔ **REMEMBER THIS**

Ozone is formed from atmospheric oxygen (O_2), which is split up by ultraviolet radiation from the Sun and then recombines as O_3. There is too little ozone to have a thermal effect as great as carbon dioxide's but as it also absorbs in the ultraviolet region, it cuts down this dangerously ionising radiation from the Sun.

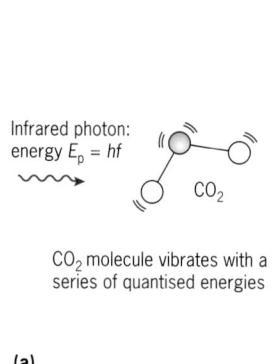

Infrared photon: energy $E_p = hf$

CO_2 molecule vibrates with a series of quantised energies

(a)

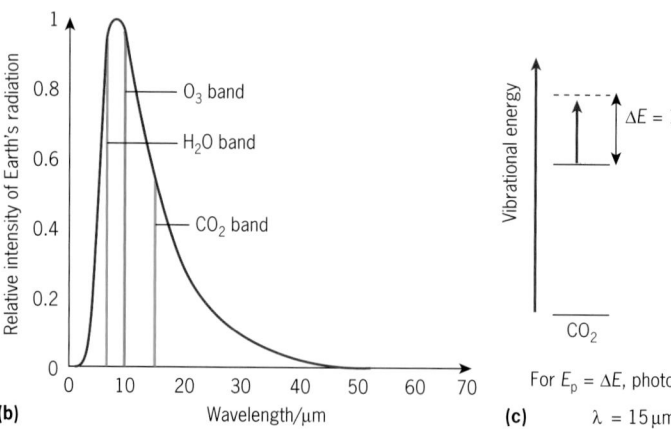

(b)

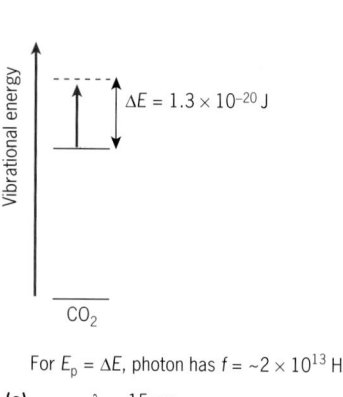

For $E_p = \Delta E$, photon has $f = \sim 2 \times 10^{13}$ Hz

$\lambda = 15$ μm

(c)

Fig. 27.3 Carbon dioxide is an effective greenhouse gas

Remember that the incoming radiation from the Sun has an energy peak in the visible part of the spectrum. The atmosphere is mostly transparent to this part. Because energy *absorption* by atmospheric gases is at the peak of the radiation emitted by the warm Earth, the atmosphere acts as a blanket. This is like the way that air in greenhouses is kept warmer than air outside: sunlight and short-wave infrared can get through the glass, but the longer wave infrared that is reradiated from the interior is absorbed within. Hence, energy absorption in the atmosphere is called the **greenhouse effect**. See Fig 27.4.

The result is that only about 60% of the thermal radiation from Earth gets through into space, that is, the **transmission factor** $b = 0.6$. The energy balance in watts can now be recalculated:

incoming power = outgoing power

From page 567:

incoming power $= S(1 - a)\pi R^2 = 947\pi R^2$

outgoing energy rate $= b \times 4\pi R^2 \times \sigma T^4$

Equating these gives:

$$T = 289 \text{ K or } 16 \text{ °C}$$

The prediction from this simple model is close to the measured value for the mean surface temperature of Earth, which is 288 K or 15 °C.

Not all gases are greenhouse gases. For absorption of infrared radiation by molecules, there need to be bonds between atoms of different elements. So carbon dioxide, water and methane are all examples. Their abundance in the atmosphere is important and so is their effectiveness. Water is 0.5% of the atmosphere and contributes 60% of the greenhouse effect. Carbon dioxide is currently 0.36% of the atmosphere but the molecules have a larger effect. The amount of methane in the atmosphere is small but the molecules are eight times as effective as those of carbon dioxide. Fig. 27.5 shows the relative amount of thermal radiation passing through the atmosphere within the infrared region as measured by an orbiting satellite. The dips in the curve correspond to absorption by greenhouse gases. Black body curves for different surface temperatures are also shown.

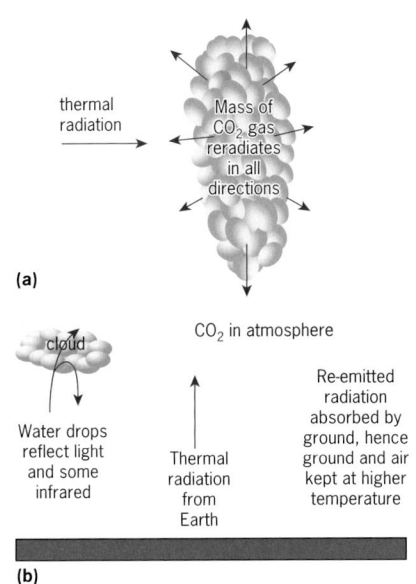

(a)

(b)

Fig 27.4 The atmosphere as a blanket, helped by clouds: the energy that carbon dioxide reradiates is much more than for other gases of the atmosphere

? QUESTION 4

4   Work through the calculation to check the value of 16 °C for the mean surface temperature of the Earth.

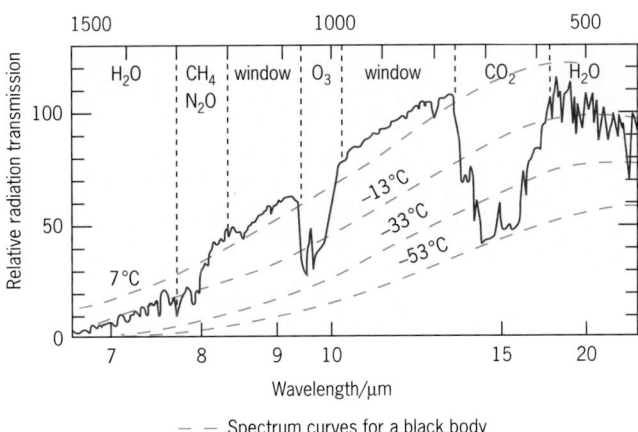

— — Spectrum curves for a black body

Fig 27.5 Thermal radiation transmission from the Earth's surface and atmosphere in the infrared region of the spectrum. Spectrum curves for a black body are shown for comparison

MORE ABOUT THE GREENHOUSE EFFECT, AND THE CARBON DIOXIDE BALANCE

Although carbon dioxide is just 0.036% of atmospheric gases, four billion years ago the atmosphere was probably 98% carbon dioxide, rather like the atmosphere of Venus today. The Earth was then cool enough for water to exist as a liquid. Carbon dioxide is water soluble, so rain washed it out of the atmosphere, and chemical processes trapped it as carbonate in rocks such as chalk, limestone and dolomite.

The oceans still contain a large mass of carbon dioxide dissolved in them. Animals in plankton, the sea organisms with the largest total mass, make their shells from carbon dioxide. These eventually fall to the sea floor and become sedimentary rocks. The oceans are therefore a **sink** for carbon dioxide – they remove the gas from the atmosphere. Over a long time, some of this is recycled as the ocean crust goes deeper into the Earth by the process of **subduction**. There, it is melted, heated carbonates release carbon dioxide, and so subduction is a **source** of carbon dioxide. The gas emerges into the atmosphere through volcanoes.

Fig 27.6 (a) shows the main stores of carbon dioxide as a gas, in solution or trapped in solid compounds on the Earth's surface. A much greater quantity is trapped in rocks of the sub-surface crust.

A quicker recycling process than plate tectonics involves organisms. Plants take carbon dioxide out of the atmosphere, use the carbon and release oxygen. The oxygen is used by most organisms in respiration and re-emerges combined with carbon as carbon dioxide.

Dead plants and animals are a sink for the carbon from carbon dioxide if they become fossilised without oxidation. This has happened many times on the Earth, providing large stores of carbon combined in the **hydrocarbons** of coal, gas and oil.

Fig 27.6 (a) Flows and reservoirs of the Earth's carbon dioxide. Figures are in gigatonnes (10^9 tonnes) of carbon

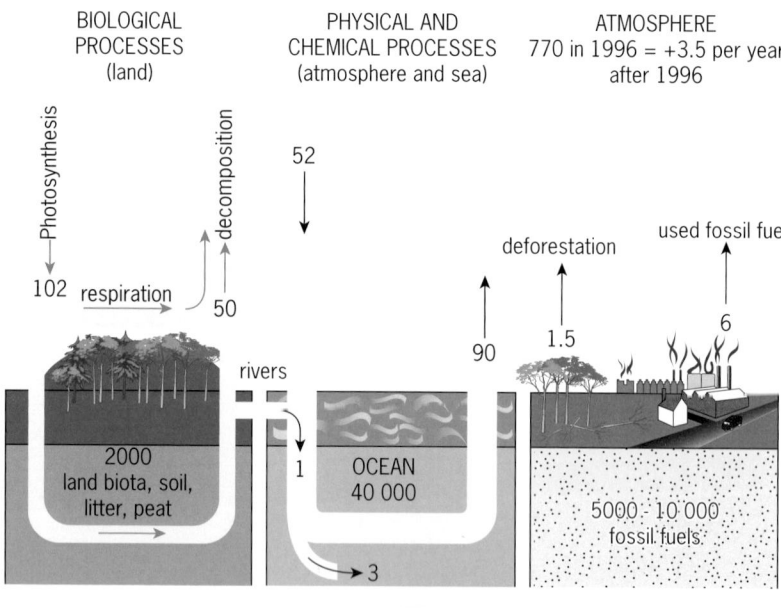

Fig 27.6 (b) Feedback control of global temperature via carbon dioxide. This assumes that CO_2 inputs and losses from other effects are a net zero

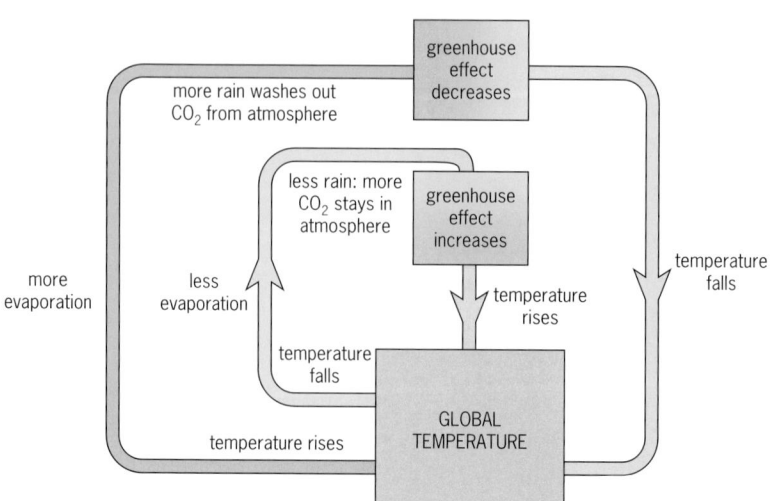

THE CARBON DIOXIDE BALANCE

About 30% of the carbon dioxide is continuously moving into and out of the atmosphere by various processes, but over long periods of the Earth's history, oxygen and carbon dioxide have been in balance, in a self-regulating feedback system. Suppose there is an excess of carbon dioxide. This is good for plant growth, so plants take up more carbon dioxide and release more oxygen, restoring the balance. If an excess of oxygen is produced, fires start more easily, so burning vegetation kill plants and put more carbon dioxide into the atmosphere as a combustion product. Fig 27.6(b) shows one of the feedback processes that helps maintain a stable temperature on Earth, via atmospheric carbon dioxide.

CARBON DIOXIDE AND GLOBAL WARMING

We are concerned nowadays about the greenhouse effect because there has been a steady *increase* in carbon dioxide levels over the last century or so (see Fig 27.7). This is largely due to human activity – the burning of fossil fuels and the increase in the number of farm animals. Both result in more carbon dioxide emission. Farm animals also produce methane, which is an even more effective greenhouse gas.

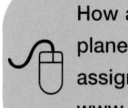

How are we going to save the planet? See the How Science Works assignment for this chapter at www.collinseducation.co.uk/CAS

The consequence of increased carbon dioxide levels is **global warming**. There has been both global warming and cooling in past ages, with warm (interglacial) periods or cool periods (ice ages) lasting for thousands to tens of thousands of years (Fig 27.8).

How do we know about these temperatures? Geological and fossil records are a good indication. However, ice cores taken deep into the Antarctic ice give a clear record of atmosphere composition and therefore of the mean global temperature. Ice cores have been drilled at the Russian Antarctic base to depths corresponding to 420 000 years.

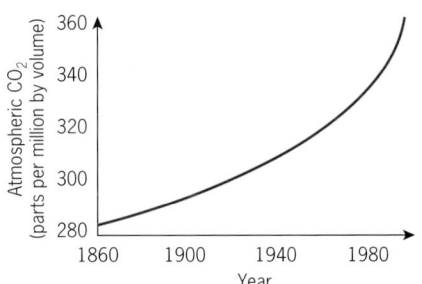

Fig 27.7 Buildup in atmospheric carbon dioxide concentration since the nineteenth-century industrial revolution

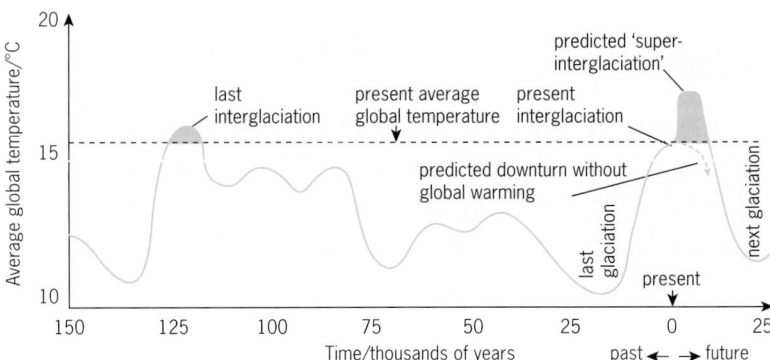

Fig 27.8 Temperature variations for the past 150 000 years and prediction for the next 25 000 years.
The causes of ice ages are not precisely known. There may be several: for example, increased volcanic activity not only produces more carbon dioxide but also more dust, so that the Earth's surface gets less solar radiation. The output of solar energy may vary with time, and the inclination of the Earth's spin axis relative to its orbit also varies. The relative positions of oceans and continents affect ocean and air currents. These currents can shift, and such changes can trigger cooling or warming processes

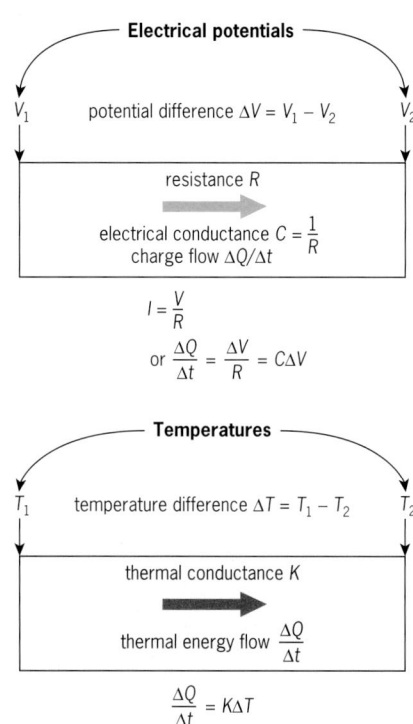

Electrical potentials

potential difference $\Delta V = V_1 - V_2$

V_1 V_2

resistance R

electrical conductance $C = \dfrac{1}{R}$
charge flow $\Delta Q / \Delta t$

$$I = \frac{V}{R}$$

or $\dfrac{\Delta Q}{\Delta t} = \dfrac{\Delta V}{R} = C\Delta V$

Temperatures

temperature difference $\Delta T = T_1 - T_2$

T_1 T_2

thermal conductance K

thermal energy flow $\dfrac{\Delta Q}{\Delta t}$

$$\frac{\Delta Q}{\Delta t} = K\Delta T$$

Fig 27.9 The analogy between electrical flow and thermal flow

3 THE ENERGY SOURCES INSIDE THE EARTH

Radioactive elements have a chemistry which tended to make them oxidise in the young Earth: they formed compounds whose density made them float to the upper layers of the molten Earth, to be concentrated in the crust. Even so, since the mantle contains so much more material, the mantle produces much more radioactive heating than the crust.

The rate of flow of this energy due to radioactive decay through surface rocks is about 80 mW per square metre. Only about a fifth of this comes from the crust, with the rest from sources deeper in the Earth. The energy is about 10 times as much as all human power sources, but 4000 times less than the Earth receives from the Sun.

THERMAL CONDUCTION AND CONVECTION

Energy released in the core and mantle moves upwards by both conduction and convection. In the rigid lithosphere (crust and outer mantle), conduction is the main steady mechanism. The movement of tectonic plates and the associated volcanic activity are other significant ways in which the hot interior loses energy.

The rate at which energy flows thermally, by conduction, through a solid is given by a simple 'heat flow' formula:

$$\text{energy flow} = \frac{\text{temperature difference}}{\text{thermal resistance}}$$

This is analogous to Ohm's law for charge flow (current), see Fig 27.9, but in thermal calculations we tend to use **thermal conductance** K rather than resistance, so we have:

$$\text{energy flow} = \text{temperature difference} \times \text{conductance}$$

As with electricity, we define conductance as:

$$\text{conductivity} \times \frac{\text{area of cross-section}}{\text{length}}$$

Thermal conductivity λ depends on the nature of the material and has units $\text{W m}^{-1}\text{ K}^{-1}$.

? QUESTION 5

5   Check that the units for thermal conductivity match those quoted.

? QUESTION 6

6   The Earth has a radius of 6.4×10^6 m. The energy flowing through surface rocks is 8×10^{-2} W m^{-2}, and is due mainly to radioactivity.

   a) Calculate how much energy is conducted per second for the whole Earth.

   b) The average energy released per second due to earthquakes is 10^{11} W. Express this as a percentage of the energy generated inside the Earth.

EXAMPLE

Q The crust is mainly composed of the igneous rocks granite and basalt. These have a mean thermal conductivity λ of 2.5 W m^{-1} K^{-1}. Estimate the temperature at a depth of 4 km.

A Thermal energy flow = 8×10^{-2} W m^{-2} = $\Delta T \times \lambda A/L$ where $A = 1$ m^2 and $L = 4 \times 10^3$ m.

Then, rearranging: $\Delta T = \dfrac{8 \times 10^{-2} \times 4 \times 10^3}{2.5} = 128$ K

Temperature difference $\Delta T = 128$ K. So, the temperature in a deep mine should be about 144 °C.

Comment on the Example

Note that the result represents a temperature gradient of about 3×10^{-2} K per metre. The measured temperature gradient is less, at 2×10^{-2} K m^{-1}. We assumed that the energy source was at a depth of 4 km. In fact, sources are spread fairly uniformly throughout the rock, some being therefore closer to the surface (Fig 27.10).

4 THE ATMOSPHERE: CLIMATE AND WEATHER

The atmosphere is a mixture of gases, see Table 27.1.

The pressure of the atmosphere at the Earth's surface is about 10^5 Pa (1 bar or 1000 millibars, as given on weather forecasts). Atmospheric pressure varies locally and depends on the temperature and humidity of the mass of gas below a height of about 15 km. This region is the **troposphere**, and is where 'the weather happens'. The pressure variation is quite small, at ± 30 mbar or so, and is caused by the differing densities of tropospheric air: cool dry air is denser than warm damp air. Fig 27.11 shows the main features of the atmosphere.

Air pressure decreases rapidly with height, following (roughly) an exponential decay law:

$$p = p_0 e^{-kh}$$

where p is pressure at height h, p_0 is pressure at sea level and k is a constant.

The pressure formula assumes that the air is at a constant temperature throughout, but this is not the case. See Fig 27.11. The air gets cooler up to the top of the troposphere, then its temperature rises in the **stratosphere**, cools in the **mesosphere** and warms up again in the **thermosphere**. This complex temperature pattern is partly due to the way that the atmosphere absorbs solar and terrestrial radiation at different levels, and partly because of a gradual cooling with height.

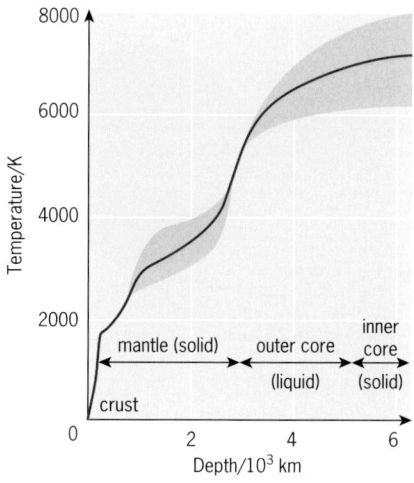

Fig 27.10 A possible geotherm for the internal temperature of the Earth. This is based on theory, and the shaded regions indicate uncertainty

Table 27.1 The gases of the atmosphere

Gas	Composition of atmosphere/% by volume	by mass
N_2	78.08	75.52
O_2	20.95	23.14
H_2O	0.1–2.8	0.06–1.70
Ar	0.93	1.29
CO_2	0.03	0.05

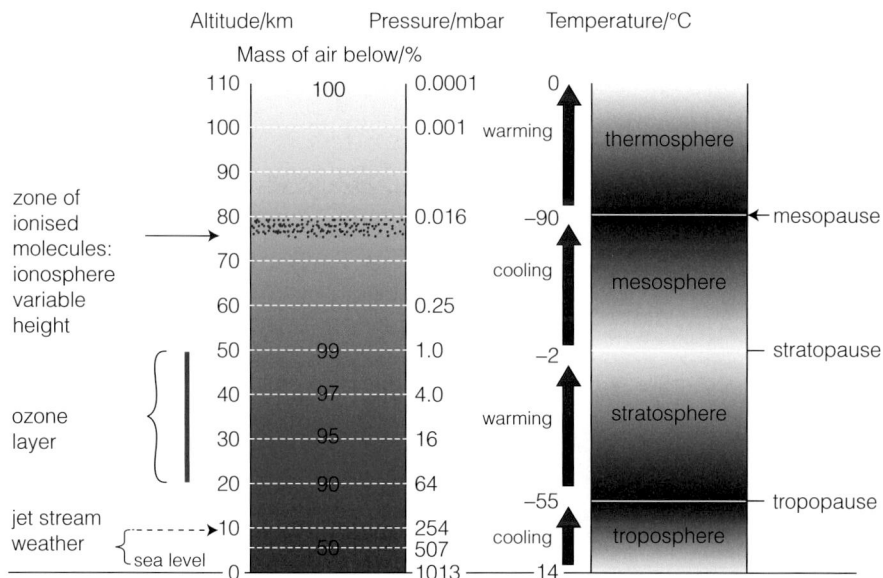

Fig 27.11 Temperature variation of the Earth's atmosphere

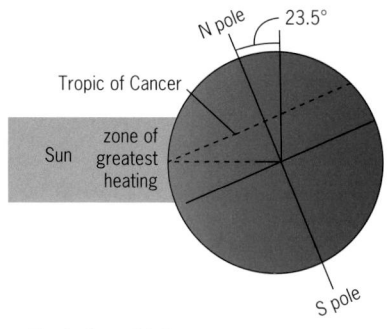

Earth tilt on 21 June

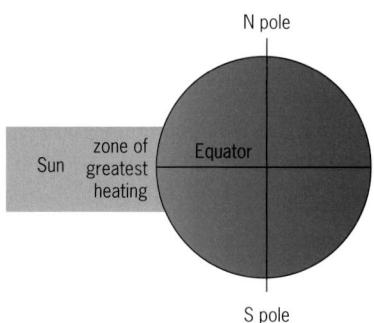

Earth tilt at equinoxes

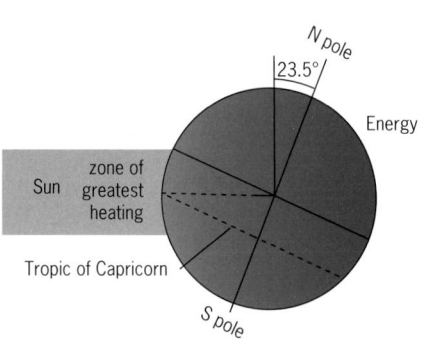

Earth tilt on 21 December

Fig 27.12 The spin axis of the Earth is tilted, so that climatic zones oscillate about the Equator as its position in orbit changes

Fig 27.13 Evolution from 1971 to 2002 of world total final consumption by fuel (Mtoe)

The overall cooling is what you would expect if a volume of gas drifted upwards into regions of *lower pressure*. Near the ground, air is heated by contact with the Sun-warmed land and seas. It expands, gets less dense and rises, carrying energy to higher levels. The gas expands, does work against its surroundings, loses energy and so cools: this process is called **adiabatic** cooling, meaning that the gas is not heated or cooled by external means.

GLOBAL CIRCULATION OF AIR

If the Earth spun vertically in its orbit, the Sun would always be overhead at the Equator. The equatorial zone would be the warmest and the poles the coolest. Thermal convection would produce a permanent circulation pattern.

Warm air rises above the Equator, cools, then falls down at about 30° latitude. This air then moves towards the Equator to replace the uplifted air, causing a more or less steady air flow called the **trade winds**.

In fact, the Earth is tilted on its axis, so that the warmest zone (and its trade winds) moves up and down with the seasons. A hemisphere gets its summer when the warm zone is furthest into it (Fig 27.12).

5 WORLD ENERGY SOURCES

Fig. 27.13 shows how the world's overall fuel consumption has risen over the period 1971 to 2002 as measured in Mtoe. The category of 'Other' includes wind, solar, geothermal, etc. but makes only a small contribution. Here the strange unit Mtoe is million tonnes of oil equivalent and its conversion factors are 1 Mtoe equals 4.187×10^4 TJ or 11 630 GWh. One million tonnes of gas releases more energy than one million tonnes of oil whereas one million tonnes of coal produces rather less. The energy density of a fuel, the amount of energy produced per unit mass, is usually measured in J kg^{-1}.

The main overall harmful effect of these fuels is the production of carbon dioxide and its influence via the greenhouse effect. Coal, oil and gas all make a significant contribution. The burning of wood and the use of other types of biomass play a much smaller part. By comparing Fig 27.13 with Fig 27.14, it is obvious that, per tonne of fuel, coal has by far the most damaging effect. This explains why coal-fired power stations are being phased

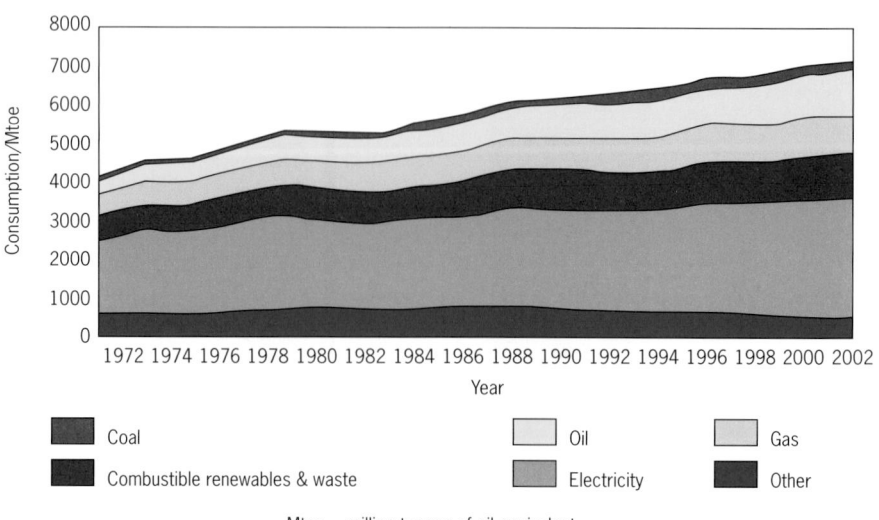

Mtoe = million tonnes of oil equivalent

? QUESTION 7

7 Using the relevant conversion factor calculate the energy density of oil.

out in the UK, although they may have a future with efficient carbon dioxide scrubbers. The figures also show why it is important for the future that alternative sources of energy are used, including nuclear energy, as these have no or little carbon dioxide emission.

Historically, much of heavy industry developed close to supplies of fossil fuel, notably of coal. The mining and open-cast digging for coal has additional environmental problems. Meanwhile, the transportation of gas and oil is generally easier and is often achieved by pipelines crossing large global distances.

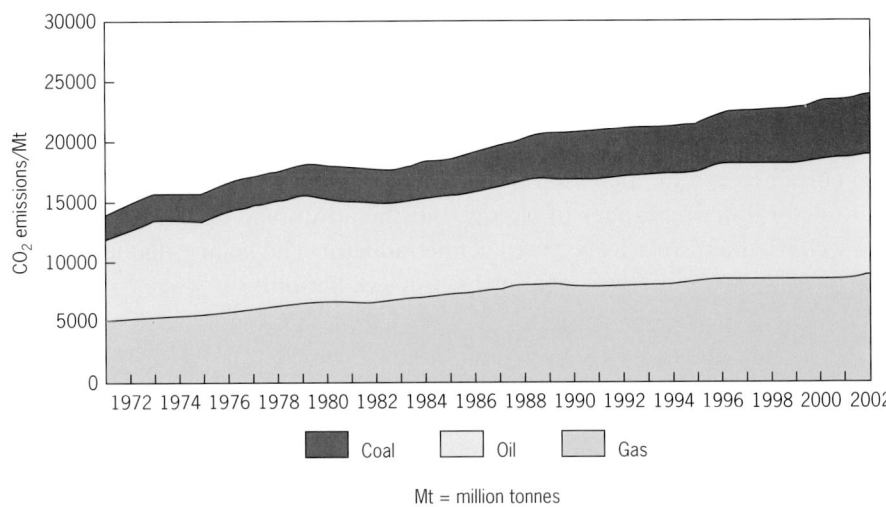

Fig 27.14 Evolution from 1971 to 2002 of world CO_2 emissions by fuel (Mt of CO_2)

Mt = million tonnes

6 POWER PRODUCTION: TRADITIONAL AND ALTERNATIVE ENERGY SOURCES

The fuels can be used for direct energy production, such as the burning of coal, gas or oil in the home for domestic heating or cooking. The thermal energy produced is low grade (it is degraded energy); it cannot then perform useful work and it is lost to the surroundings. Improvement in the thermal insulation of houses and offices is therefore an effective method of reducing the energy required for spatial heating. Much fuel is used in power stations for producing electrical energy. This is high grade energy because the production of electricity can be used to drive motors and various electrical devices. Much of the remaining fuel is used in transport, particularly for internal combustion engines (see page 273).

ELECTRICAL POWER PLANTS

The fuel used for these can be traditional, such as coal, gas or oil, or it can be nuclear. First, the consumption of the fuel (by burning or nuclear reaction) is used to produce work energy. There is a limit to the efficiency of such a process. Most power plants use steam to power turbines. Water is heated to produce the steam. The optimum efficiency can never be higher than that of a Carnot cycle and, as was seen on page 277, this depends on the incoming temperature of the superheated steam and the temperature of the condensed steam. The higher the ratio of the temperatures of the incoming and outgoing steam, the greater the efficiency. However, the turbines themselves will have a mechanical efficiency as they power electrical generators (see page 237). There will be further energy losses as a result of transmission along the power lines to the end user (page 239). In the case of hydroelectric schemes, the turbines are driven by the flow of water.

SOLAR POWER

The energy of the Sun can be used to produce electricity directly via **photovoltaic cells**. Such cells consist of a thin layer of semiconductor, which is usually in the polycrystalline form, of a suitable band gap such that the incoming light can create electron–hole pairs. These provide the electrical current. The principle is similar to that for light-dependent resistors (LDRs – see page 408). Solar cells usually use silicon doped with phosphorus or another impurity to give the best characteristics, and may consist of a sandwich of n-type silicon and p-type silicon. A contact grid is added to the top surface and a contact layer to the back surface. Silicon is highly reflective so, in order to maximise the amount of solar energy absorbed, an anti-reflective coating is added. Finally, a cover glass or similar protective layer is added (Fig 27.15). Other materials used for solar cells include gallium arsenide, copper indium diselenide and cadmium telluride. The efficiency can be increased by having a number of layers absorbing photons of differing ranges of energy, but the advantage of silicon is that it is a well-tried and relatively cheap semiconductor. The solar cells need to be oriented to take best advantage of the Sun's radiation.

Solar heating panels, on the other hand, are used for spatial heating and for hot water. The incoming solar energy directly increases the temperature of water, which is pumped around a building or supplied to a tank.

Fig 27.15 Photovoltaic cell

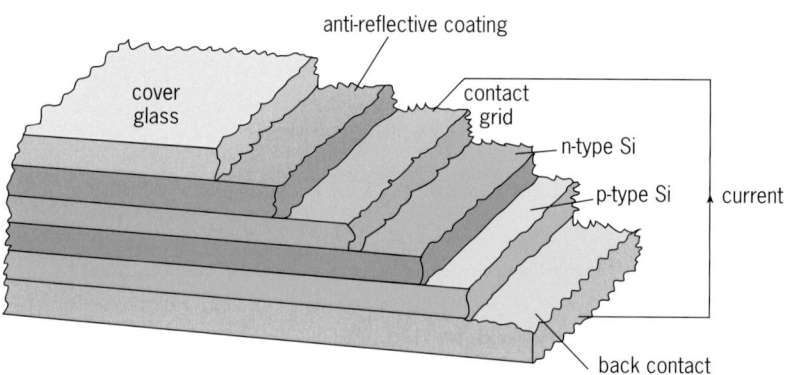

HYDROELECTRIC POWER

The flow of water that drives the turbines in a hydroelectric scheme comes from the potential energy of water retained in a reservoir to a greater height.

A mass of water m at the top of a dam, height h, has potential energy mgh.

As power is energy/time, the power P is given by mgh/t, where t is the time over which the mass of water flows through the turbines. The transfer of energy to the turbines is highly efficient, being usually approximately 90%. As an example, the Grand Coulee Dam in the USA has a height of fall of 87 metres and produces approximately 700 MW from one power plant (there are a number). Taking as a guide an output of 1000 MW from established coal burning and nuclear power stations, it can be seen that hydroelectric schemes are comparable or better.

Hydroelectric power can be obtained in conjunction with pumped storage. A notable example in the UK is at Dinorwig (North Wales). There are reservoirs at two levels and the turbines are constructed so that they can operate in either direction. When there is a heavy peak demand for electricity (and this is often associated with a concentration of household activities connected to the timetable of events such as international matches on the television), water can be released at a very high rate to produce maximum power. Under these conditions Dinorwig can supply over 1.7 GW of electricity within 90 seconds of any decision. The upper reservoir can be slowly refilled at night using power from the National Grid using power stations such as nuclear ones that operate continuously.

Similar considerations exist for tidal power stations. Here, the reservoir is filled from variation of water level due to the tides. One disadvantage is that in such systems there may be intermittent and variable filling of the reservoir, although turbines operating in both directions can be incorporated. There has been a long-standing proposal for such a scheme in the Bristol Channel but this would be likely to produce associated environmental problems.

The Example below demonstrates some typical quantities.

EXAMPLE

The table below provides some data for a turbine converting the gravitational potential energy of a head of water of 9.0 m to electrical energy. We will calculate the torque T on the turbine ($T = \Delta P/\Delta t$, see page 72) and the efficiency.

Flow rate (kg s^{-1})	Power output (kW)	Revolutions per minute	Rotational speed (rad s^{-1})
580	46	750	76

$$T = \Delta P/\Delta t = 41 \times 10^3/76 = 540 \text{ N m}$$

The gravitational power is given by

$$mgh/t = \text{flow rate} \times gh$$
$$= 580 \times 9.8 \times 9.0 \text{ W}$$
$$= 5.1 \times 10^4 \text{ W}$$

The efficiency is therefore

$$\frac{\text{power output}}{\text{gravitational power}} \times 100\% = \frac{46 \times 10^3}{5.1 \times 10^4} \times 100\%$$
$$= 90\%$$

WIND TURBINES

Wind turbines take advantage of the flow of air in the atmosphere to generate electricity directly. They operate for wind speeds between approximately 10 mph (4.5 m s^{-1}) and 65 mph (29 m s^{-1}). The low speed shaft is connected via gears to a high speed shaft to increase the rotational speeds from approximately 50 rpm to 1200 to 1500 rpm. It is this part of the mechanism that is costly and is subject to wear and possible breakdown. The pitch or angle of the blades may be altered when the wind speeds are low or high. The turbines are also designed to rotate about a vertical axis and designed to either face the wind or face away. Most current wind turbine blades rotate on a horizontal axis, these blades being not unlike aeroplane propellers. Large turbines can have a capacity of 5 MW and can have a column height equivalent to a 20 storey building. They are usually grouped as wind farms to simplify connection to the electrical grid (Fig 27.16). Wind turbines have the disadvantage that they are not supplying energy when the wind speed is unsuitable, so that storage or an alternative supply may be required.

Air pushing against the blades of the wind turbine causes the blades to rotate such that as much as possible of the kinetic energy of the wind is converted to rotational energy. As one might expect, the energy transferred increases with wind speed and with the diameter of the blades.

The maximum power that can be extracted from the air stream is given by

$$P = 0.5d^2v^3$$

where d is the diameter of the blade or blades in metres and v is the wind speed in metres per second. The feature to notice in particular is the dependence on the

 REMEMBER THIS
$P = 0.5d^2v^3$ is a "rule of thumb" expression. It incorporates a density $\rho = 1.3$ kg m^{-3} and $A = \pi d^2/4$ where A is the area intercepted by the revolving blade.

Fig 27.16 Wind turbine farm in the North Sea

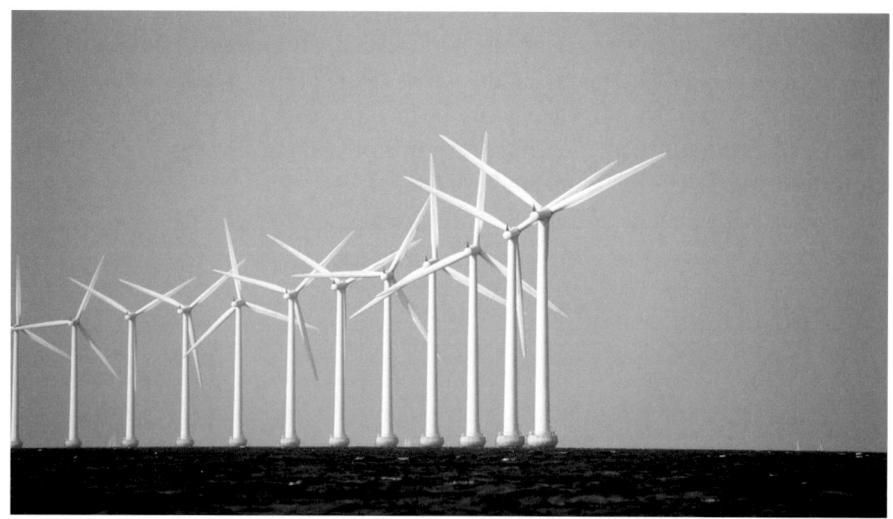

velocity cubed. This means that, operating between the speed limits suggested above, the power output will vary by a factor of nearly 300. Therefore, wind turbines need to be designed appropriately. The Stretch and Challenge box below obtains the formula for 100% efficiency of transfer.

However, not all the energy is transferred as there is still some air movement beyond the blades. Operating at optimum efficiency, the wind is only slowed by two-thirds of its original speed so that the theoretical efficiency is 0.6 and the practical efficiency rather less. Then there are losses in the gearing system and in the transfer when generating the electrical power. Although the efficiency of a commercial turbine will be higher than for a household turbine, overall efficiency may not be much more than 0.25 (that is 25%). This does not allow for periods when the turbine is not operating due to unsuitable wind speeds or because of maintenance.

STRETCH AND CHALLENGE

Maximum energy from a wind turbine

To calculate the energy obtainable by a wind turbine, we imagine a column of air in front of the turbine blade (or blades) as in Fig. 27.17. We assume the blade outlines a circular area of magnitude A so that the column of air is given this cross-section together with a length L equal to vt, where v is the wind velocity and t is the period of time under consideration. We now have:

Mass of air M within the column $= \rho AL$ where ρ is the density of the air.
Kinetic energy of the air $= \frac{1}{2}(Mv^2) = \frac{1}{2}(\rho ALv^2)$.
However, $v = L/t$.
Hence the kinetic energy is $\frac{1}{2}(\rho Av^3)t$.
But power $P = E/t$ so that $P = \frac{1}{2}(\rho Av^3)$.

Let us see what theoretical power this formula might give us under average conditions. We will take the density of air as 1.3 kg m^{-3} and assume a wind speed of 8 m s^{-1} together with a turbine blade diameter of 80 m. Then

$$P = \frac{1}{2}(\rho Av^3)$$
$$= \frac{1}{2}(1.3 \times \pi \times 40^2 \times 8^3) \text{ W}$$
$$= 1.7 \times 10^6 \text{ W or } 1.7 \text{ MW}$$

If we were to assume an overall efficiency of 25%, the turbine would produce approximately 400 kW.

However, power falls away rapidly with wind speed so that, with a wind speed of 5 m s^{-1} and again an overall efficiency of 25%, the output power falls to 50 kW. This shows the importance of siting the turbines correctly.

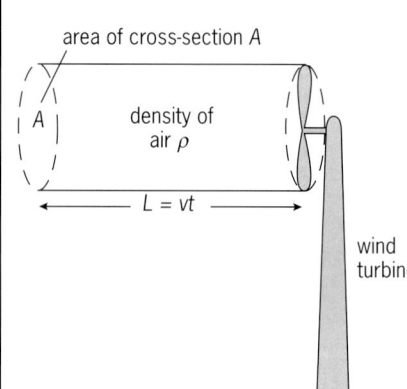

area of cross-section A

density of air ρ

$L = vt$

wind turbine

Fig 27.17 Maximum energy from a wind turbine

WAVE POWER

Although there is a large amount of energy available within sea waves, progress in harnessing the waves has been limited. The so-called Salter Duck (named after Stephen Salter of the University of Edinburgh) consists of a cam-like structure, which in small-scale tests could stop 90% of wave energy and convert 90% of that energy to electricity. Conditions in the sea are, however, more adverse. Consequently, less energy is extracted there, a complex hydraulic system is involved, and costs are high. The Duck provides a comparison for other systems.

A simpler proposed system is the oscillating water column (OWC) and the basic arrangement is shown in Fig 27.18. An incident wave builds up crests and then troughs such that a chamber (the column) is filled and emptied with water. This produces an air flow so that, with non-return valves, the air can drive an air turbine. Based on the overall principle, a number of different arrangements of the OWC have been proposed. Other systems have been tested, usually operating on similar principles to the Salter Duck in which variously designed moving parts operate hydraulic rams.

Calculating the energy that can be obtained is a complex matter. Surface water waves cannot really be described as sinusoidal as for sound and electromagnetic waves. Only a very simplified expression can be used here (see Stretch and Challenge box on next page). The key result, assuming sinusoidal waves, is that the energy transported by a wave in a medium is proportional to the square of the amplitude and to the square of the frequency. More complex calculations involving non-sinusoidal surface waves still give the energy as the square of the height of the waves but with a different dependence on frequency.

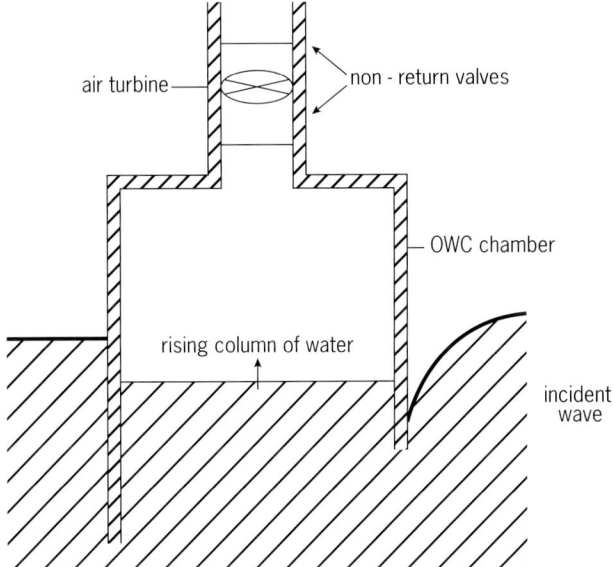

? **QUESTION 8**

8 A household sets up a small wind turbine with a diameter of blade of 5 m. Calculate the output power assuming a wind speed of 6 m s^{-1} and an efficiency of 25%. Suggest what equipment in the house the windmill generator might drive.

Fig 27.18 Schematic diagram of an oscillating water column

OTHER SOURCES OF ENERGY

What have been described so far are not the only methods of obtaining energy. For instance, geothermal plants have been built where high temperatures exist below ground. These can depend on a natural supply of steam to power turbines or water can be pumped into the ground to be heated by the surrounding hot magma deposits. Temperature gradients in the ocean can produce a source of energy and hence power. These depend on the internal energy of the Earth rather than on energy arising from the Sun.

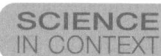

Energy of a plane sinusoidal wave

We saw (page 128) that, for a sinusoidal wave, the energy is proportional to (amplitude)^2, that is $E = \frac{1}{2}kD_M^2$ where D_M is the maximum displacement of the wave (amplitude) and k is a constant. For simple harmonic motion involving a mass m, the frequency is given (see page 126) by

$$f = \tfrac{1}{2}\pi(k/m)^{1/2}$$

so that $\qquad k = 4\pi^2 mf^2$

and $\qquad E = 2\pi^2 mf^2 D_M^2$

Now $m = \rho V$, where ρ is the density of the water and

V is volume given by $V = Al$, where A is the cross-sectional area of the wave and l is given by $l = vt$, where v is the velocity of the wave and t is time. Hence,

$$m = \rho V = \rho Al = \rho Avt$$

such that $\qquad E = 2\pi^2 \rho Avtf^2 D_M^2$

The average energy transferred per unit area (intensity) is

$$E = 2\pi^2 \rho vtf^2 D_M^2$$

The power transmitted is $P = 2\pi^2 \rho vf^2 D_M^2$ (in watts) or, assuming *unit length* of wave impacting, we have

$$E = 2\pi^2 \rho f^2 D_M^2 \text{ (in joules).}$$

7 FACING THE FUTURE

We have seen that traditional fuels produce large amounts of carbon dioxide and that carbon dioxide affects the global surface temperature, as it is a greenhouse gas. As the temperature rises, so there is melting of areas of ice which, if originating as land based, will raise the sea level. In addition, there is an expansion of water with increase of temperature, which reinforces the sea level rise. As more nations of the world become fully industrialised and wealthy, so there will be an inevitable increase in energy consumption. Clearly, this needs to be kept to a minimum.

There are various ways in which consumption can be constrained. Efficiency of power production needs to be increased and there have been recent increases in efficiency of both commercial and domestic generators and heaters. But, as we have seen, there are limitations based on principles of physics as to why the efficiency of power plants is limited. Choice of fuel affects carbon dioxide production. Replacing coal and oil by natural gas reduces carbon dioxide emission and this has been achieved on a large scale in the UK. Where carbon dioxide is emitted, the technology is developing for capturing and storing the gas. Combined heating and power systems have been operated in certain localities (for instance, heating of housing estates by the waste energy produced by electricity power stations).

But the need for energy is ever present so the contributions from renewable energy sources need to be increased. Power from nuclear fission can produce power in large quantities but the power stations are expensive and so is decommissioning. The production of radioactive waste and the possibility of a large-scale accidents reduce the popularity of the source. Power from nuclear fusion is a long way off.

The other approach is to use less energy. Many pieces of electronic equipment are left on standby, consuming electrical energy. The thermal insulation of most houses can be increased and this is encouraged by governments. The efficiency of car engines has increased (but the use of smaller cars would help) and so has the efficiency of aero-engines, together with lighter fuselages. Hybrid road vehicles can cut down carbon dioxide production. However, it is necessary to consider the full energy balance between production of the equipment and consumption of energy during use.

Both governments and the population at large need to play a role in keeping down energy production. International agreements prove difficult. The most notable negotiations have been those of Kyoto in 1997. The International Energy Agency

(IEA) was set up in 1974 by the Organisation for Economic Co-operation and Development (OECD) to implement an international energy programme. However, progress depends on scientific input including that of physics and a commitment from us all.

SUMMARY

After studying this chapter you should know and understand:

- The importance of solar energy for maintaining the average temperature of the Earth.
- Why the greenhouse effect occurs.
- The role of greenhouse gases, particularly carbon dioxide, in influencing global temperatures.
- That some global energy is released internally.
- That global temperature has a significant effect on climate.
- The main sources of energy for human use.
- Why alternative energy sources are important and

why there is a need to move away from traditional sources of energy such as coal and oil.
- How briefly such alternative energy sources such as photovoltaic cells, hydroelectric power, wind turbines and wave machines operate.
- Why both governments and individuals need to work towards reducing energy consumption and carbon dioxide production.

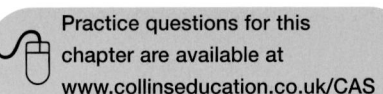

Practice questions for this chapter are available at www.collinseducation.co.uk/CAS

APPENDIX 1: ENERGY

Energy is one of the most fundamental ideas in physics. There are few chapters in this book in which the word does not appear. This appendix gives a summary of how physicists today use the concept of energy.

Defining energy

This is the simplest definition of energy:

Energy is the ability of a system to do work.

Work is done when a force moves something. The idea of work is dealt with on page 44.

A system consists of at least two parts, for example:

- A mixture of a **fuel** and **oxygen** can do work via an internal combustion engine.
- A **mass** at a height above the **Earth's** surface can do work via a machine when the mass is allowed to move downwards under the force of gravity.
- A **moving mass** can do work via a machine when slowing down relative to the machine. For example, a moving mass of water can turn a stationary turbine wheel and generate electricity. (This will not happen if the turbine is floating along at the same speed as the water.)

The **quantity of energy** is defined by the **state** of the system, for example how far apart masses or charges are, and how much mass or charge is involved. In atomic physics we often call 'state' an **energy level**.

We can rarely measure the total energy in a system. What we measure is an energy *change* as a system moves from one state to another, or an energy *difference* between one system and another.

Using energy

It is impossible to use all the energy change of a system to do work. This is sometimes for practical or design reasons – such as inefficiency due to friction or work done in moving parts of a machine other than a load. But there is also a more fundamental reason for the inefficiency that applies to **heat engines** which rely on thermal transfer, like steam turbines and car engines. There is more about this in Chapter 14 The laws of thermodynamics.

Measuring energy

The unit for both energy and work is the **joule** (J). A joule is the work done when a force of 1 newton (N) moves something through a distance of 1 metre: $1\,\text{J} = 1\,\text{N m}$. Energy is measured in the same unit since it is defined as the capacity to do work.

Forms of energy?

In elementary work and in everyday life it is often helpful to think of different *forms* of energy, such as *chemical* energy, *nuclear* energy, *electrical* energy and *heat* energy. We then talk about 'converting energy from one form to another'.

This approach to energy is less useful – and can be misleading – in advanced studies. For example, if we take a closer look at 'heat energy' we find that when a solid object is heated ('gets hotter') its particles vibrate more. The particles in a solid are held together in fixed positions by forces between them (bonds) and the particles vibrate about these positions. This means that the particles have a changing mix of kinetic and potential energy. In a gas, the extra energy that makes the gas hotter is spread amongst the particles as kinetic energy. For a body at a fixed temperature the sum of the particles' kinetic and potential energies is constant. This is called **internal energy**. Many textbooks and examination specifications still use the term *heat* or *thermal energy* to describe it.

The basic *fundamental* forms of energy that you are likely to meet (ignoring more advanced study of physics, e.g. in general relativity or quantum physics) are as follows:

- **Potential energy:** the energy of a *system* in which a body is in a force field of some kind which exerts a force on it. Gravity fields exert forces on mass itself, giving rise to gravitational potential energy. Electric fields act on charges and give rise to *electrical potential energy*. Nuclear forces act on nucleons and they have potential energy often called *binding energy*. In the simplest cases there will be *two* bodies which interact to give the *system* this energy. These kinds of potential energy are fully dealt with in the relevant chapters.

- **Kinetic energy** is the energy of a mass moving relative to the observer, measured by the work it could do by being brought to rest (i.e. to the same speed as the observer, e.g. someone at rest on Earth).

- **Radiation energy** describes the energy carried by electromagnetic waves, which are a combination of moving electric and magnetic fields. The energy is transferred by photons, each carrying its quantum of energy at the speed of light.

All other 'forms' of energy can be described more simply and fundamentally as combinations of these three basic types.

'Transferring' energy is more useful than 'converting' it

In most practical situations, energy becomes important when it is being **transferred** from one system to another. It is therefore sounder and more useful to have a good understanding of **energy transfer processes**.

Electrical transfer or electrical energy?

Instead of talking about the 'electrical energy' in a wire, it is better to think of the wire as a vehicle for the transfer of energy by an **electrical transfer** process. Think of a battery connected to a torch bulb, see Fig A1.1. The chemicals in the battery contain charged particles (ions) which are separated and so produce an electrical potential difference and hence a force which can move electrons around the circuit. When electrons move, the force does work, pushing them against other electrons, atoms and ions in a conductor to give them extra kinetic and potential energy. We say that the filament **resists** the flow of electrons. The work done in creating movement raises the internal energy and so the temperature of the filament rises. In time, a balance is achieved in the filament – the work done electrically equals the radiation energy (infrared, light) emitted, and any transfer to the internal energy of other objects by thermal conduction or convection.

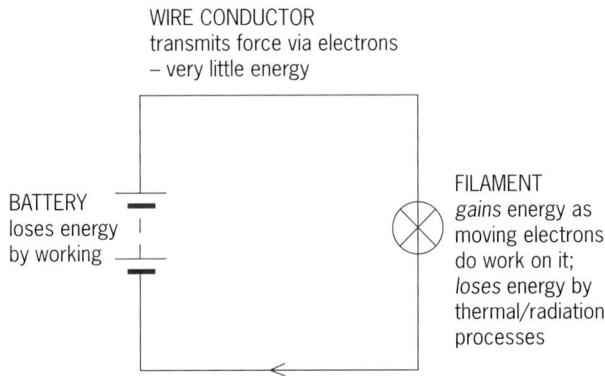

Fig A1.1 Energy in a simple circuit

The battery will 'run down', as chemicals change and the total electrical potential difference between the ions decreases. Note that the current of electrons in the wire connecting the battery to the bulb does not 'carry a load of energy' to the bulb. Although the electrons move randomly at high speeds they move along the wire with a very *small* drift speed. The kinetic energy they have due to this slow drift is also very small. The job of the electrons is to transmit a force, just like the chain in a bicycle. This is an electric force and so can do work, for example, on a machine such as an electric motor, or by interacting with charged particles in a resistor and making them move (increasing internal energy or 'heat').

Heating and working

Energy can move from one object to another via thermal processes: **conduction, convection, change of state** or **radiation**. These are random processes, because they involve the random motion of particles in the substances. Compare this with *working*, which is an ordered process where a clearly directed force acts on something.

Strictly speaking, *heating* is a process in which energy is transferred from a hot object to a cooler one via the processes described above. But of course you can heat something by a non-random process – think of sawing through a piece of metal. This is *working* (you are using a directed force), but the metal and saw get hot. In the same way, the current in a bulb filament does work to make it hot. Using 'heating' in this way is an example of physicists stealing an ordinary word from the dictionary, giving it a special meaning and so causing some confusion to students. But, unless the specification you are studying makes a special point of these distinctions, you are unlikely to lose marks by misusing the word 'heat'.

To summarise, we can increase the **internal energy** of an object by supplying energy via **working** and also by supplying it via **heating**, i.e. random thermal processes due to temperature differences.

The law of conservation of energy

This states that in any closed system or set of systems the total energy remains constant. It is also stated as:

Energy can neither be created nor destroyed.

It is one of the most fundamental laws of physics. It means that when a system loses a quantity of energy, other systems must together gain an exactly equal quantity of energy.

The law has been extended to include the idea that mass and energy are equivalent (see Chapter 24) so that a change in mass also means a change in energy, and vice versa; the changes are linked by the Einstein formula:

$$\Delta E = c^2 \, \Delta m.$$

Energy is not an easy idea to understand, but it is usually simpler to think about and describe the processes by which work is done and by which energy is transferred, rather than to worry about what energy *is*, or what *form* it may take.

APPENDIX 2: DATA AND RELATIONSHIPS

A PHYSICAL CONSTANTS AND SYMBOLS

1 Fundamental physical constants

Constant	Preferred value	Units
Avogadro constant N_A	$6.022\ 136\ 7 \times 10^{23}$	mol^{-1}
Boltzmann constant k	$1.380\ 658 \times 10^{-23}$	$J\ K^{-1}$
electron charge e	$1.602\ 177\ 33 \times 10^{-19}$	C
electron rest mass m_e	$9.109\ 389\ 7 \times 10^{-31}$	kg
Faraday constant F	$9.648\ 530\ 9 \times 10^4$	$C\ mol^{-1}$
gravitational constant G	$6.672\ 59 \times 10^{-11}$	$N\ m^2\ kg^{-2}$
light speed in a vacuum c	$2.997\ 924\ 58 \times 10^8$	$m\ s^{-1}$
molar gas constant R	$8.314\ 510$	$J\ K^{-1}\ mol^{-1}$
neutron rest mass m_n	$1.674\ 928\ 6 \times 10^{-27}$	kg
permeability of a vacuum μ_0	$4\pi \times 10^{-7}$	$H\ m^{-1}$
permittivity of a vacuum ϵ_0	$8.854\ 187\ 817 \times 10^{-12}$	$F\ m^{-1}$
Planck constant h	$6.626\ 075\ 5 \times 10^{-34}$	J s
proton rest mass m_p	$1.672\ 623\ 1 \times 10^{-27}$	kg
Stefan–Boltzmann constant σ	$5.670\ 51 \times 10^{-8}$	$W\ m^{-2}\ K^{-4}$
unified atomic mass constant u	$1.660\ 540\ 2 \times 10^{-27}$	kg

NOTE In most calculations at A-level, the above constants are used rounded off to 2 significant figures only.

2 Other useful constants and values in physics
a) General

electric force constant $\frac{1}{4}\pi\epsilon_0$	$9.0 \times 10^9\ m\ F^{-1}$
volume of 1 mole of gas at s.t.p.	$22.4 \times 10^{-2}\ m^3$
atomic mass unit u	$931.3\ MeV$
electronvolt eV	$1.60 \times 10^{-19}\ J$
Wien constant α	$2.90 \times 10^{-3}\ m\ K$

b) Earth data

Earth mass	$5.98 \times 10^{24}\ kg$
age of Earth	$\sim 4.5 \times 10^9\ y$
Earth radius (mean)	$6.37 \times 10^6\ m$
distance from Sun	$1.50 \times 10^{11}\ m$
mean gravitational field strength g	$9.81\ N\ kg^{-1}$
acceleration of free fall	$9.81\ m\ s^{-2}$
Earth constant in gravitation GM	$4.0 \times 10^{14}\ N\ m^2\ kg^{-1}$
mean atmospheric pressure	$1.01 \times 10^5\ Pa$
escape speed	$1.1 \times 10^4\ m\ s^{-1}$
solar constant	$1.37 \times 10^3\ W\ m^{-2}$

c) Astronomical data

Hubble constant H	70–$75\ km\ s^{-1}\ Mpc^{-1}$
astronomical unit AU	$1.5 \times 10^{11}\ m$
light year ly	$9.46 \times 10^{15}\ m = 6.32 \times 10^4\ AU = 0.31\ pc$
parsec pc	$3.09 \times 10^{14}\ m = 2.06 \times 10^5\ AU = 3.26\ ly$
age of Sun	$5 \times 10^9\ y$
luminosity of Sun	$3.90 \times 10^{26}\ W$
mass of Sun	$2.00 \times 10^{30}\ kg$
sidereal year	$3.16 \times 10^7\ s$
mass of Moon	$7.35 \times 10^{22}\ kg$
radius of Moon	$1.74 \times 10^6\ m$
Earth–Moon distance (mean)	$3.84 \times 10^8\ m$
mean density of Universe	$10^{-31}\ kg\ m^{-3}$

3 Standard symbols for quantities

A displacement, amplitude, area

a acceleration

B flux density

C capacitance

c specific heat capacity

d separation

E energy, e.m.f.

F force

f frequency

I current, intensity

k any constant

l length

m, M mass

n, N number (no dimensions)

P power

p momentum, pressure

Q charge, energy transferred thermally

R resistance: electrical, thermal

r radius, separation

s distance, displacement

T Kelvin temperature

t time or Celsius temperature

U internal energy

V voltage, p.d., potential

v speed, velocity, volume

W work

x distance, displacement, extension

Δ change in quantity

θ Celsius temperature, angle

λ wavelength, decay constant

ρ density, resistivity

σ electric conductivity

Φ flux

ω angular velocity/frequency

ϵ electromotive force (e.m.f.)

B FORMULAE AND RELATIONSHIPS

Refer to Section A for the identities of most symbols in the formulae and relationships in Section B. See brackets below the formulae for other symbols.

1 Motion and forces

linear momentum $p = mv$

final speed $v_1 = v_0 + at$

final speed $v_1^2 = v_0^2 + 2ax$

distance $x = v_0 t + \frac{1}{2}at^2$

force = rate of change of momentum = ma (mass constant)

impulse = $F\Delta t$

kinetic energy $\frac{1}{2}mv^2 = p^2/2m$

efficiency = energy output/energy input

power = rate of using or developing energy = $\Delta E/\Delta t = Fv$

gravitational potential energy difference = $mg\Delta h$

energy transferred (work) = force component × displacement

components of force in two perpendicular directions:

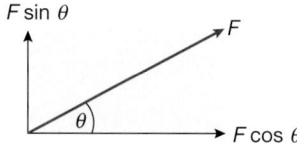

moment of force about a point = force × perpendicular distance from point to line of action of force

circular motion $a = v^2/r$

centripetal force $F = mv^2/r$

2 Rotational physics

angular velocity $\omega = \Delta\theta/\Delta t = v/r = 2\pi f$

angular acceleration $\alpha = \Delta\omega/\Delta t$

moment of inertia $I = \Sigma mr^2$

angular momentum = $I\omega$

torque $T = I\alpha$

work done = $T\theta$

kinetic energy = $\frac{1}{2}I\omega^2$

power = $T\omega$

inward acceleration (centripetal) = $a = v^2/r = r\omega^2$

3 Electricity

terminal p.d. $V = \epsilon - Ir$

current $I = AvnQ$

charge $\Delta Q = I\Delta t$

resistance $R = V/I$, $R = \dfrac{\rho l}{A} = \dfrac{l}{\sigma A}$

resistance in series $R = R_1 + R_2 + ...$

resistance in parallel $1/R = 1/R_1 + 1/R_2 + ...$

conductance = 1/resistance

capacitance $C = Q/V$

capacitance in series $1/C = 1/C_1 + 1/C_2 + ...$

capacitance in parallel $C = C_1 + C_2 + ...$

energy stored = $\frac{1}{2}QV = \frac{1}{2}CV^2$

discharge of capacitor $Q = Q_0 e^{-t/RC}$

  (RC = time constant)

power $P = IV$

4 Fields and potential

a) All fields:

field strength $E = -dV/dr \approx -\Delta V/\Delta r$

b) Electrical:

electric field $E = F/Q$

uniform field between parallel plates $E = V/d$, $E = \sigma/\epsilon_0$

capacitance of parallel plate capacitor $C = \epsilon_0 \epsilon_1 A/d$
  (ϵ_r = relative permittivity)

for point charges $F = \dfrac{1}{4\pi\epsilon_0}\dfrac{Q_1 Q_2}{r^2}$

electric field strength $E = \dfrac{1}{4\pi\epsilon_0}\dfrac{Q_1 Q_2}{r^2}$

electric potential $V = \dfrac{1}{4\pi\epsilon_0}\dfrac{Q}{r}$

c) Gravitational:

field strength $g = F/m = -GM/r^2$
  (M = mass of Earth or other body)

force $F = -Gm_1 m_2/r^2$
  (r = separation of centres)

gravitational potential energy change $\Delta E = GM(1/r_1 - 1/r_2)$

5 Matter

density = mass/volume

a) Solids: material in tension

Hooke's law: tension $F = kx$
  (k = spring constant)

stress = tension/cross-sectional area

strain = extension/original length

Young modulus = stress/strain

elastic strain energy = stress/strain

elastic strain energy = $\frac{1}{2}kx^2$

elastic strain energy per unit volume = $\frac{1}{2}$stress × strain

b) Liquids

liquid (fluid) pressure $p = \rho gh$

Bernouilli's equation: $p = \frac{1}{2}\rho v^2 + \rho gh$ = constant

power available from fluid flow $P = \frac{1}{2}A\rho v^2$

Stokes' law: $F = 6\pi\eta rv$
  (η = viscosity coefficient)

Reynolds number $R_e = \rho vr/\eta$

pressure drag force for object moving in a fluid $F = A\rho v^2$

drag force in turbulent flow $F = Br^2 \rho v^2$

Archimedes' principle: upthrust on a body wholly or partly immersed in a fluid = weight of fluid displaced

c) Gases

($\overline{c^2}$ = mean square speed, m = mass of molecule, N = molecules, n = moles, R = gas constant)

ideal gas equation: $pV = nRT$

kinetic theory of gases: $pV = \frac{1}{3}Nm\overline{c^2}$

pressure $\rho = \frac{1}{3}\rho\overline{c^2}$

for 1 mole of an ideal gas: mean kinetic translational energy = $\frac{3}{2}RT$

molar gas constant $R = kN_A$

6 Thermal physics

rate of thermal energy flow (conduction):

$$\frac{\Delta Q}{\Delta t} = -Ak\Delta\theta/\Delta x$$

power $P = k(A\Delta\theta)/l$
(k = thermal conductivity, A = cross-sectional area, l = length, $\Delta\theta$ = temperature difference)

thermal energy ('heat') transfer $\Delta Q = mc\Delta\theta$

thermal energy $\Delta Q = \Delta U - \Delta W$
(W = work done on system)

work done by a gas $\Delta W = -p\Delta V$

kinetic energy of a monatomic molecule $E_K = \frac{3}{2}kT$

change of state $\Delta Q = mL$
(L = specific latent heat)

efficiency of a heat engine $\eta = (T_{hot} - T_{cold})/T_{hot}$

entropy change $\Delta S = \Delta Q/T = k\Delta \ln W$
(k = Boltzmann constant)

7 Oscillations and waves

a) Simple harmonic motion

angular frequency $\omega = 2\pi ft$
equation of motion $a = -(k/m)x$
(k = force per unit displacement)

Displacement–time relationships:

displacement $x = A \cos \omega t$

angular frequency^2 $\omega^2 = k/m$

periodic time $T = \dfrac{2\pi}{\omega} = 2\pi\sqrt{\dfrac{m}{k}}$

frequency $f = \dfrac{1}{t} = \dfrac{\omega}{2\pi} = \dfrac{1}{2\pi}\sqrt{\dfrac{k}{m}}$

maximum velocity $V_{max} = \omega A$

velocity at displacement x, $v = \omega\sqrt{(A^2 - x^2)}$

maximum acceleration $a_{max} = \omega v_{max} = \omega^2 A$

total energy $= \frac{1}{2}kA^2$

period of simple pendulum, $T = 2\pi\sqrt{\dfrac{l}{g}}$

b) Wave speeds

general wave equation: $= A \sin(kx - \omega t)$

all waves: speed $c = f\lambda$

compression wave in mass–spring system $c = x\sqrt{(k/m)}$
(x = spacing, k = force per unit displacement)

transverse wave on string $c = \sqrt{(T/\mu)}$
(T = tension, μ = mass per unit length)

electromagnetic waves in free space $c = 1/\sqrt{(\epsilon_0\mu_0)}$

c) Radiation and light

Wien displacement equation: $\lambda_{max}T$ = constant

Stefan–Boltzmann equation: $P = \sigma AT^4$

Doppler effect $\Delta\lambda/\lambda_e = \Delta f/f = v/c$
(λ_e = wavelength emitted)

d) Diffraction and Young's slits

through narrow slit: $n\lambda = b \sin \theta$
(n = order, b = slit width, θ = angles of minima)

Rayleigh criterion: $\theta \geq \lambda/D$

diffraction grating: $n\lambda = d \sin \theta$
(d = grating spacing, θ = angles of maxima)

Young's double slits: $\Delta x = \lambda D/s$
(Δx = fringe separation, s = slit spacing)

8 Electromagnetism

a) Magnetic fields

force on current-carrying conductor $F = l/B$
($F = BTl \sin \theta$)
($F = BQv \sin \theta$)

force on moving charge $F = QvB$
(v = velocity perpendicular to field)

flux density:
– inside a long solenoid $B = \mu_0 Nl/l$
(N = turns, l = length of solenoid)
– near a long straight wire $B = \mu_0 l/2\pi r$
(r = radial distance)
– at centre of circular coil $B = \mu_0 Nl/2r$
(r = radius of coil)

reluctance $= l/\mu_0\mu_r A$
(μ_r = relative permeability, A = area)

magnetic flux $\Phi = BA$

flux Φ = current turns(Nl)/reluctance

permeance $= \mu_0\mu_r A/l = \Phi/Nl$

b) Induction

induced e.m.f. = rate of change of flux linked

induced e.m.f. $\epsilon_i = Nd\Phi/dt$
(N = linked turns, $d\Phi/dt$ = rate of change of flux)

p.d. across coil $V = Ldl/dt$
(L = self inductance)

e.m.f. induced in a moving conductor $\epsilon = Blv$

c) Transformers

e.m.f. in secondary $\epsilon_S = V_P N_S/N_P$
(V_P = p.d. across primary, N_S and N_P = turns)

in transformer: $I_P V_P > I_S \epsilon_S$

9 a.c. circuits

r.m.s. current $I_{r.m.s} = I_0/\sqrt{2}$
(I_0 = peak current)

r.m.s. voltage $V = V_0/\sqrt{2}$
(V_0 = peak voltage)

inductive reactance $X_L = \omega L$
(L = self inductance) Or we can write $X_L = 2\pi fL$

capacitive reactance $X_C = 1/\omega C$ Or we can write $X_C = \frac{1}{2}\pi fC$

impedance $Z = \sqrt{(R^2 + X^2)}$

mean power $= I_0 V_0/2$

Phase angle $\Phi = \tan \Phi = (V_L - V_C)/V_K = I(X_L - X_C)/IR = (X_L - X_C)/R$

10 Atomic, nuclear and particle physics

radioactive decay $dN/dt = -\lambda N$
(λ = decay constant)

kinetic energy of electron trapped in box of length L, $E_k = n^2h^2/8m\,L^2$

particles: number remaining $N = N_0 e^{-\lambda t}$
(N_0 = initial number)

half-life $t_{\frac{1}{2}} = \ln 2/\lambda = 0.693/\lambda$

kinetic energy of nth electron in hydrogen atom $E_k = 13.6$ eV$/n^2$

mass–energy relationship $\Delta E = c^2 \Delta m$

photons: energy–frequency relationship $E = hf$

particles: wavelength–momentum relationship $\lambda = h/p$
  (p = momentum)

radius of hydrogen atom, $r = h/kme^2$

radius of a nucleus $r \propto A^{\frac{1}{3}}$

  (A = mass number)

radius of path of charged particle moving in
  magnetic field B, $r = P/BQ$

momentum–energy relationship for relativistic particles
  $E^2 = P^2c^2 + m_0^2c^4$
  (p = momentum, m_0 = rest mass)

Heisenberg uncertainty relationships: $\Delta p\,\Delta x \geq h/4\pi$, $\Delta E\,\Delta t \geq h/4\pi$

11 Communications

sampling rate = 2 × max. frequency in signal

channel bandwidth = 2 × max. audio frequency

bit rate = (sampling rate) × (number of bits per sample)

ratio in decibels of two sounds = $10 \log \left(\dfrac{p_2}{p_1}\right)$.

12 Electronics

voltage gain in dB = $20 \log_{10}\left(\dfrac{V_2}{V_1}\right)$

op-amp inverting amplifier:

gain = $\dfrac{V_{out}}{V_{in}} = -\dfrac{R_f}{R_{in}}$

op-amp non-inverting amplifier:

gain = $\dfrac{V_{out}}{V_{in}} = 1 + \dfrac{R_2}{R_1}$

13 Special relativity

relativistic constant $\gamma = \left(1 - \dfrac{v^2}{c^2}\right)^{\frac{1}{2}} = \dfrac{1}{\sqrt{1 - \dfrac{v^2}{c^2}}}$

time dilation $\Delta t' = \gamma \Delta t$

Lorentz contraction $x = x_0/\gamma$

relativistic mass $m = m_0\gamma$

14 Astronomy and astrophysics

Kepler's laws:

$R^2\omega$ = constant

$GmT^2 = 4\pi^2R^3$

  (T = orbital period: years, R = distance from Sun)

luminosity of star $L = 4\pi R^2\sigma T^4$

  (σ = Stefan–Boltzmann constant)

apparent magnitude $m = -2.5 \log I$ + constant

  (I = intensity)

distance of star D: $5 \log D = m - M + 5$

  (m, M = apparent and absolute magnitudes)

Hubble law $v = HD$

  (H = Hubble constant)

Hubble time = $1/H$

red shift $z = (\lambda_0/\lambda_e) - 1 = v/c$

Schwarzschild radius for a black hole, $r_s = 2GM/c^2$

critical density of universe, $\rho_c = 3H^2/8\pi G$

density parameter for universe of density ρ, $\Omega = \rho/\rho_c$

APPENDIX 3: MATHEMATICS FOR PHYSICS

At A-level you are using mathematics in physics in four main roles:

Role 1: computation – to get the right (and *suitably accurate*) answers in straightforward routine problems and calculations;

Role 2: to **model** what might be sets of complicated data and relationships in a way that makes them easier to understand;

Role 3: to **prove** some of the formulae and relationships that make up the models in 2;

Role 4: to **explore and investigate** the possible consequences of models when data, factors or even the models themselves are changed: *What will happen if …?*

ROLE 1: COMPUTATION

Only rarely will a physics activity not involve **Role 1**, and every examination will test your skills in this area. This means that you will need to become fluent and confident in:

- using simple arithmetic – and powers of 10;
- using electronic calculators;
- your choice and use of significant figures;
- setting up, rearranging and solving linear equations;
- drawing and interpreting graphs;

ROLE 2 : MODELLING WITH MATHEMATICS

Role 2 will also be an important feature of your physics studies. Many definitions, laws and rules in physics are expressed mathematically. We have simple **linear relationships** such as:

distance covered = speed × time $x = vt$

hydrostatic pressure = density × gravitational
field strength × depth $p = \rho gh$

force stretching a spring
= spring constant × extension $F = kx$

Next, we have relationships in which one variable is raised to a *power*, that is, it is squared or cubed:

kinetic energy = constant × speed squared $E_K = \frac{1}{2} mv^2$

volume of a sphere = $\frac{4}{3}\pi \times$ radius^3 $V = \frac{4}{3}\pi r^3$

power generated in a resistor
= current^2 × resistance $P = I^2 R$

distance fallen from rest
= constant × (time of fall)^2 $x = \frac{1}{2} gt^2$

Inverse relationships are a special case of a 'power law', with a quantity raised to a power of –1. The classic example is Boyle's law:

volume of a fixed mass of gas at constant temperature
= constant/pressure
$$V = k/p = kp^{-1} \text{ or } \boldsymbol{pV = k}$$

TIP: Note the third version of the formula (in **bold**): it gives us a quick way to check if any relationship is an inverse one like Boyle's law.

Inverse square relationships describe some of the most important laws in physics: Newton's law of gravitation and Coulomb's law of force between charges, for example.

$$F = G\frac{Mm}{r^2} \quad F = \frac{Q_1 Q_2}{r^2}$$

where G is the universal gravitational constant and k the electrical constant (usually written as $1/4\pi\varepsilon_0$). Inverse square relationships in these two examples are linked to the fact that space is three-dimensional - see Chapters 2 and 9 for more about this.

Equally important, but a little more difficult to handle, are **exponential** relationships. These are quite difficult ideas and are best understood after you have studied the relevant physics. They are likely to appear in three forms.

1 Relationships involving the number e
$N = N_0 e^{-kt}$ (radioactive decay)
$Q = Q_0 e^{-t/RC}$ (decay of charge on a capacitor)

2 Relationships in a logarithmic form:
$\ln(N/N_0) = -kT$
where ln is logarithm to base e, also written log$_e$.
noise level in dB = 10 log (I/I_0)
where log is logarithm to base 10, or log$_{10}$.

3 Relationships in a form based on the defining physical process (change in a short time) proportional to (how much there is):

$$\Delta N = \pm kN \Delta t \quad dN/N = \pm kdt$$

Handling the formulae

You should be able to use any of these relationships (formulae, equations) to calculate the value of an unknown quantity, given the values of the others involved. This may mean rearranging the equation to make the unknown quantity the subject of the equation (*algebra*). You will need to insert the right numbers in the right places and carry out the necessary *arithmetic*, probably using an electronic calculator (see *Hints and tips for computation* on page 592). You then clearly state the result with the correct units and to the appropriate number of significant figures (*physics*).

You should also be able to analyse two sets of related numerical data to test for the relationship between them. In simple cases you can do this 'by inspection' - does one variable double when the other one does, for example. If so, the relationship is *linear*:

$$y = \text{constant} \times x$$

Simple calculation might show that when you multiply a pair of related numbers together you always get much the same answer – showing an *inverse* relationship as in Boyle's law

$$xy = k \quad \text{so} \quad y = k/x$$

A simple test for an exponential relationship

Table A3.1 shows some data which follow (approximately) an exponential relationship.

Table A3.1 The equal ratio test for exponential dependence

X	2	4	6	8	10
Y	0.8	1.2	1.6	2.2	3
ratios of successive y values		1.5	1.3	1.4	1.4

You can check this by looking for the 'equal ratio property': as one quantity increases by equal amounts the other changes, so that dividing any value by the next one

gives the same result. The *y* values increase successively by a factor of about 1.4 – a near enough agreement for such a simple test.

Graphing relationships

Graphing results or data should make it obvious whether they follow a pattern or not – and which pattern they follow. Fig A3.1 shows the types of graph given by various mathematical relationships.

As a general rule, plot the **independent** variable on the horizontal (*x*) axis and the **dependent** variable on the vertical (*y*) axis. For example, the *speed* of an accelerating vehicle changes with the *time* during which it is accelerating. We usually define time as the independent variable, speed the dependent variable.

But note that in physics it is not always sensible to obey this rule. For example, an elastic object stretches when we apply a force to it. The stretch – its extension – is the variable that depends on the force applied. But when we plot a force–extension graph we always plot the dependent variable *extension* on the *x* axis and the independent variable *force* on the *y* axis. This is because the equation linking force and extension is:

$$\text{force} = \text{constant} \times \text{extension}$$

and the constant is the *slope* of the graph, as explained next.

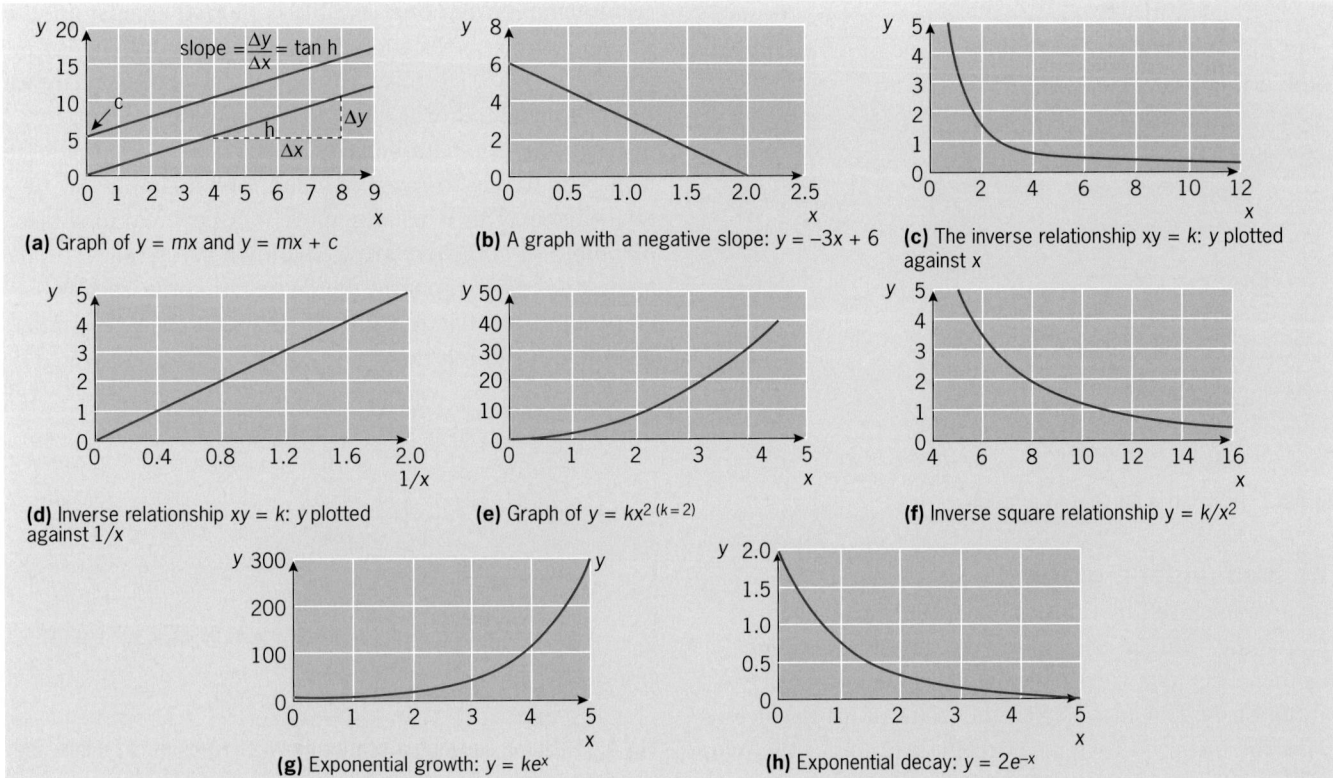

(a) Graph of $y = mx$ and $y = mx + c$

(b) A graph with a negative slope: $y = -3x + 6$

(c) The inverse relationship $xy = k$: y plotted against x

(d) Inverse relationship $xy = k$: y plotted against $1/x$

(e) Graph of $y = kx^2$ $(k = 2)$

(f) Inverse square relationship $y = k/x^2$

(g) Exponential growth: $y = ke^x$

(h) Exponential decay: $y = 2e^{-x}$

Fig A3.1 Relationships shown graphically

Slopes and tangents

The rate at which some quantity changes with respect to another variable is given by the **slope** (or tangent, gradient) of the graph line. Mathematically, the formula that gives a straight-line graph is of the form:

$$y = mx + c$$

where m is the slope of the graph and c its intercept on the y axis. The intercept occurs when $x = 0$, so here $y = c$.

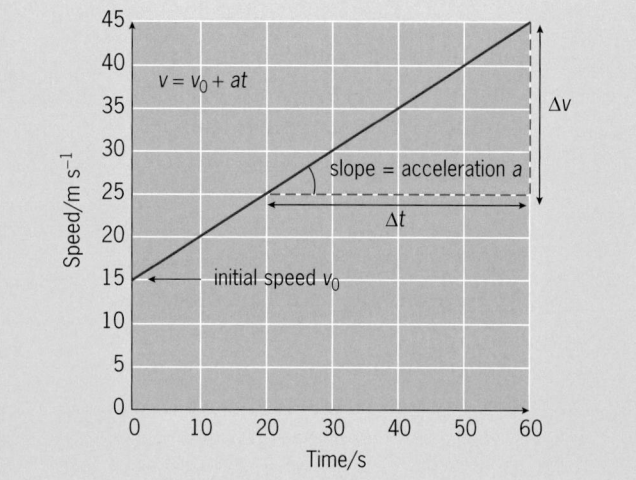

Fig A3.2 Slope and intercept: graph of accelerated motion

This idea is illustrated in Fig A3.2: speed is plotted on the y axis and time on the x axis. The slope of the line is the constant rate of change of speed, that is, the acceleration. The intercept on the y axis is the starting speed – the speed when $t = 0$.

Fig A3.3 shows how to find the slope of a non-linear graph at a point by drawing a tangent.

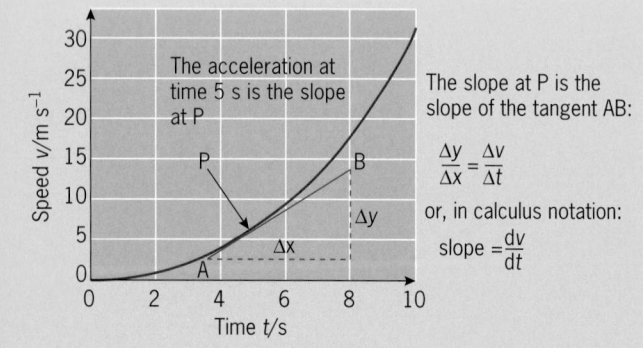

Fig A3.3 Drawing a tangent to a graph

The area under a graph

The area enclosed by ('under') a graph is a measure of the quantity you get by multiplying the two variables together. This idea works even when they are varying continuously. This area is also the result of using calculus to get the *integral* of whatever relationship links the two variables. This is shown in Fig A3.4.

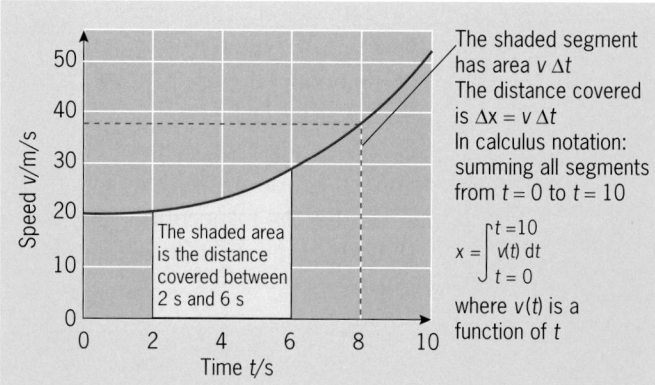

Fig A3.4 The area under a graph, with calculus

Turning curves into straight-line graphs

Plotting y against x in a relationship such as $y = ax^2$ will produce a curve. Plotting y against x^2 will produce a straight-line graph of slope a. This is a useful way of both checking that data are related by a power relationship - and for finding the value of the linking constant a.

If you don't know how one set of values (y) is related to another set (x) but suspect that it has the form: $y = ax^n$, a plot of log y against log x will help. The plotted relationship would have the form:

$$\log y = \log a + n \log x$$

and will be a straight-line graph of slope n and intercept $\log a$.

Scattergraphs

Data do not always follow a neatly obvious mathematical relationship. When one variable is plotted against another the points may be 'scattered' around a straight line or a curve (Fig A3.5). In this case we can think of the **line of best** fit as a kind of average of the way the system described by the data behaves. If the data is too scattered it may be wrong to say that it supports a simple law or relationship. This is usually more of a problem in subjects like biology, and there are well-known statistical techniques for estimating the degree of confidence you can claim for a relationship. Most spreadsheet programs give help for doing this.

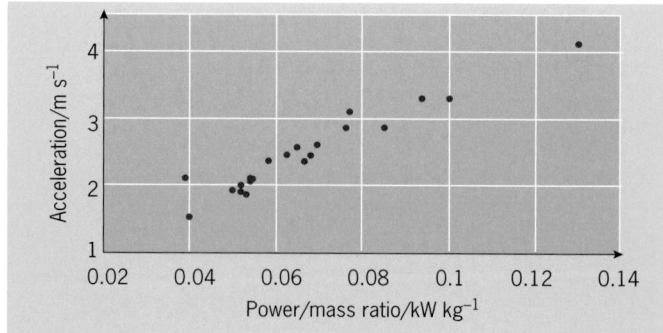

Fig A3.5 Graph showing a scatter: How 21 types of car might obey Newton's laws

ROLE 3: MATHEMATICAL PROOFS

You should be able to follow the proofs of formulae and relationships which are derived from basic definitions, such as:

- centripetal acceleration v^2/r from the basic definition of acceleration as rate of change of velocity,
- the gravitational potential energy formula $-GM/r$ from the definitions of work and the inverse square law,
- the energy stored in a charged capacitor $E = \frac{1}{2} QV = \frac{1}{2} CV^2$ by considering the area under a voltage – charge graph,
- the kinetic theory formula $pV = \frac{1}{3} Nm\overline{c^2}$ from conservation of momentum and the definition of pressure.

Very few A-level specifications expect you to reproduce such proofs in an examination – but check your own specification about this.

ROLE 4: EXPLORING AND INVESTIGATING WITH MATHEMATICS: MODELLING

Traditionally physicists have modelled 'real life' by making simplifying assumptions - such as zero friction, perfect spheres, uniform density, etc. – and used some quite advanced mathematics to describe what might happen. The result is a model of reality – which with any luck will be close enough to the real thing for useful predictions to be made - and give a better understanding of what is going on.

The most useful kind of mathematics for this has been the **calculus** – which was in fact invented by Isaac Newton (and others) to help solve the problems that arose when he was producing his models ('laws') of motion and of gravity. Calculus remains one of the most useful tools for mathematical modelling. See page 594 for a list of the main results in calculus useful at A-level.

But increasingly both working physicists and students are using more basic, numerical methods to make mathematical models – using **computer spreadsheet** programs or programmable graphical calculators. These methods allow you to change the conditions – the values of constants and variables – and calculate the effects very easily and quickly, as the electronics does all the hard work. The spreadsheet programs have most features in common, but have slightly different ways for setting up equations. It will be very worthwhile learning how to use these aids, and using them to investigate mathematical models in physics (without having to do too much maths!).

There are three main ways in which you should find spreadsheets useful:

1 Entering and storing experimental data and plotting graphs. Examples: investigating data about car performance, experimental results.

2 Using previously derived formulae with real or made-up data and constants to model what happens when data and/or constants change. Essentially all the mathematical physics has been done by whoever derived the formula. Examples: using derived equations of motion, modelling projectile motion with different speeds and air resistance, investigating simple harmonic motion, investigating the addition of sound waves of different frequencies.

3 Using numerical methods based on simple fundamental definitions to make models. This relies on repeated calculations in small steps (iterations), and no derivation of possible advanced equations is needed. Examples: modelling radioactive decay, capacitor discharge, gravitational potential near a planet, rocket motion. (See Assignments in Chapters 1 and 3, for example.)

See page 595 for suggested models that you might investigate.

Hints and tips for computation

Powers and indices
If $x = a^y$ then $y = \log_a x$ e.g. $x = 10^3$, $\log_{10} x = 3$
$$x = e^4, \log_e x \text{ or } \ln x = 4$$

Table A3.2 Powers, indices and prefixes

Sub-multiple	Prefix	Symbol	Multiple	Prefix	Symbol
10^{-1}	deci	d	10^1	deca	da*
10^{-2}	centi	c	10^2	hecto	h*
10^{-3}	milli	m	10^3	kilo	K
10^{-6}	micro	μ	10^6	mega	M
10^{-9}	nano	n	10^9	giga	G
10^{-12}	pico	p	10^{12}	tera	T
10^{-15}	femto	f	10^{15}	peta	P*
10^{-18}	atto	a	10^{18}	exa	E*

*rarely used

Scientific (or standard) notation uses powers of ten, e.g.:
$$542.3 \text{ is written } 5.423 \times 10^2$$
$$0.05423 \text{ is written } 5.423 \times 10^{-2}$$

The ^{2} and the $^{-2}$ are also called **indices**.

Computers and calculators may present standard form coded with the letter E standing for *exponent* (index), e.g.:
$$5.423\text{E}2 \quad \text{or} \quad 5.423\text{E}{-2}$$

Always give final answers and results in standard form. *Take care when plugging numbers into a calculator* – what you press is not what you see! For example, 5.423×10^2 is entered into a calculator as:

step 1 **5.432**
step 2 **EXP** (the exponent key)
step 3 **2**

In other words, follow the notation above. If you insert × 10 between steps 1 and 2 the answer will be 10 times too big. Try it and see!

When you *multiply* numbers given in powers of 10, **add** the indices:

$$3 \times 10^4 \times 2 \times 10^5 = 6 \times 10^9$$
$$3 \times 10^4 \times 2 \times 10^{-5} = 6 \times 10^{-1}$$

In general, $a^5 \times a^2 = a^7 \qquad a^m \times a^n = a^{(m + n)}$

When *dividing*, **subtract** the indices:

$$3 \times 10^4 \div 2 \times 10^5 = 1.5 \times 10^{-1}$$
$$3 \times 10^4 \div 2 \times 10^{-5} = 1.5 \times 10^9$$

You should work out that:

$10^2 = 100$, $10^1 = 10$, $10^{-1} = 1/10 = 0.1$ and
$10^{-2} = 1/10^2 = 1/100 = 0.01$.

The missing element in this sequence is 10^0. You would be correct in guessing that $10^0 = 1$. In fact, anything raised to power zero is 1: $a^0 = 1$. Try multiplying $a^2 \times a^{-2}$!

Algebra: rearranging and solving equations

Linear equations have no variables ('unknowns') raised to a power higher than 1, e.g.

$$v = u + at \qquad V = IR \quad F = ma$$

To calculate a value for one unknown you need to have the values of all the others: e.g. you need to know that $u = 0$ m s^{-1}, $a = 9.8$ m s^{-2} and $t = 10$ s to find a value for speed:

$$v = 0 + 9 \times 10 = 98 \text{ m s}^{-1}$$

To find, for example, how long it will take for an object falling from rest to reach a speed of 98 m s^{-1} you first rearrange the formula to make t the subject. You can do this in steps:

1 move u across and change its sign: $v - u = at$
2 which is the same as: $at = v - u$
3 then divide both sides by a: $t = (v - u)/a$
4 and insert the known values: $t = (98 - 0)/9.8$

$$t = 10 \text{ s}$$

Quadratic equations involve quantities raised to the power 2. Simple examples include:

$$E = \tfrac{1}{2} mv^2$$
$$v^2 = u^2 + 2as$$

You can solve these types using exactly the same technique as above for linear equations. Sometimes (but

quite rarely at A-level) you may have to solve a 'proper' quadratic equation of the type:

$$ax^2 + bx + c = 0$$

Here a and b are constants (numbers) and x is the unknown. In general, such an equation will have two solutions (i.e. give two values for x). Elementary maths courses give lots of tricks for solving such equations, but brute force uses the general solution:

$$x = \frac{-b \pm \sqrt{b^2 - 4ac}}{2a}$$

EXAMPLE

Q An object is thrown straight up into the air with an initial speed of 20 m s^{-1}. Use the formula

$$s = ut + \tfrac{1}{2} at^2$$

to find how long it will take to reach a height of 10 m. Note that a = -9.8 m s^{-2}.

A Insert the numbers into the equation:

$$10 = 20t + 0.5 \times (-9.8)t^2$$

Tidy up and rearrange: $4.9t^2 - 20t + 10 = 0$

Use the solution formula:

$$x = \frac{+20 \pm \sqrt{400 - (4 \times 4.9 \times 10)}}{2 \times 4.9}$$

$$= \frac{20 \pm \sqrt{204}}{9.8}$$

which gives two values for x: 3.5 s and 0.58 s. The object is 10 m high going up (after 0.58 s) *and* coming down (after 3.5 s).

Trigonometry

Fig A3.6 shows the three main trigonometric ratios, based upon the right-angled triangle: sine, cosine and tangent.

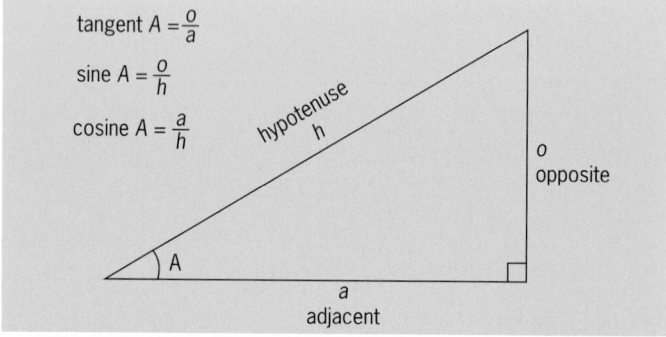

tangent A $= \frac{o}{a}$

sine A $= \frac{o}{h}$

cosine A $= \frac{a}{h}$

hypotenuse h

o opposite

A

a adjacent

Fig A3.6 Trigonometric ratios

You will occasionally come across the inverse of these ratios, the cosecant, secant and cotangent:

cosec A $= 1/\sin A$ sec A $= 1/\cos A$ cot A $= 1/\tan A$

Do not confuse these with the following terminology (as used on calculators):

$\sin^{-1} n$ meaning *the angle whose sine is n*

$\cos^{-1} n$ meaning *the angle whose cosine is n*

$\tan^{-1} n$ meaning *the angle whose tangent is n*

Looking at the triangle in Fig A3.6, you should be able to recognize that:

$$\sin A = \cos (90 - A)$$
$$\cos A = \sin (90 - A)$$
$$\cot A = \tan (90 - A)$$

As the triangle is right angled, Pythagoras' theorem gives:

$$a^2 + b^2 = c^2$$

From this it is easy to show that:

$$\sin^2 A + \cos^2 A = 1$$

Other trigonometrical identities that you might find useful are:

$$\sin 2A = 2 \sin A \cos A$$
$$\cos 2A = \cos^2 A - \sin^2 A = 2 \cos^2 A - 1 = 1 - 2 \sin^2 A$$
$$\sin(A \pm B) = \sin A \cos B \pm \cos A \sin B$$
$$\cos(A \pm B) = \cos A \cos B \mp \sin A \sin B$$

Radians and small angle approximations

The radian is a measure of angle based on a circle such that:

angle in radians = length of arc subtended
divided by the radius of the circle

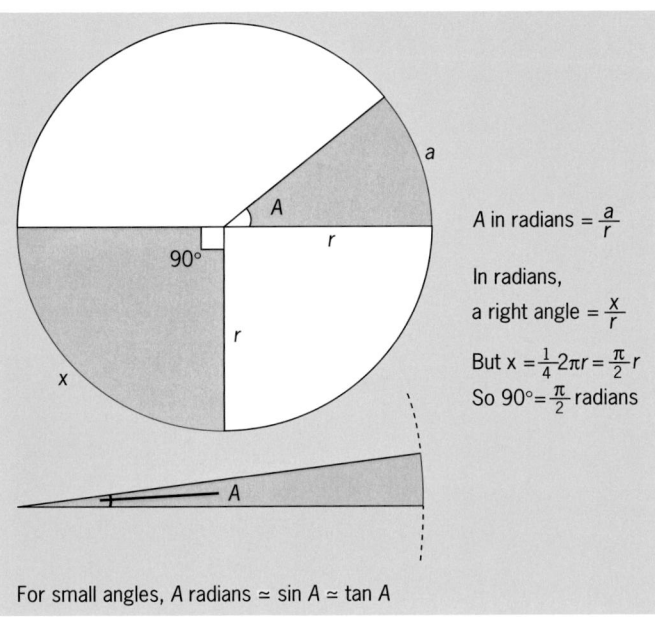

A in radians $= \frac{a}{r}$

In radians,
a right angle $= \frac{x}{r}$

But $x = \frac{1}{4} 2\pi r = \frac{\pi}{2} r$

So $90° = \frac{\pi}{2}$ radians

For small angles, A radians $\approx \sin A \approx \tan A$

Fig A3.7 Angles in radians

When the angles involved are small, the segment of the circle is very close to a right-angled triangle, and we can put:

angle A in radians $\approx \sin A \approx \tan A$

This approximation is correct to two significant figures for angles less than 5 degrees.

TIP: Calculators can work in degrees or radians (or even the unusual American system of grads) – so when using a calculator to work out trigonometrical expressions check that it is operating in the correct mode.

Useful calculus formulae

Derivatives are formed by **differentiating** a function.

Table A3.3 Integrals and differentials

y	x^n	$\sin x$	$\cos x$	$\tan x$	$\cot x$	$\mathrm{cosec}\, x$
dy/dx	nx^{n-1}	$\cos x$	$-\sin x$	$\sec^2 x$	$-\mathrm{cosec}^2 x$	$-\mathrm{cosec}\, x \cot x$

y	e^{kx}	$\ln x$	$\ln kx$
dy/dx	ke^{kx}	$1/x$	$1/x$

Integrals

These are indefinite integrals; an arbitrary constant should be added to the right-hand side in each case:

f (x) (function of x) $\int$f(x) dx

x^n	$\dfrac{x^{n+1}}{n+1}$	unless $n = -1$
$\dfrac{1}{x}$	$\ln x$	
e^x	e^x	
a^x	$\dfrac{a^x}{\ln a}$	
$\dfrac{1}{\sqrt{a^2 - x^2}}$	$\sin^{-1} \dfrac{x}{a}$	

Differentiating and integrating combinations of functions of x

Note: We use the ′ notation to show a derivative:

$$u = f(x) \qquad u' = du/dx$$
$$v = f(x) \qquad v' = dv/dx$$

Using this notation we have the following results:

$$(uv)' = u'v + uv'$$

Using spreadsheets in physics

Spreadsheets are computer programs that can handle large amounts of data and plot graphs of various kinds. They have built-in mathematical and statistical formulae and you can write your own to create mathematical models of a physical system. Such a model may contain several variables and constants and can be set up quite easily.

Once the formulae are put in, the spreadsheet can perform hundreds of calculations in a few seconds and also plot several graphs to illustrate the model. You can change some of the constants to see the consequences, which appear very quickly on the graphs.

Data is inserted in the spreadsheet in cells, labelled by their position in a grid which has letters along the top and numbers down the side.

Nowadays most common spreadsheets use the same symbols and conventions for formulae and operators. The most commonly used in physics modelling are as follows. As printed on your spreadsheets, upright lettering is given here for variables, D for Δ and PI or PI() for π.

= introduces a formula you want to construct, e.g. = B6 + C6 is the formula telling the spreadsheet to add the contents of cell B6 to the contents of cell C6

* means multiply, so 23×42 is written as 23*42

^ shows an exponent, so 3^2 is written as 3^2

E denotes powers of 10, so 5×10^4 is written as 5E4 (or as 5*10^4)

/ means divide by, so $4 \div 3$ is written as 4/3

Spreadsheet tasks

A. Data handling

This includes recording experimental data, sorting data into an order, plotting graphs and charts, taking averages, finding correlations and patterns.

B. Modelling

You can either use standard equations and formulae (e.g. from textbooks) to find out what happens when a key numerical factor or quantity is changed, or, more fundamentally, to build up a model from the basic definitions of quantities.

In the first case, somebody has already done the clever work of using algebra or geometry to analyse the situation. In the second case the spreadsheet does the work by making lots of small calculations as quantities vary by a small amount each time – the human user does not need to be expert at advanced mathematics!

Examples of both kinds are listed in Table A3.4, with hints for the formulae or basic definitions involved.

Table A3.4

Model	Hints and formulae
1. Accelerated motion	v=v+Dv, Dv=vDt, s=s+Ds, Ds=vDt
2. Motion in a uniform gravity field	g=9.8, Dv=gDt, v=v+Dv, average velocity=0.5(v′+v)
3. Projectile motion with air resistance	Modify Model 2. Set a value for angle A, initial speed V; vertical velocity = Vsin(A), horizontal = Vcos(A), vertical acceleration is −g. Calculate vertical and horizontal coordinates (height, distance). Plot appropriately
4. Simple harmonic motion (horizontal spring)	You need: spring constant k, mass m, initial disturbance x; speed v=v+Dv, a=−kx/m, Dv=aDt, x=x+vDt
5. Beats	Plot sum of waves at two frequencies defined by sin (2PIft), eg 4Hz, 6Hz with time increasing by 0.005s
6. Radioactive decay	You need: decay constant k, initial number of nuclei N, sensible time interval. N=N+DN, DN=−kNDt
7. Radioactive decay with daughter products	As above, plus daughter B (zero at start) with decay constant b, DB=+DN−bBDt
8. Rockets	You need: initial mass of rocket M, initial rocket speed V, flow rate of ejected gases R in kg/s, speed of ejected gases v, M=M−DM, DM=RDt, V=V+DV, DV=vDM/M
9. Charge and discharge of a capacitor	See example 6 above. You need Q=Q−DQ, DQ=(Q/RC)Dt
10. Analysing planetary data	Get the data from any astronomy source book; look for patterns
11. Radiations from hot objects: the Planck function	Calculate the main constant, use exponential formula in spreadsheet. Find the effect of changing temperature, check Wien's law, etc.

APPENDIX 4: EXPERIMENTS AND INVESTIGATIONS

WHY DO EXPERIMENTS?

There are a number of good reasons for doing practical laboratory work in A-level physics. They can be summarised by the following four objectives:

1 Practicals help you understand physics better – by making abstract ideas more real
2 They help you learn the skills of handling equipment safely and …
3 …well enough to get accurate and reliable measurements
4 They help you develop the more general skills of designing, carrying out and evaluating an investigation.

Doing practical work helps you understand physics and should ensure that you get better grades in examinations. The second objective is fundamental to any laboratory work: safety is an obvious necessity, and for every practical procedure you should make a risk *assessment* – see your teacher about this. Objective 3 is also fundamental: poor results tend to give rise to confused ideas, and poor techniques may lead to unsafe practice.

The fourth objective combines the other three – and more: most importantly, it tests your understanding of a theory or model by making you predict an outcome based upon that theory, that is, you form a reasoned prediction or **hypothesis**.

Next, you need to know enough about the use and availability of equipment to *design* a workable plan and then use it to take *appropriate, relevant and reliable measurements*. You then go back to the model and compare it with the outcomes: Do they support the hypothesis?

Laboratory tasks may be divided into three main categories:

A. Illustrative or learning tasks

These make abstract ideas more real and understandable.

B. Measurement tasks

These may achieve the above as well as teach you the use of basic measuring and data-gathering instruments and techniques, and give you an idea of the scale of important quantities in physics (the value of g, the Young modulus for steel, the specific heat capacity of copper, for example).

C. Investigations

These bring together the skills and ideas you have learnt in designing and carrying out the test of your own hypothesis or model.

APPROPRIATE ACCURACY

In all experiments, there is a trade-off between obtaining accurate and reliable measurements and the time and effort it would require to get them. The accuracy aimed at should match the needs of the task, which means that when planning an experiment or investigation you must think about:

- the range of measurements of a variable (enough to match an aim or test a prediction)
- the number of readings you need to take (enough to ensure reliability within the time available)
- the accuracy aimed at for each reading (appropriate to the aim)
- the choice of measuring equipment (matching the desired accuracy and range)
- whether or not some measurements or sets of measurements need to be repeated.

All measurements are inaccurate – to some extent

We can measure or estimate the accuracy of a measurement in terms of either a 'percentage error' or an 'uncertainty' in its value. For example:

$$\text{voltage across resistor } R = 11.0\,\text{V} \pm 2\%$$
$$\text{voltage across resistor } R = (11.0 \pm 0.2)\,\text{V}$$

$$\text{percentage uncertainty} = \frac{\text{estimated uncertainty}}{\text{average value}} \times 100\%$$

The value you quote should have enough significant figures to match the uncertainty. It would be wrong to quote the reading of a digital voltmeter used in this case, say, as 11.025 V, even though that is what it says. But how we do we know how accurate a measurement is?

Estimating accuracy

Measurements can be uncertain for a number of reasons:
- limitations due to the scale markings of instruments (e.g. a millimetre rule can only measure to say 0.2 mm – depending on how good your eyesight is, the thickness of a meter pointer and the size of the smallest scale divisions)
- they might be inherently variable (e.g. the speed of sound in the open air, the water pressure in a tap – even the mains voltage)
- human error: response time (e.g. timing the fall of mass or the period of an oscillation with a stopclock); reading a scale at an angle and so introducing a parallax error
- interference by other events or factors – 'noise in the system' which produces an effect similar in size to the

one you are trying to measure (e.g. the gravitational force between two masses, the Hall voltage in a slab of semiconductor)

● calibration errors – a faulty scale, often because the zero value is incorrect (e.g. thermometers whose 0 °C marking is not at the ice point).

Of these, you can usually make an estimate only of the first cause – just by looking at the instrument you intend to use. The uncertainty in the others will be revealed when you have collected the data and find that there is a range of values in a final result, or when you plot a graph and find that the points match an expected line or curve only approximately. As a rule, more than one source of uncertainty will be present.

The effect is shown in Fig A4.1, where error bars (uncertainties) have been plotted to indicate the estimated (predicted) errors in each measurement of force and extension for a stretched wire. The plot is expected to be a straight line, but the values do not fall exactly on any single line: the one plotted is a 'line of best fit'. This has been drawn by eye – but a good spreadsheet will plot an accurate best fit of data if needed.

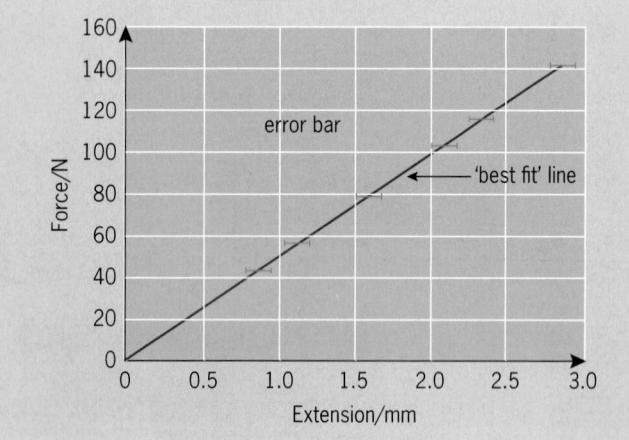

Fig A4.1 Graph of force-extension for a wire, with error bars

Combining uncertainties

The graph of force and extension in Fig A4.1 may be used to measure the Young modulus for the metal of the wire. The formula is:

$$E = \frac{stress}{strain} = \frac{\Delta F}{A}\frac{L}{\Delta L} = \frac{L}{\pi r^2}\frac{\Delta F}{\Delta L}$$

Here, A is the cross-sectional area of the wire (πr^2 where r is the radius). Radius r is measured with a micrometer screw gauge to be (0.32 ± 0.01) mm. L is the unstretched length of wire, measured to be (1.225 ± 0.002) m. The slope of the graph force-extension graph, $\Delta F/\Delta L$, is measured as:

$$100 \text{ N}/2.0\text{mm} = 5.0 \times 10^4 \text{ N m}^{-1}$$

The uncertainty in the slope is due to the uncertainty in the instruments used *plus* the inherent uncertainty in the

way the wire behaves, and perhaps some slippage in the system when heavy weights are added. We can find a reasonable estimate of the uncertainty by calculating the slopes of the most extreme lines that we could draw through the error bars. This works out to be:

$$\text{slope} = (5.0 \pm 0.4) \times 10^4 \text{ N m}^{-1}$$

When we calculate E from these values, *the percentage uncertainty of the result is the sum of the percentage uncertainties in the values used to make the calculation*, see Table A4.1.

Table A4.1

Quantity:	L	r	r	ΔF/ΔL
value	1.25 m	0.32 mm	0.32 mm	5.0 x 10⁴ N m⁻¹
% uncertainty	0.2	3	3	4

The total percentage uncertainty in the final value of E is therefore about 10 per cent. Note that r appears twice because $r^2 = r \times r$.

We calculate E from the data as 1.943×10^{-11} N m^{-2} to 4 significant figures. But how many are justified? A 10 per cent uncertainty is about 0.2×10^{-11} N m^{-2}, so we should quote the result of the experiment as $E = (1.9 \pm 0.2) \times 10^{-11}$ N m^{-2}.

Look for the critical measurement

When you become familiar with this approach to estimating likely errors and uncertainties in results based on laboratory measurements, you will be able to spot the most critical measurements. These are the ones that introduce the greatest uncertainty.

In the example above, it is the measurement of the radius r of the wire. Not only is it hard to measure but its effect is doubled because the calculation involves r^2. This means that if you want to improve the final accuracy you should look for ways of improving this measurement.

Improve accuracy by repeating readings

You can improve accuracy with an instrument of limited sensitivity (ability to make fine-scale measurements) by repeating the measurements. As a general rule, taking N measurements of the same quantity, each having an uncertainty of x per cent, reduces the error in the mean of the measurements by a factor $\sqrt{N}$, that is, the error in the mean reduces from x per cent to $x/\sqrt{N}$ per cent.

NOTE: When you obtain a value by adding two quantities, you do not add the percentage errors but take the uncertainty in the final value to be that of the least certain value.

UNITS AND DIMENSIONS

Quantities in physics may or may not have units attached to them. Those that don't may be *simple numbers*, like the number of atoms in a sample; or they may be **ratios** of quantities which have the same units, such as strain, the ratio of an extension (in m) to an original length (also in m).

Some ratios are easy to spot because they are named as relative quantities, like *relative density* (the ratio of the density of a material to the density of water) or *relative permittivity* (the ratio of an electric force constant for a material compared with that of a vacuum). These are called **dimensionless** numbers – the word 'dimensions' is used with a special meaning in physics to denote the physical factors linked together in the quantity.

The most basic dimensions are length (l), mass (m) and time (t). There is more about these in the section *Using the method of dimensions*.

The basic units in physics are defined by the *Système Internationale* or **SI** system. For example, the dimension of length is measured in the base unit the metre and the dimension of mass has the kilogram as its associated unit. All physical quantities can be measured in terms of just seven **base units** and two **supplementary units**, listed in Table A4.2.

Table A4.2 SI quantities and units

Quantity	Name of unit	Unit symbol
Base unit:		
length	metre	m
mass	kilogram	kg
time	second	s
electric current	ampere	A
thermodynamic temperature	kelvin	K
amount of substance	mole	mol
luminous intensity	candela	cd
Supplementary quantities:		
plane angle	radian	rad
solid angle	steradian	sr

Derived quantities

Other quantities are derived from the base quantities via their definitions. Table A4.3 shows examples.

Table A4.3

Quantity	Units
area = (distance)^2	m^2
speed = distance/time	m s^{-1}
acceleration = speed/time	m s^{-2}
force = mass × acceleration	kg m s^{-2}

Some of these quantities are important enough to have named units of their own, for example, force, where the unit combination kg m s^{-2} is also called a newton (N). This makes life simpler! Again, the ratio of voltage to current is called resistance, defined as $R = V/I$ and measured in ohms (Ω). In base units we would have to work out the units of voltage from its definition as joules per coulomb, where a joule is defined as a force times a distance:

$$\text{joule} = \text{force} \times \text{distance}$$

has units kg m s^{-2} × m or kg m^2 s^{-2}. But a coulomb is a derived unit too:

$$\text{coulomb} = \text{current} \times \text{time}$$

and has base units A s.

So the base units of voltage are:

$$\frac{\text{joules}}{\text{coulombs}} = \frac{\text{kg m}^2 \text{ s}^{-2}}{\text{As}}$$

which simplifies to kg m^2 A^{-1} s^{-3}; and the base units of resistance are:

$$\text{resistance} = \frac{\text{voltage}}{\text{current}}$$

$$= \frac{\text{kg m}^2 \text{ A}^{-1} \text{ s}^{-3}}{\text{A}}$$

$$= \text{kg m}^2 \text{ A}^{-1} \text{ s}^{-3}$$

This explains why so many common quantities have their own named unit!

SEE QUESTION 1 PAGE 559

Using the method of dimensions

Dimensions and units can be used to check the validity of a formula or equation - and even to derive the form of an equation. In some books you will see the basic dimensions labelled as length l, mass m, time t, current I, etc.

We can derive the form of an equation as follows. We might guess that the period T of a simple pendulum depends on its mass m, its length l and the strength of the gravitational field (or acceleration of free fall) g.

Let us say we decide T = a function of (m, l, g). On the left-hand side T has units (dimensions) of time only, in s. We observe that the longer the pendulum the slower it oscillates, and guess that a more massive pendulum swings faster and also that the stronger the gravity field the faster it will swing. We could write down the right – hand side of the equation as a combination of the quantities as follows: length/(mass × acceleration due to gravity). Inserting units gives:

$$\frac{\text{m}}{\text{kg} \times \text{ms}^{-2}} = \frac{\text{s}^2}{\text{kg}}$$

This is clearly wrong: there is no mass unit on the right-hand side, and time is measured in seconds not (seconds)^2. This means that the period does not depend on mass m. We know it depends on length l and the only combination of l and g that fits is $\sqrt{(l/g)}$. Check this! You will find that the units are now matching on both sides of the equation. But there may of course be a dimensionless factor involved. A proper physical treatment gives us the result $T = 2\pi\sqrt{(l/g)}$.

Using *l*, *m* and *t*

The left-hand side of the equation has dimension T. The right-hand side of the equation might involve length (l), g ($l\,T^{-2}$) and mass (m):

$$T = kl^x g^y m^z \text{ (where } k \text{ is a constant)}$$

The possible relationship between dimensions is:

$$T = (l)^x \times (lT^{-2})^y \times (m)^z = (l)^{(x+y)} \times (T)^{-2y} \times m^z$$

We see immediately that $z = 0$, as m is not involved. Looking at the indices we can write an equation:

$$\text{For } T : 1 = -2y, \text{ giving } y = -\tfrac{1}{2}$$
$$\text{For } l : 0 = x + y$$

and using our knowledge of y we get $x = -y = \tfrac{1}{2}$.

This means that the formula for the period of the pendulum must be:

$$T = kl^{\frac{1}{2}} g^{-\frac{1}{2}} = k\sqrt{l/g}$$

SEE QUESTION 2 PAGE 599

QUESTIONS

1 Work out the base units involved in
a) pressure
b) volume
c) angular velocity
d) density
e) the watt
f) the gravitational constant G.

2 Check that the following formulae are dimensionally matched, that is, the base units are the same on both sides of the equation:
a) power $P = VIt$
b) centripetal acceleration $a = v^2/r$
c) speed of a wave on a string $V = \sqrt{(T\,\mu)}$ where T is the tension force and μ is the mass per unit length of the string.

PHOTOGRAPH CREDITS

Every effort has been made to contact the holders of copyright material, but if any have been inadvertently overlooked the publishers will be pleased to make the necessary arrangements at the first opportunity.

The publishers would like to thank the following for permission to reproduce photographs (T = Top, B = Bottom, C = Centre, L= Left, R = Right):

The Advertising Archives, p.252; *Allsport/* Vandystadt/Klein, 2.13, M Indurain, 4.37, S Chou, 5.30, F Delecour, 6.14b, P Rondeau, 7.5; *AP/PA Photos*, D J Phillip, p.22, A Tsukada, p.120; *Ardea Photo Library/*W Weisser, 17.40; *Aviation Pictures*, 2.4, 15.6; *Biophoto Associates*, p.306R; *BT Corporate Picture Library, a BT photograph*, 21.14; *CERN Media Services*, p.208B, 24.31a, 24.31b, 24.36b, 24.37; *Collections/*B Shuel, 5.21, A Sieveking, 6.15; *Corbis/Range-Bettmann*, 6.16; *Corbis/Bettmann/UPI*, 23.5; *EEV Co*, 15.7; *European Organisation for Astronomical Research in the Southern Hemisphere (ESO)*, p.510T, p.510B; *European Space Agency*, 3.17b, 3.27; *Flight Collection*, p.222; *P Fowler*, p.194; *Genesis Space Picture Library*, 25.26; *Stuart George (Head Paramedic) Cardigan Ambulance Station*, p.418; *Peter Gould*, 2.25, 5.19R, 15.15b, 15.19a, 15.29, 16.8C; *David Grace*, 8.24, 8.26, 9.12a; *The Ronald Grant Archive*, p.452; *Hand Held Products*, 20.16; *IBM UK Ltd*, p.306L, p.402; *Instron*, 5.32; *Intelsat Global Service Corporation*, 3.22; *Istock*, 4.15, 5.8, Pierre Landry, 4.28, Brandon Laufenberg, 6.25T, Tore Johannesen, 27.16; *Dr D Jones, Dr M Catani & Dr R Howard*, 19.17; © *2008 Jupiterimages Corporation*, 18.40; *Andrew Lambert Photographs*, 2.7, 2.16, 2.22, 4.1, 4.18, 4.27, 5.19L, 6.20, 7.20, 8.20, p.194, 9.12b, 9.12c, 14.19a, 15.2, 15.25, 15.36a, 15.36b, 15.36c, 16.15, 18.25, 20.11a, 22.25; *London Features International/*D Fisher, p.438B; *Microscopix/*A Syred, 5.37; *Dr D S Moore*, 5.44; *NASA*, p.42, 3.24; *NASA/JHUAPL/NLR*, 3.2; *National Grid Company plc*, p.236; *National Maritime Museum Picture Library, London*, 1.2; *Oxford Scientific Films (OSF)/*G I Bernard, p.275; *Panos Pictures/*J Hartley, 21.13; *Polaroid International*, 15.40; *Rex Features Ltd*, p.92; *Ann Ronan Pictures/Heritage-Images*, 1.1, 7.1; *Mikaela Rose*, p.566; *Science Photo Library (SPL)*, 13.1, 15.18, 24.5b, SPL/NASA, 1.3, 3.15, 15.32a, 25.14, 25.30, 26.22, SPL/NOAO, 1.4, 16.13, SPL/C Butler, 3.3, SPL/NRSC Ltd, 3.17a, 18.41, SPL/F Sauze, p.66, SPL/M Bond, p.67, SPL/Dr J Burgess, 4.6, 5.16, SPL/R Megna/Fundamental Photos, 4.22, SPL/T Takara, 4.35, SPL/G Muller, Struers GMBH, 5.38, SPL/P Aprahamian/Sharples Stress Engineers Ltd, 5.45, SPL/B Frisch, 5.49, SPL/J Stevenson, 6.1, SPL/J Watts, 6.25B, SPL/D Parker, 7.4, 19.26, 24.33, 24.45, 24.46, SPL/F Norman, p.170, SPL/J Fielding, J Matthey PLC, 8.12b, SPL/G Garradd, 9.10b, SPL/V Steger, p.266, SPL/P Fletcher, 14.12, SPL/C D Winters, 15.8, SPL/M Meadows/P Arnold INC, 15.9, SPL/F Evelegh, 15.10a, SPL/Royal Greenwich Observatory, 15.11bL, SPL/Max Planck Institute for Radio Astronomy, 15.11bR, SPL/Space Telescope Science Institute, 15.32b, SPL/Department of Physics, Imperial College, 15.33, 16.8T, 16.8B, SPL/Dr R Schild, Smithsonian Astrophysical Observatory, p.306C, 25.43, SPL/A Bartel, p.322T, SPL/M Chillmaid, 17.1b, SPL/J King-Holmes, 17.39, SPL/C Nuridsany & M Perennou, p.354, SPL/R Ressmeyer, Starlight, 18.31, 25.27, SPL/J Walsh, 18.39, SPL/University of Medicine & Dentistry of New Jersey, 18.43, SPL/1BM, 18.44, SPL/A Pol, ISM, p.380T, SPL/M Meadows, 19.4, SPL/Zephyr, 19.14, SPL/Dr K F R Schiller, 19.19, SPL/Wellcome Dept of Cognitive Neurology, 19.24, SPL/S Fraser/Medical Physics, RVI, Newcastle Upon-Tyne, 19.22b, SPL/M Dohrn, 19.27, SPL/Dr K Sikora, 19.28, SPL/W & D McIntyre, 19.29, SPL/H Morgan, 20.11b, SPL/D Parker/IMI/University of Birmingham High TC Consortium, 20.20b, SPL/M Rain, 21.32, SPL/NASA/ESA/STScI, 23.18, SPL/Space Telescope Science Institute, Professor P Fowler, University of Bristol, 24.1a, SPL/C Powell, P Fowler & D Perkins, 24.1c, SPL/P Loiez, CERN, 24.28, SPL/Royal Observatory, Edinburgh, 25.12, 25.40, SPL/Royal Observatory, Edinburgh/AATB, 26.11, SPL/US Geological Survey, 25.18, SPL/ESA, 25.24, SPL/R Scagell, 25.28, SPL/J Hester & P Scowen, Arizona State University, 25.45, SPL/J Schad, 26.2, SPL/T Hallas, 26.4, SPL/Celestial Image Co., 26.7; *Science and Society Picture Library*, 15.10b; *Shout Pictures*, 1.10; *Stage Effects/*E Landy, p.438T; *Starland Picture Library*, 25.25, 26.5, 26.6; *M R Stringer, Department of Medical Physics, University of Leeds, Leeds General Infirmary*, p.284; *SuperStock*, 1.7; © *TomTom*, p.2; *UKAEA Photographic Library*, 19.31a; *Volvo Cars UK Ltd*, 4.14; *The Wellcome Trust*, 19.30.

Front cover: NASA Johnson Space Centre – Earth Sciences and Image Analysis (NASA-JSC-ES&IA).

Chapter contents and unit photo: Istock/Andrew Robinson.

ANSWERS TO NUMERICAL QUESTIONS

Chapter 1
1. 2.2×10^6 y
2. 1.7×10^{-4} s
7. 5 s
8. (a) 96 m; (b) 2.7 m
10. (a) 6 s
12. (a) 0.8 m; (b) 100 m
14. (b) 30 to 40 m s^{-1}
15. (a) 510 km h^{-1} at 80° N of E; (b) 8 hours (12 to 20 hours)

Chapter 2
5. (a) 2.1 N s; (b) 2.1 N s; (c) (i) 14 N, (ii) 14 N
6. (a) 5 N s
7. 2.4 kg
8. (a) 3 kg; (b) 29 N
11. (a) 0.25 m
13. 5.3 s
18. (a) yes; (b) about 1 s; (c) 3 m
19. (a) 12 m s^{-1}; (b) 2.5 s; (c) a close call! (Why?)
20. 16 m s^{-1}
22. 112 km

Chapter 3
4. (a) 196 J
5. (a) 18.5 J; (b) 18.5 J; (c) 6 m s^{-1}
7. (b) 5050 kJ
11. (b) 7.9 km s^{-1}
12. (a) 7.7 km s^{-1}; (b) 93 min; (c) 15.5

Chapter 4
1. Are you flat-footed? About 10^5 N m^{-2} (Pa)
2. 7.8 m s^{-2} (it's always μg!)
4. (a) π radians s^{-1}; (b) 47 m s^{-1}
5. 375 kg m^2
8. 3×10^4 Pa
9. 1.2 kPa
14. 100 m s^{-1}
15. about 400 km! (So what has gone wrong?)

Chapter 5
2. 8.5 units, 4.7° E of N
3. 15(.2) m
8. 53 N
9. (a) 3.5 mm; (b) 21 mm

Chapter 6
1. 800 Hz
5. 2.20; s, (a) larger; (b) smaller
8. 3 Hz, 0.33 s
9. 1.6 cm
10. (a) 700 Hz; (b) 1400 Hz
12. (a) 32 cm; (b) 16 cm
13. 258.5 Hz, 253.5 Hz

Chapter 7
2. 0.148 or 1:6.8
3. (a) 6.8 MJ; (b) 14p
5. 1
6. $\pi/4$:$\pi/2\sqrt{3}$ or 1:1.15
7. 4
10. (a) 900 m s^{-1}; (b) 0.4; (c) 0.04 (approx. values)

Chapter 8
3. 6.2×10^{18}
4. (a) 0.2 A; (b) 2 mA; (c) 40 nA
5. (a) 1.8×10^4 C; (b) 4320 C; (c) 100 µC
6. ratio 1 (drift velocities are same)
8. 100 Ω
10. 12 V bulb filament dia. 20 times larger than for 240 V bulb
11. iron:copper resistance 5.2:1. In series iron wire hotter, in parallel, copper wire hotter
12. 3240 J
13. 0.42 A
14. 1 MΩ
15. 9.009 Ω
17. voltage changes from 12.5 V to 14.3 V; that is, an increase of 1.8 V
18. 1.33 µF
22. just over 111 hours, or nearly 5 days

Chapter 9
1. 10 V
3. (a) (i) 1.6×10^{-19} J, (ii) 1.6×10^{-16} J, (iii) 1.6×10^{-13} J; (b) (i) 1 eV, (ii) 1000 eV (1 keV), (iii) 1 000 000 eV (1 MeV)
5. (a) 180 V
6. (a) ~110 m^2; (b) ~19 m^2
8. 2.3×10^{-8} N, about 10^{18} times the weight of a hydrogen atom

Chapter 10
3. 0.05 N
7. (a) 1.6×10^{-3} m s^{-1}; (b) 3.1×10^{-5} V; A 1 mm misalignment → resistance 2.7×10^{-5} Ω in direction of current. 5 A would cause p.d. of 130 µV

Chapter 11
1. 0.5 V

Chapter 12
1. 322 V
2. 11.3 V

3. (a) 1:10 (step up); (b) current reduced × 10, energy losses reduced × 100
4. (a) 159 Ω; (b) 1.6 Ω; (c) 0.16 Ω
5. (a) 6.3×10^{-3} Ω; (b) 0.63 Ω; (c) 6.3 Ω
7. 225 kHz

Chapter 13
1. 184 J,
3. 81.6 °C, 354.8 K

Chapter 14
7. 61%
8. 1500% (approx. only)

Chapter 15
5. (b) 3 cm or more
7. 2 million times
8. 6×10^{-8} radians
9. 1.3

Chapter 16
1. (a) 12 000 K; (b) 9.7×10^{-7} m
3. 160 W m^{-2}, 2×10^{16} W m^{-2}
4. (a) (i) 1×10^{-18} J; (ii) 3×10^{-19} J; (iii) 1×10^{-19} J; (iv) 2×10^{-23} J
6. 3.16×10^{15} Hz; ultraviolet

Chapter 17
1. about 12 000
3. Ca 20, Te 71
7. 250 T
8. 7×10^{-15} m
9. 5×10^{-14} m
12. (a) (i) 3.2×10^{-19} J, (ii) 6.4×10^{-13} J; (b) (i) 6.8 MeV, (ii) 1.6×10^{20} eV
14. (b) 7.2×10^{10} J

Chapter 18
2. (a) 6×10^{-7} m; (b) (i) 4×10^{-7} m (ii) 1.33
5. (a) −14.5 dioptre, +34.5 dioptre; (b) +20 dioptre; (c) 50 mm
7. 1.3 m, 0.93 m
9. 2.8 m, 1.9 m × 2.5 m
10. 0.8 cm
11. ×30
16. about 2.5 cm
18. (b) (i) 6.6×10^{-23} N s; (ii) 2.4×10^{-15} J; (c) 15 kV

Chapter 19
2. 15.4 MHz
4. 0.15

Chapter 20
1. 8 m, 4 m, 2.67 m, 2 m
3. 10^6 s, 10^{11} m
4. 1.60×10^{-19} J
5. 3×10^{-19}, 6×10^{-10}
10. 7.6 m at 110 km per hour

Chapter 21
1. (a) (i) 1500 m; (ii) 300 m; (iii) 3 m; (iv) 0.6 m; (v) 3 cm; (b) (i) 1.5 MHz; (ii) 3.75 MHz; (iii) 150 MHz; (iv) 1.5 GHz; (v) 30 GHz
2. 1.001 MHz, 0.999 MHz
3. 1.1 MHz
4. 110 stations
5. (b) 133 stations
6. (a) (i) 5 bits; (ii) 6 bits; (iii) 7 bits
9. 4.3×10^9
11. from 8 cm at 900 MHz to 4 cm at 1800 MHz

Chapter 22
5. 50 mV
6. 10^9 times
7. +10
8. 90 kΩ
9. 10 µA, 0.17 V
11. (difficult to get one value!) 0.5 MHz: $L = $ ~200 µH, 1.5 MHz: $L = $ ~60 µH

Chapter 23
2. 1.3
3. (b) (i) 600 m, (ii) 9 km
6. you get ~22 times more massive

Chapter 24
5. 3×10^{-23} s
11. 8×10^{-21} s
17. 7 times

Chapter 25
4. (b) 2×10^{30} kg
9. 6.1×10^{18} m^2
11. 5800 K
15. (a) ~100 km
18. (a) (i) 1 kpc; (ii) 2×10^8 AU

Chapter 27
6. (a) 4×10^{13} J s^{-1}; (b) ~0.25%
7. 42 MJ kg^{-1}
8. 2.7 Kw